MANUAL OF COMMUNITY NURSING AND COMMUNICABLE DISEASES

Manual of
Community Nursing
and Communicable Diseases

A Textbook for South African Students

By
MARIE E. VLOK

M.A. (Clin. Psychol.) (Witwatersrand), D.N.Ed. (Witwatersrand)

JUTA & CO, LTD

First published in 1980
Fifth edition 1996
First impression 2000
Second impression 2001
Third impression 2002
Fourth impression 2003

© Juta & Co, Ltd
PO Box 24309, Lansdowne 7779

ISBN 0 7021 3310 8

Subediting and proofreading: C Balchin, Cape Town
Cover design and typesetting: Zebra Publications, Cape Town

Printed and bound in the Republic of South Africa by
Creda Communications, Eliot Avenue, Eppindust II, Cape Town

Preface

The revision of the *Manual of Community Nursing and Communicable Diseases* took place in 1993/1994, a troubled yet joyous period in the history of South Africa. It was a time that covered the transition of South Africa from an apartheid to a democratic society in which all its citizens were freed from the restrictions of inequality. The legal inequalities which existed before April 1994 have been erased but many social, psychological, racial, economic, health services and educational inequalities remain. Nurses, and especially community nurses, can do much to stamp out the injustices of the past and to ensure harmonious sharing in our rainbow nation.

The student will notice that in this *Manual* the Health Department of the Central Government is sometimes called 'The Department of National Health and Population Development — DNHPD' and at other times 'The Department of Health — DOH'. The latter title is the one in present use and has been since May 1994. The distinction has, however, been maintained as the functions of the two departments were/are not quite the same.

Provincial names such as Gauteng, Free State, Kwazulu/Natal, Eastern Cape, Western Cape, Northern Cape, Northwest, Northern Province, Mpumalanga seem to be acceptable generally and each of these nine regions is a Health Region with a Regional Director (RD) in charge of each Regional Health Office (RHO). The ten small black national states have disappeared.

The content of the fifth edition of the *Manual* resembles that of the fourth edition in most respects. The subject matter has been rearranged into seven parts. Part I deals mainly with Community Nursing. In this part an attempt has been made to highlight the transitional structures that bridge the gap between the old and the new. New legislation for health care in the new South Africa is in the pipeline, and the transition is in a stormy phase at present, as people's expectations are dashed by over-optimistic promises — real or imagined — for a better life. There is no doubt, however, that the government of national unity (GNU) will eventually have a favourable effect on community health care.

In Chapter 1 the structure and functions of the present (1994) system of democratic government (GNU) have been outlined, and the old and new population development programmes (PDP 1983 and RDP 1994) have been juxtaposed.

Chapter 2 now deals with health care in the RSA — the national health plans of 1986 and 1994 (ANC), as well as the restructuring of nursing organisation.

Primary health care, the foundation on which the 1994 health plan is to be structured, and its infrastructure, have been given a place of prominence in this *Manual*, as has occupational health nursing.

Part II, shorn of its Part I chapters, retains the chapters on basic knowledge for community nursing. From Part III — Health Education — the chapters follow the order of the fourth edition.

Chapter 29 'The Control of Infection by Antimicrobial Agents' (AMA) contains some extracts from Chapter 26 of *Manual of Nursing Vol. 1 Basic Nursing* by ME Vlok. The inclusion of this chapter serves to remind the student of the natural and acquired resistance of microbes to antibiotics, of the opportunistic infections and the immunocompromised patient, and of the untoward side-effects of antimicrobial agents, especially the hypersensitivity reactions and anaphylactic shock to one of our most useful antibiotics, penicillin. Because of the disastrous effect syphilis may have on the unborn child, the oral desensitisation procedure for syphilitic mothers with proven allergy to penicillin as recommended by the Centers for Disease Control, Atlanta, USA, has been included.

The student will notice the reduced number of pages of the fifth edition — from 1067 to 838. The contents of the manual have not been reduced; more than 200 pages have been saved by the new format — double columns will be a boon to the studious student.

MARIE E VLOK
May 1996

Contents

PART 4
Maternal and Child Health Care

PART 5
Communicable Diseases

PART 6
Impairment and Disablement as Community Health Problems

PART 7
A Miscellany of Subjects

Part 1

COMMUNITY NURSING

1

Government of National Unity (GNU)
Community Health Care
The Community Nurse
Population Development Programmes

OBJECTIVES

A brief summary is given of the structure and functions of the present (1994) system of democratic government of the RSA. This government of national unity (GNU) will have a profound effect on the implementation of community health care.

This chapter sets the stage for the subjects discussed throughout this book. It introduces the student to the concept of community health care of both a personal and non-personal nature. The student will be introduced to the South African Population Development Programme (PDP 1983) which was aimed at stemming the tide of population growth by measures designed to upgrade the quality of life of the underprivileged masses and, in so doing, ensuring balance between the size of the population on the one hand and the socio-economic ability and available resources of the country on the other. After that the ANC's RDP 1994 will be introduced.

In this chapter reference is made to primary health care services, and primary, sec-ondary and tertiary preventive health care. Although constantly used throughout this book, these concepts have been defined in Chapter 1 to prevent later confusion in termi-nology.

The attention of the student is also drawn to the differing health problems of Third-World and First-World communities within South Africa and the priorities of health care in each type of community, e.g. comprehen-sive primary health care in Third-World com-munities, and life-style intervention in First World communities.

The student is introduced to the work of the community nurse — the nurse who works in the community, i.e. outside the hospital. Although she may specialise in any of a num-ber of fields, her approach will be comprehen-sive to include primary curative care, health education and ill-health prevention (primary health care).

IN THIS CHAPTER

GOVERNMENT OF NATIONAL UNITY (GNU)

The South African government has undergone tremendous changes since the first democratic election (in April 1994) and the inauguration of the new Government of National Unity (GNU) in May 1994.

Central government (first tier)

The central government is in place, the new interim Constitution is operative and the GNU has launched its Reconstruction and Development Programme (RDP). In the first-tier government, *legislative authority* vests in Parliament which consists of:

(1) National Assembly (400 members of parliament (MPs), mainly ANC but also from the NP and other lesser political parties);
(2) Senate (90 members, 10 from each province).

Executive authority vests in the president as the head of state, two executive deputy presidents and 27 ministers (with a variable number of deputy ministers) which together form the cabinet. Each minister has a portfolio (department of state, e.g. Health, Labour, Housing, Water Affairs, etc.) with a hierarchy of civil servants who run the country. A minister without portfolio secures co-ordination and co-operation between all the departments of state to ensure the smooth execution of the GNU's Reconstruction and Development Programme (RDP) for South Africa.

Judicial authority vests in the courts. There is a Chief Justice of the Supreme Court and a President of the Constitutional Court. The latter tests the legitimacy or feasibility of the Constitution where problems of interpretation crop up.

The Constitution is the body of basic principles according to which the state is governed. An important part of the Constitution is the fundamental rights (Bill of Rights) of all South Africans. These rights are protected in the Constitution (Act 200 of 1993) and its amendment.

The Bill of Rights includes the following: equality, life, human dignity, freedom and security, privacy, religion, belief and opinion, expression, assembly, demonstration and petition, association, movement, residence, political activities, access to court, access to information, administrative justice, economic activity, fair labour practices, property, healthy environment, language and culture, education; a number of children's rights. The Constitution is in an interim phase and is being rewritten at present. HSRC — Research for Progress.

The provincial administrations (second tier)

The nine regional (provincial) governments have been structured and their functions and powers are being negotiated with the central government (1994). The old system of provincial government, headed by a centrally appointed administrator, had jurisdiction over, *inter alia*, education, health and roads. Since the 1980s it was replaced by nominated provincial administrations — all white. They had limited powers of taxation and were financed by the central government. Since the change-over, the provincial governments are democratic institutions headed by a premier who is assisted by a provincial executive authority (provincial ministers). They are called MECs (members of executive council). The Constitution stipulates the areas of jurisdiction of regional governments.

Provincial legislature and executive powers cover many portfolios of the central government, e.g. Health, Housing, some portfolios such as regional language policy, sport and recreation, primary and secondary education, casinos, racing, road traffic regulations, traditional authorities, regional airports, cultural affairs, etc.

The Constitution does not, however, cede exclusive powers to the provinces — the central government has concurrent and overriding power over similar governmental functions, e.g. Housing. In their taxation powers, the provinces are restrained by national economic policies and interprovincial commerce and they are largely dependent on the central government for funding. Each province has to lobby MPs to secure more powers for their province. The interests of provincial governments are, however, protected by the regionally based Senate and the Constitutional Court.

The provincial governmental executive authority for local government, in turn, grants powers to local governments (authorities), according to their abilities to run their cities and towns.

Local government (third tier)

Short background history

Before 1988 there were approximately 800 local authorities (governments, municipalities, town or city councils) in South Africa. They were elected by the people on a racially segregated basis. Because of the great desire of the people (the 'civics' (see p. 199)) to end 'apartheid' and their resentment about the unequal distribution of wealth, they boycotted the polls and instituted a rent and service boycott in the black townships in 1988.

One of the main missions of the 'civics' (p. 199) has been the destruction of black local authorities. In this they have succeeded; nearly half the number of black local authorities have collapsed and hundreds of councillors have resigned country-wide since 1990. Black local authority systems in many African townships were then run by administrators. The black townships deteriorated markedly.

The 'civics' have also encouraged the building of shacks by the homeless squatters and have fought for the provision of affordable housing and for reasonable service charges.

Regional services councils

The Regional Services Councils (RSCs) established by the Regional Services Councils Act of 1985 (Department of Local Government, Housing and Works) are multiracial bodies based on racially segregated local authorities. The RSCs are horizontal extensions of local authorities, each RSC consisting of variable numbers of black, white, coloured and Indian local authorities, who nominate their representatives to serve on the RSC. As a result of the establishment of RSCs, a number of local government bodies were abolished, including the 13 development boards, the Transvaal Board of Peri-urban Areas, and the 38 divisional councils of the Cape Province.

The three goals of the RSCs are: political participation, effective rendering of services and the distribution of additional sources of income, i.e. a percentage of the wages paid by, and the turnover of, businesses and enterprises (excluding religious, charitable and educational). RSCs are required (but not compelled) to deliver bulk services to a region. These include electricity and water; sewage purification and disposal; and transport, health services and the upgrading of many other services (22 services are listed in Schedule 2 of the Act). The idea was that the supply of bulk services would no longer be the function of local authorities, once RSCs are fully operative. RSCs, therefore, helped the discredited former black local town councils.

Local authorities or RSCs purchase water and electricity from public utilities, e.g. Eskom (electricity), Rand Water Board (water in Gauteng).

The RSC Act makes provision for the establishment of rural councils in rural regions outside the areas of jurisdiction of a local authority. Rural councils have no power to impose levies or service charges and expenditure in connection with their administration is supplied by Parliament.

In 1994 no provision had as yet been made to cater adequately for local government in rural areas. Only health services in these areas have been catered for. (See Section 30 areas).

Restructuring of local government

In December 1993 the Local Government Transition Act was passed in Parliament for the transitional phase (five years plus). This Act provides for the establishment of non-racial local authority (city council) elections in November 1995.

By the end of 1994 transitional non-racial local authorities (municipalities) were formed to bridge the gap between the former racially elected local authorities (dissolved in 1994) and the democratic non-racial local authorities to be elected by all racial groups towards the end of 1995. 1994 and 1995 are the difficult years in which *TMCs* (transitional metropolitan councils) were set up to govern metropolitan areas and *TLCs* (transitional local councils) to govern towns, after the dissolution of the racially based local authorities.

The transitional local and metropolitan council members are appointees or nominees, representative of the South African population, viz. 50% are statutory (from the dissolved councils) and 50% non-statutory (representing political parties and residents' and ratepayers' associations). The administrative staff of the dissolved councils or municipalities will carry out the functions of the TMCs and TLCs.

The large metropoles, e.g. greater Johannesburg, greater Pretoria, greater Durban, greater Cape Town, will each have one TMC, cut up into several MSS (metropolitan substructures). Example: greater Johannesburg has 4 MSS.

In the smaller towns and cities, many small formerly racially segregated municipalities will amalgamate to form single non-racial transitional local councils (TLCs). In this way the former 800 local authorities will be condensed to 300 local authorities. The need for the RSCs will be eliminated.

The new local authorities (TLCs and TMCs) will have to be economically viable and represent a population mix of both rich and poor, thereby distributing the major burdens of reconstruction and ensuring racial equality. For example, in the greater Johannesburg TMC, the main suburbs of one MSS will include Sandton (rich) and Alexandria (poor). The chairman of the TMC or TLC will be the mayor of the metropole, city or town.

The TMCs and TLCs will pave the way for the first non-racial and democratically elected local governments. They have less than one year in which to prepare for the elections, e.g. establishing wards and drawing up voters' rolls. They must also run their metropoles, cities and towns until elections take place.

During this time many disputes are occuring, the main ones dealing with the rent and service charge arrears of the black townships and the TMC and TLC nominations.

Legislation is being tabled at present (1995) by local authority MECs to enable rural residents (i.e. those without local governments) to take part in the local elections scheduled for November 1995 or later. Regional Services Councils will be replaced with democratically elected regional councils.

In 1995 the first democratic municipal elections will take place. The powers of the new councils will have to be negotiated with the provincial MEC for local government and may differ from province to province and from council to council, according to their ability to use the power for the well-being of all their citizens. For example, some councils will be allowed to raise levies (rates on properties, on casinos and gambling) and will have some autonomy to control their own finances, while others will be funded by first- and second-tier governments and, therefore, have little authority.

DEFINITIONS

Much confusion exists as to the exact meaning of the terms *community medicine* or *community health* as they relate to nursing. The 'community nurse' is a loosely used term. In this chapter the scope of community nursing will be defined in terms of comprehensive community health care.

Community

In a strictly sociological sense the term may be defined as a group of interacting individuals who occupy a certain territory and who are united by commonly shared beliefs, values and norms. A community is characterised by community sentiment, community involvement and group solidarity. 'The mark of a community is that one's life may be lived wholly within it.'[1] A community may be small and clearly recognisable as such, for example a rural village, or it may be large and have few of the distinguishing features which we have described; so for our purpose we shall consider a group to be a community if its members live in a certain geographical area, share a similar physical environment and a common way of life.

According to an ANC definition, a community consists of those people who share a Community Health Centre (see p. 34).

Health

This was defined in 1948 by the World Health Organization as a 'state of complete physical, mental and social well-being and not merely the absence of disease or infirmity'. This definition is interesting because it implies that physical, mental and social health are inseparable and also because it defines health positively. It may well be that health as defined above is a dream or an unattainable ideal. This unattainable definition of health has been substituted by a more reasonable definition, viz.[2] 'A level of health that permits the people of the world to lead a socially and economically productive life', later slightly amended to read: 'A level of economically productive life that would permit people to maintain health'.

Community health

According to the WHO, this refers to 'the health status of the members of a community, to the problems affecting their health and to the totality of the health care provided for the community'. While community health is to some extent the sum of the health of its individual members,

it is also more than this, and many complex factors operate which affect the health of a community. The health status of a community is the result of the interaction between the biological characteristics of the people, factors in the physical environment, the life-style of the group and the health care system. This applies likewise to the individual.

The community health caregivers (doctors and nurses) are concerned with the management of disease and disability in a whole population or community. To quote Theron,[3] 'the clinician seeks to understand and modify abnormal health states in the psychobiological system of the individual, whereas the community health physician concentrates on the same condition in the sociopsychobiological system of man as he lives in community with his fellow-men'.

COMMUNITY HEALTH CARE

By health care we mean all the health services that are available to the community. Health services may be either personal or non-personal.

(1) Personal health services include antenatal clinics, community health centres and clinics, private practitioner care and hospital care.
(2) Non-personal health services include water supplies and purification, smoke pollution control, housing schemes, sanitation, immunisation and birth control in the interest of the community.

Service should be provided according to need; if the need is for control of communicable diseases, change in fertility pattern, health education, improvement in nutrition or environmental health and sanitation, then it must be met by the services in order of priority.

Throughout the world we find gross maldistribution of health care services. There is an

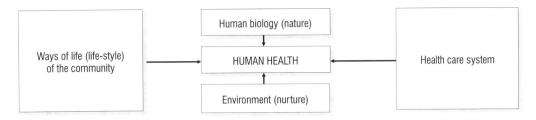

almost universal tendency to use the greatest part of the available resources to provide highly sophisticated treatment for a relatively small number of people in enormous and costly hospitals situated in urban areas. Dr Garde calls these hospitals 'little islands of excellence in the midst of unsolved health problems', while Dr J W Bodenstein wrote, 'What a far cry it is from the opulent chromium plated temples of curative medicine to the forlorn little shrines dedicated to the humble pursuit of preventive and promotive community services'. In fact, in the developing countries the possession of such hospitals may adversely affect the health of the population as a whole, for even where these hospitals have been donated to the government by generous friends, their running requires vast sums of money, and this means that there is even less available for the provision of health services at the community level. It is also in these urban areas that we find the greatest number of medical practitioners, nurses and other professional health workers. Furthermore, the training and education of these health professionals, including nurses, have always been hospital-orientated. Most of their experience has been gained on hospitalised patients and they have had little, if any, community nursing experience. Because of these factors the emphasis during their training had, in the past, been on the curative rather than on the promotive and preventive aspects of health care, and illness rather than health has been the focus of their concern. In contrast, in the rural areas, health care services are totally inadequate or completely absent and there are millions of people without access to even the most basic health care services.

Yet it is in these regions that the need for these services is the greatest because it is here that we find real poverty, lack of educational and employment opportunities, high infant and child mortality rates. Acute infections, chiefly gastro-intestinal and respiratory, parasitic infections and malnutrition, contribute heavily to mortality and morbidity rates. It is, therefore, clear that there is an inverse relationship between need and the availability of health services.

In all countries the cost of providing health care continues to increase, but this increased expenditure has not been accompanied by a corresponding improvement in the health of populations. It has become clear that what is needed is community-based and community-orientated health services which are freely available and easily accessible to all members of the community. This approach to the delivery of health care is known as 'primary health care'. (See Chapter 3.)

While accepting that health care is an important determinant of community health we must not make the mistake of thinking that it is the only one. The establishment of a health care system will not dramatically improve the health status of a group unless attention is also paid to economic progress and community development.

THE COMMUNITY NURSE

The community nurse is the nurse whose sphere of work is mainly in the community, i.e. outside the hospital. Although the emphasis in community nursing is on preventive and health promotive measures, it is essentially part of a comprehensive health service. Comprehensive health services aim at bringing health care as close as possible to the community, be it the home, the place of work, the school or a clinic situated within easy reach of the target population. Although the bulk of community health services is dispensed either from clinics or directly to the individual at home or at work, they form part of a health care system centred either in hospitals or in community health centres, where specialised care is given and administration done.

The community nurse is, therefore, any nurse who dispenses health care outside the hospital and comes into direct contact with the 'patient-in-his-environment', be it in the family, in a clinic, or in the patient's place of work. The important target group is the family and in all categories of community nursing it behoves the nurse to get to know and to feel responsible for the health of the problem-families and families-with-problems with whom she becomes associated.

The community nurse is a specialised worker in one of the following categories of health care:

(1) Community preventive health care by the Community Health Nurse (CHN), formerly called Health Visitor.

(2) Primary health care nursing usually done by the Primary Health Care Nurse (PHCN) in

day hospitals or comprehensive community clinics.

(3) District (domiciliary) general (curative) nursing by the District Nursing Sister.

The following categories of nurses also deal with people in the community, either on an ill-health preventive level, or on a primary health care level:

(4) School nursing by the School Nurse.

(5) Occupational health by the Occupational Health Nurse (OHN).

(6) Family planning nursing. Family planning is done either by a general nurse, a midwife or CHN, who has undergone special training in modern contraceptive methods.

(7) Obstetric nursing by the community midwife who does maternal and neonatal health care.

(8) Psychiatric community nursing by the Psychiatric Community Nurse (PCN) who does psychiatric clinic and domiciliary nursing.

(9) Genetic nursing done by Genetics Nurses who are attached to all levels of genetics service.

(10) Tuberculosis nursing by the community TB nurse (TB clinic sister).

(11) Hospice and hospicare nurses who care for the terminally ill patients in their homes by instructing and supporting their families.

Whatever the nature of her speciality, the basic tasks of the nurse who works in the community are related. The community nurse's tasks are comprehensive and include the following.

Preventive intervention

Preventive intervention and health promotive measures can be applied at three levels:

(1) primary,
(2) secondary, and
(3) tertiary.

1. Primary prevention

(1) Health promotive measures, i.e. health education, parent education and marriage guidance for a happy family life which promotes mental health; promotion of family planning, good nutrition, housing, recreation and pleasant working conditions.

(2) Specific protective measures, e.g. immunisation, personal hygiene and environmental hygiene, avoidance of carcinogens and allergens, genetic counselling, careful driving and wearing of seat belts, wearing of protective clothing in industry, food fortification schemes in malnourished communities, preparation for retirement, etc.

2. Secondary prevention

The aim here is to cure and prevent disease processes, to prevent the spread of communicable diseases, to prevent the complications and sequelae of diseases, thereby shortening the period and extent of disability and preventing chronicity and death. It can be done by:

(1) dealing with health crises either directly or by referral to suitable agencies;

(2) case finding and screening surveys, e.g. screening for deafness, cytological screening, breast palpation for cancer. Early diagnosis and prompt treatment are the important secondary preventive measures. Screening means identifying unrecognised diseases in people who are asymptomatic, by means of simple tests.

3. Tertiary prevention

The aim of tertiary prevention is to limit advanced disease by rehabilitation and maintenance in the community.

(1) Rehabilitation is concerned mainly with retraining and re-education after loss of ability due to ageing, illness or accident, for maximum use of remaining capacities. Employment of the rehabilitated patient by selective placement, sheltered employment and work therapy in occupational therapy departments are the main aims of tertiary prevention. The success of rehabilitation will depend on the education of the community to utilise the potential of the rehabilitated person as fully as possible.

(2) Out-patient clinics where patients with chronic diseases are treated to maintain the patient in the community and prevent complications, e.g. diabetic and hypertensive clinics, tuberculosis and sexually transmitted diseases clinics, service centres for the

aged, etc. are important agents of tertiary prevention and maintenance in the community.

The community nurse must be able to decide when her training has equipped her to deal directly with a problem and when she is not competent to do so and, therefore, must refer the patient to a specialised agency, either a hospital or an NGO helping agency or another nursing speciality. In order to be able to make a wise decision, the community nurse must have a wide spectrum of obstetric, medical and psychiatric knowledge and be cognizant of the scope of helping agencies in her community to which she can refer patients with problems beyond her ken.

The concept of life-style intervention

Life-style intervention refers to attempts by health educational/socio-political measures to change destructive, illness-producing aspects of a community's way of living (life-style). Intervention priorities are of necessity different in societies with different socio-economic levels.

In First-World societies intervention is geared to combating the environmental factors which cause preventable diseases and conditions: hypertension, coronary artery disease, obesity, certain cancers, motor vehicle accidents, bowel disorders. These factors include smoking, alcohol and drug abuse, overeating and incorrect eating (some aspects of the Western diet), reckless driving, sloth (physical inactivity) and family tensions and stress. Life-style intervention purports to temper excesses of affluence (overeating, sloth), and eliminate stress-relieving habits (smoking, drinking and drugging). These life-style interventions do not form part of the WHO global indicators of Health for All (HFA) by the year 2000, which are directed at the poor quality-of-life of developing nations.

In Third-World societies primary intervention is geared to socio-economic upgrading by whichever method is chosen by the authorities in power. In order to combat the diseases of poverty and ignorance — malnutrition and infectious diseases and especially tuberculosis, comprehensive primary health care, clinical and non-clinical, is indicated.

The poor quality of life of socio-economically oppressed people gives rise to high fertility rates and uncontrolled population growth. Overpopulation leads to the threat of starvation and competition for power over scarce resources. War, famine, poverty, unemployment and social degeneration are the wages of overpopulation through uncontrolled population growth.

THE POPULATION DEVELOPMENT PROGRAMME OF THE RSA (PDP)

This programme arose out of the President's Council's report on demographic trends in South Africa in 1983, which highlighted the alarming rate of increase of the population, i.e. 2,3 % per annum. In 1985 the population of the RSA (excluding the 10 black homelands) was 28,5 million of whom 11 million lived in rural areas. Five to six million blacks lived on 65 000 farms. If the growth rate continued at 2,3 % per annum, the population of South Africa would almost double to 47 million by 2010;[5] this rapid increase would result in malnutrition, increased unemployment, poverty and illiteracy. The primary goal of the PDP was to maintain a balance between population growth and natural resources.[4] In 1989 the fertility pattern of blacks on farms was 5,7 and in the black urban areas 2,8 children per fertile woman. Rapid population growth prevents efforts to improve quality of life.

There is a direct association between population growth and socio-economic development. The higher the standard of living, the smaller the population growth. It had, therefore, become very important for the socio-economic status of the underdeveloped section of the nation to be raised towards First-World standards.

The long-term aim of the South African Population Development Programme is an optimum, stationary population of 80 million (including the TBVC states) by the year 2100 (at the end of the next century).[15] This is possible if a fertility pattern of 2,1 children per fertile woman is achieved by all population groups. A stationary population means an equal number of births and deaths so that the population growth rate is zero.

The South African (National) Population Development Programme (PDP) was directed by the Department of National Health and Population Development but several departments, e.g. Manpower, as well as welfare organisations, churches, women's groups, youth organisations, (NGOs) co-operated on national and regional level. The Department was assisted by the Council for Population Development, which is composed of private sector population development experts.

The nine quality-of-life indicators of the PDP monitoring process are:

(1) Adult literacy rate
(2) Infant mortality rate
(3) Teenage pregnancy rate
(4) School non-attendance percentage
(5) The per capita income
(6) Economic dependency and unemployment
(7) The size of the family (total fertility)
(8) The number of people per room (room density in houses)
(9) Life expectancy at birth.

The PDP shares the following indicators with the WHO HFA/2000 (p.26) programme:

(1) Infant mortality rate
(2) The adult literacy rate
(3) The per capita income
(4) PHC as the vehicle for improving the health of the nation.

The upgrading of the quality of life of the underdeveloped people, especially a large section of the black community, is facilitated by the following strategies:

(1) Education. This includes the education and training of workers and the upgrading of the role of women, *inter alia*, by in-service training. The education of women is the most important factor in reducing child mortality. Adult education to enable illiterate adults to read and write are important PDP aims. Formal mandatory school education for all South African children for 10 years is the ideal to be aimed at.
(2) Primary health care (PHC).
(3) The extension/intensification of family planning services.
(4) Large-scale provision of low-cost housing.

(5) Creation of job opportunities. At present the informal small business sector holds enormous promise for job creation. The Department of Manpower has a job creation fund which is used for supplying small businesses with essential equipment, for example a sewing machine for a housewife who wants to supply the home market with manufactured articles.
(6) Provision of basic infrastructure.
(7) An orderly urbanisation strategy.
(8) Rural development.

The government appointed a large number of graduate community public relations officers to initiate and co-ordinate development projects in the 44 economic subregions of greater South Africa, as well as community development facilitators to raise the socio-economic level of impoverished communities. Of great importance in the development programme is the establishment of the **Rural Foundation**.

This private organisation, initiated by the South African Agricultural Union in 1982, employed more than 100 community developers in farming areas, its aim being to raise the general quality of life of farm labourers and their families. Three-quarters of the salaries of these developers is paid by the Department NHPD and one-quarter by the farmer. The Rural Foundation reaches approximately 350 000 people on 3 500 farms.

The developers do not prescribe but give advice to employers of labour. The farmers and their wives who want to become actively involved in the programme offered by the Rural Foundation are richly rewarded for their investment in human development. The developers co-operate with community leaders. The local communities must identify their own needs and form committees to fulfil these needs. The committees can get help from welfare and other development organisations, e.g. Operation Hunger. Examples of community projects: training of nursery school teachers for the large number of 'nursery schools' being built on farms by farmers or by parents; initiation and management of a crèche and play schools for the children of working mothers. Farmers are building state-subsidised schools for which the DET provides the teachers. In 1991 86 % of black children between the ages of 6 and 16 years are at school.

The Rural Foundation collects money from the private sector to build community and cultural centres in a region for a number of farms. Here the farm labourers gather for sporting and cultural activities and educational and vocational training. Farmers' wives are playing an important role in teaching the wives of their labourers crafts, e.g. sewing. Labourers are taught to build their own houses with the help of a borrowed brick-making machine. The rural population is also taught to make pit privies and vegetable gardens and the safeguarding of springs to ensure a pure water supply. It has been found that as people develop pride in their accomplishments and attain a decent standard of living, they are more prepared to accept family planning. Clinics for this purpose are readily available.

Farm labourers are being trained in the Boskop centres in the Transvaal to develop farming skills (e.g. the maintenance of tractors and the use of expensive machinery).

The developers work with trained female volunteers from the black communities, who motivate the people to improve their living standards. People are encouraged to attend literacy classes in the evenings at the farm schools.

Health is the foundation of social upgrading and on some farms basic health services are rendered by community health workers (care groups) — women from the community trained by the professional PHC workers to meet the basic health needs of people, e.g. first aid, immunisation, family planning, adequate nutrition, oral rehydration of infants with diarrhoea, personal hygiene, fly control, sanitation and the purifying of drinking water. These workers are in a position to refer cases beyond their helping capability to the PHC clinics.

NON-GOVERNMENT ORGANISATIONS (NGOs)

NGOs are voluntary organisations in civil society which, *inter alia*, extend and complement the functions of government institutions, e.g. health, education, etc. They are of great importance in the public life of a democratic society as they arise 'from the people' to work 'for the people'. There are many thousands (54 000) of NGOs in the RSA — some religious, some educational, some sporting, some civilian (the 'civics'); a great number are involved in community health projects, e.g. National Cancer Association, Heart Foundation, SA National Councils for the Deaf and for the Blind, SANCA (alcoholism and drug abuse), SANCCA (aged), SANTA (TB), Operation Hunger. Many NGOs aim specifically at development initiatives, e.g. Urban Foundation, National Progressive Primary Health Care Network.

NGOs employ a large number of people, some of them professional, paid employees, and they also raise large sums of money ('for charity'). For fund-raising they must acquire a 'WO' number or be registered as a 'trust' or 'Section 21' company which gives them a legal status to attract donors.

NGOs attract donations from the public and from overseas donors. Their combined funds during the past year were R6 billion (Development Resources Centre, Johannesburg).

There is no doubt that the proliferation of these NGOs was in response to apartheid policies which harmed the black population. Since the demise of apartheid, the future role of some NGOs and their capacity for attracting funds, especially from overseas, is in the balance. The government of national unity is bringing about social change and may well attract funding from overseas and local business. On the other hand, NGOs provide private citizens with the means of enhancing the process of reconstruction and development in our democratic society.

THE GNU'S FIVE-YEAR PLAN FOR IMPLEMENTING THE ANC'S RECONSTRUCTION AND DEVELOPMENT PROGRAMME (RDP) 1994

The ANC's five-year Reconstruction and Development Programme is people-oriented (i.e. it aims to better the lives of the people) and will cost between R80 billion and R90 billion. It is an extension of the PDP. The ANC hopes to complete this programme in 10 years.

This RDP programme plans to provide millions of jobs, 10 years' free education for every child in the RSA, health care for all (see the National Health Plan in Chapter 3), electricity, housing and water on a massive scale and a telephone service within reach of all. This programme will be intersectorally co-ordinated by the Minister-Without-Portfolio and will start off with a 100-day upliftment plan. The programme will be a combined effort by cabinet ministers, provincial governments and the community.

The success of this five-year plan depends on a partnership between the government, the private sector (i.e. business expertise) and the labour movement (i.e. unions) to get the plan working on the ground. The cabinet departments crucial to the success of the RDP are: labour, trade and industry, finance, housing, transport, telecommunications, provincial affairs, health, education and water. The priorities will be education, health, jobs and the provision of houses, infrastructure and services (electricity, sanitation). This requires the RDP team to deal directly with the communities (i.e. local government structures). NGOs will also lend their support by donating their resources.

Points of particular interest to community nurses are:

- Children under the age of 6 and pregnant women: free medical care in every state hospital and clinic.
- A nutritional feeding scheme in every primary school where such need exists.
- Provision of affordable medicines through greater use of essential drug lists and a single national price for each medicine.
- Eradication of poliomyelitis and neonatal tetanus by 1995.
- Addition of 2 541 clinics to the 2 218 public health care clinics by 2000.
- Full immunisation for 80 % of all children under 2 years by 1995, and 90 % by the end of 1997.

The President committed his government to:

- The provision of clean water.
- Addressing the housing shortage.
- Addressing the needs of the aged and disabled, the unemployed and students. Free and compulsory schooling for 10 years.
- Rural development with accessible water supplies, electricity, telephones, roads and sewage disposal, housing and schools; creation of jobs by developing industries and small business; helping small farmers to gain access to training, credit and markets for their products.

- Land reform.
- The electrification of 350 000 homes during the current financial year.
- Rebuild townships, restore services and create jobs.

The first democratic budget (June 1994) contains big increases in social spending. It supports the Government of National Unity's promise to uplift the standard of living of the millions of very poor people in South Africa. It is a 'people's' budget in which housing, education, welfare, water affairs, job creation and health have emerged as priorities in the Government's Reconstruction and Development Programme (RDP).

For success in its implementation the RDP needs the enthusiastic involvement of communities and the second- and third-tier governments.

REFERENCES

(1) MacIver RM, Page CH. *In Society: An Introductory Analysis.*
(2) *Primary Health Care (1978)* Report of the International Conference on Primary Health Care. Alma-Ata, USSR. 6–12 September 1978. Geneva: WHO.
(3) Theron ES. Putting community health into perspective. *S Afr Med J* 1983; **63**: 1018–1019.
(4) Council for Population Development. Population Growth — South Africa's ticking time bomb.
(5) Van Niekerk WA. Address to International Conference on Population Development. *PopDevNews* October 1988.

TEST OF KNOWLEDGE

The student has benefited from studying this chapter and asking knowledge-broadening questions if he/she can answer the following questions:

(1) Define the following:
  – Health
  – Secondary health care services
  – Secondary preventive health care
  – Non-personal health services
  – Community

(2) Give reasons for the statement that some indicators of poor quality of life are:
   – high birth-rate
   – high teenage pregnancy rate
   – high fertility rate
   – high infant mortality rate
   – high room density
   – high population growth rate

(3) Discuss the objectives of the Department of NHPD Population Development Programme (PDP) for promoting the health and quality of life status of a developing (Third-World) community.

(4) Write an essay on the non-government organisations you have come across in your community.

(5) Comment on the ANC's Reconstruction and Development Programme (RDP).

2

Organisation of Health Care in the RSA
The National Health Plans of 1986 and of 1994
Restructuring of Nursing Organisation

SUMMARY

The Health Act 63 of 1977 ushered in a new health care philosophy: the introduction of a comprehensive approach to health care, i.e. the addition of promotive, preventive and rehabilitative components to curative services in order to improve the health status of communities. This led to the formulation of the National Health Care Facilities Plan in 1981 and the National Health Plan in 1986. This plan has six structural levels of health services including environmental and personal primary health care. In 1994 the National Health Plan of the ANC was announced. The entire health structure will be rebuilt around primary health care with mobile and fixed clinics on the lowest rung of the ladder and the seven large academic health complexes (AHC) at the top. These independent AHCs will come directly under the central government (Department of Health) and their services will be shared across the provinces. Their service role comes under the provinces.

Restructuring of nursing organisations is also taking place with the yearning of nurses for 'mental liberation' and the striving for democratisation of nursing organisations.

HEALTH SERVICES IN THE RSA BEFORE 1994

In the Republic of South Africa, over the past 60 years, patterns of health and disease among whites, and to some extent urban blacks, have changed considerably. The changing demographic characteristics of the white population, coupled with improvements in socio-economic conditions, and consequently in nutrition, as well as the control of environmental hazards such as poor sanitation, and the extensive use of immunisation, have led to a marked decline in the incidence of the communicable and nutritional disorders. At the same time there has been a significant increase in the degenerative conditions, cardio-vascular diseases, emotional disorders and cancer in the population. Coupled with these changes, we find the development of a new philosophy concerning the delivery of

health care services. What is now needed, say the authorities, is a 'comprehensive' approach to the situation. Health care services must include promotive, preventive and rehabilitative components as curative services alone will not improve the health status of a community. Moreover, communities must accept some responsibility for their own health care; active participation by members of the community in the delivery of health care must be encouraged. It was felt that in order to implement this new approach, new health legislation was required.

The new Health Act 63 of 1977 came into effect in May 1977.

National plan for health service facilities

In 1980 the National Health Service Facilities Plan was announced by the then Minister of Health and Welfare. In 1981 the National Health Care Facilities Plan was finalised and announced and, in 1986, an extension of the above, the National Health Plan. The aim of these plans is to provide a comprehensive health service for the entire South African population.

In the National Health Care Facilities Plan the following important principles, ideal for health care in the RSA, are stressed:

(1) There should be a shift in emphasis from the sick person to the healthy person.
(2) Regard should be had for the total needs of a person.
(3) Services should be increasingly community-oriented.
(4) There should be a shift in emphasis from curative to preventive care.

The National Health Plan 1986

The National Health Plan, an extension of the above plan announced in 1986, has the following objectives:

(1) A centralised policy for achieving health goals and priorities.
(2) Centralised responsibility for the provision of health services. This rests with the Department of National Health and Population Development. This Department has the following functions:
   (a) To provide the structure for planning and co-ordinating national health.

(b) To control expenditure on health, and to allocate funds according to the shift in emphasis from curative to preventive care.

(c) To deal with general policy, disease prevention, population development for all race groups.

(d) To deal with the provincial authorities (which deal with hospital services for all races).

(3) Decentralised implementation based on the National Health Plan to render comprehensive health services. According to the National Health Plan, health services will no longer be rendered at three tiers of government. In short, tier two government (provincial) will run all hospitals, and tier three (local government) will render levels I, II and III services (primary health care).

During the apartheid era, there were 11 Departments of Health in the greater South Africa — each of the black homelands had its own Department of Health and the Republic of South Africa had its own. In 1984 a new constitutional dispensation in the RSA established a Tricameral (3-house) Parliament to provide separate health facilities for 3 population groups. Each 'house' had its own Department of Health Services and Welfare, headed by a minister. Health services were thus compartmentalised as follows:

■ House of Assembly — White 'own affairs'
■ House of Representatives — Coloured 'own affairs'
■ House of Delegates — Indian 'own affairs'

Overlapping these 'own affairs' health departments was a general Health Department—the Department of National Health and Population Development (DNHPD) under a Minister of Health. Each 'house' was responsible for health services for its own group and hospitals were segregated. The DNHPD was responsible for black level I–III services, these services being delegated to provincial administrations.

The National Health Plan was the formula for achieving the ideal of a comprehensive health service for South Africa.

Structural levels of health service according to the National Health Plan (1986)

Level I

Provision of basic subsistence needs (environmental PHC)

■ Safe drinking water and wider environmental health
■ Sewage and waste disposal
■ Food supplementation
■ Infrastructure and basic housing

Level II

Health education

■ Minimum education level
■ Training and education
■ Guidance

Level III

Primary health care

■ Self-care
■ Community nursing services
■ Community health centres

Levels IV to VI

Hospitalisation (for secondary and tertiary health care)

■ Level IV — Community hospital
■ Level V — Regional hospital
■ Level VI — Academic hospital

Arrangements for rendering health services according to levels

Levels I–III

Environmental and personal health services, i.e. primary health care, are the responsibility of local governments.

Levels IV–VI: hospitalisation

All hospitals are administered by the Provincial Administrations, who also execute delegated services, e.g. community health centres for blacks.

EXTRACTS FROM THE HEALTH ACT 63 OF 1977

Functions of the first-tier government — Department of National Health and Population Development

(1) (a) The co-ordination of Health Services and the provision of additional services towards the establishment of a comprehensive health service.

(b) The establishment of a national health laboratory service.

(c) The promotion of a safe and healthy environment.

(d) The promotion of family planning.

(e) The undertaking of research in terms of this Act and the South African Medical Research Council Act.

(f) The provision of medico-legal services.

(g) The performance of other functions assigned to it by the Minister.

(2) The Minister can delegate any function of the Department to a Provincial Administration under conditions that he may prescribe.

Health functions of the second-tier government — Provincial Administrations

(1) The provision of:

(a) Hospital facilities and services.

(b) Ambulance services.

(c) Facilities for the treatment of patients suffering from acute mental illness.

(d) Facilities for the treatment of out-patients in hospitals or in other places where patients are treated for a period of less than 24 hours.

(e) Maternity homes and services and their maintenance.

(f) Personal health services, either on their own or in the implementation of a decision by the Minister, or in co-operation with any local authority.

(2) The co-ordination of the above-mentioned services with a view to the establishment of a comprehensive health service.

Health functions of the third-tier government — Local Authorities

(a) The prevention of communicable diseases.

(b) The promotion of the health of persons, i.e. health education.

(c) The rehabilitation in the community of persons who have received treatment for any medical condition.

(d) The co-ordination of such services with due regard to similar services rendered by the Department of National Health and Population Development, and the provincial administration, e.g. the institution and maintenance of a comprehensive health centre.

Note: The Provincial Secretary of a provincial administration is responsible for personal health services in a Section 30 area.

Subsidisable health services

The following subsidisable health services conducted by medical practitioners and nurses are set out in the schedule of R2 714 (1984) for the purposes of section 26 of the Health Act 63 of 1977 (refunds in respect of health services rendered by local authorities):

(a) The prevention of communicable diseases by means of:

(i) immunisation;

(ii) the detection and treatment of persons suffering from tuberculosis or venereal diseases, or their contacts;

(iii) the detection of persons suffering from other communicable diseases and their contacts.

(b) The prevention of non-communicable diseases by means of:

(i) the detection of persons suffering from such diseases;

(ii) the diagnosis and treatment of minor ailments of indigent persons;

(iii) the supply of medicines, approved by the director-general from time to time for the treatment referred to in paragraph (b)(ii).

(c) All activities, whether at facilities run for such purpose by a local authority or during home visits, aimed at the following:

(i) the promotion of the health of and the prevention of diseases in mothers, pre-school and school-going children and aged persons;

(ii) the promotion of mental health and the rendering of psychiatric community services;

(iii) family planning as part of a health service.

(d) Health education for the prevention of diseases and the promotion of health.

(e) The rehabilitation in the community of persons cured of a medical condition.

(f) The supply of skim milk powder, or protein-vitamin-mineral mixtures to persons for the prevention of nutrition deficiency diseases.

1990 Regulations under the Health Act 63 of 1977

On 16 May 1990 the Minister of National Health and Population Development announced that all South African public hospitals would immediately open their doors to all race groups. This was part of the new government policy to rid South Africa of discriminating practices.

The Minister stressed the importance of primary health care and a more equitable distribution of funds for primary health care. She said health services are to be reconstructed on the basis of 5 principles:

(1) accessibility of services;
(2) efficacy of care programmes;
(3) affordability of services;
(4) equity in provision of services;
(5) acceptability of services.

There is a shift in health service policy from curative to preventive medicine.

Restructuring of health services by the DNHPD[*]

In order to distribute the state money allocated to health care more equitably between primary, secondary and tertiary health care services and also to make the best possible use of the available health care personnel, it was now generally accepted and was the policy of the Department of National Health and Population Development, to shift the emphasis of health care to Primary Health Care. In 1989 the Health Policy Council recommitted the public health services to the provision of PHC to all and to bring gastro-intestinal diseases in children and measles under better control. The health care force can be extended for a total onslaught on the health care of the neglected millions of poverty-stricken blacks — urban as well as rural — who have not been able to afford or reach the expensive services of urban hospitals — both private

and provincial. Besides, poverty for whatever reason causes poor health if it deprives people of basic subsistence needs (see level 1 of the National Health Plan).

Professional and auxiliary nurses, health inspectors, pharmacists, and other members of the health care team can be utilised to the full and their functions extended by using thousands of community health workers from the ranks of the black population (see p. 37). The important health care service of the future will, therefore, be Primary Health Care (see Chapter 3).

The main restructuring of health services in the RSA to date (April 1994) was the transfer of Primary Health Care (PHC) services to local authorities. This decision was taken by the government in 1991 but was still in the process of execution in 1994 and will be for some years. Much research has been done on the enormous discrepancies in the spending of the R9,2 billion spent annually on health care in the RSA. Fifty-six per cent is spent in the public sector which serves 80 % of the population. Four billion goes to the private sector — to the 20 % well-to-do people, mostly whites. The public sector is also much more dependent on the services of nurses and nearly half the country's doctors serve the private sector. In the public sector the biggest slice of the financial cake goes to the maintenance of community, regional and academic hospitals. The slice for the rural and urban poor — that section of the community dependent on PHC services, is very thin indeed.

THE NATIONAL HEALTH PLAN OF THE ANC (FROM 1994)

This plan is not yet policy. Enabling legislation is hoped to be passed in 1995.

The ANC's health plan stresses the need for change from the health plan of the previous government. All the services provided by the Departments of Health — 14 departments in all — are to be merged and rationalised. Unification will be carried out by the Government of National Unity (GNU).

The main 'reforms' of the new health plan are that the present fragmented services will be

* Up to 1994, when they started to merge with the ANC's National Health Plan.

taken apart and put together in more rational ways.

Professional health workers will go on working as and where they worked before. The main 'actors' in the rationalisation of health services will be the administrative staff. The nursing burden will be shared by a large number of community health workers (see p. 37, 43). Primary health care will be organised in small district and community structures, co-ordinated at regional level.

The emphasis will shift towards preventive health care but the curative aspect of primary health care (PHC) will remain in place. The entire health structure will be rebuilt around primary health care (PHC). At the bottom of the PHC ladder will be mobile and fixed clinics. Health care will move up to community and regional hospitals. At the top of the ladder will be the seven large academic health complexes (AHC) consisting of a medical school and its 1–5 academic hospitals. They will serve as centres of training and research, and will be shared across provinces, e.g. in one AHC, all heart transplants can be done, in another, all kidney transplants.

The ANC's National Health System (NHS)

This section has been extracted, with many direct quotations, from the ANC's National Health Plan.

The National Health System is organised on four levels — community, district, provincial, central.

(1) Community level

Community represents those people living in the geographical area served by a Community Health Centre (CHC) (see Chapter 4) — the backbone of the NHS. All communities will form intersectoral (health, housing, etc.) *Community Development Committees* to prioritise community health needs.

The CHC provides comprehensive services: promotive, preventive, curative and rehabilitative care. Each CHC will also run fixed clinics (Ch 4) and send staff to visit health posts in the area. Casualty and maternity services will be available 24 hours a day. Community health workers are part of the team (see Chapter 4).

Health posts are part-time facilities visited by clinic (stationary or mobile) or CHC teams. They bring services closer to the people who need them.

(2) District level

The development of health districts is essential to the transformation of health care and the decentralised management of the ANC's NHS. The whole of the RSA will be divided into approximately 100 health districts, each containing 200 000 to 750 000 people. A district may comprise one, two or three local authorities. All community level services, both public and private, will fall under the District Health Authority from which they will receive material and logistic support.

Each district will receive a budget for PHC services and will appoint a team *(the District Health Authority, DHA)* to manage this budget and run the services. Like at community level, the health district will have an *Intersectoral District Development Committee* comprising senior representatives (of sectors impacting on health) of local governments, to co-ordinate all development in the district.

Community hospitals (i.e. District or non-specialist) run by the DHA, will work closely with CHCs and will provide in-patient care close to where people live. They will be visited regularly by specialists from the provincial (specialist) hospital with which they are linked.

DHAs will encourage the training of community health workers (CHWs). (See p. 37, 43.)

A *District Health Advisory Body* representing all the district stake holders in health will advise the DHAs Management Committee.

Note: No decisions have as yet been taken concerning the level of government which should be responsible for the district health system.

(3) Provincial level

The National Health Authority delegates responsibility for the delivery of health services to the provinces. As on the other levels, there will be an *Intersectoral Provincial Development Committee* comprised of MECs responsible for all sectors impacting on health. The main task of the *Provincial Health Authority* (PHA) will be the support and supervision of the

DHAs, especially with regard to the provision of specialist hospitals and services, the organisation of training and the co-ordination, evaluation and planning of primary health care services. Specialists from the provincial institutions will visit district health facilities for teaching and learning purposes and to facilitate efficient referral between primary, secondary and tertiary facilities.

All specialist hospitals, including academic hospitals, will be co-ordinated by the PHA. These specialist hospitals can also support and do relevant research and have a large role to play in both basic and continuing education and training of all types of health workers.

Academic hospitals should be fully integrated into provincial health services in their service role. They are a national resource and as such will be accountable to the National Health Authority.

A *Provincial Health Advisory Body* will include representatives of stake holders in the private health sector and in civil society.

(4) Central (national) level

The single, comprehensive, equitable and integrated National Health System (NHS) requires planning, co-ordination and monitoring at the central government level. There will be an *Intersectoral National Development Committee* consisting of the ministers of all sectors affecting health.

There will be a *National Health Authority (NHA)* chaired by the *Minister of Health* and including the following: Secretary for Health, Heads of the National Divisions (Primary Health Care, Hospital and Support Services, Planning and Human Resources, Administration and Finance), representatives from the PHAs, DHAs and from the National Health Advisory Body.

The NHA will be responsible for the development and provision of all health care in South Africa.

Functions

(a) Policy formulation and strategic planning.
(b) Development of guidelines, norms and standards to apply throughout the health system.
(c) Translating policy into relevant integrated programmes in health development.
(d) Policy statements and health legislation.
(e) Co-ordination of international and donor support.
(f) Allocation of the national health budget.
(g) Co-ordination of both public and private health care.

The *National Health Advisory Body* advises the Secretary for Health and Central Management Committee of the NHA. It is comprised of representatives of the Statutory bodies (SANC, SAMDC), the national associations of health professionals (e.g. the DENOSA and MASA), NGOs involved in health and national community structures such as 'civics' and unions.

Health Educational Institutions (Medical Schools and Academic Hospital complexes (AHC) are regarded as national resources and are accountable, therefore, to the NHA.

They are responsible for comprehensive health care through service rendering, teaching, research and management at primary, secondary and tertiary levels. Their activities will be co-ordinated so that their contributions to human resource training and development are appropriate to the needs of the country.

The role of the private sector and independent practitioners

Although private practitioners and hospitals will continue to play an important role in the National Health System, in the longer term, most health care will be provided within the public health service. Expansion of the private health sector will be discouraged and will no longer be subsidised by the state.

Private practitioners will be encouraged to work in public clinics, health centres and hospitals on a regular rotational basis.

The important role played by traditional healers in the health care of a large proportion of our population is acknowledged — so too the role of the so-called 'complementary' or 'natural' therapists. Systems of repayment such as capitation fees will largely replace fee-for-service payments in order to reduce the incentive to over-service patients.

The pharmaceutical industry and suppliers of medication and equipment will be encouraged to sell their products largely, if not exclusively, to the state.

RESTRUCTURING OF NURSING ORGANISATION

Introduction

Nurses form the largest category of health care workers and, therefore, play a very important role in the health care of South Africans. Political upheavals, due to the rapid transition of South Africa from an 'apartheid' society, to a fully democratic non-racial society have caused many cracks and even rifts in the nursing profession. The SA Nursing Association (SANA) has taken a very strong lead in keeping the profession together — a united force which works for the good of the sick people entrusted to its care.

The government has removed many obstacles from the process of conciliation between white and non-white nurses by removing 'apartheid' structures and opening hospitals and nursing colleges to nurses and patients from all racial groups.

In March 1992 the Nursing Amendment Act 21 of 1992 was published. This Act made the following provisions:

(a) The constitution of the SA Nursing Council (Council) was changed by, *inter alia*,
  (i) the deletion of all reference to population groups and consequently the proportionate representation of the four population groups on the Council;
  (ii) the increase of the elected component of the Council from 10 to 15 members and the reduction of non-nursing appointed members.
(b) The necessity of a disciplinary inquiry was reduced by giving the Council the power to impose a fine.
(c) The legal prohibition on strikes in the nursing profession was deleted.

Note: Strike action by nurses still remains an ethical transgression, subject to disciplinary steps by the Council, if it can be proved that the nurse has abandoned her patients and they have been harmed as a consequence.

The South African Nursing Association (SANA)

The SANA has gone through a period of 'change, transformation and renewal' to accommodate the opinions of nurses from all the racial groups which constituted its involuntary (obligatory) membership.

In 1993 SANA asked the nurses of South Africa whether it should be managed as a non-statutory body or remain within the Nursing Act subject to laws (statutes). The nurses voted for change; the wish of the nursing profession is also for freedom of association.

High-powered members of SANA lobbied Parliament and obtained approval for an amendment to the Nursing Act, which allows for non-statutory status and voluntary membership of SANA. This amendment came into force on 1 January 1994. Nurses who no longer wish to be members of SANA lose out on all membership benefits.

Nursing Amendment Act 145 of 1993: repeal of section 38 of Act 50 of 1978

(1) Section 38 of the Nursing Act, 1978, is hereby repealed.
(2) With effect from the date on which subsection (1) comes into operation:
  (a) The South African Nursing Association referred to in the said Section 38 shall cease to exist;
  (b) All assets, rights, liabilities and obligations of the said Association shall devolve upon an organisation designated by the Minister for National Health and Welfare (sic) after consultation with the persons who immediately before that date were members of the board of the said Association.

The main reasons why SANA addressed this urgent request to Parliament are:

(a) Respect for basic human rights which includes the right of the individual to freedom of association.
(b) Voluntary membership is a prerequisite for participation by SANA on many negotiation forums, e.g. those which are implicated in the Public Service Labour Relations Act. Hereby the goal of quality nursing care is more likely to be attained.
(c) Nurses in South Africa have voted in favour of managing their professional organisations as a non-statutory body. Thus decisions taken for the nursing profession can be taken by the nursing profession.

In future, matters of importance for nurses will increasingly be debated at forums (meetings for public discussion) where nurses from all nurse interest groups meet. Thus the development of nursing in South Africa will be democratically guided by the nurses themselves.

The 'Nurses planning for the future' forum

The Nursing Act 50 of 1978, recently replaced by the Nursing Amendment Act 21 of 1992, caused many nurse interest groups to form within the profession. Apart from SANA the following nurse groups exist in the RSA: Elizabeth Fry Quaker Nurses, Communist Party (Health Desk), Concerned Nurses of South Africa, Democratic Association of South African Nurses, Women for Peace, Students' Federation of the Transvaal.

These nurse groups realised the necessity of getting together to plan for the future in a democratic South Africa. Unity of purpose is of great importance if the nursing profession is to play its major role in the health services in the country. The first nurses' forum — Nurses Planning for the Future (NPFF) — took place in March 1993. Representatives of all the nurse interest groups came together to achieve understanding and unity as they planned together for the future. Ideas gathered here were disseminated countrywide. At future forums of all nurses in South/Southern Africa, nurses will be able to debate crucial issues such as the positioning of the nursing profession in a future health care system (the new health dispensation).

Labour relations of private and public sector nurses

As trade unions became more and more involved in the private and public sectors of health care institutions, disruption of patient care started taking place. The trade unions tried to organise all health workers, even the nurses. Hospital managers could not control the situation.

Legitimate trade union activity in the private sector

SANA decided to play a more active role in employer/employee relations by acting as the third party in disputes involving nurses working in the private sector. This was done to preserve the nurse/patient relationship which is bound by the tradition of a westernised nursing profession to put the interests of the patient first.

This role as intermediary could only be accomplished by registering a 'leg' (section) of SANA as a trade union with the Department of Manpower (Labour) (in October 1993) — a mandate having been obtained from the profession. This trade union is call SANTU — The South African Nurses Trade Union. The formation of a trade union is a requirement of the Labour Relations Act for SANA to gain entry to negotiating bodies, in this case, the industrial councils for local authorities. Membership of SANTU is open only to nurses working in the private sector — local authorities, private hospitals, and old age homes. An elected Executive Committee manages the affairs of SANTU.

The Public Service Labour Relations Act 1993

This Act benefits nurses working in the public sector, *inter alia*, in the provincial hospitals. SANA represented 75 000 nurses in the public service before voluntary membership became legal.

Major provisions of the Act:

(1) Negotiations for salaries and other conditions of service. Representation of employees will be by their respective organisations, e.g. SANA for nurses.

(2) Provision is made for the settlement of disputes:
  (*a*) Individual disputes, e.g. — unfair labour practice.
  (*b*) Collective disputes for essential and non-essential services.
  Essential services: Nursing, medical and paramedical, emergency health, provision of water, power and sanitation services; services by employees of the Defence Force, etc.
  None of the essential service personnel may embark on a legal strike. Various forms of arbitration have been provided for. Nurses now have more bargaining power than they ever had before. In the past they were powerless in the event of a dispute. Now they do not have to abandon their patients to try to get a better deal.

In January 1994, the NPFF organised a National Convention of all South African nursing groups. The objectives of this convention were to discuss the concerns and needs of nurses and nursing for now and the future and to formulate principles that could be considered in addressing these concerns and needs.

Of particular importance was the organisation of nurses into an independent body, with both professional and trade union functions, by January 1995.

Other concerns were nursing education, health systems management, industrial relations, relationships with the communities and mental liberation.

The formulation of the Forum (NPFF) as the TNC (Transitional Nurses Committee) was brought about. The aim of the TNC (representing all nursing groups in South Africa) was to facilitate the process towards establishing a new democratic nurses' organisation, which will re-unite the nursing profession.

In January 1995, approximately 800 nursing delegates and observers met in Pretoria to form the new democratic organisation as planned by the TNC. The meeting was facilitated by the Independent Mediation Service of South Africa, and international independent observers monitored the procedures and provided international support. A democratic constitution was adopted. Thus a new organisation for nurses — The Democratic Nursing Organisation of South Africa (DENOSA) — was formed. This is a professional organisation (stressing professional values for all categories of nurses) with trade union components. Existing nursing organisations may dissolve and join DENOSA if they wish to do so. This seems to be the path SANA is following.

The Nursing Council

With the reunification of South Africa and the establishment of a new interim constitution, it became necessary to amalgamate the four existing nursing councils, viz. the SANC and those of Bophuthatswana, Ciskei and Transkei.

In June 1994 the four councils were requested by the Department of Health to submit regulations regarding the constitution of an Interim Nursing Council. The four councils would, however, continue to function until the first meeting of the interim council early in 1995.

The interim council will consist of 34 nominated members, 24 of whom will be nurses. It will undertake the election of a new democratic nursing council within 2 years. It will work towards the transformation of the Nursing Act and its regulations

REFERENCES

(1) *Race Relations Survey 1986. Part 2*. Johannesburg: South African Institute of Race Relations, 1988.

With acknowledgement to *Nursing News* for the section 'Restructuring of Nursing Organisation'.

TEST OF KNOWLEDGE

The student has benefited from studying this chapter if he/she can answer the following questions:

(1) Discuss the National Health Plan of the ANC (1994). Compare this plan with the National Health Plan of 1986.

(2) Discuss the restructuring of nursing organisation in South Africa since 1993. How has this process been influenced by the political struggle for a democratic South Africa?

(3) Discuss strike action by nurses: its legality, its morality and its purpose.

(4) Discuss the concern of modern South African nurses with 'mental liberation'.

3

An Introduction to Primary Health Care (PHC)

OBJECTIVE

This chapter on primary health care is intended as an introduction to the vast subject of the essential health care services which are intended to ensure the health of all the citizens of South Africa by curing the sick and injured when their indisposition is in the early stages, by preventing ill-health and especially by promoting the health of mothers and children. PHC also includes the care of those with chronic diseases for which there is no cure, as well as of the elderly.

Primary health care shifts the emphasis from the importance of curatively oriented services which provide the best possible care of the individual patient to the greater importance of preventive and health promotive services which are purported to meet the health needs of the whole of society. The term can be used interchangeably with community-based care.

The aim of the planners of PHC is to provide a better health service for all and especially for those who, through lack of privilege, have little access to the country's health promoting and ill-health curing resources. Nurses, forming the largest category of caregivers, are playing an important role in solving the problem of providing good health care for all. They are assisted by the community health workers.

In the chapters following this introductory chapter, a detailed description of the different facets of primary health care is given.

IN THIS CHAPTER

INTRODUCTION TO PRIMARY HEALTH CARE

The concept primary health care (PHC) received prominence at the Alma-Ata conference
where it was used to indicate much more than
primary care or 'first contact' care. Primary
health care constitutes a person's point of entry
into a comprehensive community health care
system; it is the first element of a continuing
health care process.

Primary care, in contrast to primary health
care, is one-to-one patient–doctor medical contact either at the office or at a clinic. Primary
health care, on the other hand, extends curative
primary care to include preventive intervention
(see p. 9). The declaration of Alma-Ata also
calls for social and economic development; participation rather than prescription; the development of a spirit of justice; the application of
research findings and public health experience;
and the tackling of the main problems in the
community.[2]

The current global trend is to move away
from curative oriented medicine to preventive
health care, i.e. from sickness and medical care
to health care. This is the most effective way of
improving the health status of countries with
limited resources, both financial and manpower
— the so-called developing countries which
include South Africa.

Although the definition of PHC formulated
at the Alma-Ata conference advocates very
comprehensive measures to ensure an improvement in global health, primary health care is
achieved mainly through maternal and child
care, family planning, immunisation and the
early treatment of minor injuries and diseases to
prevent serious complications.

Primary health care — involving a team of
health workers (see p. 42), not only doctors and
nurses — should provide a balance of promotive, preventive, curative and rehabilitative
services according to the community needs
which are most urgent. The health team helps
the community solve their own health problems
thereby enabling communities to take responsibility for, and contribute to, their own health.

The general practitioner is a key figure in
community health and, in the modern version of
community primary health care, is the leader of
the health team consisting either of nurses or of
specially trained lay persons, selected by the
community from amongst their own people. In
black rural areas doctors are often not available.

As the team leader in the comprehensive
community health programme, the doctor has
largely lost his personal relationship with patients and has delegated primary health care to
nurses, paramedical workers (where available)
and lay workers.

The community must be involved in the
planning of these health services, e.g. by the
establishment of clinic advisory committees.
Furthermore, voluntary welfare organisations
active in the community can be used to help
make the service acceptable to the people.

WHO GLOBAL STRATEGY TO REACH HFA/2000

In 1978 the World Health Organisation (WHO)[1]
declared a global strategy defined at the Alma-
Ata Conference, USSR, for 'Health for All by
the Year 2000', when the world population is
estimated to be 6 000 million. This global strategy is used for monitoring progress towards
health for all by a definite date and applies
especially to Third-World nations. The strategy
comprises 12 indicators to facilitate international comparisons and to guide countries with
community health problems to evaluate and
monitor their progress towards the ideal of
'Health for All' (HFA). An indicator is a component of the health service, whose quality is
likely to be a reflection of the quality of the
health service as a whole.

Primary health care based on scientifically sound and socially acceptable methods and technology is to be the medium of this global strategy. The purpose of primary health care is to contribute to economic and social development and to achieve the social goal of providing adequate health care for all.

DECLARATION OF ALMA-ATA[2]

'The International Conference on Primary Health Care, held in September in Alma-Ata, the capital of the Soviet Republic of Kazakh, expressed the need for urgent action by all governments, all health and development workers, and the world community to protect and promote the health of all the people of the world. The following declaration was pronounced.

(1) The Conference strongly re-affirms that health, which is a state of complete physical, mental and social well-being, and not merely the absence of disease or infirmity, is a fundamental human right and that the attainment of the highest possible level of health is a most important world-wide social goal whose realisation requires the action of many other social and economic sectors in addition to the health sector.

(2) The existing gross inequality in the health status of people particularly between developed and developing countries is politically, socially and economically unacceptable and is, therefore, of common concern to all countries.

(3) Economic and social development, based on a New International Economic Order, is of basic importance to the fullest attainment of health for all and to the reduction of the gap between the health status of the developing and developed countries. The promotion and protection of the health of the people is essential to sustained economic and social development and contributes to a better quality of life and to world peace.

(4) The people have the right and duty to participate individually and collectively in the planning and implementation of their own care.

(5) Governments have a responsibility for the health of their people which can be fulfilled only by the provision of adequate health and social measures. A main social target of governments, international organisations and the whole world community in the coming decades should be the attainment by all peoples of the world by the year 2000 of a level of health that will permit them to lead a socially and economically productive life. Primary health care is the key to attaining this target as part of development in the spirit of social justice.

(6) Primary health care is essential health care based on practical, scientifically sound and socially acceptable methods and technology made universally accessible to individuals through their full participation and at a cost that the community and country can afford to maintain at every stage of their development in the spirit of self-reliance and self-determination. It forms an integral part both of the country's health system, of which it is the central function and main focus, and of the overall social and economic development of the community. It is the first level of contact of individuals, the family and community with the national health system bringing health care as close as possible to where people live and work, and constitutes the first element of a continuing health care process.

(7) Primary health care:
 (a) reflects and evolves from the economic conditions and socio-cultural and political characteristics of the country and its communities and is based on the application of the relevant results of social, biomedical and health services research and public health experience;
 (b) addresses the main health problems in the community, providing promotive, preventive, curative and rehabilitative services accordingly;
 (c) includes at least: education concerning prevailing health problems and the methods of preventing and controlling them; promotion of food supply and proper nutrition; an adequate supply of safe water and basic sanitation; maternal and child health care, including family planning; immunisation against the major infectious diseases; prevention and control of locally endemic diseases; ap-

propriate treatment of common diseases and injuries; and provision of essential drugs;

(*d*) involves, in addition to the health sector, all related sectors and aspects of national and community development, in particular agriculture, animal husbandry, food industry, education, housing, public works, communications and other sectors; and demands the co-ordinated efforts of all those sectors;

(*e*) requires and promotes maximum community and individual self-reliance and participation in the planning, organisation, operation and control of primary health care, making fullest use of local, national and other available resources; and to this end develops through appropriate education the ability of communities to participate;

(*f*) should be sustained by integrated, functional and mutually supportive referral systems; leading to the progressive improvement of comprehensive health care for all, and giving priority to those most in need;

(*g*) relies, at local and referral levels, on health workers, including physicians, nurses, midwives, auxiliaries and community workers as applicable, as well as traditional practitioners as needed, suitably trained socially and technically to work as a health team and to respond to the expressed health needs of the community.

(8) All governments should formulate national policies, strategies and plans of action to launch and sustain primary health care as part of a comprehensive national health system and in co-ordination with other sectors. To this end, it will be necessary to exercise political will, to mobilise the country's resources and to use available external resources rationally.

(9) All countries should co-operate in a spirit of partnership and service to ensure primary health care for all people since the attainment of health by people in any one country directly concerns and benefits every other country. In this context the joint WHO/UNICEF report on primary health care constitutes a solid basis for the further development and operation of primary health care throughout the world.

(10) An acceptable level of health for all the people in the world by the year 2000 can be attained through a fuller and better use of the world's resources, a considerable part of which is now spent on armaments and military conflicts. A genuine policy of independence, peace détente and disarmament could and should release additional resources that could well be devoted to peaceful aims and in particular to the acceleration of social and economic development of which primary health care, as an essential part, should be allotted its proper share.

The International Conference on Primary Health Care calls for urgent and effective national and international action to develop and implement primary health care throughout the world and particularly in developing countries in a spirit of technical co-operation and in keeping with a New International Economic Order. It urges governments, WHO and UNICEF, and other international organisations, as well as multilateral and bilateral agencies, non-governmental organisations, funding agencies, all health workers, and the whole world community to support national and international commitment to primary health care and to channel increased technical and financial support to it, particularly in developing countries. The Conference calls on all the aforementioned to collaborate in introducing, developing and maintaining primary health care in accordance with the spirit and content of this Declaration.'

PRIMARY HEALTH CARE AND THE NATIONAL HEALTH PLAN 1986

Primary health care as proposed and accepted unanimously by 134 countries (excluding the banned South Africa) at the Alma-Ata Conference in 1978, is essential health care which is universally available for individuals and groups. The primary health principles are set out in the first three levels of the National Health Plan for South Africa (refer to p. 17). In South Africa the primary health care goals were slow to be reached, perhaps because South Africa was not a signatory to the multinational undertaking. Only in the late eighties could consensus be reached by clinicians and health administrators. In the meantime South Africa was implementing its Population Development Programme (PDP) (see p. 10). Thus the Rural Foundation (see p.11) was established to initiate and co-ordinate development projects in the farming areas.

Some PDP achievements

- Crèches on farms to care for children while their mothers work
- Education in reading and writing for illiterates
- Training of community health workers

In some local authorities many of the PHC principles were tried out, e.g. mother-and-child health, supervision of TB medication, child nutrition status, immunisation, etc. Goals were set and evaluations done annually to push up achievements in health indicators. The idea of a just dispensation for everyone — the best way of promoting the health of the family and community — was taking root in health care. Striving for HFA/2000 was inspiring health workers to move their goals for health achievements increasingly further.

HFA/2000 had become the health slogan in South Africa and was used to promote a new approach and health ethic.

In 1991 the Minister of Health announced that future health policy would embrace the principles of primary health care. This meant not only the rechannelling of health care resources but also required a change in attitude and emphasis of all health care personnel. (See Chapter 2 — Organisation of Health Care in the RSA.) The biggest changes would be community participation and involvement, and the notion that health is intimately connected with provision for basic social and economic needs.

A STRATEGY FOR PRIMARY HEALTH CARE IN SOUTH AFRICA (JULY 1992)

In South Africa, national definitions of health and primary health care were gazetted as policy for the first time on 3 September 1993 (No. R1646 to the Health Act). This regulation refers to the 'Strategy for PHC in South Africa' com-

piled by Subcommittee: Primary Health Care, July 1992. This subcommittee was appointed by the DNHPD to draw up policy guidelines for the development of PHC, in line with WHO principles.[3] The subcommittee consisted of many prominent doctors and nurses in touch with personnel presently rendering PHC services in the field, with whom they consulted. The 'Strategy for PHC' is a comprehensive manual and is available from the Department of Health (DOH).

The Primary Health Care Mission is to ensure the provision of cost-effective primary health care of all the inhabitants of South Africa. The strategy for PHC is based on the following WHO definition of PHC:[6] 'The key to attaining the goal of health for all by the year 2000 is, in the view of the Alma-Ata Conference, primary health care.'

Primary health care is essential health care made accessible at a cost the country and community can afford, with methods that are practical, scientifically sound and socially acceptable. Everyone in the community should have access to it, and everyone should be involved in it. Related sectors should also be involved in it in addition to the health sector. At the very least it should include education of the community on the health problems prevalent and on methods of preventing health problems from arising or of controlling them; the promotion of adequate supplies of food and of proper nutrition; sufficient safe water and basic sanitation; maternal and child health care, including family planning; the prevention and control of locally endemic diseases; immunisation against the main infectious diseases; appropriate treatment of common diseases; and the provision of essential drugs.[3]

ANC 'NATIONAL HEALTH PLAN FOR SOUTH AFRICA' (MAY 1994)[5]

(These extracts have been taken from Chapter 3 of the above plan. Chapters indicated in this text indicate recommended reading in this manual.)

The ANC will follow the Primary Health Care approach to the delivery of health services. PHC will form part *both* of South Africa's National Health System (NHS) and of the overall social and economic development of the community (RDP). The main aim will be the improvement of women's legal, educational and employment status together with the lowering of rates of infant mortality, maternal mortality and morbidity and teenage pregnancy.

Social welfare is closely linked with health and has a major role to play in improving health status. The areas of overlap of these two disciplines are violence, alcoholism and care of the elderly.

In alphabetical order:

- Accident, emergency and rescue services
  - Designated emergency clinics and health centers must be open 24 hours a day. Staff trained and skilled in First Aid must be on call and in communication with local hospitals. Each District Health Authority must set up an Emergency Control Centre to receive phone calls and despatch response vehicles.
  - This subject is not discussed in this manual.
- Chronic diseases (Non-communicable)
  - Many are caused by unhealthy lifestyles (smoking, substance abuse (see Chapters 15 and 42), and others are associated with contamination of the environment and food chain (see Chapters 5, 9 and 10).
- Control of communicable diseases (see Chapter 27)
  - This is a national priority and is discussed fully in Part V.
- Drugs policy
  - This subject is not discussed in this manual.
  The ANC's drug policy includes:
  - A registration process for the initial pricing of drugs to ensure their cost-effectiveness.
  - The continued and wider use of generic (non-proprietary) medicines.
  - An essential drug list with therapeutic protocols.
- Environmental health
  - A National Advisory Committee on Environmental Health will be convened with representatives from the State department concerned with the environment, plus local authorities, organised

business and labour, universities and NGOs. See Chapters 9 and 10 for a discussion of the functions of local government, environmental hygiene, health inspectors (Enviromental Health Officers) and soil and water conservation.

- HIV/AIDS and STDs
  - These subjects are discussed fully in Chapters 33 and 34.
- Laboratory services
  - This subject is not discussed in this manual.
  - ANC policy on laboratories includes the following principles:
  - Integration of laboratory services into the PHC system.
  - Provision of relevant services appropriate to South Africa's needs by laboratory personnel.
  - Appropriate training of technologists equipped to work in district laboratories.
  - Restructuring of the laboratory training institutions based on the primary health care approach.
  - Accelerated recruitment from disadvantaged and rural communities for prospective students of medical technology.
- Maternal and child health (MCH)
  - MCH is a national priority and is discussed in Part IV Chapters 20–24; as well as Chapter 19 (Problems of Adolescence). The ANC's MCH principles are included.
- Mental health
  - This subject has not been addressed in this manual. The ANC has identified the following services, *inter alia*, as priorities:
  - Supporting and developing services for all those affected by violence and civil conflict.
  - Developing preventive and promotive programmes to counter alcohol and drug abuse, poor parenting and to foster youth development.
  - Improving and supporting services concerned with the victims of rape, child abuse and family violence.
  - Provision of community care, rehabilitation services and education of mentally handicapped and disabled people,

in addition to support services for care-givers and families.
- Developing and supporting community-based mental health care services.
- Fostering liaison and co-operation with traditional healers.
- Nutrition
  - Nutrition is a national priority and is discussed in Chapters 12, 16 and 24 and includes the ANC's PHC principles.
- Occupational health
  - This is discussed in Chapter 5 and includes the ANC's PHC principles.
- Oral health
  - This is discussed in Chapter 18 and includes the ANC's PHC principles.
- Rehabilitation
  - This is discussed in Part VI and includes the ANC's PHC principles.
- Research
  - This is discussed in Chapters 6 and 7.
- Rural health
  - The principles of PHC apply in these neglected areas to the extent that the Ministry of Health should play an advocacy role in ensuring the application of all the environmental and personal PHC services. All categories of health personnel should have experience of working in rural settings.
- Women's health
  - Policy principles of the ANC are the following:
  - Emphasis on health promotion in order to enable women to make informed decisions about their health.
  - Recognition of the right to control the reproductive functions of one's body, including abortion.

    Note: The issues around abortion remain contentious and need further debating.

  - Setting priorities for the improvement of women's economic and social status.
  - Recognition of women's rights; encouraging women's participation in decision making in health; and freedom from gender oppression.
  - Giving priority to cost-effective screening programmes for diseases which affect women (e.g. carcinoma of cervix).

- Providing legal protection for women victims of violence.
- Enacting a law protecting women against rape.
- Providing access to child care, including at workplaces.
- Providing maternity benefits with job security and, where necessary, paternity benefits.

In the proposed plan the following areas of greatest need have been highlighted:

(1) Maternal and child health.
(2) Nutrition — the aim is to reduce by 40 % the prevalence of severe malnutrition, by the end of 1997.
(3) The control of communicable diseases.
(4) Measures to combat the effects of violence.

Special attention will be given to:

- Measles immunisation.
- Decreasing dehydration problems and respiratory infections in the very young.
- The major threats to public health in South Africa: tuberculosis, hepatitis and sexually transmitted diseases including AIDS will be curbed by immunisation programmes and other strategies.

The plan also includes care of the elderly and terminally ill.

Health care for children under six is already free at state hospitals and clinics (June 1994). Fifty per cent of births are to be supervised and carried out under hygienic conditions by 1995. Breast-feeding will be encouraged to such a degree that hopefully 70 % of children will be breast-fed at six months by 1995. Pregnant women will get free medical attention in every state hospital and clinic.

The first 'democratic' budget (June 1994) has increased health spending by 7 % to R14 billion. Primary health care services are allocated 25 % of the total health budget. This was made possible by restricting growth in secondary and tertiary health care.

The Health Ministry recently persuaded the academic hospitals to cut their budget by 5 % in favour of the running of new clinics during 1995/1996.

REFERENCES

(1) World Health Organisation. *Development of indicators for monitoring progress towards Health for All by the year 2000*. Geneva: WHO, 1981.

(2) Declaration of Alma-Ata. *Br Med J* 1983; **286**: 192.

(3) Subcommittee Primary Health Care. *Strategy for Primary Health Care*. Department of National Health and Population Development. July 1992.

(4) Segar J. The paper chase. *CHASA Journal* **3** (3 & 4). July 1992.

(5) ANC Health Department and WHO and UNICEF consultants. *A National Health Plan for South Africa*. Chapter 3. January 1994.

(6) WHO. *Glossary of Terms*. Geneva: WHO, 1984.

TEST OF KNOWLEDGE

The student has benefited from studying this chapter if he/she can answer the following questions:

(1) Define primary health care as conceptualised by the Declaration of Alma-Ata.

(2) Distinguish between the National Health Plan (1986) of the DNHPD and the National Health Plan (1994) of the ANC.

(3) The 'Strategy for PHC in South Africa' was gazetted as policy in September 1993 (Regulation 1646 to the Health Act 63 of 1977). Discuss the implementation of this policy in the area covered by your training school.

4

Community Health Centres and Clinics
The Primary Health Care Nurse
The Community Health Worker

OBJECTIVES

The main objective of this chapter is to introduce the student to the clinics and health centres which provide primary health care in the rural and urban areas. Curative clinic care is provided for people who do not belong to medical aid schemes and who cannot afford the services of private medical practitioners, even should they be available.

Clinics and health centres may be either comprehensive or selective (i.e. preventive or curative) to meet the needs of the communities around them and according to the resources of the caregiving agencies. In the rural areas, on the other hand, primary health care clinics and health centres are comprehensive in that they provide not only preventive, health promotive and curative functions but also promote community organisation and development.

A comprehensive primary health care (PHC) service is good if it meets the following criteria:

(1) PHC is provided by a health care team. This may not always be possible in the poor rural areas where medical and paramedical personnel are in short supply. Nurses are specially trained to fulfil a versatile PHC role, often working under indirect and remote control of a medical practitioner who is

(2) attached to a base hospital with referral facilities. The base hospital supplies personnel and materials for running the clinics.

(3) The quality of service at PHC clinics which are manned by nursing staff can be very good indeed if the nurse has been properly trained to meet the demands of her extended role.

(4) The PHC clinic is accessible to the community, i.e. within 5 km of the consumers of health care.

(5) The community participates in the PHC service through the services of its own community health worker.

(6) The primary health care service provides more than just medical care, e.g. a crèche service for working mothers and community development programmes such as the putting down of boreholes and pit privies and the making of vegetable gardens.

(7) The PHC clinic provides family planning services. The incorporation of family planning services with PHC services became state policy in August 1991. This amalgamation has doubled the number of comprehensive mobile teams in the rural areas.

For Child Health Clinics, see Chapter 22.

IN THIS CHAPTER

DEFINITIONS

A clinic in the context of community health care is a place where medical advice, examination and treatment are available, generally only during daytime hours.

A clinic may be manned by a health team (see p. 42) fully representative of all types of caregivers or the staff may be limited to one type of caregiver, e.g. various grades of nurses.

A clinic may be either preventive and health promotive, e.g. some of the clinics of urban local authorities; or they may be specialised, e.g. dental; or they may be generalised curative, e.g. day hospitals of the Cape; or they may dispense comprehensive primary health care, e.g. the rural clinics.

A clinic may be fixed, i.e. permanently domiciled in a building, or it may be mobile, i.e. set up in a vehicle which is driven to a different pre-arranged site every day. The latest mobile clinic in the RSA is a primary health care train with a number of clinics. The main aim of the train is to provide health care to peaceful rural areas (see p. 40).

A fixed clinic may be either single and small or multiple and large, in which case it is called a polyclinic.

A health centre is halfway in size and complexity between a large clinic and a small hospital. Health centres should have radio contact with a base hospital to which cases can be referred and should have a 24-hour emergency service. Community health centres supply more sophisticated services than clinics and usually have some beds for short stay obstetric and emergency cases. The health centre may be either comprehensive, e.g. the Alexandra Health Centre of the Witwatersrand University, Sandton, or curative only, e.g. the day hospitals of the Cape. Community health centres are intended to serve 50 000–100 000 people.

Community clinics are organisationally attached to hospitals or health centres. They are situated either within the parent building or at a distance, i.e. within the outlying areas serviced by the hospital or health centre. Ideally health consumers should not be more than 5 km from the nearest clinic, health centre or hospital.

Clinics which are supervised and supplied by larger clinics, health centres or hospitals are called satellite clinics.

COMPREHENSIVE COMMUNITY HEALTH CENTRES AND PRIMARY HEALTH CARE

Comprehensive community health centres are polyclinics where medical, midwifery and nursing facilities are readily available in the community, the aim being to have the health centre within a 5 km radius of each patient's home in densely populated areas. In some rural areas, small hospitals with staffing problems have been converted to comprehensive health centres. In the health centres, patients receive medical attention during normal daytime working hours only; ideally emergency care should be available at night. Midwifery staff in midwifery units are usually resident, to cater for deliveries at all hours of the day and night.

Comprehensive health centres provide curative, preventive, psychiatric and midwifery services. The health centre is connected by telephone or radio and a transport system to the base hospital with which it is affiliated; the transport system should be available even at night to cater for seriously ill patients who have no independent means of reaching the base hospital.

The following is an example of the services that can be made available at a health centre (e.g. Alexandra Health Centre and Soweto community health centres):

(1) Antenatal clinic attached to a 24-hour midwifery service. A midwife should always be on call and normal cases can be delivered at home during the day, if the mother so desires. Night deliveries should be done at the centre and emergencies are transported to the base hospital. The centre, therefore, has beds for in-patients.

(2) Maternal and child welfare or well-baby clinic. Besides providing mothercraft counselling and immunisation against infectious diseases, underprivileged mothers can be educated by nurses or members of the public in housecrafts and the cooking of nutritious meals for the family. The growth and development of the young child are supervised and timely steps are taken to prevent malnutrition.

(3) A paediatric section for the care of sick children, especially those suffering from malnutrition, chronic diseases (e.g. renal diseases), skin diseases and gastro-enteritis. There should be facilities for intravenous therapy for dehydrated children. The paediatrician should be assisted by primary care paediatric nurses.

(4) Dental clinic for both preventive (conservation) and curative (extraction) work.

(5) Clinic for chronic sick adults, e.g. those with hypertension, diabetes mellitus, cardiac and pulmonary diseases, mental disorder and epilepsy.

(6) Social assistance facilities. Patients are helped with social problems through liaison with a social welfare agency. Patients can be assessed for pensions, housing and other social aid. Food parcels, clothing and blankets collected from the public can be distributed from this centre. Social workers see patients at the centre and at home.

(7) A casualty section which deals mainly with 'Occupational Compensation' patients who

are injured at work; general minor surgery is also done for the community.

(8) Family planning clinic.

(9) Geriatric screening clinic (see p. 819) and geriatric long-term clinics.

(10) Tuberculosis clinic for medication and diagnosis.

(11) Sexually transmitted (venereal) diseases (STD) clinic; AIDS clinic.

(12) X-ray unit for the X-ray of small structures (elbows, hands, etc.) and chests.

(13) Laboratory for the common tests on blood, urine, faeces and discharges.

(14) Psychiatric (mental health) clinic staffed by a psychiatrist, psychiatric nurses and social workers.

(15) A physiotherapy clinic for diathermy, ultrasound, massage, breathing and other remedial exercises.

(16) A pharmacy for the dispensing of medicines. Ideally a registered pharmacist should be in charge.

The following domiciliary work in the area bounding the community health centre can be done by the community nurses:

(1) visiting of antenatal and paediatric defaulters;

(2) follow-up care of tuberculosis and psychiatric patients and children with malnutrition discharged from the base hospital;

(3) visiting of bedridden cases to check up on their care by friends and relatives;

(4) delivery of low-risk cases during the daytime and postnatal care where necessary;

(5) visiting by the community health nurse of crèches to weigh children and check their health charts, their teeth and immunisation status.

The community can participate in the preventive and health-promotive functions of comprehensive community health centres through the organisation of care groups (community health workers) with the help of community leaders. These groups are formed from selected volunteers in the vicinity of the health centre. The helping groups visit allocated families and bring community problems to the attention of the health care team. They stimulate the making of vegetable gardens and the erection of pit privies in areas without a communal sanitation service.

They teach the mothers the importance of family hygiene and of breast-feeding, immunisation of infants and correct eating and feeding habits. They encourage mothers to bring children to the under-fives' clinics regularly, even though the children may be perfectly well.

THE DAY HOSPITALS OF CAPE TOWN

The day hospitals described here are community health centres.

The Day Hospitals Organisation was started in Cape Town in 1969 to provide a primary health care service for the lower income group not covered by medical insurance. In 1979 there were 18 such hospitals in the Cape Peninsula, each low socio-economic area with a population of at least 50 000 qualifying to have its own day hospital to provide primary health care services for the lower income groups. The day hospitals are run by the Provincial Council and in 1974 the scheme was spreading to other parts of the Cape Province.

The registered nurses working at the day hospitals undergo a post-basic study course of four months to prepare them for the additional primary health care functions which include physical screening and history-taking. They give a primary health care service under delegated medical control and relieve the doctors of a tremendous load of work. Nurses may rotate in the following roles: district (domiciliary) visiting, physical screening and history-taking, surgical out-patient and theatre work and selected out-patient clinic work with chronic medical patients. Part of the domiciliary patient load is from the regional hospitals; this domiciliary service is an important extension of the work done at the day hospitals. The midwife obstetric units (see p. 375) of the Peninsula Maternity and Neonatal Service are attached to some of the day hospitals; they serve as short-stay labour units and antenatal clinics.

All the day hospitals belong to a day hospital organisation with central headquarters, with its own medical superintendent, matron, secretary, administrative staff, supply and transport systems, and engineering workshops. On an average, the staff of each day hospital consists of 4–6 general practitioners, 12–16 nurses and some paramedical practitioners. The emphasis is on teamwork between doctors, nurses and paramedical staff, regular seminars on medical topics conducted by experts being attended by all. The purpose of the day hospital is not only to bring primary health care services within walking distance of all the indigent peoples of the Cape Peninsula but also to relieve the tremendous patient load on the regional and teaching hospitals by diverting their former large load of patients with minor ailments. The day hospitals can also handle out-patients from these hospitals for physiotherapy, social work therapy and repeat medications. The day hospitals refer only their most urgent medical and surgical problems for secondary and tertiary health care to regional and teaching hospitals, as many of them have theatres for minor surgery. Nurock[1] writing on the first four years' experience of the Day Hospitals Organisation states that this organisation was able to cope with 95 % of its patients, only 5 % having to be referred to more specialised medical facilities. (In 1978 this number was reduced to 2 %.) He stresses that day hospitals are not satellite clinics of the general hospitals; moreover, in liaison with the hospitals, in-patients can be discharged earlier and convalesce in their own homes with the help of the day hospital domiciliary nursing and social work services.

Day hospitals fall short of the ideal requirements of a comprehensive primary health care centre in the following respects: community participation is very limited and only curative care is provided.

Preventive work is done by the Local Authority Community Health Nurses (Health Visitors), and Midwifery by the MOUs (see p. 375).

PRIMARY HEALTH CARE BY NURSES

In South Africa it is felt that there are sufficient professional nurses available to supply the PHC service and consequently additional training programmes have been developed so that nurses may function effectively in this new extended role.

Primary health care nurses (PHCNs), some specially trained for the task, supply the bulk of PHC services from fixed (residential) and mobile clinics. In 1987 there were 2 000 PHC clinics[3] in South Africa (excluding Transkei). These clinics are run by the day hospitals of the Cape, local authorities, and the Department of Health (through the hospital services of the provincial administrations).

The aspects of primary health care which may be the concern of a primary health care worker are the following:

(1) Health education.
(2) The promotion of adequate nutrition.
(3) Family planning.
(4) Immunisation.
(5) Maternal and child health.
(6) The prevention and control of locally endemic communicable diseases.
(7) The diagnosis and treatment of common diseases and injuries.
(8) The provision of essential medicines.

In the RSA PHCNs[6] work predominantly in black communities where there is a dearth of medical personnel and where basic needs of the community are poorly supplied. The black communities may be either urban or rural. The rural and urban primary health care needs which are met by PHCNs differ.

The tasks of the urban PHCNs are predominantly of a diagnostic and curative nature as preventive services are provided by city health (local authority) departments. The urban PHCN has ready access to a doctor for medical problems beyond her capability. Urban PHCNs work in a team headed by a medical officer in large community health centres which are either private or run by the Department of Hospital Services of Provincial Administrations in Soweto or in day hospitals of Cape Town.

The urban primary health care nurse is often a specialist in, for example, child and maternal health, family planning, psychiatry, paediatrics, midwifery or tuberculosis curative nursing. We can therefore speak of a paediatric primary health care nurse, for instance. She can also be called a paediatric nurse-practitioner.

Rural PHCNs work either from mobile clinics in Section 30 areas or in residential (fixed) clinics attached to community hospitals or health centres.

In the villages of the former black homelands the rural PHCN has a very comprehensive role. She must be skilled in clinical diagnostic and curative tasks as well as in preventive community health. The rural PHCN is often required to provide emergency care for difficult medical problems until her patient can be transported to the nearest hospital for secondary (hospital) or tertiary (specialist) medical care. One PHCN may be responsible for the primary health care needs of 10 000 to 15 000 people.[5]

Rural PHC nurses work as 'generalists' in polyclinics of regional or community hospitals, in community health centres and their satellite clinics and in mobile clinics. Their medical back-up services are usually remote and they may have to handle medical emergencies.

Comprehensive primary health care services must be designed to meet all the daily personal health needs of the members of a community, and should be adapted to the life-style of that particular community.

Account should be taken of the physical environment in which the community exists, and of those diseases and conditions which are most prevalent in the area. Because all communities are not similar, health services which are suitable for one community may not meet the needs of another. The provision of social welfare services is an important part of primary health care and full use should be made of existing local resources in order to solve social as well as physical health problems.

Rural black nurses also play a part in community development. The Department of Health runs regular courses in community development in Pretoria for community nurses from all the former homelands. The emphasis here is on teaching the community to attend to their own health needs. The regional hospital or health centre is used for comprehensive health care, including obstetric care, as well as for the training of community health workers.

In many of the developing countries primary health care is delivered by certain categories of non-professional workers who have been selected by the members of the community from among themselves, and who have undergone some kind of training. These community health workers are successful members of the community, either volunteers who are not paid or others paid on a fee-for-service basis for their health-promoting work. These workers are trained in the community they serve, for a specific work. They are heeded by the community they serve because they are respected for their compassionate interest in people (see p. 43 for examples of lay PHC or community health workers).

A comprehensive primary health care clinic in a rural area would be run by a 'generalist' PHCN on the following lines.

1. Curative service

The PHCN is likely to devote half her time to the diagnosis and treatment of children and adults with diseases or injuries. The curative clinic would be open daily at set times.

In diagnosing a case, the PHCN would

(1) take a full history and do a complete physical examination;
(2) make a diagnosis and prescribe treatment including medicines up to Schedule IV. Management of a case according to the signs and symptoms elicited is laid down by the doctor in charge of the service, in protocols. In some of the rural clinics doctors' visits may be spaced at weekly or fortnightly intervals.

2. Preventive care

This is essentially maternal and child health care. The following weekly clinics are essential for adequate service:

(1) Under-fives clinic at which healthy children are weighed and immunised and their mothers are educated in child care and motivated to bring their children with their Road-to-Health cards at the appointed time even though the children are well.
(2) Antenatal clinic.
(3) Postnatal clinic.
(4) Family planning clinic.

3. Chronic diseases

Chronic diseases care clinics are held once a week for sufferers from chronic diseases, e.g. a hypertension clinic alternates with a diabetic clinic, an asthma clinic and a clinic for epileptics.

Besides these clinics run by one or more PHCNs, duties also include administration,

training of staff and doing home visits in the community.

MOBILE PHC CLINICS

Mobile PHC clinics are used to render services to outlying areas, i.e. those more than 5 km from the nearest fixed clinic. In the health regions of the RSA, their main targets are farm labourers and their families — in the so-called Section 30 areas.

Note: Regulation R628 (Act 63 of 1977). With effect from 1 April 1988, the Provincial Secretary of a provincial administration shall for the purpose of Act 63 of 1977, excluding a provision of section 20(1)(*a*), (*b*), (*c*) (non-personal health services of a local authority), be the local authority within the province concerned in respect of an area referred to in Section 30(1) of the Act (rural area where there is no local authority).

There are 134 Section 30 areas in the Transvaal, Natal and Free State with a target population of approximately 4 250 000, consisting mostly of farm labourers and their families. The duties of the Department of National Health and Population Development with regard to this population previously comprised environmental hygiene, immunisation, health education and control and treatment of tuberculosis. Although the department still controls the vectors of tropical diseases (malaria, schistosomiasis) it is no longer responsible for sanitation and a pure water supply.

The Administration Commission accepted the Rheeder report which recommended the delivery of primary health care to these areas by teams of nurses using mobile units. This service was initiated in 1976; it is practically the only health care service available to this community. At present primary health care includes ante- and postnatal care and the treatment of minor ailments. Besides maternal and child welfare, geriatric problems and tuberculosis control, other special services are: control and referral of psychiatric patients, school health services, the monitoring of leprosy patients and the treatment and control of cholera.

The medical leader of the primary health care team is the district surgeon (State Health) and the regional hospital to which referrals can be made is provincial.

The primary health care nurse in the mobile clinic, therefore, has no supporting health centre to fall back on; regional provincial hospitals are frequently distant and, therefore, inaccessible, and the district surgeon may also be remote. Farm labourers do not form a homogeneous community; there is unlikely to be community organisation; community health workers are not likely to emerge in these circumstances. In such a heterogeneous, widely disseminated community it is difficult to plan health care services to meet health needs effectively, i.e. according to priorities. The latter are difficult to ascertain, as communication channels for the notification of births, deaths and disease are lacking.

The delivery of primary health care services in Section 30 areas can be a great challenge to the nurse as she works independently without direct medical coverage and with only remote control of her highly innovative nursing interventions.

Services are planned carefully to limit travelling time and to establish venues which encourage maximal attendance. These venues are frequently a shady tree, or a farm school. The co-operation of farmers must be obtained, as attendance at the mobile unit may take the labourers away from work and require the farmer to transport them. Their living conditions may also come under scrutiny and require modification by the farmer, after gentle persuasion by the primary health care nurse. She also tries to involve the farmer's wife in health projects, e.g. helping farm labourers grow their own vegetables, health education in proper nutrition and hygiene. The mobile primary health care nurse must also liaise closely with the magistrate and school principals and inspectors as their co-operation and enthusiasm help to ensure the success of this service.

The travelling PHCN brings health care to outlying areas — settlements of people and farms — by means of a mobile unit, i.e. a van with medical supplies driven by a driver. Besides the driver the team comprises a registered (preferably trained PHC) nurse, an enrolled nurse and a clerk. Non-nursing staff can help with non-specialised nursing tasks such as weighing of children.

One area of care of a regional hospital may have 10 or more mobile clinics to give a satis-factory comprehensive primary health care service. Fewer patients can be handled than at a fixed clinic as much time is wasted in travelling and packing the van before departure in the morning.

The mobile unit either stops at a prearranged time and meeting place ('point') or at a building used for the purpose of a clinic. At the 'point' or clinic the staff attend to people, mostly mothers and children, who have gathered there from the countryside.

The van is designed and furnished to enable the PHCN to carry out physical examinations, weigh children, sterilise instruments (by boiling), take histories and carry stocks of dried milks and medicines, immunising and testing materials and the record cards of the patients. Stocks are replenished when the van returns to the hospital in the afternoon. The PHCN can call on the help of a medical officer if she encounters a serious case on district and works in close liaison with the hospital, referring cases there and having cases referred to her for supervision in her area.

The main functions of the travelling PHCN are as follows:

(1) Health care of the child up to the age of 5 years. Mass (weight) charts are kept of all children and the progress of each child is discussed with his mother. The child's general state of nutrition is assessed and minor ailments (coughs, sores, rashes) are treated.

(2) Requests to supervise children discharged from hospital with some residual malnutrition are carried out by home visiting to discover if there are any social causes for the malnutrition. The mother is advised on feeding and hygiene and if necessary she is supplied with skim milk powder and vitamin syrup.

(3) Children are immunised according to the immunisation programme (see p. 494). The mothers are given the date on which they must return for further doses of vaccines. The van must be equipped with a refrigerator for the vaccines.

(4) Sick children and adults who need hospitalisation and do not have the means to get there are often transported by the PHCN

when she returns to hospital at the end of her clinic round.

(5) The PHCN discusses family planning with the mothers and dispenses either oral or parenteral steroidal contraceptives. Since 1991 PHC and family planning clinics have amalgamated. Theoretically this has doubled the number of comprehensive care mobile clinics. It is hoped that this move will enable mobile teams to reach every farm every 4 weeks.

(6) Pregnant women are given antenatal care and arrangements are made for them to be confined in the hospital.

(7) Tuberculosis patients also come to the van or clinic for their medication. Apart from giving BCG vaccine to the children, the PHCN is involved with TB prophylaxis, i.e. she does tuberculin sensitivity testing on contacts.

(8) Home visits are done, usually in the afternoons, on children discharged from hospital for whom visiting is requested. First visits to newborn babies are done as soon as their births have been notified. TB patients and patients with STD (venereal diseases) or their contacts who have failed to keep their appointments at the mobile or fixed clinics are also visited.

Note: Home visiting affords a good opportunity for health education.

PRIMARY HEALTH CARE TRAIN TO SERVE RURAL COMMUNITIES

Transnet launched a PHC train of 13 coaches on 9 January 1994. The train has 38 destinations in rural areas to reach out to the people and to provide a comprehensive primary health care service, thus enhancing the quality of life in the rural areas. The train has the following clinics: an eye clinic, an edu-clinic, a medicine clinic, a health clinic for basic screening and many more.

PRIMARY HEALTH CARE FOR SQUATTERS IN INFORMAL HOUSING (SHACKS)

The 1991 census revealed the number of South Africans living in shacks to be 2,8 million. They are the migrant squatters who are flocking to the cities and towns from the impoverished rural areas in search of a better life.

Since 1990 when Primary Health Care was officially adopted by the Health Policy Council, 200 new facilities (mobile units, community health centres, clinics and their infrastructures) have been established (1992) by public health services throughout the length and breadth of the country (see the RDP's intention of erecting 2541 PHC units by the year 2000). (See p.13.)

As some of the districts with squatter camps already had functional health services and environmental primary health care facilities (water, sanitation, refuse disposal) only those communities in greatest need were highlighted for maximal attention.

The provision of additional funding for this huge public health expenditure on PHC services was conditional on certain criteria being met, the most important being community involvement and participation through all stages of construction to the ultimate feeling by the community that they owned the facility.

These new clinics were constructed in partnership with the whole local community and provide a service for that community, and not only for the squatters in shack dwellings.

THE TRAINING OF THE PRIMARY HEALTH CARE (PHC) NURSE

As nurses may be primary health care providers in the absence of the doctor, they are being trained in primary health care nursing by their regional hospitals, to cater for the special needs of their community.

The practical education of the primary health care nurse is a continuing process and training takes place on an in-service basis, with tutors and doctors from the central (base) hospital or health centre supervising and evaluating the quality of the service. The aims of training will differ somewhat in rural and urban areas, community development being emphasised in the rural areas. The nurses in the rural areas will need a wider range of skills as they often work without doctors. In the urban areas the PHC nurse focuses on the individual patient.

Primary health care nursing is an essential part of the comprehensive health care plan of the Department of Health. Regulations for the theoretical course: Diploma in 'Clinical Nursing Science, Health Assessment, Treatment and

Care' which qualifies a registered nurse to practise as a generalist PHC nurse, were promulgated by the SA Nursing Council in January 1982. This course is offered at nursing colleges.

There are many regional training hospitals and community health centres for training PHC nurses.

The legality of the PHC course was ensured by section 38A which was inserted in Act 50 of 1978 by the passing of The Nursing Amendment Act 71 of 1981. Section 38A states that any authorised, registered nurse may . . . perform with reference to —

(1) the physical examination of any person;
(2) the diagnosing of any physical defect, illness or deficiency in any person;
(3) the keeping of scheduled medicines and the supply, administering or prescribing thereof on the prescribed conditions;
(4) the promotion of family planning.

For admission to the course, the student must be registered as a general nurse and be in possession of a matric certificate. The course extends over at least one academic year, of at least 200 days (excluding days off). The curriculum tabled must be read in conjunction with the directive obtainable from the council, and comprises: general disease conditions; clinical nursing (pharmacology and other) in health assessment, treatment and care; health care systems and research methodology. The SANC requires the following skills to be evaluated in a clinical setting: interpersonal relationships; clinical (diagnosis); practical; personal professional growth.

The SANC course is a national course and is, therefore, standardised. The emphasis is on competency in the practical situation, not so much on the theory.

The PHC nursing course is a difficult one, clinical skills being taught by doctors. These include pathology, diagnosis and prescription of medicines. Teaching is predominantly clinical, i.e. on the patient.

The PHC nurse must understand the needs and social problems of the community and must be available when needed; she must be involved in the community and be able to bridge the cultural gap between the giver and receiver of health care. In order to be effective, the nurse must be accepted by the community in which he/she works.

As the concept of PHC nursing in South Africa is new, the pioneer PHC nurses need to be experts in human relationships; they must treat the objections of people used to medical care even for minor ailments with tact and refer those patients who insist on seeing a doctor to the hospital or to a general practitioner attached to the clinic.

The primary health care nurse in training is taught to take an accurate history, do a physical examination and carry out and interpret laboratory investigations, in order to make a diagnosis. The PHC nurse is taught to recognise abnormalities and to screen patients into those she can help and those to be referred to a general practitioner, district surgeon or hospital doctor. She is also taught how to treat symptoms, how to dispense certain classes of medicines, how to counsel patients and teach health promotive principles. The initial intensive training course in the hospital takes from 2 to 4 months after which the PHC nurse mans the clinic or day hospital either as an intern or a full practising worker, meeting with the health care team regularly to discuss problems and matters of common interest and to receive ongoing education. The PHC nurse does not replace the doctor; she remains dependent upon him for referral and for consultation and the evaluation of her work.

Writing of primary health care nursing which she has done so much to pioneer, Lucy Wagstaff [6] says: 'Their approach is problem oriented and they have clear guidelines and protocols for management and referral. They issue appropriate medicines, including certain antibiotics and specified drugs up to Schedule 4, as allowed by a special permit (Health Permit 0177 in accordance with Article 22A (12) of the Drugs (Medicines) and Related Substances Control Act 101 of 1965 granted by the Director-General for Health . . . Since the medicines are given directly to the patients or relatives by the nurse, we feel that explanations might be better understood . . .' (p. 916). The implication of the latter statement is that patient compliance with his treatment may be better than in the case of patients going through the conventional channels of medicine prescription by the doctors, and medicine issue by the dispensers.

Wagstaff goes on to say: '. . . our primary health care nurses are prepared and anxious to meet this challenge (better integrated comprehensive care). Having dealt with the expressed needs of the patients (i.e. the provision of curative services), they are ideally situated to discover and attend to the requirements of the promotive and preventive aspects of health. Thus, every child is weighed, and the weight is plotted for age and sex, and nutrition advice is given if indicated. Family planning may be discussed. TB contacts and other health hazards are considered, and immunisation is ensured' (p. 916).

Irwig *et al.* state:

'Continuing evaluation and education of PHC nurses is important in the maintenance of good patient care . . . With adequate training and supervision non-physician practitioners can provide high quality health care.'[7]

The pioneer work of PHC nurses in Soweto has revealed some of the important needs of target patients.

(1) Privacy during examination by the nurses or doctors. Privacy encourages the broaching of intimate problems which worry the patient. The patient should be encouraged to ask questions.

(2) Prompt attention and the elimination of queues. Most patients who go to urban clinics work and have to account to employers for time wasted at clinics. When patients are worried about time wasted, they cannot concentrate on the instructions given with regard to medicines, etc.

(3) Friendly reception at the clinic. This is important to get the patient's co-operation.

(4) The provision of adequate and clean toilets and hand basins with soap and paper towels. The clinic must set an example in the promotion of personal hygiene.

(5) Health education. The emphasis should be on health education rather than on medicines.

THE ROLE OF THE SOCIAL WORKER IN URBAN PRIMARY HEALTH CARE

The PHC nurses should be made aware of the role of the social worker in primary health care.

(1) Orientation of community and families to accept the nurse as a PHC worker. She prepares the patient to go to the PHC clinics. If patients are suspicious they will not accept the change from doctors to nurses. If patients feel PHC is cheap treatment, their attitudes need to be changed by the social worker. Patient compliance can be prevented by lack of contact with social workers in the community.

(2) The social worker can enlighten the PHC nurse about the resources in the community. They need to co-operate and share ideas.

THE COMMUNITY-BASED MULTIDISCIPLINARY HEALTH TEAM

The community or PHC nurse does not work on her own in the community, the best way of tackling community health problems with their wide ramifications being as a member of a primary health care team.

The community or PHC nurse must be able to share in the care of the patient with the other members of the health care team: the doctor, the Environmental Health Officer, the pharmacist, occupational and physiotherapist, the community psychologist, community leaders and community health workers, as well as with the patient himself and his family.

The community or PHC nurse must be willing to share the responsibility for the health of the patient, always remembering that she is accountable for her own acts and omissions.

The nurse must know what contribution each member of the health team can make. True interdisciplinary co-operation depends on reciprocity (give and take) and on good communication and negotiation skills. The nurse plays a very important role in facilitating the role of other team members; when she recognises her own limitations she will refer the patient to the team member best able to cope with the problem. Lack of co-operation due to jealousy, selfishness and ignorance of the role of other team members, can only harm the patient and weaken the strength inherent in the true team spirit.

THE TRAINING OF THE COMMUNITY HEALTH WORKER (CHW)

Community health (or care-group) workers (CHW) play a very important role, especially in rural areas, in dispensing effective primary health care to the people. Some of these workers are illiterate, some are voluntary and others are paid by the community on a fee-for-service basis. (See p. 37.)

These workers are chosen for training by the leaders of their community after the latter have assessed and prioritised the main health problems to be treated.

The following criteria for selection of prospective CHWs are used: male or female; married with children and living in the vicinity; over 30 years old for maturity; from the local community for cultural reciprocity between worker and clients.

CHWs are trained and later supervised by either enrolled auxiliary or registered professional nurses. CHWs will be forming part of the Health Care Team. The training period ranges between 2 weeks and 6 months, depending upon the health needs of the community of origin. Training takes place at the nearest regional hospital or health centre and theory courses are interspersed with in-service education. The training concentrates on the work which the community expects from its CHWs. At the end of the course they are examined for proficiency and given a certificate as a trained CHW. Examples of skills taught: application of the GOBI-FFF principles (see p. 393).

In some communities the CHWs are taught how to grow vegetables, how to make VIP (see p. 152) and disinfect their water supplies. They are taught personal hygiene (see p. 237), especially with regard to hand-washing and other ways of preventing the spread of communicable diseases.

In Gazankulu many care-groups were/are trained at Elim hospital to combat trachoma. Their work has been described in more detail on p. 708.

The CHWs are taught the principles of good nutrition, a good diet being possible despite ethnic differences. (See Nutritional habits of people on p. 277.) The CHWs are taught how to make the home safe for children, e.g. storage of fluids in the correct containers to avoid paraffin poisoning.

The training of the CHW concentrates on the acquisition of skills. Therefore in-service education may be an ongoing process as the community makes demands for a greater variety of skills as their awareness of health increases.

The most important aspect of the training of CHWs (usually women) is female education and raising the status of women. Training and acceptance by their community give these women self-confidence and raise their self-esteem and sense of worth.

The CHWs report to a health professional supervisor in order to maintain standards of practice. This is done 2–4 times weekly, either orally or in writing, depending on the CHW's level of literacy. The supervisor, usually an enrolled auxiliary nurse, in turn compiles a report from her input and evaluates the quality of the activities of CHWs. She also guides and counsels her CHWs.

The CHWs are seen as an asset in the realisation of the goal HFA/2000. They are showing that they do contribute to an improvement in health. They are part of the culture of the community and they are available at all times.

CHWs are taught to motivate people to make vegetable gardens, to take their children for immunisation and to go for help with their health problems to the clinics and health centres, especially to give birth at the clinics.

REFERENCES

(1) Nurock R. *S Afr Med J* 1974; **48**: 1053.
(2) Wilson TD, Robb D, Ferrinho P. de L, *et al.* Insights into community participation. *S Afr Med J* 1991; **80**: 372.
(3) McNulty D. Die uitdagings verbonde aan die lewering van primêre gesondheidsorgdienste in artikel 30-gebiede. *Curationis* **4**: 22.
(4) Gumbi RV. Community health workers in developing rural areas. *CHASA* 1991; **2**(1).
(5) Buch E. *Aspects of Rural Health Services Development.* Johannesburg: University of the Witwatersrand 1986.
(6) Wagstaff L. *S Afr Med J* 1978; **54**: 916.
(7) Irwig LM, Porter B, Wilson TD *et al*. Clinical competence of paediatric primary health

care nurses in Soweto. *S Afr Med J* 1985; **67**: 92–95.

(8) The Squatters. Department of National Health and Population Development. *Epidemiological Comments* 1993; **20**(8).

TEST OF KNOWLEDGE

The student has benefited from studying this chapter if he/she can answer the following questions:

(1) (*a*) Write a short essay on clinics and health care centres in the context of a comprehensive health care service.

(*b*) Name the components of a comprehensive primary health care clinic and the criteria by which its adequacy may be judged.

(2) What is meant by the 'Day Hospital Organisation' of Cape Town. In what way does the Cape Town day hospital differ from a community health centre such as the Alexandra Health Centre of Sandton?

(3) Discuss the equipping of a mobile PHC clinic as well as the advantages and disadvantages of such a system of PHC.

(4) Discuss the training of rural community health workers.

5

Occupational Health Nursing

OBJECTIVES

To make the student aware of the large work-force in South Africa, and especially in non-mining industries, which is exposed to occupational hazards against which workers must be protected, or for which workers who are damaged by the hazards must be compensated. This chapter deals with the meaning and scope of occupational health as defined in 1950 by the joint WHO/ILO (International Labour Organisation) committee[6] as:

(1) The promotion and maintenance of the highest degree of physical, mental and social well-being of workers in all occupations.

(2) The prevention among workers of departure from health caused by their working conditions.

(3) The protection of workers in their employment from risks resulting from factors adverse to health.

(4) Placing and maintenance of the worker in an occupational environment adapted to his physiological and psychological equipment.

These four aspects of occupational health can be summed up in the last aim given by the Committee, namely:

(5) The adaptation of work to man and of each man to his job.

These principles can be elaborated and extended by an Occupational Health Nursing Service which aims:

- To persuade management to believe in sound occupational health principles and to convince them that by adopting these principles productivity will be increased and employer/employee relationships will be maintained at a high level. Management must be persuaded to appreciate the advantage of having more contented and healthy staff.
- To deal with occupational diseases and the occupational hazards which cause accidents. The promotion of the general health of the employee and the adjustment of work to man, and man to work.
- To reduce lost man-hours which result when employees have to attend outside clinics and doctors' consulting rooms.
- To give rehabilitative treatment and social and emotional guidance to injured or sick employees who are not eligible for Workmen's Rehabilitative care.

Note: Powerful unions are demanding health care for their members. Some firms view their occupational health clinics where PHC is practised as much cheaper alternatives to medical aid coverage of employees.

Occupational health covers a much broader area than its predecessor, industrial health, which was practised in factories. It applies to any place where people are employed (with certain exceptions)—in commerce, industry, supermarkets, hospitals, on farms, etc.

IN THIS CHAPTER

INTRODUCTION

Occupational health is a multidisciplinary subject comprising the knowledge and skills of
physicians, industrial hygienists, chemists, engineers, safety officers and nurses. It is the study
of the occupational hazards of the working environment and the use of methods to control
these hazards and prevent accidents. Modern
industry is complex and is becoming increasingly hazardous because of the greater number
of toxic and carcinogenic substances used, some
of which are inflammable and explosive. Environmental pollution is also increased by the
by-products of chemical processes.

A hazard is a condition which facilitates the
occurrence of injury. The hazard may arise
either from a defect in the worker who commits
unsafe acts due to, for instance, lack of skill or
impaired abilities, or from an environmental
danger (unsafe condition), for instance, faulty
equipment, exposure to toxic substances, excessive heat and noise, electricity and radiation.

The dangers of modern industries are compounded by the human problems resulting from
rapid industrialisation and urbanisation. It has
been estimated that 80 % of industrial accidents
are due to personal causes. The problems of
occupational health in the RSA are further compounded by the difference in morbidity patterns
among whites, blacks, coloureds and Asians
with special reference to the high prevalence of
tuberculosis, sexually transmitted diseases and
malnutrition amongst blacks and coloureds —
the bulk of the work-force in industry.

Occupational (industrial) health comprises:

(1) Occupational (industrial) hygiene (the field of the industrial chemist and the engineer). It is concerned with the measurement and physical control of environmental hazards.

(2) Occupational medicine (a specialised branch of preventive medicine) for diagnosing health hazards and work stresses and determining their relative importance. It includes medical services for occupational diseases (both preventive and curative) for employees in industry, as well as the treatment of accidents at work.

The prevention of occupational diseases and work accidents depends not only on legislation which makes provision for the safety and health of employees but also on the technology of ergonomics and the measures taken by the health and safety team within the organisation (factory, work or mine) to protect the health of the workmen.

OCCUPATIONAL HYGIENE

An important facet of occupational health is the adaptation of work to the worker, in order to prevent accidents and occupational diseases. This is the field of industrial chemists and engineers and comprises ergonomics and industrial hygiene.

Note: Occupational health is also promoted by adapting the worker to the job. Worker selection is an important aspect of industrial (occupational) health and is practised by most employers in order to get maximal service by placement of the right man in a post. At present hard manual labour is not required from most employees in surface industries because of mechanisation. Industry requires trained manpower, however, to man the machines. Aptitude testing can be done by industrial psychologists for the selection and placement of high-powered employees. Worker education in any occupational hazards that may be present is also important.

Ergonomics

Ergonomics, a kind of human engineering practised by the ergonomist, is a new applied science which combines biomedical and engineering skills to benefit the workman (*ergon* means work and *nomos*, law). The ergonomist designs tools and methods of work to suit the worker and his abilities. He 'fits the job to the worker', i.e. he modifies the job so as to reduce unnecessary effort, boredom and fatigue. He also tries to make the work a challenge and a source of satisfaction to the worker. The aim of the ergonomist is not to increase production but to protect the health of the worker. Any positive effects on production are fortuitous but quite possible.

In order to apply the remedy to work-induced ills, the ergonomist must first study the type of movements which tax the tolerance of a muscle, tendon or joint and cause irritation, inflammation of joints, tension in muscles and pain. When these have been defined, he makes changes in the methods of work, the work environment and the working tools (machinery). These changes are aimed at eliminating faulty movements and joint and muscle pathology.

An ergonomically designed product or tool is easy and safe to use and does its job effectively. For the guidance of the safety committee or team of an industrial concern, ergonomic instructions are finding their way into some places of work. These instructions specify how to use sitting and standing positions for a specific job and the optimal height of desks and chairs; they give advice about optimal lighting and temperatures and the necessity for noise reduction to reduce fatigue. They show how work can be planned not only to eliminate health hazards but also to suit the capacities and needs of the worker.

The ergonomic factor means any workplace or any machine, appliance, equipment or article used by or to which an employee is exposed in the performance of his duties which:

(1) may cause a psychosomatic illness in man;

(2) does not fit the anatomical and biological characteristics of man.[4]

Industrial (occupational) hygiene

Industrial hygiene is the science through which the conditions in which an employee works are made and kept reasonably free of industrial health hazards.

In 1980 there were approximately 5,5 million industrial employees in the RSA. In 1976 the Erasmus Commission of Inquiry into Industrial Health found an alarmingly high rate of occupational disease in industry and on the mines due to extremely dangerous working conditions (e.g. poor protection of industrial employees). The Commission also found that only 29 out of 66 posts of factory inspectors were filled (*Rand Daily Mail*, 8.10.1981).

Industrial (occupational) hygiene (safety) is controlled by the OHS Act 85 of 1993. Legislation is enforced by inspectors of the Department of Labour (and the Department of Mineral and Energy Affairs, by the Government Mining Engineer).

Note: Safety on the mines is not discussed in this manual.

It should be the moral obligation of employers to protect employees from occupational hazards. This principle is promoted by the International Labour Organisation (ILO), which consists of representatives of governments, employers and employees.

THE OCCUPATIONAL HEALTH AND SAFETY ACT

The Occupational Health and Safety Act 85 of 1993 (OHS Act) is intended for all employers in Commerce, Industry and Agriculture (but not for Mines and Works), particularly for those involved in technical as well as occupational health matters, to safeguard the health and safety of persons at work.

For the first time in South Africa, the occupational safety and health in the workplace has been legislated for and will fall under a single department — The Department of Manpower (Labour).

Extracts from Act 85 of 1993

'Definitions

(ii) "biological monitoring" means a planned programme of periodic collection and analysis of body fluid, tissues, excreta or exhaled air in order to detect and quantify the exposure to or absorption of any substance or organism by persons;

(iv) "chief executive officer" in relation to a body corporate or an enterprise conducted by the State, means the person who is responsible for the overall management and control of the business of such body corporate or enterprise;

(xxix) "medical surveillance" means a planned programme of periodic examination (which may include clinical examinations, biological monitoring or medical tests) of employees by an occupational health practitioner or, in prescribed cases, by an occupational medicine practitioner;

(xxxi) "occupational health" includes occupational hygiene, occupational medicine and biological monitoring;

(xxxii) "occupational health practitioner" means an occupational medicine practitioner or a person who holds a qualification in occupational health recognised as such by the South African Medical and Dental Council as referred to in the Medical, Dental and Supplementary Health Service Professions Act, 1974 (Act 56 of 1974), or the South African Nursing Council as referred to in the Nursing Act 1978 (Act 50 of 1978);

Note: The qualified Occupational Health Nurse is, therefore, an occupational health practitioner.

(xxxiii) "occupational hygiene" means the anticipation, recognition, evaluation and control of conditions arising in or from the workplace, which may cause illness or adverse health effects to persons (the old narrow term was industrial hygiene);

(xxxiv) "occupational medicine" means the prevention, diagnosis and treatment of illness, injury and adverse health effects associated with a particular type of work;

(xlvi) "risk" means the probability that injury or damage will occur;

(lv) "workplace" means any premises or place where a person performs work in the course of his employment;

2. There is hereby established an Advisory Council for Occupational Health and Safety.

Health and Safety Policy

7. (1) The chief inspector may direct —
    (a) any employer in writing; . . . to prepare a written policy concerning the protection of the health and safety of his employees at work . . .

(3) An employer shall prominently display a copy of the policy referred to in subsection (1), signed by the chief executive officer, in the

workplace where his employees normally report for service.

General duties of employers to their employees

8. (1) Every employer shall provide and maintain, as far as is reasonably practicable, a working environment that is safe and without risk to the health of his employees.

Listed Work

11. (1) The Minister may declare any work, under the conditions or circumstances specified in the notice, to be listed work.

12. (1) Every employer whose employees undertake listed work or are liable to be exposed to the hazards emanating from listed work, shall . . .

  (*a*) identify the hazards and evaluate the risks associated with such work constituting a hazard to the health of such employees . . .

  (*b*) as far as is reasonably practicable, prevent exposure of such employees to the hazards . . .

  (*c*) having regard to the nature of the risks associated with such work and the level of exposure of such employees to the hazards, carry out an occupational hygiene programme and biological monitoring, and subject such employees to medical surveillance.

Duty to inform

13. Without derogating from any specific duty imposed on an employer by this Act, every employer shall —

(*a*) as far as is reasonably practicable, cause every employee to be made conversant with the hazards to his health and safety attached to any work which he has to perform . . .

General duties of employees at work

14. Every employee shall at work —

(*a*) take reasonable care for the health and safety of himself and of other persons who may be affected by his acts or omissions;

(*c*) carry out any lawful order given to him, and obey the health and safety rules and procedures laid down by his employer or by any-

one authorised thereto by his employer, in the interest of health or safety;

(*d*) if any situation which is unsafe or unhealthy comes to his attention, as soon as practicable report such situation to his employer or to the health and safety representative for his workplace . . .

(*e*) if he is involved in any incident which may affect his health or which has caused an injury to himself, report such incident to his employer or to anyone authorised thereto by the employer, or to his health and safety representative . . .

Duty not to interfere with or misuse things

15. No persons shall intentionally or recklessly interfere with or misuse anything which is provided in the interest of health or safety.

Chief Executive Officer charged with certain duties

16. (1) Every chief executive officer shall as far as is reasonably practicable ensure that the duties of his employer as contemplated in this Act, are properly discharged.

Health and Safety Representatives

17. (1) Subject to the provisions of subsection (2), every employer who has more than 20 employees in his employment at any workplace, shall . . . designate in writing for a specified period health and safety representatives for such workplace . . .

  (5) The number of health and safety representatives for a workplace or section thereof shall in the case of shops and offices be at least one health and safety representative for every 100 employees or part thereof, and in the case of all other workplaces at least one health and safety representative for every 50 employees or part thereof:

Functions of health and safety representatives

18. (1) A health and safety representative may perform the following functions in respect of the workplace or section of the workplace for which he has been designated, namely —

(*a*) review the effectiveness of health and safety measures;

(*b*) identify potential hazards and potential major incidents at the workplace;

(*c*) in collaboration with his employer, examine the causes of incidents at the workplace;

(*d*) investigate complaints by any employee relating to that employee's health or safety at work;

(*h*) participate in consultations with inspectors at the workplace and accompany inspectors on inspection of the workplace;

(*i*) in his capacity as a health and safety representative attend meetings of the health and safety committee of which he is a member, in connection with any of the above functions.

(3) An employer shall provide such facilities, assistance and training as a health and safety representative may reasonably require and as have been agreed upon for the carrying out of his functions.

Health and safety committees

19. (1) An employer shall in respect of each workplace where two or more health and safety representatives have been designated, establish one or more health and safety committees and, at every meeting of such a committee as contemplated in subsection (4), consult with the committee . . . to ensure the health and safety of his employees at work.

(2) A health and safety committee shall consist of such number of members as the employer may from time to time determine:
Provided that —

(*a*) if one health and safety committee has been established in respect of a workplace, all the health and safety representatives for that workplace shall be members of the committee;

(4) A health and safety committee shall hold meetings as often as may be necessary, but at least once every three months . . .

(6) (*a*) A health and safety committee may co-opt one or more persons by reason of his or their particular knowledge of health or safety matters as an advisory member or as advisory members of the committee.

(*b*) An advisory member shall not be entitled to vote on any matter before the committee.

Functions of health and safety committees

20. (1) A health and safety committee —

(*a*) may make recommendations to the employer or to an inspector regarding any matter affecting the health or safety of persons at the workplace . . .

(*b*) shall discuss any incident at the workplace or section thereof in which or in consequence of which any person was injured, became ill, died . . .

Report to inspector regarding certain incidents

24. (1)Each incident occurring at work . . . in which, or in consequence of which —

(*a*) any person dies, becomes unconscious, suffers the loss of a limb or part of a limb or is otherwise injured or becomes ill to such a degree that he is likely either to die or to suffer a permanent physical defect or likely to be unable for a period of at least 14 days either to work or to continue with the activity for which he was employed or is usually employed;

(*b*) a major incident occurred; or

(*c*) the health or safety of any person was endangered . . . shall, within the prescribed period and in the prescribed manner, be reported to an inspector by the employer or the user of the plant or machinery concerned, as the case may be.

Report to Chief Inspector regarding occupational disease

25. Any medical practitioner who examines or treats a person for a disease described in the Third Schedule to the Compensation for Occupational Injuries and Diseases Act (Act 130 of 1993), or any other disease which he believes arose out of that person's employment, shall within the prescribed period and in the prescribed manner report the case to the person's employer and to the Chief Inspector.

Designations and functions of Chief Inspector

27. (1) The Minister shall designate an officer serving in the Department (Labour) as Chief Inspector for the purposes of this Act.

(2) The Chief Inspector shall perform his functions subject to the control and supervision of the Director-General of the Department and may perform any function assigned to an inspector by this Act.

Designation of inspectors by Minister

28. (1) The Minister may designate any person as an inspector to perform subject to the control and directions of the Chief Inspector, any or all of the functions assigned to an inspector by this Act.

Functions of inspectors

29. (1) An inspector may —
    (*a*) without previous notice, at all reasonable times, enter any premises which are occupied or used by an employer or on or in which an employee performs any work or any plant or machinery is used, or which he suspects to be such premises;
    (*b*) question any person . . .
    (*c*) require from any person who has control over or custody of a book . . . to produce to him . . . such book, record or other document;

(3) When an inspector enters any premises under subsection (1) the employer occupying or using those premises and each employee performing any work thereon or therein and any user of plant or machinery thereon or therein, shall at all times provide such facilities as are reasonably required by the inspector to enable him and his assistant (if any) or perform effectively and safely his or their functions under this Act.

Special powers of inspectors

30. (1)(*a*)Whenever an employer performs an act . . . which in the opinion of an inspector threatens or is likely to threaten the health or safety of any person, the inspector may in writing prohibit that employer from continuing . . .

Regulations

43. (1) the Minister may make regulations —
    (*a*) as to any matter which in terms of this Act shall or may be prescribed;
    (*b*) which in the opinion of the Minister are necessary or expedient in the interest of the health and safety of persons at work or the health and safety of persons in connection with the use of plant or machinery, or the protection of persons other than persons at work against risks to health and safety arising from or connected with the activities of persons at work . . .'

Any person who contravenes or fails to comply with a provision of the requirements of the above sections of the law, shall be guilty of an offence and on conviction be liable to a fine not exceeding R50 000 or to imprisonment for a period not exceeding one year or to both such fine and such imprisonment.

The MOS Act 1983 and all its amendments have been repealed, but not the regulations thereof.

The Act requires that an *accident register* be kept by the workplace. Where an accident happens in a factory or where building or excavation work is done, and where the worker suffers an injury which incapacitates him for more than three days, this must, under certain circumstances, be reported to the Divisional Inspector of Labour of the area. Accidents which merit an enquiry by the inspector include those causing death and unconsciousness due to heat-stroke or heat exhaustion, electric shock, inhalation of poisonous gases, as well as physical injury which may cause permanent physical defect or death.

BASIC CONDITIONS OF EMPLOYMENT ACT

This Act (Act 3 of 1983) deals with sick leave, sick certification (required from an employee who is absent from work for more than 2 consecutive days), maximum daily working hours, overtime, meal intervals, and the prohibition of employment with regard to age and pregnancy.

Knowledge of this Act is of some importance to the OHN.

OCCUPATIONAL MEDICINE

The subject-matter of Occupational Medicine is occupational disease and disability.

Occupational medicine means the medical measures which have to be taken for the prevention, treatment, research and rehabilitation of the 'medical condition' of an employee before or during his work in a workplace and the identification and evaluation of agents and ergonomic factors which may cause such a medical condition.

A 'medical condition' is defined as any physical or psychological condition in which any person is as a result of exposure to an agent or ergonomic factor in his workplace and which is of such a nature that it requires medical attention.

An occupational disease or disability is one which is acquired through an occupation or work (industry). People with occupational diseases are generally workmen, but people who live in a polluted atmosphere can also be affected, e.g. mesothelioma can develop in persons who have been exposed to asbestos fibres in their non-occupational environments. In South Africa, the main occupational disabilities are work accidents, noise-induced deafness and the scheduled occupational diseases.

The National Centre for Occupational Health (NCOH)[1] of the Department of National Health, based in Johannesburg and linked to the Department of Occupational Health of the University of the Witwatersrand, studies the problem of occupational diseases in the workplace. The Centre conducts research into the incidence and aetiology (i.e. epidemiology) of diseases which are suspected of being occupational in nature. It is hoped that by the early detection of a disease and recognition of the patient's occupation in its aetiology, timely steps may be taken to prevent premature death and permanent disability of the sufferer and the protection (i.e. primary prevention) of others exposed to the same environmental hazards.

The NCOH has a number of departments for its varied functions, viz.:

(1) Education in occupational health for medical students and doctors, and an extensive reference library for Occupational Medicine.

(2) Research facilities in occupational medicine and an epidemiology section which will assist doctors and nurses in the design of occupational health surveys.

(3) Laboratory facilities include pathology, biochemistry, immunology and microbiology departments.

(4) An occupational hygiene section does surveys on the physical and chemical quality of employees' environments.*

(5) An occupational (NCOH) medicine clinic offers a consulting service to medical practitioners, occupational health nurses, the trade unions and factory managers in the investigation and evaluation of occupational diseases.

Note:
(1) This service (occupational medicine) is also available in the rest of South Africa at medical universities.
(2) A parallel facility for the certification of lung diseases in mineworkers is also based in Johannesburg. It is called the Medical Bureau for Occupational Diseases (MBOD) and is administered by the Department of Health. Any doctor who attends a mineworker or worker must, if death occurs and permission has been given, remove the cardio-respiratory organs and forward them to the Medical Bureau for Occupation Diseases.

THE NCOH MEDICINE CLINIC[2]

The NCOH occupational medicine clinic deals with work-related medical conditions, as opposed to injuries on duty. The main criterion for attendance is significant exposure to an occupational hazard, or ill-health or abnormality with a suspected relationship to work.

The clinic is a multispecialty referral clinic which is free and open to all. It has no statutory basis. Referrals are accepted from medical personnel (doctors and nurses), employers, trade unions and even from patients themselves.

The clinic delivers a secondary preventive occupational health service by diagnosing occupational diseases mainly by history-taking, chest X-rays, spirometry and biochemical tests of blood and urine. These skills can be learned and performed by non-medical staff.

* Industrial hygiene is also the concern of the NCOH clinic and may involve contact with or visits to factories by clinic staff. The finding of a hazardous situation in the workplace may lead to investigation by an informed inspector of the Department of Labour and may involve the management in costs.

The role of the clinic is to provide an opinion on whether an occupational disease is present, on the extent of the impairment and on whether compensation should be paid. The clinic does not dispense therapy; the patient is referred to his usual health service. The clinic personnel may, however, suggest action which may improve the prognosis and the comfort of the patient.

As the aetiology of occupational diseases is detectable, they are essentially preventable and thus fall within the realm of community health.

NOTIFICATION OF OCCUPATIONAL DISEASES AND INJURIES FOR COMPENSATION PURPOSES

Occupational diseases and injuries must be notified for compensation purposes: diseases under the Occupational Diseases in Mines and Works Amendment Act 208 of 1993 to the Department of Mineral and Energy Affairs; disease under the Compensation for Occupational Injuries and Diseases Act 130 of 1993 to the Compensation Commissioner of the Department of Labour. Notification is the responsibility of the management of the mines and works (scheduled works, e.g. Iscor, Armscor and plants processing raw rock or ore), and of the management of occupations which fall under the Occupational Health and Safety (OHS) Act 85 of 1993.

In this manual only the injuries or diseases contracted in the course of employment under the OHS Act 85 of 1993 will be discussed.

Compensation for Occupational Injuries and Diseases Act*

Compensation for disablement caused at work is paid to employees who suffer from injury, noise-induced deafness or a scheduled occupational disease.

An employee means a person who works under a contract of service . . . with an employer. The Act excludes certain categories of police and military personnel, a contractor who engages other persons to perform work and domestic employees who work in a private household.

An employer means any person, including the state, who employs an employee.

Every employer must register with the Compensation Commissioner and furnish him with particulars about his employees and his business. He must keep a record of wages and keep the record for at least four years after the date of the last entry.

Compensation to disabled employees is a right and is paid from a **Compensation Fund**. This fund consists of, *inter alia*, the assessments of the employers by the Commissioner, calculated on the basis of a percentage of the annual earnings of their employees. Certain employers are exempt from assessment, e.g. the state and provincial authorities, certain local authorities, and employers who have a policy of insurance (mutual associations) to cover the disability needs of their employees.

The Minister of Labour appoints an officer, the Compensation Commissioner and his helping staff.

The functions of the Commissioner include receiving notices of accidents and occupational diseases and claims for compensation and paying compensation in respect of an award made by him, after considering the merits of the case. The Commissioner is also concerned with the prevention of accidents or of any disease which is due to the nature of a particular activity and the promotion of health or safety of employees.

The Act provides for the establishment of a Compensation Board consisting of the Commissioner, the Chief Inspector of Occupational Health and Safety, members of mutual assurance companies, members of the medical council (SAMDC), persons representing the interests of employees and of employers, to advise the Minister of Labour regarding matters of policy arising out of the application of the Act.

Injuries and scheduled occupational diseases that have caused employees in non-mining industry to be absent from work for 3 days or longer, or have caused disability, are notifiable to the Compensation Commissioner by the employer.

An employee who claims compensation must submit to an examination by a medical practitioner designated by the Commissioner, the employer or the mutual association concerned — who pay the examination fees.

* Act 130 of 1993 (in place of WCA, 30 of 1941).

A claim for compensation shall be lodged within 12 months after the accident or 12 months of the date of death, otherwise the right to benefits will lapse.

An employee must notify his employer or the Commissioner in writing as soon as possible after the commencement of a scheduled disease. The employer must also notify the Commissioner or mutual association of the disease.

Medical aid

An employer shall furnish and maintain equipment and services for first aid to employees injured in accidents. He should also make the necessary conveyance available and pay for the service.

The Commissioner, or employer individually liable or mutual association concerned, shall for a period of not more than 2 years pay the reasonable costs incurred by or on behalf of an employee in respect of medical aid necessitated by such an accident or disease.

Further medical aid will be paid for if further treatment will reduce the disablement.

A medical practitioner or chiropractor must supply a medical report to the employer within 14 days. Further reports may be requested. A copy of the report may be furnished to the employee. The employee is prohibited from paying towards the costs of medical aid.

Note: Any person affected by a decision of a Commissioner or a trade union or employers' organisation of which that person was a member at the relevant time may, within 90 days after such decision, lodge an objection against that decision with the Commissioner in the prescribed manner.

If the Commissioner cannot get support from his assessors, he must submit the dispute to the Supreme Court for decision.

COMPENSATION FOR OCCUPATIONAL INJURIES AND DISEASES

The list of compensable diseases is contained in Schedule 3 of Act 130 of 1993 and therefore known as 'scheduled diseases'. They are listed in the table on page 55.

Compensation for occupational injuries

The percentage of permanent disablement through occupational injury has been laid down in Schedule 2 of the Act, e.g.:

- loss of two limbs — 100 %
- loss of four fingers — 40 %
- loss of eye: whole eye — 30 %
- loss of hearing: both ears — 50 %

The manner of calculating compensation has been laid down in Schedule 4 of the Act. The nature of the disablement may be temporary, permanent or the outcome may be fatal. The nature of the benefit may be either periodical payments (for temporary disablement), a lump sum or a monthly pension (to the dependants in case of death) and the funeral costs in the case of death. The compensation may not form part of the deceased employee's estate.

Benefits for injuries and diseases

(1) Medical aid, including the supply and repair of prostheses and other aids. Reasonable medical expenses will be paid by the Compensation Commissioner. Since 1974, compensation for noise-induced hearing loss can be claimed.

(2) The employee is also entitled to a percentage of his wages for the period of his temporary disablement for work. There are certain conditions for payment, e.g. the accident should not have been caused by wilful misconduct; however, if the injury causes death or serious disablement, the Commissioner may waive refusal to pay the disabled person or his dependants (in the case of his death).

(3) If the employee is permanently disabled through an injury or scheduled disease, he is entitled to a compensation which is based on his monthly earnings and the degree of his disablement as determined by the Compensation Commissioner. An employee may appeal against the decision of the Commissioner. For disability below 30 % a lump sum is awarded; above 30 % a monthly pension.

When an employee suffers a compensable disability, he must bring this to the notice of his employer, who must then notify the

SCHEDULED OCCUPATIONAL DISEASES	WORK
	(a) Any work involving the handling of or exposure to any of the following substances emanating from the workplace concerned:
Pneumoconiosis-fibrosis of the parenchyma of the lung	organic or inorganic fibrogenic dust
Pleural thickening causing significant impairment of function	asbestos or asbestos dust
Bronchopulmonary disease	metal carbides (hard metals)
Byssinosis	flax, cotton or sisal
Occupational asthma	the sensitising agents — (1) isocyanates (2) platinum, nickel, cobalt, vanadium or chromium salts (3) hardening agents, including epoxy resins (4) acrylic acids or derived acrylates (5) soldering or welding fumes (6) substances from animals or insects (7) fungi or spores (8) proteolytic enzymes (9) organic dust (10) vapours or fumes of formaldehyde, anhydrides, amines or diamines
Extrinsic allergic alveolitis	moulds, fungal spores or any other allergenic proteinaceous material, 2,4 toluene-di-isocyanates
Any disease or pathological manifestations	beryllium, cadmium, phosphorus, chromium, manganese, arsenic, mercury, lead, fluorine, carbon-disulfide, cyanide, halogen derivatives of aliphatic or aromatic hydrocarbons, benzene or its homologues, nitro- and amino- derivatives of benzene or its homologues, nitroglycerine or other nitric acid esters, hydrocarbons, trinitrotoluol, alcohols, glycols or ketones, acrylamide, or any compounds of the aforementioned substances
Erosion of the tissues of the oral cavity or nasal cavity	irritants, alkalis, acids or fumes thereof
Dysbarism, including decompression sickness, baro-trauma or osteonecrosis	abnormal atmospheric or water pressure
Any disease	ionising radiation from any source
Allergic or irritant contact dermatitis	dust, liquids or other external agents or factors
Mesothelioma of the pleura or peritoneum or other malignancy of the lung	asbestos or asbestos dust
Malignancy of the lung, skin, larynx, mouth cavity or bladder	coal-tar, pitch, asphalt or bitumen or volatiles thereof
Malignancy of the lung, mucous membrane of the nose or associated air sinuses	nickel or its compounds
Malignancy of the lung	hexavalant chromium compounds, or bis chloromethyl ether

SCHEDULED OCCUPATIONAL DISEASES	WORK
Angiosarcoma of the liver	vinyl chloride monomer
Malignancy of the bladder	4-amino-diphenyl, benzidine, beta naphthylamine, 4-nitro-diphenyl
Leukaemia	benzene
Melanoma of the skin	polychlorinated biphenyls
Tuberculosis of the lung	(1) crystalline silica (alpha quartz) (2) mycobacterium tuberculosis or MOTTS (mycobacterium other than tuberculosis) transmitted to an employee during the performance of health care work from a patient suffering from active open tuberculosis
Brucellosis	brucella abortus, suis or melitensis transmitted through contact with infected animals or their products
Anthrax	bacillus anthracis transmitted through contact with infected animals or their products
Q-fever	*Coxiella burnettii* emanating from infected animals or their products
Bovine tuberculosis	*Mycobacterium bovis* transmitted thorugh contact with infected animals or their products
Rift Valley fever	virus transmitted by infected animals or their products
	(b) Any work involving the handling of or exposure to any of the following:
Hearing impairment	excessive noise
Hand-arm vibration syndrome (Raynaud's phenomenon)	vibrating equipment
Any disease due to overstraining of muscular tendonous insertions	repetitive movements

Commissioner on prescribed forms. If the firm employs an Occupational Health Nurse, she deals with the claims made under the Act.

After initial treatment at work in the case of an accident, employees are allowed to choose their own doctors for treatment except if the employer has an approved medical aid scheme for the treatment of his employees. All practising doctors, general practitioners as well as specialists, have to comply with the provisions of the Compensation for Occupational Injuries and Diseases Act, if and when they render services to injured employees.

Compensation according to the Act is akin to a state insurance scheme to provide for employees injured on duty (or suffering from a compensable occupational disease), or for their dependants if death should ensue, and for the payment of medical expenses. The Act requires all employers of labour to register with the Compensation Fund (with certain exemptions).

The Compensation Fund also subsidises NOSA (see p. 791) and the Rehabilitation Association for injured employees that provides facilities for treatment and rehabilitation for injured employees in the Johannesburg and Durban areas.

The diagnosis of a scheduled disease, e.g. occupational asthma, may be very difficult to make. Claims for compensation may be submitted but the onus is on the doctor who made the occupational diagnosis to prove the latter. In this case, the NCOH medicine clinic in Johannesburg provides excellent reference and consultation facilities for all doctors in the RSA.[5] Other facilities for the diagnosis of occupational diseases are: the Environmental and Occupational Clinic at Groote Schuur Hospital and the Industrial Health Unit at the University of Natal.

OCCUPATIONAL HEALTH NURSING (OHN)

The great surge of knowledge and progress in occupational medicine which occurred during both world wars bears testimony to the fact that a good occupational health service means greater productivity. Occupational medicine is a vital ill-health preventive and health promotive service, indispensable to industry. The occupational health nurse is the kingpin of occupational medicine in South Africa.

Nurses in the field of occupational medicine were formerly referred to as 'industrial' or even 'factory' nurses, as the majority were employed by industry and factories. The title was changed to 'Occupational Health Nurses' (OHN), as it is not only the industrial field which is concerned with the health of the employees (workers) but also commerce, the building trade, shipping, railways, mines, forestry, agriculture, etc. Being interested in the health of the worker really means being closely involved with his occupation. Occupational health nursing, therefore, appears to be a more appropriate title for the type of work an OHN does.

The scope of the OHN is virtually unlimited. Apart from dealing with health problems in the work situation, the OHN dispenses primary health care to employees of occupational health clinics. There certainly appears to be a very real need for specialised training in this field of nursing in which there are only a handful of experts.

THE TRAINING OF THE OHN AND OTHER OCCUPATIONAL HEALTH PERSONNEL

1. Post-basic training of the OHN

The integrated community health course of the SANC (of one year's duration on a full-time basis) makes provision for the academic needs of the OHN. Registered nurses already in employment in industry, but without specialised post-basic training as OHN, find it very difficult, however, to persuade their managements in the private sector to release them on a year's study leave.

Eskom offers an in-service training course for occupational health nurses at Megawatt Park. The annual training programme is presented during the first full week of each month over a ten-month period and is undertaken in collaboration with the Rand Afrikaans University which approves the academic standards and curriculum.

They also offer refresher training for those who have completed the above OHN course. This refresher course includes ECG interpretation, research, epidemiology, management skills and primary medical care.

Note: A qualified (certificated) occupational health nurse is, according to the OHS Act 85 of 1993, an Occupational Health Practitioner.

A part-time two-year post-registration diploma course in 'industrial' nursing was started by lecturers of the Department of Nursing at the Potchefstroom University (PU for CHE) in 1982. The course includes theory and visits to many industrial centres. The theory course consists of lecture periods of a week each, four times a year.

2.   In-service training of the OHN

A primary treatment service by the OHN at the medical centre (OH Clinic) of the company can be effective only when given with first-hand knowledge of the occupation and work environment of the employee, the quality of the supervision and the interpersonal relationships between employees and between supervisors and employees. Regular and frequent visits by the OHN to the locus of work and discreet observation of the employees are essential for the gaining of knowledge.

It is essential that the OHN receive adequate training in such areas as types of machines being used, specific hazardous substances that employees will be exposed to and the working conditions. The in-service training should be ongoing as new machines may be installed and new procedures introduced. The OHN must know about the guards used on machines and the various precautions used in danger areas. Only with this knowledge will the OHN be aware of the danger areas and what type of responsible precautions should be taken.

The OHN and the company doctor must know the types of employment used in the company so that a new employee can be suitably placed; they must be able to help fit the right man to the right job especially if the worker has a medical or mental handicap.

The OHN must know the employer's attitude and legal responsibility before making recommendations for placement. With proper knowledge of the work environment, the OHN will be able to detect any problems which may be due to hazards or working conditions.

3.   Training of non-professional medical assistant staff

The OHN is frequently responsible for the selection and training of medical assistants. She must teach them in such a way that they are able to maintain a high level of morale amongst the employees who come for attention to the medical centre (OH Clinic) either because they are unhappy and need understanding or because they are physically sick or injured. Every procedure must be clearly taught to the assistant and a job description compiled so that the assistant knows what specific tasks are required of him. He must know to whom he is responsible and lines of communication must be clearly defined.

4.   First-aid training of employees

First-aid training of employees should be organised by the OHN. On her tours of the factory or workshops, the OHN must check first-aid boxes to ensure that the employees who are trained in first aid have the proper equipment available when an accident occurs. With more and more employees being trained in first aid, the severity of accident damage should decrease.

Note: The registered nurse who works in the Occupational Health field, whether certificated or not, should become a member of the S.A. Society of Occupational Health Nurses (SASON), in order to remain in touch with developments in this field.

THE SUPPLY OF SCHEDULED MEDICINES (SCHEDULE 1–SCHEDULE 4) TO AND BY OCCUPATIONAL HEALTH CLINICS

The sale or supply of medicines and scheduled substances is governed by section 22A of the Medicines and Related Substances Control Act 101 of 1965.

However, section 22A(12) of the Act authorises the Director-General of the Department of Health to issue a permit which authorises an organisation performing a health service to acquire, possess, use or supply any specified schedule 1, 2, 3 or 4 substance after consultation with the Pharmacy Board. This permit is subject to the conditions specified by the Director-General. This permit makes it possible to render effective primary health care at the work site.

In order to facilitate the issue of permits to occupational health clinics, a number of requirements have been decided upon by the Department of Health in consultation with the South African Pharmacy Board.

Prerequisites for granting of permits

(1) The appointment of a medical practitioner (full-time or part-time).
(2) The clinic must be registered with the Department of Health.
(3) A registered nurse, who should preferably be in possession of a National Occupational Health Certificate, should be on duty full-time. The doctor is, however, fully responsible for the medicines.
(4) There must be efficient internal control of medicine in respect of: (i) patient cards; (ii) registers with details of type, quantity and strength of medicine; and (iii) monthly balancing of the stock of medicine, which balance must be signed by a medical practitioner or a pharmacist.
(5) The clinic must provide satisfactory lock-up facilities for medicines (excluding first-aid requirements).
(6) The medicines applied for shall be listed generically.
(7) The service must be rendered without any cost to the patient.
(8) The permit must be renewed annually.

The prerequisites listed above were decided upon because it was felt that they were necessary in the interest of the patient, and that correct storage and balancing of records are in the interest of medicine control in this country, as well as providing information, which may be required by the medical practitioner, about the patient's medication regimen.

The medicines to be stocked must be listed generically. The reason for this is to enable the clinic to buy different brands of the medicine.

THE CHOICE OF AN OCCUPATIONAL HEALTH AND SAFETY SERVICE

The type of work of a particular company, factory or firm, the size of its labour force, the nature of materials used, together with other factors such as hazards likely to be encountered and the policy of the management, are taken into account when deciding on the kind of health and safety service which would be most suitable for the company, factory or firm. The OHN is the hub around which this medical service revolves. Sometimes a doctor is in full-time employment of the company, but at other times the company doctor works on a part-time basis.

Of paramount importance in organising a health and safety service based in a medical centre (OH Clinic) is the amount of money allocated to it by management. The financial side of the health and safety service must be controlled by a budget system. The programme must be planned in co-ordination with other departments because without the full co-operation of senior personnel, the employees and their supervisors, the programme will surely fail.

Conditions for the successful running of an occupational health and safety service

Ideally, the management, the company medical officer, the OHN, the medical assistants, the safety representatives, must form a collaborative team which is geared to protect the health of the employee and to prevent occupational diseases and accidents.

The OHN must be recognised by all employees and the employer as a mature, responsible person who has to make decisions which could affect the welfare of employees. The medical centre should be a neutral area between management and employee. The OHN must at all times have access to the company doctor for the medical needs of her patients and the employee must be free to seek help from his own general practitioner.

The OHN must attach great importance to her working relationships with (1) management; (2) the employees; (3) the medical profession.

Management

The ideal situation is for the OHN to be responsible to the company medical officer for the nursing aspects of her role and to the personnel manager for the administrative side of the medical service. The OHN must have access to all top senior managers, as a situation may arise which could necessitate her having to discuss a matter with a person in authority.

The OHN should be involved in decision-making on occupational safety, the monitoring of environmental hazards and the maintenance of standards of environmental hygiene.

The employees

There must be a good relationship between the OHN and the employees. The employee must get to know the OHN not only in the medical centre but also as a visitor on the job. The employee must feel that the OHN is interested not only in his health but also in him as a person. The OHN must get to know about the employee's family, social background, outside stresses, as well as the employee's ambitions and hopes, frustrations and failures.

The confidential nature of personal information given to the OHN by the employee must be respected by the OHN. The OHN has a moral responsibility to the employees to ensure that they return home 'whole' at the end of each working day.

The medical profession

The observance of certain ethical rules is mandatory when dealing with the medical profession, these rules applying to all members of the health team, viz. management, company doctor and OHN, who are likely to have a working relationship with the medical profession.

Note: According to the Occupational Health and Safety Act 85 of 1993, an 'occupational health practitioner' means an occupational medicine practitioner or a person who holds a qualification in occupational health recognised as such by the . . . South African Nursing Council as referred to in the Nursing Act 50 of 1978 (i.e. a certified OHN).

The following ethical rules apply to the occupational health practitioner.

(1) If an employee has been treated at his place of work, his own doctor must be notified.

(2) If an employee is unfit to work, he must be sent to his own doctor.

(3) If an employee is being treated by his own doctor, and this treatment needs to be continued at the company medical centre, the doctor's permission must first be obtained. This treatment includes the taking of blood pressure.

(4) If the employee is examined for pension or retirement purposes, any relevant facts must be forwarded to his own doctor.

(5) Except in an emergency or at the request of the employee, the OHN or company doctor should not treat an employee for a condition which could normally be treated by his own doctor.

(6) A company doctor should not use his position to influence an employee to become his own private patient.

(7) An occupational health practitioner should not treat members of the family of the employee at the company medical centre.

(8) An occupational health practitioner may not, unless it is an emergency, send a patient directly to hospital. If it is an emergency, his own doctor and his family must be notified.

(9) If, by request of management, the occupational health practitioner is asked to investigate the absence of an employee who is being treated by his own doctor, the occupational health practitioner must first communicate with the employee's own doctor.

(10) The occupational health practitioner must respond wherever possible to the invitation of a private doctor to discuss a patient. The local practitioners should get to know the occupational health practitioner and, where possible, discuss patients with him.

(11) The occupational health practitioner should not do preventive treatment and experimental work on any employee without the consent of the employee's own doctor, e.g. flu vaccinations and mass X-rays.

(12) Personal records are confidential documents. No one has the right to inspect these without the permission of the company doctor who is responsible for the safe custody of the records. Should the doctor leave the employ of the company, the records should be handed over personally to his successor.

(13) If, as a result of pre-employment examination, employment has been denied, the company doctor may inform the applicant of his findings and should inform the applicant's private doctor.

Note: The company doctor and the OHN have a moral obligation to the company not to disclose the details of any industrial process to anybody outside the company except if permission has been granted by management or except if they have been ordered to do so by a court of law.

AIMS AND FUNCTIONS OF AN OCCUPATIONAL HEALTH SERVICE

The aim of OH care is to keep the employees at work and to prevent them from becoming ill. To achieve this aim the following services are required:[20] correct placement of employees, industrial hygiene, health care of the employees and their dependants by PHC curative, preventive and rehabilitative services, catering amenities and environmental control outside the workplace.

In fairness to both the employer and the employee, the employee is subjected to the following planned activities.

Medical examination

Medical examination by the company medical officer, assisted by the OHN to whom the doctor may delegate certain technical procedures.

The following kinds of examinations may be done.

1. Pre-employment examination to establish a base-line

A routine occupational history should be taken in order to elicit evidence of occupational risks. The following screening questions can be asked:

(1) Family history of illnesses.
(2) A record of medical problems, accidents and operations.
(3) A history of allergies, e.g. asthma, hay fever, eczema.
(4) Past history of chronic bronchitis, epilepsy, hypertension, diabetes mellitus, and back problems.
(5) Smoking and drinking habits and details of medication.
(6) Previous exposure to the following environmental factors: dust, bases, chemicals and noise.

A full physical examination should be carried out on each prospective employee; this includes urinalysis, mass and blood pressure. Lung function tests and large plate roentgenography are done where the employee is going to work in a dusty department. Eye-testing for motor vehicle drivers is essential. All employees should undergo chest roentgenography for the screening of tuberculosis. Prospective employees should then be monitored for TB symptoms and mass loss.

At the end of the pre-employment examination, the doctor should be able to answer the following questions:[7]

(1) Has the employee got an infectious disease (e.g. TB) or epilepsy, diabetes mellitus, poor vision or a personality disturbance which may increase his accident-proneness?
(2) Is the prospective employee suitable (vocationally and medically) for the type of work applied for?
(3) Is the prospective employee suitable for other available work?
(4) Is the prospective employee acceptable for the company's disability insurance and medical aid schemes?

Regulations of the OHS Act (see p. 48) make it legally incumbent upon the doctor to inform the prospective employee of potential risks in the job for which he has applied.

The pre-employment examination is of great benefit to the management; the ideal employee is the one who is 100 % fit, but in practice this ideal is not always obtained. Management usually employs those whose disability or malady is treatable or for whom certain jobs are suitable. Those who fail the pre-employment examination are advised to seek further medical investigation; the OHN should make suitable referrals in this regard.

2. Periodic

This examination is usually aimed at finding out whether certain factors in the work area are affecting people, e.g. lead fumes, X-rays, asbestos, noise. Audiograms, lung function tests and eye tests may be required. Employees in dusty departments should be examined six-monthly so that a deterioration in health can be detected early. Rigorous annual medical examination should be arranged for all drivers, with blood pressure checks, mass, urinalysis and eye tests. Food handlers should undergo quarterly medical examinations to check for carrier conditions in throat, urine and stools.

3. On termination of service

This should be done to detect an occupational disease or injury for which claims may be made at a later date.

4. After a long illness or accident

The employee should be examined to ascertain if he is really fit to return to his earlier job; if not, suitable employment should be found for him.

Control of environmental hazards — occupational hygiene

See OHS Act and safety legislation p. 48.

High environmental temperatures

These must be controlled in places of work to prevent heat-stroke and heat exhaustion.

Doctors will be expected to certify that a new employee is fit to work in a specified warm atmosphere.

The cooling power of the atmosphere is measured with a Kata thermometer. This wet and dry bulb thermometer indicates air movement, temperature and humidity, i.e. the cooling capacity of the air.

Prospective employees required to do hard manual labour at a Kata thermometer measured temperature of over 25 °C must be medically screened for physical fitness and must be of normal mass.

They must have no history of heat intolerance.

In the mines where the underground atmosphere is hot and humid, new employees are subjected to a special acclimatising programme to teach the body to retain salt.

Early signs of heat-sickness are exhaustion, nausea and muscle cramps. A hot, dry skin and aggressiveness may herald an attack of heat-stroke which requires rest and rapid cooling of the body.

Air pollutants

These must be removed by special means; if necessary the inspector may require the use of ventilators by employees. Regulations require that protective appliances and clothing be provided and maintained by the employer where employees are exposed to wet working conditions, or where the skin or clothes of the employees are likely to come in contact with injurious substances such as corrosive dyes and poisons. Nobody may deliberately damage or misuse protective clothing or appliances which must be used by the employee when specifically supplied for the health and safety of the employee and his co-workers. No one is allowed to imperil the welfare of others.

In dusty departments

Dust counts should be carried out to ensure that a strict control is kept on the dust load in these working areas. Ventilation should be adequate to reduce the dust in the air. If possible, damp cleaning, such as the use of wet sawdust, rather than air hoses should be used.

In noise zones

The source of the noise must be effectively isolated and the different noise levels on all boundaries demarcated.

Employees must wear SABS-approved earmuffs as protectors when working in a noise zone. These muffs are to be provided free of charge and for the sole use of the employee, unless special exemption to the latter requirement has been obtained. The employer must have his premises noise-zoned, demarcating the different noise levels on all boundaries and at entrances and exits with notices understandable to the various language groups. Where the equivalent sound level exceeds 85 dBA, noise must be reduced to a level below 85 dBA, or to a level as near thereto as possible.[7]

With regard to **hearing conservation**, the Act requires that any employee connected with a 'Specified Activity' be audiometrically assessed at intervals not exceeding 6 months, according to certain definite criteria by a person competent to do so. Nurses can become audiometrists by attending a course at a technikon lasting 2 weeks.

(Specified activity in this case is an activity which is excessively noisy and which has been specifically enumerated.)

A noise zone is any area in a factory where the equivalent noise level is equal to or exceeds 85 dBA (see p. 66).

Food-handling hygiene

In factories manufacturing processed foods, clean clothing should be supplied on a regular basis, the company bearing the cost. Hand-washing facilities and soap dispensers should be easily accessible; hot air for instant drying of hands in the place of towels would be an advantage. As there should be no smoking in a food-handling department, special bays should be provided for periodic smoke breaks. Spot checks for cleanliness of hands, clothes, utensils and working areas can be carried out by the OHN or company doctor, and reports regularly submitted to management.

In like manner, the hygiene (personal and environmental) in company canteens should be supervised by the OHN or company doctor. Regular immunisation of the food handlers against typhoid should be carried out and mass checked quarterly. A mass loss of 3 kg or more should be investigated as this might be an early sign of tuberculosis.

Nutrition

There should be safe and adequate *canteen facilities* to ensure optimal nutrition of the employees.

Screening

There should be routine *screening* for evidence of non-occupational diseases.

Safety precautions

The OHN must keep an alert eye on the safety aspects of workshop housekeeping, e.g. on the amount of scrap lying about, on the regular servicing of fire extinguishers, etc. First-aid equipment must be adequate and personnel trained to use it must be readily available.

Curative

Treatment of occupational diseases.

First-aid treatment for accidents

Employees trained in first aid apply emergency treatment on site and this prevents the escalation of physical damage, e.g. by hypoxia or blood loss.

Speedy and efficient treatment of minor accidents and ailments can be carried out at the medical centre. A great advantage of having a well-equipped medical department is the early first-aid treatment and resuscitation of life-threatening accidents.

Treatment of chronic non-occupational diseases

The chronically sick patient who suffers from either tuberculosis, diabetes mellitus, hypertension, sexually transmitted diseases, obesity, epilepsy or asthma, can be effectively controlled by the OHN. It must be noted that the chronically sick patient has a choice: whether he is treated at the medical centre by the company doctor or whether he attends a hospital clinic or general practitioner surgery. Irrespective of who controls his disease, the OHN should check with the employee that his medication is taken correctly and regularly. If the patient requests treatment by the company doctor, the OHN is involved in follow-up treatment, e.g. medication and blood pressure checks.

In treating the tuberculotic patient, it is essential to work in close liaison with the local authority. Once the number of tuberculotics on site has been established through periodic mass miniature roentgenography, a service can be brought into operation.

Medication is supervised, the patient is regularly weighed and a suitable high protein diet prescribed. The reason for these measures is carefully explained to the patient and the measures are painstakingly enforced by the OHN. Ignorance on the part of the employee with tuberculosis can lead to lapses in treatment and to consultations with *sangomas*. The affected employee must be assured of financial support and continued employment even if admission to a tuberculosis hospital becomes necessary. The affected employee is a breadwinner and unless he can be assured of an income for his family, he may abscond from the hospital in a desperate bid to find a means of supporting his family. Should an ambulant patient in employment request leave, the OHN should issue sufficient medication and supply a covering letter clearly stating the nature of his treatment. This is done in case there is a breakdown in health during the leave period to ensure suitable assistance at a hospital or TB clinic. Many of the black employees go to the rural areas for their annual vacation and, with such a letter of explanation for the local authority, a lot of misunderstanding can be avoided.

Alcoholism in the employee

Alcoholism is a condition where a person has lost control over his drinking habits. As a result, he cannot comply with acceptable standards of interpersonal behaviour and exposes himself to possible damage of his physical and mental health. The OHN must be able to recognise some of the symptoms of alcoholism — noticeable avoidance of supervisors and colleagues, dubious reasons for, and repeated, absenteeism, seediness at work, shaky hands, and red, bloodshot eyes. She must be aware of the problems that an unstable work record, loss of productivity, and accidents at work, cause for the employer of the alcoholic, as well as the material and financial distress, social embarrassments and tense, disintegrating family relationships. Both the alcoholic and the family need her understanding, help, and support to face up to the facts of the condition — which is the first and most difficult step along the road to recovery.

The second step is to make use of expert help in the form of professional advice, and out-patient or in-patient treatment. Early recognition, and the fact that treatment is available, should make her realise that communication with the employee is the most important aspect of professional help. Being able to talk about the problem comes through education, which must be carried through into the working environment.

Note: SANCA employs an industrial consultant at SANCA headquarters in Johannesburg, to advise industry on the problems of alcoholism. The OHN can make use of this service, in whatever part of the RSA she finds herself.

Health education

The OHN can play a vital role in the health education of employees, e.g. it can be brought to their attention that *smokers in dusty environments* are more likely to contract lung cancer than non-smokers. Nearly half of all employees in industry smoke. Health education programmes can be introduced where necessary by using visual aids.

The OHN can *counsel vulnerable groups*, e.g. the aged, the disabled, the young inexperienced employees and those being rehabilitated after illness or accidents. Women in industry form a vulnerable group as many women who work also run homes and carry the responsibility of children. The double function often leads to fatigue and strain with the inevitable absenteeism. The OHN must counsel a stressed woman on community help which is available, e.g. crèches and marriage guidance services, to lighten her burden. She must also be knowledgeable about maternity benefits and sick leave regulations. The OHN can become the confidante and counsellor of the troubled woman in industry and help her to fulfil her occupational and domestic roles.

The establishment of a *family planning clinic* and programme is an important aspect of the work of the OHN. She can also make arrangements for the showing of films and the giving of lectures on personal hygiene, sexually transmitted diseases and the prevention and early detection of cancer.

Health education with regard to *cancer* can be a valuable service of the OHN to the community. The high-risk female employees can be incorporated in a screening programme for carcinoma of the breast and cervix/corpus uteri, in collaboration with the National Cancer Association (see p. 795). The causes of occupational cancers (mesothelioma) and the role cigarette smoking plays in aggravating pneumoconiosis can also be brought to the attention of the at-risk population.

Preparation for retirement (see p. 819) comes within the ambit of the OHN.

Safety education of the employees. All employees should be instructed in the hazards they may meet at work.

Health education concerning *nutrition*. The control of mass of employees in sedentary occupations, e.g. drivers, is important. The OHN can play an important role in stimulating interest in the employees, in correct nutrition, especially in companies that provide canteen services for its employees. The obese employees can be given diet sheets and arrangements can be made with the canteen to provide low energy dishes.

High protein diet for the undernourished should be discussed and encouraged and the employee can be educated in the planning of well-balanced diets for the family.

Health education on the *prevention, symptoms and curability of tuberculosis* is an important function of the OHN. The body mass of those employees at risk should be regularly checked.

Research and keeping of records

Research is made possible by keeping records. The medical department should be a centre for epidemiological research. Examples: notice should be taken of the effect on employees of new processes in the factory or workshop; if there is a high sick record pertaining to any particular area, investigations should be made to ascertain whether new processes are being used and with what detrimental effects. Accurate recording of attendances at the medical centre may help to detect early signs of an occupational disease.

Personal record cards and treatment cards should be kept for every employee. The date and nature of illness or injury, treatment given, outcome and discharge of the patient, must be recorded diligently, as the OHN may have to give evidence in court. All absences from work due to sickness as well as their duration should be recorded. An important objective of the medical centre should be to reduce absenteeism by a certain percentage. By analysing the figures, the OHN can try to establish why certain employees require more sick leave than others.

The success of the medical programme must be evaluated and areas defined where research is warranted in order to improve the health care of the employees. The medical programme should be altered to keep in step with changes in the programme of the company. All injuries should be reported to the medical centre for assessment and treatment. In this way the OHN can become aware of a sudden increase in the accident rate which would call for an investigation.

A summary of the activities of the medical centre should be sent periodically to the personnel manager. In this way he will be aware of the type of service being offered to the employees.

Rehabilitation

Where employees have been involved in major injuries, the OHN should be able to assess when and where these injured employees could be suitably placed, either on a temporary or a permanent basis. The OHN must be fully conversant with the handling of Compensation for Occupational Injuries and Diseases documentation. It is the duty of the OHN to see that those injured at their place of work are, firstly, treated adequately and, secondly, that their reports are sent to the Compensation Commissioner and, finally, that if and when compensation is awarded, the employee receives it.

SOME COMPENSABLE OCCUPATIONAL DISABILITIES

Hearing loss

Continuous noise — loud undesirable sound — causes many damaging effects on the body, such as irritation, tension, insomnia, loss of efficiency in work, disturbances in verbal communication and hearing impairment.

The perception of sound waves

Sound waves are perceived by the human ear with regard to their intensity (loudness) and their frequency (pitch).

The loudness of a sound depends upon the number of hair cells in the organ of Corti which are stimulated by the transmitted pressure of the sound waves. Noise causes intensive stimulation of the delicate hair cells which vary in sensitivity, being more sensitive in the high frequency range. Prolonged intense stimulation damages the hair cells and causes hearing loss. The loudness of a sound is measured in units called decibels (dB). A decibel is not an absolute measure of pressure (such as, for instance, a microbar) and is not related in a linear fashion to the intensity of the noise. Example: doubling the pressure (loudness) of a sound, say, 70 dB, adds only 3 dB to its decibel power, making it 73 dB, while halving the intensity of the sound reduces its sound power by 3 dB, thus making the 70 dB sound 67 dB. A decibel is, therefore, a measure of the ratio of sound intensities. The decibel unit of measurement is used in audiometers which measure sound perception, i.e. the hearing threshold of the ear for sound. The decibel is also the measurement unit of sound-level meters which measure the noise level of a steady noise, e.g. in industrial concerns.

The pitch of a sound depends upon the frequency of a sound wave; high frequency sound waves are interpreted as high tones and vice versa. Pitch is perceived as a range between high and low tones, the perception of tones being measured in octaves. Each octave represents a doubling of sound wave frequency, the actual size of waves being measured in units called hertz (Hz). Audiometers make use of the Hz measure to determine at which pitch hearing loss has occurred. Perception of pitch depends upon which hair cells have been stimulated. The organ of Corti is more sensitive in the high frequency range; when an ear is exposed to damaging noise it becomes deaf to high tones before the hearing of low tones is affected. Noise-induced deafness first shows at 6 000 Hz, later at 4 000 Hz.

Hearing loss for speech is audiometrically estimated by measuring hearing thresholds at different frequencies and taking the average. If the mean is 26 dB and higher, significant hearing loss has occurred. Audiometry is also used to detect those people who are particularly susceptible to noise-induced deafness and who should, therefore, avoid exposure to critical noise levels.

Exposure to damaging noise

The damaging consequences of noise depend not only upon the overall average noise level (dBA), which may be 75 dBA in city traffic and 95 dBA in a factory, but also upon the duration of daily exposure to noise and total exposure time during a lifetime. The overall sound level to which employees in industry are exposed gives an indication of its hearing damage potential. A sound level of 80 dBA for 8 hours a day (40 hours a week) during a full working life of 45 years is considered safe. As the sound level in industrial concerns is not steady during the whole working day, an equivalent dBA can be computed from the total sound energy to which employees are exposed during the whole day. Noise damage depends upon the total sound energy to which the employee is exposed, therefore daily exposure to a sound level of 83 dBA for 4 hours only carries no risk. The equivalent

sound level in this case would be 80 dBA for a period of 8 hours. Daily exposure to 92 dBA for 3 hours carries the same risk as 86 dBA for 8 hours.

In employees exposed to risk, hearing loss will depend upon exposure duration in years — the longer the exposure, the greater the hearing loss. The hearing loss is greater during the early years of exposure.

Full-time exposure to damaging noise has the same effect; a sound level of 90 dBA for 8 hours daily will cause considerable hearing damage during 10 years of exposure. Loudness of a sound, e.g. a sound-pressure level of 135 dB or more during short periods, even though it does not exceed an equivalent noise level of 80 dBA for 8 hours, may do damage to an unprotected ear.

Hearing damage risk criteria

Employees who are likely to be exposed to critical noise levels should be assessed audiometrically before employment in order to acquaint those who are particularly susceptible to noise of the dangers. The common criteria for safety (80 dBA, 40 hours a week for 45 years) do not guarantee that all employees thus exposed will escape hearing loss after many years of exposure; they apply only to the average employee. Warning signs that the noise to which an employee is exposed is dangerously high for him are:

(1) head noises or ringing in the ears after exposure to high level noise;
(2) muffled hearing for a few hours after such exposure.

A safe noise level in industry can be judged:

(1) subjectively, by the ability to hear conversational speech at a distance of at least 300 mm;
(2) objectively, by taking sound level readings over a period of 8 hours to compute the overall average noise level; the equivalent noise level should not exceed 85 dBA.

The SA Bureau of Standards (SABS) suggests that a hearing conservation programme is required whenever the equivalent noise level exceeds 85 dBA and whenever audiometric tests on the employees show a deterioration of hearing despite maximum protection. OHNs can be trained as audiometrists at technikons.

Hearing conservation programmes in industry

The objective of hearing conservation programmes (by which noise is limited) is the preservation of hearing ability for speech. The facilitation of communication by audible speech is the most important function of hearing in man. Measures to control the noise which impinges on the hair cells of the organ of Corti are:

(1) the reduction of sound at its source by modification of machinery;
(2) isolation of the source of the noise in a sound-insulating compartment.

The aim of these measures is to bring the equivalent noise level down to 85 dBA. If this reduction cannot be obtained, then the employee at risk must be protected either by the wearing of ear-muffs or ear-plugs or by reducing his noise-exposure time. Education of the employee and instruction in the proper use of protective equipment are of the utmost importance because the employee is likely to co-operate only when he understands the hazards of occupational noise and the importance of prophylactic measures.[9]

Pneumoconiosis

The most important scheduled occupational diseases are the dust diseases, collectively called pneumoconioses. Pneumoconiosis is characterised by fibrosis of the lungs due to irritation caused by the prolonged inhalation of dust. It is usually an occupational disease occurring in industries with a dust risk. In the case of asbestos dust it can, however, be caused by prolonged exposure to an asbestos-dusty atmosphere unrelated to occupation.

In South Africa the main kind of pneumoconiosis is silicosis, caused by the inhalation of silica (stone) dust. People liable to get silicosis are stonemasons, miners in gold and diamond mines and people who work in dusty conditions in factories and earthworks.

Other pneumoconioses include:

- *Anthracosis:* from inhaled smoke and coal dust;
- *Asbestosis:* from inhaled asbestos fibres; a serious complication of asbestos inhalation

is cancer of the lung and mesothelioma (cancer) of pleura and peritoneum;
- *Siderosis:* (steelgrinder's disease) from exposure to iron dust in iron mines;
- *Byssinosis:* from inhaled cotton dust during ginning (removing seeds from cotton).

Combination of dusts may cause conditions such as: anthracosilicosis, silicosiderosis. Bronchiectasis, cor pulmonale, lung cancer and pulmonary tuberculosis may supervene in all dust diseases. Tuberculosis combined with silicosis, i.e. silicotuberculosis, is known as miner's phthisis.

Tobacco smoking exacerbates all forms of pneumoconiosis.

In pneumoconiosis fibrous hardening of the lung occurs gradually, fibrotic nodules coalescing to produce large masses. The first signs of pulmonary disability are: chronic cough with sputum, and haemoptysis. Later dyspnoea and cyanosis appear as the vital capacity of the lungs becomes reduced. This eventually leads to fatigue after slight exertion and cor pulmonale.

Primary prevention

Primary prevention of pneumoconiosis can be achieved in the following ways:

(1) Ventilation in dust-laden work environments can be improved by the use of fans (air-conditioning).
(2) Dust can be settled by dampening it with spraying or sawdust.
(3) A respirator should be worn by the employee if the dusty atmosphere cannot be controlled.
(4) Employees at risk should not smoke.

Secondary prevention

This involves taking the following precautions:

(1) Lung function tests should be done regularly on employees at risk, in order to detect early signs of pneumoconiosis.
(2) Any employee who has developed signs of pneumoconiosis should be removed from the dust-laden atmosphere and given an occupation 'above ground' in a dust-free environment. An exact assessment of the damaged employee's future work capacity

should be made and employment arranged accordingly.

(3) Employees who are found to be in the first stages of pneumoconiosis could be kept in a state of relative health by —

    (a) not allowing a cold to develop into pneumonia;

    (b) stopping smoking;

    (c) preventing further exposure to the dust.

Pneumoconiosis in non-mining industries

Pneumoconiosis can also occur in non-mining industries. In a study done by the NCOH the following industrial dusts were found to be some of the main hazards:

- asbestos in asbestos/cement manufacture and fibre milling and handling;
- silica in brick (furnace) laying;
- ceramic and glass manufacture, stone crushing and sand blasting and trenching by dry drilling tunnelling;
- iron dust in cast grinding and trimming;
- wood dust in carpentry and timber handling;
- cotton dust in textile factories.

The asbestos hazards in mines and processing industries

Asbestos is much used in industry, being an important component of cement, insulating materials, textiles and paper and plastic products. The blue and brown types, which are produced in the RSA, are the most dangerous fibres in the induction of mesotheliomas and lung cancer. Employees in the insulation industry who are liable to inhale fibres over a long period are most at risk of developing asbestosis.

Permissible atmospheric levels[11]

In the UK

- 1 fibre per ml for chrysotile (white) — 90 % of world production
- 0,5 fibre per ml for amosite (brown)
- 0,2 fibre per ml for crocidolite (blue)

In the USA (1976)

- 2 fibres per ml for all fibres

In the RSA[12] (Mines and Works Industry)

- 2 fibres per ml averaged over 8 hour period

Note: There is biological evidence that the risk for ill-health effects is greater in the secondary uses and applications of asbestos than in mines and works.[12]

Workplace standards are enforced by the inspectorates of the Government Mining Engineer and the Department of Manpower (Labour). South Africa still produces crocidolite (the most dangerous asbestos particularly in terms of mesothelioma production)[12] of which importation is banned in the U.K.

Asbestos-related diseases usually take 20 years to develop, although primary mesothelioma of the pleura and peritoneum may occur in employees who have been constantly exposed to visible floating asbestos fibres for a minimum period of four months.[10] Because of the long incubation period, asbestos-related diseases diagnosed in the 1980s are likely to be the consequences of exposure in the 1960s and 1970s. At that time the number of employees at risk was greater and the exposure levels very much higher. Environmental fibre concentrations in South African mines and mills fell from 120 fibres/ml air in the 1940s to below 2 fibres/ml in the 1980s. Moreover, the number of employees exposed to the inhalation of fibres has decreased, due to decreased world demand for asbestos. Asbestos-related diseases should, therefore, abate in the future.

There is ongoing health surveillance for exposed employees in mines and scheduled works through the provisions of the Occupational Diseases in Mines and Works Amendment Act (208/1993). This kind of organised monitoring is not available for non-mining employees in asbestos processing industries.

The NCOH medicine clinic (see p. 52) offers a consultative service to medical practitioners and can also facilitate the submission of the documentation to the Commissioner for Compensation when asbestos work-related disease is diagnosed.

Primary prevention of asbestos associated diseases is through education, dust (asbestos fibres in the atmosphere) control and the enforced use of protective masks. Employees and management must be educated about the dangers of inhaling asbestos fibres and especially with regard to the combined effects of smoking and asbestos exposure. It has been suggested that public posting in factories of records of monitored environmental levels of asbestos fibres for scrutiny by employees might lead to improved workplace practice.[12]

Lead intoxication

Lead is probably the most intensely studied occupational toxic agent. Lead poisoning is notifiable to the Department of Health and in 1989 six such cases were notified. In 1992, two cases were notified and none in 1993.

Approximately 86 000 tonnes of lead are produced annually in South Africa and 14 500 persons are occupationally exposed to lead.

The sources of lead poisoning in industry are: white lead oxide used in the manufacture of batteries, pipes, paint and solder, lead glazing in pottery, lead used in the printing industry. Lead can be discharged into the environment by a lead-handling factory and become an environmental hazard. Lead smelting causes the release of lead fumes; so does petrol.

Petroleum and battery industries are the greatest users of lead. Ninety-eight per cent of atmospheric lead in cities comes from petrol. People at greatest risk of developing lead poisoning are: employees engaged in industries utilising lead, motor mechanics and city street newspaper vendors. When metallic lead is exposed to air, it becomes coated with a dusty layer of lead oxide which can be inhaled by labourers shovelling scrap lead. Non-occupational exposure is usually from food, drinking water, dust ingested by young children, and petrol fumes in the air. Although lead can be ingested — for the population at large, food and water are important sources of baseline exposure to lead — practically all industrial lead poisoning is due to inhalation of dust and fumes. Lead circulates in the blood and is excreted in the urine; it is also eliminated by gastro-intestinal secretion (lead line on gums). Lead passes through the placenta and across the blood-brain barrier, although the brain does not secrete lead.

Absorbed lead in the body is distributed as follows:
(1) Exchangeable fraction in blood and soft tissue. Blood level will vary with exposure. The blood level of lead (Pb-B) is the best available indicator of current exposure of individuals to lead.

(2) Stable fraction in bones and teeth (90 %). This fraction is the result of long-term absorption. As lead accumulates in the dentine of children, their deciduous teeth can be assayed for lead concentration. This finding is used in research as a marker of the amount of lead absorbed in a community.

There is a difference in the Pb-B level of occupationally and non-occupationally exposed persons. It is important for an industry using lead to screen new employees (pre-employment screening) in order to prevent the additional exposure of individuals, especially women during their reproductive life, with high Pb-B levels.

Recommended health-based limits of lead are obtained by:
(1) *Biological monitoring:*
   (a) Blood tests done in specialised laboratories. The total blood content is an important test because of the adverse effects of lead on the body.
   Pb-B of 30 µg/dl for males and for females over reproductive age.
   This is the upper limit which has been reported for different population groups throughout the world. Pb-B above 70 µg/dl is the lead level at which symptoms of lead poisoning (intoxication) became apparent.[14]
   Pb-B of less than 25 µg/dl for children. Pb-B of less than 25 µg/dl for females of reproductive age, to protect the foetus.
   Baseline blood lead levels can be inferred from the blood lead level of adolescent children living in an unpolluted (by lead) 'rural area', viz. mean Pb-B of 3,4 µg/dl.[14]
   It must be remembered that lead serves no metabolic function in the body hence there is no lower limit to its presence in the blood.
   (b) The ZPP (zinc protoporphyrin) screening test, for lead absorption, done every 2 weeks by the OHN, on a drop of blood (from ear lobe). The test measures interference with haematopoiesis, and iron deficiency anaemia. The results are read off on a haematofluorometer. The ZPP level serves as a warning that something

is wrong. The result is expressed as µg ZPP/gHb; 18–20 µg/gHb correlates with a Pb-B level of 60 µg/dl.

Alarm criteria used are: ZPP 16 µg/gHb as an alert. Two readings of 18 µg/gHb–further blood test.[13]

(c) Haematocrit and haemoglobin tests, if ZPP test results are suspect.

(d) The amount of lead in urine.

(2) *Environmental monitoring:*

(a) Lead-in-air measurements of air in the work situation.

The correlation between Pb-B and lead in air is weak. The level of lead in the air is used as a guideline for engineering purposes in factories. If the level is kept low enough, the Pb-B level will not rise to toxic limits, unless there are other sources of contamination. The level of lead in air should not exceed 30 µg/m³ for populations with an average Pb-B of 25,00 µg/dl. A range of 30–60 µg/m³ is generally acceptable.

(b) Inspection of prescribed work practices to ensure that there is no unnecessary exposure to lead.

(c) Personal hygiene to prevent ingestion of lead.

Signs and symptoms of lead poisoning are the result of an incremental accumulation of lead in the tissues.[14]

The clinical features of lead intoxication are:

(1) Elevated blood lead and ZPP and urine lead levels. Although the recommended health-based limits of lead in the blood is 30 µg/dl for adults and 25 µg/dl for children, these limits are constantly being lowered in the light of modern findings of lead toxicity at lower blood levels.

(2) Inhibition of haemoglobin synthesis with resultant anaemia and pallor. Women and children are more sensitive than men to the toxic effects of lead on haemoglobin synthesis.

(3) Abdominal colic and constipation; the lead line on the gums and on X-ray films of the long bones (at epiphyses).

(4) Peripheral neuritis, an early manifestation being paralysis of the extensor muscles of the wrist. There is evidence that increased lead blood levels cause neurological damage to developing children (learning difficulties, behavioural changes and mental retardation) who have no history of encephalopathy. It appears that the developing CNS of the foetus and infant is more sensitive to the toxic effects of lead than the CNS of adults.

(5) Non-specific nephropathy.

Primary prevention of lead intoxication involves the following precautions:

(1) Employees handling lead oxide, e.g. employees in battery factories, must wear face masks.

(2) In a factory handling lead, the blood of the employees must be monitored at regular intervals to detect evidence of excessive lead absorption before the nervous system is affected.

(3) The effluent from a lead-handling factory must be controlled so as not to become an environmental hazard. The safe disposal of industrial waste is a very important community health measure.

(4) The source of lead poisoning must be ascertained so that further poisoning may be avoided.

In the RSA only voluntary action by an employer will lead to this preventive action. The Chief Inspector can, however, intervene as he has the authority to prohibit an employer from endangering the life of an employee in a 'specified activity' for a period determined by him. The inspector is guided by a medical report.

After removal from exposure, the employee should be monitored for another 6 months. When all blood tests have reverted to normal, he may return to similar work.

Childhood lead exposure causes a preventable disease. Childhood lead poisoning is defined as' blood lead ≥ 30 micrograms per decilitre (1,448 µg/dl) in children under 14 years of age'.[21]

The reduction of the lead content of petrol, paint, tins for canned food and drinking water is a community matter which can be solved by legislation and other community measures.

Recently the initial steps were taken to lower the lead content of South African petrol which used to have one of the highest levels of lead in the Western world.

Efforts could also be made to site schools and crèches away from major roads and heavy traffic.[15]

Scleroderma (PSS)

(PSS — Progressive systemic sclerosis)
This is a collagen disease which is possibly linked, in the gold-mining industry, to exposure to silicates, vinyl chloride and welding. These chemicals probably cause damage to chromosomes. There may be an inherited predisposition to PSS.[17]

Scleroderma is characterised by a thickening of the skin due to swelling and thickening of fibrous tissue. The disease affects internal organs, e.g. causing renal failure, as well as atrophy of the epidermis with loss of hair.

Occupational contact dermatitis

Industrial dermatitis is a non-infective inflammation of the skin, of exogenous origin. It is caused by contact of the skin with either irritants or allergens. In some cases the allergic and the irritant reactions appear only after exposure of the sensitised skin to ultraviolet light (photosensitivity).

Occupational dermatitis is the most commonly reported occupational disease in terms of the Compensation for Occupational Injuries and Diseases Act.[8]

There are two kinds of contact dermatitis.[18]

(1) Non-allergic irritation contact dermatitis is caused by prolonged or intense exposure of a dehydrated dry skin to chemicals which damage the skin, e.g. soap and water, solvents, acids, alkalis, phenols, washing powders, petrol, metals and cements. Damp skin, e.g. under rings, aggravates the inflammation. The inflammation may progress to oedema, papules, vesicles and pustules and even necrotic bullae. After 48 hours healing starts. In order for the skin to recover, the irritant must be avoided for some weeks; as non-allergic dermatitis is mostly confined to the hands, contact with strong irritants must be avoided by wearing gloves. To prevent maceration of the skin under waterproof gloves, inner absorbent gloves can be worn. Creams can be used to moisturise and soften the dry skin of sensitive hands. Barrier creams are of value only to prevent the adhering of dirt which then requires traumatising scrubbing for removal. As soiled protective clothing may irritate the skin, it must be washed regularly.

(2) Allergic (hypersensitivity) contact dermatitis involves the sensitisation of small lymphocytes and their circulation in the blood (cell-mediated localised immune response). After sensitisation has occurred, any further skin contact with the allergen — even years later — will elicit eczema after a latent period of a few days. Circulating antibodies do not play a role and there is no direct damage to the skin (as with irritants). Some people are genetically predisposed to develop hypersensitivity reactions to certain specific substances such as chrome, nickel, cobalt, rubber, epoxy, acrylic and formaldehyde resins, plasticisers, turpentine, tar, mercury and many others.

In allergic contact dermatitis there may be a generalised spread from the area of contact to the whole body, especially the eyelids.

The diagnosis of contact dermatitis is made by means of patch tests, applied to the back or to the inside of the upper arm for 48 hours.

Prevention of allergic (contact) dermatitis is the avoidance of contact with known sensitisers by the use of protective clothing. Employees who suffer from eczema or a dry skin should not be employed in industries requiring contact with water and chemicals.

As skin sensitivity to a specific allergen is usually permanent, the employee should be moved to an occupation where contact with it is unlikely.

Pesticide poisoning

In terms of the Fertilizers, Farm Feeds, Agricultural Remedies and Stock Remedies Act 36 of 1947 (as amended), poisoning from any agricultural or stock remedy registered in terms of the Act is notifiable to the Department of Health. In 1989, 119 cases of agricultural and stock remedies poisoning were notified thus. In 1992, 142 cases were reported and in 1993, 100. Some deaths occurred.

Pesticides are included in these remedies. All pesticides must be considered toxic. Pesticide employees at risk include farm labourers, crop sprayers, research students and pesticide manufacturers.

The main pesticides which can be a health hazard through occupational exposure are:

(1) Organophosphates, e.g. malathion, brom-chlorphos (DBM), parathion. They are highly toxic to mammals. Poisoning occurs from accumulation of acetylcholine in the body due to the inhibition of cholinesterase. They are used especially in anti-malaria programmes, replacing DDT and γ-BHC to which mosquitoes are becoming resistant (see p. 657 for uses of organochlorides (DDT) and organophosphates). Occupational exposure is due to inhalation and mixing of spray and ingestion of sprayed food. Cases of acute organophosphate poisoning require treatment in an ICU with continuous IV atropine infusions and symptomatic treatment of respiratory depression and electrolyte, fluid and acid-base imbalances.

In 1977 Perold and Bezuidenhout[19] investigated an epidemic of chronic organophosphate poisoning among staff members (and their families) of an agricultural college. They recommended the following precautions:

(a) personnel handling pesticides must be instructed in their dangers and their proper usage;

(b) dilutions should be strictly in accordance with manufacturer's recommendations;

(c) spraying should be carried out only on wind-free days;

(d) the user must wear gloves, mask and protective overalls;

(e) any skin contamination must immediately be washed off;

(f) all containers must be effectively destroyed;

(g) while the poison is being used, no food or fluids should be taken and smoking should be forbidden.

(2) Carbamates such as Carbaryl are also cholinesterase-inhibiting pesticides, e.g. Doom, Sluggem, Karbadust. Cholinesterase inhibition is easily reversed by the injection of atropine.

(3) Gamma-HCH (lindane) and γ-BHC (gamma-benzene hexachloride). They are general agricultural pesticides, also useful in malaria control, and on human beings against pediculosis and scabies. In human beings poisoning affects mainly the CNS. Non-occupational poisoning may result from incorrect application to the skin or from accidental ingestion. Occupational exposure during the manufacture and application of γ-HCH may cause dermal and respiratory absorption and acute poisoning (convulsions and muscle cramps).

(4) Organochlorides, e.g. Dieldrin, DDT and its derivatives, are effective contact pesticides; they are stable chemicals which are sprayed on to surfaces likely to come into contact with insects. Their long-lasting effect because of their stability, unfortunately, also causes environmental pollution. For this reason the use of DDT is prohibited in many countries. In the RSA this cheap and effective pesticide is still used in house-spraying for malaria control.

Legally enforced general precautionary measures

Regulations (1981) under the Foodstuffs, Cosmetics and Disinfectants Act 54 of 1972, lay down the maximum limits for pesticide residues that foodstuffs may contain.

This is a community safety precaution against poisoning through non-occupational exposure. Likewise DDT and its derivatives are not for sale to the public.

All agricultural remedies offered for sale in the RSA must be registered with the Department of Agricultural Technical Services. This department ensures that the label on the container bears no unsubstantiated claims for efficacy. The label carries 'Warning' and 'Precautionary' statements.

In terms of the Hazardous Substances Act 15 of 1973, the empty containers and the remaining contents of all pesticides must be disposed of in a responsible manner. Containers are either securely closed if returnable and, if not, must be perforated and flattened and then buried in the ground or disposed of in any other safe manner. They may never be used as containers for any foodstuffs or cosmetics.

REFERENCES

(1) Davies JCA. The National Centre for Occupational Health: Functions and facilities. *S Afr J CME* 1986; **4**: 125–128.

(2) Ehrlich RI. The occupational medicine clinic of the National Centre for Occupational Health. *S Afr Med J* 1989; **75**: 227–230.

(3) Baker MD. Legislation on occupational health in South Africa. *S Afr J CME* 1986; **4**: 103–110.

(4) Department of National Health and Population Development Occupational Medicine Bill. *Government Gazette* Notice 20, 1984.

(5) Myers JE, Garisch D, Cornell JC. Compensation for occupational diseases in the RSA. *S Afr Med J* 1987; **71**: 302–306.

(6) Recommendation 112 of the International Labour Organisation. *International Labour Conventions and Recommendations 1919–1981.* Geneva: ILO, 1959; p. 345.

(7) Swiegers WRS. Periodieke en aanstellingsondersoeke. *S Afr J CME.* 1986; **4**: 24–27.

(8) Zwi AB, Ehrlich RI. Occupational history-taking in the RSA. *S Afr Med J* 1986; **70**: 601–605.

(9) Mets JT. *S Afr Med J* 1971; **46**: 935.

(10) Cochrane, JC, Webster I. *S Afr Med J* 1978; **54**: 279.

(11) Benatar SR, Bateman ED. The asbestos hazard. *S Afr Med J* 1982; **62**: 881.

(12) Becklake MR. Control of asbestos-related disease in the RSA. *S Afr Med J* 1987; **71**: 208–210.

(13) Mets JT. Biological monitoring of occupational exposure to lead with a zinc protoporphyrin (ZPP) meter. *S Afr Med J* 1981; **60**: 891.

(14) Grobler SR, Rossouw RJ, Maresky LS. Blood lead levels in a remote, unpolluted rural area in South Africa. *S Afr Med J* 1985; **68**: 323–324.

(15) Von Schirnding YER. Reducing environmental lead exposure — time to act. *S Afr Med J* 1989; **76**: 293–294.

(16) Davies JCA. Lead toxicity in South Africa. *S Afr Med J* 1985; **67**: 833–834.

(17) Bernstein R, Prinsloo I, Zwi S, *et al.* Chromosomal aberrations in occupation associated PSS. *S Afr Med J* 1980; **58**: 235.

(18) De Beer HA. Kontakdermatitis in die bedryf. *S Afr Med J* 1980; **57**: 1091.

(19) Perold JG, Bezuidenhout DJJ. Chronic organophosphate poisoning. *S Afr Med J* 1980; **57**: 7.

(20) Maluleke FRS. Strategies for integrating primary health care and occupational health. *CHASA* 1991; **2**(1).

(21) Ehrlich RT. Recommendations for changes in the method of notification of lead poisoning in the RSA. *Epidemiological Comments* 1993; **20**(5).

TEST OF KNOWLEDGE

The student has benefited from studying this chapter if he/she can answer the following questions:

(1) Discuss the main functions of an Occupational Health Nurse (OHN) in a factory and the conditions for the successful running of an occupational health and safety service.

(2) Why is a knowledge of the Occupational Health and Safety Act 85 of 1993 important for the OHN?

(3) (*a*) What legalised steps are taken to conserve hearing in a noisy factory?

(*b*) Discuss the causes and prevention of hearing loss due to damaging noise.

(4) Discuss briefly the benefits for industrial employees of the Compensation for Occupational Injuries and Diseases Act.

(5) What are the advantages of a pre-employment medical examination by the company medical doctor or his deputy, the OHN?

(6) Write notes on:
The OHN as health educator
The handling of alcoholism amongst employees by the OHN
The supply of scheduled medicines to and by Occupational Health Clinics
The dangers of occupational lead intoxication and the primary prevention of childhood lead exposure.

Part 2

BASIC KNOWLEDGE FOR COMMUNITY NURSING

6

Demography and Biostatistics

OBJECTIVES

Demography is the study of human populations by statistical methods. Biostatistics (vital statistics) is concerned with numbers derived from scientifically gathered data of births, health, disease and deaths. The objectives of the study of demography in this chapter are to introduce the student to concepts about differences in populations which affect their life-style and quality of life. The student will be looking first at world statistics of population size, distribution and composition, and then at the biostatistics of birth, death and population growth. With the world population rising to over 6 billion, the danger of a global population explosion in Third-World countries should become obvious to the student. World demographic problems are well represented in South Africa, where the majority of the population have the problems of a Third-World country, viz. poverty, overcrowding, poor housing, poor sanitation, poor water supplies, low educational standards and low productive capacity. Added to this, Third-World countries have high fertility and infant mortality rates, and short life expectancies.

By studying demography, the student will understand the importance of demographic data in enabling the authorities to set objectives when planning national health strategies, e.g. the PDP of the National Government and the RDP of the GNU aimed especially at improving the health of the great mass of the South African population living under Third-World conditions.

The student will be introduced to the concept of 'loss of potential years of life', i.e. premature death before the age of 65 years, in both Third-World and First-World sectors of the population, and the need for preventive health care during the productive years. The student must understand that, with an improvement in health care and a reduction in the high infant mortality rate (IMR) in Third-World countries, there will be an increasing number of non-productive old people. High growth rates, due to falling death-rates in developing countries, threaten to cause a population explosion with its attendant dangers: overcrowding, increased environmental pollution, violent competition for scarce resources, and starvation. But the objectives of curative and preventive health are not only to decrease the death-rate but also to bring down the birth-rate by planned and involuntary birth control, and to raise the quality of life of the underdeveloped masses by education and by instilling the First-World ideal of zero population growth in our already overcrowded world.

The big problem caused by improving the health status of everyone ('All') is the lengthening of life expectancy and the great increase in numbers of old people past the so-called retirement age. The student who understands the problems of an ageing population will encourage and enable old people to remain productive in the community. The student must understand that as the Third-World sectors of the RSA adopt First-World life-styles and respond to the government's health strategy plan, a large non-productive aged black population will be added to the large elderly white population. This will place a tremendous burden on the productive capacity of the younger members of the community. The Health Plan is aimed at reducing mortality and disability, and especially the IMR due to low birth mass and infections. Reduction in the IMR will reduce the high fertility rate which saps the energy and resources of Third-World populations. Reducing the growth rate will enhance the quality of life of Third-World communities; thus Health for All by the Year 2000 can become a reality.

Another objective of the study of demography and biostatistics is to understand the differences in the mortality rates, their causes in the different population groups in the RSA, and the fact that black and coloured children die largely of preventable causes.

The analysis of mortality patterns in a heterogeneous population has, therefore, tremendous implications for health care which will ensure acceptable health standards and productive capacity for all members of the population.

IN THIS CHAPTER

INTRODUCTION TO DEMOGRAPHY

Demography is a social science which makes use of statistical methods for the study of human populations. Demography is derived from the Greek work, *demos* — the people. In order to illustrate conditions of life in a community, the subject-matter of demography comprises the characteristics of a community (its size, distribution and composition), as well as its biodata — the biostatistics of births, deaths and disease. Demography is a basic component of community medicine and epidemiology.

Demography had its origins in the work of John Gaunt who studied the 'Bills of Mortality' in London. These were lists of baptisms and deaths which were printed weekly in London. Gaunt made use of these lists in order to calculate sex ratios and to compare births with deaths. (It may be of interest to note that at that time deaths exceeded births in London.) He published some of his work in 1662.

Thomas Malthus, a British clergyman and economist, also made an important contribution to demography when he published an *Essay on the Principles of Population* in 1798. In this essay he stated that all populations had a tendency to increase faster than their means of subsistence unless checked, and this was true of human populations as well. The increase in the human population would outstrip any increase in food supplies and this would lead to war, starvation and disease; for this reason there would never be a happy society, or Utopia. Malthus studied rates of increase in various populations and postulated that although population growth could be checked by measures such as late marriages and abstinence from sex (which Malthus thought was the only acceptable way to avoid pregnancy), he did not think that people would make use of these means to limit their numbers, so 'war, famine and pestilence' would continue to exist in the world and in this way population increase would be held in check. There were developments, such as the colonisation of North America, advances in agriculture, improvement in transport and the Industrial Revolution, which Malthus could not foresee, which prevented the occurrence of starvation on a global scale. Malthus thought that the increase in the size of Britain's population was due to increasing birth-rates which he blamed on the introduction of various kinds of social assistance, but this was not so, and the increase in the size of the population was in fact due to the falling death-rates. We find a similar situation in countries in Asia, Africa and South America today where the rapid increase in population which they are experiencing is not the result of increasing birth-rates but of the fall in death-rates which started in these countries soon after the Second World War.

Demographers study the **characteristics of populations** such as their size, distribution and composition, and the changes which take place in these characteristics over time. They attempt to explain why these changes have occurred and to predict future trends.

GLOBAL DEMOGRAPHIC DATA

Size of population

In the modern world the size of a population is established by carrying out a census. A population census is the total enumeration of the people in a certain area or country. Clay tablets found in Babylon show that the ancient Babylonians compiled lists of people more than five thousand years ago. We know as well that as early as 435 BC the Romans established a Censorate whose function was to count the Roman citizens every five years. These early inventories differ from the modern census in that they were confined to counting only sections of the population, usually in order to identify those

members who were eligible for forced labour, military service or taxation. Today many countries conduct censuses at regular intervals, usually every ten years. Some governments have been doing this for hundreds of years. Sweden has been carrying out a regular census since 1750, the United States of America since 1790 and Britain since 1801. The Cape Colony carried out a census in 1865.

The census not only indicates the number of people in a population but supplies a great deal of information about the individual members of the population such as their age, sex, marital status, income, occupation, etc. In the years between censuses population figures are kept up to date by adding the numbers of births and immigrants to the census figures, and subtracting the number of deaths and emigrants.

TABLE 1
Some world population figures

Estimates in millions for	1974	1978
World	3 900,00	4 222,00
United States of America	211,91	218,06
UK (England and Wales)	55,93	49,18
Netherlands	13,54	13,94
USSR	252,06	261,00
South Africa	24,92	27,70
Zambia	4,75	5,45

Source: Demographic Year Book, UN (1974) and World Health Statistics (1981).

Some of these figures may not be accurate because to date not all the people in the world have been counted; also many countries have not yet enumerated their populations or have done so only at very irregular intervals. The accuracy of population figures depends on the recency of the last census as well as the facilities available for the registration of births and deaths. Nevertheless, the census remains the demographer's most important source of data.

Distribution

This refers to the manner in which a population is dispersed throughout a territory. The urban-rural distribution of a population concerns the division of its members between the towns and cities on the one hand and the country on the other. This characteristic of a population has important consequences for a society. Over the last 150 years there has been a steady drift of the world's population from the rural areas to the towns and cities; 150 years ago about 2 % of the world's population lived in urban areas. This figure is now over 30 %. In the highly industrialised countries, such as those of Western Europe, over 80 % of the population are to be found in the towns and cities. This movement of people to the towns is the trend in South Africa as well.

It is an almost universal phenomenon that the young, able-bodied, better educated males migrate to the towns in search of employment, leaving behind women and children, the elderly and the sick or disabled.

This affects agricultural production because it results in fewer people being employed in this important activity. A report released in1978 by the International Labour Organisation, which is a specialised agency of the United Nations, indicates that between 1950 and 1970 the agricultural labour force of the developed countries has decreased by sixty million, and they predict that this trend will continue. Agricultural production is not the only aspect of social life which is affected; there is often severe poverty in these areas due, in part, to the fact that young men who start off by sending money home to their wives and dependants frequently form attachments in the city and set up another home there so that there is no longer any money available to send. On the other hand, the slum areas of the cities become overpopulated and we find large numbers of unemployed young men living in congested areas, a situation which gives rise to a great deal of social deviance, especially violence.

Composition

The age and sex composition of a population may be depicted by means of a histogram, which is known as a population pyramid. Males form the left side and females the right. Age categories are placed along the vertical axis. The youngest, that is the 0–4 year category, forms the base of the pyramid and the oldest category the apex. A population pyramid will show us the percentage distribution of both sexes at five-year intervals.

Age composition

Figure 6.2 is the population of a developing country (blacks in the RSA). Notice that it has a broad base and tapers off rapidly towards the apex. In developing populations birth-rates are high with the result that children make up a large part of the population; nearly 40 % of the population are under 15 years of age and this is reflected in the broad base of the pyramid. Death-rates are relatively high and this is reflected in the fairly rapid tapering off of the pyramid. There are few old people in these populations. Only 2 to 3 % of the population are over 65 years.

In developed populations (whites in the RSA) birth-rates are low and there are relatively fewer children in the population; only 25 % are under 15 years of age. Death-rates are also low and 10 to 15 % of the population are over the age of 65 years. We speak of these populations as being 'ageing' populations. These factors are responsible for the shape of the pyramid in figure 6.4 with its narrow base.

The age composition of a population affects fertility rates, mortality rates, and patterns of health and disease in societies.

TABLE 2
Age distribution of RSA population 1991

The corresponding population pyramids (figures 6.1–6.4) illustrate the very different age distributions of the various population groups. Some age groups of specific interest are:

Age in years	Percentage of total population
Under 1	2,53 %
Under 5	12,33 %
Under 15	34,64 %
Females 10–19	10,38 %
Females 15–44	23,69 %
Females 15–49	25,85 %
Persons 65 and older	4,29 %

Source: Epidemiological Comments, 1994; **21**(2).

Sex composition

In the developed countries males outnumber females at birth, the ratio being 105:100, but because male mortality rates are higher than those for females at all ages, this ratio soon begins to change, and by the time the 50 to 54 age category is reached females outnumber males. This excess of females over males becomes progressively greater as the more ad-

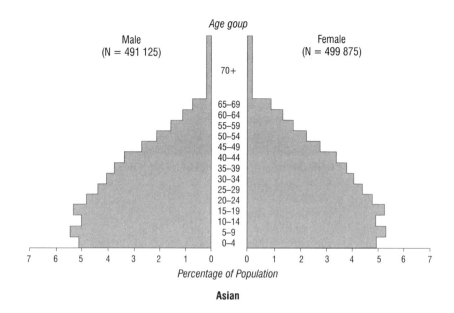

Figure 6.1

(Source: Population Pyramids RSA, *Epidemiological Comments* **21**(2), February 1994
Estimations based on 1991 census)

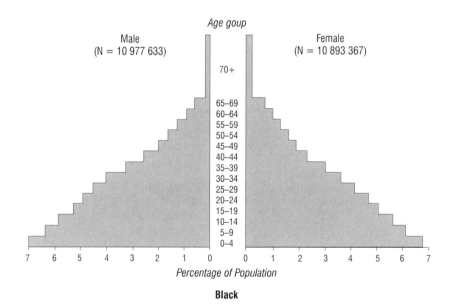

Figure 6.2

(Source: Population Pyramids RSA, *Epidemiological Comments* **21**(2), February 1994
Estimations based on 1991 census)

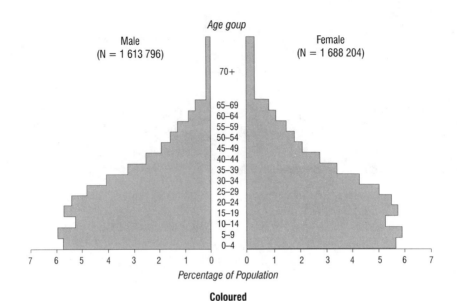

Coloured

Figure 6.3

(Source: Population Pyramids RSA, *Epidemiological Comments* **21**(2), February 1994
Estimations based on 1991 census)

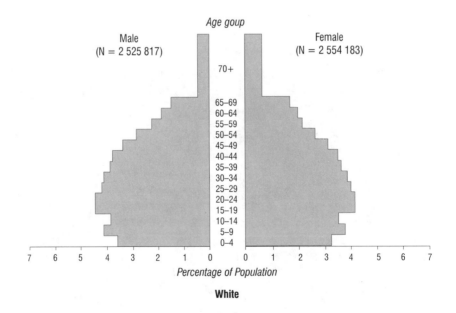

White

Figure 6.4

(Source: Population Pyramids RSA, *Epidemiological Comments* **21**(2), February 1994
Estimations based on 1991 census)

vanced ages are reached and, in some countries, by the age of 70 years females outnumber males by four to one. There are some countries where this situation is not found, for example in India, where women are subjected to many pregnancies and maternal mortality rates are high, males outnumber females.

The sex ratio may also be affected by wars which usually result in the death of more males than females, and by emigration, where often the males are the people most likely to emigrate. The shape of the population pyramid will be affected by these events.

BIOSTATISTICS (VITAL STATISTICS)

The demographer also obtains data for his study of human populations from the registration of 'vital events' such as births and deaths and the recording of diseases. Vital statistics (biostatistics) deals with data concerning human births, health, disease and death.

In most countries data and information concerning vital statistics can be obtained from government departments. In South Africa such information can be obtained from the Central Statistical Service in Pretoria. The information is also available in a publication of the Department, *South African Statistics*, which is published every second year. The demographic division of the United Nations compiles world statistics and publishes a *Demographic Yearbook*. WHO publishes *World Health Statistics*.

When dealing with vital statistics it is customary to make use of rates rather than whole or absolute numbers. Rates relate the number of the observations or events (the numerator) to the size of the population (the denominator). It is of little value to know that there were 89 596 live white births in South Africa and 783 155 in the United Kingdom in 1971 unless we take the difference in the size of the two populations into account, South Africa 4 million, United Kingdom 55 million. If we do this we find that the white population of South Africa had a crude birth-rate of 23,1 per 1 000, while the crude birth-rate in the United Kingdom was 16,0. The use of rates, therefore, enables us to compare the frequency of events in different places or at different times or between different groups.

Fertility rates

Crude birth-rates

These are computed as follows:

$$\frac{\text{Number of live births in a calendar year}}{\text{Estimated population at mid-year}} \times 1\ 000$$

This measure is known as the **crude** birth-rate because it does not take the age and sex composition of the population into account, but it is a measure which is commonly used because it is fairly easy to compute, provided certain information is available; for example, it can be used in countries where provision is made for the registration of births. In those countries where births are not registered it is possible to estimate crude birth-rates by carrying out a simple survey.

TABLE 3
Some crude birth-rates

	1971	1979
United States of America	17,1	15,8
United Kingdom (England and Wales)	16,0	13,0
Netherlands	17,2	12,5
USSR	16,9	18,2
South Africa		
— Asian and Coloured	35,2	25,5
— White	23,1	16,3
Zambia	49,8	—

Source: Demographic Yearbook, United Nations, 1974, and WHO, *World Health Statistics* (1981).

Age-specific fertility rates

$$\frac{\begin{array}{c}\text{Number of live births in a calendar year to}\\ \text{women in a certain age category}\end{array}}{\begin{array}{c}\text{Number of women in the population in the}\\ \text{same age category, e.g. 24–29 years}\end{array}} \times 1\ 000$$

Total fertility rates

$$\frac{\text{Number of live births in a calendar year}}{\begin{array}{c}\text{Number of women aged 15–49 years in the}\\ \text{population}\end{array}} \times 1\ 000$$

Factors affecting fertility rates in populations

(1) The age structure of the population. The developed countries such as those of Western Europe which have an 'ageing' population, with relatively few young people in the population, and therefore relatively few women of childbearing age, have low crude

birth-rates, in the region of 15 per 1 000.

In contrast, the developing countries have a high proportion of young people in the population, and consequently many women of childbearing age, so their crude birth-rates are high, being in the region of 39 per 1 000.

(2) The age at which marriage takes place. The younger the age at which marriage takes place in a society, the higher the fertility rates will be. Late marriage is an effective way of reducing birth-rates, and in countries such as Russia and China where governments are concerned about their growing population, late marriage is actively encouraged.

(3) The number of people in a population who marry. Fertility rates are higher in countries where almost all people marry than in those where a relatively large number remain single; in Ireland this was a factor which contributed to the decline in the fertility rates.

(4) The structure of the family. In a society where the extended family is the dominant family form, fertility rates are high. There are many reasons for this; couples marry young and have many children because they are assisted by the other members of the family; children are not an economic burden, rather they are looked upon as assets; also the main desire of the family is to perpetuate the family, so young couples are encouraged to have many children.

(5) Infant mortality rates. High fertility rates are associated with high child mortality rates because women have many children to ensure that at least some of them will survive into adulthood.

(6) The cultural values. There are some societies, such as the Indian, in which a woman occupies an inferior status. Her position in the family and her status are closely linked to the number of sons she will bear. She is, therefore, under considerable pressure to continue having children until she has produced the required number of sons.

(7) Religious factors. Societies in which ancestor worship is a part of the religion have large families because there must be sufficient children to pray to the ancestors.

Life expectancy

This is the average number of years an individual who has attained a certain age can still expect to live. Expectation of life at birth is the probable number of years which an individual born today may expect to live. These figures can be read off on life tables which are constructed by insurance companies and are based on mortality rates and census data. Expectation of life at birth has increased dramatically in the developed countries since the nineteenth century due mainly to the decrease in infant and child mortality. Man's life expectancy in ancient Rome was probably in the region of 20 years; in Britain, in the first half of the nineteenth century, it was 40 years; today in Western Europe it is approximately 70 years for males and 75 for females.

The average for Africa is 49, for Asia 60, and for South American countries 64. (*Rand Daily Mail*, 24.03.1983.)

Factors influencing life expectancy

Heredity

Longevity appears to be influenced by genetic factors, and generally the lifespan of offspring will be similar to that of the parents and the grandparents.

Sex

In almost all human populations females have a greater life expectancy than males. This appears to be due partly to biological and partly to environmental factors and life experiences. In most societies women lead a less stressful and more sheltered life, although this is beginning to change in the industrialised countries.

Socio-economic status

There is a relationship between socio-economic class and life expectancy; mortality rates are highest in the lowest socio-economic classes and fall steadily as the higher income groups are reached. This is probably due to the better housing, nutrition and medical care which are available to these groups.

Occupation

Occupation may influence life expectancy directly or indirectly. Mortality rates are highest in unskilled workers and lowest in those engaged in professional or business occupations. These mortality rates may reflect the hazard of the work, for example, mortality rates are higher among miners than among clerical workers, or they may be the result of economic factors. To a great extent occupation and income are linked and unskilled workers are found in the lowest income groups, where mortality rates are higher.

Mortality (death) rates

Crude death-rates

$$\frac{\text{Number of deaths in a calendar year}}{\text{Estimated population at mid-year}} \times 1\ 000$$

TABLE 4
Some crude death-rates

	1971	1979
United States of America	9,3	8,7
UK (England and Wales)	11,6	12,1
Netherlands	8,5	8,0
USSR	8,2	9,7
South Africa		
— Asian	6,8	5,9
— Coloured	13,1	9,3
— White	8,5	8,0
Zambia	20,6 (1967)	

Source: Demographic Yearbook, United Nations, 1974, and WHO, *World Health Statistics,* 1981.

Factors which influence crude death-rates

(1) The age structure of the population. In developed countries which have an 'ageing' population, crude death-rates are sometimes higher than in some of the developing countries where there are fewer old people in the population. In these countries the higher death-rates are not the result of environmental factors or standards of medical care and are unlikely to fall in the future.
(2) Child mortality rates. High infant and child mortality rates contribute to the high mortality rates which are found in some of the developing countries.
(3) Adverse environmental conditions, such as lack of sanitary facilities, poor nutrition, and the presence of insect vectors, will increase crude death-rates in a community.

Standardised mortality rates

The comparison of the death-rates of different countries whose populations do not have the same age structure is not valid. If we wish to make such comparisons, the death-rates have to be adjusted to allow for these differences. These death-rates are then said to be standardised.

Cause-specific mortality rates

It is possible to calculate how many people in a population die from a certain condition or disease because the cause of death has to be entered on the death certificate. The cause specific death-rate is calculated as follows:

$$\frac{\begin{array}{c}\text{Number of deaths due to a certain disease}\\\text{(tuberculosis) in a calendar year}\end{array}}{\text{Estimated population at mid-year}} \times \begin{array}{c}10\ 000\\or\\100\ 000\end{array}$$

It is important to remember that the cause of death as entered on the death certificate may not be correct. The following are some of the reasons why this may be so.

(1) A correct diagnosis is not always made even in the most sophisticated institutions where all the facilities for diagnosis are available, so how much more likely is it that an incorrect diagnosis may be made in some small rural centre where none of these diagnostic facilities is available!
(2) Vague causes of death may be entered on the death certificate, such as 'stroke' or 'gastroenteritis'.
(3) Where a condition is common in a community it is more likely to be given as a cause of death than any other condition, e.g. ischaemic heart disease.
(4) For many reasons a 'socially acceptable' cause of death may be given, particularly where the diagnosis is in doubt, or where there is a desire to spare the feelings of the relatives. In some countries this may be done for political reasons.
(5) Where multiple pathology is present, as in the aged, the choice of the actual cause of death may be arbitrary.

Maternal mortality rates

These may be expressed in a number of ways: the denominator used may be the number of live births, or the number of registered births, or the number of confinements or even the number in the population. The following is the most common way of computing maternal mortality rates.

$$\frac{\text{Number of deaths due to a pregnancy, childbirth or the puerperium in a calendar year}}{\text{Number of deliveries in that year}} \times \frac{10\ 000}{\text{or}} \\ 100\ 000$$

Maternal mortality rates can also be expressed per number of the population, e.g.

TABLE 5
Some maternal mortality rates
(per 100 000 of the population) 1975

United States of America	0,4
Netherlands	0,1
United Kingdom (England and Wales)	0,3
Egypt	6,7
Mauritius	5,7

Source: World Health Statistics, 1978, WHO, Geneva.

Maternal mortality rates have been declining steadily in all the developed countries in the world during the last 50 years. This decline has been due to improved antenatal and obstetric care, and also to the improved economic conditions and nutrition. The main causes of death in these countries are abortion, toxaemia of pregnancy and haemorrhage; infections, such as puerperal sepsis, are no longer an important cause of death. Although maternal mortality rates are low in these countries, a certain number of preventable deaths do still occur. In the developing countries, on the other hand, maternal deaths are still unacceptably high.

The women in any community at greatest risk during pregnancy and childbirth are those under 16 years or over 40, those who suffer from some systemic disease such as diabetes mellitus or chronic nephritis, those who have had four or more previous pregnancies, unmarried mothers and those who come from the lower socio-economic groups.

Age-specific death-rates

These mortality rates may be computed for any age group, e.g. 20–24 years or 60–64 years as follows:

$$\frac{\text{Number of deaths in a particular age category, e.g. 20–24 years}}{\text{Number of persons in the population aged 20–24 years}} \times 1000$$

The following are examples of age-specific death-rates.

Neonatal death-rate

$$\frac{\text{Number of deaths occurring within the first 28 days of life, in a calendar year}}{\text{Number of live births in that year}} \times 1000$$

The risk of an infant dying is greatest during the first four weeks of life and more than half of all infant deaths occur within the first month of life. Important causes of death are: congenital abnormalities, prematurity, birth injuries and infections. To some extent the neonatal death-rates are a reflection of the maternity services in an area.

Infant mortality rate

$$\frac{\text{Number of deaths occurring in infants during the first year of life, in one calendar year}}{\text{Number of live births in that year}} \times 1000$$

TABLE 6
Some infant mortality rates, 1972

United States of America	18,5
UK (England and Wales)	17,2
Netherlands	11,7
Portugal	41,4
USSR	24,7
Lesotho	114,4

Source: Demographic Yearbook, 1974, United Nations, N.Y..

Infant mortality rates are a very important epidemiological indicator. High infant mortality rates are associated with large families, poor infant care, poverty, unsatisfactory environmental conditions, high illegitimacy rates, uneducated mothers and lack of medical care services. The most common causes of death are undernutrition and malnutrition, and infections, especially respiratory and gastro-intestinal infections.

Important as infant mortality rates may be in reflecting socio-economic and environmental conditions, they do not tell the whole story. In the rural areas of the developing countries many children survive the first year of life because they are breast-fed, only to fall prey to malnutrition and infection once they have been weaned; the under-5 mortality rate probably gives a better picture of the health status of children in these areas, where nearly half of all children born die before they reach the age of five. Twelve million healthy children in the world die annually because of want.

The case-fatality rate or ratio (CFR)[4]

The case-fatality rate refers to the proportion of deaths that occur in any particular disease, in any given community over a specified time interval, e.g. a year. Thus:

$$CFR = \frac{\text{Number of deaths}}{\text{Number of cases}} \times 100$$

The CFR is an estimate of the probability of dying of a disease contracted. The CFR of diseases varies, symptomatic rabies usually having a CFR of 100 % and the common cold having a CFR of less than 0,1 %.

The growth rate

The annual natural growth rate is the difference between births and deaths expressed per 1 000 or 100 of the population (i.e. percentage). Growth rate is also affected by emigration and immigration.

TABLE 7
Some rates of natural increase, 1970–4

World	2,0 %
Asia	2,2 %
Africa	2,7 %
Europe	0,6 %
South Africa (1972)	
— Whites	1,4 %
— Asians	2,7 %
— Coloureds	2,2 %

Source: Demographic Yearbook, 1974, United Nations, N.Y.

A low rate of natural increase is found in countries which have a low crude birth-rate and a low crude death-rate, such as Western Europe, and we notice that they have a rate of natural increase of less than 1 %. Low rates of natural increase were also found in countries which had a high crude birth-rate and a high crude death-rate as well. This was the position in Africa a century or so ago.

A high rate of natural increase occurs in countries with a high crude birth-rate and a falling crude death-rate. This is the situation which exists in Africa today and which accounts

for the rate of natural increase of 2,7 % which we notice above. The rapid increase in the size of the world's population, which has been called the 'population explosion', is a fairly recent phenomenon and is not due to increasing birth-rates as some people mistakenly believe, but rather to falling death-rates. Population growth in Africa and Asia was probably zero until a couple of hundred years ago, due to the very high death-rates. At first death-rates fell slowly and these populations started increasing gradually, but the increase became far more rapid after the Second World War when immunisation techniques, insecticides and antibiotics were introduced into these countries from the developed countries.

A population increase of 3 % means that a population will double itself every 24 years, one of 2 %, every 35 years and one of 1 % every 70 years. Although there are some countries which may be able to support a higher population density than they have at present, the world cannot support such numbers; not only are the world resources, such as fuel, minerals, land, food and water finite, but services such as educational and medical services would be overwhelmed by such numbers. Pollution and the degradation of the environment could reach disaster levels. For all these reasons it is essential that the rate of population growth be slowed down. There is some evidence that this has already commenced. The latest issue of *Population Bulletin*, which is a publication of the Population Reference Bureau in the United States, reports that fertility rates in some countries, such as China, India and Indonesia, declined by 10 % between 1968 and 1975.

Morbidity (sickness) statistics

Morbidity statistics indicate the amount of ill-health which is present in a community; this information may be obtained from the following sources:

(1) Hospital records. However, to some extent the number of persons admitted to a hospital for treatment depends on the accessibility and the availability of such services, and there may be a considerable amount of ill-health in a community in which the rates for hospital attendance are low.

(2) Clinic records.

(3) School health service records.

(4) Notification of disease. In this connection we must be aware that generally speaking there is more likely to be under-reporting of a condition than over-reporting, and sometimes the number of diseases notified represents only a small proportion of the actual number of cases occurring.

(5) Reports of district surgeons, medical officers of health, and others in similar positions.

(6) Registers of chronic diseases, such as carcinoma.

(7) Information from private medical practitioners.

(8) Medical records of employees, which may be kept by the larger industrial and commercial organisations.

(9) Information and health statistics from insurance companies.

(10) Epidemiological, or health surveys.

Incidence and prevalence rates

Two important rates which are used in epidemiology are the *incidence rate* and the *prevalence rate*.

The *incidence rate* indicates the number of **new** cases of a disease arising in a population during a certain time, which may be a day or a month or a year. For example, the list of notified diseases which are submitted by medical officers of health to the Department of Health every week would indicate the incidence of these conditions in a district in that week. Incidence rates are computed as follows:

$$\frac{\text{Number of new cases of a condition occurring during a certain time, e.g. a week}}{\text{Population at risk}} \times 1\ 000$$

The multiple 1 000 is arbitrary, and 10 000 or 1 000 000 may be used instead. This would depend on the frequency of the condition under discussion. It is important that in one's reading one should take note of the multiple which is being used.

The 'population at risk' may also vary. If we were interested in an outbreak of measles in a particular school, then the population at risk would be all the children attending that school,

while in another case it might be all the children in the city who attend school.

Prevalence rates indicate the amount of **chronic** disease which is present in a population; for example, we speak of the 'prevalence of hypertension among urban blacks'. Prevalence rates are computed as follows:

$$\frac{\text{Number of cases of a condition existing in a population at a given time}}{\text{Population at that time}} \times \begin{array}{l} 1\ 000 \\ or\ 10\ 000\ or \\ 100\ 000 \end{array}$$

Prevalence rates are affected by two factors, the incidence of the condition and its duration. A chronic condition such as hypertension will have a high prevalence rate but a relatively low incidence rate, while an acute condition will usually have a low prevalence rate, excepting during an epidemic when the incidence rate will be high and for a short time the prevalence rate will be high too.

Conclusions

The demographic characteristics and biostatistics of the developing and the developed countries have been discussed and compared and certain differences have been noted.

(1) The developed countries are largely urbanised and industrialised. The majority of the population are adult, and between 10 and 16 % of the population are over the age of 65 years. Rates of natural increase are low, and some countries in Western Europe have reached zero population growth. Cardiovascular disease, neoplasms and violence (such as motor vehicle accidents) are the most important causes of death, and degenerative conditions are common.

(2) The developing countries are predominantly rural. Fertility rates are high and, because of this, the population is a young one, and children make up a large proportion of it. Although death-rates are falling, infant mortality rates are in the region of 150 per 1 000 live births, while nearly half the children die before they reach the age of 5 years. Life expectancy is shorter than in the developed countries, due to high child mortality, and there are few old people in the population. Malnutrition and infections such as typhoid fever and other gastro-intestinal in-

fections, tuberculosis and malaria contribute heavily to the high mortality rates. Although death-rates are high they are falling and in these countries the population is increasing rapidly, most having rates of natural increase between 2 % and 3 %.

SOUTH AFRICAN DEMOGRAPHIC DATA

South Africa has a heterogeneous population of great ethnic diversity. The population had the following composition in 1991: blacks form 70 % of the population, whites 16,4 %, coloureds 10,5 % and Asians 3,1 %. (The proportion of blacks in the population is increasing, as blacks have a high fertility rate.) There are more than four times as many blacks as whites in South Africa.

In South Africa all demographic data have been collected, computed and published along ethnic lines. Information concerning the blacks is frequently not available because many births, particularly in the rural areas, are not registered. Blacks have demographic characteristics similar to those of the other developing countries, viz. high fertility rates, a young population and, because of this, falling death-rates, in spite of adverse economic and environmental conditions. Blacks in the rural areas still have a high fertility motivation and, coupled with this, a large number of women of childbearing age in the population; birth-rates will, therefore, decline only gradually in the foreseeable future.

The white population, on the other hand, is similar to those of the developed countries (Western Europe for example) with low fertility rates and low mortality rates and a long life expectancy.

Statistics are collected in the RSA by the Central Statistical Service on a continuous basis. Much information is supplied by the censuses held in the RSA every 10 years (i.e. 1980, 1991), but an interim census was held in 1985. The registration of births and deaths is compulsory in the RSA but enforcement of registration laws is not always possible, especially in the black rural areas. Since 1978, information on deaths amongst blacks has become available for the whole RSA.

BIRTHS AND DEATHS REGISTRATION ACT 51 OF 1992

This Act was passed to regulate the registration of births and deaths. It applies to all South African citizens, whether in the RSA or outside, and includes persons who are not South African citizens but live permanently or temporarily in the Republic of South Africa.

'Registration of births

Notice of birth

9. (1) In the case of any child born alive, any one of his parents or, if neither of his parents is able to do so, the person having charge of the child or a person requested to do so by the parents or the said person, shall within seven days after the birth give notice thereof in the prescribed manner.

(2) Subject to the provisions of section 10, the notice of birth referred to in subsection (1) of this section shall be given under the surname of the father of the child concerned.

(3) Where the notice of a birth is given after the expiration of seven days from the date of birth, the Director-General may demand that reasons for the late notice be furnished and that the fingerprints be taken of the person whose notice of birth is given.

(4) No registration of birth shall be done of a person who dies before notice of his birth has been given in terms of subsection (1).

(5) The person to whom notice of birth was given in terms of subsection (1), shall furnish the person who gave that notice with a birth certificate, or an acknowledgement of receipt of the notice of birth in the prescribed form, as the Director-General may determine.

(6) No person's birth shall be registered unless a forename and a surname have been assigned to him.

Notice of birth of illegitimate child

10. (1) Notice of birth of an illegitimate child shall be given —
(a) under the surname of the mother; or
(b) at the joint request of the mother and of the person who in the presence of the person to whom the notice of birth was given acknowledges himself in writing to be the father of the child and enters the prescribed particulars regarding himself upon the notice of birth, under the surname of the person who has so acknowledged.

(2) Notwithstanding the provisions of subsection (1), the notice of birth may be given under the surname of the mother if the person mentioned in subsection (1)(b), with the consent of the mother, acknowledges himself in writing to be the father of the child and enters particulars regarding himself upon the notice of birth.

Amendment of birth registration of illegitimate child

11. (1) Any parent or guardian of an illegitimate child whose parents married each other after the registration of his birth, may, if such child is a minor, or such child himself may, if he is of age, apply to the Director-General to amend the registration of his birth as if his parents were married to each other at the time of his birth, and thereupon the Director-General shall, if satisfied that the applicant is competent to make the application, the alleged parents of the child are in fact his parents and that they legally married each other, amend the registration of birth in the prescribed manner as if such a child's parents were legally married to each other at the time of his birth.

(2) If an illegitimate child's parents marry each other before notice of his birth is given, notice of such birth shall be given and the birth registered as if the parents were married to each other at the time of his birth.

Notice of birth of abandoned child

12. The notice of birth of an abandoned child which has not yet been given, shall be given, after an enquiry in respect of the child concerned in terms of the Child Care Act, 1983 (Act 74 of 1983), by the social worker or authorised officer concerned: Provided that in the event of any parent of the child being traced after the registration of the birth and the particulars in any document or record in respect of the child not being reflected correctly, the Director-General may on application amplify and correct the said particulars.

Birth outside the Republic

13. If a child of a father or a mother who is a South African citizen is born outside the Republic, notice of birth may be given to the head of a South African diplomatic or consular mission, or a regional representative in the Republic.

Registration of deaths

Death due to natural causes

14. (1) In the case of a death due to natural causes any person who was present at the death, or who became aware thereof, or who has charge of the burial concerned, shall give, as soon as practicable, by means of a certificate mentioned in section 15(1) or (2), notice thereof to a person contemplated in section 4.

(2) If the person contemplated in section 4 is satisfied on the basis of the certificate issued in terms of section 15(1) or (2) that the death was due to natural causes, he shall complete the prescribed death register and issue a prescribed burial order authorising burial.

(3) If, before a prescribed burial order has been issued, a person contemplated in section 4 has reasonable doubt whether the death was due to natural causes, he shall not issue a burial order and he shall inform a police officer as to such doubt.

(4) If, after a prescribed burial order has been issued, a person contemplated in section 4 has reasonable doubt whether the death was due to natural causes, he shall inform a police officer as to such doubt, and before the police officer acts in terms of the provisions of section 16, he shall, if the corpse has not yet been buried, withdraw and cancel the burial order.

Certificate by medical practitioner

15. (1) Where a medical practitioner is satisfied that the death of any person who was attended before his death by

the medical practitioner was due to natural causes, he shall issue a prescribed certificate stating the cause of death.

(2) A medical practitioner who did not attend any person before his death but after the death of the person examined the corpse and is satisfied that the death was due to natural causes, may issue a prescribed certificate to that effect.

(3) If a medical practitioner is of the opinion that the death was due to other than natural causes, he shall not issue a certificate mentioned in subsection (1) or (2) and shall inform a police officer as to his opinion in that regard.

Death due to other than natural causes

17. (1) After an investigation as to the circumstances of a death due to other than natural causes in terms of section 3 of the Inquests Act, 1959 (act 58 of 1959), the medical practitioner concerned shall, as soon as he is satisfied that the corpse concerned is no longer required for the purposes of an examination mentioned in the said section 3, issue a prescribed certificate to that effect and deliver it to the police officer concerned.

(2) After the certificate referred to in subsection (1) has been issued, the police officer concerned, or any person contemplated in section (4), as the case may be, without stating a cause of death, and the police officer concerned or the person contemplated in section 4, as the case may be, may issue the prescribed burial order authorising burial.

Still-birth

18. (1) A medical practitioner who was present at a still-birth, or who examined the corpse of a child and is satisfied that the child was still-born, shall issue a prescribed certificate to that effect.

(2) If no medical practitioner was present at the still-birth, or if no medical practitioner examined the corpse of a still-born child, any person who was present at the still-birth shall make a prescribed declaration thereof to any person contemplated in section 4.

(3) The certificate mentioned in subsection (1) or the declaration mentioned in subsection (2) shall be deemed to be the notice of the still-birth, and a person contemplated in section 4 shall, on the basis of such notice and if he is satisfied that the child was still-born, issue under the surname of any parent concerned a prescribed burial order authorising burial.

(4) If, before a prescribed burial order has been issued, a person contemplated in section 4 has reasonable doubt whether the child was still-born, he shall not issue a burial order and he shall inform a police officer as to such doubt.

(5) If, after a prescribed burial order has been issued, a person contemplated in section 4 has reasonable doubt whether the child was still-born, he shall inform a police officer as to such doubt, and before the police officer acts in terms of the provisions of section 16, he shall, if the corpse has not yet been buried, withdraw and cancel the burial order.

Definitions

1. In this Act, unless the context otherwise indicates —
    (i) "birth", in relation to a child, means the birth of a child born alive;
    (ii) "burial" means burial in earth or the cremation or any other mode of disposal of a corpse;

(iii) "burial place" means any public, private or other place which is used for a burial;

(iv) "corpse" means any dead human body, including the body of any still-born child;

(v) "Department" means the Department of Home Affairs;

"Director-General" means the Director-General: Home Affairs;

(vii) "fingerprints" includes palmprints;

(viii) "forename" means the word or words by which a person is designated as an individual and which precede his surname;

"major" or "person of age" means any person who has attained the age of 21 years or who has under the provisions of section 2 of the Age of Majority Act, 1972 (act 57 of 1972), been declared to be a major, and includes a person under the age of 21 years who has contracted a legal marriage;

(xviii) "still-born", in relation to a child, means that it has had at least 26 weeks of intra-uterine existence but showed no sign of life after complete birth, and "still-birth", in relation to a child, has a corresponding meaning ... '

Population size

TABLE 8
Estimated SA population figures for 1994
(*Epidemiological Comments* 20(2), February 1993).

Asians	2.5 %	(1 037 000)
Blacks	58 %	(23 584 000)
Coloureds	8.5 %	(3 451 000)
Whites	13 %	(5 184 000)
RSA total	82 %	(33 256 000)
TBVC	18 %	(7 330 000)
SA TOTAL	100 %	(40 586 000)
Blacks total	76 %	(30 914 000)
Estimated illegal aliens		(8 000 000)

At the present rate of increase (2,44 %) the population of the RSA will be 80 million in 2020 (Dr R Venter on TV 27.03.1990).

Geographic distribution

It is estimated that 93 % of whites, 86 % of coloureds, 92 % of Asians and 75 % of blacks will live in urban areas in 2000. In keeping with a universal trend and also because of the former influx control of blacks in the RSA, women and children, the elderly and the sick or disabled are

TABLE 9
RSA population by age and sex, 1985[7]
See age distribution of the 1991 census of the SA population (p. 80).

Age group (years)	Asian		Black		Coloured		White	
	Male	Female	Male	Female	Male	Female	Male	Female
0–4	45 000	43 400	1 516 500	1 507 700	170 800	168 800	199 200	191 400
5–9	45 000	45 100	1 265 200	1 264 000	160 800	158 000	192 600	184 200
10–14	50 000	49 000	1 105 600	1 100 100	180 000	178 300	229 800	221 400
15–19	45 200	45 200	1 038 700	960 500	171 000	171 600	219 800	212 000
20–24	42 600	42 700	994 300	855 300	154 600	160 900	208 700	203 200
25–29	39 400	39 400	891 500	739 300	129 400	134 400	205 000	199 600
30–34	36 700	36 600	728 900	599 900	99 800	107 800	192 200	187 400
35–39	32 200	32 500	578 300	480 800	77 600	85 100	193 100	185 200
40–44	25 600	26 500	461 300	391 800	61 800	68 100	169 500	160 300
45–49	20 100	21 300	381 700	329 600	54 200	58 300	142 200	135 400
50–54	15 300	16 700	302 700	266 100	44 700	49 000	113 200	112 800
55–59	11 200	12 600	235 900	210 800	31 400	35 100	95 900	104 100
60–64	7 900	9 200	174 300	159 800	24 200	29 700	81 700	93 900
65–69	5 300	6 100	111 000	116 300	17 600	21 000	62 600	79 100
70–74	2 900	3 500	68 800	79 400	11 600	16 100	50 000	70 300
75 and older	3 000	3 300	58 000	77 400	11 700	18 800	89 300	162 000

left behind when job-seeking males move to the cities.

The Human Sciences Research Council (HSRC) (*The Star*, 1982) found that despite the government's attempt to decentralise jobs and to use influx control, there has been a massive move of people, especially blacks, from the rural areas to the cities, i.e. there is an ongoing depopulation of the 'platteland' as a result of urbanisation.

BIOSTATISTICS

Birth-rates

The birth-rate in the RSA has shown a downward trend but despite that, the population of the RSA increased by 27 % (5 million) between 1970 and 1980 (census findings). The coloured birth-rate dropped from 4,66 % to 2,72 % between 1960 and 1976. This is a decrease of nearly 42 %. Blacks have shown a decline of 8,4 % in their birth-rate. The rate of natural increase of the white population is declining towards zero, being 0,83 % per annum.

The fertility pattern

This statistic refers to the number of children born to a woman. The generation replacement of children per woman is 2,1 during her reproductive years. According to the Human Sciences Research Council, the average number of children per woman has dropped by a third since the 1960s. The average number of children has dropped from 6 to 4 among African women, from 6,3 to 2,4 among coloured women, from 6,4 to 2,3 among Indian women and from 3,3 to 1,7 among white women. (*Fast Facts*, May 1994, SAIRR)

Life expectancy

Table 11 shows the mean life expectancy at birth in years for the major population groups in South Africa.

The findings of a study done for the subcommittee on Ageing of the HMAC (Health Matters Advisory Committee) on increased life expectancy, warned that between the years 1980–2000 the numbers of elderly of all races in the RSA will increase as follows:

Whites by 40 %   Asians by 185 %
Coloureds by 44 %   Blacks by 336 %

This does not mean that people are living to an older age, but that more people will survive the younger years to reach man's allotted life span.

Mortality rates

Crude Mortality Rate (CMR)

The trend of the crude mortality rates from 1938–1980 shows a drop for blacks, coloureds

TABLE 10
Crude birth-rates for major population groups
(per 1 000 population) for 1938, 1975 and 1980 in SA

Population Group	Year		
	1938	1975	1980
White	25,0	18,9	16,5
Coloured	45,5	28,5	27,8
Asian	37,3	27,9	24,0
Black	42	39,6*	39,1
*Estimated			

TABLE 11
Mean life expectancy at birth in years for the major population groups in South Africa

YEARS	POPULATION GROUP							
	White		Coloured		Asian		Black*	
	Male	Female	Male	Female	Male	Female	Male	Female
1945–1947	63,8	68,3	41,7	44,0	50,7	49,8	39,1	39,2
1959–1961	64,7	71,7	49,6	54,3	47,7	59,6	47,9	53,7
1969–1971	64,5	72,3	48,8	56,1	59,3	63,9	49,0	55,6
1979–1981	66,6	74,2	54,3	62,6	62,3	68,4	—	—
*Estimated								

and Asians; whites maintained a fairly constant CMR from 1938 onwards.

TABLE 12
Crude mortality rate per 1 000 population of the major population groups in South Africa

YEAR	POPULATION GROUP			
	White	Coloured	Asian	Black
1938	9,5	23,6	13,9	22,0*
1975	8,3	11,7	06,6	11,0
1980	8,3	9,2	5,9	11,0
*Estimated				

TABLE 14
Comparison for age group 15–64 years of mortality rates (per 100 000) in whites with those in Asians, coloureds and blacks
(Age-adjusted to MOSU age-distribution of whites in 1970, by ICD cause groups[9])

	Whites		Asians		Coloureds		Blacks	
	MRs	%	MRs	%	MRs	%	MRs	%
Infective diseases, etc.	7,0	1	36,3	4	110,4	10	104,2	11
— Gastro-enteritis	0,8		4,2		10,0		15,7,	
— Tuberculosis	2,9		21,9		90,5(3)	8	78,2(3)	8
Neoplasms	102,8	18	68,9	8	144,0	13	104,9	11
— Digestive system	28,2(4)	5	30,6(8)	4	57,5(7)	5	55,6(7)	6
— Lungs	20,2(7)	3	7,3		22,7		9,6,	
— Genito-urinary organs	13,3		10,8		25,6		16,8,	
Endocrine, etc.	6,1	1	40,0	6	16,1	2	17,6	2
— Diabetes	5,0		37,1(7)	4	10,4		10,5,	
— Nutritional defics.	0,1		2,2		3,0		6,2,	
Circulatory diseases	259,1	45	405,7	46	369,2	34	201,9	21
— Chronic rheumatic heart disease	6,4		12,4		15,7		8,5,	
— Hypertensive disease	7,9		51,2(4)	6	144,3(10)	4	33,9(9)	4
— IHD	167,5(1)	28	184,8(1)	21	93,5(2)	9	11,9	1
— Other forms of heart disease	14,2(10)	2	36,7		60,9(6)	6	62,9(6)	7
— CVA	41,2(3)	7	110,2(2)	13	120,4(1)	11	70,8(4)	7
Respiratory diseases	54,5	9	124,4	14	144,4	13	127,3	15
— Pneumonias	21,0(6)	4	55,2(3)	6	74,2(4)	7	82,9(2)	9
— Bronchitis, etc.	22,0(5)	4	49,9(5)	6	45,3(9)	4	17,4,	
Digestive system	25,3	4	46,5	5	42,7	4	39,7,	
— Liver diseases	16,5(9)	3	37,3(6)	4	28,1		25,4(10)	3
Symptoms, etc.	7,9	1	29,6	3	37,9	4	127,0	13
— Ill-defined diseases	7,9	1	29,6(9)	3	37,9		122,3(1)	13
Accidents, etc.	101,6	18	82,8	9	187,6	17	186,8	19
Motor vehicle accids.	56,3(2)	9	25,7(10)	3	69,7(5)	6	47,3	5
— Other accidents	7,8		12,9		22,6		12,6,	
— Unspecified violence	3,3		1,6		5,4		24,6,	
— Suicide	18,1(8)	3	17,1		6,5		7,2,	
— Homicide	3,4		7,9		49,0(8)	5	70,3(5)	7
Population	2 388 550		370 930		1 064 020		2 258 860	
All causes (MRs)	579,8		872,7		1 080,5		958,0	

*In brackets are given the rank order of the 10 leading causes of death.
†The black population is that estimated to be in the 34 'selected' magisterial districts.

TABLE 13
The 1984 mortality[1]

MALES	White	Coloured	Asian	Black
Total number of deaths	21 226	14 974	3 006	61 497
Crude death-rate/1 000	8,8	10,8	6,8	6,5

FEMALES	White	Coloured	Asian	Black
Total number of deaths	16 949	10 935	1 980	40 468
Crude death-rate/1 000	7,0	7,6	4,4	4,5

Note: The lower crude death-rate in blacks is a reflection of the small proportion of elderly in this group and the falling infant mortality rate.

Potential years of life lost[1]

A useful statistic used by the Institute for Biostatistics of the SAMRC is 'Potential Years of Life Lost'.

It is assumed that death is premature if it occurs before the age of 65 and potential years of life are lost thereby. Example: if a person dies at the age of 40 years he has lost 24 (64–40) potential years of life.

To exclude the great intergroup infant mortality rate differences, only deaths after the age of 1 year are used in calculations. This statistic is calculated as the sum total for each population group of potential years lost each year, and then as a percentage for each major 'cause of death' category, there being 17 categories according to the ICD classification of diseases.

It was found that blacks lost the largest number of 'potential years of life' and that 'death due to non-natural causes' accounted for the most potential years lost in all groups, 49,8 % of whites' 'potential years of life lost' being from this cause. After that comes circulatory diseases and neoplasms in whites and Asians, and infections/parasitic and respiratory diseases in coloureds and blacks.

This statistic provides an indication of the preventive potential of health care strategies.

Child mortality in 1984[1]

The infant mortality rate (IMR) has always been an indicator of the state of health care services of a country and of the quality of its social, economic and physical environment. Recently this statistic has been broadened to include age-specific death-rates for the first 5 years of life.

UNICEF (in *The State of the World's Children*, 1986)[1] estimated that 15 million children under the age of 5 years die every year in the world.

TABLE 15
Deaths in childhood according to age-specific categories

Age	Whites	Coloureds	Asians	Blacks
0–6 days	477	1 328	219	5 281
7–27 days	118	566	44	2 043
1–12 months	294	2 356	100	10 928
1–5 years	314	1 332	78	6 902

Age-specific categories

- *Perinatal period*: 28 weeks gestation to first 7 days.
- *Neonatal period*: from birth up to the 28th day.
- *Post-neonatal period*: 1 month to 1 year.
- *Infancy*: 0–1 year.
- *Early childhood*: 1–4 years.
- *Late childhood*: 5–14 years.

Main risk factors of death

- *Perinatal deaths*: poor quality of antenatal and perinatal care, poor health status of the pregnant woman.
- *Neonatal deaths*: low birthmass, i.e. less than 2 500 g.
- *Post-neonatal deaths*: low socio-economic status and environmental factors, e.g. infections, especially gastro-enteritis.
- *Early childhood*: the above, plus the dangers of the physical environment.

In infant mortality (0–1 year) the greatest proportion of deaths in whites and Asians occurs during the neonatal period (0–1 month), while in coloureds and blacks, the greatest proportion occurs during the post-neonatal infancy period (1–12 months), when death is due mainly to gastro-enteritis, respiratory illness and malnutrition. These are preventable causes of death.

Note: The IMR in whites is as low as is possible, i.e. according to First-World standards.

TABLE 16
IMRS (/1 000) for whites, coloureds and Asians, 1981–1985

Year	Whites	Coloureds	Asians
1981	13,3	59,2	18,8
1982	13,5	58,4	17,6
1983	13,5	55,0	20,1
1984	11,7	46,5	17,4
1985	9,7	40,4	15,6

Estimated IMR for blacks in 1985 was 60,6 (HSRC).

This shows a substantial decrease in IMR in these three groups, the IMR in 1985 for whites dropping below 10/1 000 births for the first time.

Average infant mortality rates

TABLE 17
Average infant mortality rates (per 1 000 live births) (IMR) in the RSA for the years 1981–1985[1]

Whites	12,3
Coloureds	51,9
Asians	17,9
Blacks	94–124*

*Estimated: there is under-reporting of births as well as deaths.

In some rural and urban black areas where health services are well developed, the black IMR is much lower, approaching the WHO IMR indicator of less than 50 required for 'Health for All by the Year 2000'.

The infant mortality rate was reduced in 1979 amongst the coloureds and blacks in Cape Town. The MOH ascribed it to the improvement in the environmental conditions as well as to the promotive and preventive services, both at hospital and clinic level. Family planning had been successfully promoted, immunisation coverage had increased and specialised clinics to combat malnutrition had been established. Successful efforts had been made to encourage community organisation and participation and to promote cultural and social upliftment to meet the ends of urbanisation.

The growth rate

TABLE 18
Average annual natural growth rate
(Expressed in numbers per 1 000 of the population and as a percentage)

	1960/70	1970/80	1980	1981
All population groups	31,4 3,14 %	27,6 2,76 %	23,1 2,31 %	23,1 2,31 %
Whites	13,1 1,31 %	13,2 1,32 %	8,6 0,86 %	8,3 0,83 %
Coloureds	32,3 3,23 %	24,8 2,48 %	18,5 1,85 %	18,5 1,85 %
Blacks (estimated)	28,0 2,8 %	28,0 2,8 %	28,0 2,8 %	28,0 2,8 %

The growth rate is also affected by immigration and emigration. In the past the white population has increased its number considerably through immigration from other countries, gaining about 30 000 members a year from this source. These figures declined in 1977 and 1978 to a net loss of immigrants following the riots. Migration* of whites has been as follows:

	Immigrants	Emigrants	Net immigrants
1975	50 312	9 916	40 396
1976	46 071	15 302	30 769
1977	24 724	25 519	–795
1978	18 565	20 078	–1 513
1979	18 568	15 171	3 307
1980	22 161	10 955	11 206

*Source: SA Statistics, Department of Statistics, 1981.

TABLE 20
White growth rate (natural plus net immigration)
(Expressed in number per 1 000 of the population and as a percentage)

1960/70	1970/80	1980	1981
20,9	18,6	12,5	14,1
2,09 %	1,86 %	1,25 %	1,41 %

At the present rate of natural growth, the black population is growing three and a half times as fast as the white population, the growth for coloureds being in between.

Morbidity data

The findings of morbidity data collected in the RSA by the Central Statistical Service from 1977–1981[5] allow the following conclusions to be drawn.

There is no correspondence between mortality rates and admission (morbidity) rates to hospital for specific diseases. (For cause-specific mortality rates, see p. 85.)

For example, cardio-vascular diseases are the highest killers in whites, yet the admission rate to hospitals and other in-patients establishments places these diseases in the 7th position when disease categories are ranked in descending order of frequency. The highest admission in whites occurred for diseases of the genito-urinary system, followed by diseases of the digestive system, respiratory system, musculo-skeletal system and complications of pregnancy and childbirth.

Amongst the coloureds, complications of pregnancy and childbirth had prior claim to hospital beds, followed by accidents, poisoning, violence and diseases of the respiratory system. Admissions due to infective and parasitic diseases came in the 8th position.

These seeming anomalies are repeated in the Asian and black groups. In the psychiatric, nervous system and sense organ disorders, the admission rate for whites is respectively four and five times higher than for the other groups; in diseases of the respiratory system, twice as high; and in diseases of the digestive and genito-urinary systems, five times as high.

Answers to these findings have not been found and beg epidemiological research. The cause could possible be over-utilisation by whites and under-utilisation by the other groups, of existing facilities.

The admission rate of infective and parasitic diseases amongst blacks and coloureds is quite low, but higher than in whites. The incidence of diabetes mellitus is high among Asians. Black children suffer more than any other group from malnutrition.

In motor vehicle accidents, blacks show the highest admission rates. (The close on 400 000 motor vehicle accidents per annum yield 100 000 casualties and 10 000 deaths.)

Admission rates for accidents, poisoning and violence are close to one another in all the population groups.

REFERENCES

(1) *Review of South African Mortality (1984).* Institute of Biostatistics South African Medical Research Council. Parow. 1987.
(2) Central Statistical Service. *Deaths 1985 — Whites, Coloureds, Asians.* Pretoria: CSS, 1985.
(3) Central Statistical Service. *Births of Blacks — 1979.* Pretoria: CSS, 1981.
(4) *Epidemiological Comments.* Department of National Health and Population Development. March 1984; **11**(3).
(5) *Epidemiological Comments.* Department of National Health and Population Development. November 1984; **11**(11).
(6) *Epidemiological Comments.* Department of National Health and Population Development. March 1986; **13**(3).
(7) *Epidemiological Comments.* Department of National Health and Population Development. January 1987; **14**(1).
(8) *Epidemiological Comments.* Department of National Health and Population Development. June 1987; **14**(6).
(9) Wyndham CH. The loss from premature death of economically active manpower in the various populations of the Republic of South Africa (1981). *S Afr Med J* **60**: 411 (Table II).
(10) *Epidemiological Comments.* Department of National Health and Population Development. February 1993; **20**(2)
(11) *Epidemiological Comments.* Department of National Health and Population Development. September 1992; **19**(9).

TEST OF KNOWLEDGE

The student has benefited from studying this chapter if he/she can answer the following questions:

(1) Discuss the age and sex composition of developing and developed communities with regard to:
(*a*) percentage productive and non-productive members by age;

(b) the differences in the population pyramids;

(c) the effects of relatively high infant mortality and birth-rates of the black population of the RSA on the shape of its population pyramid; and

(d) the shape of the population pyramid of an 'ageing' population.

(2) Define the following:
- biostatistical rates
- crude death-rate
- perinatal death-rate
- cause-specific death-rates
- morbidity data
- total fertility rate
- crude birth-rate
- the case-fatality rate
- the population explosion
- First and Third-World countries

(3) State the factors which affect fertility rates.

(4) State the importance of compulsory registration of births and deaths and the holding of population censuses.

(5) State the causes of high infant mortality rates.

(6) Write notes on:
(a) developed and developing countries and their demographic differences;
(b) factors influencing life expectancy; and
(c) the demographic consequences of a rapidly falling IMR (leading to an increased life expectancy) amongst blacks and coloureds in the RSA in the next century.

(7) Discuss the looming population explosion in the RSA by the year 2010 — its causes and the preventive strategies contained in the Population Development Programme (see p. 10, 29).

(8) How is the annual growth rate of a community assessed? Discuss the trends in the growth rates of the different population groups in the RSA.

(9) Define the following:
(a) morbidity statistics;
(b) incidence rate; and
(c) prevalence rate.

7

Epidemiology

OBJECTIVES

Epidemiology, the study of the distribution, causes and control of community health problems, is an applied science which is basic to the study of community medicine and nursing.

The objectives of this chapter are to introduce the student to the work of the epidemiologist, who uses demographic and biostatistical data and who contributes to this data by doing epidemiological research.

The student will be given some insight into the different research methods so that he/she may be able to comprehend how the extent of health problems and their impact on a community are investigated. The student must understand how the life-style of a community can be linked by means of research to the risk factors of chronic diseases, for instance, smoking to lung cancer and ischaemic heart disease.

The student must become aware that preventive and therapeutic community health programmes are based on demographic and biostatistical data and on intervention epidemiological research, the latter also evaluating the effectiveness of the health care interventions applied by local authorities.

INTRODUCTION

Epidemiology is the method of study of the distribution and causes of ill-health in populations and the evaluation of the effectiveness of health care. Its goal is to improve the health of human populations, and to this end it involves the politico-economic arena. Epidemiology is one of the basic components of community medicine and as such it is concerned with the health of populations rather than individuals.

'Epidemiology' was formerly defined as 'the science of epidemics'. This was because it had its origin in the study of, firstly, the great epidemic diseases such as cholera, plague and smallpox, and later, the other communicable diseases which were so prevalent at the time. Epidemiologists studied the frequency and the distribution of these diseases and tried to discover the ways in which they were transmitted, and to develop methods of prevention. They were often remarkably successful in their efforts to reduce the incidence of such diseases, when one considers that frequently even the causative organism had not yet been identified. Later epidemiologists widened their scope to include the study of nutritional disorders such as scurvy, beriberi and pellagra, as well as the institution of disease control measures.

Today changing patterns of disease, especially in the developing countries, have caused epidemiologists to extend their field of study still further; consequently a great deal of attention is being devoted to the non-communicable conditions such as cardio-vascular disease and cancer, which contribute so heavily to morbidity and mortality in the Western world. Modern epidemiology concerns itself with all the factors influencing the health status of populations.

Because the health of a community is to some extent affected by the availability, the organisation and the utilisation of health care services, epidemiological methods are now being applied to the study of this important area of community health.

The Medical Research Council (MRC) recently established the Centre for Epidemiological Research in Southern Africa (CERSA). The purpose of this centre is to co-ordinate epidemiological research, and is especially concerned with the health effects of increasing urbanisation in the RSA. The Institute of Biostatistics of the MRC helps with the planning of epidemiological research.

Modern epidemiology differs from the older discipline in its approach. Modern epidemiology adopts an ecological approach, that is, it studies populations against the background of their total environment, social and cultural as well as physical.

OBTAINING EPIDEMIOLOGICAL DATA

The modern epidemiologist obtains his data from two main sources, discussed below.

Disease surveillance (see p. 481)

The incidence and prevalence of diseases in a community are supervised by studying demographic data, morbidity and mortality trends (see Chapter 6) and disease notification (see Chapter 27). '*Surveillance, when applied to a disease, means the continued watchfulness over the distribution and trends of incidence through the systematic collection, consolidation and evaluation of morbidity and mortality reports and other relevant data.*'[3] Routine disease surveillance is carried out by the Epidemiology Directorate of the Department of Health.

Note: Notification of notifiable diseases and biostatistical trends extracted from '*Epidemiological Comments*', a monthly publication of the Department of Health, will be included in the relevant chapters of this book.

The new disease AIDS was discovered in the USA by means of the special surveillance activities of the US Centres for Disease Control, which employ epidemiologists to interpret surveillance data. It was noticed that two diseases characterised by immunodeficiency, Pneumocystis carinii pneumonia and Kaposi's sarcoma, occurred in previously healthy homosexual men in certain regions over a circumscribed period of time (1980–1981). These somewhat unusual morbidity data led to the search for and discovery of a common aetiological agent, the Human Immunodeficiency Virus (HIV).

AIDS and HIV-infection data are obtained by surveillance systems which involve both active and passive surveillance.

(1) Passive surveillance, for instance, the routine screening of blood donors for HIV infection. The findings will be artificially low because of voluntary self-exclusion of homo-bisexual donors. Passive surveillance data may also be obtained through reports by health care providers who may or may not be conscientious and cannot be legally obliged to do so. For instance, Anonymous AIDS reports (filled in on DNHPD forms by medical practitioners and dentists for AIDS cases) which are to be forwarded to the regional offices (see p. 481) of the DOH.

Note: Many AIDS patients do not see a doctor or dentist and are, therefore, not reported.

(2) Active surveillance of sentinel sites or subgroups may be more accurate and reliable than passive surveillance but requires more resources, for instance, seroprevalence HIV surveys in a defined population group such as STD attenders, or pregnant women attending antenatal clinics, carried out by designated persons. In this case blood samples for HIV-antibody tests are taken from a representative sample of patients.

Note: A national HIV survey of the prevalence of HIV infection in women attending antenatal clinics has been carried out annually by the DNHPD since 1990 and is discussed on p. 608.

Passive surveillance information is thus complemented by findings of epidemiological research studies, which are ideally conducted by trained epidemiologists.

Epidemiological research

Epidemiological research is co-ordinated in the RSA by the Centre for Epidemiological Research in Southern Africa. Chronic disease, e.g. tuberculosis, malnutrition and ischaemic heart disease, and new diseases likely to assume epi

demic proportions, e.g. AIDS, are the most frequent subjects of epidemiological research.

'In the RSA approximately 100 disease outbreaks or epidemics requiring investigation and control can be anticipated each year.'[4]

Epidemiological research makes use of three research methods, viz. descriptive studies, analytical (comparative) studies and intervention studies, to reach its goal of improving the health of the local authority districts, regional services councils regions, or whole nations. The control of any disease must begin with a description of its occurrence, i.e. where, when and in whom it occurs. After this, causal factors are established; when therapeutic agents have been synthesised in the laboratory or a disease-preventive strategy has been devised, then the outcome of therapeutic intervention is tested.

Epidemiological studies are thus undertaken for the following reasons:

(1) To determine the extent of health problems in the community.

(2) To investigate the causes of diseases, especially the risk factors involved in diseases which appear to be related to the life-style of a community.

(3) To study the natural history of a disease from the premorbid, health state of subjects at risk, to the morbid state and eventual outcome. The epidemiologist studies the interaction of the susceptible host with the suspected disease-causing agent in the disease-facilitating environment.

(4) To develop the rationale for a preventive or therapeutic community health programme.

(5) To evaluate the effectiveness of preventive or therapeutic programmes.

Note: The epidemiologist studies health problems which require solution by the decision-makers (administrators, politicians). The epidemiologist, therefore, does not solve the health problem; he supplies the data on which wise decisions may be based.

Descriptive research

Community-based descriptive studies are used to investigate health problems and to describe the impact of disease on the community.

This type of study is based on scientific observations. It makes use of mortality and morbidity statistics to describe accurately the fre quency of a condition in a population. This type of study will not only indicate how many people are suffering from a condition at a given time but will also describe the characteristics of these persons in terms of age, sex, occupation, socio-economic class, level of education, as well as certain relevant cultural factors such as smoking habits, use of drugs such as alcohol, and dietary habits. Descriptive studies may also include details of geographic and climatic conditions, as well as the time of the year or the season of the year when the condition is most prevalent. These studies are of great value in identifying those persons in the population who are at greater risk. For example, epidemiology has given us a detailed description of the person most likely to suffer from ischaemic heart disease. He is a white male, over the age of forty, from the higher socio-economic groups, who has close relatives who died from 'heart attacks', who smokes cigarettes, who has a sedentary occupation and who is slightly overweight. However, epidemiology deals in probabilities, not in certainties, and not every person who fits the above description will develop ischaemic heart disease. The epidemiologist says only that such a person is more likely to do so than other persons in the population. Descriptive studies are also useful because they enable the epidemiologist to estimate the extent of a health problem, to predict future trends in the area and to formulate hypotheses concerning causation.

Types of questions that can be asked in a descriptive epidemiological study:

(1) What were the age-specific annual tuberculosis incidence rates during the years 1980–1985 in the RSA?

(2) How good was the compliance to therapy for hypertension in Soweto during 1988?

(3) What is the seroprevalence of the HIV/AIDS epidemic in South Africa?

The research design includes the method by which the subjects will be selected and the procedures which will be followed in order to obtain data.

A cross-sectional research design is used when some characteristics of a community are studied. The time period of the survey or field study is of short duration. Uncontrolled settings, such as the natural environment, are used for conducting a field survey of, for example, the incidence of a disease in a locality.

The sampling units will be determined by the purpose of the research. Method of sampling is important to avoid the unconscious selection of a biased sample. Sometimes a representative sample of a population is randomly chosen, but at other times the entire population (community) is studied, e.g. all the children between the ages of 1–5 years.

Note: In descriptive research there are no control groups. Descriptive studies have no hypotheses; here the phenomena to be investigated must be clearly stated. The 'why' and 'how' of the phenomena are not studied, only the 'what' and the 'how many'.

Measurement and data collection

Scientifically gathered data can be in the form either of words (verbal data) or of numbers (numerical data). The researcher may use measures of physical magnitude, e.g. mass for height, or observations of vital signs, or of quality (which is rated), or he may gather verbal data by means of structured interviews and paper and pencil questionnaires. Some questions may be open-ended, allowing the respondent to express an opinion or an attitude. Answers to questions require coding for statistical analysis.

Raw scores can be grouped, summarised, transformed and displayed in ways that make them easier to handle and understand, by:

(1) arranging them in classes or categories and counting the class frequency in order to draw up frequency distribution tables;

(2) computing measures of central tendency and variability;

(3) transforming raw scores to percentile ranks and standard scores;

(4) computing measures of correlation;

(5) constructing graphs; and

(6) constructing statistical tables.

Analytical (comparative) research

The purpose of analytical research is to test a hypothesis regarding an assumed causal or an associative (correlational) relationship between variables, for example, to determine which risk factors are likely to be causally related to the outcome (result) being measured, e.g. ischaemic heart disease, lung cancer.

Analytical studies attempt to explain why certain persons in a community suffer from a certain condition and others do not. Epidemiologists do not believe that disease occurs by chance or that it is haphazardly distributed in populations; they believe that disease is the result of a complex interaction between the individual with his genetic predispositions, and his environment, physical and social. It is the aim of the epidemiologist to unravel the multiplicity of causal factors which may be involved.

Examples of questions asked which give rise to analytical studies:

- How much of South Africa's high cardiovascular mortality rate can be explained on a genetic basis?
- What factors (e.g. age, sex, level of education, knowledge imparted by doctors and nurses, socio-economic status) affect the likelihood of a patient not complying with treatment?

Analytical studies make use of the range of life-styles of the unique South African population to determine particular risk factors for disease and to study the effects of the risk factors on chronic diseases. In the case of skin cancer such a relationship has already been demonstrated between the disease, the amount of pigment in the person's skin, and the number of hours of exposure to sunlight over a period.

Comparative research may be either non-RCT (not randomised controlled trials) or RCT, the common feature of the two kinds being the comparison of two or more groups of subjects: the research and the control groups.

Non-RCT, analytical, comparative research may also be called correlational research as it purports to find out how variables go together or are associated. The groups here are not randomly selected by the researcher; they are self-selected or defined by nature, e.g. smokers and non-smokers. For this reason causality cannot be proved. The higher the strength of association, however, the greater the likelihood that the independent and dependent variables will be causally related. To test for causality, consistent results from a number of different studies should be obtained. It is on this basis that cigarette smoking and lung cancer have been causally linked.

Types of analytical, non-RCT research designs:

(1) *Cross-sectional studies called surveys or field studies.* Here some characteristic of people who differ in, for example, age is observed once only by observing the characteristic in different age groups. In this way predictions can be made about the way in which people change with age.

Both descriptive and non-RCT comparative studies make use of cross-sectional research designs. The aim of cross-sectional studies is to discover the frequency of a characteristic in a defined population at a given time. If an epidemiologist were interested in the frequency of dental caries in black children under the age of 6 years, living in Soweto, he would select a representative sample of the population in which he is interested. Each child in the sample would be examined to establish the presence and the extent of dental caries. All the children would be examined during a certain period of time, and each child would be examined once only.

(2) *Longitudinal studies.* In these studies groups are studied at two or more points in time. Longitudinal studies are not only interested in the frequency of a condition but also in the possible aetiological factors which they try to establish by following up the sample over a period of time, sometimes for many years.

There are two main types of longitudinal studies: (1) prospective studies, and (2) retrospective field and case studies.

1. Prospective studies, also called follow-up and cohort studies[1]

Note: A **cohort** is a group with some common attributes or experience, e.g. all children born in a certain year; residence in a certain area. An 'inception cohort' refers to a group of patients who were identified at an early and uniform point in the course of their common disease,[1] e.g. patients with coronary risk factors.

Follow-up studies start with the cohort at a point in time and continue into the future, to see what effect a present phenomenon (e.g. smoking or hypercholesterolaemia or assumed causes of dental caries) will have on a future phenomenon, called an 'outcome'. The outcome and the period of follow-up must be clearly defined and laid down.

In analytical follow-up studies, baseline measurements to detect the characteristic being studied (e.g. risk factors, early signs of disease) are made on a sample of the population, usually chosen because their drop-out rate is likely to be low. The measurements will define the inception cohort and the control group, i.e. those who do not suffer from the characteristic to be studied. The whole sample is then followed up for a predetermined period of time to estimate the outcome. An example of a predetermined outcome could be the incidence rate of an expected disease, e.g. lung cancer in a group of smokers.

In the Soweto example, the sample of children selected from the population of black children under the age of six years living in Soweto would be examined every six months or every year for many years, and the development of dental caries over the years recorded. At the same time note would be taken of such factors as sugar intake, type and source of water, diet, brushing of teeth, etc. In this way the natural history of the disease is determined.

Follow-up analytical studies are, therefore, used to determine:

(1) particular risk factors for the diseases described;
(2) the natural history of a disease; and
(3) the prognosis of patients with existing disease.

2. Retrospective field and case studies

Retrospective field and case studies start at a point in time and then trace back events in time which may have a causal or correlational (associative) relationship to the phenomenon being studied in the present, e.g. the association between lung cancer and smoking. It can also be called a non-concurrent (historical) prospective study.

For example, if we wish to establish whether the birth mass of infants born to mothers who smoke is lower than that of infants born to mothers who do not smoke, we would select two groups of pregnant women and match them for all important variables, such as socio-economic class, race, age, height, etc.; in other words, we try to ensure as far as possible that the two groups differ only in this one important aspect, i.e. smoking. We would then weigh all the infants at birth, ensuring that our weighing technique was standardised and that the scales were accurate. Then, using certain statistical techniques, we would compare the birth masses of the two groups and decide whether there was a statistically significant difference between them.

Intervention research

Intervention studies are done to evaluate the outcome of therapeutic interventions in community problems. The success of interventions can be assessed in a number of ways, the ideal method being the use of randomised control trials (RCTs).

In random or probability sampling, neither the researcher nor the sampling unit has an influence over who will be drawn. This avoids the selection of a biased sample.

In RCT intervention research with comparison groups, randomly drawn subjects are randomly assigned to these groups. By the double process of randomisation the extraneous (i.e. organismic and socio-psychological) variables of the research group are equated with those of the control group and the target population. The control group serves as proof that the observed effects of the intervention (i.e. manipulated independent variable) on the outcome (dependent variable) are a true reflection of a relationship of 'cause' and 'effect' between variables, i.e. that artefacts have not been responsible for the observed effects.

Special statistical techniques, called tests of significance, can be applied to two or more randomly drawn samples from the same target population. These tests are based on the fact that the sample is not exactly the same as the target population, this small 'sampling' error causing a slight 'insignificant' difference between the different samples drawn from the same target population. Tests of significance are devised to find out if the difference in results found between alternative groups is due to chance or is due to the intentional manipulation of the independent variable, i.e. the intervention applied to the research group.

Interventions are often aimed at amenable risk factors, especially where diseases are of multifactorial causation. In this case research information for risk factor intervention programmes should come from community-based studies and not from RCTs conducted on highly selected hospital/clinic-based studies.

Opportunities for experimentation do arise in epidemiology, frequently in connection with the evaluation of treatment or the testing of drugs or vaccines. If we were interested in the effectiveness of a new drug in the treatment of an infection such as tuberculosis, we would select a sample of persons suffering from tuberculosis, who would then be allocated, by randomisation technique, to two groups. The new drug would then be administered to one group (this is known as the research group) while a known medicine would be administered to the other group (the control group). The course of the disease in these two groups would then be compared and, in this way, it is hoped that the effectiveness of the new drug would be established.

The types of interventions applied either during RCT or non-RCT therapy and clinical drug trials and before-and-after studies may be:

(1) Drugs, especially for tuberculosis and hypertension. The question asked is: does a specified new medicine have a superior therapeutic effect to known medicines on a chronic disease?

(2) An integrated primary health care approach such as UNICEF GOBI-FFF (see p. 393) for improving childhood survival. The outcome is the child mortality rate, which is compared with the CMR during previous years. This is a before-and-after study.

(3) Disease eradication programmes by immunisation of mono-cause infections, e.g. measles, poliomyelitis, on the model of the smallpox eradication programme.

(4) Socio-economic upliftment (housing, water, sanitation, income, employment and education) to improve the general health standards of Third-World populations). The upliftment is aimed especially at reducing the incidence and prevalence of tuberculosis in the RSA.

(5) Testing a new compliance-improving strategy, e.g. reminding out-patients of their appointments. The research question asked is: is compliance improved by applying this time-consuming strategy?

(6) Eliminating a risk factor (e.g. inactivity) in a group of selected patients (i.e. with coronary risk factors) by prescribing therapeutic exercise. The research group but not the control group of similar patients complies with the prescription. The question asked is: does compliance with the prescription of therapeutic exercise affect the premature death-rate of the research group of patients; i.e. is the premature death-rate (potential years of life lost) lower than in the non-compliant control group?

CONTRIBUTIONS OF EPIDEMIOLOGY

Epidemiology makes great contributions to the health status of populations. It does this in many ways.

(1) It supplies the numerical data which make it possible to determine whether a health problem exists and, if it does, what the extent of the problem is. The epidemiologist is also able to predict future trends in the area.

(2) The information gathered by epidemiologists assists in defining areas of need and assists in the planning of the organisation and delivery of health care services by the administrators and/or the politicians.

(3) Epidemiology supplies objective criteria for the evaluation of health care.

(4) Epidemiologists formulate hypotheses concerning disease causation and undertake research in order to test these hypotheses, and by doing so add greatly to the store of knowledge of community medicine.

(5) Epidemiologists may be responsible for the detection of environmental hazards such as the presence of insect vectors, contamination of water supplies and other more subtle environmental factors which may affect health.

(6) Epidemiologists can assist the authorities concerned with the provision of health care services to allocate their limited resources rationally and according to the findings of community-based research.

National epidemiological research programmes will be launched in the near future to study rapid urbanisation and its impact on health and health services in the RSA. This information is urgently needed for the development of effective community-based health services.

A national research programme on trauma is being carried out, as trauma is the prime cause in the RSA of potential years of life lost.

Epidemiology is an applied science; this means that it is essentially a practical discipline. It is, therefore, not interested in accumulating knowledge merely for the sake of knowledge; rather, the aim of epidemiology is to use the findings of its research to prevent disease, improve treatment and advance the health of populations.

To the health planner, risk factors which are amenable to change at either the primary, secondary or tertiary level of prevention, are of prime consideration (p. 134).[2]

Yach and Botha[2] describe the epidemiological rationale of health planning thus:

'A descriptive study is used to describe the impact of disease in a particular community, analytical studies are used to determine particular risk factors for the disease described, interventions are applied by the local health authority to reduce the impact of the risk factors and subsequent disease on a community.' (p. 633)

REFERENCES

(1) Yach D, Botha JL. Epidemiological research methods (Part V). *S Afr Med J* 1987; **72**: 266–269.

(2) Yach D, Botha JL. Epidemiological research methods (Part VII). *S Afr Med J* 1987; **72**: 633–636.

(3) Langmuir AD. The surveillance of communicable diseases of national importance. *New Engl J Med* 1963; **268**: 182–192.

(4) Strebel PM, Küstner HGV. Disease outbreak investigations — objectives, methods and importance. *S Afr Med J* 1988; **73**: 334–336.

TEST OF KNOWLEDGE

The student has benefited from studying this chapter if he/she can:

(1) Define epidemiology in its modern sense and state the sources from which the epidemiologist obtains his data.

(2) State the ways in which an epidemiologist uses data obtained to contribute to the improvement of the health status of a community.

(3) Name the research methods used by epidemiologists and explain the role of each type of research in yielding data which can be used to improve the health of a community.

(4) Define the following terms:
– disease surveillance
– biostatistical trends
– disease incidence and prevalence
– hypothesis
– cohort
– prospective studies
– randomised control trials (RCTs)
– risk factors

8

Medical Genetics

GENERAL OBJECTIVES

The recognition of the hereditary nature of disease is an important aspect of community health. Genetic disorders not only place a heavy economic burden on the health resources of a nation, but also exact a heavy toll in terms of the quality of life of some 3–5 % of the population. In South Africa from 700 000 to 1 000 000 people suffer from a handicap due to a genetic disorder. Although not common as individual disorders, as a group they comprise over 5 % of paediatric hospital admissions.[11] Genetic disorders are for life and affect not only the individual but also his family, the local community and the wider national community. South Africa has a comprehensive, active national genetics service employing primary, secondary and tertiary preventive measures to help affected individuals and families cope with problems inflicted on them by nature, aided in some cases by nurture.

STUDY OBJECTIVES

(1) The student must revise the anatomy and physiology of the human cell, especially with regard to mitosis, meiosis and fertilisation.

The student will be introduced to:

(2) The study of cytogenetics: chromosomes, genes, DNA and RNA, genetic inheritance, mutations and teratogenesis.

(3) Clinical genetics, the common genetic disorders being classified according to their modes of inheritance.

(4) The organisation and functions of the National Genetics Programme, some genetics diagnostic procedures, the principles of genetics counselling and the scope of practice of the genetics nurse.

IN THIS CHAPTER

INTRODUCTION

Genetics is defined as the 'science of breeding'; it deals with genetic inheritance, i.e. that which is transmitted from one generation to another by means of the genes contained in the gametes of the parents. Medical genetics is an important branch of human genetics and is concerned with the transmission of diseases and abnormalities from one generation to another. Medical genetics may be divided into the following specialised branches.

(1) Clinical genetics deals with the diagnosis, prognosis and treatment of genetic diseases.

(2) Cytogenetics is concerned with the study of chromosomes.

(3) Biochemical genetics deals with inborn errors of metabolism and the process by which the genetic code is translated into normal and abnormal protein synthesis.

(4) Immunogenetics deals with the way in which antibodies (immunoglobulins) are formed in response to an antigenic stimulus and react specifically with this antigen in order to eliminate it.

(5) Pharmacogenetics is concerned with the way in which an individual deals with a drug introduced into the body. Pharmacogenetics includes all genetically determined variations in reactions to drugs.
Examples:
Scoline apnoea is due to an abnormal gene which produces abnormal cholinesterase; in porphyria variegata, the patient responds abnormally to the introduction of a normal dose of barbiturates.

(6) Ecogenetics is the science dealing with the role environmental risk factors play in genetic diseases.

(7) Population genetics deals with mutations, gene frequencies of a population and the effects of inbreeding and isolation.[1]

The main concern of population genetics is the behaviour of genes in different populations. Population genetics deals with genetic variations among population groups and between different populations. Modern genetic techniques are being used to study the origin and migrations of populations and the mixing of races. Population genetics also studies genetic variations among population groups which may cause certain inherited diseases to be more prevalent in certain ethnic groups than in others, the so-called founder effect.[1] This is of great importance in South Africa where the different population groups have their own genetic diseases, e.g. sclerosteosis, porphyria variegata and Oudtshoorn skin disease in Afrikaners, Huntington's chorea in the English group, Tay-Sachs and Gaucher disease amongst the Jews and thalassaemia in the Greek community. Population geneticists attempt to find out what factors affect gene frequencies and why some genes favour certain population groups.

CYTOGENETICS—THE STUDY OF CHROMOSOMES

Note: For background knowledge on the following subjects, the nurse is referred to a textbook of anatomy and physiology: the cell and its functions; mitosis and meiosis; gametogenesis (oogenesis and spermatogenesis); fertilisation of the ovum and embryonic development.

The nucleus of the human cell contains the nucleolus and 23 pairs of chromosomes: 22 pairs of autosomes and 1 pair of gonosomes (sex chromosomes). The chromosomes which pair during fertilisation and are identical are called homologous chromosomes. The chromosomes are lengthy filaments of DNA (deoxyribonucleic acid); they contain the genetic code according to which the human being develops.

Interphase examination of nuclei

Interphase (i.e. non-dividing) nuclei are examined for sex chromatin in females and fluorescent F bodies in males. The nuclei of female cells contain a small condensed mass of chromatin under the nuclear membrane; this is inactivated X material (see p. 113). This so-called sex chromatin is referred to as the Barr body. Stained cells from buccal mucous membrane, skin or blood are used for the detection of Barr bodies, approximately 200 being examined in an attempt to establish their presence or absence with absolute certainty (for significance of Barr bodies, see p. 113). Cells can also be stained with quinacrine to establish the presence of fluorescent F bodies which indicate the presence of the Y chromosome.

Metaphase examination of nuclei

Dividing, cultured chromosomes, made visible by a special staining technique, can be studied under a high-powered microscope which magnifies 1 500 times. Chromosome microscopy is successful only during the metaphase of cell division, when the fine filaments of the chromosome contract into thick, stick-like structures split down the middle but held together during the metaphase by the centromere. The incompletely split chromosome forms two chromatids. Complete splitting into two daughter chromosomes is prevented, for the purpose of studying the chromosomes, by the addition of a small amount of colchicine to the culture of cells. The cells studied are obtained by scraping the buccal (mouth) mucosa or by taking a sample of blood—the usual method. The red cells are removed and the remaining white cells are incubated for 3 days in a special culture medium which stimulates cell division. Then colchicine is added to stop mitosis at the stage of the metaphase and hypotonic saline is added to spread the chromosomes. The resulting chromosome spread is photographed through the microscope and the photograph is enlarged. The individual chromosomes are cut out and arranged in pairs in decreasing order of size. They are numbered from 1 to 22 in 7 groups, labelled A to G. The sex chromosomes, 2 tall X chromosomes in females and 1 tall X and 1 short Y in males, complete the 23 pairs. This arranging of chromosomes is called *karyotyping*.

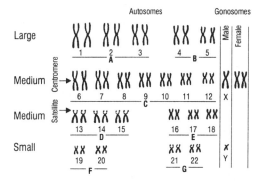

Figure 8.1

Karyotyping—a schematic idiogram of human subject
The difference between male and female is illustrated under 'gonosomes'.

Note: Karyo- refers to nucleus.

Chromosomes can be identified according to their length, the position of the centromere and the presence or not of a stalk and a small globular satellite. With special staining, specific horizontal banding patterns show up which make the precise identification of chromosomes possible.

The molecular structure and function of a chromosome

The chromosome contains a large molecule of *DNA (deoxyribonucleic acid)* which is the gene carrier of the cell. All the hereditary information needed for the development and maintenance of the organism is encoded in the genes, every nucleated cell in the body carrying a full complement of this information. Only the gametes can transmit this information from parent to offspring, however.

There are approximately 200 000 genes in a chromosome. A genome is the total gene complement of a set of chromosomes.

The DNA molecule is a double spiral (helix) that looks like a coiled ladder. Each side of the ladder is composed of a sugar (deoxyribose) and a phosphate group and half the rung of a nitrogenous base; this combination is called a *nucleotide*, the nucleic acid (DNA) consisting of many nucleotides. The nitrogenous bases are: adenine, thymine (replaced in RNA by uracil), guanine and cytosine. Each rung of the DNA ladder is formed by two nitrogenous bases, adenine joined to thymine and cytosine to guanine by means of hydrogen bonds. DNA is present in every nucleated cell and the DNA in every cell contains the same hereditary information as the zygote from which the organism developed. By some mechanism not yet known, those sections of the DNA ladder not used in a particular cell are covered up.

The DNA molecule stores vast quantities of information in the form of a triplet code—a sequence of three nucleotides—known as a codon. A codon is, therefore, a triplet of nucleotides; it codes for one amino acid or for a punctuation mark. Codons vary according to the sequencing of their nucleotides, there being more than 20 variations, one for each kind of amino acid and some for punctuation signs between genes, e.g. to indicate where to terminate a polypeptide chain. A single fault in the sequence of nucleotides in a codon may alter the nature of the genetic code; for example, it may cause 'glutamic acid' to be read as 'valine' or 'leucine' to be read as 'stop' thus cutting off the

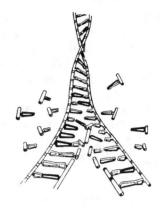

Figure 8.2
The splitting of a DNA filament during mitosis

polypeptide chain prematurely. These faults are called mutations. The usual faults are insertions, deletions or exchanges of nucleotides. This is the origin of inborn errors of metabolism. The different codons are arranged in different sequences along the DNA molecule in order to form the *template* (guide) for a large number of different *polypeptide chains*. That section of the DNA molecule which carries the code for the synthesis of one polypeptide chain is called a *gene*. A gene is, therefore, that bit of DNA that codifies for one polypeptide chain. There are approximately 200 000 genes in a human chromosome. Genetic mutations are invisible under the microscope and are studied biochemically.

DNA never leaves the nucleus but directs the cell's activities, i.e. the manufacture of cell proteins and enzymes which are protein in nature. This is done by means of molecules which are similar to DNA, called *RNA (ribonucleic acid)*, which carry the coded messages for the synthesis of polypeptide chains from the nucleus to the *ribosomes* (protein factories) in the cytoplasm of the cell. The polypeptides (portions of proteins) are specific to each kind of cell and will determine its functional and structural characteristics. A protein is composed of a number of polypeptide chains which undergo up to 4 foldings in order to fit into the site where it is to perform its function, e.g. enzyme action.

When the cell divides (mitosis), the long DNA filaments which form the chromosomes contract into stick-like structures and split in their entire length, each half forming a new spiral ladder from materials available in the cell and brought there by the blood. Each daughter cell will have a complete set of genetic instructions. The DNA filaments can be photographed under an electron microscope which magnifies 40 000 times.

As has been mentioned, DNA does not leave the nucleus but forms the template for RNA (ribonucleic acid) which carries the genetic code to the ribosomes of the cytoplasm where the polypeptides are made. There are two main kinds of *RNA, messenger (m-)* and *transfer (t-)*. They are formed as a complement to a segment of DNA. RNA is a single chain (strand) with ribose instead of deoxyribose as sugar, and uracil instead of thymine as one of the nitrogenous bases. The process whereby information is transmitted from DNA to RNA is called *transcription*. A unique feature of retroviruses (e.g. HIV) is their ability to transcribe their RNA genome into DNA, each by a similar enzyme, **reverse transciptase**. This has profound implications for the host for it is the means by which these viruses may become integrated into the host genome and establish chronic infection. On entry into a cell, a complementary DNA strand is produced from the viral RNA which can then be converted into double-stranded DNA and integrated into the host DNA. Thereafter, control over cell function is exercised by both host and viral DNA.

Each m-RNA can be conceptualised as a coded bar which latches on to a group of ribosomes (polysomes). It is punctuated by 'stop' and 'start' codons which signal where one

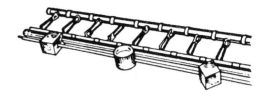

Figure 8.4

t-RNA locks onto the m-RNA bar.
Amino acids joined to form part of a polypeptide chain.

polypeptide chain stops and another one starts. It has all the directions needed to make several kinds of polypeptides; it bears the genetic message as sequences of triplets (codons). This is the template for sequencing the amino acids brought to it by t-RNA. A particular triplet on the m-RNA is related through t-RNA to a specific amino acid. The m-RNA determines the sequence of the amino acids in the polypeptide chain. The process whereby genetic information is transformed from m-RNA into the synthesis of polypeptide chains is called *translation*.

The t-RNA can be conceptualised as units of 3 nucleotides on a protein (clover-leaf) base. In each one the sequencing of the nucleotides is derived from the DNA template. There are more than 20 different kinds of t-RNA, each one able to recognise one of the 20 different kinds of amino acids as well as punctuation signs. These units carry the amino acids towards the coded bar of the m-RNA for correct sequencing in the polypeptide chain they are to form. When the amino acids are lined up according to genetic instructions on the m-RNA, they are joined together by a 'zipper-like' action (peptide linkage) as the m-RNA and amino acids move onwards through the ribosomes. In the illustration only three amino acids are shown, but in reality a polypeptide chain contains hundreds of amino acids. Therefore the m-RNA will be a long thread, resembling a split portion of the DNA molecule but with only one strand. After the chain emerges from the ribosome, the polypeptide chain separates from the m-RNA.

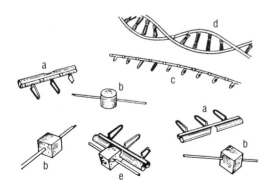

Figure 8.3

Manufacture of polypeptide

(a) t-RNA; (b) amino acids; (c) m-RNA; (d) DNA;
(e) amino acid latched on to t-RNA

CHROMOSOMAL ABERRATIONS

Morphological abnormalities in chromosomes can usually be seen under a microscope and may be due to either numerical or structural changes. Some of these aberrations are outlined below.

Numerical changes

Numerical changes occur when there is nondisjunction of one pair of autosomal chromosomes of the primary oocyte during meiosis. There is a failure of the paired homologous chromosomes to separate at anaphase and to move to opposite poles of the cell prior to cell division. If these abnormal cells, i.e. one with 2 homologous chromosomes and one with none of a particular chromosome, are fertilised by a normal sperm, the result will be a *trisomic* (3 chromosomes instead of the homologous pair) zygote in the first case and a *monosomic* (one chromosome) zygote in the second case.

The latter is incompatible with life. In trisomy 21, the foetus will develop to term and it will be a mongol (Down syndrome). This is the commonest type of chromosomal abnormality (98 %) in mongolism and is commonly found in the advanced maternal age group, especially where the pregnancy occurs over the age of 40 years. Nondisjunction may also apply to sister chromatids in the zygote during mitotic cell division. This gives rise to the *mosaic* who has some normal cells and some trisomic cells, i.e. two populations of cells 46/47 trisomy 21.

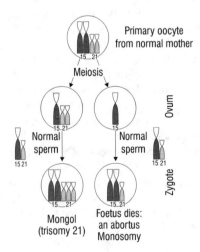

Figure 8.5

Nondisjunction during meiosis causes trisomy 21 (Down syndrome).

The greater the proportion of normal 46 chromosome cells, the nearer the child will approach normality.

Note:
(1) One extra or one less chromosome in the nucleus is known as *aneuploidy*. Down syndrome is, therefore, characterised by aneuploidy.
(2) A mosaic is a person with two or more different kinds of chromosomal constitutions derived from a single genetic source following normal fertilisation. Mosaics commonly occur with the sex chromosomes, e.g.

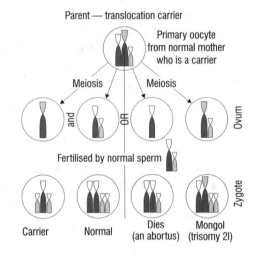

Figure 8.6

Translocation carrier 15/21 trisomy

46XY/47XXY.

Structural changes

Structural changes can occur in chromosomes, most of them resulting in breaks in either the short arm (p) or the long arm (q) of the chromosome. Two of a number of consequences of breaks are:

(1) Deletion, i.e. loss of a portion of a chromosome. This can cause a profound disturbance in the affected child, for example, the *cri-du-chat* (cat's cry) syndrome with mental deficiency, microcephaly as a result of the deletion of the short arm of one chromosome 5 (5p-).
(2) Translocations, i.e. the transfer of a segment from one chromosome to another. Translocations can be inherited, i.e. either the mother or the father can be a carrier. During

meiosis, translocation causes problems as it is impossible for the affected chromosome to divide equally, thus giving rise to extra chromosomal material (akin to a trisomy) in the zygote that survives. Translocations can occur between two homologous chromosomes or between adjacent chromosomes, the commonest translocations occurring between 21/21, 15/21 and 22/21. This is another cause of Down syndrome with a predictable risk of transmission if one parent is a carrier; the offspring may be either a carrier or a mongol, or may be normal. The risk is higher if the mother is the carrier. This type of Down syndrome can occur in any age group and is strongly suspected if a young mother gives birth to a child with Down syndrome.

Clinical features of Down syndrome (mongolism):

(1) mental retardation and friendly personality;
(2) epicanthic folds and slanting eyes giving the characteristic facies (mongoloid appearance);
(3) short stature, stubby hands and feet, brachycephaly (short head), low-set ears;
(4) large space between 1st and 2nd toes; short 5th finger permanently bent; transverse single palmar crease;
(5) protruding large tongue (macroglossia) and mouth held open constantly;
(6) poor physique with hypotonia and, frequently, congenital heart abnormality. Mongols used to die early but with modern medical care, are surviving into adulthood;
(7) sterility in males and reduced fertility in females.

Sex chromosomes and their aberrations

The nuclei of the cells of males and females differ in the following ways:

(1) Both have 22 pairs of similar autosomal chromosomes but male cells have one X and one Y sex chromosome and female cells have two X chromosomes. The presence of the Y chromosome is responsible for the male sexual characteristics. The X chromosome is much larger than the Y chromosome and has somatic functions as well as female

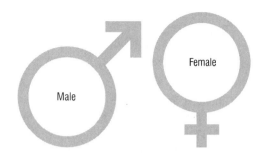

Figure 8.7
Universal signs for male and female

sexual functions; it appears to be necessary for essential enzyme systems. Early in embryonic development (12th day) the extra X material contained in the female cell is inactivated, each sex retaining one functional X chromosome.

(2) Female cell nuclei contain a Barr body and male cell nuclei a fluorescent F body. By suitable staining of interphase (i.e. non-dividing) cell nuclei, these bodies can be identified and a person's sex chromosome constitution defined without preparing a karyotype after cell culture.

(a) The *Barr body* in female cell nuclei is a small condensed mass of chromatin under the nuclear membrane; this is the inactivated X material mentioned above, hence it is referred to as *sex chromatin*. In polymorphonuclear leucocytes, the sex chromatin looks like a drumstick projecting from the nucleus. The number of Barr bodies in a nucleus is one less than the number of X chromosomes. Therefore a normal male genotype has no Barr body and a normal female genotype has one.

(b) The *Y chromosome* can be detected in male nuclei which have been stained with quinacrine to make the Y chromosomes fluoresce. These are referred to as *fluorescent F bodies*.

Sex chromosome aneuploidy (incorrect number), e.g. XO/45 and XXY/47, does not affect the body as profoundly as autosomal aneuploidy. As in Down syndrome (non-carrier type), sex chromosome aneuploidy is caused by nondisjunction of the sex chromosomes during gametogenesis (meiosis). When nondisjunction occurs during mitosis in the zygote, *mosaicism* (see p. 112) results, e.g. XX/XO (mosaic Turner's) or XY/XX (mosaic Klinefelter's).

The important sex chromosome aberrations are the following:

(1) Klinefelter syndrome in males who have one, two or three extra X chromosomes, thus XXY or XXXY or XXXXY, the common form being XXY which presents as follows:
  (*a*) testicular dysgenesis with sterility and small testes;
  (*b*) gynaecomastia;
  (*c*) tall stature;
  (*d*) sometimes mental retardation, especially in males with an XXXY constitution.

  Note: Persons with multiple X chromosome aberrations always have more than one Barr body, one less than the number of X chromosomes in their cell nuclei. Example: the XXXY genotype will have two Barr bodies despite a male phenotype. The superfemale with XXX chromosomes will also have two Barr bodies in the nuclei of her cells.

(2) Males with an *XYY sex chromosome genotype*. These men are usually tall and are sometimes subnormal. They may be aggressive and exhibit antisocial behaviour.

Sex chromosomal aberrations in women are either one more or one less X chromosome.

  The XXX and XXXX female who is referred to as the '*superfemale*' is mentally defective. She can reproduce and her female children are normal.

Turner syndrome is an XO female with a 45/XO chromosomal constitution. She presents as follows:

(1) ovarian agenesis with sterility and primary amenorrhoea;
(2) short stature;
(3) webbing of the skin on either side of the neck;
(4) cardiac abnormalities;
(5) sometimes mental retardation.

Note:
(1) A YO pattern is not seen and is probably lethal.
(2) Very voluptuous women often have an XY genotype and female phenotype. This anomaly is called *testicular feminisation* and is caused by the inability of the genotypically male to use testosterone. These women have external female genitalia but they cannot menstruate and they are sterile. They do have testes which are hidden in the groin. They are sometimes called *male pseudohermaphrodites*.
(3) The *adrenogenital syndrome* (genotype XX) is called *female pseudohermaphroditism*. Here the virilisation of the genotypical female is due to adrenal hyperplasia.

True *hermaphrodites* usually have a female genotype (XX) and less commonly are mosaics, XX/XY, XX/XO. Phenotypically they vary from those who appear almost fully male to those who appear almost fully female. There are varying degrees of bisexuality in the genitalia and internally their gonads may be a mixture of ovary and testis.

GENETIC INHERITANCE

Biological traits are transmitted from parents to offspring through the genes (see p. 110) which are situated on the chromosomes of the gametes, one of the pair of the chromosomes from the mother and one of the pair (23) from the father. Genes which occupy the same site (locus) on a pair of homologous chromosomes are called *alleles*. Alleles for a specific locus affect similar parts or processes of an organism. If the pair of alleles have the same effect on a genetic trait, the individual is said to be *homozygous* for the gene. Mutation can, however, take place in one of a pair of alleles so that the effects of the two genes on the trait they mediate will not be the same; then the organism is said to be *heterozygous* for the gene. In this case there is a normal and a mutant gene; the latter is either dominant or recessive to the normal gene. Some genes exist in more than two allelic forms in the population although one individual will have only two of these multiple alleles. Such *multiple alleles* mediate antigens which are found on erythrocytes to form the ABO blood groups. Here there are at least 4 alleles: A_1, A_2, B and O. An individual possesses any two of these alleles which may be different or the same; thus there can be 10 ABO genotypes (A_1A_1, A,O, A_2B, etc.) but only 6 ABO phenotypes, viz. A_1, A_2, B, O, A_1B and A_2B. The O, being a recessive allele, is not expressed in the phenotype unless it occurs in double dose, viz. OO(O).

Dominance and recessivity

Only one of two alternative alleles can be expressed at a time in the phenotype, although both are present in the heterozygous genotype. (An exception occurs in the rare instances of codominance as demonstrated in the ABO blood groups where both the A and B alleles are expressed in the phenotype.) In the heterozygote, the mutant gene which is expressed in the phenotype is called the *dominant* one and the mutant one which is not expressed is called the *recessive* one. Because the recessive gene is not expressed, i.e. is not manifest in the biological trait mediated by the gene, the person carrying it is not aware of its presence. The concepts of dominance and recessiveness refer only to the phenotypic (see p.117) manifestation of one of a pair of alleles in a heterozygote.

Expressivity and penetrance

Expressivity is the degree to which a particular dominant gene is expressed. The *expressivity* of a particular dominant gene may be modified by the action of other genes, so that the gene is either not expressed or is incompletely expressed; in this case we say that the *penetrance* of the dominant gene has been reduced. When a dominant gene is not expressed at all, we speak of non-penetrance.

Mutations

A mutation is a permanent change in inherited material, i.e. chromosomes and genes. Mutations may have either harmful or beneficial effects; in the latter case they give rise to new characteristics. They are probably the origins of every form of evolutionary development.

If a harmful mutation occurs in the gametes, the offspring will suffer deleterious effects. When a disease which is known to be hereditary in nature appears in a family for the first time, it may be due to a fresh mutation; the offspring will differ genetically from the parents.

Note: A disease which appears in a family for the first time may also be due to a double dose of an autosomal recessive gene (see p. 119).

Mutations which occur in the genetic material of somatic cells will not be transmitted to the offspring of the parent, but will occur in all cells derived from the mutated cell. Mutations which affect offspring occur in the gametes of parents either while they are still in the gonads or after

they have been discharged and are being transported in the reproductive canals.

Mutations may be of two kinds:

(1) Chromosomal mutations when breaks, deletions, nondisjunctions and translocations occur. These mutations can be seen under the microscope when karyotyping has been done. The aberration is usually gross as many genes are involved; often the woman will have a spontaneous abortion as the foetus is not viable.

(2) Point mutations occur in a single gene locus or in a few adjacent genes. These mutations cannot be seen under the microscope. In gene mutations there is either a rearrangement, or an insertion, or a deletion of one or more of the nucleotides of the DNA molecule. This interferes with the correct synthesising of polypeptide chains used for the making of enzymes and cell proteins, thus causing metabolic defects. (See nucleotides, p. 110.)

Mutations may be either spontaneous or they may be induced by **mutagenic agents**. Overmature gametes are suspected of harbouring damaged chromosomes. The following are the two most important mutagenic agents:

(1) Chemicals, e.g. cytotoxic drugs.

(2) Ionising radiations. No matter what part of the body is being irradiated, other parts, i.e. the gonads, will get a small dose. Even the smallest dose of radiation may produce a mutation, successive doses having an additive effect. If the head is X-rayed at one time and the thorax at another, the gonads and the gametes will receive two minute doses which add up to a bigger dose. The total number of mutations will depend upon the total gonad dose. Greater amounts of exposure, e.g. due to direct irradiation of the gonads, will cause sterility and even greater exposure will destroy the sex cells.

The genetic effects of mutagenic agents will not be manifest in the generation of people exposed to them, but in their offspring, inheritance occurring according to Mendelian laws in the case of single gene mutations. Recessive autosomal mutations are unlikely to manifest for some time—only when two similar heterozygous individuals mate by chance. All persons probably carry 5 to 8 'bad' genes of which they are not aware as they are either recessive or part of a polygenic consortium.

TERATOLOGY AND TERATOGENESIS

Teratology is the science which deals, *inter alia*, with the aetiology and development of monsters, the 'monster' being a congenitally damaged child. A teratogen is an environmental agent that causes the abnormal development (dysmorphogenesis) and may include mutagens, i.e. agents which cause damage to genes and chromosomes.

Congenital defects

A congenital defect is one present at birth. The foetus may have been damaged *in utero* or the defect may have been inherited. It is important to understand that an inherited defect is transmitted through the genes and may manifest either at birth (i.e. it may be congenital) or later in life; porphyria variegata appears at puberty and Huntington's chorea only at the 4th or 5th decade of life, while Down syndrome is obvious at birth.

Teratology deals with abnormal development (malformation) caused by damage either to the zygote in the Fallopian tube or to the zygote or embryo in the uterus, the implication being that this damage is not inheritable because the teratogenic damage is not to genetic material in gametes. Neither somatic mutations nor teratogenic damage are transmissible through the genes.

It may be difficult to distinguish between the inherited and teratogenic nature of foetal malformations. At this early stage in development, the interaction between nature and nurture is very important, the effect of teratogens differing from genotype to genotype. For example, in some mothers cigarette smoking harms the foetus, while in others no damage is evident. The susceptibility to a teratogen, therefore, depends on the genotype. Teratogenic effects are greatest in early pregnancy, i.e. between the 18th and the 55th day, the most vulnerable period for the embryo being on the 30th day.

The common teratogenic agents are:

(1) Radiation.
(2) Chemical agents, e.g. cigarette smoke, industrial solvents, alcohol, heavy metals, e.g. lead, pesticides and any dangerous medicine, e.g. ergometrine, thalidomide, phenylhydantoin, diethylstilboestrol, anti-cancer drugs and Warfarin.
(3) Infection, especially virus infections, e.g. megalovirus, rubella and mumps.
(4) Some incompatibilities between mother and foetus, e.g. endocrine and blood.
(5) Hyperpyrexia.

The severity of malformations induced by a teratogen depends upon the gestational age of the foetus, the dose of the teratogenic agent and the genotype. Embryos at different stages of gestation can have dissimilar responses to the same teratogen. For example, the rubella virus affects heart development between the 4th and 9th week, lens development between the 5th and 8th week and inner ear development between the 6th and 12th week, an overlapping of sensitive periods occurring in the 8th week. After organs have been formed, the same teratogen can still cause defects in cell growth, throughout pregnancy, especially in the nervous and reproductive systems.[2]

The defects produced by a teratogen may be modified by pollutants, diet, (other) drugs, climate, maternal age. Thus the congenital malformation depends on the interaction of several environmental factors in a genetically vulnerable embryo at a time when the embryo or foetus is at a susceptible stage of development—the so-called multifactorial cause of congenital malformations.

Examples of developmental aberrations are mental retardation, microcephaly, hydrocephalus, microphthalmus, chorioretinitis with blindness, deafness, congenital heart anomalies, spina bifida and myelomeningocele, phocomelia (missing limbs), absence of bones, hemi-hypertrophy—unequal size in the two halves of the body.

A condition known as *Poland syndrome* is caused by the ingestion of ergometrine early in pregnancy, in an attempt to procure an abortion. There is complete absence of the pectoral muscle and the arm on the same side is shrunken.

A condition known as *foetal alcohol syndrome* appears in a large number of infants of chronic alcoholic women suggesting that alcohol is a true teratogen.

Alcohol crosses the placental and blood-brain barriers of the foetus and reaches the same level in the foetus as in the mother. The foetal brain is damaged during the first trimester. The infant may be premature and/or small-for-gestational-age and exhibit tremulousness. There may also be cardiac abnormalities, limb defects and craniofacial anomalies, e.g. flat upper lip. Infants fail to thrive as a result of their impaired ability to grow normally. The major teratogenic effect of alcohol is mental retardation.

The *foetal hydantoin syndrome* sometimes occurs in the offspring of epileptic women. It is characterised by mild to moderate mental retardation, cleft lip and palate and cardiac and skeletal abnormalities.

GENOTYPE AND PHENOTYPE

Each person's genetic make-up or constitution—*his genotype*—determines largely how he reacts to chemical, physical and psychological stimuli from his environment. Nature, the inherited genotype, and nurture, the influence of the environment, interact to produce the final product, the *phenotype*.

Twin studies are used to determine the roles of genetic and environmental (intra-uterine) factors in the aetiology of congenital defects. If the same defect appears in both monozygotic twins, the cause is probably genetic, and if there is discordance, the cause is environmental.

The same conclusions can be drawn from studying monozygotic twins, apparently normal at birth, who are then separated and subjected to different environmental influences during subsequent growth and development.

Twin studies supply very strong evidence for genetically and environmentally related variation in man—it helps us to get an understanding of the relative importance of nature and nurture in the end product: the phenotype.

The phenotype is thus an expression of the individual's life experiences as expressed within the limits of response set by his genotype. We inherit our genotype biologically; it gives us our hereditary potential for physical, emotional

and intellectual development. The final product, the phenotype, will depend, however, upon the interaction between our nature and our nurture. For instance, a child born with a potentially high intelligence into an intellectually unstimulating environment, will not be able to develop this potential; the final product may be the same as that of a child born with a lower intellectual potential into an intellectually stimulating environment which allows the full development of his potential. Not only intelligence but also temperament, special talents, physical appearance and physical and emotional health are determined by the unique interaction between the environment and the inherited constitution. The interrelationship between nature and nurture is very complicated, especially where more than one gene is responsible for the production of a specific trait—the so-called *polygenic inheritance*.

At one extreme, genetic abnormalities and disorders, e.g. Crouzon's disease (craniofacial dysostosis), cystic fibrosis, haemophilia, will manifest regardless of environmental influence, while at the other extreme, genetic disorders will manifest only in the presence of special environmental stimulation, e.g. schizophrenia, atherosclerotic cardio-vascular disease. Even our immunity to infection has a genetic basis, as the formation of antibodies is genetically determined. Because of the different genetic constitutions of different families, we find that specific diseases run in families, thus some families are prone to diabetes mellitus in middle age whilst others are prone to cancer.

Monogenic inheritance is the manner of inheritance in which one pair of genes (two alleles) is responsible for different manifestations of a single trait, for example, colour of eyes. Inheritance cannot be traced along simple monogenic Mendelian lines, however, when a trait is determined by a number of genes, some of these genes modifying others so that penetrance and expressivity can be variable. Many traits, e.g. intelligence, stature (height), blood pressure, skin colour, probably have a *polygenic origin*, the phenotype being the product of these multiple genes and environmental facilitation of their expression. The expression of this multifactorial inheritance has a normal distribution in the population. Few people fall in the extremes of 'muchness' and 'littleness' or 'highness' and 'lowness'—the majority cluster about the mean.

The laws of *monogenic biological inheritance* were formulated in 1865 by a Moravian monk, Gregor Mendel. He postulated that the genes of the parents were not mingled equally at conception to make each child a blend of its mother and father, but that parents transmitted some of their dominant genes (e.g. for brown eyes, (A), to some offspring and some of their recessive genes (e.g. for blue eyes, (*a*)) to others. Hence the following genotypes are possible in the offspring of two heterozygous parents:

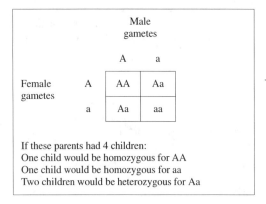

If these parents had 4 children:
One child would be homozygous for AA
One child would be homozygous for aa
Two children would be heterozygous for Aa

Three of the progeny would have brown eyes and one would have blue eyes, brown eyes being a dominant trait. The brown eyes would be present in the genotypes Aa and AA.

If both parents are homozygous for A, all the progeny would be likewise and all would have brown eyes. If only the mother is homozygous and for A, the following genotypes can be expected:

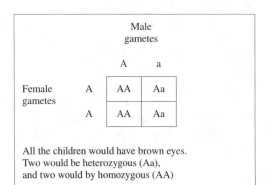

All the children would have brown eyes.
Two would be heterozygous (Aa),
and two would by homozygous (AA)

If the father is heterozygous for A and the mother homozygous for a, the recessive allele, the outcome illustrated in the following diagram could be expected.

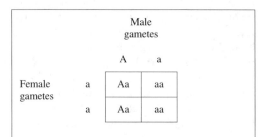

Two of the children would have brown and two blue eyes. Two will be heterozygous like the father, and two would be homozygous for a, like the mother.

If both parents are homozygous, the father for A and the mother for a, all the children would be genotypically heterozygous and would phenotypically have brown eyes.

The predictions given above have been presented in a rigid fashion for the sake of clarity. What is really meant when we say, for example, one out of 4 children will have blue eyes and 3 out of 4 will have brown eyes, is that every child born of such a union will have a 25 % (1 in 4) chance of having blue eyes and a 75 % (3 in 4) chance of having brown eyes.

THE INHERITANCE OF MONOGENIC DISORDERS

Not only normal traits but also abnormal traits causing deformities and mental and physical ill-health may be inherited. Abnormal genes are caused by gene *mutations,* i.e. changes in the chromosomes and genes by agents called *mutagens.*

Mutated genes are usually harmful but the reverse may be true. We are usually not aware of enhancing mutations as only the mutations which harm the body are obtrusive. In monogenic inheritance a mutated gene may be either dominant or recessive with regard to its allele, according to whether the trait it expresses is manifest or not. In addition, the mutated gene is situated either on an autosomal chromosome or on an X (sex) chromosome.

A large number of metabolic disorders are of genetic origin; more than 4 000[3] of these **inborn errors of metabolism** are known, some widely distributed geographically and ethnically and others rare. Many of them are inherited recessively and in some cases (e.g. Gaucher and Tay-Sachs) the heterozygous carrier can be recognised by finding a reduced activity of the affected enzyme on doing a blood test. In the metabolic disorders there is either an absence of an enzyme necessary for the metabolism of a nutrient or there is a deviation in function of one or more enzymes so that a metabolic sequence is adversely affected. Some of the metabolic disorders manifest soon after birth and are incompatible with normal development unless treated with special diets, drugs, or replacement of the deficient enzymes or proteins.

Autosomal recessive inheritance

If the effect of a mutated gene is not expressed, it is recessive. Autosomally recessive traits can be expressed in the offspring only if the abnormal recessive alleles are carried by both parents, so that the offspring has a chance of being homozygous for the abnormal gene. Examples: cystic fibrosis, phenylketonuria, galactosaemia, glycogen storage disease, sickle cell anaemia, sclerosteosis, thalassaemia, familial cretinism with goitre, Tay-Sachs disease, albinism, Hurler syndrome. There is an autosomal recessive type of achondroplasia.

The recessive gene will find expression only if the individual is homozygous for it. This accounts for the sporadic nature of autosomal recessive diseases. Blood relatives are more likely than unrelated persons to carry the same recessive alleles, therefore the children of consanguineous marriages are more likely to be homozygous for a hitherto unsuspected abnormal recessive gene.

SINGLE MUTANT GENE INHERITANCE

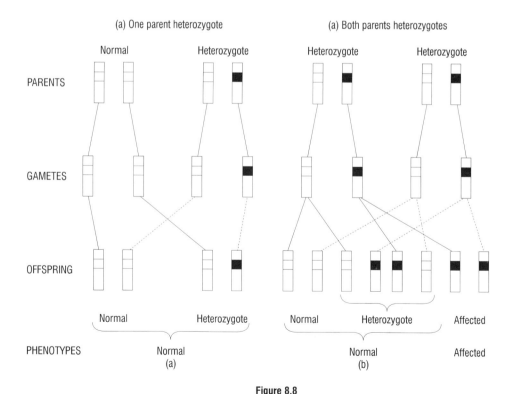

Figure 8.8

Autosomal recessive inheritance

(a) All children normal; 50 % chance of children being heterozygous carriers
(b) 25 % chance of children being affected; 50 % chance of children being heterozygous carriers

Autosomal recessive disorders

The muco-polysaccharidoses (MPS) (gargoylism)

(Hurler and Hunter syndromes)
The MPS are a group of rare genetic disorders in which there is a deficiency of an enzyme which is necessary for normal connective tissue metabolism. This deficiency causes the partially degraded metabolites to accumulate in the cells and to cause the abnormal development of the tissues.

The main MPS are Hurler and Hunter syndromes. Hurler syndrome has an autosomal recessive mode of inheritance and Hunter an X-linked mode. Hurler syndrome is more common, occurring in 1/100 000 births, and is better understood. Except for the corneal pathology, their symptoms and prognoses are similar.

FEATURES OF HURLER SYNDROME (MPS IH)

(1) Mental retardation with coarse facies, commonly referred to as gargoylism;
(2) dwarfism;
(3) enlarged liver and spleen;
(4) corneal opacity;
(5) flaccid muscles and protruding tongue.

The disorder is progressive and ends fatally in childhood from respiratory infection or cardiac failure.

PREVENTION OF HURLER SYNDROME

This is possible through antenatal diagnosis (amniocentesis) and termination of pregnancy. Prevention is possible if a woman who has had a child with Hurler syndrome comes for genetic counselling.

Phenylketonuria (PKU)

The incidence of PKU in the RSA has not yet been established but some 20 affected families are known.[12] The world-wide incidence of PKU is 1:11 000 white infants.

Phenylketonuria is a congenital abnormality which causes mental retardation unless diagnosed and treated in early infancy. In phenylketonuria, phenylalanine (an essential amino acid comprising approximately 5 % of protein) cannot be metabolised fully to tyrosine because of the absence of the enzyme, phenylalanine hydroxylase, thereby causing harmful metabolites (phenylpyruvic acid and phenyllactic acid) to accumulate in the blood.

SIGNS AND SYMPTOMS IN CHILDREN

(1) Irritability, convulsions and EEG abnormalities;
(2) eczema; fair skin, mental retardation;
(3) musty odour of urine due to the presence of phenyllactic acid. Phenylpyruvic acid is detected in the urine from third week of life by means of Ames' Phenistix reagent strips (which are impregnated with ferric chloride).

MANAGEMENT OF PHENYLKETONURIA

(1) Early diagnosis, i.e. during the neonatal period. If detected by a urine screening test, diagnosis is confirmed by means of a blood test, i.e. phenylalanine above 10 mg %.
(2) Feeding infants and older children (i.e. during the growth period) with a diet low in phenylalanine. Infants who have been on this type of diet from the first few weeks of life have shown normal physical and mental development, but once cerebral damage has developed, it cannot be corrected by treatment.

Galactosaemia

Galactosaemia is an inborn disorder of galactose metabolism in which galactose accumulates in the blood and tissues. The child fails to thrive and, if dietetic treatment is not instituted early, will become mentally deficient. The condition is diagnosed by finding sugar in the urine; this sugar can be identified as galactose in the laboratory.

If the blood level of galactose rises to above normal, poisoning of the liver, brain and kidneys takes place and the child develops cataracts. The condition eventually leads to fatty infiltration of the liver with cirrhosis and jaundice. The treatment is to exclude lactose from the diet. Cow & Gate Low Lactose Food or Sobee can be used for this purpose. The former is made from coconut and maize oils, glucose, demineralised casein and mineral salts. Trace elements and vitamins must be added to the infant's diet. Mead Johnson Sobee contains proteins and oils from soy beans, maltose, sucrose, dextrins, as well as mineral salts and vitamins.

Early diagnosis and treatment are essential if the severe complications of galactosaemia are to be prevented. There is no way of detecting heterozygous carriers.

Tay-Sachs disease (amaurotic family idiocy)

This is a disorder of lipid metabolism caused by lack of the enzyme, hexosaminidase. The child appears normal at birth but starts deteriorating from the age of 3 to 6 months and dies by the age of 3 to 4 years. Deterioration affects the nerves, intelligence and eyes, leading to blindness, paralysis and idiocy.

Tay-Sachs disease is especially prevalent amongst Jews of Ashkenazi stock.[13]

The following are well-known facts:

(1) among every 25 members of the local Ashkenazi Jewish community, 1 will be a carrier for Tay-Sachs disease;

(2) out of every 625 marriages, 1 will be between two carriers;

(3) in these marriages 1 in 4 or 25 % of the children will have Tay-Sachs disease.

Note: Only 1 in 250 non-Jewish people will be carriers.

A blood test can be done to detect the Tay-Sachs disease carrier state. The faulty gene does no harm when it occurs in 'single dose'. If both parents are carriers the possibility is 1:4 that each pregnancy will be affected. The expectant mother should, therefore, undergo an amniocentesis at 16 to 18 weeks.

If the biochemical test on the amniotic fluid cells shows the foetus to be affected, pregnancy can be terminated legally. As the woman has 3 in 4 chances of producing a normal child, there is no reason why she should not become pregnant again.

Gaucher's disease

Gaucher's disease[14]—cerebroside lipidosis—is caused by a deficiency of the enzyme beta-glucosidase; this causes an accumulation of cerebrosides in various organs.

Gaucher's disease occurs in three forms: the acute infantile cerebral variety, the juvenile form and the chronic 'adult' form.

The *infantile variety* is fatal at an early age, being characterised by hepatosplenomegaly, failure to thrive and neurological complications.

The *juvenile variety* progresses to dementia and cerebellar ataxia.

The *'adult' form* is chronic and neurological changes do not occur; it is characterised by splenomegaly, dyshaemopoiesis and skeletal involvement. Later there may be hepatic and pulmonary complications, causing death from cor pulmonale. The chronic form of the disease may be diagnosed in childhood; it is progressive, the course being variable. Diagnosis is confirmed by finding an absence of the enzyme, beta-glucosidase, in peripheral blood leucocytes and skin fibroblasts. In normal heterozygous carriers of the recessive gene there is a partial deficiency of the enzyme. Carriers can thus be identified.

The chronic non-neuropathic form of Gaucher's disease occurs among Ashkenazi Jews and Afrikaners in the RSA. In the Jews the condition is relatively mild but in the Afrikaner the condition manifests early and has serious complications.

Unfortunately the family has usually been completed before chronic Gaucher's disease is diagnosed in one of the children of two heterozygous carriers of the disease; therefore, it is possible that more than one child will develop the disease. The parents and offspring of affected individuals are usually not affected. Gaucher's disease can be detected prenatally by doing amniocentesis and examining cultured amniotic fluid cells biochemically.

The chronic form of the disease is managed symptomatically, e.g. splenectomy may relieve abdominal distension (in splenomegaly) and haematological complications, and orthopaedic care is given for bone complications.

Cystic fibrosis (CF)

Cystic fibrosis is also known as mucoviscidosis (viscid, sticky thick mucus). Cystic fibrosis is a common recessive autosomal disease, predominantly of white peoples, being especially prevalent amongst Namibian Afrikaners. Super (1975) gives its incidence in Namibia as 1 in every 622 babies born to Afrikaner parents.[15]

Cystic fibrosis is considered to be the most common serious genetic disorder among whites.[18]

The most generally found incidence figures amongst whites is 1/2 000–2 500 live births, incidence rates being much lower in coloureds; it is hardly known amongst blacks.[16] It has been known to run in families and mothers with CF have produced infants with CF (father of unknown genetic status).[18]

Cystic fibrosis is a generalised disorder of exocrine glands, especially mucus-producing and sweat glands. The organs especially affected are the pancreas and the lungs. Heterozygous carriers (established to be 1 in 20 in whites and 1 in 12 in Namibian Afrikaners) cannot be detected as no biochemical tests for carriers have as yet been devised. Parents and offspring of affected persons are usually normal, but siblings have a 1 in 4 chance of being affected. The prenatal detection of a homozygous foetus is not possible, the disease being diagnosed in infancy—sometimes as late as the 6th year—by the following tests:

(1) In high-risk populations the meconium of neonates is screened with either Albustix (green colour reaction) or BM meconium test (blue colour reaction) for the presence of an increased amount of albumin.

(2) The 'sweat' test or the pilocarpine sweat iontophoresis test is at present the only reliable method of diagnosing CF.[16] This test requires the stimulation of sweating by pilocarpine iontophoresis, the careful collection of at least 100 mg sweat on gauze and the subsequent treatment of this specimen in the laboratory, to quantify the sodium and/or chloride content of the sweat. A value greater than 70 mmol/ℓ for either electrolyte measured on two separate occasions is diagnostic of cystic fibrosis.[17]

THE CLINICAL SIGNS OF CYSTIC FIBROSIS

(1) Meconium ileus—bowel obstruction by masses of meconium—is present in 15 % of affected neonates. This condition is usually fatal but can be relieved by surgery. An ileostomy is done and faeces-liquefying medications, e.g. Gastrografin and N-acetyl cysteine, are injected into the bowel prior to evacuating the meconium.

Beyond the neonatal period, even into adolescence, there is danger of bowel obstruction by dried impacted faeces, usually in the distal ileum. This is caused by dehydration,

fat-free diet and failure to take digestive enzyme medication.

(2) Infants usually present with chronic lung disease, failure to thrive and diarrhoea or steatorrhoea. The mean age of onset of symptoms in a Cape Town study was 4,2 months.[16]

(3) Affected persons often suffer from salt-losing crises: this is characterised by heat prostration with pyrexia and dehydration which may be fatal if not treated with salt, fluids and cooling, especially in a hot climate. During a crisis, laboratory sodium estimations will reveal a hyponatraemia.

(4) Lack of pancreatic enzymes leads to impaired digestion, steatorrhoea and failure to thrive. The bowel symptoms are similar to those of coeliac disease, but the child has a good appetite. Malabsorption causes poor physique and delayed onset of puberty.

(5) Obstructive lung disease and chronic bronchitis due to blockage of the respiratory tract with viscid, thick secretions. There are recurrent severe pulmonary tract infections which may cause death. Few affected children survive into adulthood, although recently life expectancy has increased and a CF child now has a reasonable chance of reaching adulthood and even of having children, provided treatment is conscientiously applied.

The Johannesburg Hospital has recently established a multidisciplinary, adult cystic fibrosis clinic to cater for the increasing number of patients, often misdiagnosed as having chronic bronchitis or bronchiectasis, who survive into adulthood.

(6) The fertility of the adult with CF is poor, males usually being sterile.

Note: Either the pulmonary or the gastro-intestinal component of the disease is the commonest cause of ill-health in those who survive to adulthood.

TREATMENT

▪ Dietary treatment is prescribed and may vary as follows:

  (*a*) Full diet supplemented by medicinal pancreatic enzymes, up to 20 tablets per meal; if this diet causes steatorrhoea, a low fat diet is given. Snacks between meals must also be accompanied by enzymes, e.g. 2 tablets before 1 glass of milk.

(b) Predigested foods such as glucose and protein hydrolysates can be given without medicinal enzymes; so too the Allen diet which is a suitable, imported liquid diet. The use of the latter is, however, not encouraged as it is very expensive and is not gratifying to the palate.

(c) Babies are fed on Portagen, a powdered skim milk with sucrose, medium chain triglycerides, modified corn starch and sunflower oil, plus vitamins and mineral salts. Up to 3 tablets of pancreatic enzymes are given before each feed.

▪ Pancreatic enzymes, obtained from hog's pancreas, are given to replace the missing digestive juices, e.g. Viakase, Pancrex-V, Cotazym. This expensive medication is essential for physical development and to prevent impaction of the bowel with faeces. The prescribed number of tablets are swallowed with water immediately before starting the meal.

▪ Pulmonary infection is kept under control with antibiotic therapy as soon as the child shows any signs of infection; daily postural drainage and aerosol inhalations are used to get rid of thick mucus secretions.

▪ Children and especially adolescents with CF need emotional support as their chronic physical handicap with problems of growth failure and delayed puberty, their fear of a fatal lung infection and their physical and social frustrations cause psychological stress. Adolescent rebellion against fate and the exacting demands of medical treatment may cause poor co-operation in therapy. CF families also need support and guidance.

A Southern African Cystic Fibrosis Association (member of the International CF Association) has been established and some of its objectives are as follows:

(1) dissemination of information to patients and families as regards recent advances in the field;

(2) increased public awareness of the prevalence of the condition;

(3) sponsorship of research into cystic fibrosis;

(4) emotional and financial support for families.

Sclerosteosis

Sclerosteosis is an autosomal recessive disease found in South Africa only amongst Afrikaners. It is a progressive disorder of bone in which there is bony overgrowth leading to cranial nerve entrapment and elevation of intracranial pressure. The disease begins in childhood with facial nerve palsy; deafness develops later. Facial distortion takes place and death usually occurs in young adulthood.

It is associated with syndactyly and gigantism develops.

Congenital hypothyroidism

This genetic metabolic deficiency of the thyroid hormone has a world-wide incidence of approximately 1:4 000. Although it can be diagnosed clinically within the early months of life, the screening of all neonates by blood tests to assess thyroid function has been found to be cost-effective. Blood is taken from either the umbilical vein or from a heel prick within the first 5 days of life and tested for FSH and/or free thyroxin. Those infants found to be hypothyroidic are immediately started on a lifelong programme of thyroid replacement therapy. Follow-up control, by community clinics if necessary, is mandatory for a good prognosis. If therapy is not started within the first few weeks of life, permanent damage to the central nervous system occurs.

The effects of failed or non-treatment are mental and motor retardation and stunted growth (cretinism).

Autosomal dominant inheritance

In dominant inheritance, the affected individuals are either heterozygous or homozygous for the abnormal gene. The abnormal trait is either familial, being carried through each successive generation, or the abnormal gene is a new mutation which is subsequently passed on to the next generation. Examples of autosomally dominant diseases are: porphyria variegata (familial); osteogenesis imperfecta; achondroplasia; Huntington's chorea (familial).

SINGLE MUTANT GENE INHERITANCE

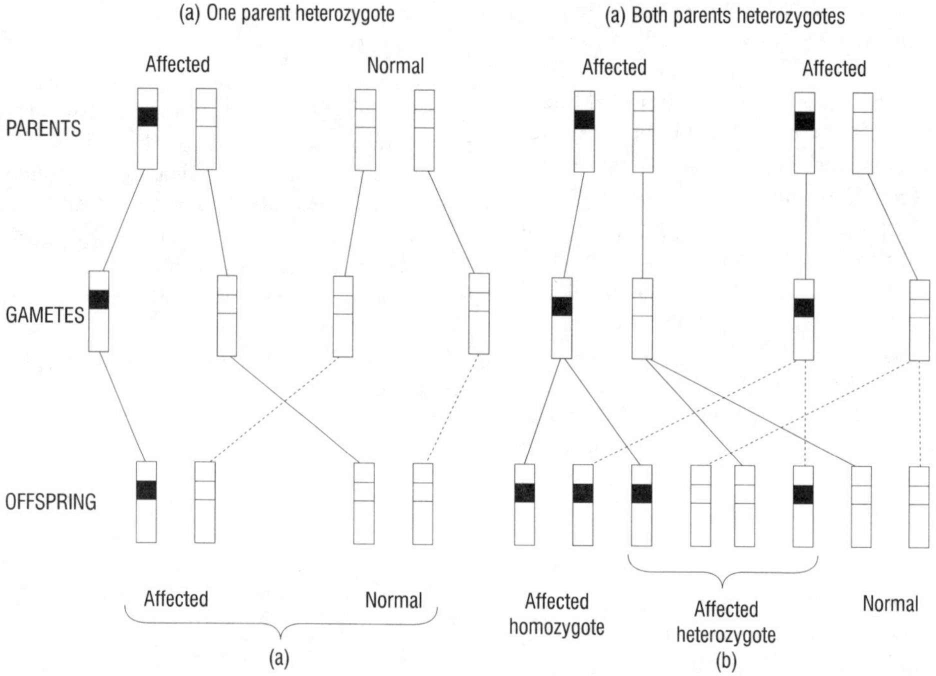

(a) One parent heterozygote   (a) Both parents heterozygotes

Affected   Normal   Affected   Affected

PARENTS

GAMETES

OFFSPRING

Affected   Normal   Affected   Affected   Normal
                                      homozygote   heterozygote
            (a)   (b)

Figure 8.9

Autosomal dominant inheritance

(a) 50 % chance of the children being affected
(b) 75 % chance of the children being affected

Note: The above statements can be confounded by *genetic heterogeneity;* this indicates the possibility that a person who has inherited an abnormal dominant gene does not exhibit all the signs of the inherited syndrome, autosomal dominant traits being extremely variable in expression. It often looks as if the aberration has skipped a generation but on closer inspection a few mild stigmata of the syndrome will usually be present. In this case the mutant gene is not fully penetrant, i.e. the expression of the genotype is less than 100 %.

Autosomal dominant disorders

Huntington's chorea

Huntington's chorea is an autosomal dominant, degenerative disease of the nervous system, which is known to run in certain families, including those of South African blacks. It appears in successive generations and offspring have a 50 % chance of inheriting the disease. Unfortunately the disease seldom manifests until the third to fourth decade of life with chorea and dementia, by which time the affected person has had his family. Thus this terrible genetic disease is perpetuated from generation to generation.

Rare cases of childhood Huntington's chorea are known.

There used to be no satisfactory ways of detecting heterozygous carriers (and eventual sufferers) at the premorbid stage of the disease. By means of modern molecular genetic techniques, however, the disease can be discovered presymptomatically and antenatally.[3] The average duration of the manifest disease is 10 to 15 years, death usually taking place before the age of 60 years. The patients can often not be maintained at home and frequently die in mental institutions.

The mean age of onset with choreic symptoms is 35 years. Early onset chorea is characterised by rigidity. The patient may become irritable, hypersensitive and moody or he may deteriorate rapidly and become apathetic, slow and slovenly. Involuntary jerking choreic movements usually commence in the upper part of the body, the face being contorted as the muscles twist uncontrollably. Speech becomes staccato. The dementing process is heralded with apathy, inertia and distractability while engaged in conversation. The effect is usually fatuous and euphoric but sometimes the patient appears depressed and is liable to commit suicide, especially if he has insight into his condition. With progressive dementia there is memory and intellectual loss, and the patient becomes a vegetable prior to death, which is caused by either wasting due to difficulty in swallowing, infection or accident.

Osteogenesis imperfecta

Osteogenesis imperfecta—a defect in the biosynthesis of collagen—is a congenital disorder with brittle bones, also called *fragilitas osseum*, which is inherited in either an autosomal dominant or recessive mode. The disease may be mild or severe and is characterised by repeated fractures on slight trauma because of the abnormal fragility of the bone. Long bones become deformed and the child may develop otosclerosis with deafness. The sclerae of the eyes have a bluish colour and, in cases where the mutant gene is not fully penetrant, the sclerae are blue but the bones are not brittle. A mother with a partially penetrant abnormal gene can, none the less, transmit the disorder to her offspring, each child having a 1 in 2 (50 %) chance of inheriting a fully penetrant abnormal gene. New dominant mutations can occur. Antenatal diagnosis is possible and parents can be counselled as to the risk of producing further affected offspring.

Multiple neurofibromatosis

Multiple neurofibromatosis (Von Recklinghausen's disease) is an autosomal dominant disorder characterised by hyperplasia of the fibrous structures of the peripheral and central nervous systems. It presents as multiple soft tumours, either within the brain or in the skin. These tumours can become malignant. This disorder is also characterised by large, flat, pale markings on the skin, known as 'café au lait' spots. Fi-

brous lesions of bone can lead to severe deformity.

The porphyrias

The porphyrias are diseases of porphyrin metabolism. Porphyrins are organic substances widely distributed in nature which do not have any biological function in man except when bound to iron to form the haem part of haemoglobin. When bound to magnesium they form the chlorophylls of plants and when bound to cobalt they form vit. B_{12}.

Haem is synthesised from porphyrins and iron in the liver and bone marrow, eight enzymes being involved in this process. The presence of large amounts of free porphyrins in the blood, urine or faeces indicates a partial abnormality in one or more of the eight enzymes.

Note: Excess porphyrins do not indicate a haem deficiency in the body. Porphyrias are common hereditary diseases in the RSA but there is an acquired variant which is temporary and has skin lesions. The acquired or symptomatic porphyria is due to impaired liver function and it is thought that alcohol precipitates an attack.

The hereditary prophyrias

The hereditary porphyrias usually have a dominant inheritance (50 % chance of inheritance) and the disease presents for the first time at puberty. The porphyrias can be classified according to enzyme defects, tissue of origin of the porphyrins (liver or bone marrow) or according to the presence or absence of acute attacks.

The three important hereditary porphyrias in the RSA are:

▨ variegate porphyria (VP);
▨ acute intermittent porphyria (AIP); and
▨ non-acute porphyria cutanea tarda (PCT).

Their tissue of origin is the liver.

In AIP there are acute attacks but skin lesions are absent. In PCT acute attacks do not occur but skin lesions are always present. In the so-called South African porphyria variegata (VP or PV), both the acute attacks and the skin lesions are present, the latter not in all cases.

The acute attack of hereditary porphyria is precipitated by certain drugs (e.g. barbiturates, sulphonamides and many more), steroids and other hormones, alcohol, infection, fasting and stress. If the porphyric patient is not exposed to any of these precipitants, then he may be unaware of his disease, e.g. in AIP in which there are no skin lesions, and in PV in which the skin lesions are sometimes minimal.

Porphyria variegata is a very common familial disease of whites, especially Afrikaners.[6] It affects approximately 1 in 200, i.e. 20 000 white South Africans. It is also common amongst the coloured population group.[7] It is generally known as 'the Van Rooyen skin' if skin lesions are present.

CUTANEOUS MANIFESTATIONS OF THE PORPHYRIAS

The photosensitive skin blisters easily on parts exposed to the sun. Where there has been infection, scars form when the blisters heal. The skin is usually pigmented and facial hairiness is common. Combined lesions usually occur on the face, V of the neck and back of the hands, the lesions ranging from fresh blisters to pigmented and depigmented scars.

Note: This must not be confused with Oudtshoorn Skin Disease (Keratolytic Winter Erythema), a dominantly inherited dermatosis not involving other systems. It is unique to Afrikaners due to the founder effect.

CHARACTERISTICS OF ACUTE PORPHYRIC ATTACKS

These attacks occur in AIP and PV if precipitating factors are present. Most attacks occur between the ages of 20 and 40 years and attacks may be recurrent. Combinations of the following may occur: severe abdominal pain (resembling an acute abdomen), diarrhoea or constipation, pyrexia, tachycardia, leucocytosis, and vomiting. The patient may become confused, hysterical and violent; he may have convulsions and exhibit other neurological signs. He may either die from cardiac failure or recover slowly.

DIAGNOSIS OF PORPHYRIA

(1) By screening a small specimen of *stool* shaken up in a solvent, in ultraviolet light, porphyrins can be detected in both the quiescent and the acute phase of the disease. The porphyric stool will show a brilliant pink fluorescence. The amount of porphyrins in these stools is often 10 to 20 times as much as in normal stools.
    This is merely a screening test since strongly positive test results may be found in many other conditions, including severe constipation and hookworm infestation.

(2) The urine is examined for excessive porphyrins during the quiescent and the acute stages by ultraviolet light screening as for stools. In an acute attack the urine is portwine in colour either when passed, or after standing a while. This sign can, however, be elicited in many other conditions, e.g. symptomatic porphyria and diffuse liver disease.

Note: Quantitative analysis of porphyrins in the urine and faeces is important for correct diagnosis of porphyria. This diagnostic service is offered free of charge to all doctors in the RSA by the Genetics Services at their laboratories and by the Porphyria Research Unit of Groote Schuur Hospital.

(3) Porphyria determination in the blood.

(4) The patient is examined for signs of skin sensitivity, for example, blisters and scars on the back of the hands.

A family history is taken to discover the presence of the 'Van Rooyen skin' in other members of the family.

Note:
(1) The porphyric skin condition is also found in symptomatic (acquired) porphyria, but not in AIP.
(2) Blood, urine and stool must always be sent to laboratories in protective tinfoil to prevent porphyrin degradation.

PREVENTION OF ACUTE ATTACKS OF PORPHYRIA

(1) No patient who suffers from this condition must ever be given barbiturates or sulphonamides. Any other precipitating factor must be treated, e.g. infection.

(2) At-risk families can be advised to have their children tested when they reach adolescence for evidence of excessive porphyrins in blood, stools and urine. If present, the at-risk person must avoid precipitants.

(3) All patients about to undergo an operation must be questioned about the possibility of having porphyria in the family. If there is uncertainty, the appropriate tests must be done to exclude the presence of the disease.

TREATMENT OF AN ACUTE ATTACK

(1) Nausea and vomiting and psychiatric symptoms are treated with phenothiazines, e.g. chlorpromazine.

(2) Fluids and electrolyte balance is maintained by intravenous infusions.

(3) A high carbohydrate diet is given orally or by nasogastric tube to reduce the overproduction of porphyrins.[7]

AVOIDANCE OF CUTANEOUS PORPHYRIA

The abnormal photosensitivity and fragility of the skin are similar in PCT and PV (if present in the latter).

PREVENTION OF SKIN LESIONS IN PCT AND PV

(1) Exposure of the skin to sunlight must be avoided.
(2) When exposure to sunlight is unavoidable, the patient must either wear opaque clothing or use an opaque barrier cream containing titanium dioxide or zinc oxide. Ordinary sun-tan lotions are of no value as they allow penetration of the ultraviolet light wavelengths to which the porphyric skin is sensitive.[8]

The muscular dystrophies

This is a group of inborn abnormalities of muscles associated with dysfunction and eventual deterioration of the muscles. The term *dystrophy* means defective nutrition.

Myotonic dystrophy is the commonest muscular dystrophy of adult life;[9] it may also present in childhood and at birth. It is transmitted through a dominant autosomal gene. In the adult form the affected individual has already parented children who have a 50 % chance of inheriting the disease.

'Myotonic' means tonic spasm of a muscle, the muscle being unable to relax after contraction. Apart from the myotonia, the patient suffers from muscular weakness and cataracts. There may also be dementia, testicular atrophy and cardiac arrhythmias and conduction defects. In its congenital form the neonate may be paralysed and hypotonic.

There are some other childhood muscular dystrophies which are relatively mild and localised. They have either an autosomal dominant or autosomal recessive mode of inheritance.

Duchenne's muscular dystrophy is caused by an X-linked recessive gene (see below).

Sex-linked inheritance (SL or XL)

Sex-linked inheritance occurs almost exclusively through the X chromosome of which the female has two and the male one. It differs somewhat from autosomal inheritance in that the female plays the major role in transmitting the disorder while the male is the major person affected by the disorder. (The majority of abnormal genes transmitted in this way are recessive, but one known disorder, vit. D-resistant rickets, is caused by a dominant X-linked gene.) When a female who is heterozygous for a recessive sex-linked disease mates with a normal male, four types of progeny may be produced:

(1) a normal male with the mother's normal X chromosome;
(2) an affected male with the mother's abnormal X chromosome (the recessive gene expresses itself because its allele is not carried on the much smaller Y gene of the male);
(3) a normal female with two normal X chromosomes;
(4) a female carrier (normal phenotype) with one normal and one abnormal X chromosome.

If the carrier daughter, in turn, mates with an affected male, the following offspring can be expected.

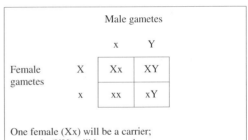

One female (Xx) will be a carrier;
one male (XY) will be normal.
One male (xY) and one female (xx) will be affected.
Note: x = abnormal recessive chromosome

Examples of recessive X-linked disorders are: Duchenne's muscular dystrophy, Lesch-Nyhan syndrome, non-specific X-linked mental retardation (Martin-Bell syndrome), haemophilia and colour blindness.

X-linked recessive disorders

Duchenne's muscular dystrophy (DMD)

Duchenne's or childhood muscular dystrophy is caused by an X-linked recessive gene. Only males are clinically affected; the genetic defect

SINGLE MUTANT GENE INHERITANCE

Mother heterozygous for a recessive X (sex) -linked trait

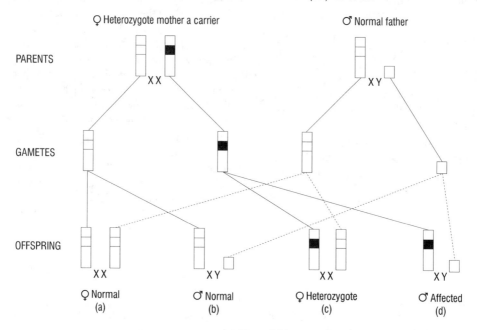

Figure 8.10

X (sex) -linked recessive inheritance

(a) 25 % chance of a normal female child; (b) 25 % chance of a normal male child;
(c) 25 % chance of a female heterozygous carrier; (d) 25 % chance of an affected male child

is transmitted in families by asymptomatic female carriers, the incidence of DMD in the RSA being about 1:3 000 newborn males.[10]

CLINICAL PRESENTATION OF DMD

The muscles become enlarged and weak (pseudohypertrophy) due to the deposition of fat and fibrous tissue. The enlarged calves are characteristic of the condition. One-third of affected persons are mentally retarded. The muscle weakness first appears between the ages of 2 and 6 years in the pelvic girdle and spreads peripherally. Affected persons eventually become confined to a wheelchair. The disease is progressive and fatal from respiratory failure before adult life. There is no effective therapy.

Prevention of Duchenne's muscular dystrophy (DMD) is by aborting a male foetus in a couple at risk. This method of prevention cannot, however, distinguish between affected and non-affected male offspring. Recently a successful method of prenatal diagnosis was discovered; it involves taking blood from the at-risk four-month-old foetus through an amniocentesis. The blood is tested for the enzyme creatine kinase (CK) and the diagnosis of DMD made if the level is elevated.[4]

Moreover, modern molecular genetic techniques using DNA probes are available in the RSA for accurate carrier detection and antenatal diagnosis.[3] Pregnancy can be terminated if the condition is diagnosed.

Lesch-Nyhan syndrome

The Lesch-Nyhan syndrome with an X-linked recessive mode of transmission is a metabolic disorder which affects only males. The child is mentally retarded and suffers from compulsive self-mutilation and choreo-athetosis. He must be restrained and sedated.

The Martin-Bell syndrome

In 1980 the first cases (in the RSA) of Martin-Bell syndrome (non-specific X-linked mental retardation) associated with a marker X-chromosome (with fragile site) were demonstrated. In affected families unaffected females carry the marker X-chromosome. It manifests as the Martin-Bell syndrome in males only.

The marker X-chromosome is found in all racial groups, predominating amongst the whites and Indians. Features of the Martin-Bell syndrome are: males only, low IQ (30–50 Wechsler), macro-orchidism (enlarged testes), large thin pinnae of the ear, thin slightly beaked nose and long narrow face and, sometimes, epilepsy and articulation disability.

Several recent studies and surveys carried out at care and rehabilitation centres (CRC) and at special schools in the RSA on 2 054 subjects found, on average, 18,2 % of chromosomal abnormality associated with mental retardation.

The most common type was Down syndrome (76 %), and the Martin-Bell syndrome was the second most common (4,2 %). Other rarer chromosomal abnormalities with mental retardation are: *cri-du-chat* syndrome, Klinefelter syndrome and females with one or more than two X-chromosomes.[19]

Haemophilia[20]

Haemophilia, a disease with a tendency to bleed spontaneously, is transmitted by X-linked recessive inheritance. In approximately one-third of all haemophilic patients the cause is ascribed to gene mutation, i.e. it is not familial, nor is there

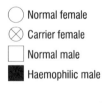

○ Normal female
⊗ Carrier female
□ Normal male
■ Haemophilic male

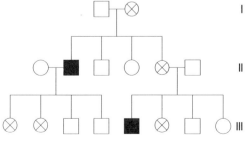

Figure 8.11
Inheritance of haemophilia

sufficient knowledge of the family history to rule out gene mutation.

Haemophilic bleeding in the newborn (e.g. from circumcision or separation of the cord) is rare, the disease usually manifesting in infancy.

The incidence of haemophilia in its severe form is 1 in 25 000 births. It is not possible to diagnose haemophilia in the foetus *in utero*.

TRANSMISSION

When a haemophilic male marries a normal female, his daughters will be obligate carriers and his sons will be unaffected. A carrier female who marries a normal male will produce sons with a 50 % chance of being affected and daughters with a 50 % chance of being carriers of the gene, i.e. 1 in 4 children may be carriers and 1 in 4 children sufferers. If an affected male marries a carrier female, their daughters have a 50 % chance of being haemophilic. This is an extremely rare occurrence.

There are a number of bleeding disorders in which there is a deficiency of a specific blood clotting factor, but only haemophilia and the related Christmas disease are sex-linked hereditary disorders which usually affect males only and are transmitted by the females of the family. Twenty-five to thirty per cent of patients give no family history of the disease. Women carriers of the disease may bleed more than normal women. In these disorders there is a deficiency of clotting factors: factor VIII in haemophilia A and factor IX in haemophilia B (Christmas disease).

There are other congenital clotting factor disorders which appear also in females and are caused by deficiencies of factors V and X. In Von Willebrand's disease a deficiency of factor VIII is associated with an abnormality of platelet function, but the achievement and maintenance of satisfactory factor VIII blood levels are easier than in true haemophilia. It is inherited as an autosomal dominant gene and affects females slightly more often than males. All these bleeding disorders are managed in the same way as haemophilia.

Haemophilia may occur in three degrees of severity.

(1) Those in the severely affected group have practically no functional clotting in their plasma, i.e. less than 1 % of the normal.

They suffer predominantly from repeated and frequent spontaneous haemorrhages into muscles and joints.

(2) The moderately severely affected group with 1 % to 5 % of the normal factor VIII or factor IX in their plasma.

(3) The mildly affected group with 5 % to 30 % of the normal factor VIII or factor IX in their plasma.

The mildly affected group do not usually experience spontaneous bleeds, but patients in this category are at risk when exposed to trauma and surgery. In order to stop spontaneous bleeding into joints of the severely affected group, the circulating clotting factor level must be raised to at least 5 % of the normal by the regular intravenous infusion of fresh plasma or plasma concentrates rich in the appropriate anti-haemophilic factor.

For a minor bleeding episode, factor VIII level is raised to 10–20 % for up to 4 days and for major bleeding, a plasma level of 10–30 % factor VIII is required. Severe haemorrhagic conditions require greatly augmented plasma levels of factor VIII, a major surgical operation being done under 50–70 % coverage.

The four plasma preparations used to control haemophilic bleeding are:

(a) Cryoprecipitate (cold precipitate). This is an extract of factor VIII and fibrinogen prepared from plasma. It is available as both a wet and dry preparation. The volume required for the equivalent number of units of factor VIII is much less than when using plasma, which is a big advantage. It is also associated with fewer transfusion reactions.

(b) Fresh frozen plasma (FFP). This is rich in factor VIII but may be associated with volume overload problems, especially in the severely ill or very young. It is dispensed in 250 ml amounts in plastic bags. Freezing fresh plasma allows most of its anti-haemophilic activity to be retained for prolonged periods. Before use the frozen plasma is thawed.

(c) Dried fresh plasma (DFP). When required, each unit is reconstituted with 200 ml sterile water. The coagulant activity of factor VIII and factor IX in the reconstituted DFP is 0,6 to 0,7 units/ml.

(d) Plasma fractions rich in factor VIII (e.g. Hemofil concentrate) are commercially available. Factor IX concentrates can also be produced, but are very expensive.

Note:
(i) Cryoprecipitate and Hemofil are of no value in the treatment of haemophilia B as they do not contain appreciable amounts of factor IX.

(ii) Patients who have received many infusions of plasma preparations, especially those imported and prepared from a large number of donors, are at risk of developing serum hepatitis and AIDS.

When factor VIII is infused into a patient, it retains its potency for only 6 to 12 hours. Repeated infusions may, therefore, be necessary, especially during the post-operative healing phase. Maintenance therapy is very expensive but is given free at provincial teaching hospitals.

SPONTANEOUS BLEEDING

The commonest lesions in haemophilia are bleeds from synovial membranes into the joints (haemarthroses), especially the knee, elbow, ankle and shoulder joints. Muscle haematoma also occur and may lead to Volkmann's ischaemic contractures. These joint and muscle bleeds often commence during sleep; once it has started in a joint, the cavity fills with blood and this results in a warm, exquisitely painful swollen joint with surrounding muscle spasm and loss of movement. If inadequately treated, haemorrhages into joints and muscles may lead to crippling deformities. Other bleeding sites are the abdomen and within the cranium, sometimes as a result of injury.

The major cause of death from bleeding in haemophiliacs results from Central Nervous System bleeds.

Treatment of acute haemarthroses:

(1) Control of bleeding. The deficient factor is replaced by intravenous plasma or cryoprecipitate infusions. Usually FFP 750 ml (in adults) and 500 ml (in children) is required to effect haemostasis in acute haemarthrosis. There may be non-haemolytic systemic reactions (urticaria, pyrexia, rigors, oedema) to the plasma; they require treatment with an antihistaminic.

(2) Orthopaedic care. Immobilisation of the joint is achieved with a POP back slab or Robert Jones bandage for 24 to 48 hours, followed by night splints for a week. The

joint must be in its functional position to prevent fixed deformities due to flexor spasm and contraction of intra-articular tissue.

(3) Pain is controlled with analgesics, but aspirin, phenacetin and intramuscular injections must be avoided. Paracetamol and propoxyphene are useful analgesics. Aspirin has an adverse affect on platelet function.

(4) Physiotherapy

    (*a*) Ice packs are applied to the affected joint to reduce swelling;

    (*b*) 'special risk' non-bleeding joints must be exercised to strengthen them, even while the infusion is taking place;

    (*c*) once bleeding and pain have been arrested, the affected joint is put through a full range of movements to prevent muscular atrophy; this is gradually followed by:

    (*d*) static muscle exercises around the joints;

    (*e*) strong exercises applied to the limb by increasing resistance with weights or springs;

    (*f*) no weight-bearing is allowed until the muscles are strong enough to protect the joint, usually after 5–7 days. To this end the physiotherapist teaches the patient special ways of walking.

(5) Aspiration of joints is seldom done—only when the joints are very tense—and only under cover of the missing factor.

BLEEDING ASSOCIATED WITH SURGERY

Dental extraction. Dental extraction of permanent teeth is done under general anaesthesia. The plasma level of the missing factor is brought up to 20 % to 40 % by means of an immediate pre-operative dose of FFP. This is followed by an administration of a fibrinolytic inhibitor such as epsilon-aminocaproic acid (EACA) or tranexamic acid. If the latter is continued orally for ten days, no further haemostatic therapy is required as EACA delays the natural process of clot destruction in the tooth socket. Further clot-preserving precautions are taken by giving the patient iced drinks and a bland soft diet for a few days.

Major surgery. A minimum of 300 bags of plasma is required for most major surgical procedures, provided there are no complications. To reduce volume, the cryoprecipitate is used. To date, none of the clotting factors has been synthesised chemically and supplies are obtainable only from human plasma. Combination therapy with FFP, cryoprecipitate and plasma fractions rich in factor VIII is usually resorted to for a few weeks post-operatively. The most commonly performed operations are for the correction of deformities, i.e. synovectomies, arthrodeses and total hip replacements.

PSYCHOLOGICAL EFFECTS OF HAEMOPHILIA

The haemophiliac lives a very troubled life; children withdraw from peer group activities for fear of physical trauma and often attend irregularly at school. They are occupied by self-doubts and insecurities and may be overprotected at home. Parents often carry a load of guilt and resentment because of the restrictions imposed by bleeding crises on the mobility of the family. A recent advance in the field of haemophilia has been the introduction of home infusions of plasma.

Home therapy. Freeze-dried fresh plasma, cryoprecipitate and fresh frozen plasma are used by all haemophilic families who are able to master the technique of intravenous therapy and who have proper storage facilities. Home infusions ensure that bleeding episodes are controlled before much damage can be done, and that a haemophilic family can take their treatment with them when they go on holiday.

The patient (or his family) who treats his bleeding successfully should also be entrusted with his own physiotherapy, the most suitable active sport being swimming. Contact sport should be avoided because of the danger of injury.

The genetic counselling and management of proven haemophilic carriers still remains a social and personal problem.

THE SOUTH AFRICAN HAEMOPHILIA FOUNDATION

This Foundation was formed in 1970 under the auspices of the South African Society of Haematology. Later that year it became a full member of the World Federation of Haemophilia (WFH). The Foundation has established five branches in the major cities of South Africa and is at present busy with the registration of all haemophiliacs, white as well as non-white. In South Africa there are some 1 500 known haemophiliacs (1982).

The aims of the Haemophilia Foundation are:

'To provide a fellowship for sufferers of haemophilia and similar disorders, for their families and those concerned in their health and welfare. To promote the interests of sufferers of haemophilia and similar disorders by whatever legal means available.'

Membership is voluntary and is obtained by writing for information to:

The Secretary
PO Box 87642
Houghton
2000 Johannesburg

The Foundation is not a welfare organisation and funds have been obtained by the efforts of Management Committees which consist of laymen and medical personnel. Most haemophiliacs are entitled to free medical services in specified wards of provincial hospitals. Families and patients are encouraged to support the Haemophilia Foundation, which is intended not only to encourage haemophiliac families to help themselves but also for the establishment of a fund to send South African doctors overseas to contribute to international congresses on haemophilia, to gain information about advances in treatment and for bursary schemes. Research in haemophilia is being done all over the world and international congresses are held in different countries each year.

The Regional Branches of the SA Haemophilia Foundation are at present concerned with the organising of:

(1) haemophilia identification cards and bracelets through the services of the Medic-Alert Foundation;

(2) rapid out-patient and in-patient treatment at provincial hospitals in the larger centres, for acute bleeding episodes;

(3) the compilation of a register with medical data of all persons in South Africa who suffer from haemophilia;

(4) haemophilia clinics for medical treatment, physiotherapy and genetic counselling for haemophiliacs and their families;

(5) studies to elucidate the social and psychiatric problems which attend the haemophiliac patient.

Note: This section has been taken from: *Manual of Advanced Nursing* (Schreiber & Vlok, 5th ed. 1987).

Heterogeneous inheritance

Some genetic diseases are heterogeneous, i.e. they are characterised by multiple forms of inheritance, variable penetrance and clinical expression, e.g. the muscular dystrophies and retinitis pigmentosa.

Retinitis pigmentosa (RP) is an inherited disease of the retinal pigment which progresses to blindness. It is the most common form of genetic blindness.

In a study done by Oswald *et al.*,[30] the following genetic distribution was found:

(1) autosomal dominant—14 %;

(2) autosomal recessive—9,5 %;

(3) X-linked—6 %.

The other 70 % of RP were either part of a 'syndrome' or could not be classified into any specific genetic category.

Although the different genetic types differ in their age of onset, clinical course and severity (penetrance), all can be diagnosed by the following symptoms:

(1) Night-blindness (nyctalopia). Nocturnal vision decreases gradually.

(2) Visual-field defects which start peripherally and spread centrally until only a small central area of the retina affords 'tunnel vision'. When this part eventually dies, the patient is blind.

There is no therapy to halt the progression of RP. The condition can be controlled only by genetic counselling.

Group support can be obtained by joining the Retinitis Pigmentosa Foundation of South Africa. This group supports research on carrier screening and antenatal diagnosis for all genetic forms of RP.

SPECIFIC CANCERS WITH A GENETIC BASE

In a few specific cancers, the primary cause of the cancer is an abnormal gene or genes.

Polyposis coli (polyps in the colon)

There are several types of polyposis coli but only one type is transmitted as an autosomal dominant trait. It occurs in a few Afrikaner families and is inclined to become malignant even in adolescents.

It is ironical that by the time the affected person is dying of cancer of the colon, he has had his family and there is a 50 % chance that each of his children has inherited the disorder. The polyps usually develop at adolescence and, if the condition comes to the attention of a medical practitioner, a 6-monthly sigmoidoscopy can be done for the purpose of preventing the development of a fatal outcome by timeous removal of the colon.

Colectomy is done before carcinoma develops. All family members must be examined every 2 years, starting at the age of 10 years and terminating at the age of 50 years.

Note: Male-limited hereditary non-polypotic colonic cancer occurs in the absence of polyps and other pre-malignant lesions, and appears to have an autosomal dominant mode of inheritance, despite being limited to young males.

Several cancerous tumours of young children arise in primitive embryonic tissue: *neuroblastoma, retinoblastoma, nephroblastoma (Wilms tumour)*.

Chondrosarcoma may occur in patients with hereditary multiple exostosis, an autosomal dominant disorder.[21]

MENTAL RETARDATION

In a proportion of mentally retarded persons, the cause of the low intelligence is either a chromosomal aberration or a genetic defect.

Causes of mental retardation

Chromosomal aberrations (11–15 %)

These are either autosomal trisomies (Patau, Edward, Down) or autosomal deletions (*cri-du-chat* syndrome).

Single gene defects (7 %)

Autosomal Dominant

- Apert syndrome
- Epiloia (tuberous sclerosis)

Autosomal Recessive

- Hurler syndrome (mucopolysaccharidosis)
- Phenylketonuria
- Lawrence Moon-Biedl syndrome
- Microcephaly (some types)

Sex-linked Recessive

- Hunter syndrome (mucopolysaccharidosis)
- Duchenne's muscular dystrophy
- Martin-Bell syndrome

Polygenic defects (15 %)

Cornelia de Lange syndrome and the bird-headed dwarf of Seckel.

Environmental and unknown causes (63 %)

Foetal alcohol syndrome (congenital), lack of stimulation due to poor socio-economic conditions, perinatal trauma, anoxia and infections account for the majority of cases of mental retardation.

ECOGENETICS

Ecogenetics deals with the alleviation of genetic diseases by the modification or exclusion of environmental risk factors.[22]

A few serious genetic conditions or predispositions of great medical importance in the RSA can be avoided if the at-risk genotype can be identified and suitable avoidance therapy applied.

For these secondary preventive measures to be applied, the offending risk factor must be known and the sensitive genotype or predisposing genetic condition identified pre-symptomatically.

The common ecogenetic conditions in the RSA are:

- Phenylketonuria (see p. 120)
- Hereditary porphyrias (see p. 126)
- Familial hypercholesterolaemia (see p. 293)

It is possible that smoking and alcohol consumption may also be environmental risk factors which wreak havoc in sensitive predisposed genotypes.

Atopic allergies (familial hypersensitivities) and asthma can be greatly helped by avoidance of known allergens.

THE RISK OF OCCURRENCE AND RECURRENCE OF INHERITED DISORDERS

A large number of genetic disorders—approximately 4 000—are known, but only a few occur with sufficient regularity for them to be recognised with ease. Comparatively few genetic diseases are 'familial', the majority occurring sporadically, either because the disease is due to a new mutation or because it is caused by an autosomal recessive gene. In the latter case the mating of two unrelated people both carrying the same defective recessive gene is remote. Many genetic diseases have a multifactorial aetiology, being the product of a number of faulty genes (polygenic) and the appropriate environment for their expression.

In *single gene (monogenic) disorders,* the risk of producing affected and carrier offspring by parents known to be either carriers or affected is as follows:

Autosomal dominant inheritance of single gene-dose disorders

(1) One parent affected (heterozygous):
1 in 2 chance of each offspring being affected.
(2) Both parents affected (heterozygous):
3 in 4 chances of each offspring being affected.

Autosomal recessive inheritance of double gene-dose disorders

(1) One parent heterozygous carrier:
All offspring normal; 1 in 2 chance of each offspring being heterozygous carrier.
(2) Both parents heterozygous carriers:
1 in 4 chance of each offspring being affected.
1 in 2 chance of each offspring being a carrier.

If one child is born with the disease, his subsequent siblings have a 25 % chance of contracting the same disorder. His children will be normal if he marries a person with dominant genes.

X-linked recessive inheritance

(1) Mother a heterozygous carrier; father normal:
1 in 4 chance of a normal female offspring
1 in 4 chance of a carrier female offspring
1 in 4 chance of a normal male offspring
1 in 4 chance of an affected male offspring
(2) Mother heterozygous carrier; father affected:
1 in 4 chance of a carrier female offspring
1 in 4 chance of an affected female offspring
1 in 4 chance of an affected male offspring
1 in 4 chance of a normal male offspring
(3) Mother normal; father affected:
All female offspring will be heterozygous carriers
All male offspring will be normal

X-linked dominant inheritance

(1) Mother affected (heterozygous); father normal:
1 in 2 chance of female offspring being affected
1 in 2 chance of male offspring being affected
(2) Mother affected (heterozygous); father affected (heterozygous): All female offspring will be affected
1 in 2 chance of male offspring being affected

Sometimes these predictions are confounded by the fact that some inherited disorders have different modes of inheritance, i.e. dominant, recessive and X-linked. This applies especially to inherited deafness, blindness (retinitis pigmentosa), mental retardation and muscular dystrophy.

It must be remembered that single gene disorders are clear-cut in their appearance and their recurrence in families can be predicted fairly accurately, but they are not as common as polygenically inherited disorders with a multifactorial aetiology.

The following common *congenital conditions* have a multifactorial aetiology: neural tube disorders such as anencephaly and spina bifida. There is a relationship between these disorders and raised alpha fetoprotein levels in the amniotic fluid. Neural tube disorders occur more frequently than the following congenital disorders: congenital pyloric stenosis; cleft lip with or without cleft palate; dislocation of the hip; heart anomalies; talipes equinovarus.

The multifactorial aetiology is due to the fact that many genes are involved to cause a genetic predisposition towards the congenital disorders. If this predisposition exceeds a certain threshold or if certain maternal environmental factors exacerbate the genetic predisposition, the anomaly will become manifest. In this case nature and nurture interact to cause the multifactorial aetiology. Predisposing genes are heritable and run in unsuspecting families. When the precipitating environmental factor (e.g. certain medicines, viruses, radiations) is present, the congenital anomaly appears 'as out of the blue'.

In these congenital conditions, inheritance does not follow simple Mendelian laws; in counselling parents about the possibility of recurrence in subsequent offspring, the clinician makes use of empirical risk figures. The recurrence risk is increased after the birth of an affected child.

Neural tube disorders: there is a *1 in 20* risk that siblings of affected persons will be born with a neural tube disorder. After two affected children the risk increases to *1 in 8*. If the woman is pregnant with a 'high-risk' foetus, an amniocentesis can be done between the 14th and 16th weeks of pregnancy for alpha fetoprotein levels. Termination of pregnancy is advised if these levels are raised.

The Genetic Services of DNHPD recently (1993) recommended the use of dietary folic acid supplementation for all women of childbearing age to reduce the risk of neural tube defects in their offspring. Prophylactic folic acid is especially important in a woman who has a child with a neural tube defect, or who has a close relative with this defect, if she is contemplating having another child.

Cleft lip and palate: there is a *1 in 30* risk that siblings of affected persons or their offspring will be born with this condition. After 2 affected children, the recurrence risk rises to *1 in 10*.

In *chromosomal disorders*, prediction of occurrence and recurrence is also very difficult, the following empirical risk figures being used in Down and Klinefelter syndromes:

In *non-disjunction trisomy 21* (regular Down) there is a *1 in 100* risk for the siblings of affected persons.

In *translocation type trisomy 21* (Down), the risk is greater.

In any chromosomal disorder, where one parent is a *translocation carrier*, the risk for each child is *1 in 5*. In practice, the risk seems to be lower, especially if the father is the carrier.

In women aged *35 to 39 years*, the risk of producing a child with a chromosomal disorder is *1 in 100*, and in women over the age of *40 years* the risk is *1 in 33*.

As a rule, however, chromosomal defects occur sporadically. The overall risk is one child with Down syndrome in every 1 000 births.

Every individual carries some bad genes, i.e. recessive genes which in single dose do no harm but which cause an inherited disease if two carriers produce an offspring with a double dose of the gene. The frequency of a particular faulty gene in a population is usually low, approximately 1 in 300 persons being carriers. The chances of two carriers mating randomly are very small, hence the low incidence of the majority of monogenically inherited disorders. Frequency rates of 1 in 20 (carriers of Tay-Sachs gene among Ashkenazi Jews) and 1 in 12 (carriers of cystic fibrosis gene among Namibian Afrikaners) indicate 'high-risk' populations. In these populations it may be worthwhile screening the population for carriers where this procedure is at all possible.

THE NATIONAL GENETICS PROGRAMME

This programme is aimed at preventing or coping with the problems of congenital and hereditary disorders. The genetics services of the Department of Health are part of a co-ordinated and comprehensive health service in the RSA, available for every individual, irrespective of community status and population group.

Each of the nine regional offices of the department is responsible for providing and/or co-ordinating genetic services in its region and has access to the services of at least one full-time genetics sister.

Referrals can be made to genetics sisters who are the field workers of the genetic services of the Department of Health. The genetics sisters co-ordinate a comprehensive network of free genetic services to the public. Genetics sisters can be contacted at every regional office. They liaise with families, the genetic counselling clinics, laboratories, private practitioners, health authorities and various social, educational and welfare facilities, and they identify high-risk patients. The genetics sister is, therefore, specially equipped to deal with all aspects of a community-based comprehensive genetic service.

Genetics sisters are trained in this speciality at courses run by State Health. They take full family genetic histories where required, take blood for chromosome studies and urine specimens for chemical analysis, record significant findings during clinical examinations by a geneticist and do follow-up care of patients and their families, after counselling by the doctor.

The genetics sisters in the regional offices are equipped to present lectures and audio-visual material to interested groups. The head of Genetic Services (Pretoria) may be consulted on any problems encountered in connection with genetic and congenital disorders.

The genetics sister thus serves as a central referral point within the community and endeavours to co-ordinate the wide network of genetic services for the public.

The Department of Health offers free laboratory services for the following genetic and/or congenital disorders:

(1) 'haemolytic disease of the newborn';
(2) 'all other genetic and/or congenital diseases . . . to identify chromosome or metabolic disorders . . . irrespective of whether such tests be carried out before or during pregnancy or after birth, provided that prior authority be obtained from the director-general . . .'.

Correct diagnosis: a priority in genetic services

In the RSA special diagnostic facilities are available for specific conditions. A list of 205 inherited metabolic diseases (IMD) is available from the Genetic Services of the Department of Health, with details of where diagnostic facilities are available.

Note: Before diagnostic screening is done on carrier parents, foetus or neonate, informed consent must be obtained. The parents must know the nature and purpose of genetic screening.

Diagnosis consists of 2 stages:

(1) deciding whether the illness is indeed due to an inherited metabolic disorder (IMD), and
(2) determining which IMD. This entails definition by a team of paediatricians, geneticists and chemical pathologists or biochemists, precisely which enzyme or protein is defective.

Recognition of inherited disorders

Whereas infection and malnutrition used to be the main causes of infantile morbidity and mortality, in developed countries congenital malformations and inherited disorders are assuming increasing importance. Retief[23] states that 4–5 % of live-born infants suffer from genetic or partly genetic disorders and that 20–30 % of paediatric in-patients have genetic diseases, the majority being polygenic disorders with a few single gene or chromosomal anomalies. The recognition of the hereditary nature of diseases is an important aspect of promotive and preventive health.

The nurse who deals with children must be alert to the possibility of congenital and familial abnormalities which may have a genetic origin. The following points may help her recognise signs of a genetic disorder which may require the services of a genetic clinic and genetic counselling service.

(1) The clinical picture which the patient presents. A newborn baby should be examined for congenital dislocations of the hips and for any other physical anomalies. The open mouth and protruding tongue of infants with hypothyroidism and Down syndrome can be recognised at an early age.
(2) A genetic disease is often diagnosed when there are no obvious environmental aetiological factors to account for an aberration, e.g. inborn errors of metabolism.
(3) The fact that the same type of disorder appears in more than one generation is clear evidence of a familial inherited disease.

Where an autosomal dominant or recessive X-linked disease is suspected, the taking of a generation-spanning history is very important. The nurse must remember that the person who has inherited an abnormal dominant gene may not exhibit all the signs of the inherited syndrome and unless a careful examination is done and history is taken, the familial nature of the disease may be missed.

Genetic diagnostic procedures

(1) A full family history is taken; this must span several generations. A nurse who has good contact with a family is invaluable in obtaining the required information.

(2) The doctor does a thorough clinical examination and if mental retardation is suspected and facilities for testing are available, the child's IQ should be measured.

(3) Sex chromatin (Barr body, see p. 109) counts may be done to establish the true genotype of persons suffering from sex chromosomal aberrations (see p. 111).

(4) Chromosomal studies are done on specimens of either blood, skin or buccal mucosa taken at a genetics laboratory.

    (a) Karyotyping for Down syndrome to discover whether mongolism is due to non-disjunction or translocation trisomy 21. In the latter case the parents are also tested for possible carrier status. This is done in all trisomy aberrations.

    (b) Karyotyping for sex chromosome abnormalities in cases of suspected sex genotype aberrations (see p. 113).

    (c) In cases where sex chromatin count is not consistent with sex phenotype.

    (d) In cases of multiple congenital abnormalities of unknown origin, especially if the child is mentally deficient; chromosomal studies are done on the parents as well.

    (e) In cases of cryptorchidism (undescended testes).

    (f) A specially modified cytogenetic technique to detect the fragile site on the long arms of the X-chromosome (marker X-chromosome) to detect female carriers and male patients with Martin-Bell syndrome in at-risk families.

(5) Specific biochemical tests for metabolic screening are done on cultured leucocytes, for detection in parents of carrier status in Tay-Sachs, Gaucher's and Lesch-Nyhan disease.

Note: By measuring enzyme levels in blood or skin cells, carriers of nearly 60 metabolic disorders can be identified.

(6) Neonatal screening for diseases amenable to secondary preventive therapy, e.g. phenylketonuria (PKU), hypothyroidism, and galactosaemia. The urine of large numbers of neonates is tested and those with positive results are put on special diets (see p. 120) or medication. Neonatal screening for PKU has been done on a small scale in South Africa.

(7) A population screening programme has been instituted for the common South African genetic disorder, porphyria variegata (see p. 126).

(8) Antenatal screening for serum alpha-feto-protein is done routinely in the UK at 4–5 months gestation. In South Africa the routine antenatal screening of pregnant women for alpha-fetoprotein (AFP) level in blood, in order to detect severe CNS defects and congenital nephrosis in the foetus, has been started. (See AFP level in amniotic fluid, p. 138.) The mother's AFP blood level reflects the level in the amniotic fluid; if found to be raised, an amniocentesis can be undertaken to confirm the diagnosis of severe CNS defect in the child.[24] The diagnosis can also be confirmed by doing endoscopy of the uterus and viewing the foetus directly (foetoscopy). Any external defect in the foetus can be detected in this way, e.g. spina bifida, anencephaly, cleft lip.

(9) Cordocentesis.[25] This means withdrawing blood from the umbilical vein during the 2nd or 3rd trimester. It is a prenatal diagnostic procedure still in the experimental stage. The needle aspirating cord blood is guided sonographically.

Cordocentesis can be used for rapid karyotyping during the 3rd trimester when foetal malformation, intra-uterine growth retardation or hydramnios is suspected.

(10) On special recommendation, an amniocentesis is carried out by an obstetrician between the 15th and 20th weeks of pregnancy. At this time the amniotic sac is large enough to permit the aspiration of fluid and pregnancy not so far advanced that its termination poses a threat to the mother's health and life.

Note:
(1) Amniocentesis carries a small risk of foetal loss (2 %). It is a safe procedure when monitored by ultrasound.
(2) Amniocentesis can be done at near term to detect foetal abnormalities unrelated to genetic disorders.

Amniocentesis

A second trimester amniocentesis is always preceded by an ultrasonic examination to locate the placenta (so that it may be avoided by the investigating needle), to diagnose gross structural anomalies such as anencephaly and to accurately determine gestational age, thus obviating failure of culture due to too few cells.[26] Informed consent is required before amniocentesis.

Protocol for genetic amniocentesis

(1) The patient voids.
(2) Ultrasound examination is done to determine gestational age (approximately 2–3 minutes).
(3) The patient is counselled to confirm genetic referral and that the date for amniocentesis is correct.
(4) The patient is scanned again to locate the pool of liquor amnii (another 2 minutes).
(5) The appropriate spot on the abdomen is marked by pressing a coin on the skin.
(6) The abdomen is sterilised. No local anaesthetic is used.
(7) A 75 mm 22-gauge spinal needle is inserted into the uterine cavity. A plastic disposable syringe is attached and 10 ml of amniotic fluid is withdrawn.
(8) The syringe is removed from the needle and the contents put into a sterile plastic bottle.
(9) The needle is withdrawn.
(10) The patient is again scanned to check the foetal heart beat.
(11) The patient is discharged and told to rest for the remainder of the day.

The specimen is sent to the laboratory for tests on the amniotic fluid and cells derived from the foetal mucous membranes. Chromosomal and biochemical studies comprise the following.

(1) Karyotyping of the amniotic fluid cell chromosomes, after the cells have been cultured:
   (a) in elderly mothers (i.e. those over 35 years) at risk of producing a mongol;
      (*Note:* In the RSA amniocentesis for advanced maternal age is accepted at the age of 40 and over to qualify for state-aided support.[27])
   (b) in a woman who has had a previous child with a chromosomal defect (Down, Edwards, Patau, *cri-du-chat*) or with a suspected marker X-chromosome;
   (c) to determine the sex of the foetus—if the mother is a carrier of an X-linked recessive trait, e.g. haemophilia, Duchenne's muscular dystrophy;
   (d) in the case of repeated abortions, which may be explained by the demonstration of chromosomal abnormalities in the extruded products of conception.

Chromosome results are available within 4 weeks. This allows termination of pregnancy at 20 to 22 weeks if an abnormality is detected.

(2) Biochemical tests on cultured amniotic fluid cells for antenatal diagnosis of affected foetus in cases of Tay-Sachs, Gaucher's and Lesch-Nyhan diseases and Hurler syndrome. These tests can be completed within 6–8 weeks. Some 100 biochemical disorders are detectable before birth.

(3) Biochemical tests on cell-free amniotic fluid for alpha-fetoprotein estimation. This is done in cases where a woman has had a child with a severe neural tube abnormality such as anencephaly and spina bifida or where her AFP blood level is raised at 4 months gestation. There must be an open lesion in the foetus for the AFP to be detected.

AFP results are available within a week. The AFP content of amniotic fluid gives an antenatal detection rate of over 95 %. Amniocentesis is done for one of the above indications to prevent the birth of a grossly handicapped child.

Note: There is no prenatal test for the majority of genetic disorders.

To use resources frugally, amniocentesis should be done only if both the doctor and the parents agree that the pregnancy will be terminated if it is found that the foetus is affected. Amniocentesis should be done only to test for those handicaps for which an abortion is justified. Amniocentesis should, therefore, be preceded by genetic counselling.

A therapeutic abortion is not done until the 19th to 24th week of pregnancy; this advanced gestational age precludes the use of a simple dilatation and curettage procedure because the placenta has formed and is securely attached to the uterine wall. A single injection of prostaglandin E_2 is instilled into the amniotic sac. A few hours later uterine contractions (labour pains) commence and usually within 12 hours the foetus is expelled. The procedure is obstetrically supervised in a designated hospital, after permission for a legal abortion has been obtained.

A therapeutic abortion thus defined is a primary preventive measure in human genetics. Primary prevention is facilitated by genetic counselling.

Genetic counselling

The diagnosis of inherited disorders and genetic counselling to impart the knowledge thus obtained to parents, are done by a family doctor, a paediatrician or a clinician with special knowledge of inherited disorders. They are often assisted by a cytogenetics laboratory and by paramedical staff (nurses, social workers and psychologists) because genetic counselling involves more than just predicting the risk of occurrence and recurrence of a specific inherited disorder. The counsellor takes the responsibility for influencing decisions not only about a single affected case but also about future progeny.

People request genetic counselling for the following reasons:

(1) After the birth of an abnormal child. Parents want to know the risk of producing another affected child and if there is something that can be done to enable them to have a normal child.

(2) Couples who are as yet childless and who have a familial defect come for counselling to find out the risk of producing an affected child. Their fears and the real danger may be compounded if they are related.

(3) Middle-aged couples who still want children and fear the possibility of producing a child with Down syndrome come for counselling and help to produce a normal child.

(4) A pregnant woman who has had German measles or teratogenic drugs or has been exposed to radiation comes for counselling and possible permission to terminate pregnancy because she fears that her foetus has been damaged.

(5) Parents may also want to know about the reproductive future of their normal (or abnormal) child if there is a genetic defect in their family, e.g. haemophilia.

(6) Mental retardation.

(7) Three or more spontaneous abortions.

(8) To be reassured of the non-genetic aetiology of their child's congenital abnormality.

(9) Consanguinity.

(10) At-risk families due to presence of marker X-chromosomes with fragile sites (Martin-Bell syndrome).

The main object of genetic counselling is to prevent birth defects and inherited disorders. Many of these disorders are preventable and couples can be recommended for a therapeutic abortion if the risk to the foetus has been proven. Genetic counselling does not mean that parents are forced to carry out the recommendations of the counsellor; they need expert advice on the likelihood of producing an abnormal child—the final decision about whether or not to have the child is theirs.[28]

Seventeen genetic clinics have been established in all the major centres in South Africa. They form part of a comprehensive national genetic service. Satellite clinics around the major centres, with facilities for genetic diagnosis, will soon be established, to deal with less complicated genetic problems. A trained clinician and a trained genetics nurse could staff such a satellite clinic. Patients are referred to these clinics by private practitioners, hospital doctors and clinics. As good genetic counselling will depend on accurate diagnosis, which may be difficult because of the rarity of the inherited disorder, the first function of the clinic is diagnosis.

When the genetic counsellor is in possession of all the facts to enable him to make a sound diagnosis in an affected person and a prognosis in a pregnancy under way, he is ready to counsel the parents.

(1) He states the risk of having an affected child and explains to the parents what this means. The parents must know the nature of the birth defect or inherited disorder. Often parents need a second visit to the genetic counsellor after they have discussed the implications of the advice so that any queries can be ironed out. The services of a social worker who does home visits may also be required to support the parents. The parents must make up their own minds as to whether they are going to risk having a child. Genetic counselling raises many ethical questions for the parents and for society.

(2) Couples may need counselling about birth control and sterilisation.

(3) If amniocentesis shows the foetus to be affected, termination of pregnancy is recommended. The abortion laws make provision for legal therapeutic abortions (see p. 349). Ethical and religious considerations may, however, cause insuperable conflicts for the parents.

(4) In the case of X-linked, recessive disorder (Duchenne's muscular dystrophy, haemophilia), foetal sexing (by amniocentesis) followed by therapeutic abortion of a male foetus can be offered to carrier mothers.

(5) An important task of the genetic counsellor is to allay anxiety and dispel feelings of guilt. Very often the fears of clients who come to genetic clinics are groundless; these clients need to be reassured.

Op't Hof describes four phases of the psychosocial processes which every family or affected person goes through when the occurrence of a handicap in a family is first learned:

(1) a reaction of shock and disbelief;
(2) pre-comprehension phase of chronic sorrow;
(3) non-acceptance phase of 'shopping around';
(4) phase of comprehension and acceptance.[29]

Help for the parents of a child with a genetic disorder

The genetics sister can play a very important role in helping parents cope with the problem, using existing community facilities such as community health clinics, parents' support groups. Parents need to know where to go for medical help (e.g. for surgically correctable conditions) and about specialised clinics, e.g. cystic fibrosis clinics.

To help families cope with the loss of their belief of invulnerability, a psychosocial support system is needed. This support system can be facilitated by the genetics nurse who encourages affected parents to join parents groups where people can obtain mutual support and fellowship.

Mutual-support groups have been formed to help parents of children afflicted with the following disorders: Down syndrome, cystic fibrosis, cleft lip and palate, spina bifida, osteogenesis imperfecta, haemophilia, dwarfism, food allergies and intolerances.

The addresses of the various associations and foundations can be obtained from the genetics sisters at one of the nine regional offices of the Department of Health and Welfare.

In South Africa at present great efforts are being made by the Department of Health to bring to the attention of doctors, nurses, paramedical staff and the public, the growing importance of inherited disorders. Educational booklets on the common inherited disorders can be obtained from the Department of Health; this is part of an extensive education programme in which the prevention of inherited disorders is stressed. Neonatal screening is done for cystic fibrosis in high-risk populations. At present, the department is subsidising a pilot scheme (Johannesburg and Pretoria) in which tests are done free in laboratories of the SAIMR and State Health for the following:

Porphyria variegata: stools and urine; Tay-Sachs carriers: blood; thalassaemia: blood; karyotyping of cells obtained by amniocentesis in case of advanced maternal age; amniocentesis for, *inter alia*, alpha-feto-proteins.

In 1973 the *South African Inherited Disorders Association* (SAIDA)—a lay medical organisation—was formed for the purpose of educating in the field of inherited diseases.

SAIDA's aims are:

■ To educate the medical and paramedical professions, and the lay public, about inherited disorders. To provide a fellowship for sufferers from these disorders, for their families and those concerned with their health and welfare.
■ To support research into the causes, treatment and prevention of hereditary disorders in southern Africa.

SAIDA has branches in Cape Town, Durban, Johannesburg, Windhoek and Pretoria.

For further information, the Secretary of SAIDA can be contacted at: Human Sero-Genetics Unit, SAIMR, PO Box 1038, Johannesburg 2000.

A child referral centre was started in Pretoria in 1978 to deal with family problems highlighted by the community-based genetic service and to direct parents to the facilities available to help their affected child.

The author wishes to acknowledge indebtedness to the Genetic Services, Department of Health, for information supplied.

REFERENCES

(1) Emery AEH. *Elements of Medical Genetics.* Edinburgh and London: Churchill Livingstone, 1975.

(2) Department of Health and Welfare. *Guide to Genetic Disorders—Teratogenic Agents.*

(3) Beighton P, Goldblatt J, Wallis G. Genetic disease in South Africa. *S Afr Med J* 1987; **72**: 766–769.

(4) From *SAIDA News* 1978; **4** (1).

(5) Jordaan HF. Inherited disorders in the RSA which commonly present with dermatological signs. *S Afr J Cont Med Educ* 1984; **2**: 115.

(6) Dean G. *The Porphyrias.* London: Pitman, 1963.

(7) Meissner PN, Meissner DM, Sturrock ED *et al.* Porphyria—The UCT experience. *S Afr Med J* 1987; **72**: 755–761.

(8) Gordon W. Photosensitivity in porphyria (Letter to the Editor). *S Afr Med J* 1988; **73**: 372.

(9) Lotz BP, Van der Meyden CH. Myotonic dystrophy. *S Afr Med J* 1985; **67**: 812–817.

(10) Ball R, Goldblatt J, Beighton P, Wallis G. Duchenne's muscular dystrophy: Molecular management. *S Afr Med J* 1989; **75**: 76.

(11) Harley EH. Awareness of inherited metabolic disorders. *S Afr Med J* 1985; **67**: 746.

(12) Op't Hof J, Hitzeroth HW. Phenylketonuria (PKU) in the RSA. *S Afr Med J* 1987; **71**: 538.

(13) Jenkins T, Lane AB & Kromberg JGR. *S Afr Med J* 1977; **51**: 95.

(14) Beighton P, Sachs S. *S Afr Med J* 1974; **48**: 1295.

(15) Super M. *S Afr Med J* 1975; **49**: 818.

(16) Hill ID, Macdonald WBC, Bowie MD, Ireland JD. Cystic fibrosis in Cape Town. *S Afr Med J* 1988; **73**: 147–149.

(17) Reef I, *et al.* The sweat test in the diagnosis of cystic fibrosis. *S Afr Med J* 1985; **67**: 441.

(18) Lewis MI, Zaltzman M, Reef I, *et al.* Experience at an adolescent and adult cystic fibrosis clinic. *S Afr Med J* 1984; **65**: 641–648.

(19) Venter PA, Op't Hof, J. *S Afr Med J* 1982; **62**: 947.

(20) Getaz EP, Staples WG, Lurie A. Haemophilia. *S Afr Med J* 1977; **52**: 595.

(21) Solomon I. *S Afr Med J* 1971; **48**: 671.

(22) Hitzeroth HW. Ecogenetics: The role of environmental risk factors. *Rehabilitation in SA* 1984; **28**: 105–111.

(23) Retief AE. *S Afr Med J* 1978; **52**: 745.

(24) Editorial. *S Afr Med J* 1977; **52**: 745.

(25) Muller I. Cordocentesis: percutaneous umbilical blood sampling. *S Afr Med J* 1989; **75**: 79.

(26) Swart RD, Nelson MM, Coetzee EJ. Ultrasound examination before amniocentesis. *S Afr Med J* 1981; **59**: 599.

(27) Op't Hof J. Juggling with lives. *Nursing RSA.* 1987; **2**: 13.

(28) Jenkins T. *S Afr Med J* 1973; **47**: 1834.

(29) Op't Hof J. Primary prevention of physical and mental handicaps. *Curationis.* 1982; **5**: 49.

(30) Oswald AH, Goldblatt J, Sampson G, Clokie R, Beighton P. Retinitis pigmentosa in South Africa. *S Afr Med J* 1985; **68**: 863–866.

TEST OF KNOWLEDGE

The student has benefited from studying this chapter if he/she can answer the following questions:

(1) Define the following pairs of words:
- Chromosomes and genes
- Barr body and fluorescent F body
- Transcription and translation (with respect to the transference of genetic information)
- DNA and RNA
- Aneuploidy and mosaicism
- Turner and Klinefelter syndromes
- Homozygous and heterozygous alleles
- Dominance and recessiveness with regard to the phenotype
- Genotype and phenotype

(2) Write an account of:
- (a) Autosomal recessive inheritance
- (b) Mutagenic and teratogenic agents and their locus of action
- (c) Congenital defects
- (d) X-linked inheritance
- (e) The diagnosis of, and prognosis in, cystic fibrosis
- (f) Ecogenetics and its role in coronary heart disease
- (g) The primary and secondary prevention of genetic conditions
- (h) Retinitis pigmentosa

(3) Give an account of the counselling role of the genetics sister after she has broken the news to the parents of a child with:
- (a) Cystic fibrosis
- (b) Congenital hypothyroidism
- (c) Down syndrome
- (d) Duchenne's muscular dystrophy

(4) Discuss the uses of the following diagnostic techniques:
- Chromosomal studies
- Neonatal screening
- Antenatal screening for alpha-fetoproteins
- Amniocentesis

9

Environmental Hygiene (Air and Soil) Soil Conservation

OBJECTIVE

The main objective of Chapters 9 and 10 is to make the student aware of the importance of the sanitary control of the environment in order to ensure the health of communities. Environmental health is essentially the responsibility of local government in its area of jurisdiction. All tiers of government can, however, be involved in the care of the environment, be it the air, the soil, water or food.

According to the Environment Conservation Act 73 of 1989, the Minister of Environment Affairs and the Premier of the province have the power to assume such responsibility in case of default by a local authority (section 31 of the Act), thus providing for effective protection and controlled utilisation of the environment.

STUDY OBJECTIVES

The student must get an understanding of:
(1) Environmental health and human welfare.
(2) The Environment Conservation Act 73 of 1989, especially its role in controlling environmental pollution.
(3) Air pollution, its causes, unfavourable effects and the main prescriptions of the Atmospheric Pollution Prevention Act which empower local authorities to define and enforce smoke control zones.

(4) The increasing pollution of the earth's surface by liquid and solid waste and the functions of a local authority under the Health Act 63 of 1977 to maintain its district in a clean and hygienic condition.
(5) The principles of sanitation as applied to the disposal of household refuse, domestic waste water and human excreta.
(6) The principles of soil conservation.

IN THIS CHAPTER

ENVIRONMENTAL HEALTH FUNCTIONS OF A LOCAL AUTHORITY (HEALTH ACT 63 OF 1977)

The functions of a local authority are governed by by-laws and regulations made by the local authority. By-laws are applicable in the area of jurisdiction of a specific local authority. There may be public health by-laws dealing with food handling and vending, production and sale of milk, restaurants and cafés. Building by-laws deal with lighting, ventilation, size of habitable rooms, etc.

The local authority may appoint a medical officer of health for the district of the local authority; if no such officer is appointed, the district surgeon is appointed as the medical officer of health (MOH). The local authority may also appoint one or more Environmental Health Officers and one or more registered nurses to assist the MOH in safeguarding the health of the inhabitants of its district. They work under the supervision of the MOH.

ENVIRONMENTAL HEALTH OFFICER (EHO) (HEALTH INSPECTOR)

The Health Inspector is an important member of the primary health care team and, therefore, works in the public sector: local, provincial or central government (Directories: Public Hygiene of the DOH). The training duration is four years at a technikon and the trained EHO must be registered with the professional board for Health Inspectors of the SA Medical Council (SAMDC).

The main sphere of activity of the EHO is the health of the environment and especially the impact on the latter caused by rapid urbanisation (e.g. squatter settlements on the periphery of cities), water and food pollution and the wastes generated by production and consumption (soil and air pollution).

The effective application of environmental health principles by health inspectors is of great importance to the success of the primary health care services. The training syllabus includes:

(a) The preventive health education and training of street food vendors and other food handlers in places that serve the public.

(b) Primary health care with regard to basic subsistence amenities (Level 1 of the National Health Plan, see p. 16), by the upgrading of basic facilities and the development of communities and populations.

(c) Health education.

(d) Prevention of endemic diseases.

e) Epidemiological research by health surveys.

According to the Health Act 63 of 1977, local authorities are charged with the provision of non-personal health services which include *environmental health.*

The following are the statutory functions under the Health Act of a local authority:

(1) The maintenance of hygiene and clean conditions in its district.

(2) The prevention of nuisances (see 'nuisance' p. 148), unhygienic and offensive conditions, and any other health hazards, such as the pollution of water supplies.

Environmental health services of the local authority (waste, water supply, communicable diseases, inspection of premises for nuisances and business premises e.g. for food and its handling, pest control, food poisoning, food, cosmetics and disinfectants, hazardous substances) are subsidisable provided they are conducted by medical officers of health, by regional medical officers of health, by health inspectors, by veterinary surgeons, by analytical chemists or by bacteriologists.

For subsidisable personal health services rendered by local authorities, refer to p.18.

ENVIRONMENTAL POLLUTION

Man is polluting his environment to an extent which is giving cause for anxiety about the continued existence of life on this planet. The increased production of the modern industrialised world is essential for the feeding and clothing of the vast population of the world, but the benefits of industrialisation are offset by the pollution of air, land and water, the earth's most important natural resources.

Research into the effects of environmental pollution on health is becoming increasingly important. In the RSA, research into environmental diseases is carried out by the Research Institute of Environmental Diseases (RIED) in Pretoria.

The Environment Conservation Act

In 1989 the Environment Conservation Act 73 of 1989 was passed (Department of Environment Affairs). The Act deals, *inter alia*, with government policy for environment conservation; the protection of the natural environment; the control of environmental pollution by prohibiting littering and prescribing waste management; the control of activities which may have detrimental effects on the environment (*inter alia*, water use and disposal, agricultural and industrial processes, transportation, waste and sewage disposal). The Act therefore provides for the effective protection and controlled utilisation of the environment.

'Prohibition of littering (section 19)

(1) No person shall discard, dump or leave any litter on any land or water surface, street, road or site in or on any place to which the public has access, except in a container or at a place which has been specially indicated, provided or set apart for such purpose.

(2) Every person or authority in control of or responsible for the maintenance of any place to which the public has access shall at all times ensure that containers or places are provided which will normally be adequate and suitable for the discarding of litter by the public. (Act 73/89)

Waste management (section 20)

(1) No person shall establish, provide or operate any disposal site without a permit by the Minister of Water Affairs and except subject to the conditions contained in such permit.

(6) Subject to the provisions of any other law no person shall discard waste or dispose of it in any other manner, except —

(*a*) at a disposal site for which a permit has been issued in terms of subsection (1); or

(*b*) in a manner or by means of a facility or method and subject to such conditions as the Minister (of Environment Affairs) may prescribe.'

The Act defines a 'disposal site' as follows: a site used for the accumulation of waste with the purpose of disposing or treatment of such waste.

'Litter' is defined as: any object or matter discarded by the person in whose possession or control it was.

'Waste' is defined as: any matter, whether gaseous, liquid or solid, or any combination thereof, originating from any residential, commercial, industrial or agricultural area, and identified by the Minister as an undesirable or superfluous by-product, emission, residue or remainder of any process or activity.

AIR POLLUTION

Pollution of air by products of combustion is of prime importance, but metal particles and dust in the air also cause much ill-health in our metropolitan areas. Air pollution in the form of smog causes damage to vegetation by screening all the ultraviolet rays of the sun. CFCs in the air damage the ozone layer.

Smoke

In South Africa coal is an important source of energy; coal stoves, hand-operated furnaces and open fireplaces which burn coal slowly at a low temperature so that it smoulders, emit black smoke with carbon particles and CO. These are important polluters of the environment. Fortunately fungi, e.g. *Aspergillus penicillium*, in the air metabolise CO to carbohydrates and protein, so CO pollution is not important. Mechanically operated furnaces do not emit black smoke but add SO_2, grit and ash to the air. The worst air pollution in the RSA occurs in Soweto.[2] In this city smoke from local fires exceeds WHO smoke recommended limits – sometimes doubling these limits – for more than a quarter of the year during the cold Highveld winters.

Industrial dust

Industrial dust includes silica, asbestos fibres, cement and fertiliser.

Metals

Lead is a dangerous atmospheric pollutant, the source being petrol fumes and lead-using industries (e.g. batteries, paints).

Iron dust and iron oxide fumes are emitted into the air from iron and steel industries. Many other metals used in industry may become occupational health hazards through inhalation as dust and fumes.

CFC (chlorofluoro-carbon)

CFC (Chlorofluoro-carbon) is a very useful industrial chemical. This chemical is used globally as follows:

(a) 50 % in aerosol spray cans.
(b) 20 % for refrigeration and air-conditioning units as coolant gases, especially on the mines.
(c) 30 % to produce polystyrene (foam plastic) containers.

Apart from certain cosmic events, human activities such as nuclear explosions, supersonic aircraft and the release of CFCs at surface level, destroy the ozone molecules, thereby thinning the ozone layer.

Ozone (O_3) — a powerful oxidising agent— is found in the atmosphere of the earth, either mixed with other gases near the surface, or as a dense layer (1 000 times the concentration of surface ozone) at a vertical height of 20–30 km in the stratosphere. This stable ozone layer which starts forming 10 km above the surface of the earth is formed by photochemical action on the atmospheric oxygen. The ozone layer does not mix with the surface ozone; it absorbs most of the solar ultraviolet radiation (UVL), thus protecting human and other forms of life.

Note: Too much UVL on the unprotected human skin, especially white skins, causes skin cancer.

The ozone layer is thinnest at the equator and therefore allows more UVL radiation to reach ground level.

Recently, we have become aware of damage to this layer in the form of regional thinning ('hole in the ozone layer') by the dissociation of ozone (O_3) to oxygen (O_2).

Unfavourable effects of some pollutants, and their prevention

(1) *Lead pollution* (of air and water) causes chronic nephritis, peripheral nerve damage, anaemia, abdominal colic and constipation. Children chronically exposed may develop hyperkinesis and lowering of intellectual potential. Dangerous blood levels are: 40,00g/dl for males and females past reproductive life, and 30,00g/dl for females of reproductive age.

Preventive measures (community):

(a) Lead pipes used for water reticulation systems should be replaced, as soft water flowing in lead pipes causes the pollution of water by lead.
(b) Petrol with low lead content should be used. In the RSA since 1986 the allowable lead content of petrol has been decreased from 0,8 g/ℓ to 0,6 g/ℓ. In the USA lead-free petrol is supplied. This is the ultimate intention of the RSA government.

Preventive measures (in lead-using industries):

(a) environmental control, e.g. adequate ventilation with extraction equipment;

(b) education of the workers in order to prevent avoidable pollution;

(c) adequate protective clothing, including respirators;

(d) regular blood and urine tests to screen those working in hazardous areas for early damage;

(e) air tests for lead content.

Note: Lead poisoning is a notifiable condition.

(2) *Iron pollution* causes siderosis of the tissues, chronic bronchitis, pneumoconiosis and diseases of the eyes. Preventive measures are as above.

(3) *The combination of dust, SO$_2$ and carbon particles* cause respiratory diseases which may become chronic and lead to premature death.

(4) *CFCs*

The destruction of the upper atmospheric protective ozone layer is a world problem which must be prevented by taking global measures to stop the production and use of CFCs. South Africa has signed the 1986 Montreal Protocol, which is binding on its sixty signatories, to phase out the manufacture and use of CFCs by the year 2000.

Ninety-six per cent of all aerosols used in the RSA are already free of CFCs (i.e. they are ozone-friendly). However, CFCs are still used for underground cooling in the mines because substitutes are more flammable.

Air pollution can be measured by passing air through a filter. The SO$_2$ dust, smoke (carbon particles) thus entrapped can be measured and expressed either as parts per million (ppm) or as micrograms per cubic metre air.

Acid rain

This term refers to the deposit of acid pollutants from the air in rainwater. These pollutants are:

(a) Dry: SO$_2$, nitrogen oxide and surface ozone.

(b) Wet: Sulphuric acid and nitric acid.

The pollutants issue mainly from the burning of coal and oil in industry, power stations and from vehicle exhaust. The pollutants may be deposited far from their course, carried there by the wind.

Apart from respiratory damage caused by inhaling the pollutant, the acid water damages life in the soil and in acidified lakes and rivers. Thereby these pollutants alter the ecological balance of nature and damage the means of producing food.

Prevention of general air pollution

The government has taken steps to minimise air pollution. The Atmospheric Pollution Prevention Act 45 of 1965 leaves the control of domestic smoke to local authorities, while the Department of Health is responsible for controlling the air pollution caused by industry.

According to the Atmospheric Pollution Prevention Amendment Act 17 of 1973, a local authority may declare an area within its jurisdiction to be a Smoke Control Zone and prohibit the emanation or emission from any premises in that zone of smoke of a darker colour or greater intensity or content than would obscure a certain percentage of light, usually 20 % but sometimes 10 % and at other times up to 40 %.

The local authority may appoint smoke control officers to enforce compliance with its rules. The law can prescribe the requirements with which any particular kind of fuel burning appliance shall comply.

If noxious or offensive gases are emitted from a vehicle, the local authority may stop and inspect the vehicle and take steps to prevent this. The local authority may prohibit the use of a public road by any vehicle from which noxious or offensive gases of a darker colour than permitted in the area are emitted.

In the domestic sector, coal stoves and open fireplaces can be replaced by electric and oil heaters or an anthracite burner. There are several smokeless coal stoves available to those who have no access to electricity. The local authority may give approval for the installation of any make, type or model of household fuel burning appliance, provided it is satisfied that such an appliance is capable of preventing smoke pollution.

No person shall burn any waste material on any premises, except in an approved fuel burning appliance, which shall be suitably provided with effective means of filtering and arresting all grits of a half mm and more in size, measured across any plane.

According to the Atmospheric Pollution Prevention Amendment Act 21 of 1981, no person shall manufacture or import –

(1) any fuel-burning appliance for use in a dwelling-house which does not comply with the requirements prescribed by regulation under section 44; or
(2) any part for such an appliance which does not comply with the requirements so prescribed, unless he has previously obtained written authority for the manufacture or import thereof from the chief officer.

Where chimneys are provided for the final emission of products of combustion of any liquid fuel, the chimneys shall be so constructed as to prevent the emission of particles carrying condensed sulphuric acid.

In industry, appliances (filters and electrostatic precipitators) can be built into chimneys to keep back dust and other impurities. Dirty industries, i.e. those in which air pollution cannot be prevented, must be built outside areas of human habitation.

The electrification of the majority of homes in South Africa, as part of the GNU's RDP, will do much to alleviate the problem of air pollution.

LAND POLLUTION BY LIQUID AND SOLID WASTE

The production of waste is a natural consequence of man's activities and the disposal of waste in urban communities is a very onerous and important task of the local authority. Adequate waste disposal to prevent pollution of the environment is becoming increasingly difficult for the following reasons:

(1) Rapid growth in the size of populations. The more people there are, the more waste they produce. Many modern industrial societies are very affluent and produce relatively greater amounts of waste.
(2) The trend towards urbanisation during the past 150 years has burdened towns and cities with a tremendous amount of solid waste.
(3) As cities grow and spread, it becomes more and more difficult to find land which is suitable for waste disposal within reason-

able distance of the dwellings and factories producing the waste.
(4) Industrialisation contributes to the problem of waste disposal by producing wastes which are either non-biodegradable (e.g. plastic material) or highly toxic and harmful to man, animals and plants, e.g. radioactive wastes, herbicides and pesticides.

In towns, cities and villages with local governments or their extensions, the RSCs, the latter are responsible for providing the services necessary for dealing with household and industrial waste.

The Health Act 63 of 1977 lays down in section 20 that:

'Every local authority shall take all lawful, necessary and reasonable practicable measures —
(a) to maintain its district at all times in a clean and hygienic condition;
(b) to prevent the occurrence within its district of —
  (i) any nuisance;
  (ii) any unhygienic condition;
  (iii) any offensive condition; or
  (iv) any other condition which will or could be harmful or dangerous to the health of any person within its district . . .'

The Act defines a *'nuisance'* as

'(a) any stream, pool, marsh, ditch, gutter, watercourse, cistern, water closet, earth closet, urinal, cesspool, cesspit, drain, sewer, dung pit, slop tank, ash heap or dung heap so foul or in such a state or so situated or constructed as to be offensive or to be injurious or dangerous to health;
(b) any stable, kraal, shed, run or premises used for the keeping of animals or birds and which is so constructed, situated, used or kept as to be offensive or to be injurious or dangerous to health;
(c) any accumulation of refuse, offal, manure or other matter which is offensive or is injurious or dangerous to health;
(d) any public building which is so situated, constructed, used or kept as to be unsafe, or to be injurious or dangerous to health;
(e) any occupied dwelling for which no proper and sufficient supply of pure water is available within a reasonable distance;

(*f*) any factory or industrial or business premises not kept in a clean state and free from
offensive smells arising from any drain,
water closet, earth closet, urinal or any other
source, or not ventilated so as to destroy or
render harmless or inoffensive as far as
practicable any gases, vapours, dust or other
impurities generated, or so overcrowded, or
so badly lighted or ventilated as to be injurious or dangerous to the health of those
employed therein or thereon;

(*g*) any factory or industrial or business premises causing or giving rise to smells or efflu-
via which are offensive or which are injurious or dangerous to health;' etc.

In areas which do not come under the jurisdiction of a local authority, the disposal of waste is
the responsibility of the individual.

The adequate disposal of waste, i.e. sanitation, involves dealing with it in such a way that
the quantity is reduced, pollution of land, air and
water is prevented and potentially dangerous
substances are rendered harmless. While the
quantity of waste in a large city may create a
problem, the main hazard of inadequate waste
disposal, particularly excreta, in the rural areas
is microbial contamination of the environment,
chiefly of water supplies.

The waste that has to be dealt with by all communities will include some or all of the following:

(1) household refuse;
(2) domestic waste water;
(3) human excreta (the drainage and disposal of
sewage and refuse from houses is called
sanitation);
(4) industrial waste;
(5) agricultural waste.

SANITATION (ENVIRONMENTAL HYGIENE)

Household refuse

This is solid waste and consists of left-over
food, peels, leaves, flowers, dust, eggshells, paper, cardboard, bottles, tins, plastic, etc. If not
adequately stored, regularly collected and disposed of, it can become a danger to health
because it attracts flies and rodents, decom-
poses, gives rise to odours and is unsightly, i.e.
it becomes a nuisance. Every household should

have a container with a lid in the kitchen to
receive refuse. This container is emptied into a
refuse bin with close-fitting lid to exclude flies,
cockroaches and rodents, in the backyard. Each
local authority will supply a regulation bin and
prescribe rules for collection of refuse and
maintenance of the bin. The householder pays
for these services. Some local authorities require that the bin be lined with a thin plastic bag
(supplied by the LA). The bag with the refuse is
removed from the bin, securely tied and put out
for collection on the stipulated day. This method
prevents the worker from coming into direct
contact with the refuse during collection and
also makes it easier to keep the refuse bin clean.
The refuse is usually collected once a week in
closed vehicles and taken for disposal.

Reducing the quantity of refuse for disposal

The quantity may be reduced in the following
ways.

(1) Householders should be encouraged to discard only the absolute minimum into their
refuse bins by keeping bottles and papers
separate and by making compost with all
vegetable matter. It is important, though,
that compost heaps be made correctly or that
the vegetable matter be buried in trenches,
so as to prevent flies breeding and smells.

(2) Sorting of rubbish and recycling useful material. Paper, aluminium, cardboard, tins and
glass should be removed before using the
refuse for land filling, either by getting the
householder to place these articles separately for collection, or by letting the refuse
disposal workers handsort the articles which
are later sold to factories for reuse. The
money received in this way goes towards
meeting the cost of the operation.

(3) Pulverisation of the solid waste to fine particles by special electrical machines is
sometimes done. Pulverisation is done
either by the householder, in which case the
waste is disposed of down the sewer, or by
the refuse disposal department of the local
authority, in which case the waste is tipped.

(4) Large hospitals with infectious waste sometimes use incineration as a means of disposal, but where smoke pollution becomes
a nuisance (e.g. from plastic syringes) infec-

tious waste, e.g. plastic syringes, needles and dressings, is first autoclaved. Bottles are removed. All waste is then compressed in large compressors. The greatly reduced quantity is then disposed of by the local authority by means of controlled tipping.

Final disposal so as to prevent pollution of air, land and water

The local authority disposes of the refuse by two common methods.

(1) *Incineration* in specially constructed furnaces at temperatures which are so high that pollution of the air by smoke and odours is obviated. Incineration causes complete destruction only of combustible material, hence the need here for pre-incineration sorting. The heat generated can be used for heating purposes and the ash and cinders for road building, the construction of cinder building blocks and for covering the refuse disposed of by controlled tipping. Incineration by the private householder in rural areas is not recommended as incinerators are not available, therefore burning is likely to be incomplete, thus causing a nuisance through smoke creation, smouldering heaps which are a danger especially to children and the blowing about of incompletely burned refuse.

(2) *Controlled tipping and land filling* is the method most frequently used by local authorities for the disposal of solid wastes. After ripping open the plastic bags to allow for decomposition of their contents, the refuse is deposited on carefully selected sites in layers of a specified depth, usually not more than two metres. Waste or derelict land, or land which has been excavated for some reason in the past, is used for the purpose. Care must be taken that contaminated water which filters out of the rubbish will not pollute underground or surface waters. The area is fenced off during the period when tipping takes place to prevent unauthorised visitors on the site and the blowing about of papers to the neighbouring areas while a tipping procedure is in operation. Useful articles are removed by the workers and tins are flattened to discourage rodents

breeding. Vehicles are used to spread the refuse evenly and to compact it firmly. Each day's refuse is covered with approximately 20 cm of earth or ash and cinders. This is done to prevent rodents, flies, and other insects gaining access to the refuse, to minimise the danger of outbreaks of fires, to prevent the escape of odours and to encourage water to run off the tip. At the end of the day, no refuse should remain uncovered. Some decomposition of organic material takes place and the tip gradually sinks down. Seven years after completion of tipping at a site, the ground should be sufficiently compact to be put to some useful purpose. In cities, playing-fields, sports grounds and parks have been laid out on such sites.

Both controlled tipping and incineration in furnaces are excellent methods of preventing the pollution of air, land and water, and of rendering potentially dangerous substances harmless. The judicious sorting of the refuse before disposal and the recycling of reusable material are economical ways of using rapidly dwindling resources and financing refuse disposal operations. Where refuse disposal is the responsibility of the individual, burying of the sorted refuse and using the organic material for land enrichment are the only practical methods of refuse disposal.

Domestic waste water

This comprises water which has been used for bathing, cooking, laundry and other domestic purposes. Where a town is served by a municipal sewerage system, the waste water is carried by the house drains into the sewers and then to the sewage disposal works. In rural areas, however, the householder has to dispose of it on his property. He should be educated to do this in such a manner that it will not attract flies, give rise to unpleasant odours or encourage the spread of disease. For these reasons it is most undesirable that waste water be discarded by throwing it out of the door or by letting it run in an open furrow into the garden or veld. Waste water may be used for irrigation purposes provided the soil is not waterlogged and the top layer is kept loosened so that the water may drain away and not accumulate in offensive puddles on the surface. A more satisfactory method of disposal is by means of the French drain.

The French drain (figure 9.1)

This is a trench dug in porous, sandy soil not nearer than 10 metres from the homestead or from a septic tank, filled with stones, broken

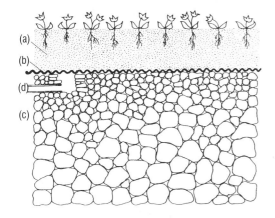

Figure 9.1

Section of a French drain

(a) Layer of soil
(b) Corrugated iron sheet
(c) Trench filled with stones
(d) Water inlet pipe

brick, and rubble and covered over with a sheet of corrugated iron and a layer of soil.

Waste water is led by means of pipes into the trench and percolates through the stones and rubble into the surrounding soil. As it seeps through the soil it is purified and the organic matter is broken down by aerobic and anaerobic bacteria. Grease must be removed from kitchen water before it enters the French drain to prevent clogging of the porous elements of the drain. A very simple grease trap may be constructed using an empty tin with holes in the bottom covered over with straw. Grease in the water flowing through the tin clings to the straw. The grease trap must be cleaned at intervals and the straw burned and replaced.

The disposal of human excreta

The safe disposal of human excreta is essential for the health of a community. Where sanitary amenities are lacking or inadequate, or where facilities for the treatment and disposal of excretion sewage are unsatisfactory, human excreta pose a grave threat to the health of individuals and communities. Excreta contain large numbers of pathogenic microbes as well as the ova of parasites, may attract flies and encourage their breeding, pollute the land and contaminate water and food.

The World Health Organisation estimates that about 1 400 million people in the less developed countries have no facilities for the disposal of excreta.

Rural black, developing, 'Third-World' areas of the RSA lack a potable (drinkable), adequate, reticulated (piped) water supply and, therefore, also a sewerage system. The lack of clean water and the inadequate disposal of excreta were responsible for the recent cholera epidemics in the rural areas of the RSA. It stands to reason that if these deficiencies could be redressed, the health of people would improve.

Yet for these amenities of a developed country to function adequately in preventing infectious disease, the community must accept and practise personal hygiene and understand the role of pure water in preventing disease, i.e. even pure water can be contaminated by unhygienic carriers. Moreover, the water reticulation and sewerage systems must be adequately maintained by the population. The sewerage system is liable to break down owing to blockages if not properly maintained; for correct functioning, it needs a liberal supply of water which is lacking in large parts of the RSA.

Education in personal hygiene in addition to a pure water supply and alternatives to a sewerage system for the safe disposal of excreta are, therefore, the main requisites for the prevention of waterborne gastro-intestinal diseases in Third-World countries.

Human excreta are disposed of either with or without the aid of water. When human excreta are mixed with water, including industrial and domestic waste water, it is called **sewage**. Sewage consists of 99,9 % water and 0,1 % organic, inorganic and microbial solids. The liquid sewage (effluent) flows in sewers (covered underground drains) to central sewage disposal works, or into individual household septic tanks.

The small room or closet where evacuation of bowel and bladder should ideally take place is called a **latrine** or a **privy**. The latrine may be either an earth-closet (i.e. over a hole in the ground), or pail-closet or a water-closet (lavatory or loo) over a porcelain bowl (pan) connected to a water cistern, the water being used to flush excreta some distance away for disposal.

In South Africa most urban communities in cities and towns are served by sewage disposal works, but in black rural areas, on farms, in small villages and temporary camps, the householder or camp manager is responsible for the disposal of excreta on a small scale. This can be done in one of the following ways.

The pit privy

A simple, removable superstructure is placed over a hole (pit) dug in the earth, size approximately 3 metres deep and 1 metre square. On ground level, a concrete slab with hole in it is placed over the pit and the slab is surmounted with a wooden seat with lid. The tight-fitting lid should be kept closed to prevent flies reaching the contents of the pit. The solids in the pit are broken down by the action of anaerobic bacteria and the liquids seep out of the pit into the surrounding soil. In order to preserve the anaerobic bacteria, no disinfectants should be used, but the contents may be covered with ash or soil, a supply of which is kept in the privy for periodic use. Such a privy will serve a family for about 8 to 10 years. When the contents have risen to within 1 metre of the top, the slab is removed and the pit completely filled in with soil. A fresh pit is dug and the superstructure relocated on a new pit.

The Ventilated Improved Pit (VIP) latrine is a great boon in rural areas. It is used throughout the world and is odourless and fly-free.

The Phungalutho VIP latrine is a waterless toilet invented by the Institute of Natural Resources of the University of Natal. The pit is sited behind the latrine superstructure to prevent collapse of the toilet pedestal into the pit.

The pit has an elevated dome-shaped cover on top, the latter being perforated by an air vent pipe which allows the circulation of air through the pedestal opening into the pit; the air and odorous gases escape through the air vent pipe to the atmosphere. The opening of the pipe is covered with gauze to prevent the escape of flies from the pit.

The outhouse and elevated pit cover are constructed by stamping a mixture of cement and subsoil/or sand into bought moulds, using chicken wire for support.

Pit and bored hole privies (earth-closets) are the simplest and least expensive method of disposing of human excreta, provided the privy is carefully sited and constructed. The most important dangers associated with the use of earth-closets are the contamination of underground water supplies and fly-borne infection. An earth-closet should be sited at a safe distance from any underground water supply, but it is difficult to specify what a 'safe distance' is, as this depends upon the nature of the soil. In some soil formations, seepage from an earth-closet will be rendered free from microbes after it has filtered through the soil for only a few centimetres, while in others, e.g. dolomite formations, microbes may be carried many metres. For this reason it is wise to site the earth-closet at least 30 metres from a well. Wherever possible, waterlogged ground should be avoided and the privy should be on a lower level than the well or borehole.

Pail privy

These privies are sometimes used in semi-rural areas where stands are too small to allow for the use of earth-closets, or in new suburbs before the houses are connected to the town sewers.

Two pails should be provided for each privy so that the full pail with well-secured lid can be removed, ideally through an aperture at the back of the superstructure, for cleaning and repair after emptying, and the second pail left in its place.

Where the local authority arranges for the removal of the pails, usually twice a week at night (hence the term 'night soil'), the contents are emptied either into the town sewers (if these are available) or into long trenches dug in a selected site on the outskirts of the village, fresh trenches being dug for each night's collection and filled no deeper than 60 cm from the top before being filled in with soil. Care should be taken that seepage does not contaminate the surface of the soil.

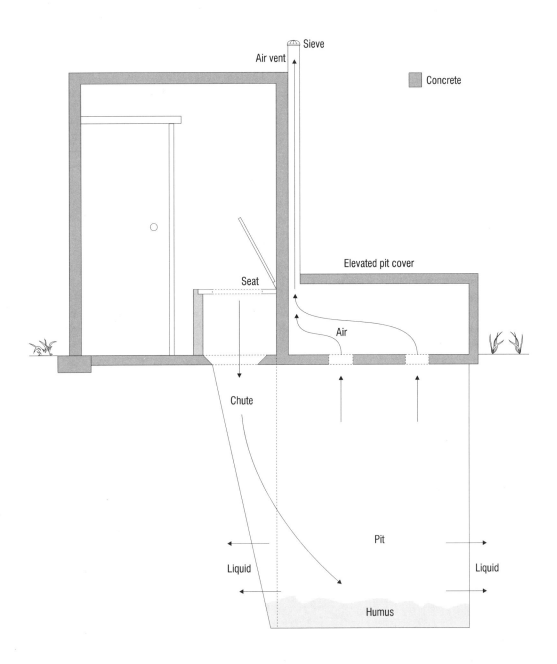

Figure 9.2
VIP (Ventilated Improved Pit) latrine

The use of pail privies and the burial of excreta in trenches is not a satisfactory method of dealing with human excreta and, for the following reasons, should not be used if alternative methods are available.

(1) It is impossible to prevent flies reaching the contents of the pails.
(2) If the pail is not correctly positioned beneath the seat, the space between the seat and the pail becomes soiled and offensive.
(3) If pails are not frequently removed, they become offensive.
(4) Pail privies involve the handling of fresh excreta by the workers who have to remove and empty the pails.

Chemical closets

These consist of specially designed pails or tanks which receive the excreta and a device which delivers a chemical into the pail. These chemicals break down and liquefy the contents of the pail, destroying all the microbes. Chemical closets are used on aircraft and in caravans.

Water-closets

Water-closets are used where septic tanks or sewers and a sewage treatment plant are available. The outlet pipe of a water-closet pan is in the form either of a p-trap or an S-trap, depending upon whether the pipe goes through the outside wall of the building or through the floor. The trap ensures that a water seal remains at the bottom of the toilet pan. This seal prevents gases from the sewer or septic tank from entering the building. The outlet pipe connects to the house drain which is extended upwards as the air vent pipe to allow for the escape of gases. In the house drain, before it enters the septic tank or sewer, there is an 'Inspection Eye', covered with a removable concrete slab, which gives access to the drain in case of blockage.

The septic tank

The septic tank is a method of sewage disposal which is being used by an ever-increasing number of private homes, holiday camps, hotels and motels in rural areas. As water is necessary to flush the contents of the pan into the septic tank,

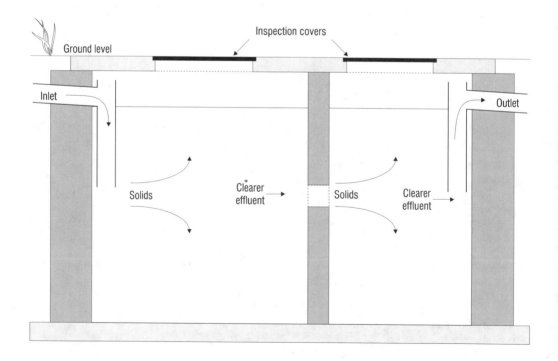

Figure 9.3
Septic tank

this method requires the building to have a piped water supply. The sanitary fittings in the toilet (water-closet) are of the conventional type.

A septic tank is an underground tank built of brick and plastered on the inside to make it airtight. It has an inlet pipe which conveys sewage into the tank and an outlet pipe which carries the liquid effluent to a French drain situated approximately 10 metres from the septic tank.

Note: Waste water from the laundry, bathroom and kitchen must not be run into the septic tank. Inspection covers are fitted on the tank for cleaning purposes; this may become necessary if anaerobic breakdown of excreta is interfered with (see later). A layer of scum (sludge), 10 cm thick, forms on the surface of the effluent, thus excluding air and providing ideal conditions for the growth and multiplication of anaerobic bacteria which are responsible for the breakdown and liquefaction of the solids in the sewage. The clear effluent which flows from the septic tank to the French drain has been partly purified. As it percolates into the soil from the drain, further purification takes place.

A septic tank will function efficiently for many years if it has been properly constructed and cared for. The following precautions must be meticulously followed in caring for a septic tank, in order to facilitate the breakdown of solids:

(1) No disinfectant may be used as it may kill the anaerobic bacteria.
(2) No cigarette butts or sanitary pads may be flushed down the toilet.
(3) Only toilet paper may be used in the toilet.

The sewage pit

This pit is like a septic tank and has the same aboveground fittings. It has no outlet into a French drain, however, and requires to be emptied by a municipal vacuum tank weekly to monthly, depending upon the use made of the pit. The contents of the vacuum tank are treated at a sewage treatment (disposal) works.

The sewage treatment (disposal) works

Sewage — domestic and industrial effluent — is carried by underground channels, called sewers, to the sewage disposal works which, of necessity, are situated outside the boundaries of the city or town, on a level lower than the latter to facilitate the flow of the sewage.

Principles

Treatment of the incoming raw sewage

(1) The sewage is first passed through *screens* to remove larger solid matter such as rags, paper and numerous other objects which people throw into sewers. Screens are constructed of parallel metal bars set at an angle to the flow of the sewage. The solids which accumulate against these bars are removed and either burned or buried.

(2) After screening, the sewage passes through *grit chambers called detritus (gravel) tanks.* Here the rate of flow of the sewage is slowed down to allow smaller solids such as coarse sand and gravel, which would cause damage to the plant, to settle out.

(3) From the grit chambers the sewage passes to large conical tanks, the *primary settlement tanks*, where the separation of the finer solids from the liquid takes place. In the primary settlement tanks, the sinkable solids, as well as a large amount of suspended solids, are removed. The solid material which sinks to the bottom is known as *sludge*, while the liquid which remains on top is called the *effluent*. Both the sludge and the effluent contain pathogens and must be subjected to further treatment to render them harmless.

Treatment of sludge

The raw sludge from the primary settlement tanks undergoes 'digestion' for three weeks in large metal tanks, known as *digestors*. The digestors are closed and heated to a temperature of 27 °C to 32 °C. Here the sludge is broken down by anaerobes and facultative aerobes to a blackish, harmless, granular material with a characteristic but not unpleasant odour. During the process of digestion gases, mainly methane, are released. Methane is used for many purposes, including the heating of the digestors. At the same time, nitrogen-containing substances are converted to nitrites and then to nitrates and carbohydrates and substances containing cellulose are broken down to carbon dioxide and water.

The wet sludge is removed from the digestors after three weeks and spread out on sludge drying beds to allow for the evaporation of water. The *dried sludge* is finally disposed of either by burning, tipping on selected sites or by using it for the fertilisation of farm lands. Sludge should never be used on gardens where animals and human beings may become infested with parasitic ova. It is used for fertilising vegetation such as trees and maize.

Note: Parasitic ova can resist the digesting process in the digestor.

At some sewage purification works the '*activated sludge*' method of sewage treatment is used. In this method, activated sludge is mixed with the incoming raw sewage and the mixture is thoroughly aerated, either by allowing compressed air to bubble through it from the bottom of aeration tanks or by means of mechanical surface aerators which keep the liquid in the tank continually violently agitated. Aeration of the liquid not only supplies the necessary aerobic conditions but also keeps the material in suspension, thereby allowing the activated sludge to come in contact with all the incoming sewage. The 'activated sludge' method offers some hope of meeting the requirements for purity of effluent of the Water Act of 1956.

The Water Act 54 of 1956 makes it unlawful for effluents (from sewage plants) which have not been subjected to treatment and which do not meet certain requirements to be run into rivers and/or streams.

Treatment of effluent

The effluent is led to a *biological filter* — a big circular tank filled with little stones on which live millions of maggots of a small fly, harmless to human beings. The effluent is spread over the surface of this filter by a revolving, perforated arm; as the effluent trickles through the stones, the maggots feed on the substances in colloidal suspension in the effluent and add humus (excreta) to the effluent which is led from there to secondary settlement tanks. Here the humus settles to the bottom and is returned to the primary settlement tanks and from there to the digestor.

The effluent is further purified either by being run on to *sand filter beds* or subjected to *land filtration in reed beds*, or by being used for *surface irrigation* on the farm lands belonging to the sewage works. The undesirable qualities of effluent include over-enrichment of the water with nutrients, especially nitrogen and phospho-

rus which can, however, be removed by a biological process.

Sewage purification usually reduces the pathogenic microbial content to 1 %. Chlorination reduces the content even further.

Effluents which meet certain standards may be discharged into rivers and streams. Sometimes the effluent is *chlorinated* before being run into streams. Effluent from sewage purification works may be recycled, i.e. subjected to intensive treatment and then used for industrial or other purposes such as cooling plants at power stations. In Windhoek use is made of recycled water for domestic purposes.

For the recycling of sewage effluent in South Africa, see p. 177.

THE PRINCIPLES OF SOIL CONSERVATION

Soil conservation means the building up of the productive potential of the top layers of the soil. Survival of all life on earth is dependent upon the productive capacity, i.e. the potential, of the crust of the earth. The soil supports the growth of vegetable matter and is the source not only of our food but also of our clothing, raw materials for our industries and food for our slaughter animals. Concern with the conservation of the top layer of the earth's crust implies that there is danger of losing this precious layer of soil.

The blowing and the washing away of the vital topsoil is called *soil erosion*. If erosion is allowed to continue unhampered, bare rocks eventually become exposed and networks of dongas are created. Not more than a quarter of the soil lost annually comes from dongas — the rest is from the ground surface. This loss is more serious than that from dongas as it comprises the finest and most fertile particles of soil which support growth, leaving behind the unproductive and heavier sand, gravel and stone. In South Africa there is an alarming annual loss of topsoil which is carried away by the wind and water to the sea; the danger is especially great because of inconsistent rainfall and poor soil. Whereas the natural vegetation conserves the topsoil for thousands of years, soil denuded of vegetation is carried away by the wind and water within a few years. Soil erosion and drought are interrelated problems, drought arising in areas which have become denuded of their covering layer of vegetation, thereby creating deserts which cannot support life.

Apart from the loss of productive potential, soil erosion causes other damage. Part of the solids carried by flood waters may be deposited *en route* and may silt up rivers and dams. This eventually leads to flooding of river valleys and a reduction in the storage capacity of dams. In the interest of water conservation, this necessitates the constant building of new storage dams. The growth of vegetation depends upon the moisture content and fertility of the soil. If the top layers of soil are exploited without being nurtured, their productive potential is destroyed. Soil potential is virtually irreplaceable as the repair costs of mismanaged, exhausted soil are prohibitively high. Soil fertility depends, in the first place, on the texture of the soil which must allow for the entrance to the plant roots of oxygen and nitrogen from the air. In the second place, fertility depends on the presence of organic matter — humus and bacteria. In the third place, it depends on the minerals: phosphorus, calcium and potassium, as well as trace elements: copper, boron, iron, cobalt, magnesium, manganese, zinc, molybdenum, iodine, fluorine, etc. Deficiencies and imbalances of these trace elements caused by inexpert farming practices affect the plant metabolism and the quality of the food grown for man and beast. There are even indications that low soil fertility, due to deficiency of trace elements, may be associated with cancer of the oesophagus, a disease which is common amongst Transkeian blacks.

The roots of plants bind the top layer of the soil and prevent it from being blown and washed away. The presence of vegetation impedes the progress of running water, thus allowing it to penetrate into the soil. South Africa has relatively small areas of arable land suitable for the cultivation of crops, almost 80 % of all agricultural land being utilisable as pastures only. Some crops, such as maize and sunflowers, afford poor protection for the topsoil. Continuous maize production causes rapid soil erosion; a sloping field of maize could lose 80 tons of soil per hectare a year if the rainfall is heavy. If maize is grown in rotation with other crops, however, the topsoil is bound effectively and soil loss is reduced.

The most important cause of soil erosion in South Africa is overgrazing and poor pasture management. Cattle have a very important social function among the black peoples and the running of large herds of cattle on exhausted veld has done irreparable harm to large tracts of veld. Overstocked pastures cause not only malnourishment of the animals but also close cropping of the vegetation by the starved animals. Consequently the soil cannot hold nor absorb the rain-water, the natural grasses die out, bare patches appear and weeds which are unpalatable to the animals take over.

In South Africa there is a tremendous need for the education of the general public with regard to the need for, and methods of, soil conservation. Vast quantities of valuable, irreplaceable soil are carried away to the sea annually, deterioration of pastures and denudation of large tracts of agricultural land continue despite efforts at conservation of the soil which started before the last war. The government is trying by appropriate legislation and education of farmers to halt the destruction of our soil potential. The judicious use of our greatest natural asset, our soil, is important to everyone, farmer and city dweller alike. Farmers, however, assume the greater responsibility for the task. For the past 50 years an Agricultural Extension Service has been in operation; extension officers are available to advise farmers on what to grow and on how to contour sloping ground in order to prevent the washing away of soil during heavy rains.

The following measures protect the current potential of the soil and restore damage done in the past:

(1) Soil conserving practices such as crop rotation with soil-binding crops (lucerne, teff and wheat); the addition of humus to the soil in the form of manure and compost and by the planting of green manure (lupins, Sunn hemp and cowpeas) which is ploughed into the soil, thus enriching it with nitrogen and water-holding humus.

(2) Prevention of flood damage to crops and to lands by the contouring of sloping ground and by the construction of furrows to control the flow of flood water.

(3) The adjustment of livestock numbers to co-incide with the grazing capacity of the pas-tures. The rotation of natural pasture lands (veld) enables the farmer to rest and increase the carrying capacity of the veld. With good veld management, sheep and beef cattle can live on the veld for most of the year, requir-ing only minimal supplementary feeding. To arrest the early deterioration of the veld by propaganda and education is more impor-tant than vast impressive schemes to reclaim land which is in an advanced state of dete-rioration with dongas and invasions of use-less weeds.

(4) The special care of vulnerable tracts of land, e.g. mountain slopes, denuded and eroded surfaces and water courses.

The Soil Conservation Act 45 of 1946 empow-ers the Division of Soil Conservation and Ex-tension of the Department of Agricultural Eco-nomics and Marketing to expropriate land and/or proclaim soil conservation districts, elect soil conservation district committees and assist farmers with the constructing of conservation works. The duties of the division include: pas-ture research, weed eradication and erosion con-trol.

Weed control: the encroachment of useless or noxious weeds on both arable and grazing lands is the full responsibility of the govern-ment, as laid down in the Weeds Act 42 of 1937.

The battle against soil erosion, weed en-croachment and water shortage has not been won despite heroic measures by the state to conserve the soil and build dams. During the war years (1939–45) the National Veld Trust came into being. The primary objective of this body of public-spirited men and women is to arouse public interest in the conservation of the soil. It is as important now as it was then to be aware of the need to conserve our natural re-sources and to take active measures, either by disseminating propaganda or by taking practical measures, to make the conservation ideal a prac-tical reality. The land belongs to the people of a country and poor farming practices constitute a threat to all, because they threaten the country's food supply and health. All the mineral wealth contained below the layer of topsoil will not save the people from starvation and indifferent health due to poor nutrition if the soil is not enriched and able to hold water. We must sup-port the vital covering layer of vegetation — our guarantee against the encroaching desert which does not support life, no matter how rich the subterranean mineral deposits may be.

REFERENCES

(1) Shaun Mackay. Fast Facts. *SAIRR* No. 3/1994

(2) *Race Relations Survey* 1992/1993 p. 151.

TEST OF KNOWLEDGE

The student has benefited from studying this chapter if he/she can answer the following ques-tions:

(1) Give a brief account of the laws in the RSA which deal with environmental health.

(2) Discuss subsidisable health services ren-dered by local authorities.

(3) Write notes on:
   The pit privy and the VIP latrine
   The septic tank and the sewage pit
   A French drain
   A nuisance (as defined by Act 63 of 1977)
   Controlled tipping of solid refuse

(4) Discuss the prevention of general air pollu-tion.

(5) Define:
   (a) litter (Act 73 of 1989)
   (b) waste (Act 73 of 1989)
   (c) sanitation
   (d) sewerage
   (e) soil erosion
   (f) sludge
   (g) sewage
   (h) organic farming

(6) Enumerate the methods by which solid re-fuse can be condensed and finally disposed of so as to prevent air, land and water pollu-tion.

(7) Describe the respective treatments of sludge and effluent at a sewage disposal works.

(8) Describe national measures that can be taken to conserve tracts of agricultural land for food production and animal husbandry.

10

Environmental Hygiene (Food and Water)
Water Conservation

OBJECTIVES

To make the student aware of the importance for health of a supply of pure food and water, how these commodities can be polluted and how their quality can be ensured.

STUDY OBJECTIVES

The student is first introduced to the legal aspect of food control. The microbial and chemical pollution of milk, as well as the toxic, chemical and microbial contamination of food, are discussed. Meat carries the special hazard in that certain diseases of animals can be transmitted to man through the consumption of meat.

The student is then introduced to extracts or summaries of regulations of food-related laws. These regulations control the safety of milk and its production in milking sheds, as well as its transport to the depots for sale to the public. A brief summary of the food-handling regulations is given.

The student must know how diseases spread by infected meat are controlled and the new regulations with regard to the transport of meat and the microbiological standards for cooked poultry, one of the most popular 'fast foods', especially in urban societies.

The student must become familiar with South Africa's water problems and the sources of water. The subject of water pollution is an important study objective. Since cholera became endemic in South Africa, especially among rural blacks, the purification of water for a single household has become an important education topic for the community nurse. The nurse must also grasp the principles of the purification of water at large regional water purification works.

Lastly, the subject of water conservation needs careful study, especially the recycling of sewage effluent, as the nurse needs to believe in its safety if her task is to persuade a water deficient urban community of the acceptability of such a source of water for domestic needs.

IN THIS CHAPTER

INTRODUCTION

It is of the utmost importance that food and milk be produced, processed, stored and prepared in such a way that their consumption will not endanger health. To ensure the safety of food and milk in the RSA, the following Acts of Parliament have been passed.

The Fertilisers, Farm Feeds, Agricultural Remedies and Stock Remedies Act 36 of 1947, as amended, controls the use of substances which may result in excessively harmful residues in agricultural products.

The Foodstuffs, Cosmetics and Disinfectants Act 54 of 1972 empowers the Minister of National Health and Population Development to prohibit the sale of foodstuffs which may be dangerous to health, or which contain a harmful substance or which do not conform to certain standards which are laid down. The Act allows for the appointment of inspectors who may inspect foodstuffs and take samples for analysis.

Regulations under this Act make it an offence for any person to sell milk which contains pathogenic micro-organisms of more than a specified number of 'colony-forming bacterial units' per 1,0 ml. A local authority health department may take samples of milk or milk products to be tested bacteriologically in order to ascertain the purity or impurity of the products. Where it is found that the milk does not conform to these standards, the responsible person may be prosecuted.

Whereas the Department of Health is responsible for controlling the bacteriological content of milk, the Department of Agricultural Economics and Marketing is responsible for controlling the composition of milk. In terms of regulations under the *Marketing Act 59 of 1968*, nothing may be added to milk or removed from it except cream; different classes of milk, for example skimmed milk, low-fat milk, fresh milk and high-fat milk, are defined and certain compositional standards are laid down. It is the function of the Department of Agricultural Economics and Marketing to ensure that the composition of milk complies with these requirements.

THE POLLUTION OF MILK

The safety of milk is threatened by the presence of chemicals secreted by the cow and by the introduction at source and subsequently of microbes which multiply rapidly in this ideal medium for microbial growth, particularly when it is warm.

Milk-borne infections

There are many important diseases which may be transmitted by infected milk. Milk products such as cream, ice-cream and cheese may also be the vehicle of transmission of these diseases. Milk is defined by the Health Act (1977) as: 'milk derived from cows, ewes, goats, mares or asses, and includes skimmed milk, buttermilk and cream, but does not include powdered milk or condensed milk contained in hermetically sealed receptacles'.

Pathogenic microbes may gain entry to the milk at any point along the line from the source to the consumer.

(1) If a *cow is diseased* the causative organism may be present in the milk and infection in man results from the ingestion of raw milk. The most important pathogens transmitted in this way are the following:
   (a) *Mycobacterium bovis* which is responsible for non-pulmonary tuberculosis in man;
   (b) *Brucella abortus* which is the causative organism of undulant fever in human beings (in cows it causes contagious abortion);
   (c) Streptococci of various types which are responsible for mastitis in cows and cause sore throats and scarlet fever in human beings;
   (d) Staphylococci which may be the cause of food poisoning;
   (e) Salmonellae — if cows are suffering from salmonellosis or diarrhoea which causes food poisoning in human beings.
(2) *Pathogens may gain access* to milk if the milkers or dairy workers are sufferers from or carriers of diseases such as typhoid fever, cholera, tuberculosis, diphtheria, streptococcal infections of the throat, dysentery and infective hepatitis.

(3) The use of *unclean utensils or impure water* and the exposure of milk to flies and dust may also result in bacterial contamination.

The chemical pollution of milk

The presence of pathogenic micro-organisms is not the only danger associated with the consumption of cow's milk; *antibiotics* may be present in the milk of cows which have been treated for infections, and *pesticides* and other chemical substances may pollute pastures or feed and find their way into the milk.

The use of pesticides has increased recently because of the urgent need to control insect-borne epidemics and to prevent the destruction of crops. The discovery of the indestructible chlorinated hydrocarbon insecticides, DDT and dieldrin, in the tissues of human beings, especially in human milk, has caused much alarm. Their everyday use by the householder has been discontinued by law in South Africa. DDT was not at first considered dangerous for animals and human beings, provided certain precautions were taken to prevent massive absorption into the body. It is a contact poison for insects, especially useful for the destruction of mosquitoes in malarious areas (see p. 72) and, for this reason, indispensable for large-scale malaria eradication programmes. The resistance of the chlorinated hydrocarbon insecticides to destruction, however, causes them to accumulate in the environment and in human and animal bodies. As they are nerve poisons, their long-term effects are not yet known.

LEGAL CONTROL OF MILK AND MILK PRODUCTS

In terms of section 15(1) of the Foodstuffs, Cosmetics and Disinfectants Act 54 of 1972, read with section 15(7) of the said Act, the Minister of National Health and Population Development made regulations R. 258 (February 1985) and R. 1256 (June 1986) relating to:

(1) restrictions on the sale of milk and milk products;
(2) milking sheds;
(3) milk containers and milking machines;
(4) dairy stock and milk;
(5) milkers and handlers of milk, and
(6) transport of milk.

Many restrictions are placed on the sale of milk and milk products. Only the restrictions of importance for the community health nurse will be quoted from R. 258.

'No person shall sell any:

2. raw milk intended for further processing
3. raw milk, cream, skim milk, reconstituted milk, reconstituted skim milk
4A. pasteurised milk, reconstituted milk, skim milk, reconstituted skim milk, cream
4B. sterilised cream, milk, reconstituted or UHT cream or milk
5. milk products or composite dairy products which contain —
   (*a*) antibiotics or other antimicrobial substances
   (*b*) pathogenic organisms, extraneous matter or any inflammatory product or other substances which for any reason whatsoever may render such product unfit for human consumption.

which are not packed in a closed package (2, 3, 5) or hermetically sealed package (4A, 4B, 5) when sold to the ultimate consumer.

Additional restrictions in the case of 3, 4A, 4B, 5

which do not meet the compositional standards prescribed for such products in the regulations under the Marketing Act 59 of 1968.

Additional restrictions in the case of 3

which are not derived from herds certified by a veterinarian as free from Brucellosis (undulant fever) or tuberculosis . . .

Additional restrictions in the case of 5

which in the case of milk powder or skimmed milk powder contain more than 50 000 colony-forming units of viable bacteria per gram.
   6. No person shall sell any milk product or composite dairy product which contains any additive not permitted by regulation.'

To ensure that milk is free from harmful pathogens, it must be subjected to one of the following processes before it may be supplied to the public.

Pasteurisation

This is a process whereby all pathogenic micro-organisms in the milk are destroyed by means of heat. Pasteurisation will not alter the taste or the appearance of the milk.

One of two methods may be used.

(1) In the first, the milk is heated to a temperature of at least 63 °C and kept at that temperature for at least 30 minutes, then cooled. This is known as the 'holder' or the 'batch' method.
(2) The second method is the 'High Temperature Short Time Method' which involves heating the milk to 72 °C for 15 seconds and then cooling it rapidly to below 10 °C (5 °C).

There are various tests which may be carried out by health authorities to determine whether milk has been adequately pasteurised.

After pasteurisation, milk is sealed in approved containers, or bottled and capped by mechanical means, and then distributed.

All milk shops in a municipal area must be in possession of a licence from the local authority and must comply with certain requirements.

Ultra-high temperature treatment (UHT)

Milk may be subjected to a temperature of above 135 °C for one or more seconds; this is known as '*ultra-high temperature treatment*'. It is aseptically packed and should still be free from spoilage by microbes after 14 days incubation at 30 °C.

Sterilisation

Milk can also be *sterilised*; this means that it has been 'rendered free from viable organisms' by exposure to temperatures of over 100 °C, usually after it has undergone preheating and bottling or hermetic sealing in a package.

Extracts from regulation R. 258 of February 1985 (Act 54 of 1972)

'(xxvi) "sterilisation" shall mean the process whereby a product in its hermetically sealed package is subjected to heat treatment to such a degree as to remain free from viable micro-organisms, and the terms "sterilise" and "sterilised" shall be construed accordingly; and

(xxvii) "UHT" or "ultra-high temperature treatment" shall mean the process whereby the milk or milk product concerned is exposed for one or more seconds to temperatures above 135 °C and is aseptically packed so as to ensure that the finished product, after being incubated for not less than 14 days at a temperature of 30 °C ± 1 °C, is free from spoilage by micro-organisms.'

SUMMARY OF MILK-HANDLING REGULATIONS (R. 1256)

Cows

Cows should be *healthy* and free from disease or lesions on the udders. A medical officer of health, a veterinarian, or health inspector employed by a local authority may inspect any dairy stock and a person who owns dairy stock may be required to have cows examined by a veterinarian. Animals which are diseased should be removed from the rest of the herd and the milk from such animals must be destroyed. It is the responsibility of the owner of a dairy herd to have the animals inoculated against certain diseases such as anthrax, brucellosis and any other diseases for which a medical officer may prescribe. The animals should also be clean and well groomed. The hair on the flanks and round the udders should be kept clipped. Cows should graze on uncontaminated pastures and an adequate supply of clean water should be available.

Workers

Milkers and dairy workers should not be *sufferers* or *carriers* of any disease. A medical officer of health or medical practitioner may examine any person working on the premises of a dairy farm, dairy or milk shop in a municipal area and carry out any tests which he may think necessary. No person who refuses or fails to submit himself to such examination may be employed in such a capacity; neither may anyone who is suspected of being a carrier of typhoid or any other disease which may be transmitted by milk.

All persons handling milk or milk products must be supplied with clean overalls of a light colour which must be kept in a locker when not in use. The highest standards of personal hygiene must be maintained at all times, hands must be washed and nails scrubbed before starting work and after going to the toilet. Employers must provide sufficient change-rooms, wash basins and showers with hot and cold running water, soap, nail-brushes and clean towels.

Premises

Premises used as a milking shed must include a *milk parlour*, a milk room, a scullery, and change-rooms and latrines for the employees.

The *milk parlour* (cowshed) shall at all times be maintained in a clean and sanitary state and in good repair, manure must be removed after milking sessions and the floor must be washed down. The milk parlour must comply with the requirements laid down in R. 1256 (1986) with regard to size, materials used in construction, lighting and ventilation. Walls must be smooth and painted with light-coloured washable paint, and the floor must be of an impervious material which should be readily cleanable. There should be an adequate supply of pure, piped water. Satisfactory arrangements must be made for the disposal of the manure which may not be allowed to accumulate for more than 24 hours within 15 metres of any place where milk is handled. In addition, steps must be taken to prevent fly breeding.

Method of milking

Cows may be milked by hand or machine. Before milking, the udders and teats must be thoroughly washed and dried. If the cows are being milked by hand, the milkers' hands must be washed and the teats lubricated with an approved lubricant. The practice of dipping hands into the milk for lubrication must not be allowed. The milk-pails should be clean, in a good state of repair and seamless. When full they should be covered and removed to a milk room as soon as possible. If milking machines are used, steps should be taken to ensure that they do not become a source of infection.

The *milk room* should be separate from the milk parlour, the only communication between them being by means of 'an aperture of minimum size necessary to accommodate the apparatus used for the transfer of milk from the milk parlour to such milk room'. The milk room should be fly proof and adequately lighted and ventilated. In the milk room, milk must be strained and cooled down to not more than 5 °C, as quickly as possible. All utensils used for milk must be cleaned immediately after use and sterilised.

The milk may now be *pasteurised and bottled* on the premises or transported in cans or stainless steel milk-tankers to a central depot, for pasteurisation or sterilisation and distribution to milk shops or direct to homes.

CARE OF MILK IN THE HOME

Milk should not be left standing in the sun (e.g. if it is delivered to the house). As soon as the milk is received, the outside of the container should be washed and the milk placed in a cool, dark place, preferably a refrigerator. Where this is not possible (and it should be remembered that by far the greatest proportion of the population do not own refrigerators) it can be placed in a basin of cold water, covered with a wet cloth and kept in the draught in front of an open window.

If milk has not been pasteurised, it should be boiled for a few minutes to ensure that it is free from pathogens. Boiling does not, however, prevent future contamination of the milk, and boiled milk should be used as soon as possible.

Milk should be poured into clean containers before use and kept covered at all times to prevent flies and dust gaining access to it.

Where there are no facilities for keeping the milk fresh and pure, the use of powdered milk should be encouraged. When reconstituted according to the directions on the packet, this milk has the same composition as fresh milk and the same nutritive value, except for the deficient vitamin content. (For this reason it is important to impress upon mothers who are using powdered milk for infant feeding that vitamins, particularly vitamin C, must be supplemented.) Powdered milk has some advantages:

(1) the processes to which the milk is subjected during drying ensure that it is free from pathogens;

(2) only sufficient milk for immediate use need be prepared, so the risk of contamination is reduced;

(3) powdered milk will keep a long time.

Effective health education is necessary to impress upon all who handle food, especially mothers, that milk can become infected in the home as readily as it can elsewhere.

FOOD POISONING

The term 'food poisoning' is usually associated with those infections and toxaemias that follow the ingestion of food contaminated with certain pathogenic micro-organisms. Infections are, however, not the only ill effects which may result from eating spoiled food.

Noxious plants and fish

Naturally occurring *poisonous substances* may also cause food poisoning, e.g.:

(1) *Plants*, some of them commonly found in our gardens or in the veld. Sometimes the whole plant is poisonous, at other times only certain parts such as the berries or the roots. Examples: the stems of the rhubarb are edible while the leaves are toxic as they contain oxalic acid. Poisonous toadstools can be mistaken for edible mushrooms with disastrous results.

(2) Some *sea foods* are always poisonous, such as the 'puffer fish', while others become poisonous only after they have ingested certain toxic marine substances, e.g. mussels off the Cape and Natal coasts at certain times of the year. Toxin-producing species of dinoflagellates which cause 'red tides' cause paralytic shellfish (mussel) poisoning in man.

By far the greatest cause of food poisoning is the contamination of non-poisonous food either by chemicals or by pathogenic micro-organisms.

Chemical pollution of food

Serious illness and even death may result from eating food which has been polluted by chemicals such as lead, mercury, arsenic, insecticides, fungicides, herbicides, etc. Such pollution may take place in a number of ways.

(1) Fruit and vegetables which have been treated with *poisonous sprays* and dusts in

order to control pests and diseases may contain unacceptable residues of such substances when they reach the consumer, if proper precautions have not been taken and the directions which accompany such sprays and dusts have not been strictly adhered to.

Note: Insecticidal poisoning is a notifiable condition in South Africa. (See p. 72 for DDT and malathion poisoning.)

(2) Foodstuffs such as flour, beans and cereals, if placed *adjacent to poisons during storage* or transportation, may become contaminated. From time to time deaths are reported due to the consumption of foods poisoned in this way.

(3) *Industrial effluents* containing toxic materials are sometimes disposed of in rivers and seas, thereby polluting the water. Fish and other creatures living in such waters become contaminated, thus causing serious disease in people who eat their flesh. An outbreak of mercury poisoning which occurred in Japan in 1968 was traced to the consumption of fish caught in Minimata Bay, containing high levels of methyl mercury. Poisoning occurred because of the disposal of mercury-contaminated waste into the bay.

(4) Many chemical substances are added to food to preserve it or to improve its taste, appearance, texture or colour. Although the use of such *additives* is strictly controlled in most countries, including South Africa, it is possible that many of them — previously thought to be harmless — may have long-term effects on human health. The main dangers associated with additives are their mutagenic, teratogenic and carcinogenic effects. Although only small amounts of additives are used, the total amount consumed by individuals in countries using many processed or 'instant' foods may be large. It is estimated that in the USA individuals consume, on an average, 4,1 kilograms of food additives per year. Apart from the above-mentioned long-term effects, some chemicals may be toxic; fatal cases of cobalt poisoning have been reported from countries where cobalt is used in the brewing of beer.

(5) *Hormones and antibiotics* may be given to animals to stimulate growth or treat disease.

These substances are retained in the tissues and can give rise to toxic or allergic reactions in human beings eating the flesh of the contaminated animals.

(6) An extremely dangerous practice is that of *storing poisonous substances in empty food and drink containers*. In this way, the accidental ingestion of poisons becomes possible.

Biological contamination of food

Food may be contaminated by fungi, viruses, protozoa and bacteria.

Fungal contamination of food

In Africa, south of the Sahara, foodstuffs such as maize, groundnuts, dried beans, rice and cassava are often contaminated by fungus, the *Aspergillus flavus*, which produces a toxin called aflatoxin. Research has shown that there is a definite relationship between the amount of aflatoxin consumed and primary carcinoma of the liver. The incidence of the latter is highest in those areas where foodstuffs are most likely to become contaminated with this fungus, i.e. where they are stored in a humid atmosphere. Insufficient drying before storage will also encourage the growth of the fungus. Regulations made under Act 54 of 1972 prohibit the sale of any foodstuff containing more than a certain amount of aflatoxin or any other fungus-producing toxin (mycotoxins).

Microbial contamination of food

Contamination of food by bacteria, viruses and protozoa may cause either communicable diseases or food poisoning.

Many diseases can be transmitted through the medium of food, e.g. typhoid fever, infective hepatitis, cholera, dysentery (refer to the section on communicable diseases).

The preparation and serving of food offer endless opportunities for pathogens to gain access to it if the requirements of hygienic food handling are not met.

Contamination of food may occur through:

(1) food-handlers who are sufferers from or carriers of communicable diseases and whose standards of personal hygiene are poor;

(2) flies and dust settling on uncovered food; cockroaches and rodents contaminating the food by contact and excreta;

(3) food left unrefrigerated: room temperature provides the ideal conditions for the growth and multiplication of micro-organisms;

(4) impure water or unclean utensils used during the preparation and serving of food;

(5) sewage-polluted water used for irrigation purposes, particularly above-ground vegetables eaten raw, such as cress and lettuce.

Note: Shellfish such as oysters and mussels may contain pathogens if collected from sewage-polluted waters.

Bacterial food poisoning

The incidence of this type of food poisoning is highest where standards of personal and environmental hygiene are poorest and where facilities for the refrigeration of food are lacking. The bacteria most commonly responsible for bacterial food poisoning are: *Salmonella, Shigella, Escherichia, Staphylococci* and *Clostridia*. Food provides the perfect medium for growth of the microbes.

Note: Food contaminated by the above-mentioned bacteria does not appear 'bad'; the food looks, smells and tastes quite normal.

Salmonella food poisoning (salmonellosis)

Infection with *S. typhimurium* and *S. enteritidis* causes an acute gastro-enteritis after an incubation period of 12 to 24 hours. The patient suffers from pyrexia, abdominal pain and diarrhoea, but vomiting is not marked.

The principal reservoirs of infection are infected animals such as pigs, cattle and poultry. Human infection results from eating infected meat which has not been adequately cooked. The eggs of infected hens may also transmit the organisms.

Some processed foods may also be contaminated, e.g. dried eggs and milk, coconut, and vegetable protein concentrates.

Rats and mice are often carriers and contaminate uncovered food through their excreta. Food may also become infected by a human food-handling carrier. Small outbreaks may occur among people who have shared a meal, while larger outbreaks occur in institutions such as boarding-schools, barracks and hostels, as well as in hotels and restaurants.

Salmonellae proliferate rapidly in food kept at room temperature or in warming ovens.

The only treatment required is the maintenance of fluid and electrolyte balance, usually by oral therapy. The infectious stools may be disposed of in water-borne toilets and strict hand-washing after the use of the toilet must be observed. Sufferers should not handle food or care for infants while they are ill.

Staphylococcal food poisoning

This is a toxaemia and not an infection, the food poisoning being caused by an enterotoxin produced by the *Staph. pyogenes*. The enterotoxin is heat stable and is, therefore, not destroyed by cooking. Man is the chief reservoir of infection and food becomes contaminated by droplets from a carrier or by the discharges from a skin lesion such as a boil, carbuncle or abscess. Cold meats, milk and milk products such as butter, cream, ice-cream and custard are the foodstuffs most frequently responsible for the transmission of the infection. Profuse vomiting follows from 1 to 6 hours after the ingestion of the infected food and is usually accompanied by abdominal cramps and diarrhoea. The temperature may be subnormal and the blood pressure falls. The illness usually lasts for a couple of days only, but the person may be acutely ill. Treatment is as for salmonellosis.

Botulism

This is a rare kind of food poisoning, usually not found in South Africa, which is caused by the exotoxin of the anaerobic, spore-bearing *Cl. botulinum*, a normal inhabitant of the intestines of animals and fish and sometimes found in soil and water. The powerful exotoxin affects the nervous system causing visual disturbances, difficulty in swallowing, bulbar paralysis and, later, death due to respiratory failure. Botulism is a serious condition with a high mortality rate.

Note: There was an outbreak of botulism among cattle in the RSA in 1994.

The foods most frequently implicated in the transmission of the *Cl. botulinum* are those from which air has been excluded, such as tinned meat and fish and large sausages.

At Tygerberg Hospital in 1981 there was a confirmed case of non-fatal botulism. Four other cases of botulism have recently been recorded in the RSA. The origin of the exotoxin could not be clearly established in any of these cases, but a certain brand of imported tinned salmon was suspected. Remaining stocks were withdrawn by the manufacturers and no more cases were reported.

Clostridium perfringens (welchii) poisoning

Spores of this organism can be found in meat and poultry. They survive ordinary cooking and then grow rapidly in warm food (between 15 °C and 60 °C).

Signs and symptoms of poisoning which may occur after a banquet include nausea, abdominal cramps and diarrhoea 12–18 hours after exposure.

Recovery takes place without specific treatment.

Bacillus cereus poisoning

Any food contaminated with this common soil microbe and stored in a warm place for several hours can cause *B. cereus* poisoning.

Signs, symptoms and recovery are as for *Cl. perfringens* poisoning.

Note: Food poisoning comprising outbreaks of more than four persons is a notifiable medical condition.

INFECTED MEAT

Cold or reheated meat, as a vehicle for the transmission of infections such as typhoid, paratyphoid and bacterial food poisoning, has been discussed and this section of the chapter will be confined to those diseases which may be transmitted to man as a result of the ingestion of the flesh of diseased animals.

An infection which is transmissible from animals to man is known as a zoonosis and may be either enzootic or epizootic. A condition which is enzootic is one which is endemic among certain animals, such as jungle yellow fever in monkeys, while one which is epizootic occurs as an epidemic in animals, such as plague in rodents. Six conditions which may be transmitted to man through the flesh of diseased animals are:

(1) taeniasis (tapeworm);
(2) anthrax;
(3) actinomycosis;
(4) foot-and-mouth disease;
(5) tuberculosis; and
(6) trichinosis.

Taeniasis (tapeworm)

See p. 631.

Anthrax

See p. 679 for anthrax in human beings.

Intestinal anthrax may follow the ingestion of contaminated meat which has not been adequately cooked. Abdominal pain and pyrexia occur after an incubation period of two to five days. The causative organism is the *Bacillus anthracis* — a large, aerobic, spore-forming organism.

Actinomycosis

This is uncommon in man but occurs in cattle, horses, pigs and other animals and may, theoretically, be transmitted to man when he eats the flesh of diseased animals. The causative organism is a ray fungus.

Foot-and-mouth disease

This is a disease which occurs most commonly in cattle, but other animals such as pigs may be affected. Man may become infected through the ingestion of meat of an infected animal or by drinking infected milk. Sore throat, pyrexia and vesicles in the mouth present the characteristic clinical picture.

Tuberculosis

Non-pulmonary tuberculosis is not commonly spread by the ingestion of meat, but the condition is included here because regulations require the destruction of the whole carcass if signs of generalised tuberculosis are found.

Trichinosis

This condition follows the ingestion of raw or inadequately cooked meat containing the cysts of the *Trichinella spiralis*, which is a roundworm. The condition occurs in many animals but is transmitted mainly by pork and pork products such as sausages. Man ingests the larvae (which form the cysts) which develop into mature adults in the small intestine. Following mating, the female passes the larvae which pass through the walls of the intestine and are carried to the muscles where they form cysts. This condition, while fairly common in the USA, does not occur in the RSA.

LEGAL CONTROL OF FOOD HYGIENE

Prevention of microbial contamination of food

This can be done by legal control of food hygiene and by education of the public in the principles of personal and environmental hygiene.

Health education

Only by insisting on the highest possible standards of personal and environmental hygiene in all places where food handling takes place, including the home, will it be possible to avoid microbial contamination of foodstuffs. Health education has a vital role to play in this connection and should be used to motivate the community, in particular those involved in the preparation of food for consumption by other people, to raise their standards of personal hygiene and to ensure that their surroundings are kept clean. The elementary health rules to be observed are: washing hands after defaecating and blowing the nose and before handling food, keeping food covered at all times and protected from flies, vermin and dust, refrigerating all perishable food, wherever possible, ensuring adequate refuse disposal and sanitation and waging a continuous war on flies and rodents. Food poisoning is frequently caused by the use of food which has been reheated. It is essential that all cooked food kept for later consumption should be refrigerated immediately. When reheating the food, the temperature attained should be at least 70 °C, as a moderate temperature encourages the growth and multiplication of microbes.

Regulation R. 185 of 1987, made in terms of sections 35 and 40 of the Health Act 63 of 1977, controls the hygiene standards of food for sale to the public.

THE CONTROL OF DISEASES SPREAD BY INFECTED MEAT

Various regulations and by-laws control the slaughtering of animals and the sale of meat.

(1) All abattoirs and slaughter houses have to be registered with the local authority and must meet certain standards which have been laid down regarding the water supply facilities for the disposal of waste and other structural requirements.

(2) Dogs, cats or birds are not allowed on the premises.

(3) No one suffering from a communicable disease is allowed on the premises.

(4) Meat inspectors are appointed by local authorities. Meat inspectors may examine animals before they are slaughtered. They examine the carcasses according to standard procedures which have been laid down.

(5) The whole carcass or parts of it may be condemned if certain conditions such as generalised tuberculosis, anthrax, foot-and-mouth disease and many others are present.

(6) All condemned carcasses must be adequately disposed of, for example by incineration.

(7) No person who is not clean or who is suffering from a communicable disease may handle carcasses.

(8) All abattoirs or slaughter houses must have adequate cold storage facilities for the carcasses.

(9) Farmers and others who do their own slaughtering should be taught to recognise conditions which would make the meat unfit for human consumption; in these circumstances the carcass must be completely destroyed or buried.

(10) Preparation of meat for consumption. Most microbes, as well as the larvae of parasites, will be destroyed by adequate cooking of meat. The meat should be cooked at a high temperature to ensure that these organisms are destroyed. Meat which has been cooked must be handled hygienically to prevent contamination by pathogens.

Regulations concerning transport of meat and sale of cooked chicken

Regulation R. 1540 of 1986 to the Health Act 63 of 1977 relating to the transport of meat. Carcasses (from the abattoirs and other meat suppliers) must be transported in an upright, free-hanging position (except poultry and frozen meat) in a cargo hold which is impenetrable to dust and liquids and is corrosive-proof on the inside. The cargo hold must be cooled so that the temperature of the carcasses does not exceed 7 °C for longer than 2 hours, or 3 °C in the case of offal. The cargo hold may not be used for any other purpose. The hygiene of the cargo hold and the meat handler and the protective clothing of the latter are strictly prescribed.

Regulation R. 106 of 1985 of the Foodstuffs, Cosmetics and Disinfectants Act 54 of 1972 prescribes the microbiological standards for cooked poultry. No person may sell cooked poultry which contains anti-microbial substances, added hormones and the following organisms: *Salmonella, Shigella* and *Escherichia*, and more than a stipulated number of the following organisms: *Staphylococcus aureus, Clostridia perfringens* and other organisms.

It is the function of local authorities through their health inspectors to ensure that such regulations are adhered to in their wards.

BRIEF SUMMARY OF FOOD-HANDLING REGULATIONS

(1) All food-handling premises must be kept in a clean and sanitary condition at all times. All rooms should be adequately cross-ventilated and, where this cannot be achieved by natural means, artificial ventilation or air-conditioning must be provided. All rooms must have adequate lighting. Walls, floors and ceilings must be constructed of impervious material and finished with a light-coloured, smooth material such as paint. All shelves, tables and working surfaces must be constructed of stainless steel or similar material.

(2) There must be sufficient basins, supplied with hot and cold running water, nail-brushes, soap and disposable towels, for the use of food-handlers. Nails, hands and overalls must be kept clean. Clothes may not be washed on food-handling premises.

(3) Premises must be kept free from flies, cockroaches and other insects as well as rodents. No birds or animals except guide dogs are allowed on such premises. The premises

must have a pure and adequate water supply as well as facilities for the disposal of refuse.

(4) Crockery, cutlery and other equipment should be free from chips and cracks and scrupulously clean. All such equipment should be washed in hot water, to which a suitable detergent has been added, and allowed to dry on a rack. The use of cloths for drying should be discouraged as they rapidly become soiled and a source of infection.

(5) Food containers must adhere to high standards. Newspapers, periodicals or used paper may not be used as such, except in the case of fruit and vegetables.

(6) Exposed food for sale must be screened from the public.

(7) Food must be transported hygienically and no poisons, persons or animals may be in the cargo holds used for the transport of meat.

(8) Perishable food is stored at a temperature below 10 °C in cases where spoilage due to room temperature is possible.

(9) There may be no pail or pit latrines in or near food-handling premises.

(10) All food-handlers should be free from any illness, sores or injury liable to contaminate the food. They must submit themselves to regular medical examinations and allow swabs, blood samples or other specimens to be taken if this is requested.

(11) The appointment of health inspectors by the local industry. A health inspector's duties involve inspecting all establishments where food is prepared, served or sold, taking samples of food and drink, as well as swabs from articles such as cups, glasses, spoons and various surfaces with which food is likely to come into contact, for bacteriological examination.

Only constant vigilance and the effective supervision of all who handle food in restaurants or other food-handling establishments can prevent the spread of diseases by infected food.

CARE OF FOOD BY THE HOUSEWIFE

The Nutritional Services of the Department of Health Services and Welfare, House of Assembly, has advised the housewife to take the following hygiene precautions.

Purchasing food. Cans of food must not be bought if the tins leak, are dented or blown (i.e. have convex lids). Other risky buys are dirty or cracked eggs, frozen vegetables which are lumpy — a sign of refreezing after thawing. Thawing, e.g. during shopping, must be avoided as this allows any microbes which are present to multiply. The student must remember that freezing does not kill microbes; it merely stops them from multiplying.

Storage. Left-over foods must be refrigerated in a closed container and reused within 48 hours. Dry foods must be protected against insects and rodents, and perishable foods kept cool and used before they wilt or rot. Flies, cockroaches and rats are dangerous carriers of disease in a storeroom and kitchen.

Food must be *prepared* hygienically, giving due attention to the cleanliness of the uncooked food, the utensils, work surfaces and hands of the cook. Foods to be eaten raw, e.g. fruit and vegetables, must be well rinsed before use. The cook should not smoke in the kitchen, or cough and sneeze over the food. Open lesions on hands must be kept covered with waterproof material.

Crockery, cutlery and cooking utensils are washed either in a dishwashing machine — the ideal — or by hand in hot, soapy water, after which they are rinsed in clean water and placed on a rack to drip-dry. Dishcloths — a source of infection — are avoided unless they are frequently laundered or are disposable.

WATER RESOURCES OF SOUTH AFRICA

South Africa has an inadequate, unreliable and unevenly distributed supply of water. Massive losses of soil and water to the sea occur during floods; devastating droughts threaten the production of food and cause selective water restrictions to be imposed at times on cities and towns when their stored sources of water reach low levels. In 1984 the Minister of Environmental Affairs and Fisheries said there was water for only 65 million people in South Africa. He predicted a catastrophe, not in terms of food but of water, if the population growth is not reduced. The Department of Water Affairs estimates that the demand for water will equal its supply in the year 2000.

The amount of water considered sufficient for the needs of a population varies tremendously from country to country. In modern industrial societies it is in the region of 300 to 500 litres per person per day. In some countries, e.g. the United States of America, the per capita consumption of water greatly exceeds this amount. Generally, approximately 50 litres per person per day for personal and domestic use is considered to be the minimum amount required for the maintenance of health. During the 1983 drought each household in Durban was limited to 400 ℓ per day. Even this amount is often not available to communities in arid areas, e.g. amongst the Bushmen of the Kalahari Desert. The present Minister of Water Affairs aims to create a national water and sanitation programme which would help all households to secure a clean and safe daily water supply of 20–30 litres per day within 200 metres for each person (*The Star*, 20 May 1994).

Another difficulty which has to be overcome by many rural communities is the inaccessibility of the water supply which may be many kilometres from the village or dwelling. In many parts of Africa, and even in South Africa, the women and children spend a large part of each day carrying water.

Water is necessary not only for drinking, cooking and personal and domestic hygiene but also for animal husbandry and agricultural and industrial development. It is, therefore, essential for the economic development of a community, as well as for the health of its members.

Dr CF Garbers, president of the CSIR, maintains that the importance of safe water supplies and sanitary disposal of waste products is often not appreciated by the public in developing countries. The recent cholera epidemic showed that many rural blacks preferred to drink dirty water from muddy pools rather than safe chlorinated water supplied by the authorities. Dr Garbers highlighted the following facts:

(1) Barely 20 % of the rural population in developing countries have safe drinking water, while only about 15 % have sanitary waste disposal facilities.

(2) About 80 % of illnesses in developing countries are related in one way or another to water.

(Quoted in part from *Rand Daily Mail*, 8.9.1982.)

A safe, reliable supply of water is thus an essential requisite for community health.

THE SOURCES OF WATER

Rain is the origin of water on earth. It may be the only direct source of water for a community or a household, but in South Africa there are very few areas where rain alone will ensure an adequate supply of water throughout the year. Falling rain-water is free from pathogenic microbes and, as it contains no mineral salts, it is soft, i.e. it readily allows soap to lather. As the rain-water falls through the air, CO_2 and O_2 are absorbed and add 'flavour' to the water. In industrial areas it may gather impurities as it passes through the sooty atmosphere and it may become polluted if the surface on which it falls is unclean. As rain-water percolates through the soil, it is filtered of organic material and microbes, but acquires dissolved mineral salts from the soil and rocks, i.e. it becomes 'hard'.

Rain-water run-off from roofs is often collected in galvanised-iron, concrete or brick tanks for household water supply in rural areas where fresh water is scarce.

Water for large-scale domestic and agricultural purposes is, however, derived from two other sources.

Surface water

Surface water comes from:

(1) *Lakes and dams* which may be natural or man-made. They collect water from streams which are fed by rain and melting snows from high mountainous areas. Where such lakes and dams are situated far from human

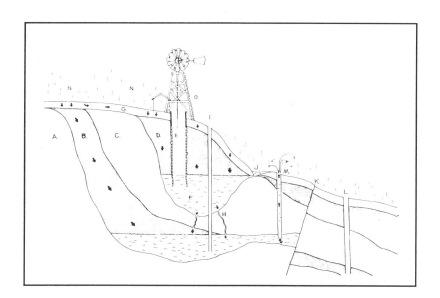

Figure 10.1

Underground water supplies

A. Impermeable layer of shale; B. Permeable layer of sandstone; C. Impermeable layer of shale; D. Permeable layer; E. Shallow well; F. Trapped water; G. Top layer of earth; H. Fissure in impermeable layer; I. Successful borehole; J. Shallow spring; K. Geological fault; L. Dry (unsuccessful) borehole; M. Artesian well; N. Rain; O. Wind-pump

habitation and the catchment area is fenced off to prevent animals and human beings gaining access to it, the water is safe for consumption.

(2) *Rivers*. In South Africa most of the larger towns and cities obtain their water supplies from rivers. River water is usually turbid and should never be considered safe for human consumption because it is always polluted; the more densely populated the area through which the river flows, the more grossly contaminated the water will be. All river water has to be subjected to intensive treatment before distribution to the consumers.

Underground water tapped by wells, boreholes and springs

This is water which has seeped down through the soil and cracks in rocks and collected above an impervious (impermeable) layer of rock. Water which lies above the first impervious layer is known as *subsoil water* and a well which taps this source as a *shallow well*, while a *deep well* or *borehole* is one which draws water from below the first impervious layer of rock. An *artesian well* (or borehole) is one in which water rises spontaneously to the surface when a hole is sunk, because the water is under pressure. This happens when the permeable layer of soil is enclosed by two impermeable layers of rock.

Springs are found where an impervious layer comes to the surface of the soil and allows the water to flow out of the soil at this point. Springs may also be shallow or deep. The water from deep wells and springs may be considered safe, provided the area is fenced off to prevent contamination by animals and human beings.

The *quality of underground water* depends upon the characteristics of the soil. In some soil formations bacteria and other impurities are filtered out of the water after it has travelled only a short distance, while in others impurities may still be present in the water after it has percolated through the soil a kilometre or more. Unfortunately the appearance of the water is no indication of its purity and water which is crystal clear may be heavily contaminated with pathogenic bacteria.

The *source of a water supply* is important because it will determine the quantity and the quality of the water. Not only the purity of the water but the kind and the amount of its constituents, such as the dissolved mineral salts, are affected by the source of a water supply. According to the World Health Organisation, water is considered polluted when its 'composition or condition has been affected to such an extent that it is no longer suitable for the purpose for which it was suitable in its natural state' (WHO 1972).

THE POLLUTION OF WATER

Life is not possible without water and an adequate and pure water supply is a prerequisite for health and, indeed, for the continuation of life on earth. It is, therefore, paradoxical that the life-giving water can at times be the carrier of death and disease.

The World Health Organisation estimates that 1 200 million people in the developing countries, where we find two-thirds of the world's population, have no safe water supply, while 1 400 million have no facilities for the disposal of excreta. Water supplies cannot be discussed meaningfully without considering the disposal of excreta at the same time, for in these underdeveloped countries the greatest danger to health is the faecal contamination of water. Dramatic improvements in the health of communities will follow the provision of a safe water supply and adequate sanitation.

All water intended for domestic use should first be tested to make sure it is not polluted.

Water quality tests

(1) *Physical tests*. The appearance, taste and odour of water are checked.
(2) *Chemical tests*. These tests will indicate the amount of dissolved and suspended solids, the degree of hardness of the water and the presence or absence of nitrites, sulphates and chlorides, the presence of which indicates possible faecal contamination of the water.
(3) *Bacteriological tests*. These tests are used mainly to detect those micro-organisms which, while themselves not pathogenic,

will indicate whether or not the water has recently been contaminated by faecal material. The coliform organisms are usually used as the 'indicators' of faecal contamination of water.

The following are some of the impurities which may be present in polluted water.

Biological pollutants

Pathogenic bacteria, viruses and the ova and larvae of parasites, many of which are present in urine and faeces of human beings and animals. These organisms gain access to the water when untreated or inadequately treated sewage is allowed to enter rivers and streams, or when excreta are washed into the streams or rivers by rain. Seepage into an underground water supply from a pit privy, septic tank or French drain may also be responsible for such contamination. People become infected through drinking the water, bathing in it or eating food which has been irrigated or washed in polluted water.

Note: All rivers in the RSA which flow into the Indian Ocean east of Plettenberg Bay are contaminated with the schistosoma.

Typhoid fever, para-typhoid fever, amoebic dysentery, cholera, infective hepatitis, schistosomiasis and helminthic infestations can be transmitted by water, while malaria, river blindness (in Central Africa), sleeping sickness and filariasis are some of the conditions in which water is implicated because the vectors of these diseases are found in close association with water.

Chemical pollutants

Chemicals used in agriculture, such as fertilisers, insecticides, fungicides and herbicides, may be present in water either because they have been washed into the river or stream by the rains or because the factories which produce them have discharged effluents containing the chemicals into rivers or seas. Industry is responsible for much pollution of both inland water and of the sea. Numerous chemicals are to be found in industrial waste and many of them are toxic. Heavy metals such as mercury, arsenic, cyanide, detergents and dyes are a few of the chemicals which may be found in water contaminated in this way.

Metals such as copper, lead and iron may be dissolved out of the pipes in which water is conducted. Today lead water pipes are no longer used, but in some of the older cities of Europe, unacceptably high levels of lead have been found in drinking water because of this.

Radioactive pollutants

Pollution of water by radioactive substances may be due to radioactive fall-out following the testing of nuclear devices, or the disposal of industrial wastes containing radioactive material. At present, radioactive pollution of water in the RSA is not a problem.

Silt

Silt is the sediment deposited by moving water.

The silt content of most rivers in the RSA is high, particularly in the rainy season when the water appears turbid and muddy. Although silt does not actually cause disease, it is unattractive and it has to be removed before water is delivered to the consumer.

Mineral salts

The dissolved mineral salts which cause the *hardness* of water are the bicarbonates of calcium and magnesium (causing temporary hardness) and the sulphates or chlorides of calcium or magnesium (causing permanent hardness). These minerals have been leached from the earth when the pure rain-water flows over or percolates through it. Very hard water does not yield a lather when agitated with a soap solution, whereas very soft water, e.g. pure rain-water, lathers freely. The minerals dissolved in water give it taste and are a source of minerals for the growth and development of man and animals. In the process of water purification, hard water is treated to get rid of excess minerals which may form deposits in pipes and boilers and hinder the action of soap. Temporary hardness is removed either by boiling water or by adding slaked lime; both processes cause insoluble calcium carbonate to form and to precipitate. Permanent hardness can be removed by the addition of sodium-aluminium-silicate or sodium carbonate (washing soda).

In South Africa the provision of pure water is controlled by the Health Act. Section 37 of the Health Act 63 of 1977 reads:

'The Minister may, after consultation with the Minister of Environment Affairs make, in respect of water intended for human use or food processing, regulations relating to

(b) The protection of catchment areas of rivers, water courses, dams, lakes and above-ground sources of water against pollution . . .

(c) The control etc. of water-purifying works, methods of purification and substances which may be added to the water during the processes . . .

(e) The registration of water purification works and of persons employed at such works.

(h) The requirements water must comply with, with respect to purity, chemical composition and quality.

(i) The reporting of pollution or suspected pollution of such water.'

Note: This extract of the law has been greatly abbreviated.

Section 20(1) of the Health Act 63 of 1977 lays down that local authorities shall take all lawful, necessary and reasonably practicable measures to 'prevent the pollution of any water intended for the use of the inhabitants of its district, irrespective of whether such water is obtained from sources within or without its district, or to purify such water which has become polluted'.

Note: The responsibility for a supply of pure water to a community has devolved upon regional services councils.

PURIFICATION OF WATER

Natural purification

The pollution of water has not always been a problem. From earliest times man has disposed of his wastes into rivers, streams and the sea. While the amount of waste disposed of in this way was relatively small, the water purified itself. As the heavier particles gradually settle to the bottom, algae and other plant and animal life ingest microbes and organic material and the oxygen which is liberated by algae and plants oxidises microbes. If the water is clear the ultra-violet rays of the sun also destroy microbes. Fish ingest the ova and larvae of animal parasites. The whole process of natural or self-purification

is dependent on there being sufficient oxygen in the water. Anything which reduces the amount of oxygen present in water will interfere with the processes of self-purification.

Necessary precautions to preserve the safety of underground water supplies

In rural areas where underground water obtained from *wells and springs* is a common source of supply, people must be taught by effective health education to protect the source from pollution by man and animals. Wells are dug in soil which can easily be excavated and have a diameter of 1 to 2 metres. The area around the well or spring should be fenced and the underground source must be situated on higher ground than a likely source of pollution, e.g. a nearby pit privy. The well must be lined with stones or bricks where the soil is inclined to cave in. The upper 3 metres of the well should be lined with some impervious material such as cast concrete to prevent seepage of contaminated surface water into the well from the sides. The mouth of the well should be surrounded by a coping of concrete which slopes away from the mouth so that rainwater or any water which is spilled near the well may drain away from the well, not into it. A well should, therefore, be constructed in such a way that opportunities for pollution of the water are minimal. Ideally the water should be brought to the top by means of a pipe connected to a windmill and the mouth of the well closed to protect the contents. Where any mechanical means of withdrawing water from a well is not available, the water is withdrawn manually.

The Division of Water Technology, CSIR, distributes a video tape to teach people how to protect a natural spring in order to improve the quality of the water and make water collection easier.

Precautions taken with manual withdrawal and transport of well water

The container used for drawing the water from a well and the hands of the person drawing the water should be clean and some kind of water-tight cover placed over the well at all times when it is not being used. During transport of the container — often on the head of a woman or child — and during storage, it should be covered to protect it from dust and human contact. Water for use must be removed from the container by means of a clean cup or jug kept for the purpose.

Where there is doubt about the purity of the water it should be purified.

Boreholes are drilled mechanically to a depth of up to 150 metres; water from this source is usually safe for domestic use. Boreholes should be provided with a casing to prevent the sides from caving in and the top three metres should be lined with an impervious material to prevent surface seepage. The water from the borehole is brought to the surface by means of *electrical or wind-pumps.*

Purification for a single household

This should be done if the purity of the source of the water is uncertain or if the water is known to be polluted. Methods of purification are:

(1) *Boiling.* This method is used by householders even in large communities where the communal source has been polluted by floods or earthquakes, e.g. the floods in Lisbon in 1979. Boiling water for 10 minutes removes the air and the salts which cause temporary hardness. This makes the water tasteless and dull in appearance and causes the deposit of 'fur' (insoluble calcium carbonate) on the inside of kettles. The sparkle can be restored by repeatedly pouring cooled, boiled water from container to container, to reintroduce air.

Note: The cost of fuel makes boiling impractical in Third-World societies.

(2) *Filtration.* Domestic filters made of various substances, such as unglazed porcelain, are obtainable and will remove bacteria and larger particles from the water, but the filterable viruses will pass through the filter. Bacteria are, however, inadequately removed by filtration without effective prior coagulation and flocculation.

Household and community slow sand filters which are used without chemicals have been designed, the design criteria being available from the Water Technology Department of the CSIR. At least 90 % turbidity and more than 99 % bacteria and viruses are removed.

The filter can be made in a 200 litre drum and construction materials cost R20,00 (1989).

(3) *Distillation.* This is a process whereby water is obtained from the condensation of steam. Distilled water is absolutely pure but tasteless.

(4) *Chemicals.* The addition of very small amounts, i.e. a few drops of iodine or chlorine, to water will destroy pathogens and will not have any harmful consequences.

The amounts necessary are: 1 teaspoon (Jik, Nomisol, Javel) to 1 litre of water (left overnight) or 5 drops/ℓ allowed to stand for 30 minutes; tincture of iodine 2 %, 6 drops/ℓ of water left to stand for 30 minutes.

(5) *Chlor-Floc drinking water tablets.* This is an inert flocculating agent with chlorine, which removes soil and dirt, bacteria and viruses from water and renders turbid infected water clear and free of microbes within 5 minutes.

Method of use: One Chlor-Floc tablet is added to 1 litre water which is then shaken for 1 minute. It is left to sediment and then strained through a cloth, e.g. piece of towel used only on one side. The strained water is ready for drinking. Chlor-Floc can be bought at retail chemists.

Purification of the water supply of a community

Distillation

This is an expensive and time-consuming method of purifying water which is used at Lüderitz to obtain domestic water from sea water, because of the total absence of fresh water. Apparatus has been designed in which the sun's heat is used to distill the water.

Storage

Storage of water in lakes, dams and reservoirs allows for the sedimentation of impurities in suspension. Most human pathogens do not survive for long in clear water, the water being free from bacteria after storage for a week.

Purification by storage is practicable only if several reservoirs are available and if the pollution of the water is minimal. In order to effect this, the source of the water — the catchment area — springs, streams, wells, boreholes, artesian wells — as well as the storage facilities, should be fenced and no unauthorised persons should be allowed to enter the area. The water should be conveyed to the storage dams and to the consumers in closed pipes.

Borehole chlorinators

Borehole chlorinators have been developed by the CSIR for use in the developing countries where water supplies come from boreholes or hand-operated pumps (wells). These sources of water need disinfection when pit privies have been sunk injudiciously in their vicinity, thus contaminating the water. These chlorinators are commercially available.

Purification works

It is seldom possible to store large quantities of water for long enough to bring about purification by natural means. The natural process is hastened by artificial means at the purification works (treatment plants) with pumping stations, situated on the banks of a river which is usually dammed back at the site to ensure a good supply of water even during the dry season. River water which flows over inhabited lowlands contains many impurities and is usually turbid.

The principles of the process of purification will be described. Purification takes place in stages, the process being continuous and automatic.

Stage 1: Coagulation and flocculation

This is the stage in which coagulation and flocculation of the impurities take place by the addition of the chemical, aluminium sulphate, to the water. Slaked lime is added if the water has a high acid content. Sodium-aluminium-silicate (permutit) is added to reduce the hardness of the water. The coagulum (floc) will eventually settle to the bottom, carrying with it microbes and other suspended matter in the next stage of the purification process.

Stage 2: Sedimentation

Precipitation and sedimentation of the solids formed during coagulation and flocculation take place in large tanks in which most of the solids sink down to the bottom when the slowly moving water is brought to a standstill for 12 hours. From here the water flows into filters.

Stage 3: Filtration

The residue of the solids is removed by filtration in filters of which there are various kinds.

(1) *Slow sand filters.* These are beds consisting of a layer of gravel at the bottom, covered by a layer of sand. Water is led on to these filter beds and then percolates through the sand and the gravel to be collected from the bottom of the filter bed by means of pipes which will lead it to the storage reservoirs for chlorination. The efficiency of this type of filter depends upon a 'vital layer'. This is a slimy layer of algae, protozoa and other biological life which forms on the surface of the sand. When this layer becomes too thick the rate of filtration slows down; the layer has then to be removed. While this is being done another filter bed has to be used.

(2) *Rapid gravity sand filters.* This type of filter is commonly used in water purification schemes in developed areas today. They also consist of beds of gravel and sand, but they filter a greater volume of water in a given time than the slow sand filters described above.

(3) *Mechanical filters or pressure filters.* These are similar to the rapid gravity sand filters, but the gravel and sand are contained in a steel tank and the water is filtered by pressure, i.e. it is forced through the sand and not allowed to run through by gravity.

Stage 4: Disinfection

The filtered water is then disinfected. Chlorine is the chemical most commonly used for the disinfection of water. It is a powerful oxidising agent and quite small amounts (i.e. 1 part chlorine in 5 million parts of water) destroy most microbes. It may be added to the water in the form of chloride of lime (bleaching powder), chlorine gas or chloramine. The chlorine will oxidise any organic matter present in the water, but large amounts of organic matter reduce its efficiency; therefore, the water should be clear and as free from organic matter as possible before the chlorine is added to it.

A combination of the methods described is used for the purification of water, the particular combination used depending upon the source of the water as well as its quality. Water from upland surface areas usually requires less treatment than river water. The processes described will render the water free from pathogens, but it is usually subjected to further treatment such as aeration and dechlorination.

Stage 5: Aeration and dechlorination

Bubbling air through the water and removing the chlorine is sometimes done to make sure that it is free from chlorine taste and odour and that it is palatable.

It is also important to make sure that the water contains a reasonable amount of mineral salts, not only for taste but also to ensure the mineralisation of bones and teeth of the consumers, especially developing children.

Delivery pumps pump the purified water via booster pumping stations to supply the various closed reservoirs from where the water is delivered via water towers or pumps to the community. The network (reticulum) of pipes must be designed to avoid cross-connections, leaks and stagnation of water. Each community should have adequate storage facilities to cater for peak demands and emergencies.

WATER CONSERVATION

Water conservation means the prevention of loss of water supplied by nature or discarded by man. It is done by storing rain-water in dams when the soil can no longer absorb the downpour of rain, or by recycling used water which has become polluted. New freshwater supplies can be created by the desalination of sea water. This process has not yet been used on a large scale because of the expense. The Water Research Commission (WRC) is doing research aimed at reducing desalination costs.

Water conservation schemes have been undertaken by the Department of Water Affairs since 1934 and include the building of the massive HF Verwoerd and PK le Roux dams on the Orange River, with the object of opening vast tracts of arable land in the interior. Vast afforestation schemes have been launched; all vacant state land on mountains which are of value for water catchment conservation are being planted to forests (Forest Act 122 of 1984).

In 1987 the Lesotho Highlands Water project was commenced in the Maluti mountains of Lesotho. This co-operative project between Lesotho and South Africa will not only supply electricity from hydro-electric dams for the use of Lesotho but will also supply water to Gauteng. This massive scheme involves the building of four dams and diverting water to South Africa to ensure that the Gauteng area does not run out of water in the near future.

Recycling sewage effluent[1]

Water is used to convey waste products, mainly body excreta, from the site of production to the site of disposal. Approximately 60–70 % of water used for industrial and domestic purposes eventually becomes sewage[1] (see p. 151 for sewage). This water can be reclaimed for reuse once the waste products and micro-organisms have been removed. See p. 155 for the treatment of sewage.

Once the treated effluent has been chlorinated, it is fit for reuse under certain conditions. Recycled water is a readily available source of water which can be mixed with the conventional water supply of a community.

Water can thus be conserved by using it over and over again. Water is used for many purposes, including drinking. The reason why so much research is done into the safety of the recycled water is the fact that the water must be potable (drinkable) with regard to its taste and its safety from microbes and chemicals which may be mutagenic.

The following bodies do research on the health aspects of reclamation of water:

(1) National Institute for Water Research (NIWR) of the South African CSIR, at Windhoek and Pretoria.

(2) Water Research Commission (WRC) of the Department of Water Affairs in Cape Town.

(3) The Department of Health.

Recycled sewage effluent for potable use can be used to supplement the conventional water supply either by indirect reuse or by direct mixing.

(1) Indirect reuse takes place by discharging the purified effluent from the sewage disposal

works into a river. An example of a recipient river is the Vaal River from where the Rand Water Board gets its water supplies. The effluent is thus purified twice. Large European cities, e.g. London and Amsterdam, use recycled water over and over again.

(2) Direct reuse occurs after the sewage effluent has been treated by more than one process in a special reclamation plant. In Windhoek, tertiary treated sewage effluent has been used to supplement the conventional water supply since 1969.

In Cape Town, the WRC of the Department of Water Affairs is operating a research pilot plant at the Cape Flats sewerage works to study the feasibility of recycling the sewage effluent in that region to supplement its water supply.

The Department of Health is responsible for the final approval of direct recycling and reuse and has stipulated that:

(1) The conventional water supply must be inadequate.

(2) The treated effluent must be of domestic origin with a minimum of industrial effluent.

(3) The special reclamation plant attached to a sewage disposal works must use more than one process for the removal or inactivation of hazardous substances and pathogenic organisms, e.g. sand filter and carbon column filtration with chlorination (chlorine contact time: 30 minutes).

(4) Storage of reclaimed water for 48 hours.

(5) Not more than 20 % reclaimed water must be thoroughly blended with the conventional, treated water.

(6) The ratio of the blend should be kept as constant as possible to prevent undue variations in the taste of the water.

(7) Epidemiological surveys (of infections like diarrhoeal diseases and viral hepatitis, and chemical compounds such as pesticides) must be done in the area before and after the introduction of the reclaimed water. The microbes most commonly found in the effluent before chlorination are the enteroviruses of the *Reoviridae* family.

(8) The chemical, microbiological and virological quality of the final product, potable purified sewage effluent, must conform to the criteria for potable water.

(9) The public concerned must be educated about the necessity for using reclaimed water and reassured about its safety.

The following techniques can improve the water supplies of a rural community:

(1) Protection of watersheds (catchment areas).

(2) Building of conservation dams.

(3) Spring protection programmes (capping and improvement of springs).

(4) The construction of rain-water and storage ferro-cement tanks.

(5) High consumers of water should be persuaded by social pressure to use less water for domestic purposes. This applies especially to wasteful unattended garden sprinklers, leaking taps.

(6) Domestic water can be conserved by the following practices:

▪ use of the shower instead of the bath for reasons of personal cleanliness;

▪ the planting of indigenous trees and shrubs which are acclimatised to South Africa's dry climate;

▪ the use of hoses and watering cans, instead of sprinklers, for the maintenance of gardens;

▪ the use of modern cistern controlling devices to toilets;

▪ the covering of swimming pools when not in use to prevent evaporation.

REFERENCE

Hattingh WHJ, Bourne DE. Research on the health implications of the use of recycled water in South Africa. *S Afr Med J* 1989; **76**: 7–10.

TEST OF KNOWLEDGE

The student has benefited from studying this chapter if he/she can answer the following questions:

(1) Enumerate the diseases of animals spread by meat consumption and discuss the measures taken to control diseases spread by infected meat.

(2) Enumerate the legal restrictions on the sale of milk and milk products.

(3) Define the following terms:
   – undulant fever
   – chlorinated hydrocarboni insecticides
   – milk room
   – milk parlour
   – potable water
   – surface water
   – biological pollutants of water
   – chlorination of water

(4) Describe the following processes purported to ensure the safety of milk:
   (*a*) sterilisation of milk;
   (*b*) ultra-high temperature treatment (UHT);
   (*c*) pasteurisation of milk.

(5) Enumerate how food supplies may become polluted and describe in some detail microbial food poisoning.

(6) Give an account of the main points of a talk you would give to a group of housewives on the subject of milk and food hygiene in the home.

(7) Write notes on:
   (*a*) The hardness of water.
   (*b*) An artesian well (or borehole).
   (*c*) The importance of an adequate supply of pure water.
   (*d*) The Lesotho Highland Water project.
   (*e*) The chemical pollutants of water.
   (*f*) Section 37 of the Health Act 63 of 1977.
   (*g*) Natural purification of water.
   (*h*) Purification of water with Chlor-Floc tablets.

(8) Give an account of the main points of a talk you would give to a group of people from an urban community whose water supply is about to be supplemented by recycled sewage effluent.

11

Housing
Urbanisation

OBJECTIVES

General objectives: to give the student an understanding of the importance of adequate housing for the biopsychosocial health of a nation and the dangers of rapid urbanisation which overwhelms the capacity of the authorities to deal effectively with the greatly increased demands for housing.

STUDY OBJECTIVES

The student must know:

(1) Why the erection of new buildings in cities and towns is controlled by a local authority, especially with regard to ventilation, lighting, heating and cooking facilities.

(2) The legislation geared to the prevention of slums and control of African urbanisation.

(3) The precautions against the dangers of electricity.

(4) The current general policy and strategies used to solve the crisis in the supply of non-white housing.

(5) What is meant by urbanisation and the particular nature and consequences of current urbanisation in the RSA.

(6) The problems caused by informal squatter settlements.

(7) About the organisations formed by black civilians and hostel dwellers to redress their unacceptably poor living conditions.

HOUSING

THE IMPORTANCE OF HOUSING

The provision of adequate housing for an entire population, particularly in towns and cities, is a problem which most governments, including that of the Republic of South Africa, have to face. In almost all countries of the world there is an urgent need for more housing, particularly for the lower socio-economic groups. At a United Nations conference on the problems of the human environment, held in 1972, it was estimated that more than 1 000 million people in the world live in substandard housing conditions.

Reasons for the growing demand for low-cost housing in urban areas are:

(1) The ever-increasing drift of the rural population to the towns and cities. The WHO estimates that in many regions of Africa, Asia and Latin America the urban population has doubled in the last ten years; this trend is expected to continue. Generally these migrants from the rural areas move into already crowded squatter camps and shanty towns on the periphery of the cities.

(2) The rapid increase in the size of populations of the developing countries which has resulted from the falling death-rate, no doubt due to the control of internecine wars and the global preventive measures against infectious diseases.

(3) The presence of oscillating migrants, i.e. workers from the rural areas in South Africa, who leave their families behind and work in the cities for a limited period of time, usually on contract to the mines, municipalities and industrial concerns.

Substandard housing conditions are, however, not confined to urban areas. The traditional dwelling units found in the rural areas of the less developed countries often do little to promote the physical health of the occupants. They are often dark, poorly ventilated, crowded and shared with domestic animals; satisfactory sanitary arrangements are frequently non-existent, squatting in the bush being the accepted way of dealing with eliminatory functions. Poor housing is found not only in the tropics but also in the Arctic regions. For example, studies on the health status of Eskimos in Alaska show high rates of tuberculosis, bronchiectasis, pneumonia and upper respiratory tract infections. This is due not only to the cold climate but also to badly ventilated dwellings with polluted air, the pollution exaggerated by cigarette smoking. In the highlands of New Guinea, the high prevalence of chronic pulmonary disease appears to be due to the burning of smoky wood fires as a method of heating the small closed huts.

Definition of the term *housing:* in a limited sense, this term refers to the erection of structures for human habitation. A *housing scheme* refers to the establishment of an entire new township, usually in close proximity to the old established town or city. The report of the Expert Committee on Housing and Health (WHO, 1974) includes under 'housing' not only the actual dwelling units but also the immediate environment, the so-called infrastructure: sanitation, facilities for refuse disposal and pure water supplies, electrification, amenities such as schools, shops, parks, streets and recreational facilities. Great dissatisfaction is experienced in communities where there has been a delay in providing community and recreational facilities after 'housing schemes' have been completed.

THE CONTROL OF HOUSING TO ENSURE ITS ADEQUACY

In cities and towns the building of new dwellings is controlled by the local authority, which requires the submission of plans by the builders.

The following conditions for adequate housing must be satisfied:

(1) ventilation must be adequate; no back to back buildings may be erected and floor and window space must adhere to certain specifications;

(2) the building site must be well drained; damp-proof courses are placed in the walls above ground level to prevent earth dampness rising from the ground into the house;

(3) all large public buildings are liable to special ventilation requirements and must be rat-proofed;

(4) dwellings must be built of lasting materials and must be maintained in a good condition;

(5) all dwellings should be supplied with running water, facilities for washing and sanitation, electricity and cooking facilities.

The local authority should provide the necessary facilities for the disposal of excreta and household refuse and an adequate supply of pure water should be available. Premises should be kept clean and no house owner may harbour a nuisance (see p. 148). The house should protect its occupants against noise and other types of atmospheric and environmental pollution.

The United Nations plays an important role in the development of international housing projects. It assists member states with their housing programmes through its Regional Economic Commissions, the Centre for Housing, Building and Planning and special agencies such as the Food and Agricultural Organisation (FAO) and UNESCO. Advice is given on the design of houses and the use of locally available building materials. Technical assistance from member states is also available on request. National housing programmes vary with the needs of each country and must take into account the economic status of the country and the existing resources in terms of manpower, skills and the availability of suitable building materials. The design of dwellings in developing countries is influenced by culture, custom and religion. As urbanisation is occurring very rapidly in developing countries, the needs of the people are changing rapidly too. Old values and customs will, therefore, not make new housing unacceptable.

In many countries hurricanes, tornadoes and earthquakes occur and this has to be taken into account when designing and building houses. Ventilation is very important in tropical areas. Care should be taken to avoid judging the adequacy of housing by conventional Western standards. A fairly simple dwelling, favourably sited with a safe water supply and satisfactory sanitary services is far better than a more sophisticated house without such facilities.

When assessing the adequacy of a dwelling, the WHO Expert Committee on housing considers the following factors:

(1) the number of persons or dwelling units in a defined area; this will indicate the density of the population;

(2) the number of people living in each room; this gives a measure of crowding;

(3) the presence or absence of facilities such as sewerage, hot water, electricity;

(4) the state of repair of the dwellings.

VENTILATION

Ventilation may be defined as the exchange of stale, polluted, warm, humid air in a closed space for fresh, pure, cooler, drier moving air from outside. Adequate ventilation occurs without a draught and is necessary to ensure that cooling of the body takes place under normal climatic conditions.

The composition of air

Oxygen 20 %; nitrogen 79 %; CO_2 0,04 %; a variable amount of water vapour; some dust and other impurities such as non-respiratory gases, soot (smoke) and microbes.

The pollution of air in a closed space, such as a room, is caused by the presence of breathing living beings, by combustion of fuel in furnaces, stoves and fireplaces and by dust and gases. As exhaled air is saturated with moisture and warmed to body temperature, respiration heats the air and adds moisture to it. Exhaled air contains a large amount of microbes from the upper respiratory tract; the microbes are discharged into the air when people talk, cough and sneeze; they float on sputum droplets and particles of dust. Although the processes of respiration and combustion constantly use oxygen and add carbon dioxide to the air, the respiratory gases remain in balance. Air which circulates between the inside and outside of buildings is *purified* by the following natural processes:

(1) green plants use CO_2 and give off O_2 by a process known as photosynthesis; by this process the excess CO_2 is removed from stale air and its depleted O_2 stores are replenished;

(2) organic impurities are oxidised and rendered harmless;

(3) wind dilutes the impurities in the air and blows them away;

(4) rain washes the air and removes particulate matter;

(5) the ultraviolet rays of the sun destroy microbes;

(6) the sun dries the air; the cooling power of dry air is greater than that of moist air.

Moving, circulating air also has a greater cooling capacity than stagnant air. *Badly polluted* and *overheated* air to which human beings are overexposed may cause disease and death.

(1) *Heat exhaustion and heat-stroke* may occur if a number of people are locked in a room with inadequate ventilation holes. A historical example of this type of catastrophe is the infamous Black Hole of Calcutta (1756) where many British prisoners suffocated in a prison dungeon with one small window; they died of heat-stroke, i.e. hyperthermia.

(2) Dust consists of fine hairs, pollen, microbes, fibres and fine sand. The main industrial dusts are silica and asbestos fibres. In workers who are constantly exposed to these types of dust, *pneumoconiosis* and *cancers* may develop (see p. 67).

(3) Large amounts of noxious gases, soot and smoke may be added to the atmosphere by factories and by communities which use open coal and wood fires for cooking and heating purposes. Pollution of the atmospheric air affects an entire community, contributing to ill-health in the form of *sinusitis* and *chronic bronchitis*. The murky atmosphere also prevents the penetration of the ultraviolet rays of the sun and thereby causes damage to plant life. Smog is a mixture of smoke and fog and is the harbinger of much respiratory ill-health.

(4) In a closed space, the greatest danger from incomplete combustion is the formation of the poisonous gas, *carbon monoxide (CO)*. This odourless, colourless gas, when inhaled, combines with haemoglobin, thus displacing oxygen and causing asphyxiation. People who sleep in poorly ventilated rooms in the winter, in front of a drum of glowing coals, become the victims of fatal carbon monoxide poisoning.

(5) Domestic gases, either piped municipal coal gas or bottled petroleum gas used for cooking, heating and lighting, can be lethal if released in a closed room for a protracted period. There is also danger of an *explosion* if a match is struck in a room filled with gas. Poisonous gases from gas stoves or from the

exhaust pipe of a running car engine are sometimes used by people who wish to commit *suicide*.

Poor ventilation, especially in places where many people gather, may cause *headaches, listlessness and lethargy,* feelings which are not conducive to efficiency, especially in the learning situation. In order to judge whether an occupied room is being adequately ventilated, certain guidelines may be used.

Signs of poor ventilation are:

(1) The smell of the room. A poorly ventilated room smells stuffy and muggy.

(2) The temperature and humidity of the room. Ideally the temperature in a room should be approximately 16 °C to 20 °C, i.e. low enough to cool the body but not so low that it causes discomfort and shivering.

(3) The space allocation per occupant and the number and size of windows and other openings. The minimum legal cubic space in the sleeping quarters of a person over the age of 10 years is 12 cubic metres; half that amount is required for a child under the age of 10 years. The floor space must be 4 and 2 square metres respectively. The size of the windows must be $\frac{1}{12}$th of the floor space and the windows must open fully or halfway. The air must be in slight movement in order that both the temperature and humidity may be maintained at optimum levels.

Note: The effectiveness of ventilation can be measured with the Kata thermometer. This thermometer, with a wet and a dry bulb, indicates air movement, temperature and humidity. It therefore measures the cooling capacity of the air.

The aims of ventilation are not primarily to supply sufficient oxygen to the air in the room because, under normal circumstances, lack of oxygen is not a problem. Adequate ventilation is aimed at maintaining a comfortable body temperature, at reducing the microbial content of the air, at removing noxious gases, smoke and odours and at providing a dust-free atmosphere. Poor ventilation is closely associated with overcrowding and a room in which the ventilation is satisfactory when it contains 10 people may be poorly ventilated when it contains 20.

Methods of ventilation

Natural ventilation

In natural ventilation — the usual method of ventilating a building — an exchange of air takes place between the inside of the building and the outside through ventilating openings such as windows, doors, chimneys, fanlights above doors, ventilation or air bricks and cracks and spaces around doors and windows. The window area must be at least $\frac{1}{12}$th of floor area and the windows must open either completely or half-way. The natural ventilating openings must be sited on opposite walls in order to facilitate cross-ventilation. Louvre windows are very useful to exclude draughts and rain. Exchange of air between the inside and the outside, through ventilating openings, is brought about by the following *physical forces:*

(1) *Diffusion of air.* Diffusion refers to the process which takes place when differences in the composition of the air inside and outside a room causes the air to intermingle through the porous material of which the dwelling is constructed. This process is too slow to be of much value in ventilation. It does, however, take place through open windows when the air is completely still.

(2) *Natural movement of the outside air*, such as *breezes and winds,* may ventilate a building either by: (i) *perflation* or (ii) *aspiration.*

    Perflation takes place when air enters a room through one opening and a corresponding amount of air leaves the room by another opening, the ideal aimed at being the placement of openings so that cross-ventilation can take place.

    Aspiration occurs when air is sucked out of a room by wind blowing over an opening such as a chimney. In modern houses which are electrically heated, chimneys are fast disappearing; aspiration is, therefore, no longer an important natural way of ventilating a room.

(3) *Convection currents* generated in a room when air is heated near the floor. Warm air expands, becomes lighter and rises to the ceiling. Air is commonly heated either by under-floor heaters in winter, people, open fires in fireplaces and other types of heaters, as well as the sun shining in through win-

dows. Convection causes the air to circulate, warm air from the bottom finding an outlet through ventilating bricks situated near the ceiling.

Artificial ventilation and air-conditioning

Where it is not possible to achieve ventilation by natural means, e.g. in cinemas and theatres, in large hospitals, in underground buildings and in the mines, and in closely crowded high-rise buildings, rooms must be ventilated by artificial means, i.e. by using large electrical fans placed in walls, either near the ceiling or near the floor. The fans may be placed at a distance from the rooms, the air being moved along ducts (conduits) and entering the room or being extracted from the rooms through vents in the walls. When air is forced into a room it is taken from the outside atmosphere and *conditioned* (i.e. heated or cooled and purified) before it is introduced into the room. Windows must be kept closed and are installed to provide light and a view of the surroundings.

The following systems of *artificial ventilation* are used:

(1) *The plenum system:* Fans force conditioned air into the rooms through a system of conduits and stale air is squeezed out through natural openings, e.g. doors.
(2) *The vacuum system:* Air is extracted from each room in the building, thus creating a relative vacuum which is filled by air sucked in through chinks and doors or through specially built inlets.
(3) *The balanced system:* Conditioned air is forced in and stale air is extracted to balance the volume of incoming air.

There are some *disadvantages* to the artificial ventilation of buildings: air-conditioning plants may harbour microbes and promote their dissemination throughout the building; the degree of ventilation cannot be altered at will by, for instance, opening a window, as this upsets the smooth functioning of the system. Overheating of rooms in winter is possible, especially the rooms on the sunny side of the building. Thus, if a building is artificially ventilated and air-conditioned, individual needs cannot be catered for and some people experience great discomfort.

LIGHTING

Adequate lighting is almost as important as satisfactory ventilation in ensuring the health and happiness of the occupants of a dwelling. During the hours of daylight, natural lighting is usually sufficient for most of the daily tasks which have to be carried out in a home, especially in South Africa where most days are bright and sunny. Adequate lighting does depend to some extent upon the design and the siting of the dwelling, but many of the laws and regulations which aim at promoting adequate ventilation ensure good lighting as well. For example, legislation which stipulates the size of windows, the minimum distance one building must be away from another, the prohibition of back to back dwellings, ensures good natural lighting of rooms during daylight hours. Natural lighting promotes health as it encourages the housewife to keep her house clean; sunlight, if allowed to enter rooms through open doors and windows, will help to destroy microbes.

Good lighting is necessary at all times while a person is awake, for the following reasons:

(1) it promotes efficiency and prevents accidents;
(2) it prevents eye-strain when visual activities are followed;
(3) it promotes cheerfulness.

Lighting may be either natural or artificial.

Natural lighting comes from the sun and in buildings with adequate window space which is not obscured by adjacent buildings should be adequate during daylight hours. Daylight is not as bright as sunlight as the rays of the sun are obscured. If sunlight is too bright it causes a glare which may harm the eyes. Direct sunlight falling on the macula of the eye, caused by looking directly into the sun, causes central blindness.

Artificial lighting is used at night and sometimes also during the day in dark rooms. Artificial lighting can come from two sources: (*a*) burning of fuel; (*b*) electricity.

Criteria for good lighting media are:

(1) They should not be a fire hazard.
(2) They should not add products of combustion (CO_2, heat, water vapour) to the atmosphere.
(3) They should not cast shadows.

(4) They should not produce glare.

(5) They should not flicker.

These criteria are not met by the lighting media which burn fuel such as candles, paraffin lamps, petroleum and coal gas. Some of the gas and pressure paraffin lamps give a good light which does not flicker, but they produce heat and other products of combustion and are a fire hazard. In areas without electricity, they are of sufficient intensity for close eye-work.

Electricity provides the ideal medium for artificial lighting, being safe and adequate for all purposes. It is, unfortunately, not yet within the reach of all South Africans. Electric bulbs and fluorescent tubes produce a good light in comparison with the amount of heat produced. No oxygen is used and no air pollution is caused. There is no fire hazard and it is immediately available.

Requirements for adequate lighting are:

(1) There must be a good source of light. Window area must be at least $\frac{1}{12}$th of the floor area and must reach as near to the ceiling as possible. Unless made of light coloured sun filter material, curtains must be pulled open during the day.

(2) While doing visual work, the source of the light must be behind the reader or worker and must come from the opposite side of the hand being used, so that no shadow is cast on the work or on the book.

(3) A bright light must not fall on the eyes and bright lights must be suitably shaded. A glare and shiny pages must be avoided as they cause eye-strain.

HEATING

The body constantly produces heat through metabolic processes and the contraction of muscles, especially during exercise. Heat production is automatically augmented in conditions of hypothermia by shivering and heat loss counteracted by peripheral vasoconstriction. Normally the body gets rid of excess heat by peripheral vasodilatation, radiation of heat from the skin, conduction of heat to the clothes and evaporation of perspiration, thus maintaining the normal temperature. The lethargy one experiences in very hot weather is a safeguard against excessive heat production by vigorous muscle contractions. In the normal person, there is a constant relationship between heat production and heat loss so that the normal body temperature varies between 36,4 °C and 37 °C. This is the temperature at which the body functions best. In conditions of hypothermia, the person feels uncomfortable and sluggish. In conditions of hyperthermia, discomfort is also experienced, metabolism is speeded up and the brain cells are damaged. Sweating causes dehydration and extreme thirst results to counteract the excessive fluid loss by encouraging fluid intake. Although hypothermia and hyperthermia are usually caused by pathological conditions in the body, extremes of atmospheric temperature may cause freezing and heat-stroke which cause death.

An atmospheric temperature of 16 °C to 20 °C is comfortable for most people who are adequately clothed. When the temperature rises much above 22 °C, *the body can be helped to cool* down by:

(1) Wearing fewer clothes and choosing the lighter colours. White and the pastel shades, which reflect the rays of the spectrum, are the coolest colours. Dark colours allow the rays to penetrate and are especially hot when worn in the sun.

Cool materials (e.g. cotton and linen) are good conductors of heat and allow the heat from the skin to be dissipated.

(2) Promoting ventilation, if people have the protection of buildings. Opening windows and switching on electric fans are simple ways of cooling a room.

(3) Deflecting the rays of the sun by making use of blinds and sunshades.

(4) Making use of air-conditioning where buildings are artificially ventilated.

When the atmospheric temperature falls to such an extent that the wearing of extra and warm clothes no longer allows people to feel comfortably warm and shelter in buildings is not adequate to protect against the cold caused by winds, rain, snow, then artificial methods of heating the air in dwellings and public buildings are resorted to.

A room is warmed by means of the following *physical forces:*

(1) *Convection currents*, i.e. warm air expands and rises and the cooler air from the top sinks to the bottom to be warmed in turn. The source of the heat should, therefore, be placed near the floor.

(2) *Conduction of heat* from one molecule to another. Heating appliances which make direct contact with the body warm by conduction of heat.

(3) *Radiation of heat* from a heated object to a distant object to be heated, without heating the space between the objects. The sun warms the earth by radiation of heat.

Artificial heating is brought about by:

(1) *Fuel-burning heaters and stoves,* such as open fires in fireplaces, closed coal stoves, gas stoves, oil burners, drums of glowing coals.

Open fires which emit smoke and require chimneys to conduct the smoke out of the room are seldom used today in middle-class suburbs because of the rapid proliferation of Smoke Control Zones (see p. 147).

Anthracite burners, smokeless coal stoves and gas stoves are household fuel burning appliances suitable for the warming of living-rooms of dwellings during cold winter days. Gas fires are inclined to dry the air, but the heat can be regulated and they cause no extra work. A bowl of water in front of the gas fire prevents the nose stuffiness caused by the drying of the air. Anthracite stoves also dry the air but require little attention and can be installed in such a way that several rooms are warmed evenly during the whole day.

The main disadvantages of fuel-burning appliances are the dangers of fire-setting, the drying of the air (except where there are open fires), O_2 consumption and CO_2 and CO emission, and the labour required for their upkeep. Pollution of the atmosphere, especially in the poorer areas where smoke control measures have not yet been applied because of the absence of electrification, may create smog conditions in winter, with resultant chronic respiratory disorders.

(2) *Electrical heating appliances* are very useful for the warming of a small room, as they are clean, easy to handle, easy to control and can be made fireproof. Those supplied with a fan can push warmed air into the room, thus warming the entire room. Strip heaters attached to the bottom of a wall heat the room by convection, and are left switched on permanently during very cold days to create a warm room atmosphere. Electrical appliances do not pollute the air but they do cause drying of the atmosphere in the room. Some electrical appliances work by heating an asbestos plate to a non-dangerous temperature; they are, therefore, safe, especially where children are concerned. A form of central heating by incorporating electrical units in the floors of houses is becoming popular in newly built prestige houses in areas with a cold winter climate.

(3) *Central heating.* This method is generally used for the heating of large buildings, although the temperature can be regulated in each room by control switches. Use is usually made of hot water or superheated steam which is led by means of pipes from a central boiler to heating appliances situated in each room of the building. The boiler is situated in a cellar of the building and the pipes run in the walls. The heating units may be one of the following:

(a) Steel heating appliances placed below the windows which heat the room by convection.

(b) Panels in the wall or ceiling; the room is heated by radiation.

(c) Coils of pipes can be placed under the floor or on top of the ceiling and heat the room by convection or radiation.

Central heating is the best and most economical way of heating a large building which is not artificially ventilated. It is commonly used for the heating of hospitals.

(4) *Air-conditioning.* In buildings which are artificially ventilated, the air is conditioned before it is circulated. Conditioning includes regulation of the temperature. Each room is warmed in winter by blowing in (plenum and balanced systems) warm air through vents which are usually placed near the ceiling. The disadvantage of this method is that the temperature cannot be regulated in each room. On sunny winter days, the

temperature in the sunny rooms may be much warmer than in the shady rooms.

GLOBAL WARMING

Global warming, i.e. increase in the temperature of our earth and its atmosphere, appears to be happening very gradually; scientists are not quite sure if the present trend in observed warming is a permanent phenomenon. They ascribe the warming to the 'greenhouse effect' caused by the ever-increasing amounts of gases (CO_2 and CFCs) released into the earth's atmosphere. The destruction of the vast forests in the Amazon basin is also cited as a cause of the increased CO_2 in the air. Loss of so much of the earth's green plants diminishes global photosynthesis — the removal of the CO_2 and production of O_2. This surfeit of gases (CO_2 and CFCs), like the glass of a greenhouse, traps the heat by reflecting the radiated heat (from earth) back to earth, thus preventing its dissipation into the stratosphere. It was estimated (Race Relations Survey 1992/1993, p. 151) that South Africa produces 2 % of the gases responsible for global warming. Not only is the heat uncomfortable but it causes expansion of sea water and the melting of land ice and snow, with resulting flooding of the lower lying plains. A warmer atmosphere will also affect the climate and disturb the present ecological balance on which our food production depends.

ELECTRICITY AND ELECTRIFICATION IN TOWNSHIPS

South Africa produces 60 % of the electricity of the African continent, yet almost two-thirds of the total population (80 % of all blacks) do not have access to electricity for their household requirements.[6] As energy for cooking, lighting and heating are basic human requirements, energy must come from burning fuel such as paraffin, coal, candles, dried cow dung and wood. Gathered wood is becoming a scarce commodity as the natural forests are dwindling without being replaced. Burning fuels are not only a fire hazard but they also add impurities to the air, thus causing chronic respiratory diseases, especially where house ventilation is poor or where smoke is emitted from densely situated houses.

Many townships around the major South African cities have recently been electrified at tremendous financial cost, the Soweto project costing R250 million. A total of 105 754 homes were supplied with electricity and 101 934 houses rewired, the average cost of wiring a house being R400. Money for the projects was raised by the administration boards of the townships. Subsequently residents were required to pay an increasing monthly levy (added to the rent) to pay off the loan and interest, irrespective of whether electricity was used or not.

In addition, monthly accounts based on consumption have to be paid. At present, therefore, the use of electricity is an expensive necessity for township households and the advantages of electrification are somewhat dampened by high costs. Bulk electricity is bought from Eskom which is considering ways of supplying Third-World consumers at a reduced cost by, for example, providing overhead cables in future, therefore compromising safety and security somewhat.

Since 1992 Eskom has secured rights from black local authorities to supply electricity directly to township residents, thereby ensuring improved electricity payment. Pre-payment meters are being installed to cut electricity consumption and thereby making it more affordable.

The National Electrification Forum (NELF) (May 1993) intends to provide domestic electricity to the 23 million people without it. This number represents 60 % of the population of South Africa,[8] i.e. 23 % in the metropolitan areas and 92 % in the rural areas (former TBVC states).

Consumers who have never used their own electrical appliances before, need to be instructed in the economical and safe use of lights and appliances, viz:

- Unnecessary lights must not be left burning.
- A stove oven or plate must not be heated for lighting a cigarette.
- A hot plate must be turned down to its lowest working power, once food is cooking.
- Except for ordinary lighting, the use of flexes with three wires, i.e. an additional 'earth' wire, must be used. This is to prevent dangerous shock.

- All appliances must be supplied with plugs which fit into wall sockets. An appliance flex must never be connected to a light fitting, e.g. by bare wires wound around matches.
- No faulty equipment should ever be used. Electrical flexes should never be patched or have interposed switches. Joints in flexes must be covered carefully with insulation tape and their points of connection with the apparatus covered with insulation tubes.
- Electrical flexes and apparatus should never be wet, or be touched with wet hands.
- 10- or 15-ampere fuse wires must never be used in a 5-ampere circuit.
- No untrained person should ever repair a plug or fuse wires.
- No heaters or electric irons may be plugged into a light socket.
- The user must switch off the current after use of an appliance.

THE ILL EFFECTS OF INADEQUATE HOUSING

Much has been written about the harmful effects of unsatisfactory housing on the health of the members of a community, but the association between health and housing is by no means clear. There are many unfavourable factors associated with poor housing such as poverty, lack of education, poor job opportunities, poor nutrition, inadequate medical services, a hostile environment and crowding. It is difficult to assess the relative effect of each disease-contributing variable. It can be said with certainty, however, that morbidity and mortality rates are higher amongst those whose housing conditions are unsatisfactory. Squatter camps and shanty towns are a definite health hazard. In these slums migrants build temporary shacks of packing-cases, sacks and corrugated iron and grossly overtax sanitary facilities and water supplies. The environment becomes polluted and insects such as flies, fleas, bugs and lice are rife, while rodents thrive in the accumulated waste and refuse. The greatest health hazards are epidemics of infectious diseases.

On the other hand, research has shown that the rehousing of a community does not necessarily lead to a dramatic improvement in the health of its members. The new houses may cause financial hardships as the rent may be higher and the location may be further from the area of work (thus causing higher transportation costs); this may lead to a fall in the nutritional status of the community. In this case improved housing may cause a deterioration in health. On the other hand, economic advancement, better nutrition, more satisfactory environmental conditions and more adequate medical care and social services may improve the health of a community, in spite of the fact that the houses or dwellings *per se* are far from adequate.

Poor housing with overcrowding in dwellings and schools may have the following effects on health.

Physical health

(1) *Communicable diseases* such as tuberculosis, non-tuberculotic respiratory infections and meningitis (see p. 554) have the highest incidence where there is overcrowding, poor ventilation and pollution of indoor air. Overcrowded conditions in schools lead to an increase in streptococcal throat infections and rheumatic heart disease (see p. 545).

(2) *Helminthic infestations and enteric infections* are associated with poor environmental hygiene inside and outside the house, as well as with inadequate facilities for the disposal of excreta. The provision of such facilities, however, will do little to decrease the frequency of these diseases unless accompanied by improved personal hygiene, especially hand-washing after elimination and before the handling of food.

(3) *External infestations* such as scabies and lice are rife in overcrowded communities as these parasites are spread when people live in close, intimate proximity to one another.

(4) *Dangerous exposure* of the occupants. A house can be considered inadequate if it cannot protect its occupants against exposure to environmental dangers and rigours:
   (*a*) insects which are vectors of disease, e.g. flies, mosquitoes;
   (*b*) rodents and their fleas which may be carriers of plague;
   (*c*) excessive heat leading to heat exhaustion and heat-stroke;

(d) excessive cold which may cause hypothermia and lowering of resistance to infection;

(e) rain, hail and lightning.

(5) *Accident hazards.* Poor housing and overcrowding offer many opportunities for accidents in the home.

Mental health and social well-being

Little is known of the relationship between housing and mental and social well-being. Although numerous studies have been carried out on the effects of variables such as crowding, life in high-rise flats, rehousing and relocation of persons, the results have generally been confusing and even contradictory.

In high-rise buildings without play facilities, the social well-being of children is adversely affected. Slum conditions with overcrowding are conducive to *juvenile delinquency,* often the result of boredom because of lack of recreational facilities. Crowded living conditions make it impossible for people to satisfy *their need for privacy.* Overcrowding usually leads to *slum conditions* and people who live in slums lose their self-respect and their motivation to create beauty around them. Their *standards of hygiene are poor,* often because it is impossible to keep a place clean if people are milling around all the time. Children who grow up in these unhygienic conditions cannot grasp the necessity for personal hygiene.

Ideally, housing should not only provide the occupants of a dwelling with shelter against the elements but should also be a haven of security. A dwelling should be a home, i.e. the abode of a family in which the functions of a family can be carried out. As the family is the basic unit of a society, housing which is not conducive to the maintenance of the unity of the family *cannot* be considered satisfactory, as the society itself is harmed thereby.

Housing which *disrupts family life* causes grave social problems. Extreme poverty and crowding which cause people to take in lodgers, thereby forcing more than one family to live in a small house, lead to *family disintegration* and all its attendant evils: prostitution, alcoholism, child neglect, delinquency.

The provision of single ('bachelor') accommodation in hostels and compounds for migrant labourers, a practice which is common in all South African cities and large towns (see p. 195), effectively excludes wives and children from the abode of the head of the family and causes disintegration of family life. As most of the migrant workers are men — the women and children remaining in the rural areas — *the balance between the sexes is disturbed* in the cities as well as in the rural areas. Thus the men in the cities cannot form stable heterosexual relationships; the rural areas are depleted of a strong labour force to develop their potential, yet overpopulated with women, children and elderly people.

THE SLUMS ACT 76 OF 1979

The Slums Act of 1934 and all its amendments were repealed and replaced with the Slums Act 76 of 1979.

The objective of the Slums Act is to make better provision for the elimination of 'slums' within the jurisdiction of certain local authorities. This Act originally applied to the eight largest towns of the RSA, but today (1979) 180 towns fall under its control. The Act defines a *slum* as 'any premises or part thereof which has been declared a slum'. *By 'premises'* the Act implies a dwelling and the land on which it is built. A *dwelling* is a structure in which people live and sleep. A slum may also refer to a poor, overcrowded, dirty, ill-kept district of a city or town — a blighted area in which people no longer maintain decent standards of living; a whole area may thus be declared a slum. In such an area buildings are often in poor repair, unpainted, with rickety staircases which pose a danger to the inhabitants of tenement buildings.

The Slums Act makes provision for a medical officer of health to report to the Slums Clearance Court that a slum nuisance exists on certain premises. On receipt of such a report, the owner of the premises (or his representative) is subpoenaed to appear before the court to show reason why the dwelling should not be declared a slum. If the premises, or part thereof, is declared a slum, the owner may be ordered to remove the nuisance and to take the necessary steps to prevent it recurring. The owner is responsible for thereby the costs incurred. On the other hand, the property may be expropriated, permission being obtained from the Minister of Community Development, or the local authority may take steps to rectify the nuisance and reclaim the costs from the owner. Where overcrowding is the reason for the premises being declared a slum, the occupiers may agree amongst themselves which of them shall cease to occupy the slum.

The owner shall not permit prohibited occupancy of the slum. A local authority may acquire any land comprised in a slum to prevent injurious conditions from arising out of the existence of unhygienic or overcrowded premises.

When any person is convicted of occupying or entering or being upon a slum, the court convicting him shall, in addition to imposing a penalty, order his ejectment from the slum. There are no exemptions on the ground of lack of other accommodation. If the local authority notifies the owner or any occupiers of the slum of other accommodation available to the occupiers of the slum affected, the local authority shall not thereby become liable to provide such accommodation or any other accommodation for such occupiers of a slum.

Any of the following conditions may be considered to be a *nuisance in terms of the Slums Act:*

(1) premises which, because of the presence of 'vermin', are dangerous or harmful to health or likely to facilitate the spread of communicable diseases;

(2) premises or part thereof which, because of their construction and state of repair, are not safe;

(3) land or buildings which are congested or overcrowded;

(4) any room which does not allow 12 cubic metres of free air space and 4 square metres of floor space for each person over the age of 10 years sleeping in the room and half that amount of space for each person less than 10 years of age;

(5) premises without an adequate and safe water supply within a reasonable distance;

(6) any premises in which latrines, passages, staircases, landings, bathrooms, cupboards, outbuildings, garages, stables, tents, store-

rooms, cellars or lofts are being used for sleeping purposes without the permission of the local authority;

(7) a dwelling which does not have facilities for the segregation of the sexes where this is necessary;

(8) premises which do not have the necessary number of latrines or facilities for washing or bathing, or have inadequate facilities for cooking;

(9)

any dwelling which fails to comply with the local by-laws governing lighting, ventilation, height of room.

Note: These are abbreviated extracts from the Slums Act 1979 and its Schedule 3.

GENERAL POLICY FOR HOUSING

▨ Self-help housing and privatisation of housing provision.

▨ Help for those who need help with loans and rent subsidies.

▨ Loans to local authorities for urban renewal.

▨ Welfare housing is considered, via loans to local authorities, for subeconomic and economic housing schemes.

▨ As part of the government of National Unity's Reconstruction and Development Programme (1994), institutional funds will be freed to help the government build 2,5 million houses over the next 10 years. To meet this target, R90 billion is needed. This money will come from the government, the private sector and communities. The present housing backlog is 1,5 million houses; to this must be added the annual requirement for a further 200 000 housing units (houses and/or flats). Some of these houses will be subsidised and some will be rental housing stock. In order to build approximately 100 000–370 000 houses a year, 10 000 men and women must be trained in building skills over the next 2–3 years (*The Star*, June 1994; interviews with the Minister of Housing).

Subeconomic housing schemes are designed to supply reasonably attractive and adequate housing for the most economically deprived members of the community. Housing supplied under such a scheme is intended only for persons who cannot afford to pay economic rentals and, therefore, a ceiling is placed on the income of the family.

Frequently persons occupying such housing are not employed, either because they are sick or disabled, or elderly, or because they are the mothers of young families whose husbands are deceased or have deserted them. Such families are dependent on social pensions or maintenance grants (see p. 773). They can, therefore, afford only the very lowest rentals.

Economic housing schemes are designed for that section of the population whose income exceeds the maximum limit for subeconomic housing, but who are not in a financial position to obtain a loan from a building society or similar organisation.

Dwellings in such housing schemes may be rented or sold to individuals who qualify, without profit. Only the cost of the building and the land is included in the price. The local authority is not meant to subsidise this type of housing.

A ceiling is placed on the gross income of persons who qualify for economic housing. In South Africa, people who earn more than the ceiling income are expected to supply their own housing, which they may do with the assistance of loans obtained from building societies or banks.

HISTORY OF NON-WHITE HOUSING PROBLEMS IN THE RSA

In *A History of Black Housing in South Africa,* Pauline Morris says that the present black housing crisis is rooted in the long history of segregation and the SA political ideology which determined all major housing policies. In 1923 an Act of Parliament decreed that blacks in urban areas could not be given freehold rights (the right to own property) and that there would be strict control over their movement into urban areas — the so-called 'influx control'. Leasehold rights were at first allowed and then withdrawn in the 1960s. Blacks thereby became temporary sojourners in white urban areas without social and political rights. The right of black women to acquire housing was withdrawn in the 1960s. Township managers had the power to evict and trading rights were restricted. White local authorities were hesitant to spend much

money on black township development. But with rapid industrialisation in the 1960s in South Africa, the 'reverse flow' of blacks from the urban to the rural areas could not be sustained. Despite stricter attempts at influx control, blacks streamed to the cities. This caused an increase in informal shanty town or squatter settlements on the periphery of cities.

Influx control was abolished in 1986. This exacerbated the problem of urban squatter settlements (see 'Urbanisation' on p. 196 below).

In 1986 the Black Communities Development Amendment Act granted freehold rights in black urban areas in white-designated South Africa to blacks who are South African citizens. The 99-year leasehold was retained as an alternative form of tenure. This opened the way for the private sector to develop and sell property in black townships. The government accepts responsibility for ensuring that lower income blacks are able to obtain housing and concentrates on the provision of land and infrastructure for low-cost housing schemes.

The Constitutional Laws Amendment Act (1987) amended several laws affecting blacks; for example, it provides for black women to acquire ownership of property in the same way as black men, i.e. black women acquired full property rights for the first time.

Housing shortages are enormous and have been estimated in various ways, the results ranging from 340 000 to 2 million housing units, and the number of people living in informal settlements and backyard shacks in 1992 ranging from 3,5 to 10 million.

Coloureds and Indians had freehold rights in their own areas, i.e. they could own their homes and pass them on to their children. The development of townships (suburbs) is the responsibility of local authorities and the private sector. Despite current increases in subeconomic and economic housing developments, the waiting list for coloured housing in the Johannesburg area stood at 7 599 in 1981. People are on the waiting list from 1–6 years before they can be accommodated. In the mean time, it is common for two families to share one house. Overcrowding is a health hazard.

Standards of living have been steadily rising for the urban Indian and coloured groups and so has the demand for better housing. With the scrapping of all apartheid legislation, people can live in any suburb of their choice, if they can afford to do so.

SOME SOLUTIONS FOR NON-WHITE HOUSING PROBLEMS

In 1982 the government decided it would no longer take primary responsibility for the provision of housing; it funds the housing development by private developers and provincial administrations. The government budgeted R2,15 billion for 1992/1993 for housing and related infrastructure, an increase of 41 % on the previous year.

The following are some of the ways in which the private sector, local authorities and the state attempted to solve the almost insurmountable housing problems.

(1) The special sale at a price below market value of 345 000 state-owned houses to all population groups was introduced in 1983.

This virtually came to a halt in 1992 after 38 % (129 398) units had been sold. Instability in the townships was given as the main cause of the lack of interest in buying these houses.

(2) Encouragement of the private sector to help people to acquire houses.

The following approaches are currently being tried:

(a) Self-help housing with site and services (water, waste removal) and loans provided. The land must be properly laid out by a town planner and the building stands must be clearly defined so that the owner can develop pride of ownership. The owner lives in a temporary shelter (e.g. a tent) while he builds his house.

(b) Self-help scheme in which a 'wet-core' of one room, toilet and basin is built. To this the owner must add rooms with his own labour, on a pre-planned basis and at a pace which he can afford. The government supplies the infrastructure.

The present government is opposed to these 'site-and-service' schemes. Most blacks, however, simply cannot afford to build a house privately.

Consumer services and urban infrastructure creation generally account for 50 % of developmental costs of a new township. Consumer services are: electricity in the home, waste removal, water laid on in the home, sanitation, clinic services, schooling, postal deliveries, police protection.

Urban infrastructure comprises: tarred roads, street lighting, electric cabling, water reticulation, waterborne sewerage, storm water drainage, post office, schools, sports stadium, clinic.

(c) Self-help. The owner arranges his own loans (from a building society, bank or employer) and makes plans for constructing the dwelling, e.g. building contractor or subcontractors.

(d) Speculative housing built by a developer. The home-owner selects his own design from a small range offered by the developer. He gets a housing loan from a building society, bank or his employer.

Some building societies are lending money to non-whites for low-cost housing, with new criteria for granting loans, including lower housing specifications. In addition the salaries of all members of the family could be taken into account. Loans are also obtainable from the SA Housing Trust.

(e) Employer-assisted housing is at present enjoying much interest, as company employers begin to realise that the security derived from home ownership results in greater stability of the work-force.

(3) Many companies build houses for their employees. The house does not become the property of the employee.

The government has a first-time home-buyers subsidy scheme (for new and old living units costing less than R40 000) for all population groups. Government loans are available to farmers for the erection of houses for full-time black farm labourers.

Since the repeal of the Group Areas Act (1966) in June 1991, there has been a steady demand by blacks for houses in so-called 'white' suburbs. Thus middle-class blacks who can afford the more expensive houses in 'white' suburbs are enabled to improve their living standard with little protest from their white neighbours.

The immediate solution to the housing problem by the blacks who are streaming to the cities from the impoverished rural areas, especially since the abolition of influx control, is to move into any available gap within reasonable distance of employment opportunities. There they put up temporary shacks (informal houses) made of available materials: sacking, packing cases, corrugated iron, wood poles from surrounding trees. Urban slums are thus created by the squatter settlements. Slums are created not only because the housing is inadequate but also because of gross overcrowding and lack of infrastructure. This results in pollution of the environment.

The Urban Foundation[3] has appealed for slum improvement instead of slum clearance, with minimal public facilities, e.g. water taps, lavatories, open street drains, minimal paving of walkways, minimal lighting and the strategy of accepting lower standards of service and facilities than those regarded as minimal in middle-class society. The standards adopted must be in line with the community's capacity to pay.

The squatter problem will be discussed below under 'Urbanisation'.

THE HOUSING OF MIGRANT LABOURERS IN CITIES

Oscillating migration for the purpose of finding employment occurs when men's homes are so far from their work that they cannot go home at night, home visits occurring either weekly, monthly or yearly. These men come from rural areas and employment is in towns and cities. Migrant labourers usually do contract work on the mines, in agriculture, in industry, in hospitals, in the municipalities and the railways and in the domestic sector. According to official statistics in 1969, it was estimated that there were 1 305 000 oscillating migrants.

In South Africa the families of the migrant workers did not accompany the men; therefore, oscillating migratory labour causes disruption of family life. The men live in single-sex hostels or compounds near their places of work; the women and children live on their own in the country. Very few family houses have been built for the labourers and their families near the place of employment. The gold-mines were, until 1969, allowed to provide family housing for not more than 3 % of its South African black labour force. Through the years, mining and industrial employers have become increasingly dependent on migrant labourers who are housed on a temporary basis in hostels and compounds which are springing up in ever-increasing numbers in all the industrial centres of the RSA.

The Johannesburg municipality distinguishes between *hostels* and *compounds. Hostels* are legally proclaimed as black areas for the housing of single men or women. *Example:* Alexandra township, outside Johannesburg, a 'hostel' complex for 60 000 migrant labourers housed in 15 hostels. One hostel may accommodate up to 6 000 people, the age of the boarders varying from 18 to 70. The hostel bedrooms house from 4 to 8 people. Most hostels are provided with ablution blocks with hot and cold showers and washing facilities, cooking facilities, a community hall, an outdoor tribal dancing arena and a beer hall. In the higher class hostels, there is a beer garden and restaurant which are open to women. Large hostels also have a chapel and shops and recreational facilities.

Compounds, on the other hand, are for workers on the mines and essential services, the men in one compound generally working for the same employer. Any employer may build a residence for his employees on allocated ground. An employer wishing to house 50 or more black workers must employ a full-time manager.

Mine compounds may be very large. Some old mine compounds may have rooms housing 50 or more men sleeping in double-decker concrete bunks, while modern mine compounds house between 12 and 20 men in dormitories. Washing facilities are available and in the new mine compounds there are dining-rooms. The mines provide a balanced diet, the food being wholesome and abundant.

Non-mining compounds are usually smaller than mine compounds. Old mine compounds are sometimes taken over by large firms, e.g. municipalities, the railways, to house large numbers of workers who feed themselves. In some compounds, film shows are provided and sport organised over the weekends, but no women are allowed in the compound.

As there is not enough accommodation for migrant workers in Johannesburg, people on the waiting-lists for hostel accommodation live as lodgers with black families in Soweto and elsewhere.[5]

Note: Henceforward the term 'hostels' will include compounds. Compounds are really privately owned hostels.

URBANISATION

Urbanisation is the process by which people move from the countryside (rural areas) to the towns and cities. *Urbs* is the Latin word for town and *rus* for country. Rural and urban are complementary words, 'urbanisation' denoting the growth of a town at the expense of the countryside.

Urbanisation may cause the individual to lose his primary contacts, especially his family, so that he becomes an isolate without a reference group in an unknown society with unexpected temptations. His new contacts may be multiple and superficial. The (im)migrant may become unstable, mobile and rootless. In this anonymous world the social norms are unable to exert their behaviour-controlling functions; this may lead to pathologically irresponsible behaviour which causes misery to the (im)migrant and his dependants.

In 'white' South Africa the distances between the countryside and towns have shrunk due to rapid means of communication. The pathological effects of urbanisation among whites are not as striking as they were earlier in this century when the urbanisation of the rural Afrikaner was at its height; today urbanisation can no longer be considered a social problem amongst the whites.

Industrialisation is the process of acquiring a technology which is based on the machine; industrialism is an economy characterised by the prevalence of manufacturing and trading industries or activities. Industrialism and scientific agriculture are the foundations of modern Western societies — the so-called developed and advanced nations of the world, e.g. those of North America, Europe and Japan. Industrialism is closely associated with the nuclear family which is independent of the wider kinship group and allows for individualism and competitiveness.

An essential accompaniment of industrialisation is the development of towns and cities. People generally flock from the poorer rural areas to the centres of industry in the cities in order to improve their circumstances — economic, health and recreational. The urban environment in South Africa has a Western-type First-World culture; people coming to the cities from the black rural areas with their dominant traditional African-type, i.e. Third-World, culture are exposed to pressures which result in culture change and the process of acculturation. Technological advance, industrialisation and urbanisation accelerate cultural and social change.

URBANISATION OF BLACKS IN SOUTH AFRICA

Urbanisation of blacks in the RSA has been rapid since 1951. Various estimates have been made, *inter alia*, between 1951 and 1987 the urban black population increased from 5,1 million to 10,6 million.[3] The Human Awareness programme[4] has given the following proportions of populations in urban areas:

	1987	Projected to 2000
Black	40 %	75 %
Coloured	70 %	86 %
Indian	93 %	92 %
White	90 %	93 %

There has been a significant influx of blacks into the cities since the promulgation of the Abolition of Influx Control Act in 1986. Blacks with South African citizenship have, since 1986, had complete freedom of movement in any region of the RSA.

Local authorities and provincial authorities both play a role in urbanisation. Local authorities are expected to provide infrastructural services and facilities to ensure that the process is orderly and to take steps to combat undesirable conditions. A recent function of provincial administrations is the upgrading of underdeveloped urban areas, especially black towns.

INFORMAL SQUATTER SETTLEMENTS

During the past decade the urban housing problems have assumed alarming proportions as millions of blacks have moved from the rural areas to the cities in search of work and a better life. Rapid urbanisation has serious consequences for cities which have to provide basic shelter and domestic services, employment and medical services. The impoverished migrants move into the hostels increasing their bed occupancy to 3 or even 6 persons per bed, changing the unisex hostels into family accommodation and causing the evils of gross overcrowding: disrepair, accumulation of waste, blocked sewerage systems, inadequate cooking facilities and violence. Other unmet demands for shelter result in crowding of township backyards and the uncontrolled building of shacks on any available piece of vacant land — illegal squatting of homeless people in squatter settlements on the periphery of our cities, sometimes adjacent to established black townships (i.e. peri-urban) and sometimes free-standing, e.g. Zevenfontein, north of Johannesburg.

Squatter settlements are huge urban slums without urban infrastructure and services. The building units are called shacks. These squatter camps have been described as ghettos of African poverty.[4] The squatter problem of blacks in urban areas is assuming alarming proportions. The squatter problem sometimes causes the government and even private landowners to forcibly remove thousands of people and their self-built shacks on unauthorised land to more inadequate accommodation in tents in emergency camps. This urban accommodation crisis is causing thousands and thousands of people to live under the most miserable, unhygienic conditions, under constant harassment from the police for illegal squatting and trespassing.[4]

It is the responsibility of every landowner to ensure that his land is not occupied illegally. Should this happen he can call on the authorities for help to remove the illegal squatters.

Dangers. The great dangers and disadvantages of informal settlements are:

(1) the outbreak of disease (see the ill effects of inadequate housing);
(2) fires;
(3) violence, and
(4) crime, both internal and across the borders.

The uncertainty and impermanence of settlements cause inability on the part of the squatters to put down roots and improve the environment. Failure to upgrade private property leads to squalor and infestation and pollution of the environment. Due to the uncertainty of impermanence small businesses cannot grow. The inhabitants of squatter camps are generally seen by settled black and white communities as outsiders and are rejected as such.

OFFICIAL ATTEMPTS AT CONTROLLING AND ACCOMMODATING THE SQUATTER PROBLEM IN CITIES

The government's White Paper on Urbanisation affirms the power of the central government to set urbanisation policy, determine development priorities, distribute financial resources and release or designate land for industrial and residential development; the financial responsibility for low-cost housing, transport and social services and the monitoring of urbanisation is, however, the responsibility of local authorities.

In order to attempt to control the squatter problem, the Prevention of Illegal Squatting Amendment Act 104 of 1988 was promulgated in 1989.

Some of the provisions of Act 104 of 1988 are:

'to increase the prescribed penalties . . . to regulate the right of certain persons to demolish certain buildings or structures . . . to assign certain powers from first tier to second tier government . . . to further regulate the administrative powers of a magistrate to effect the removal of squatters . . . to provide for the declaration of transit areas (in squatter camps) in lieu of the establishment of emergency camps . . . to do away with controlled squatting and to provide for the designation of land for development of residential areas.' (*Government Gazette*)

This, in essence, means that a squatter settlement could be proclaimed, by the premier of a provincial parliament, as a transit camp outside the jurisdiction of the local authority with the government upgrading it, i.e. providing services and administration on a temporary basis, while a 'designated area' is in the process of being prepared for habitation. There the people could buy their own plots and erect informal housing, i.e. reside permanently.

In 1991 the *Less Formal Township Establishment Act 113 of 1991* was passed to provide for shortened procedures for the designation, provision and development of land, and the establishment of townships for less formal forms of residential settlement. In terms of the Act provincial administrators and local authorities are empowered to establish townships on any land at their disposal. Settlement can take place as soon as the land has been surveyed. Other legal procedures for formal township development are bypassed. This Act helps to deal with the acute needs of urbanisation.

The disadvantages of permanent resettlement areas are:

(1) they may be further from work, thus increasing the cost of transportation;

(2) moving means a change of address; this may cause hardship to prospective pensioners who must have a formal address.

In some areas squatters are arrested and removed and their shacks demolished whenever a complaint is received. This does not resolve the problem, however, as squatting is resumed elsewhere. Jammine[4] believes that, if serviced land and basic building materials were made available, squatter families could build their own houses and the informal settlement could be upgraded into reasonably satisfactory living environments.

Urbanisation: the consequences for health in South Africa

Rapid urbanisation, if adequately accommodated, can improve the health of Third-World populations in that it creates opportunities for an improvement in the social, educational, economic and health status of the people. Children of migrant families always suffer, though, as they are subjected to stresses and pressures which have an adverse effect on psycho-social development.

Rapid urbanisation, with concomitant housing problems and the mushrooming of informal squatter settlements without amenities for healthy living, causes many social and health problems.

Rapid urbanisation is liable to give rise to:

(1) Diseases of poverty — infectious diseases and malnutrition with high infant mortality rates.

(2) Social instability which causes an increase in sexual promiscuity and sexually transmitted diseases, as well as crimes of violence such as homicide and rape. Teenage pregnancy and street children are caused by the breakdown of traditional family structures.

(3) The effects of industrialisation, viz. occupational (scheduled) diseases, ischaemic heart disease and lung cancer because of the se-

vere air pollution in the absence of electrical installations.

Uncontrolled urbanisation can, therefore, create great problems for the local authorities of cities. Yach[7] quotes Relly, chairman of Anglo American: 'Squatting should be seen as the first stage in the necessary process of urbanisation, and the squatter's shack as an initial form of housing needing upgrading in due course — not demolition.'

It is important that governments in developing countries accept the desirability and inevitability of rapid urbanisation and make some provision for basic shelter and services to improve the health status of people flocking to the cities in search of a better future for themselves and their children. It has been estimated that the proportion of blacks living in urban areas in South Africa will double from about 40 % in 1988 to nearly 80 % by the turn of the century.[7] (See p. 196.)

The squatters and Health Services[9]

At the 1991 census, the squatter population (shack dwellers) of South Africa was approximately 2,8 million people (9 % of the population). They were counted by magisterial districts in order to, *inter alia*, enable the health authorities to plan health services according to population needs. In 1994 it was estimated that 5–7,5 million people live in shacks in South Africa.

Early in 1990, 200 projects (mostly fixed and mobile clinics) began to be built (or provided) throughout the length and breadth of the country, in line with the commitment, in 1989, of the Health Policy Council to provide Primary Health Care Services for all. These facilities have been sited to provide a service not only for the settled formal townships but also for the shack dwellers. Government conditions for providing funds for this service were:

- certification that a need indeed existed;
- community involvement and participation to give the community a sense of ownership of the facility (clinic);
- maximal use of local labour for construction of the facility;
- community-based evaluation of the health benefits of the clinic.

BLACK CIVIC COMMUNITY ATTEMPTS AT ADDRESSING THEIR PROBLEM OF HOUSING SHORTAGES (AS WELL AS OTHER NEIGHBOURHOOD PROBLEMS)

Formally housed residents of crowded, poorly serviced townships and informally housed squatters have organised themselves into voluntary associations — called civic associations — which make demands for better housing with permanency of tenure (for squatters) and some of the basic services necessary for survival in a city: a steady supply of potable water, sanitation and waste removal.

Note: The 'Civics' are the counterparts of the white Residents and Ratepayers' Associations of local authorities

Local civic associations ('Civics') may be affiliated to larger regional or even national associations. Each association is represented by an elected executive committee. Before demands are made on authorities, the committee elicits the needs of its association. The efficiency of a committee and/or its chairman is judged by whether it can muster support for mass action and whether an interested audience turns up at report-back meetings.

The civic associations are primarily concerned with improving the living conditions of their members, i.e. they are not political associations, although a sympathetic and helpful political party will win their allegiance. They claim to be independent of political parties, although the intensity of their survival needs may moderate this claim somewhat.

There are hundreds of civic associations (NGOs) in the RSA, each one with a variety of developmental civic functions, e.g. to get adequate housing, water, etc. Some are alert and strident in their demands, and others (those without skills and resources) are non-assertive and compliant.

Sanco (South African National Civic Organisation) is a national umbrella body for civic associations (as well as some hostel dwellers' associations) launched in March 1992. It deals with broad developmental issues and the restructuring of local government.

The Cape Housing Action Committee (Cahac) is an umbrella civic organisation representing the interests of coloured people in formal houses in the Cape.

There are associations which deal solely with squatters' survival problems, viz. Western Cape United Squatters Association (Wecusa). Wecusa sees itself as independent of civic associations, as the needs of the homeless (squatters) are not the same as those of the formally housed people. All spontaneous free-standing shack settlements in the Transvaal have residents' committees which may or may not work closely with nearby civic associations, or with political parties.

HOSTEL RESIDENTS' ASSOCIATIONS

The urban hostels are a very sensitive issue because they are often seen as the focal point of violence. Their suggested abolition or isolation by fencing is perceived as a direct attack on migrant workers. In June 1992 there were 240 hostels for blacks in the RSA, of which 177 were owned by local and provincial authorities. There are, officially, nearly $\frac{1}{2}$ million hostel beds, but with the recent rapid urbanisation and the influx of women and children, the ratio of beds to occupants has increased from 1:1 to 1:3 or perhaps even 1:6.

With overcrowding and lack of maintenance, hostels have deteriorated to such an extent that some are hardly habitable. The authorities realise that these hazards to peace and health must either be demolished, isolated from the communities around them by security fencing, upgraded to habitable single quarter accommodation, or converted to family units.

In 1992 the government set aside R295 million from the 1992/93 budget for the upgrading and/or conversion of black hostels, which started towards the end of 1992.

The hostel residents are ambivalent about the changes initiated, some wanting single quarter hostels and others wanting family units to house their families.

Although essentially non-party political, fear of eviction and physical harm (violence) have caused residents to become politicised and hostels to become known as either ANC or IFP strongholds.

Like the civic associations formed by the homeless squatters and residents of under-serviced townships, hostel residents have organised themselves into associations with elected executive committees.

(a) The SA Hostel Dwellers' Association (Sah-da) was formed, May 1991, in Durban where the hostel population is estimated at 70 000. It is a non-political organisation whose aim it is to improve the living conditions of hostel residents and to prevent the demolition of hostels.

(b) The Transvaal Residents' Association was formed in September 1991 to represent the interests of 22 hostels in the Gauteng region in the face of calls for demolition by local civic associations which saw the hostels as a source of the violence on the Reef in 1990. Most of the residents favoured the upgrading of single quarters hostels, although separate (either permanent or temporary) family units are also an option. The ANC tends to favour family units, while the IFP supports the single quarters option. The two upgrading options may have become politicised.[10]

(c) In 1991 hostel dwellers in the Cape started to organise in order to improve their lot. The hostel residents' association, Umzamo Development Project, aims to transform government-owned hostels into family units.

THE PRESENT (1994) HOUSING STRATEGIES

At the Housing Summit in October 1994, consensus was reached by the delegates, who signed a Housing Accord, to deliver on the government's promises of shelter for all. The delegates were members of the construction industry, regional and central government, Ministries of Housing, banks, the civic movements and the federation of the homeless. The aim of the consensus reached was to build 1 million houses in 5 years with money loaned by banks and from other resources. Thus agreement was reached on South Africa's first truly national housing policy under the RDP.

Mass housing construction will be a people-centred development — a shared responsibility of the government, the private sector and the homeless, the emphasis falling on the efforts of the latter.

The building of renting stock by the government is another option for housing the very poor and migrant workers, but this is a long-term strategy. Rental stock will of necessity be limited, so only a few will gain access to this housing.

The homeless poor will be helped by the government in yet another way which is akin to the site-and-service scheme. It is called the 'starter' home. The government gives a subsidy of R12 500 to cover the cost of a serviced stand and one room. This unit will be extended by the owner as he can afford it, helped with low-cost housing loans.

The ANC spokesman stated on SABC that, for every R1 million spent on building houses, 120 jobs are created. Housing stimulates the provision of infrastructure and houses need decoration with furniture and gardens. People with jobs will be able to pay the rentals, electricity, water and sewerage costs.

These huge housing programmes should, therefore, give a good kick-start to the South African economy.

REFERENCES

(1) Keeble L. (1959). Principles and practice of town and country planning. *Estate Gazette Ltd.*

(2) SA Institute of Race Relations. *Race Relations Survey.* Johannesburg: SA Institute of Race Relations. 1985.

(3) SA Institute of Race Relations. *Race Relations Survey* Part 1. Johannesburg: SA Institute of Race Relations, 1986.

(4) SA Institute of Race Relations. *Race Relations Survey.* Johannesburg: SA Institute of Race Relations, 1987/1988.

(5) Wilson F. *Migrant Labour in South Africa.* Johannesburg: SA Council of Churches and SPROCAS, 1972.

(6) Wilson F, Ramphele M. *Uprooting Poverty.* Cape Town: David Philip, 1989.

(7) Yach D. Urbanization in South Africa — consequences for health. S *Afr Med J* 1988; **74**: 479.

(8) SA Institute of Race Relations. *Fast Facts* 1/1994.

(9) The Squatters. National Health and Population Development. *Epidemiological Comments* 1993; **20**:123

(10) Murphy S. *Housing, Politics and Civil Society. Spotlight.* Johannesburg: SA Institute of Race Relations. 3/1993.

TEST OF KNOWLEDGE

The student has benefited from studying this chapter if he/she can:

(1) Discuss the advantages of electrification of black urban townships.

(2) Write an essay on the dangers and ill effects on health of informal urban settlements (squatter camps).

(3) Give an account of the dangers and signs of poor ventilation and the way in which poor ventilation can be structurally and functionally prevented:

(*a*) in a dwelling, and

(*b*) in a large hospital.

(4) State how safe and adequate lighting and a comfortable temperature can be maintained during midwinter and during midsummer in a family home with schoolgoing and younger children.

(5) Discuss South Africa's acute housing crisis with regard to:

(*a*) the history with regard to the development of the problem;

(*b*) attempts by the government of the day to combat the problem;

(*c*) attempts by the people affected to resolve the problem;

(*d*) the viability of the plan of the present government (1994) to find a quick solution to the housing problem.

12

Global and South African Food Problems
Malnutrition
Poverty in South Africa

OBJECTIVES

The objectives of this chapter are to introduce the student to poverty and its effects on people and communities. Many community nurses will be dealing with diseases associated with poverty. They will be gaining first-hand knowledge of the many social evils and misery caused by conditions of chronic want. It is hoped to give the student some insight into the social and political forces which shape people's lives; some are destined to belong to privileged groups, while others are relegated to groups which struggle to survive in a country where there is enough for all.

Other objectives are to introduce the student to global and national food production and distribution problems which are the prime causes of malnutrition, especially the undernutrition which is rife amongst the underprivileged sections of our society, especially the children. Malnutrition in children is discussed in Chapter 24.

The student must realise that undernutrition is a direct consequence not only of material want but that it also correlates with all the parameters of lack of privilege: chronic community deprivation, lack of intellectual stimulation, overpopulation and overcrowding, ignorance and superstition, and the social disorganisation caused by the migrant labour system. Undernutrition is more prevalent in the rural areas from which many adult males have migrated to the cities in search of work, leaving their wives and children behind. In the rural areas medical (clinic) services are also much more limited than in the urban areas, hence health education is not abundantly available.

The Government of National Unity has embarked (1994) on a 10-year programme (RDP) to root out poverty in South Africa.

IN THIS CHAPTER

GLOBAL FOOD PROBLEMS

The Food and Agricultural Organisation, the United Nations body responsible for implementing solutions to the world food problem, was founded in 1945. In 1974 the world food famine, especially in the countries south of the Equator (Third-World countries), was brought to the attention of the rich, industrialised countries in the north. It was estimated that 800 million people go hungry. Targets agreed upon for alleviating the world food crisis have not yet been met — the number of people in the world who are undernourished continues to increase. Droughts are increasing the misery of the hungry.

The problem of hunger is not so much due to insufficient global production as to distribution problems. Approximately half the food produced is wasted due to destruction by insects, birds and rodents. Poor roads and long distances cause uneconomical transport costs; thus hungry people may be cut off from supplies because no one is prepared to pay the distribution costs. Free gifts of food from one country to another are not entirely satisfactory as this may have the effect of reducing local production.

Global food production increased in 1981 by 2,9 %, the 'North' producing more than twice its requirements; even India has become self-sufficient in cereals. Yet 50 % of the sub-Saharan African people are undernourished. The Director-General of FAO ascribes this predicament to the progressive impoverishment of these countries (1981, 1982). It is the only region where food production per head has declined over the past 20 years. This means that more land needs to be brought into cultivation and more cultivated lands need to be irrigated. The problem is that increased production needs the kind of money lacking in the Third World which has already borrowed so much from the industrialised countries that they cannot pay their yearly interest dues. Moreover, the poor countries cannot afford to buy food from the surplus stocks of the 'North'.

SOUTH AFRICAN FOOD PROBLEMS

The present (1994) population of the RSA is estimated to be 40 586 000 (*Epidemiological Comments* **20**:2). With a growth rate of 2,31 %, the South African population is increasing by approximately 1 million per year, of whom 800,000 will be blacks. The projected total in the year 2020 at the same growth rate will be about 80 million.

At present the RSA is producing sufficient food for its needs and is even exporting food, although the available food is unevenly distributed so that there is widespread malnutrition.

The question that concerns the future generations is whether the available agricultural land will be able to nutritionally support a population of 80 million in the year 2020. The capacity of available land to produce is limited by the rainfall which is low and erratic over large parts of the country. Much of the soil is too stony or the terrain too mountainous to farm. Only about 15 % of the land surface can be used economically for crop production. Massive irrigation schemes have enabled skilled farmers to practise intensive farming, thereby enhancing the very limited amount of arable land. Almost half the cultivated land is used for maize production.

Approximately one third of the maize crop is normally exported, one third is fed to animals (yellow maize) and one third is used for human consumption.

As the amount of land available cannot be increased, it is important that the yield per hectare be increased.

Pastures cover almost 80 % of the agricultural land surface and partly support the animals which provide us with milk, cheese, butter and meat. They vary in productive capacity, some being grasslands with high potential and others being bush and scrub with low potential.

MALNUTRITION

Definition

Malnutrition means incorrect or poor feeding. It is due either to excess or to a deficiency of one or more food constituents. In nutritional health education we are aware of diseases caused by both dietary excess and dietary privation. These diseases can be prevented or markedly reduced. In affluent societies poor nutrition is more likely to be caused by overnutrition than by undernutrition.

NUTRITIONAL SURVEILLANCE

Nutritional surveillance can be done to enable health authorities to define the nutritional problem.

Nutritional surveillance refers to the regular collection of data with regard to the nutritional status of a population, with particular reference to the population subgroup at risk. In South Africa, the black and coloured subgroups with low socio-economic status, and especially the children of these subgroups, are at risk of suffering the effects of undernutrition: PEM, intellectual backwardness, tuberculosis, gastro-enteritis and pneumonia. Example: in a nutritional survey done in 1975 by the Johannesburg City Health Department, it was found that one-third of the Indian, one-quarter of the coloured and one-fifth of the black children falling under its jurisdiction suffered from malnutrition.

Nutritional surveillance of population subgroups at risk has the following specific objectives:[1]

(1) to provide information that will help to analyse the cause of malnutrition, thereby permitting the application of preventive measures;

(2) to promote decisions by governments concerning nutrition priorities;

(3) to enable predictions to be made on the basis of current trends, and

(4) to monitor nutritional programmes and to evaluate their effectiveness.

Nutritional surveillance must, therefore, detect and define the nutritional problem; it is essential for the formulation of a corrective policy and for the planning and evaluation of action programmes. An example of the latter is the policy followed by the state health department to combat malnutrition and nutritional disease through nutritional education and the distribution of supplementary foods through its clinics, the main object being to combat PEM among young children. It is also involved in the scheme of the enrichment of maize meal to combat pellagra (see p. 212).

Faulty nutrition, be it malnutrition, overnutrition or undernutrition, has an adverse effect on the development of the child. Kotze[2] has estimated (from the number of children who benefited from a government-subsidised skimmed milk powder scheme) in 1979 that 90 000 children in the RSA are at risk of developing protein energy malnutrition (PEM).

In a study done among coloured people[2] in western Johannesburg, it was found that malnutrition was often caused by lack of knowledge and lack of motivation to use existing knowledge, alcohol being a contributory factor. One-third of the children between the ages of 1 and 6 years suffered from mild PEM (WHO first-degree PEM). The criterion used is mass for age under the third NCHS percentile, i.e. less than 80 % of expected mass.

Richardson's comparison of population groups, with regard to body mass and height below the third percentile (PEM)[3]

Whites	Coloureds	Indians	Blacks	
Children under the age of 1 year				Measured during 1975
2 %	12,9 %	4,6 %	8,5 %	
Children at the age of 12 years				Measured between 1971 and 1973
11 %	44,7 %	61,2 %	49,1 %	
Adolescents at the age of 17 years				
2,6 %	14,9 %	32,8 %	15,8 %	

These percentages decreased from 1969 to 1975, i.e. the nutritional status of all children improved without any direct dietary intervention.

Primary schoolchildren appear to have the highest incidence of undermass. Little has been done for this age group in the form of supplemental feeding. Richardson's findings indicate the desirability of school feeding schemes for underprivileged children. This is being done at present. Operation Hunger claims that they can feed one child per year for R25 — 7 cents per day, the food they use being maize, fortified high protein soup powder/stew and milk powder (for the very young).

CHANGING PATTERNS OF MALNUTRITION WITH RISE IN PRIVILEGE

With rise in privilege, which is almost synonymous with migration to and assimilation of the socio-economic structure of the cities, there have been changes in the way of life and in the pattern of disease. People in developing countries consume a diet consisting largely of cereals and vegetable matter; as soon as there is a rise in privilege, there is a decrease in the intake of cereals and starchy vegetables and an increase in the intake of animal proteins, fats and sugar.

The main killers among the underprivileged people (e.g. rural blacks) are undernutrition, tuberculosis and other infections, violence and certain types of cancer; coronary thrombosis is a rarity. The main killers amongst the privileged people are degenerative diseases (coronary thrombosis, diabetes mellitus and cerebral vascular accidents), obesity, hypertension, cancer of the colon and lung and vehicular accidents. The three important attributes of enjoyable living — smoking, overeating and speed, decrease life expectancy in affluent societies. Generally the life expectancy in underprivileged communities is lower than in privileged communities, because of the high infant mortality rate in the former. The changes in the pattern of disease can be ascribed to many factors: dietary change due to the availability of new foods and labour-earned wealth, a decrease in physical activity, the acquisition of competitive values in order to acquire and maintain privilege, the loosening of family ties giving rise to social pathology and the anxieties of alienation, and, lastly, cigarette smoking and exposure to air pollution.

Dietary changes play an important role in changing the pattern of disease. People who have improved their economic status are eating more processed and refined foods, more animal proteins and fats and more sugar.

In the middle and upper income groups malnutrition is caused by high fat and salt intake and the injudicious use of refined carbohydrates and sugar with consequent lack of fibre in the diet. There is epidemiological evidence that fibre-depleted diets are the basic cause of the increasing prevalence of several degenerative diseases (see p. 208, 284 for a discussion of the role of fibre (roughage) in the diet). High fat diets not only cause obesity and hyperlipidaemia but are also linked with a greater risk of developing certain kinds of cancer (see p. 284). Although the link between high salt intake and hypertension has not been proved unequivocally, it is a fact that rural blacks amongst whom hypertension is relatively rare also have a low salt intake. Too much protein involves extra work for kidneys and liver and can thus be harmful in infants or in adults with diseases of the kidneys or liver. It may also cause loss of body calcium.

Hunger and undernutrition lead to riots (civil unrest), socio-economic disorganisation, delinquency, ill-health and disruption of family life. This, in turn, places an increased financial burden on the state. In the RSA, the daily hospitalisation costs for a child admitted with malnutrition can be compared to the cost of a bag of maize. A rise in the cost of basic foodstuffs will, naturally, lead to great food deprivation among the underprivileged and a greater number of children who need treatment for malnutrition at state cost — a vicious cycle in that measures to combat inflation lead to greater inflation.

DISEASES OF OVERNUTRITION

Atherosclerosis

There appears to be some association between high intake of animal fats, a raised level of serum cholesterol, breast cancer and atherosclerosis. The association between raised serum cholesterol and atherosclerosis is probably triggered by other factors, *inter alia*, hereditary predisposition towards atherosclerosis and heart disease, smoking, tension and a sedentary life which favours obesity. When these triggering factors operate, the blood level of cholesterol and other lipids shoots up despite dietary reduction of animal fats. Doctors do not normally restrict the animal fat intake of their patients (except in the interest of mass reduction), but will do so if the serum total cholesterol (TC) level is raised above normal levels and other predisposing causes of coronary thrombosis are present, in which case the animal fats are reduced to a maximum of 30 grams daily.

Cholesterol is not found to any extent in vegetable matter; fats which are derived from the vegetable kingdom and fish are usually in the form of oils which contain a preponderance of unsaturated fatty acids in contrast to animal fats which contain mostly saturated fatty acids. The important vegetable oils used in dietetics are derived from: olives, soya beans, maize, groundnuts and sunflower seeds. It has been found that if these unsaturated fats are used in the diet of patients with elevated serum lipid levels, dangerously high levels (which may trigger coronary thrombosis) are reduced. The main dietary sources of unsaturated fats are cooking oils, nuts (especially groundnuts), millet and soy beans.

Note: The process of converting vegetable oils to margarine, converts most of the unsaturated fatty acids in the oils to saturated fats, unless the oils are subjected to a special process. Ordinary 'hard' margarine, therefore, contains saturated vegetable fats and cannot be used for the purpose of reducing serum cholesterol.

Overdosage with vitamins A, D and C: see p. 275, Chapter 16.

Obesity

Obesity is the most important nutritional disease in affluent societies. Rise in privilege usually leads to less physical activity because of car ownership and sedentary occupations, as well as to the consumption of richer diets. The enjoyment of food may become the goal of eating. In an affluent pleasure-oriented society there is a great temptation to overindulge. Obesity is, however, also a problem in Third-World societies with a high carbohydrate diet.

A person is deemed overmass if he is more than 10 % heavier than standard mass for persons of his height, sex, age and race. Examples: a white man aged 25 years, height 1,83 metres (6 feet) should weigh 72 kg. If he weighs 80 kg or more, he is overmass. A white woman aged 40 years, height 1,25 metres (5 feet) should weigh 55 kg. If she weighs 60,5 kg or more, she is overmass. The term obesity is usually reserved for a state of gross mass excess.

The cause of obesity is the intake of kilojoules in excess of the body's requirements for energy. Excess energy is converted to fat and deposited in the body's fat depots. The fault usually lies in the consumption of rich foods containing 'empty' kilojoules from sugar, refined starches and animal fats. Excessive intake of animal fats also raises the cholesterol level of the blood, i.e. it causes hypercholesterolaemia — always a serious risk factor for coronary artery disease.

Hunger — the body's demand for kilojoules — is a sensation which is so powerful that almost anything will be eaten to assuage the energy deficit; as kilojoules are taken in, so the sensation of hunger diminishes. Some people need more kilojoules than others. Appetite, on the other hand, is the demand for a particular food. Appetite can grow with eating and with sensory stimulation by food (taste, texture and sight). Appetite is acquired and is affected by, for instance, moods. Thus worry or depression may either stimulate or suppress appetite. Children acquire certain taste sensitivities, e.g. 'sweet-tooth', revulsion for cabbage, from their feeding experiences at home. Eating habits acquired in childhood (e.g. overeating) endure into adulthood. People do not eat and do not require the same amount of food. Both hunger and appetite are halted by satiety. People who habitually overeat and become obese are insensitive to physiological cues of satiety and are oversensitive to food-related cues.

Slimming diets are of value if they meet certain criteria; they must:

(1) be low in kilojoules in order to reduce mass;
(2) be nutritionally adequate (i.e. balanced) in order to maintain health;
(3) satisfy the palate to prevent boredom and abandonment of the diet;
(4) not be so expensive that they impoverish the dieter;
(5) be potentially permanent so that loss of mass can be maintained after it has been achieved.

Obesity is a precipitating factor in the most important degenerative diseases of affluent societies: coronary thrombosis, diabetes mellitus and hypertension. These three killer diseases improve greatly when mass is reduced either by restricting the consumption of 'empty' kilojoules and/or by increasing body activity to use up the excess energy.

Obesity due to overfeeding may also occur in infants and in children. A rejecting mother frequently overfeeds her child, especially with ice-cream, biscuits and sweets. In this way she is giving him 'goodness' in substitution for the love and acceptance of which she is depriving him. Overnutrition in infancy leads to increased appetite and the laying down of excess numbers of fat cells; these cells are permanent and subsequent attempts to lose weight merely cause a temporary shrinkage of excess fat cells. Health educators should recognise obesity in children and try to prevent its occurrence by propagating

simple health principles, e.g. encouragement of breast-feeding, late introduction of cereals and a moderate sugar intake. If the health educator is able to restrict the energy intake of the obese infant or child, she will be increasing his life expectancy.

DISEASES OF UNDERNUTRITION

The nutritional deficiency diseases are caused by a deficiency of one or more food constituents, the so-called protective foods. In affluent societies deficiency diseases may occur in food faddists and compulsive dieters (anorexia nervosa), but they are much more prevalent in underprivileged societies where they occur in infants and children, as well as in pregnant and lactating women. Breast-feeding can be successfully carried out by poorly nourished mothers, the nutritional state of the mother hardly affecting the quality of the milk. Pregnancy and lactation may, however, precipitate deficiency diseases in an underfed mother; the nutrients which she gives to her parasitic child cannot be replaced by her defective diet.

Lack of dietary fibre

Faecal stasis in the large intestine — constipation

With rise in privilege and the consumption of refined foods, there is a great reduction in the dietary intake of crude fibre (roughage). Whereas the stools of people on a diet composed mainly of unrefined cereals and vegetables are bulky, the stools of those on a refined diet with lots of animal protein and fat are small. Bulky stools stimulate peristalsis, and constipation can be expected when stools are small. As diseases of the large intestine — appendicitis, diverticular diseases, carcinoma of the colon, ulcerative colitis, and haemorrhoids are common in people consuming a westernised diet and uncommon among rural blacks, it seems likely that these diseases are related to low fibre intake with consequent stasis of faeces in the large intestine.

Recent studies[4] have shown that there are major differences in bowel function between whites and blacks (who seldom have chronic non-infective bowel diseases). Blacks defaecate more frequently and their stools are less formed; faeces have shorter transit times and are more acid. The colonic surface area of blacks is greater than that of whites.

Urban blacks of Soweto at present consume a low fat, low fibre diet.[4] These new discoveries cast some doubt on, but do not discard, the dietary-fibre hypothesis in respect of chronic, non-infective bowel diseases.

Deficiency of minerals and vitamins

Some deficiency diseases are not confined to poor people; they may be due to lack of certain nutrients in the environment or to abnormal losses by the body. Example: iron deficiency causes anaemia.

The cause of iron deficiency may be nutritional or it may be due to excess loss of blood (menstruation, accidents, operations, childbirth) and the subsequent rapid haemopoiesis to make good the loss. The body needs iron, protein, vitamin B_{12} and folic acid and its salt, folate, for its haemopoietic functions; if the stores in the body are depleted and the diet cannot supply the building materials, anaemia, usually iron-deficiency anaemia, will result.

Iron deficiency

The balanced omnivorous diet contains approximately 15 mg iron daily. Of this iron, men absorb 1,3 mg and women and children 2,5 mg. Before iron is absorbed, it must be freed from its attachment to organic molecules in the food, as it is absorbed in ionic form. For this release gastric HC1 is needed. Vitamin C is also necessary for iron absorption in the small intestine. In the gut epithelium the iron combines with apoferritin to form ferritin. Ferritin is important for the storage (in many organs) and transport of iron in the blood plasma. As the body needs the iron, it is released from ferritin and transported in linkage with the protein, transferrin. Serum iron, transferrin and ferritin levels can be measured by special blood tests, low levels indicating iron-deficiency anaemia. These levels are also useful to assess the anaemic patient's response to iron therapy.

Rural blacks generally have an excessively high iron intake, the source of iron being the iron pots used in cooking or the iron in fermented beer prepared in iron utensils. This may cause iron-storage diseases — haemochromatosis and haemosiderosis — often superimposed upon a liver which is chronically diseased. On the other hand, urban children of the lower socio-economic class, especially coloureds and blacks, need supplementary iron in their diets to prevent nutritional anaemia, unless the home diet contains iron-rich and vitamin B_{12}-rich foods such as egg yolk and meat, especially heart, kidneys and liver. Milk, fruit and vegetables contain very little iron, but the following cereals and vegetables are fairly rich sources of iron: barley, millet, sorghum, soy beans, black-eyed peas, pigweed and turnip leaves. Maize is a poor source of iron.

Folic acid and vitamin B_{12} deficiency

Megaloblastic anaemia, characterised by abnormal erythropoiesis with macrocytic, hyperchromic red cells, is commonly caused by folic acid (folate) and/or vitamin B_{12} deficiency.

Folate is a B-group vitamin found mainly in green leaves (peas, spinach).

Folic acid and vitamin B_{12} deficiency have many causes, including severe malnutrition.

Vitamin B_{12} deficiency anaemia (pernicious anaemia) is nearly always due to lack of the intrinsic gastric factor associated with achlorhydria. This factor is essential for its absorption in the terminal part of the ileum. A deficit may also occur in those on a strict vegetarian diet, as its source is liver, kidneys, meat, milk and eggs. The enrichment of soya milk with vitamin B_{12} is at present being investigated.

Note: Only very small amounts of animal protein in the diet are required to maintain adequate vitamin B_{12} nutrition.

An excess supply of vitamin B_{12} is stored, especially in the liver, thereby postponing the effects of a deficit in the diet for up to a year.

Although folic acid replacement therapy will cure the macrocytic, hyperchromic anaemia caused by both folic acid and vitamin B_{12} deficiency, it does not cure the neurological symptoms which are caused by the inability of the body to absorb vitamin B_{12}. Pernicious anaemia is, therefore, treated by the parenteral administration of vitamin B_{12} (cyanocobalamin).

Several studies were done in the RSA between 1984 and 1988 on nutritional deficiency anaemias. The commonest deficit found was iron, but folate and vitamin B_{12} deficiencies sometimes occurred concomitantly.

(1) The rural population of Mseleni (northern Natal) subsist on a diet of maize, locally grown vegetables and wild fruit, but seldom eat meat. Their tap water is without iron, and they drink palm beer which contains no iron. Iron deficiency was found to be the main cause of the anaemia commonly found, but low levels of vitamin B_{12} frequently co-existed with the low serum ferritin levels. In some cases bacterial infection and liver disease were additional aetiological factors.[5]

(2) Deficiency of nutritional haemopoietic factors was found to be prevalent in black preschool children in the Letaba area of the Northern Transvaal. A large number of children were iron and folate deficient.[6]

(3) Lamparelli *et al.*[7] found a high degree of iron-deficiency nutritional anaemia in pregnant coloured women in Johannesburg. Many of these women were iron deficient in the first trimester, suggesting a high level of nutritional anaemia in this population group.

(4) Lamparelli *et al.*[8] did a nutritional anaemia survey of 11-year-old coloured, black and white children in the Western Cape and found only the coloured group to have low haemoglobin and serum ferritin levels.

(5) Baynes *et al.*[9] found a significant folate deficiency in pregnant black women in Gazankulu. Iron deficiency occurred less frequently.

Note: Folate deficiency tends to mask concomitant iron deficiency.

The role of folate in the diet of women of childbearing age, to prevent intra-uterine neural tube defects, has recently been discovered (see p. 135).

Iodine deficiency

Iodine deficiency results from a lack of iodine in the ground and consequently in the drinking water. There are many iodine-deficient areas on earth and people who do not make good the iodine deficit in their drinking water, by eating fish and iodised salt, may develop endemic goitre.

Vitamin D and calcium deficiencies

Metabolic bone diseases caused by the above deficiencies include rickets and osteomalacia. They are fairly common and preventable diseases. In both diseases there is an impairment or failure of mineralisation (with calcium and phosphates) of bone.

Rickets is a disease of growing children that affects the modelling (formation of shape) of bone; osteomalacia occurs in adults and affects bone remodelling.

Rickets/osteomalacia used to be synonymous with vitamin D deficiency caused either by dietary lack or by non-exposure of the skin to sunshine. The latter is necessary to convert the provitamin 7-dehydrocholesterol in the skin to vitamin D. It has recently been discovered (in the RSA) that nutritional rickets/osteomalacia may be due to dietary lack of calcium in areas where there is little calcium in the water and children do not drink milk. In these cases there may be no vitamin D deficiency.

Modern research has broadened the range of aetiological factors of rickets/osteomalacia into three major classes.[10]

(1) Primary calcium deficiency in the blood (hypocalcaemia) due to a deficiency of dietary calcium and/or vitamin D.

(2) Phosphate deficiency (hypophosphataemia), including dietary deficiency of phosphates and increased renal loss.

(3) Local inhibition of mineralisation of bone due to fluoride excess.

The subdivisions of the classes are legion, but for the sake of simplicity only those causes which are of preventive community health importance are mentioned.

Where there is a primary calcium deficiency in the body (rickets/osteomalacia) the body cannot maintain a normal calcium blood level (hypocalcaemia); this leads to secondary hyperparathyroidism in the effort of the body to raise the calcium level in the blood to supply minerals to bone and to prevent tetany. The increased parathyroid hormone concentration leads to increased bone resorption (absorption of tissue in the body), hence the osteopenia (decreased density of bone) of rickets. Hyperparathyroidism causes increased excretion of phosphates by the kidneys; this causes secondary hypophosphataemia.

In rickets/osteomalacia there is thus an impairment in mineralisation of bone, a secondary resorption of bone (causing osteopenia) and hypophosphataemia, the latter contributing to the mineralisation defect. This causes softening of bones and deformation of the weight-bearing bones.

Primary prevention of rickets

Rickets occurs commonly during the infancy period of preterm infants. Robertson[11] found, in Cape Town, the incidence of clinical rickets to be 24 % in preterm infants and 16 % in full-term infants, in a low socio-economic group. These figures were considered to be unacceptably high.

In a prospective study done in 1984 in Cape Town by Heese *et al*[12], the prevalence of nutritional rickets at the age of 12 months in a group of low birthweight preterm infants in the lower socio-economic group was found to be nil. These encouraging findings are ascribed to the full utilisation of available community health services of the City Health Department, viz. community clinics and nurses who dispense not only health education and encouragement of the mothers to attend clinics but also vitamin D fortified milks and multivitamin syrup introduced after the revelations of the Robertson[11] study. Good compliance was obtained from the mothers.

Secondary prevention of rickets/osteomalacia

This comprises diagnosis and treatment. The diagnosis of rickets/osteomalacia:

Clinical signs of rickets

(1) Fractiousness and insomnia. In the early stages, clinical signs of hypocalcaemia (i.e. convulsions, tetany) may be the only presenting symptoms.

(2) The head: Excessive perspiration; bossing of the frontal bones (square head) and failure of the fontanelles to close, should the disease start in infancy. There may be craniotabes, i.e. areas of thinning and softening of the skull.

(3) Lower limbs: Softening of the bones so that the child has marked and varied deformities

of the lower limbs, e.g. bow-legged or knock-kneed should he be at the walking stage. Pathological fractures may occur.

(4) The spine: Curvature of the spine, resulting in kyphosis and scoliosis.

(5) The joints: (*a*) Enlargement of the joints; (*b*) beading of the anterior extremity of the ribs, at the junction of the rib with the cartilage, which is known as the 'rickety rosary'.

(6) The teeth: (*a*) Late dentition; (*b*) the teeth come out crooked and are weak and irregular.

(7) Muscles and ligaments: (*a*) Flaccidity of musculature and ligaments; (*b*) during inception and recovery from rickets, signs of tetany (spasmophilia) are often in evidence.

Radiological signs of rickets/osteomalacia confirm the clinical signs, which are sometimes overdiagnozed if not confirmed by radiography. X-rays of the wrists and knees may show poorly developed epiphyses and abnormal epiphyseal plates.

Biochemical signs of rickets/osteomalacia: low serum calcium and phosphorus. If the disease is due to calcium deficiency in the diet, vitamin D levels in the blood will be high. These levels will be low if the disease is due to vitamin D deficiency.

Note: The method of measuring the amount of vitamin D in the blood was only recently established in the RSA. This measurement cannot be carried out at all laboratories. The test was developed at the MRC/University of the Witwatersrand Research Unit for Mineral Metabolism, Baragwanath Hospital, Johannesburg.

Treatment of diet and sunshine dependent rickets/osteomalacia

(1) The fortification of processed and evaporated milk with 400 IU vit. D per litre of reconstituted milk when these milks are used for infant feeding.

(2) Vitamin D and calcium administered medicinally.

(3) Exposure of infants to a moderate amount of sunlight.

(4) It is important to increase the consumption of dairy products. The calcium intake of strict vegetarians can be increased by including green leafy vegetables, peanuts, almonds, sesame seeds, molasses and soya milk in the diet. The enrichment of soya

milk with calcium is at present being investigated in South Africa.

Tertiary prevention

Rehabilitation for the after-effects of rickets/osteomalacia consists of corrective surgery for bone deformities. Surgery must be delayed until the rickets/osteomalacia is under control and is always done in consultation with the physician handling the metabolic bone disease.

Vitamin B deficiency

In South Africa the most common vitamin B deficiencies are those of riboflavin and niacin because the staple diet of the poorly nourished section of the community is maize. Whole maize contains very little riboflavin, niacin and tryptophan. Thiamin deficiency occurs most commonly in the Far East where the staple diet is rice, but is also found in South Africa, especially among male migrant workers who drink heavily.

Niacin deficiency

The overt form of niacin deficiency is called pellagra. The Department of National Health and Population Development estimated that at least 100 000 people with pellagra are treated as in- and out-patients annually. The stigmata of nutritional pellagra are:

(1) Desquamation dermatitis with dark discoloration of areas of skin exposed to the sun, i.e. the arms, the legs and face, with a typical butterfly distribution over the bridge of the nose and cheeks. The skin is finely cracked in a mosaic pattern. Desquamation (shedding of the top layer of the skin) leaves areas of depigmentation. The skin lesions may ulcerate and form thick crusts.

(2) Glossitis with fiery-red, painful swollen tongue, progressing eventually to atrophy and insensitivity. There may be angular stomatitis and ulceration of the mouth and throat.

(3) Diarrhoea.

(4) Dementia with confusion.

In its pure form pellagra is not characterised by anaemia. Pellagra can be diagnosed biochemically by the *plasma tryptophan test*.

The purely nutritional form of pellagra seen in children is limited to skin lesions, but in the severely malnourished adult alcoholic, the well-known triad — *dermatitis, diarrhoea, dementia* (3 Ds) — is demonstrated. In these chronically malnourished adults there are usually multiple deficiencies of pyridoxin (with convulsions), folic acid (with anaemia), thiamin (with peripheral neuritis), riboflavin.

Riboflavin deficiency

The signs of riboflavin deficiency (ariboflavinosis) often occur in combination with niacin deficiency:

(1) Cheilosis, a condition marked by fissuring and dry scaling of the vermilion surface of the lips and angles of the mouth, the latter being known as angular stomatitis.

(2) Fissures around the nostrils.

(3) Glossitis — inflammation of the tongue. It is characterised by a smooth tongue which has a purplish-red or magenta hue.

(4) Conjunctivitis — inflammation of the conjunctiva, characterised by excessive dryness, burning and photophobia.

(5) Greasy, seborrhoeic dermatitis of the face and scalp and scaly, greasy desquamation around the nose and ears.

Prevention of pellagra and riboflavin deficiency (as well as protein deficiency)

Experimentation with maize breeding in which the maize proteins are genetically manipulated to produce hybrids with high lysine and tryptophan content, is going on in South Africa at present. The human body is able to make niacin from tryptophan. These hybrids are, therefore, not pellagragenic.

Pellagra can also be prevented and treated by the selective enrichment of maize meal with riboflavin and niacin during the milling process.

Treatment of pellagra

For quick relief of the condition niacin and vit. B complex are given daily in addition to a normal diet. If there is confusion (due to dementia), parenteral dextrose and electrolytes are administered initially.

Thiamine deficiency

Thiamine deficiency, which causes beriberi, is not as common in South Africa as riboflavin and niacin deficiency, but it may develop within a few weeks in a malnourished alcoholic or vomiting patient. Nutritional beriberi is rare in South African children, probably because of the high thiamine content of maize, but may develop in children with severe gastro-enteritis. In adults multiple vitamin deficiencies and the pathological effects of the primary condition (chronic alcoholism, gastric carcinoma or hyperemesis gravidarum — pathological vomiting of pregnancy) may cloud the clinical picture of beriberi.

The following forms of thiamine deficiency occur: peripheral neuropathy, beriberi heart disease (high output failure, Shoshin beriberi), and Wernicke's encephalopathy. Either one form or combinations of two of three forms may occur to give a confusing clinical picture of the disease beriberi.

Peripheral neuropathy (polyneuritis) is sometimes called dry beriberi, because of the absence of oedema. The patient presents with emotional hypersensitivity and depression, anorexia, insomnia, fatigue and muscle weakness. There is muscle wasting, loss of sensation and of tendon reflexes in the affected muscles; there may be gangrene of the extremities.

Beriberi cardiac failure accompanied by generalised oedema and a hyperdynamic circulation, plus the history of chronic alcoholism, can be diagnosed clinically as wet or cardio-vascular beriberi. A hyperdynamic circulation is characterised by high output (high systolic pressure) and low diastolic pressure with resultant high pulse pressure (Corrigan pulse). The cardiac failure may be superimposed on cardiomyopathy. Wet beriberi may progress to acute fulminating (pernicious) beriberi heart failure, characterised by severe lactic acidosis (caused by disturbed carbohydrate metabolism) and dyspnoea (hyperpnoea) due to the acidosis. This so-called Shoshin beriberi culminates in circulatory collapse (shock) due to a fall in cardiac output as the heart dilates and eventually fails because it is starved of energy. The patient may die in cardiac failure; the failure is rapidly reversible, however, by the prompt intravenous injection of thiamine. Further management includes inotropic support with a dobutamine and sodium bicarbonate infusion. Although the thiamine usually induces diuresis, the aid of an intravenous diuretic may be required.[13, 14]

Note: Before glucose is administered to a malnourished or alcoholic patient in a comatose state, the patient should be given an intravenous injection of thiamine, in case there is a thiamine deficiency. In thiamine deficiency the patient cannot metabolise glucose; should the latter accumulate in the blood, it can lead to the development of acute Wernicke's encephalopathy, circulatory collapse and death.[13, 15]

In *Wernicke's encephalopathy* the upper part of the midbrain is affected by thiamin deficiency, the patient presenting with mental confusion and delusions. If an alcoholic or other type of malnourished patient has an acute psychotic attack, the diagnosis is probably Wernicke's encephalopathy.

Vitamin A deficiency

The stigmata of nutritional vitamin (antixerophthalmic vitamin) deficiency may complicate the clinical picture of the vitamin B complex deficiencies. As enough vitamin A is stored in the liver (under normal conditions) to last a few years, deficiency of this vitamin is indicative of longstanding malnutrition. There is not as much vitamin A deficiency in South Africa as in other parts of the world. Each year 250 000 children in Asia and Latin America lose their sight as a result of xerophthalmia.[16]

Even when food is readily available, the following may contribute to an insufficient intake of vitamin A:

(1) Lack of appetite amongst the elderly or the depressed.
(2) Poor food choices of people on fad or slimming diets.
(3) The regular use of mineral oils and other laxatives which influence the absorption of vitamin A.
(4) Injudicious diet consisting of fast-foods which provide little vitamin A.
(5) Acute or chronic alcoholism.

Signs of vitamin A deficiency

(1) Xerophthalmia. In this condition the lacrimal glands stop functioning so that the eyes become dry and sensitive to light (photophobia); there is conjunctivitis and corneae become discoloured and soft; corneal ulcers

may develop. The corneal condition is called keratomalacia. Xerophthalmic blindness is permanent.

(2) Night blindness due to lack of visual purple.
(3) Dryness and scaliness of the skin with sebaceous plugs in the pores (follicular hyperkeratosis).
(4) Unhealthy mucous membranes with lowered resistance predispose children to infections of the airways and gastro-intestinal tract.
(5) Poor dental development in children.

Prescribed treatment

(1) A water-soluble vitamin A preparation (10 000 U/kg/day) is given by injection for a few days followed by daily oral vitamin A medication for a few weeks.
(2) For corneal drying or ulceration atropine 1 % and antibiotic ointments are applied topically and the eyes are lightly covered with pad and bandage.

Note:
(1) Refer to p. 706 for large-scale prevention of xerophthalmia.
(2) Overdosage with vitamin A may cause toxicity, hypervitaminosis A with hypercalcaemia. The condition may result from taking massive doses of vit. A for the treatment of acne and the prevention of sunburn. To prevent overdosage, beta-carotene may be used instead of vitamin A.

Vitamin C deficiency (avitaminosis C)

Ascorbic acid (vitamin C) deficiency causes scurvy, a deficiency disease which is rare in South Africa. It may, however, be found among the elderly living alone and subsisting on tea and bread, in alcoholics and drug addicts, in those who survive prolonged famine, and in infants who are fed inadequate formula diets. A major function of ascorbic acid is the synthesis of collagen fibres of the various forms of connective tissue, *inter alia*, tendons and fascia, the matrix of calcified tissue (bones and teeth), and the endothelial cells of the entire vascular tree including capillaries. Vitamin C has many other metabolic functions including conversion of folic acid to its active form in the body and the formation of steroids by the adrenal glands.

The adult vitamin C reserve of the body is approximately 1 500 mg.[17] Any excess vitamin C in the blood is excreted in the urine. When the normal reserve is reduced to 300 mg the following signs of generalised scurvy will be manifest:

(1) Swelling, tenderness, redness, bleeding and, later, ulceration of the gums, if teeth are present. The teeth become loose and carious and there is halitosis, especially if oral hygiene is poor.

Note: Bleeding gums are seldom caused by avitaminosis C. Other causes are: acute leukaemia, acute necrotising ulceromembranous gingivitis, haemorrhagic diathesis (predisposition), viral haemorrhagic diseases and periodontal disease.

(2) Bleeding due to spontaneous rupture of capillaries (purpura) of the following structures leads to anaemia:
   (*a*) in the skin and subcutaneous tissues, especially around the eyes and in the conjunctivae;
   (*b*) in the mucous membrane of the mouth, alimentary canal and urinary tract;
   (*c*) in the muscles and joints and under the periosteum causing joint effusions and aching limbs.
(3) Increased susceptibility to infection and poor wound healing with secondary infection causing necrosis and ulceration.
(4) Weariness and lethargy.
(5) The hair follicles may become distended with blood and keratin and will then be prominent.

Scurvy will develop after 60 days on a vitamin C-free diet in the person who had normal vitamin C reserves.

Assessment of vitamin C levels in the blood is reliable only if the levels in the leucocytes are assessed.

Treatment of scurvy

Apart from correcting the diet to include food rich in vitamin C, the patient is given medicinal L-ascorbic acid in large doses to build up the body's reserves.

Effective treatment will stop the bleeding and lead to a near complete reversal of symptoms.

Vitamin K deficiency

Vitamin K deficiency, which causes hypoprothrombinaemia, is not usually classified as a dietary deficiency, as vitamin K is manufactured in the intestine by the normal intestinal flora.

The cause of vitamin K deficiency which is characterised by purpura is, therefore, not nutritional; it is caused by the administration of oral antibiotics which destroy the intestinal flora, or diseases which cause the absence of bile salts which are essential for the absorption of vitamin K. Children can be born with vit. K deficiency, especially if their mothers have become depleted of this vitamin due to repeated use of liquid paraffin during pregnancy.

Treatment

(1) The use of oral antibiotics must be controlled with due regard for the damage it may do to the intestinal flora; the concomitant use of plain yoghurt milk helps to maintain the intestinal flora.

(2) Vitamin K can be replaced parenterally. Premature infants are given vitamin K routinely as they are lacking in prothrombin which is formed from vitamin K.

Protein-energy malnutrition (PEM)

A chronic severe lack of protein in the diet accompanied by starvation of energy foods causes the condition called famine oedema in adults. This condition was very prevalent in the Nazi concentration camps during World War II and claimed numerous lives. The main deficiency diseases of people whose staple diet is maize are protein deficiency and pellagra. Maize is not a complete food as it is low in certain essential amino acids (tryptophan and lysine) and B vitamins (riboflavin and nicotinic acid (niacin)). It has a relatively high thiamin content. Protein deficiency and pellagra are especially prevalent amongst malnourished children under the age of six, but both pellagra and beriberi (thiamin deficiency) can occur in poorly fed adults who are heavy drinkers.

Pregnant and lactating women and labourers are also prone to protein deficiency.

For a discussion of malnutrition in children and nutritional rehabilitation, see Chapter 24.

POVERTY IN SOUTH AFRICA[20]

This section relies heavily on a report for the second Carnegie Inquiry in Poverty and Development in Southern Africa as contained in: Wilson F, Ramphele M. *Uprooting Poverty — The South African Challenge*.

David Hamburg,[20] president of the Carnegie Corporation of New York, describes poverty thus:

'Poverty is partly a matter of income and partly a matter of human dignity. It is one thing to have a very low income but to be treated with respect by your compatriots; it is quite another matter to have a very low income and to be harshly deprecated by more powerful compatriots. Let us speak then of human impoverishment: low income plus harsh disrespect. To speak of impoverishment in this sense is to speak of human degradation so profound as to undermine any reasonable and decent standard of human life.'

While poverty is not confined to any one particular group, in South Africa it is concentrated mostly among coloured and black people, being worst in the rural platteland on white-owned farms and in small villages, as well as in the former black homelands. South Africa is a country of extremes — the division between the rich (generally whites) and the poor (generally blacks) is greater than in any other country in the world for which there are statistics. The most striking feature of poverty in the RSA is the degree of inequality of wealth distribution; in 1970 the richest 20 % of the population owned 75 % of the wealth.

Poverty in the RSA is a profoundly political issue. The fact that politics is not discussed in this manual does not deny its central importance in the causation of poverty and in the curative strategies for this iniquitous social evil.

Measuring the extent of poverty by income

Various poverty levels are used in the RSA to define the extent of poverty.

HSL (household subsistence level) and PDL (poverty datum line)

When income is above these two levels, it covers food, clothing, fuel/lighting, washing/cleansing, rent, transport. In 1985 this was R345 per month for a 5–6 person urban family. Dire poverty exists below this level of income. Africans constitute 95 % of the 18 million people in South Africa existing below the MLL, with 60 % of this group living in total poverty.[22]

MLL (minimum living level)

As above, plus tax, medical expenses, education, household equipment, replacement. In 1985 this income level was R350 and in 1994 R750 [22] per month for a 5–6 person black urban family.

SLL (supplementary living level)

This is equal to the MLL plus 30 %. It includes more for each item, plus recreation, entertainment, personal care, pension, UIF and medical aid contributions.

In the rural areas cash required for subsistence is not much less, despite lower costs for housing and transport and some food production by the family.

In South Africa, including the homelands, in 1980, 50 % of the total population was living below subsistence level (as measured by urban MLL). This percentage rose to 81 % in the homelands and 60,5 % for blacks throughout the country.

Poverty is a state of chronic want and material deprivation. Many of the consequences of poverty are also its causes. Those who are poor remain vulnerable to the ongoing process of impoverishment, hence poverty is difficult to eradicate.

Some of the main features of poverty are sickness (especially tuberculosis), hunger and malnutrition. These features are not primarily due to a lack of resources in the society as a whole. South Africa produces enough food to adequately feed the entire population and has some of the best medical facilities in the world. Yet these problems continue unabated.

FACTORS ASSOCIATED WITH POVERTY

Land exhaustion, overpopulation and lack of fuel and water in rural areas

Much of South Africa is arid; South Africa has neither the soil nor the climate to be a natural grain-basket. Floods and droughts make farming an uncertain means of livelihood. Bad land management plus overstocking have led to heavy erosion by wind and water. Soil erosion and the accompanying deterioration of vegetation from sweet pastures to inedible sour scrub — the encroaching desert — is a very serious problem facing South Africa. When the land is destroyed, those who have nowhere else to live have no means of making a living. Gradual impoverishment of badly managed soil is one of the causes of rural poverty which is further exacerbated by high population density, especially in the black rural areas.

Some comparative examples:

	Rural population density (persons/km^2, 1980)	Percentage urbanised
Transkei	55	5 %
KwaZulu	76	22 %
QwaQwa	298	9 %
Transvaal province	11	71 %
Natal province	22	57 %
Cape province	2	75 %
All white areas	6	67 %
Total South Africa	13	46 %

Source: *Saldru Handbook*, 1986

Urban areas: those having some form of local authority.
Rural areas: some mines and other places where there is no proclaimed local authority.

In spite of the overpopulation of rural areas, the land available is underutilised due to insufficient labour and insufficient capital.

Shortage of labour is due to demographic maldistribution, i.e. able-bodied men and young women migrate to the cities in search of work leaving women, children and old people to work the land according to their meagre capacities. The land is, therefore, not used to full capacity.

In the rural areas firewood and water are also scare commodities. Unless there is enough money for buying paraffin, women and children spend hours per day collecting firewood, the source of which is moving further and further away from human habitation. Primeval forests are being relentlessly plundered and not replaced. The mutilation of the environment is a consequence of the energy crisis in underdeveloped rural areas.

Note: The burning of discarded storage-battery casings in open braziers for fuel has led to a new hazard for children — lead encephalopathy.

As forests regulate our water supplies by their sponge effect after rains, their destruction leads to the drying up of springs and the washing away of top soil after heavy rains. The great paradox is that, while the RSA produces 60 % of all the electricity on the African continent, almost two thirds of the total population of South Africa (and 80 % of blacks) do not have access to that energy for their household requirements.

The purity of drinking water has a significant effect on the health of children. The problem of contaminated drinking water is exacerbated among poor people who live outside local authority boundaries as it needs time, effort and money in arid areas to acquire and carry water from a distant source and more money for chemicals to render contaminated water potable. Not all poor people have problems with water supplies, but it is none the less a major problem facing black rural communities. The water position becomes untenable in times of drought. The help of the army may be required to transport water to parched communities, both urban and rural.

Note: The WHO goal is 50 litres per person per day. In areas without proper water resources, people have to do with much less in times of drought, or in areas where every drop of water has to be carried many kilometers.

Illiteracy and poor learning ability[21]

Schlemmer *et al.*[21] are of the opinion that 'the most telling resource disadvantage of the poor is often interlinked with the social psychology of family life and child socialisation' (p. 190). Black family life has been weakened by the migrant labour system and rapid urbanisation. 'Incomplete, female-headed families are now estimated to constitute some 54 % of families in metropolitan townships . . . In these families, absence of male reference figures and simple material stress create problems beyond health policy alone' (p. 216).

According to the South African census of 1980, 33 % of blacks over the age of 15 years judged themselves to be illiterate and 30 % of those older than 20 had not had 6 years of schooling and so were functionally illiterate. It is estimated that there are 6–9 million post-school illiterates in the RSA.

Illiteracy is a major dimension of poverty all over South Africa, but particularly in the rural areas. Many organisations are at present under-taking literacy training, but their manifest success and combined efforts have helped only about 25 000 persons. The extent of the illiteracy problems has no doubt been influenced by the comparatively low funding of black education by the state.

Present schooling and learning problems

The number of black children going to school has risen sharply over the past decade, but it is generally agreed that the quality of education provided is low with overcrowding of classrooms and poorly qualified and motivated teachers.

While more black pupils than whites passed standard 10 at the end of 1987, the pass rate for blacks was only 56 % compared to 95 % for white and 93 % for Indian pupils. In 1987, 46 % of DET teachers did not have standard 10 qualifications.[21]

Note: The government is at present attempting to address problems in black education. There are at present (1989) some 14 000 black pupils at 'white' private schools. This represents a core of quality education for the future.[21]

It will take years, however, before black education reaches parity with white education. Sheer hunger (physical deprivation) often causes learning problems. The child who is ill-fed and hungry when he goes to school in the morning, sometimes also exhausted by long distances walked, lacks the energy and enthusiasm to do his school work; he may drop out of school to become functionally illiterate. In addition, children drop out because of the cost of education (relative to parents' income) or because the child must look after young siblings while the mother works. For the children of farm labourers the opportunities for continuing education may be lacking. Thus many children do not acquire the basic education needed to escape poverty.

CAUSES OF POVERTY

(1) Lack of education for many reasons (e.g. lack of opportunity, learning disability).

(2) A social system which entrenches privilege for certain sections of the population and withholds equal opportunities from other sections.

(3) Physical disability and low intellectual endowment which limit earning capacity.

(4) Cultural, food and/or emotional deprivation in childhood which stunts the development of personal resources (work and learning capacity).

(5) Poor physical and mental health (including alcoholism and drug addiction) which prevents employment or the proper utilisation of income.

(6) Natural catastrophes which destroy resources and homes and rob people of the chance to make a living: earthquakes and tornadoes, droughts, pestilences, wars and revolutions (nation-wide cause of poverty).

(7) Lack of natural resources and lack of expertise to run a successful industrial, urban society with many job opportunities (nation-wide cause of poverty).

(8) Large families and overpopulation.

(9) Unemployment through lack of job opportunity, lack of skills and education and rapid urbanisation, economic recession, rapid population growth, the use of foreign unskilled labour, the trend towards increasingly capital-intensive production, in an attempt to improve productivity.

The Central Statistical Service collects data on unemployment, particularly among blacks, and publishes these regularly in the Current Population Survey (CPS). Unemployment has risen alarmingly over the past two decades. Some people choose not to work because of the low level of opportunities available. Some would work if wages were higher. Some simply do not look for work. Unemployment is, therefore, not always unavoidable. Generally, however, the number of workseekers exceeds the jobs available. The number of workseekers coming onto the market continues to grow faster than job creation. Retrenchment because of disinvestment by overseas firms played a role in the rising unemployment rate.

Those people especially vulnerable to the ravages of unemployment are: women, young people leaving school, able-bodied men with families affected by economic recession and those whose worklessness is compounded by resettlement or drought.

Unemployment not only causes sickness and starvation but also increases alcoholism. The frustration of unemployment accounts for an increase in shebeens and excessive drinking to dull the pain. Unemployment robs people of their feelings of self-worth and causes boredom and depression; for some it is a death sentence, especially if they have no reserves or families to tide them over the crisis.

(10) Low wages of unskilled and semi-skilled labourers. Many households simply do not have the income that would enable them to rise above a low level of poverty. In the modern industrial urban sector of the economy, wages for black unskilled labourers are low — below the SLL; some workers are paid less than the MLL. Wages on farms are even lower, although farm labourers receive payment in kind (housing, rations) and in money. From their low wages migrant workers send remittances home to support their families. These remittances are often the primary cash income of a household. Should the worker fail to support his/her dependants, they are plunged into dire poverty. There is very little income from home production or local jobs. State old-age pensions are small and apply only to people who have no private means and can no longer work because they have reached the pensionable age limit. This pittance is frequently shared by a family.

SOME CONSEQUENCES OF POVERTY

Crime

People who cannot rise above their poverty are powerless to change their circumstances, unless they resort to crime and violence, i.e. assume power in a destructive, antisocial way. Crime can, therefore, be a social consequence of poverty. Where there is acute poverty and unemployment, people are more likely to rob and assault others in order to survive or out of sheer frustration. In South Africa the crime rate is extremely high. The murder rate in Cape Town (530 murders per 1 million inhabitants in 1985) was nearly three times that of New York (*Cape Times* 12.8.1987). There is a correlation between levels of crime and socio-economic environments — the poorer the socio-economic circumstances, the higher the crime rate. Although violent crime has in the past been associated with overcrowded urban areas, it is now also prevalent in rural areas, especially in the poorer, more densely populated parts of the former homelands. There is a direct correlation here between density of population, high rate of unemployment and crimes of violence and robbery committed by roaming gangs of tsotsis, frequently the children of the neighbourhood. Power is passing from the elders into the hands of the youth, who are learning to survive by illicit means and to wield authority (i.e. become powerful) by violent 'might is right' tactics. People exposed to gang violence live in constant fear of their lives. Younger children learn to model themselves on these powerful gangsters and are no longer restrained by law-supporting moral values. Communities which are divided against themselves deteriorate into breeding grounds for criminals.

Alcoholism

The insecurities and fears of the powerless poor are further exacerbated by alcohol. Alcoholism is at present wreaking havoc in disorganised communities, both urban and rural. Because the poor are more vulnerable, the effects of alcohol abuse are more devastating than in well-off communities with their organised social services. The alcohol trade is flourishing in black rural areas where many bottle-stores are owned by tribal and other community leaders.

Lack of food

Lack of food causes malnutrition, hunger and starvation. South Africa exports food, yet there is widespread malnutrition because of poor food distribution.

Inadequate housing

Inadequate housing causes:

(1) exposure and overcrowding with all its evils; lack of security and the establishment of shanty towns;
(2) blighted neighbourhoods which become hotbeds of crime;
(3) family disintegration with consequent damage to children;

(4) discouragement and lack of motivation for self-help to make the best use of resources.

Lack of education

Lack of education and lack of time and opportunity for recreation cause:

(1) lack of cultural stimulation;
(2) lack of skills with consequent poor earning capacity;
(3) inability to maintain health.

Major infectious diseases

The major infectious diseases relate to poor socio-economic conditions. These diseases include:

(1) the gastro-intestinal diseases with particular reference to acute infantile diarrhoea (AID) of the under-fives;
(2) respiratory infections such as measles and tuberculosis;
(3) vector-borne parasitic and viral infections;
(4) sexually transmitted diseases.

Poor hygiene standards

Poor hygiene standards are due to:

(1) poor education in personal hygiene and in the causes of ill-health;
(2) inadequate housing (e.g. shacks) and overcrowding;
(3) poor sanitation.

Poor physical and mental health

Poor physical and mental health; poor manpower potential if food and cultural deprivation is nation-wide or community-wide.

Envy

Envy of the 'have-nots' for the 'haves', resulting in civil unrest.

Social disorganisation

Social disorganisation occurs through overcrowding, delinquency and alcoholism where there is chronic community deprivation.

The Theron Commission[18] found the existence of chronic community deprivation amongst the coloured people. Forty per cent of the population thus identified are characterised by: 'work failure, lack of motivation and sense of personal responsibility and an overwhelming concern for present advantage'. There is a corresponding lack of concern for family and community and a tendency towards deviant behaviour.[19]

MEASURES AGAINST POVERTY[20]

It is not enough to merely understand the features, causes and consequences of poverty if the understanding ends there. There is consensus amongst all thinking persons that poverty is an evil that must be rooted out: indeed, that it can be rooted out. It is important for the community nurse who works in poor communities to know that it is not helpful in the long run to 'give to the poor' in order to alleviate chronic want. Charities which are based on 'handouts' are doomed to be ineffective as they merely perpetuate 'the lack of motivation and sense of personal responsibility' to take positive steps to change the *status quo*. Whites have for many years been acutely aware of impoverished black communities; their collective guilt feelings have given rise to philanthropic actions, like giving charity to the poor, usually blacks. Many blacks have reacted reciprocally by developing habits of dependency and apathy, passively accepting charity. They have learned to expect whites to take the lead in helping them. Today we realise that this attitude may actually exacerbate poverty in that it does not help people to help themselves in reconstructing and developing their communities and in gaining the skills and power to change their miserable living circumstances.

Power lies at the heart of the problem of poverty in South Africa, yet political democracy for all the inhabitants (empowerment of the masses) is not a guarantee of equal privileges for all.

Trade unions

At present trade unions are making a contribution in shifting the balance of forces within South African society in favour of the poor. Before 1979 black industrial workers were not allowed to be members of registered trade un-ions. Since then black membership has rocketed to 511 000 in 1985, the total for all races being 1 391 000. Trade unions are independent and democratically organised. South Africa's modern industrial economy needs workers' organisations to articulate workers' rights, grievances and demands in the ongoing conflict between capital and labour — in the industrial bargaining process between employers of labour and employees. Thus successful negotiating for higher wages has become a powerful tool in the struggle of industrial workers to uproot a major cause of poverty. This empowerment of manual workers has become possible through the education and training of labourers to acquire the skills which give them the bargaining leverage in a strike action.

Periodic relief measures

In times of distress such as floods and drought periodic relief measures are necessary for all sectors of the society, not only the chronically poor. Independent coping must, however, be re-established as soon as possible to prevent the crippling of people's self-help efforts.

In order to be able to develop, people need self-respect. Oppressed people need to develop a sense of identity and dignity for the release of their social energies. This was indeed the message of the Black Consciousness movement which emerged in the 1970s. The movement identified blackness in terms of dignity, self-respect and self-reliance. This is important to help people rise above the degradation of their powerlessness and sense of despair.

Self-help projects

In many Third-World countries, especially Latin America and Asia, rural and urban collective action in community projects to uproot poverty have been employed with much success. These community projects are as important for the poor as have been the trade union movements for the exploited industrial workers.

In South Africa genuine community developmental programmes are needed to empower members of communities to work together to deal with their problems such as, for instance, water shortage, illiteracy, inadequate preventive health care. Examples of ongoing projects centred on health needs are the Valley Trust at Botha's Hill (see p. 444) and Ithuseng Community Health Centre in the northern Transvaal. Operation Hunger not only feeds the hungry, but will assist self-help projects on request (see p. 443). Local organisations of people involved in business ventures support their members materially and emotionally and bring about change in their low self-image and sense of hopelessness. The powerless become empowered to control their own lives and map out a future by forward planning.

See p. 778 for the DPSA and SHAP.

Non-governmental organisations (NGOs)

The Urban Foundation

The Urban Foundation was founded in 1977 to improve the quality of life in South Africa's black townships. It functions largely by raising money from the private sector to initiate and stimulate self-help projects among black communities.

The aims of the foundation are:

(1) equal opportunity and the advantages of the free enterprise system available and accessible to all;
(2) recognition of the dignity of the individual stimulated and sustained by appropriate social structures;
(3) elimination of discrimination based on colour and sex;
(4) the development of the value of self-sufficiency and the capacity for self-help.

The Urban Foundation is liberally supported by companies, institutions and individuals. It mobilises and administers projects in the following fields: housing, education and training, community facilities, health services and research and feasibility studies.

The Rural Foundation

See p. 11, 29.

The business sector

Business concern with socio-economic reform is expressed at many levels, e.g. through the Private Sector Council on Urbanisation. Leading corporate business is attempting to secure stability by working for major socio-political change to empower blacks in the social and economic field.

The state

The state bears a huge responsibility to redress the unequal investment during the past century in infrastructure (sanitation, water supplies and reticulation, electricity) and housing in Third-World sectors of South Africa.

Some government socio-economic reform initiatives (before the democratic elections) are:

▪ Promoting small businesses in the 'informal sector' with the help of the Small Business Development Corporation and the deregulation of constraint on entrepreneurship (business undertaking). This stimulus to entrepreneurship is aimed at creating a larger black middle class and a rise in black socio-economic status.
▪ Training of the unemployed.
▪ State strategies for upgrading rural areas include afforestation schemes, especially the planting of trees which have multiple uses and benefits. Without state financial backing, the re-establishment of forests and programmes of water and soil conservation are doomed to failure. The encroaching desert is a threat to all South Africans, no matter what their socio-economic status is.
▪ Funding trusts, whose main concern is the provision of residential units and housing infrastructure for the poor, i.e. SA Housing Trust and the Independent Development Trust.

See the GNU's Reconstruction and Development Programme (RDP) for combating poverty in South Africa in Chapter 1.

REFERENCES

(1) *WHO 1976 Technical Report Series* 593.
(2) Kotze JP. Facts regarding malnutrition in South Africa. In: Griesel RD (ed). *Malnutrition in Southern Africa*. Pretoria: UNISA, 1979.
(3) Richardson BD. Underweight — a nutritional risk? *S Afr Med J* 1977; **51**: 42–48.
(4) Segal I. The geography of chronic digestive disease in Southern Africa. *S Afr Med J* 1988; **73**: 649–652.

(5) Mayet FGH, Schutte CH, Reinach SG. Anaemia among the inhabitants of a rural area in Northern Natal. *S Afr Med J* 1985; **67**: 658–462.

(6) Van der Westhuizen J, *et al.* Iron, folate and vitamin B_{12} nutrition and anaemia in black preschool children in the Northern Transvaal. *S Afr Med J* 1986; **70**: 143–146.

(7) Lamparelli RDV, *et al.* Nutritional anaemia in pregnant coloured women in Johannesburg. *S Afr Med J* 1988; **73**: 478–481.

(8) Lamparelli RDV, *et al.* Nutritional anaemia in 11 year old school children in the Western Cape. *S Afr Med J* 1988; **73**: 473–478.

(9) Baynes RD, *et al.* Iron and folate status of pregnant women in Gazankulu. *S Afr Med J* 1986; **70**: 148–151.

(10) Pettifor JM. Rickets and osteomalacia. *S Afr J of Cont Med Educ* 1988; **6**: 27–37.

(11) Robertson I. Survey of clinical rickets in the infant population in Cape Town, 1967–1968. *S Afr Med J* 1969; **43**: 1072–1076.

(12) Heese H de V, *et al.* Prevalence of rickets at age of 12 months. *S Afr Med J* 1984; **66**: 604–607.

(13) Naidoo DP. Beriberi heart disease in Durban. *S Afr Med J* 1987; **72**: 241–244.

(14) Naidoo DP, *et al.* Cardiac beriberi. *S Afr Med J* 1987; **72**: 283–285.

(15) Van der Heyden CH. Koma. *S Afr J Cont Med Educ* 1985; **3**: 77–84.

(16) Rowland W. *Curationis* 1978; **1**: 5.

(17) Touyz LZG. Vitamin C, oral scurvy and periodontal disease. *S Afr Med J* 1984; **65**: 838–842.

(18) *Report of the Commission of Enquiry into Matters Related to the Coloured Population* p. 469. Pretoria: Government Printer, 1976.

(19) Quoted from: Bowie MD, *et al.* A prospective 15-year follow-up study of kwashiorkor patients. *S Afr Med J* 1980; **58**: 681.

(20) Wilson F, Ramphele M. *Uprooting Poverty. The South African Challenge*. David Philip: Cape Town, 1989.

(21) *Policy Perspectives 1989 of Centre for Policy Studies*. Johannesburg: Graduate School of Business Administration, University of Witwatersrand.

(22) *ANC's National Health Plan for South Africa*. Socio-economic profile.

TEST OF KNOWLEDGE

(1) Define the following pairs of words to emphasise their differences:
   (*a*) rickets/osteomalacia
   (*b*) calcipenia/hypocalcaemia
   (*c*) hypochromic anaemia/hyperchromic anaemia
   (*d*) beriberi/pellagra
   (*e*) xerophthalmia/night blindness

(2) Discuss the aetiology and clinical picture of scurvy, as encountered in South Africa.

(3) What are the objectives of nutritional surveillance? What methods can be used to realise these objectives and what measures have been taken in the RSA to combat malnutrition?

(4) Discuss the manifestations of overnutrition which can be considered to be aspects of malnutrition.

(5) Describe the importance of dietary fibre in the diet with reference to Chapters 16 and 17.

(6) Discuss the prevention (all phases) of rickets/osteomalacia.

(7) Discuss the recognition of beriberi in the chronic alcoholic patient.

(8) Define and comment on the abbreviations HSL, PDL, and MLL.

(9) What are the relationships between:
   (*a*) Poverty and crime
   (*b*) Poverty and illiteracy
   (*c*) Poverty and ill-health
   (*d*) Poverty and lack of concern for family and community
   (*e*) Rural poverty and the migrant labour system

(10) Discuss the root causes of poverty among Third-World communities in South Africa and the possible measures for its uprooting.

(11) Discuss David Hamburg's description of human impoverishment with reference to the factors associated with rural poverty in the RSA.

Part 3

HEALTH EDUCATION

13

The Principles of Health Education

OBJECTIVES

The objective of this chapter is to help the nurse understand his/her role in promoting the health of the community in which he/she lives.

The ability to raise the health standards of others depends firstly on knowledge of what health is, and of what promotes health and prevents or corrects ill-health, and secondly, on the ability of the educator to relate to people in need of health education in a way that makes them receptive to health education.

IN THIS CHAPTER

THE IMPORTANCE OF HEALTH EDUCATION

The aim of health education is the promotion of good health, i.e. physical, emotional and social well-being and the prevention of ill-health; the role of the nurse in health education is to motivate the community to participate actively in improving its health status.

The WHO defines health education as an active learning process aimed at health promotion; it is successful if it helps people to change behavioural patterns and habits.

Health education is the basis of preventive medicine. It must not be confused with the authoritarian imposition of rules for desirable health behaviour on the people whose attitudes to health and disease need to be changed. It is not just the giving of lectures nor the showing of films or slides in order to disseminate information either, although this health propaganda may be a useful adjunct to health education where people's attitudes are such that they are ready and willing to absorb the relevant information. Effective health education changes attitudes and behaviour which cause ill-health. A community has benefited from health educative programmes when the people actively and voluntarily participate in health promotive and ill-health preventive action. An important objective of health education is self-care by the population. The health of a nation is not entirely

dependent on the nature and excellence of its health care services. Man's environment, i.e. everything impinging on or taken into the body, plays a greater role in his physical, emotional and social well-being than even the best possible health care service, no matter how well organised the latter may be. The health of a community is related to its level of development with regard to housing, education, agricultural production, nutrition and income. Kriel and Beuster[1] postulate that the decline in rheumatic heart disease among white South Africans is more directly related to improved nutrition, better housing and school accommodation than it is to more effective antistreptococcal therapy. The more developed a community is, the more enlightened its citizens are with regard to health matters.

With the Health Service Facilities Plan announced by the Minister of National Health and Population Development in November 1980, the accent shifted from sickness to health, i.e. away from the idea that medical care is responsible for the health status of a country.

In a poor community, lack of food, poor housing, a polluted water supply and inadequate sanitation cause the type of ill-health for which medical care can only offer first-aid treatment to prevent premature death. South Africa's scourge of tuberculosis, which is rife amongst all blacks, will not be stemmed by chemotherapy and symptomatic treatment. For the eradication of these problems the ravages of poverty, overcrowding in inadequate houses and poor personal and environmental hygiene must first be eliminated.

The responsibility for the health of a nation rests with both the government and the individual. Individuals and voluntary organisations are expected (according to the Health Services Facilities Plan) to help the community health services (launched by the Department of National Health and Population Development) with the realisation of a healthy nation. Individual responsibility can be awakened by health education given by health professionals at the community level.

THE MAJOR COMMUNITY HEALTH HAZARDS

Major community health hazards:

(1) human infestations and infections;
(2) malnutrition;
(3) family pathology and family disintegration leading to child neglect and abuse;
(4) social pathology and social disorganisation;
(5) smoking and drug and alcohol abuse;
(6) pollution of land, air, food and water — poor environmental hygiene, and
(7) sloth and an atherogenic diet.

Health hazards are exacerbated and precipitated by:

(1) poverty due to lack of natural resources, lack of natural endowment and privilege; and lack of early human stimulation and opportunity;
(2) ignorance and misuse of the natural resources of the community;
(3) overpopulation and overcrowding;
(4) wars and natural disasters such as earthquakes, droughts and floods, and
(5) rapid social change implicit in urbanisation and industrialisation.

Health hazards increase the amount of ill-health (morbidity) present in a community.

The morbidity rate is the proportion of patients with a particular disease during a given year per given unit of the population, e.g. 100 (percentage) or 1 000. Morbidity rates are difficult to compute as accurate figures can be obtained only from national registries of chronic diseases such as cancer, or from the notification of acute infectious diseases. But even with the compulsory notification of diseases, there may

be underreporting, hence the difficulty with getting accurate morbidity rates.

Morbidity rates are to a limited extent related to mortality rates; the latter will be used below to suggest the amount of ill-health in the RSA. The reasons why the mortality rate is not an exact reflection of the morbidity rate are:

(1) acute diseases with a fatal prognosis may be converted to chronic conditions by modern medical techniques, e.g. heart operations and pharmacotherapy, enabling people to survive to old age;
(2) many chronic diseases are not usually fatal, e.g. rheumatoid arthritis, psychiatric diseases.

Because of the prevalence of chronic diseases, especially in developed societies, the following mortality rates are, therefore, mere approximations of, at best, and unrelated to, at the worst, the morbidity rates. These mortality rates can, however, guide the health educator with regard to the content of health education which purports to prevent the premature death of economically active members of the population.

Rates of preventable (premature) deaths

The reduction of mortality in the economically active age group of the population in the RSA will require different health-promotive and disease-preventive strategies. Whereas the privileged groups (mostly whites and Asians) need to be educated to modify their self-destructive life-styles, the underprivileged groups (mostly coloureds and blacks) need the provision, at a community level, of public facilities such as adequate housing, clean and adequate water supplies and proper sanitation, especially in the

Percentage of deaths in the Republic of South Africa (with rank order in brackets) from causes related to destructive life-styles (age group 15–64 years, 1970)[2]

Diseases	Whites		Asians		Coloureds		Blacks	
Ischaemic heart disease	28,9 %	(1)	19,5 %	(1)	7,6 %	(3)	1,0 %	(5)
Cerebral vascular accident Hypertensive disease	8,5 %	(3)	16,7 %	(2)	13,5 %	(1)	9,2 %	(1)
Bronchitis and lung cancer	7,3, %	(4)	6,2 %	(3)	5,5 %	(4)	2,4 %	(3)
Cirrhosis of the liver	2,0 %	(6)	3,1 %	(5)	1,3 %	(5)	1,6 %	(4)
Motor vehicle accidents	9,7 %	(2)	4,2 %	(4)	8,0 %	(2)	6,0 %	(2)
Suicide	3,1 %	(5)	2,8 %	(6)	0,7 %	(6)	0,9 %	(6)
TOTAL PERCENTAGE	59,5 %		52,5 %		36,5 %		21,1 %	

Percentage of deaths in the Republic of South Africa (with rank order in brackets) from causes
which are common in less developed communities (age group 15–64 years, 1970)[2]

Diseases	Whites		Asians		Coloureds		Blacks	
Infective	1,2 %	(3)	4,2 %	(2)	10,6 %	(1)	11,1 %	(3)
(Tuberculosis)	(0,4 %)	(6)	(2,5 %)	(4)	(8,6 %)	(2)	(8,3 %)	(4)
Chronic rheumatic heart	1,1 %	(4)	1,8 %	(5)	1,8 %	(6)	1,0 %	(6)
Pneumonias	3,6 %	(1)	6,2 %	(1)	6,7 %	(3)	8,2 %	(5)
Ill-defined diseases	1,4 %	(2)	3,6 %	(3)	3,5 %	(5)	12,1 %	(1)
Homicide and unspecified violence	1,1 %	(5)	1,3 %	(6)	6,4 %	(4)	11,5 %	(2)
TOTAL PERCENTAGE	8,8 %		19,6 %		37,6 %		52,2 %	(5)

Note: 'Ill-defined' cause of disease on a death certificate indicates an uncertain diagnosis. This is most common
amongst the blacks.

black rural areas, as well as education in the proper utilisation of improved facilities and food, and in water conservation and soil cultivation. Above all, they need education and socio-political upliftment in order to overcome poverty and rise above their underprivileged status.

The improvement in health, which is the aim of health education, is likely to increase life expectancy and the incidence of degenerative diseases associated with the terminal years of a long life.

High infant mortality rates are associated with large families, poor infant care, poverty, unsatisfactory environmental conditions, uneducated mothers and lack of medical care services. Improved health and death prevention should, theoretically, increase the population. The converse is, however, the case. As the health and socio-economic circumstances of a community improve, so the birth-rate comes down and the quality of family life improves. Educated parents who have the confidence and the means to raise healthy families will have fewer children, mindful of the importance of giving every child a good start in life and also of conserving the limited fuel and food resources of the world. They will make use of health education which includes education in family planning. In order to practise contraception effectively, people must understand and accept the urgency of the need for human beings to curb their reproductive potential. The need for population control measures is a very difficult health-promotive principle for educators to put across to uneducated people who, in the first place, are

not concerned with world population problems and, in the second place, still value large families as a labour force and as an investment against economic insecurity in old age. Health education is geared towards improving the quality of human life, not the quantity, if quantity alone is the purpose of prolonging life.

Educated people are also able to grasp the threat of AIDS and, if necessary, will adapt their sexual life-style to combat the spread of this disease.

People are generally inclined to resist change, especially change of customs and beliefs. A person's security is often tied up with his traditions as they provide known and trusted ways of coping with his environment. In health education an attempt is made to change people's beliefs about the aetiology of disease, especially nutritional and communicable diseases, and their customary way of treating disease. People do not change their traditional beliefs and customs simply because they are offered a new set of beliefs and customs, even if the dispenser of the latter is a respected person in the community. The new 'facts' must be related to the old in such a way that they are convincing and can be assimilated. In every cultural group there are patterns of behaviour, e.g. methods of preparing food, to which new information can be linked. The person to be educated must be given proof of the superiority of the modified pattern of behaviour. Any educator who ignores established beliefs and customs, either because he is smug and insensitive to people's feelings and therefore treats them with contempt, or because he is ignorant of their customs and beliefs, is likely to meet with resistance and failure in his efforts to disseminate health-promotive principles.

Man's beliefs are very closely related to his social values and both belief and value systems depend to a remarkable degree on the social organisation and structure of the community to which he belongs.

The successful educator is the person who has understanding of the culture of the people to be educated, especially the role beliefs and value systems play in the accepted norms of behaviour. Beliefs which have been inculcated from early childhood are accompanied by positive feelings that they are good and right. The beliefs to which people have been conditioned from childhood tend to transcend newly acquired knowledge even in educated and socially advanced persons, especially when they are under stress and crave the comfort and security of childhood. Any strongly held beliefs are intellectually incomprehensible to the non-believer who regards them as superstitions.

It is essential for the health educator to know and to accept the importance of the belief systems which support the erroneous ideas about nutritional and other preventable diseases. In health education it is wise to start with what people believe and to guide them gradually towards greater enlightenment. In traditional black societies it is important, for instance, to elicit the support of the diviners and herbalists to get people to come to the health clinics and to report notifiable diseases. People who come for help to the health clinics can be guided or effectively persuaded to accept alternative rational regimes of treatment. If the treatment is successful and the patient has acquired confidence in the health team, the advice of the latter about prevention of recurrence is likely to be followed. In this way the health educator can change people's concepts about disease and especially the role they themselves can play in preventive and promotive health.

In practice, however, health education which is diametrically opposed to people's cultural habits is unlikely to be implemented unless the whole community can become involved to support those who have been educated to change their life-style, to maintain the altered life-style. One enlightened individual in a community has little chance of spreading his light; health education must be organised at a community level, as the following examples will demonstrate.

EXAMPLES OF THE PROCESS OF HEALTH EDUCATION

Nutritional rehabilitation units in Transkei

Nutrition rehabilitation units (NRUs) near hospitals that see a large number of severely malnourished children have been operating in Transkei since 1973.[3] Doctors had become disenchanted with curative in-patient treatment and the aim of these units was to demonstrate to the mothers, who were steeped in traditional tribal culture, that kwashiorkor can be cured by correct feeding without necessarily admitting the child to hospital for injections and medicines.

The mothers and their children were admitted to a village-like unit near the hospital for a small weekly fee. Ideally, women respected in their community, active, highly motivated and sociable were selected for the study, in the hope that when they went home they would teach their neighbours about the causes of kwashiorkor and its prevention.

The NRU comprised thatched huts, the living conditions resembling those at home. The unit was run by an enrolled assistant nurse, housekeeper and gardener/animal keeper. The mothers had no luxuries, like jam, but they and the children had a well-balanced diet consisting of eggs from the local fowl run, home-grown vegetables, skim milk powder, soup, ProNutro, soy beans, brown beans, plus the basic maize products. No expensive meat, fish or eggs were bought from the local stores. In summer the women gathered wild spinaches from the veld and dried some for the winter. They were taught the following: how to budget ahead, how to grow vegetables, how to rear chickens, how to grind mealies out of doors (to prevent Transkei silicosis), how to cook nutritious meals and how to do sewing and knitting. The use of pit latrines and enclosed mud stoves was encouraged, the latter to minimise the risk of toddlers burning themselves on open fires.

Mothers who stayed the course went home with a healthy child and some subsidised protein foods, instructions being given for them to return to replenish their supplies. On follow-up, results were not good but encouraging; return visits for supplies seldom took place, however. Since that time, many NRUs have been operating at hospitals in Transkei. In a study done four years later, Frankish comes to the following conclusions:

> 'While the NRUs have been effective in providing nutrition education to the guardians and in bringing about some changes in home practices, the condition of the children at follow-up casts doubt on their immediate practical benefit. The study highlights the totality of the problem of malnutrition where economic, social, agricultural and other factors tend to outweigh the small progress achieved through health education. The study has however, provided information on which recommendations concerning NRUs may be based.' (p. **511**)

Frankish[4] makes a very pertinent recommendation, viz. that 'some form of follow-up and support service for children and their guardians is necessary after discharge and that nutrition rehabilitation programmes need to be community-based'. It would seem that without encouragement and help at home, the teaching given at the NRU is not carried into effect and mothers slip back into their old nutrition habits.

Ill-health-promoting habits are difficult to break; despite great efforts by health authorities to overcome overpopulation, malnutrition and the smoking habit, these three prime causes of ill-health persist unabated. Giving health-promoting facts to people will not necessarily result in an improvement in the health status of a community. People will change their attitudes to health as well as disease-promoting habits only through interpersonal relationships which influence their lives.

Health education has been found to be most effective when it has involved the community. Involvement and motivation can be achieved only if the educator establishes a good interpersonal relationship with his clients so that they trust his sincerity and judgement and are willing to try to change old customs.

Community-based trachoma control programme

(See p. 708.)

The battle against trachoma amongst the blacks in the northern Transvaal is being waged with the help of public-spirited community members. All blacks in the trachoma-endemic area know trachoma, but they interpret its aetiology according to their own magico-religious beliefs which cause them to be fatalistic and unwilling to accept the help of clinics and hospitals. They believe that every child must go through a stage of discharging eyes in order to be able to see properly in later life. They also believe that the sequelae of trachoma in adulthood (entropion, trichiasis and blindness) are caused by evil spirits which leave the hut of the witch at night and enter the hut of the victim to plant the seeds of eye destruction.

It was found that only villagers can change the attitude of the people to disease, including trachoma. Scientific explanations are greeted with derision. With the help of chiefs, headmen and nurses in touch with the people, unpaid groups of women volunteers (including teachers and other community leaders) were recruited to help raise the standard of hygiene of the people whose standards, because of ignorance and lack of water, leave much to be desired. These groups gather regularly for instruction by nurses and social workers and are taught the elements of personal and community hygiene. The latter includes the construction of pit privies, refuse disposal, the making of compost with garbage, the washing of cooking utensils, in order to eliminate the fly menace. The making of a garden is taught for a supply of fresh vegetables. The helpers are taught to recognise trachoma and to instil tetracycline ointment. The black educators convey to these highly motivated women an idea of how infection is spread by flies and the communal family face-cloth. The women, in turn, go into the huts of the village to spread the gospel of hygiene and good nutrition. They distribute eye ointment to families in infected huts and teach the adults how to care for the infected eyes.

This community approach to trachoma control seems to be making tremendous headway in an area where mass treatment of school children during the past 25 years has had little effect in eradicating the disease.

Health education depends very much on basic education and methods of health-educating well-informed, literate people differ markedly from methods of educating poorly educated people; when dealing with illiterate people, community involvement and personal supervision to ensure the carrying out of health care instructions are the only effective ways to ensure that health educative efforts bear any results.

The nurse must be aware of the importance of adapting the health education programme to the needs and the educational level of the community she serves. Health education is directed not only towards the less developed members of the community but also towards the educated, affluent sections whose anxieties, emotional hungers and greeds may cause them to ignore the health-promotive information to which they are constantly exposed, for instance, facts about the dangers of smoking and overeating. Health education programmes are important in urban communities to curb air pollution, transportation accidents and noise, and to promote the psychological health of people who feel rootless and alienated. Diseases of affluence no less than diseases of poverty form the subject-matter of health education.

HEALTH EDUCATION TOPICS (HEALTH NEEDS) OF SPECIAL IMPORTANCE

For the less developed section of the South African population:

(1) overpopulation and the need to curb population growth;
(2) environmental and personal hygiene (cleanliness and infection control);
(3) desirability of breast-feeding; malnutrition and health needs of children and pregnant women;
(4) communicable diseases, especially tuberculosis, gastro-enteritis and measles;
(5) the origins of common disease processes.

For the more developed section of the South African population:

(1) psychiatric ill-health, especially emotional disorders, occupational stress, and psychosomatic diseases;
(2) diseases caused by self-destructive lifestyles, especially those caused by the self-indulgent habits of affluence, e.g. smoking, overeating, lack of exercise and speeding in fast cars;
(3) preparation for old age;
(4) genetics;

(5) sex education and child-rearing skills.

For all sections of the population:

(1) cancer;
(2) alcoholism;
(3) nutrition.

The public, especially schoolchildren, should be educated to appreciate health and to recognise that ill-health is abnormal and preventable. Social awareness can be created by community health education, especially by the media (newspaper, radio, TV) and schools, so that people generally know about the most important factors which promote health and improve unsatisfactory health standards, viz.:

(1) education and preparation for employment (training of skills) in order to ensure a satisfactory socio-economic standard;
(2) adequate sanitation;
(3) adequate and pure water supply;
(4) adequate nutrition;
(5) adequate housing;
(6) preservation of the family unit which is so often disrupted by divorce, alcoholism and by the migratory labour system operating in the RSA.

THE ART OF THE HEALTH EDUCATIONIST

The art of health education lies in communicating meaningfully with people so that they will change that part of their life-style which causes preventable ill-health out of conviction that comes through insight and, perhaps, through a wish to feel well and enhance the quality of life. The health educator must remember that clients are not necessarily educated when they have memorised the facts presented to them. True education has taken place when there has been a change of attitude and belief and the client acts in accordance with learned facts. A successful health educator is one who has the knowledge, can impart this knowledge by word of mouth and by means of educational aids — which any enterprising teacher can devise *ad hoc* — and, above all, is able to motivate people to change their health-destructive behaviour.

Nurses are generally accepted and respected by the community and therefore their role as health educators is of inestimable value to the country. South Africa is a land of contrasts with extremes of wealth and poverty. Urban areas are usually considered 'developed' and rural black areas as 'developing'. The nurse health educator may belong to any of the South African population groups and those to be educated, likewise. Black and white professional nurses receive the same basic training and learn the same basic facts about the causes and treatment of diseases. These facts are based in scientific research and give rise to the practice of rational scientific Western medicine which is characterised by constant endeavours to disentangle the mysteries of nature in order to prevent premature death and to enhance the quality of life. Black and white nurses are required to apply their common pool of skills and knowledge in communities which differ greatly in cultural values, beliefs about the causes of ill-health, customs and resources and even in the nature of the prevalent disease.

Although it is important for the professional nurse to become knowledgeable during her training, it is just as important for her to continue her education by learning about the culture of the peoples among whom she works (if the culture is alien to her) and to add to her basic store of scientific facts by reading professional journals and by making use of opportunities to attend post-basic courses and professional congresses. The body of medical knowledge is not static and the nurse who ceases to study loses her effectiveness as a health educator, although she probably retains her worth as a dispenser of basic curative nursing care.

In order to educate, the nurse must have the knowledge to carry over to the group to be educated; what is more, she must believe this knowledge to be scientifically valid and worth transmitting to the group about whose health status she is concerned. The nurse who does not really believe that diseases are caused by natural causes — either physical or chemical agents, lack of essential nutriments, or stress — will not be able to teach her clients how to prevent disease and promote health, as her clients will sooner or later find out that she merely pays lip-service to that which she professes to 'know'. The nurse who teaches the

dangers of cigarette smoking and continues to smoke has not assimilated the gospel she is teaching; she feels ambivalent about the 'facts' and passes this ambivalence on to her confused audience. In order to be an effective educator, the nurse must believe sincerely in what she is teaching.

It is, therefore, important for the health educator to believe in and have knowledge of the causes of and the pathological processes that operate in sickness, before she can presume to teach others the principles of health promotion. One's attitudes to preventive and curative treatment rest on one's conception of health and disease. In South Africa the nursing profession subscribes to Western scientific medicine which is progressing at a phenomenal rate as research brings new insights to light. Medical science does not claim to be all-knowing, but no one can deny that great progress in medical treatment and health preservation has taken place during the past 50 years, just as no one with any scientific insight will doubt that great scientific discoveries which may change man's conception of health and disease will be made during the next 50 years.

It therefore behoves the nurse who has joined a scientific health profession to keep up to date with the ever-expanding body of scientific knowledge upon which the treatment of her patient is based.

Methods of teaching the principles of health promotion and ill-health prevention will depend very much on the basic education of the client-pupil. A group of illiterate clients is hardly likely to derive any benefit from a didactic lecture, especially if it is illustrated with the trappings of a sophisticated Western culture, e.g. posters, films, flannelgraphs, microscopic slides. People who have not had a literate education are not even able to recognise depth and perspective in a picture which depicts a three-dimensional scene — hence their inability to understand such a picture. Such persons are more likely to benefit from a practical demonstration of objects and activities indirectly concerned with health, e.g. the making of a vegetable garden and the conversion of vegetable refuse into compost; ways of preparing meals without destroying the essential nutriments; methods of destroying the fly menace to health.

Communication of medical knowledge transculturally, i.e. from those steeped in the scientific traditions of Western medicine to those who believe in the magical causation of misfortune, is a difficult task. Black women who train as professional nurses have generally had a Western-type education and have attained the same academic educational level as their white, coloured and Indian counterparts. They therefore have the same conceptual tools with which to grasp the concepts of scientific medicine. Theirs is the important task of educating large masses of their own people who have not yet had the privilege of an enlightening education. Numerically, the most potentially effective group of health educators in the RSA are the black nurses. Likewise, the largest group of people to be health educated are blacks.

Success as a health educator depends on many factors: the personality of the educator, his/her knowledge, the opportunities for educating and the audience to be educated. Educative activities may range between the following extremes: getting a community involved in concrete health-promoting projects which are geared to specific needs, in the case of an intellectually unsophisticated, illiterate or semi-illiterate community, to appealing to the intellect and interest of people who are knowledgeable about the functioning of their bodies and are health conscious, by means of the public communication media such as TV, radio, newspaper articles and public lectures.

No health educator is versatile enough to meet the health educational needs of all types of communities; the health educator should, therefore, be cognisant of the educational and intellectual level of his/her clients and their special health needs and gear the teaching accordingly.

There are, however, certain principles of teaching which are common to all health educating. Educational aids such as posters, pamphlets and models help to hold interest and to illustrate a point which may be difficult to grasp on a verbal conceptual level, but if the educator cannot establish rapport with her audience, she will not be able to communicate health education effectively, despite the most elaborate educational material imaginable.

EDUCATIONAL ERRORS

Health education has very little chance of succeeding if the following *educational errors* are committed:

(1) Teaching transculturally without first learning the language and culture of the people to be educated, where there are large cultural gaps between teacher and pupil.

(2) Teaching without the necessary knowledge of the subject, a deficiency which cannot be hidden under verbiage and outdated 'folksy' remedies and solutions to problems when well-informed members of the audience start asking questions.

(3) Giving double messages which confuse the audience. For example, a health educator who smokes or over- or under-eats or who punishes her body or mind in ways which are obvious to the audience, and feels ambivalent about her interest in health promotion, is not likely to persuade an audience to change their habits for habits advocated by one who obviously does not believe wholeheartedly in the advantages of being healthy.

(4) Adopting a rigid, authoritarian attitude, or one of contempt and intolerance towards the people to be educated. Talking down at people and condemning their present life-style, merely antagonises them and discourages two-way communication, i.e. the asking of questions and discussion of controversial or unacceptable statements by the health educator. Unless the educator can get feedback from the audience, she will have no idea if the teaching is effective or not. When there is discussion and two-way accommodation, small gains may be made as people become willing to experiment with new ideas gleaned at a health education session. The educator must gain the trust and respect of her pupils before they will be willing to change their attitudes.

(5) Impatience and intolerance of the slow or resistant learner. The educator must be patient and willing to explain over and over again, for instance, where she is trying to improve patient compliance in treatment at out-patient clinics. Patients must not be made to feel foolish and guilty if understanding comes slowly and if memory

lapses cause incorrect medication at home. The nurse educator must encourage questioning and give the patient the confidence to report truthfully on what actually happens at home. Problems can then be ironed out by devising methods of helping the patient find ways of complying with treatment demands.

(6) Authoritarian teaching encourages placatory behaviour in clients who feel dependent on the health educator, e.g. for favours received. Placatory, compliant behaviour in the presence of the educator does not mean that this behaviour will be adhered to in the absence of the educator. People who comply through fear (of rejection, of punishment) have not been educated as their basic attitudes to health-promoting behaviour have not been changed.

REFERENCES

(1) Kriel JR, Beuster DJ. *S Afr Med J* 1977; **52**: 167.
(2) Wyndham CH. The loss from premature deaths of economically active manpower in the various populations of the Republic of South Africa. *S Afr Med J* 1981; **60**: 411.
(3) Beach H, Lwana P. *S Afr Med J* 1974; **48**: 2177.
(4) Frankish JGS. *S Afr Med J* 1978; **53**: 507.

TEST OF KNOWLEDGE

The student has benefited from studying this chapter if he/she can answer the following questions:

(1) Write about sound educational principles and contents of an educational session which you would use for the health education of a group of underprivileged women during the second trimester of pregnancy.

(2) How can a health educator who smokes best serve a group of adolescents sent to her by their school for a talk on a healthy life-style to prevent premature coronary artery disease?

(3) What are the special skills of a successful health educator in a community plagued by gastro-intestinal infections?

(4) What educational aids would be helpful in putting across health education on the following topics:
   (*a*) Tuberculosis
   (*b*) Cigarette smoking
   (*c*) Substance abuse
   (*d*) Venereal (sexually transmitted) disease
   (*e*) Malnutrition

The student should consult the relevant chapters in this book.

14

Health Education for a Healthy Life-style
Personal Hygiene

Hygiene is the science of health; personal hygiene is the term used for the steps taken by an individual to ensure that he/she remains healthy.

OBJECTIVES

In order to dispense health education to others, the nurse must know what constitutes healthy living and apply health principles to her own life-style.

In this chapter on personal hygiene all aspects of healthy living will be discussed, some by reference to other chapters, and some directly.

PERSONAL HYGIENE FOR A HEALTHY LIFE-STYLE

The following are the main subjects related to
the maintenance of health.

Adequate nutrition

The body can be harmed by overnutrition as
much as by undernutrition; if the diet has sufficient kilojoules but is not well balanced, the
body may likewise suffer from malnutrition. For
a discussion of the principles of correct feeding,
refer to Chapter 16.

Note: A healthy life-style includes the maintenance of ideal
body weight.

Care of the eyes and ears

For the prevention of avoidable blindness and
deafness, refer to Chapters 39 and 40.

Accident prevention

This applies especially to those accidents occurring in the home. Refer to Chapter 45.

Control of mental stress by mental hygiene

Mental hygiene is purported to prevent not only
psychiatric illnesses but also psychosomatic
diseases, i.e. those diseases with both a physical
and a mental component. Personal mental hygiene has to do with the maintenance of gratifying and rewarding interpersonal relationships,
job (including study) satisfaction, adequate recreation and continuous personal growth from a
state of dependency and emotional immaturity
to a state of emotional maturity, autonomy and
mature, human interdependence in which concern is felt for others and the individual feels
adequate, secure, loved and lovable. These are
some of the characteristics of the mentally
healthy, adult person.

Mental health and physical health are inter-
dependent states of personal well-being, and a
person's state of mental health is as important
as his state of physical health in considerations
of personal hygiene. The subject of mental hygiene is a vast one which involves the mental
health of families and communities, in the same
way as environmental hygiene involves the
physical health of families and communities.

(Refer to Fisher E *Psychology for Nurses
and the Health Team.* Juta & Co. Ltd.)

Harmful habits

Smoking and the misuse of alcohol and drugs
harm the body; their avoidance and cure are
important aspects of personal hygiene. For a
detailed discussion of harmful habits, refer to
Chapters 15 and 42.

Sexual intercourse

As coitus is so closely bound up with human
emotions and as it plays a prime role in intimate
interpersonal relationships, the subject-matter
of sexual personal hygiene is hedged in by
moral issues, guilts, prohibitions, interpersonal
jealousies, fears and recreational and procrea-
tional needs. Personal hygiene with regard to
sexual functions thus involves physical and
mental health.

For the prevention of sexually transmitted
diseases, refer to Chapter 33.

For the prevention of unwanted pregnancies, refer to Chapter 20.

For the prevention of cancer of the cervix, refer to Chapter 46.

Psychosexual functioning is discussed in M E Vlok *Manual of Nursing* Volume II.

Elimination

Regular bowel action promotes physical comfort as constipation may cause flatulence, haemorrhoids and anal fissures. On the other hand, purgation may cause dehydration and hypokalaemia due to loss of these substances in the watery stools. Constipation should be avoided as far as possible by natural means, such as a high fluid and fibre diet, exercise, abdominal massage and regular visits to the toilet. If the use of laxatives is unavoidable, bulking agents should receive preference. The washing of the hands after the use of the toilet and before meals is important to prevent the spread of pathogens.

Treatment of common infections

Certain common infections should be treated to prevent complications. These are:

(1) common cold, that may lead to sinus infections and bronchitis;
(2) sore throat, that may lead to rheumatic heart disease, and
(3) streptococcal skin infections, that may also cause rheumatic disease with heart complications.

Sufficient sleep and avoidance of physical exhaustion

These are important for the promotion of efficiency, for creating a sense of well-being and to promote the general resistance of the body to infection. People vary in their sleep requirements and sufficiency of sleep is judged subjectively; the person who is not getting enough sleep looks and feels tired during normal waking hours and lacks zest for life. 'Burning the candle at both ends' causes premature ageing as vital energy is spent prematurely.

Exercise

The body needs exercise in order to function normally. Exercise is necessary to increase muscle tone, induce low serum lipid levels and enhanced glucose tolerance, prevent constipation, prevent the accumulation of excess body mass and to prevent cardio-vascular diseases. Exercise is usually associated with recreational sport which not only promotes friendly interaction with other people but also relaxes the mind and reduces workaday worries.

Persons who exercise regularly tend to be happier and more stress-resistant and less tense, anxious and depressed than those who do not exercise.[1] Activities of high energy expenditure (40 kJ/min for average person) are jogging, running, cycling, squash, aerobics and swimming. Walking is an activity of lower energy expenditure (20 kJ/min) at a speed of 5 km/h.

The more vigorous the exercise, the shorter the exercise period required for protection against heart disease.

The length of exercise periods required may, therefore, vary from 3,5–12 hours per week.

The protective effect of exercise in youth does not continue in slothful middle and old age.[1]

Oral hygiene

For the care of the teeth and the mouth, refer to Preventive Dentistry, Chapter 18.

Safety of the immediate environment

In order to prevent contamination of the skin and mucous membranes:

(1) food and liquids for consumption must be safe, i.e. not poisonous and not infected, and must be handled by the consumer with clean cutlery or hands;
(2) fresh air is needed at night during sleep and while working indoors during the day to prevent the inhalation of polluted air and to allow sufficient cooling of the body; heat exhaustion and heat-stroke may result from inadequate ventilation, and
(3) bilharzia-polluted waters and hookworm-infested latrines must be avoided.

Care of the hands and nails

Our hands are our most efficient implements and are used for a multitude of purposes. They are also very important carriers of disease. For these reasons the skin must be kept supple and without cracks and tears, especially around the nails where infection may enter to cause parony-chia. Dirty nails are especially liable to spread infection and nails must, therefore, be cleaned regularly. Hands exposed to chemicals and hard work need extra care in the form of hand creams which are rubbed in at night and after washing the hands. Hands should never be placed in or rubbed with strong disinfectants as the skin will sooner or later become sensitive and develop contact (eczematous) dermatitis. If sensitive skin is constantly exposed to soap and water, waterproof gloves should be worn to prevent chronic paronychia caused by *Monilia albicans* (thrush) which flourishes in damp nail folds. It may also cause intertrigo (moniliasis), *inter alia*, in the folds between the fingers.

Care of the feet

Aching feet cause the body to feel tired. Badly fitting shoes or shoes which are not supporting the ligaments of the tarsal and metatarsal bones and their arches are usually the cause of foot problems. If human beings did not wear shoes they would not develop corns, calluses, bunions or ingrowing toe-nails. Flat feet are common in young children who usually outgrow them but if they occur later they may be due to poor posture or obesity. Hallux valgus may start as a slight congenital malformation which becomes exaggerated due to the wearing of pointed shoes and tight stockings which push the big toe to the middle of the foot.

Structural foot abnormalities should be treated by an orthopaedic surgeon and severe pressure defects by a podiatrist. Regular podia-try care is especially important in the aged and in diabetics. Onychogryphosis (very thick big toe-nails) caused by peripheral ischaemia oc-curs in the aged and requires podiatry care.

Ordinary preventive foot care includes the wearing of well-fitting and supporting shoes, changing shoes frequently to prevent feet from becoming tired, avoiding high-heeled shoes for walking and standing purposes and avoiding blisters on the feet by wearing either socks, stockings or shoe liners. The skin of the feet can be kept supple and free from thick, hard skin by rubbing in cream or skin lotion after the bath. Toe-nails must be kept short and ingrowing

toe-nails prevented by judicious cutting out of the corners, if necessary by a podiatrist.

Note: Some podiatrists prefer cutting out a V-shaped piece of nail in the centre, to allow the nail to grow inwards from the corners.

Menstruation

This is a normal body function and should be treated as such. Cleanliness and frequent change of pads or tampons are important to avoid un-pleasant smells, chafing and soiling of clothes. The average person baths daily and washes hair once weekly or more often and this routine should not be interrupted because of menstrua-tion. Swimming is usually avoided during men-struation to avoid embarrassment and soiling of pool water with blood, but where swimming is unavoidable because of commitments, a tampon can be used to seal the vagina. Great care should be exercised with the use of tampons; they must be changed frequently and the wearer must make sure that tampons are not left in the vagina inadvertently, as the retention of this foreign body may cause infection and unpleasant smells.

Menstruation should not be treated as the reason for being 'unwell', as dysmenorrhoea can be treated in consultation with a gynaecol-ogist.

Care of the hair

Care with regard to cleanliness and styling of the hair is part of body grooming and is a reflec-tion of the personality. Styles vary with age and sex. In nursing short styles are generally pre-ferred as long hair can be a source of cross-in-fection, especially if it is allowed to become dirty and untidy. Cross-infection hazards can be avoided by wearing a tight-fitting 'theatre' cap in the vicinity of infection-prone areas. Thor-ough brushing of the hair cleanses it and stimu-lates its growth and is an important aspect of personal hygiene; brushes and combs should be washed frequently if they are to contribute to the cleanliness of the hair.

Infestation of hair with lice is a fairly com-mon occurrence and is by no means confined to the lower socio-economic classes. It occurs in epidemics in schools, usually in pre-primary and primary schools, and any child found to be infested is excluded from school until he has been certified free from lice and nits by the medical inspector of schools or his deputy, usually a school nurse.

Legal aspects: it is a criminal offence to be infested with lice. Any infested person can be deloused by a government, provincial or municipal official and can be prosecuted if such treatment is refused. These drastic measures are taken to prevent the spread of typhus.

For the treatment of lice, see M E Vlok *Manual of Nursing* Volume I.

Care of the skin

Regular bathing and change of clothing are important to prevent unpleasant smells, infections and infestations. These latter conditions are especially liable to arise where there is overcrowding.

In middle and upper class society the daily bath and change of clothing are considered essential for an acceptable standard of personal hygiene. This high standard of personal cleanliness is, however, not universal, nor is it essential for the maintenance of health. Standards of skin cleanliness are to a large extent culturally determined and this in turn depends on the availability of water, especially hot water on tap, and housing with bathrooms.

Body smells *per se* do not cause ill health. The strict avoidance and abhorrence of offensive body odours by constant washing and the use of deodorants are standards set by certain westernised cultures which set great store by the perfumed body. Absence of body odours and their replacement by perfumes likewise do not promote health, i.e. they are not essential for personal hygiene.

The *essential requirements for the personal hygiene* of the skin are:

(1) Body odours must not be so offensive that they cause the individual to be a nuisance. Noxious smells may lead to avoidance of people and give rise to social prejudices which prevent co-operation between different groups of people.

(2) Dirt and discharges must not be allowed to accumulate on the skin. Dirt which is allowed to accumulate on the skin is attractive to flies which are the carriers of many kinds of diseases, e.g. trachoma. Trachoma is endemic in dry areas in the RSA where standards of skin cleanliness are poor. Flies sit on dirt encrusted faces and carry chlamydia and pyogenic organisms to other faces, thus spreading disease.

(3) The washing of hands after the use of the toilet and before eating.

(4) The absence of infectious and parasitic lesions.

Note: The teaching of personal cleanliness may be difficult where the educational background is such that the concept of microbes and infection cannot be comprehended.

Impetigenous lesions can form from scratching the lesions in scabies and from the bites of lice, bedbugs, mosquitoes and fleas. These conditions and insects are associated with poor standards of personal and home cleanliness. Impetigo is uncommon amongst people who keep their skins and their homes clean. Standards of personal cleanliness must therefore be of a standard which will prevent the skin from being assaulted by ectoparasites.

Sunbathing and sun abuse

Excessive exposure to sun, as in prolonged, chronic unprotected sunbathing, is harmful as it causes premature ageing of the skin, solar keratoses and squamous and basal cell skin cancer, the most common kind of cancer of white skins in South Africa. Acute exposure causes sunburn, varying from erythema to blistering.

The dangerous rays of the sun are the ultraviolet (UV) rays which are divided into UVA, UVB and UVC according to wavelength. UVC is absorbed by the ozone layer of the earth's atmosphere.[2] UVB causes tanning of the skin and with acute exposure causes sunburn. UVA causes degenerative and disease processes in the dermis and epidermis.

White skins vary in their susceptibility to ultraviolet radiation, some skins tanning easily while others burn without tanning — the so-called sensitive skins. Dark skins are not easily affected by exposure to sun due to the pigment layer in the epidermis; deeply pigmented skin never burns.[3]

White skins need protection against the ageing effects of UVA. Protection may be achieved by suitable clothing and sunshades or by using sunscreen products in the form of sunscreen preparations which contain sun protective factors (SPFs). These preparations attenuate UVA and UVB rays to avoid the acute and chronic ill effects of solar radiation. They are not tanning agents. Several varieties meet the varying needs of different skins,e.g. Piz Buin Sun Block cream is used for sensitive areas such as the lips.

Sunscreen preparations are labelled with their SPF values which are, however, only a test of UVB effects.[3] An SPF value of 12–15 is adequate, although reapplication is necessary with prolonged exposure to sun or after swimming if it is not water-resistant. Most products used in the RSA screen only UVB, while some screen both UVA and UVB. These details must appear on the package label and should be studied by the health-conscious user.

Note: Sunscreening should be commenced in childhood to prevent skin damage in adulthood.

Scabies

The *Acarus scabiei (Sarcoptes scabiei)* is an external metazoal parasite which causes scabies. It is a mite which burrows into the epidermis and is strictly parasitic. The burrows cause incessant itching. Scabies is a contagious infestation which is associated with over-population and lack of personal cleanliness.

Treatment of scabies

In scabies the bedding and clothes will also be infested, as well as other people who live in close proximity to the index patient. It is therefore important to treat all members of the 'family' and to disinfect and wash all clothes which have been in contact with the infested people. After completion of treatment it is important for all treated persons to wear clean clothes.

The modern treatment is with Gamma Benzene Hexachloride (Gamma BHC). The two common lotions used are: Skabex (Gamma BHC 1 % in cetrimide 0,5 %) and Quellada Lotion (Gamma BHC 1 % in a water-dispersible base — a thin white cream).

Method of application: a thin layer of the Gamma BHC lotion is applied to the whole body except the scalp and face. The lotion is left for 24 hours and then washed off. Usually one application is sufficient to eradicate the parasite, but a second or a third application may be made at weekly intervals.

For special precautions consult the product inserts.

IMPROVING HYGIENE PRACTICE IN THIRD-WORLD POPULATIONS

In an article in the *South African Journal of Epidemiology and Infection* (1989), the global problem of poor personal and domestic hygiene, water supply and sanitation in Third-World populations is discussed. Startling Third-World statistics: diarrhoea afflicts up to 1 billion children annually and nearly 3,5 million infants and young children die from acute gastro-enteritis every year. Gastro-enteritis is still rampant in South Africa, especially in its rural areas. Ignorance of hygiene principles plays a major role in the prevalence of gastro-intestinal sicknesses, i.e. they are not due only to poor water supplies and sanitation. Evidence for the following statements comes from investigations.[4]

> 'Superior water and sanitation facilities may not protect families from infection if the overall level of faecal contamination of the environment remains high.'

> '. . . as with water supply, even the value of satisfactory toilets may be offset by the presence of uniformly poor hygiene and widespread faecal contamination.'

> 'In an enquiry into the profile of intestinal parasitic infestation in Assam, India, observations were made on three groups of persons who differed in hygienic conditions, in monthly income and in educational level. The living environment was more or less alike in the different groups (from better state to poor). All had pure water for drinking and had latrines of their own. The only observable differences in these groups were personal hygiene, literacy and monthly income in the family. In the mostly illiterate group with poor personal hygiene and very low income, the overall prevalence rate of parasites was 56 %; in contrast, in the more favoured group infestation rate was 12 %.'[4]

A primary factor which prevents progress in the control of water-borne and intestinal infections is ignorance. Example: few of the Third-World populations studied make any attempt to improve the quality of drinking water. Even amongst the 'educated' section of the study populations, the prevalence of intestinal infestations is high. An ignorant mother who breast-feeds her infant may none the less transmit gastro-intestinal diseases to him if she fails to wash her hands after defaecating. Another primary factor preventing disease control is socio-economic status. Even if health education levels are raised, poverty and lack of facilities to apply health principles will hamper progress in controlling intestinal diseases.

It was found that little money is spent by Third-World countries on health education. While the slow process of water and sanitation upgrading takes place, much can be done by improving personal hygiene, especially in relation to hand-washing after defaecation, the building of fly-proof pit latrines, clean food preparation and preventing the fly menace by cleaning cooking and eating utensils immediately after use. This can be taught by community nurses at primary health care and other community health clinics and at schools. These simple health education principles of good personal and domestic hygiene, well put across to the target populations, will do much to lighten the burden of gastro-intestinal diseases in Third-World countries.

REFERENCES

(1) Noakes T D. How much exercise is needed to keep healthy? *S Afr Med J* CME 1988; **6**: 25–34.

(2) SAMJ News. *S Afr Med J* 1987; **72**: xi

(3) Summers R S, Summers B. Sun-induced skin damage — Where do we stand? *S Afr Med J* 1987; **72**: 519–520.

(4) Comment and opinion. Can't we improve hygiene practice in Third-World populations? *The Southern African Journal of Epidemiology and Infection* 1989; **4**: 21.

TEST OF KNOWLEDGE

(1) The nurse has benefited from reading this chapter and the reference chapters if he/she can outline the main principles of a healthy life-style in a First-World community, of:

(*a*) A six-year-old schoolboy.

(*b*) An adolescent girl aged 15 years.

(*c*) A married successful businessman aged 40 years.

(*d*) An elderly woman aged 75 years.

(2) (*a*) What are the dangers of chronic, moderate sunbathing in South Africa?

(*b*) What advice would you give a white mother who is taking her children to the seaside, about care of the skin?

(3) Prepare a talk you would give to a group of rural black women about hygiene in the home.

15

Health Education and Smoking

OBJECTIVE

This chapter is intended as a special information chapter for nurses who are interested in their own health and the health of the community for which they care. The World Health Organisation states that the control of cigarette smoking is the greatest priority for ill-health prevention in developed countries and amongst developing people who adopt an urban life-style.

People generally start smoking when they are young. If they continue the habit, they start paying the price of their drug (nicotine) dependency when they enter middle age: chronic cardio-vascular diseases, male impotence, chronic respiratory diseases, including cancer of the lung and larynx, premature ageing of the skin. The pregnant woman who smokes does incalculable harm to her foetus.

The attention of the nurse is also drawn to the unwholesome atmosphere created by the smoker whose hair is impregnated with the fumes, whose breath smells of stale tobacco smoke and whose home or office is permeated by an offensive smell. Smokers pollute the environment of non-smokers and expose them to the passive inhalation of noxious fumes. Smoking takes the glamour out of romance, although clever advertising may suggest the opposite. Inconsiderate smokers leave a trail of cigarette butts for others to dispose of.

The community nurse who smokes cannot be an effective health educator. By committing this deed he/she is telling the public that smoking is not harmful and that medical research done world-wide to expose the hazards of smoking, should be ignored. He/she has indeed become a 'traitor' to the cause of health.

IN THIS CHAPTER

INTRODUCTION

According to the World Health Organisation, smoking is the most important cause of ill-health in the world. Smoking-related diseases are the single most avoidable cause of morbidity and mortality at present.[3]

SMOKING AND THE MRC[2]

The South African Medical Research Council (MRC), the most influential body for medical research in South Africa, spoke out against smoking in its 1985 statement on Smoking and Health. The statement is supported by 30 000 studies world-wide, showing the relationship between smoking and disease and death.

The MRC pointed out the following ill effects of smoking; it is harmful not only to smokers but also to those around them.

(1) Respiratory diseases: lung cancer, chronic bronchitis and emphysema.

(2) Myocardial disease. Cigarette smoking in combination with hypercholesterolaemia and hypertension are considered the most important risk factors for ischaemic heart disease.

(3) Cigarette smoke potentiates the toxic effects of industrial irritants, e.g. silica dust, asbestos fibres.

(4) Cigarette smoke has deleterious effects on passive smokers, i.e. non-smokers in close contact with smokers, such as the spouse and children of a smoker. The risk of developing lung cancer and chronic bronchitis is increased in passive smokers.

(5) Infants of mothers who smoke during pregnancy are at a disadvantage.

THE HEALTH HAZARDS OF SMOKING

Much has been said and taught about the dangers of smoking, yet the smoking habit is acquired and maintained with unabated vigour.

The following statement on the health hazards of smoking is included by kind permission of S Zwi, S S Hurwitz and J Kallenbach.

'There can no longer be any doubt that tobacco smoking (especially of cigarettes) is a major health hazard. It has been conclusively demonstrated that certain diseases occur more frequently in smokers than in non-smokers and a causal relationship has been established between smoking and these diseases.

'Premature deaths and disabling illnesses caused by cigarette smoking have reached epidemic proportions and present the most challenging of all opportunities for preventive medicine in developed countries (Royal College of Physicians, 1971). The World Health Organisation Expert Committee on Smoking concluded that smoking-related diseases are such important causes of disability and premature death in developed countries that control of cigarette smoking could do more to improve health and prolong life in these countries than any other single action in the whole field of preventive medicine.

'*Smoking and Cardiovascular disease*

'The most important specific health consequence of cigarette smoking in terms of the number of people affected is the development of premature CHD. Liability to CHD is approximately twice as great in cigarette smokers as in non-smokers and is related to the number of cigarettes smoked, to smoke inhalation and to an early age of starting to smoke. Raised serum cholesterol, hypertension and cigarette smoking are the most important known risk factors for CHD.

'Smoking is a very strong risk factor for peripheral vascular disease and aortic aneurysm and a much stronger risk factor for myocardial infarction than angina pectoris. Women who smoke and also use the contraceptive pill have a considerable risk of developing CHD. Strokes (cerebrovascular accidents) are also related to cigarette smoking.

'Nicotine and carbon monoxide (CO) are probably the chief causes in tobacco smoke of CHD and vascular disease. Nicotine stimulates catecholamine secretion and thereby increases the work of the heart. CO in inhaled smoke leads to carboxy-haemoglobin levels of up to 15 %, thus reducing the amount of oxygen available to the myocardium. Coronary artery atheroma and fibrous intimal thickening are closely related to smoking. Both nicotine and CO increase the tendency to thrombosis (by increasing platelet stickiness) and reduce the threshold for ventricular fibrillation during an episode of myocardial ischaemia (Aronow 1976).

'Smoking and Cancer

'Expert committees in many countries are agreed that cigarette smoking is the cause of the modern epidemic of lung cancer. Overall, approximately 90 % of all primary lung cancer cases occur in people who smoke cigarettes. In regular cigarette smokers, the commonest form of cancer is that affecting the lung (*Brit. Med. J.* 1976). The risk of developing lung cancer is 10 times greater for smokers than non-smokers, and is increased by smoking more cigarettes, inhaling, starting to smoke at an early age, or smoking for many years. Pipes and cigars play a small part in causing lung cancer, as does general air pollution. However, cigarette smokers exposed to certain occupational hazards have a high risk of developing lung cancer; asbestos workers who smoke have 90 times the risk of non-smokers in the general population.

'In South Africa, cancer of the lung is the second most common cancer among men of all racial groups, the most common being cancer of the skin in whites, of the oesophagus in blacks and of the stomach in coloureds and Indians.

'The tar (particulate matter) from cigarette smoke has been found to induce malignant changes in the skin and respiratory tract of experimental animals and a number of specific chemical compounds contained in smoke have been established as potent carcinogens or co-carcinogens.

'Besides lung cancer, smoking is associated with malignancy in other organs. Smoking any kind of tobacco predisposes to the development of cancer in the oropharynx, larynx and oesophagus. Cancers of the pancreas and urinary bladder are more common in cigarette smokers than non-smokers.

'Smoking and non-malignant respiratory disease

'Chronic obstructive lung disease (COLD) is a major cause of temporary and permanent disability. It includes chronic bronchitis and emphysema (B & E) from which over 30 000 men and women die in the United Kingdom each year, after years of disability. Cigarette smoking is the most important cause of B & E; this has been demonstrated in many countries though other causes such as air pollution and dust play a role. For example, exposure to silica, coal dust and cotton fibre is related to chronic bronchitis but if combined with cigarette smoking, the incidence of bronchitis is much increased. "Smoking cigarettes may cause an apparent accelerated ageing of lungs by producing both airways obstruction and emphysema which in turn may lead to disability and death." (*Brit. Med. J.* 1975)

'Cigarette smokers are more frequently subject to, and require longer convalescence from, many different respiratory infections, from lobar pneumonia to the common cold (*Brit. Med. J.* 1974). If smokers require general anaesthesia, they are more likely to develop postoperative respiratory complications. In addition, chronic cough predisposes to and aggravates hernia.

'Smoking and Pregnancy

'Pregnant women who smoke cigarettes during the last two trimesters have babies with a lower average birth weight than non-smoking mothers. There is also a greater risk of having a stillbirth and the foetal and neonatal death-rates are

increased. These risks are exaggerated if there is a high risk pregnancy for other reasons.

'Possibly smoking may reduce the blood flow to the placenta and thereby impair the nutrition of the foetus. Also, CO passes freely across the placenta and is readily bound by foetal haemoglobin, thus decreasing the oxygen-carrying capacity of foetal blood.

'Smoking and the Digestive Tract

'Many studies have shown that smokers are more liable to various inflammatory conditions of the gums, e.g. Vincent's gingivitis. This may account for the finding that smokers have more often lost all their teeth than have non-smokers.

'Cancers of the upper gastro-intestinal tract and pancreas are more common in smokers. Smoking does not cause peptic ulcers, but delays their healing so that ulcers are more persistent and more fatal in smokers than in non-smokers.

'Smoking and Physical Fitness

'No serious athlete should be a smoker. Smoking impairs the capacity for strenuous exercise and abstinence improves performance. Endurance, maximum exercise capacity and improvement on training are impaired in proportion to the number of cigarettes smoked daily and the duration of smoking.

'Smoking and Miscellaneous Conditions

'In a study of 1 104 men and women, the severity of facial skin wrinkling correlated with smoking after adjustment for age and outdoor exposure. Smokers in the 5th decade were as likely to be prominently wrinkled as non-smokers who were 20 years older (Daniell 1971). Smokers are more prone to accidents than non-smokers. This applies to industrial as well as traffic accidents and of course to fires. A lighted match or a live cigarette dropped from an old person's shaky fingers can be just as lethal as lung cancer.

'Involuntary or Passive Smoking

'This refers to the inhalation of tobacco combustion prod'ucts from smoke-polluted atmospheres by the non-smoker. Several minor symptoms (such as conjunctival irritation, dry throat) are caused by cigarette smoke. Serious allergic-like reactions may occur in sensitive individuals but the major concern about atmospheric contamination by cigarette smoke has been due to the production of significant levels of CO, enough to cause slight deterioration in tests of psychomotor performance, especially attentiveness and cognitive function.

'Children of parents who smoke are more likely to have bronchitis and pneumonia during the first year of life and this may risk the life of the child or leave it with residual lung damage for the rest of its life (*Brit. Med. J.* 1977).

'Benefits of Stopping Smoking

'There is no doubt that the smoker who gives up cigarettes will feel much better and breathe with less effort. Symptoms such as sputum production, cough and dyspnoea improve when smoking stops, probably due to decrease in bronchoconstriction, improved lung clearance and lessened respiratory tract irritation. The risk of developing the major smoking-associated diseases declines so that after 10 years without smoking, the death-rates of ex-smokers approach those of non-smokers. A woman who stops smoking by the fourth month of her pregnancy obviates the harmful effects on her unborn child.

'The death-rate from ischaemic heart disease (especially sudden death) declines rapidly in the first year after stopping cigarette smoking. The risk of developing cancer declines relative to the continuing smoker in the first few years after cessation and after 10 to 15 years approximates the risk of the non-smoker. It is never too late to give up smoking.'

COSTS OF SMOKING TO SOUTH AFRICA

In terms of health care costs and lost productivity of the labour force, smoking cost the RSA between R362,8 and R396,9 million in 1985, possibly R584,4 to R652 million, if the loss of productivity of those outside the labour force not earning a monthly salary, such as housewives, is included.[1]

In 1987, R55 million was spent on advertising by the tobacco industry, 5,3 % of total advertising expenditure. With the exception of television, the tobacco industry uses all other South African media extensively for advertising: 16 % of radio advertising, 16,3 % of billboard advertising, and 56,3 % of cinema advertising come from tobacco and associated products. Even on television indirect advertising is done on sports and news programmes during sport coverage of cigarette-sponsored sporting events.

McIntyre and Taylor state that smoking-related health care costs and disability grants (social costs) would be imposed on smokers and non-smokers alike were it not for the special taxation (excise duty) on tobacco. Increasing the taxation on cigarettes has the greatest potential as a deterrent to smoking. The impact of the current tobacco taxation has not been determined and may, indeed, not cover the social costs of smoking; smoking-related health care costs could, therefore, be subsidised by non-smokers through income tax payments.[1]

THE EPIDEMIOLOGY OF THE SMOKING HABIT IN SOUTH AFRICA

Prevalence rates (i.e. people who have smoked continuously for at least a year):

- 71 % in men
- 37,9 % in women

Professor Coetzee (UP) says R400 million is spent every year by hospitals on smoke-related diseases.

Smoking accounts directly or in part for about 40 % of patients at Groote Schuur Hospital.[6]

The Royal College of Physicians (London) has found that 80 % of smokers start smoking before the age of 20. In the RSA about 19 000 adolescents of both sexes leave school every year as smokers, 43 % of them being confirmed smokers (Baird). In a survey done on smokers in Bloemfontein schools, Olivier et al.[4] found that in the sample group studied 16 % smoked. In comparison with the prevalence of smoking in other schools, this is a low figure. Most of these Bloemfontein schoolchildren started smoking between the ages of 12 and 18 years.

It is believed that nearly half of all white schoolchildren are smoking by the time they leave school, and that 33 000 youngsters start smoking each year.

A South African survey[5] found that as the level of education increased, so did the proportion of smokers decrease.

Men are generally heavier smokers than women, especially among blacks; few black women smoke. In adult black males smoking rates are high and highest in those who have lived in the urban environment for more than five years.[3]

Some of our hospitals are aiming to become smoke-free. In many, smoking is forbidden in the wards, a concession being made for nicotine addicts in the form of a special room set aside for their smoking use.

PRIMARY PREVENTION OF SMOKING

In South Africa the problem of cigarette smoking is assuming epidemic proportions. Smoking is a social problem in that every smoker can create another smoker. Despite the free availability of information regarding the hazards of smoking, there has been no abatement of the problem. Even doctors and nurses continue to smoke and use the common rationalisations offered by those addicted to the habit:

(1) I am healthy and I am a moderate smoker, therefore, smoking will not harm me.

(2) We all have to die of something.

(3) People who stop smoking get fat and obesity is worse for health than smoking.

(4) I've smoked for so many years — it's not worth stopping now.

(5) I can give up smoking if I want to — but I enjoy it and it calms my nerves.

Smoking is a major killer amongst developed nations; it is generally considered the most serious form of personal pollution in the world, people becoming more addicted to cigarettes than to alcohol or drugs.

In discussing urinary bladder cancer, Fichardt et al. state: 'Smoking related diseases are such important causes of disability and premature death that the control of cigarette smoking could do more to improve health and prolong life than any other single action (including jogging) in the whole field of preventive medicine.'[7]

Yach et al.[8] make the plea to give the highest research priority to community-wide interventions aimed at changing social norms, as over 90 % of people who quit smoking do so outside of specific programmes aimed at individuals.

The reasons why schoolchildren start smoking are peer group pressure and the example of parents and teachers, and the marketing industry. The findings of Olivier et al. indicate that the optimal age for starting a primary preventive programme against smoking in schools appears to be 11 years, i.e. when children are in Std. IV. The age of onset of smoking seems to be coming down, however, as more and more junior school children are starting to smoke. Most experts concerned with the problem of smoking are of the opinion that the best way of fighting the problem is to educate children and adolescents in the hazards of smoking.

School programmes directed at pre-primary and primary school children need to be developed.

The MRC[2] made the following recommendations in 1985:

(1) Smoking should be banned in all public places, as well as on public transport.

(2) The harmful consequences of cigarette smoking must be made more widely known, the important target population being young children and adolescents. The message to the youth should destroy the glamorous picture of the smoking culture hero.

(3) A limit must be placed on the advertising of cigarettes.

It is impossible to legislate against smoking but restrictions on smoking can be enforced and have been, in some instances, in public places. Some public-spirited doctors forbid smoking in their consulting-rooms. SATV has decided that tobacco advertising will not be screened on television.

Benatar et al.[9] feel that the government (State Health) has a moral obligation to play a leading role in disseminating information about the health hazards of smoking. They feel that only if the social attitudes to smoking change so that it becomes an unacceptable habit (like dagga smoking) will there be any success. These authors state:

'The Department of Health [which] is as morally responsible for the prevention of loss of lives from smoking as for the control of infectious diseases . . .'

At present the policy of the Department of Health regarding the health hazards related to smoking is to follow an approach which is aimed at preventing people, especially children, from ever taking up the habit. The Department of Health is actively pursuing the following programme:

(1) at the request of the Department, the Human Sciences Research Council has undertaken a comprehensive survey on the smoking habit in the RSA;

(2) pamphlets published by the Department are available free of charge on request;

(3) movie films, especially geared for use by high schools, universities and youth organisations may be borrowed for screening from the Department, free of charge;

(4) voluntary organisations and other bodies which strive to publicise the health hazards of smoking and which actively promote opposition to the smoking habit, are encouraged and advised by the Department; provision has even been made to subsidise their authorised health-education programmes.

MASA: Statement on smoking[10]

'The Medical Association of South Africa (MASA) believes that the time has come when there can no longer be any equivocation about the ill effects — medical and social — resulting from smoking.

'With this in mind the MASA wishes to make clear its strongly felt beliefs about smoking and the steps which should be taken to curb it in South Africa. In taking this standpoint the MASA is aware that it is incumbent on it, as the representative body of the medical profession, to offer guidance on this important question.

'The MASA believes that the weight of scientific evidence linking cigarette smoking to the excessively high incidence of many serious diseases is beyond question. Various forms of cancer, heart disease and chronic respiratory disease have an excessive incidence related to tobacco consumption. And the MASA believes that it should be made clear that attempts to dilute this scientific evidence by various interest groups verges on the "immoral".

'Only a concerted and whole-hearted effort will break the hold which cigarette smoking has on South Africa's population as a whole. Such steps are vital if we are to prevent future generations from suffering a similar fate.'

The MASA does not hesitate in calling for the following legislative action:

(1) A total ban on all tobacco advertising in all media.
(2) All purchases should bear a clear health warning ensuring that the public is told that tobacco smoking damages health.
(3) A ban on all cigarette-vending machines.
(4) The removal of tobacco products from open display shelves in supermarkets.
(5) The discontinuation of allowing tax relief on any form of tobacco promotion.
(6) A ban on sale of cigarettes to minors — to be strictly enforced.
(7) The maximum permitted nicotine and tar yields should be established by law and enforced.

The MASA is aware that the implementation of such legislation would result in certain potential areas of hardship.

Additionally, the MASA seeks the support of important influence groups:

Doctors and other health professionals — to assist and encourage education campaigns promoted by various organisations including the Department of Health to actively discourage patients from smoking — and give up smoking themselves where they have not done so.

Department of Health — to set a target of reducing tobacco consumption by at least 3 % per annum; to begin a major and continuous health education campaign against smoking among schoolchildren with the active participation of the teaching profession.

Sportsmen and entertainers — to avoid being directly and indirectly involved in promoting smoking and never to be seen smoking in public.

Insurance companies — to continue the trend towards offering reduced premiums for non-smokers on life insurance policies and to advertise the fact.

Industry and commerce — to be encouraged to actively promote anti-smoking campaigns in their establishments.

Nurses and doctors have a grave responsibility with regard to smoking and the public. If the public sees members of the health profession smoking, they are not likely to be influenced in a positive way by anti-smoking health education. No doctor or nurse who is health conscious, in possession of the facts and figures with regard to the hazards of smoking and is concerned about the health of his/her patients, will smoke, especially not in front of patients who might follow his/her example, reassured by the apparent accepting attitude of the health professional to their addiction.

Likewise, no schoolteacher or university lecturer should ever smoke in front of his students as the example set by people in authority is often followed. The social responsibility for the health education of the public is mainly the work of voluntary organisations who do so with the blessing and help of the Department of Health.

Women can act as pressure groups to prevent advertising of tobacco products on the media, such as the radio and television. They can encourage the dissemination of facts on the health hazards of smoking by health authorities in hospitals, clinics and the civil service.

By widely disseminated health education, people are given the prudent option to smoke or not to smoke. If a non-smoker is convinced that smoking is dangerous to health, he is unlikely to risk his health in order to acquire a habit with dubious advantages, especially if this habit is economically taxing.

In the nation-wide campaign against cigarette smoking, the health education of the group at risk of starting the smoking habit — the school-going child — should receive priority. As many of these children are too immature to make a prudent decision to smoke or not to smoke, their parents and teachers who may be setting the example also need to be made aware of the dangers of the habit. Parents and teachers are the 'oracles', the source of standards of right and wrong. If a child defies his authority figures and becomes receptive to health educative influences he is, in fact, registering a vote of no confidence in the wisdom of his authority figures. The odds against health education influencing children with this kind of familial handicap are heavy indeed.

NON-SMOKERS' 'BILL OF RIGHTS'

The Council on Smoking and Health has issued the following non-smokers' 'Bill of Rights'.

Non-smokers help protect the health, comfort and safety of everyone by insisting on the following rights:

The right to breathe clean air

Non-smokers have the right to breathe clean air, free from harmful and irritating tobacco smoke. This right supersedes the right to smoke when the two conflict.

The right to speak out

Non-smokers have the right to express — firmly but politely — their discomfort and adverse reactions to tobacco smoke.

They have the right to voice their objections when smokers light up without asking permission.

The right to act

Non-smokers have the right to take action through legislative channels, social pressures or any other legitimate means — as individuals or in groups, to prevent or discourage smokers from polluting the atmosphere and to seek the restriction of smoking in public places.

SECONDARY PREVENTION — THE CURE OF THE SMOKING HABIT

The National Cancer Association is concerned with the dangers of cigarette smoking and declares an annual 'smokeless day', asking all smokers to stop and think, on that day, before they light up. This is to encourage people to stop smoking, by arousing their feelings of anxiety (most people know smoking is harming their health) and jogging their resolve to do something about it.

In 1976 the Council on Smoking and Health (a country-wide association for non-smokers) was formed in Johannesburg. It consists of prominent doctors and lay people and has a full-time director who acts in a consultative and educational capacity throughout the entire RSA. The main aims of the Council on Smoking and Health (CSH) are: 'to curb the present epidemic of tobacco-related disorders experienced by all population groups in South Africa by preventive and therapeutic programmes'.

The following are subsidiary aims of the Council:

(1) to have regular programmes on radio and TV on the detrimental effects on health of smoking;

(2) to prevent the advertising of tobacco products on all public media (radio, TV, newspapers and magazines, buses, neon lights, hoardings);

(3) the establishment of smoke-free zones, for instance, in doctors' consulting-rooms, clinics and hospitals, in cinemas, theatres, lecture halls, buses, trains, food stores, etc.;

(4) to educate medical students, nurses and general practitioners on the hazards of cigarette smoking, using films and research material made available by overseas countries;

(5) to give advice regarding what to do to stop smoking; the CSH issues a booklet on 'How to stop smoking without gaining weight', and

(6) to persuade legislators to require the tobacco industry to:

(a) affix a warning notice on every packet of cigarettes, stating that smoking is dangerous to health, and giving the tar and nicotine content of the product, and

(b) regularly publish in the media the constituents of all brands of cigarettes on sale.

There is epidemiological evidence (not proof) that, by lowering the tar and nicotine content of cigarettes, the death-rate from lung cancer will be lowered. The safer cigarettes are those with low tar and nicotine content. There are many different ways of reducing the total particulate matter (TPM) (including tar and nicotine) of cigarettes, such as the use of filters and cigarette holders, increasing porosity of cigarette papers, the use of low TPM tobaccos to which is added non-toxic flavour additives. It is the stimulation by nicotine and the smell and taste of smoke, however, which have the addictive properties and give the smoker gratification. In spite of knowing that cigarettes with low tar and nicotine content are safer, few smokers have been found to change to less carcinogenic kinds of cigarettes. During the past 25 years, however, the tar and nicotine levels of cigarette tobacco have dropped off steadily in overseas countries. In South Africa, the tar and nicotine content of cigarettes is amongst the highest in the world.

The dangers of smoking depend upon the depth of inhalation; as pipe and cigar smokers generally puff and seldom inhale deeply, these forms of smoking are less dangerous than cigarette smoking. One of the risks of using low TPM tobaccos is that smokers may inhale with increasing depth in order to get satisfaction and thereby inhale other harmful substances such as carbon monoxide.

There is no such thing as a 'safe' cigarette. Smokers of low-tar cigarettes usually smoke more, so cancelling out any possible benefit.

Giving up smoking is much more difficult than resisting the inception of the habit. Some smoking cures depend on cutting down the inhalation of tar and nicotine gradually, either by reducing the number of cigarettes smoked daily, or by the use of cigarettes with increasingly low tar and nicotine content, or by the use of filters in cigarette holders which hold back tar and nicotine to an increasing extent. In this way the subject's ability to tolerate nicotine deprivation is catered for. In practice this method of helping a smoker to stop his addiction has been found futile. The subject fails to see himself as a 'non-smoker' and succumbs to his addiction as soon as a stressful situation causes stress and tension, conditions of dysphoria which the smoker has in the past relieved by the inhalation of nicotine.

Many abrupt smoking cures have been advocated, from unassisted self-denial to temporary medicine — or hypnosis-assisted cures, which nevertheless may lead to complete cessation of smoking. In both cases the motivation and incentive to stop smoking must be high, and social support and encouragement adequate. The person who eventually gives up the habit must be able to see himself as belonging to the non-smoking section of the community. The Council on Smoking and Health offers prospective clients who wish to give up the habit a behaviour modification programme at its withdrawal clinics. As the recurrent need for the 'stress dummy' is very persistent in the months after stopping, ex-smokers who join the withdrawal clinics attend group meetings for as long as they need group support.

Nicotine-containing chewing gum (Nicorette)[11]

This Schedule 3 preparation is obtainable on doctor's prescription in the RSA. It is used as a temporary aid for those who wish to stop smoking. It must be used in conjunction with a behaviour modification programme in order to be effective.

As the gum merely alleviates the withdrawal symptoms in nicotine addicts, it should be used only by persons strongly motivated to stop smoking and who, therefore, suffer from the effects of nicotine withdrawal. It must not be used by those who are gradually cutting down on cigarettes as the nicotine level in their blood will then remain high and strengthen the addiction.

Dosage: 6 pieces of gum, containing 2 mg nicotine each, are chewed intermittently, tapering off slowly after 2 months. The gum may cause a temporary local irritation and dyspepsia and must not be used by children and pregnant women.

The Government of National Unity of South Africa (1994) plans to ban or severely restrict smoking in all workplaces and public buildings. The Minister of Health feels it is the duty of the government (through employers) to protect those who do not want to be exposed to smoking, either through persuasion or through legislation.

Note: In terms of clause 29 of the Interim Constitution and the Occupational Health and Safety Act (see p. 48), people are entitled to a healthy working environment. There is thus a legal obligation for employers not to allow smoking in the workplace.

Draft regulations (under the Tobacco Products Controls Act (1993)) for health warnings on tobacco products and advertisements have been published in the *Government Gazette* for comment by the public.

The new warnings take up at least a quarter of the space on the front of cigarette packets and half the back. Smoking advertisements on cinema screens also carry warnings against the dangers of smoking.

Tobacco Products Control Act 83 of 1993, *GG* No. 14916 of 2 July 1993.

Major provisions

'This Act provides that the Minister of Health, by notice in the *Gazette* can prohibit the smoking of tobacco products, or determine the conditions under which smoking may occur, in public places including public transport . . . The Minister can also delegate this power to a local authority in certain instances.

'Any tobacco product which is sold or advertised must reflect (in the advert or on the package):

- the prescribed health hazard warning
- the quantities of hazardous substances

'No person may sell or supply tobacco products to a person under 16 years of age – whether for his personal use or not.'

Surveys amongst those who have given up, indicate the importance of the following in their success:

(1) They wanted to stop smoking. Unless the addict wants to give up smoking, he is not likely to succeed.
(2) They stopped smoking 'cold turkey', i.e. they did not switch to milder cigarettes to cut down on the number smoked daily; they stopped completely on a target day (CSH booklet).

(3) They were 'frightened' into giving up smoking when they were confronted with the medical diagnosis of smoking-related symptoms, e.g. chronic cough, myocardial ischaemia, intermittent claudication.

REFERENCES

(1) McIntyre DE, Taylor SP. Economic aspects of smoking in South Africa. *S Afr Med J* 1989; **75**: 432–435.
(2) MRC. *Statement on Smoking and Health.* Cape Town: South African Medical Research Council, 1985.
(3) Yach D, Strebel P, McIntyre DE, Taylor S. Time to ban tobacco advertising. *S Afr Med J* 1989; **75**: 40.
(4) Olivier LR, *et al. S Afr Med J* 1977; **52**: 607.
(5) Van der Burgh C. *S Afr Med J* 1979; **55**: 975.
(6) Opie LH. Smoking — what you can do. *S Afr Med J* 1989; **75**: 409.
(7) Fichardt T, Sandison AG. *S Afr Med J* 1978; **54**: 738.
(8) Yach D, Steyn K, Albrecht C. Priorities for research on smoking and health. *S Afr Med J* 1989; **75**: 158–159.
(9) Benatar SR, *et al. S Afr Med J* 1977; **52**: 870.
(10) Medical Association of South Africa. *S Afr Med J* 1981; **59**: 471.
(11) Editorial. Nicotine chewing gum. *S Afr Med J* 1985; **67**: 953.

TEST OF KNOWLEDGE

The student has benefited from studying this chapter if he/she can answer the following questions:

(1) Discuss the health hazards of smoking.
(2) Discuss the concept of 'passive' smoking and the non-smokers' 'Bill of Rights'.
(3) Name the benefits, both material and physical, of stopping smoking.
(4) Discuss the uses of nicotine-containing chewing gum and relatively 'safe' cigarettes in smoking cures.
(5) What are the main motivating forces which lead to success in giving up the smoking habit?
(6) Discuss the pros and cons of allowing smoking in hospitals.

16

Health Education in Nutrition

OBJECTIVES

Nutrition covers all the processes whereby food is ingested, digested, metabolised and assimilated and whereby waste products are excreted. The principles of good nutrition will be discussed in this chapter; in addition, the chemical composition and nutritional values of some common basic foods and some special foods will be given.

Another objective of this chapter is to introduce the student to the planning of balanced diets — both mixed omnivorous and vegetarian — according to the basic food groups which comprise each kind of diet.

An important objective is the introduction of the concept of the 'prudent' diet. The prudent diet is a mixed, balanced diet which does not have the atherogenic properties of the so-called, normal diet of westernised South Africans. The prudent diet has the health advantages of the balanced vegetarian diet without any of its possible disadvantages.

The regulations with regard to the sale of milk, milk products and milk substitutes are discussed to aid the student in his/her health educating role.

Nutrition is a very important subject in health education; it therefore behoves the health educator to be conversant with the essential knowledge about good nutrition and the effects of malnutrition.

The nurse educator is introduced to fallacies about certain foods and diets which are elevated to the status of a cult and which may be harmful and are certainly costly. The nutritional habits of some of the South African cultural groups are discussed and the chemical composition of foods preferred and available to those people not following the typical westernised diet is given for comparison purposes.

Although indigenous articles of diet may be wholesome if used correctly, the nutrition health educator must be aware that the unenlightened often do not see a connection between food and health and thus may allow beliefs and food preferences to cause malnutrition, even where enough food is available.

The health educator is also made aware of the dangers of the westernised diet with its excesses of refined carbohydrates, fat and salt and its low fibre content.

INTRODUCTION

Six classes of nutrients fulfil man's metabolic
needs: carbohydrates (CHO), fats, proteins,
water, vitamins and minerals.

Metabolism is the process by which nutritive material is
built up into living matter (anabolic or constructive metabolism) or is broken down into simpler substances (catabolic
metabolism) for a variety or purposes. Basal metabolism
refers to these living processes taking place with the body
at complete rest.

The specific functions of food are:

- *Anabolic.* Minerals, CHO, fats and proteins
  are used as building materials to synthesise
  cells, tissues and enzymes, not only for the
  growth of the body to maturity but also to
  continually repair and replace worn or damaged tissues and to supply the catalysts of
  specific chemical reactions for the functioning of the living body.
- *Catabolic.* CHO, fats and proteins — the
  fuel foods — are broken down (burned or
  oxidated) to release energy in various forms:
  to maintain basal metabolic functions, to
  drive the biochemical reactions, to heat the
  body (Kilojoule energy) and generate
  movement (Kinetic energy).

  Kilojoule (kJ) energy of fuels:
  – 1 g CHO – 17 kJ
  – 1 g protein – 17 kJ
  – 1 g fat – 38 kJ.
- *Vitamins and minerals* are essential for life
  and health but are not broken down to release energy. They are regulators of the bio-

chemical reactions required to build up tissue and release energy from the fuel foods.

- *Water* makes up 60 % of the mass of adult males and 52 % of the mass of adult females.[17] Children have more. Water and its solutes is known as tissue fluids. Water serves as a coolant, solvent and transport medium in which chemical reactions take place.

Note: Dietary fibre (see pp. 284, 261)

THE COMPOSITION, SOURCES AND FUNCTIONS OF FOOD

Food is composed of the constituents (nutrients) discussed below.

Carbohydrates (CHO)

The elements forming carbohydrates are C, H and O.

Source

Starch (complex carbohydrates): All kinds of grain, dried legumes and potatoes.
Glycogen: Meat (muscle) and liver.
Sugars: Cane, beetroot, fruit and honey. Sugar may be in the form of sucrose, glucose, fructose or lactose.

Functions

(1) Chief source of energy;
(2) prevention of excessive breakdown of body protein and fat with attendant weakness, emaciation, ketosis and acidosis.

Complex carbohydrates are the most important sources of energy.

Starch, disaccharide sugars and glycogen are digested to monosaccharides (mainly glucose, but also fructose and galactose) in the small intestines, before they are absorbed. Insulin is needed for the utilisation of glucose, the main source of energy in the muscle cells of the body.

While the body requires dietary carbohydrates for energy, pure sugar (sucrose, fructose and glucose) is not an essential food and is often referred to as 'empty kilojoules'. The sugars found in combination with other nutrients in vegetables, fruit and milk supply enough supplementary kilojoules to satisfy the body's needs under normal circumstances.

If fuel consumption exceeds energy needs, the body converts the excess CHO to fat which is laid down in the subcutaneous tissues and causes obesity. The danger in taking in empty kilojoules lies in the fact that they may satisfy energy needs before the need for other nutrients (found in combination with energy-providing foods) has been satisfied. In this way the excessive intake of sugar may cause malnutrition.

Example of two meals which supply the same number of kilojoules (2000)

Meal grossly deficient in all the essential nutrients:

- 1 bottle of cold drink (300 ml)
- Small piece (20 g) milk chocolate
- A sandwich of white bread and jam.

Meal in which kilojoules are balanced with all the other essential nutrients:

- 1 glass of milk (250 ml)
- 1 medium-sized orange
- A sandwich of whole-wheat bread and peanut butter.

Sugar substitutes

(Artificial sweeteners)
Sugar is a palatable food, the high consumption of which has become habitual in the RSA. Nutritionists are of the opinion that our sugar intake should be cut by half. To satisfy the acquired need for a sweet taste, the following sugar substitutes can be used:

(1) Sorbitol (a polyalcohol). This has the same energy value as sugar but is absorbed more slowly and does not require insulin for utilisation.
(2) Saccharin and cyclamate products. They are sweeter than sugar and have no energy value.
(3) Aspartame (Nouvelle, NutraSweet). This is a low-kilojoule sweetener, much sweeter than sugar, which leaves no bitter aftertaste. It contains phenylalanine; for table use, package units shall not exceed the sweetening equivalent of 2 teaspoonfuls of sucrose.
(4) Acesulfame K.

Note: Sweeteners are controlled by law and only 'permitted' sweeteners may be added to a foodstuff prior to the sale of such foodstuff.

Average amount of carbohydrates in 100 grams of a variety of foods

Less than 6 %

- avocado
- asparagus
- beet tops
- broccoli
- cabbage
- cauliflower
- celery
- cucumber
- egg fruit
- gem squash
- green beans (young)
- lettuce
- marrow
- mushrooms
- parsley
- radishes
- rhubarb
- spinach
- sweet peppers
- watercress

6 to 10 %

- cantaloupe
- grapefruit
- lemons
- mulberries
- naartjies
- pawpaw
- peaches
- strawberries
- beetroot
- Brussels sprouts
- butternut squash
- carrots
- hubbard squash
- leeks
- onions
- pumpkin
- turnips

11 to 15 %

- apples
- apricots

- cherries
- gooseberries
- granadillas
- guavas
- litchis
- mangoes
- oranges
- pears
- pineapples, plums
- prickly pears
- quinces
- youngberries
- green peas
- parsnips
- Brazil nuts
- pecan nuts
- walnuts
- porridge

16 to 20 %

- grapes
- figs
- potatoes
- almonds
- peanuts
- ice-cream

21 to 25 %

- bananas
- sweet corn
- sweet potatoes
- cooked rice
- cooked dry pulses

30 to 35 %

- soy beans

50 to 55 %

- bread
    - brown
    - raisin
    - white

60 to 65 %

- dry pulses
    - beans
    - lentils
    - peas
- cake

66 to 75 %

- dried fruits
  - dates
  - prunes
  - raisins
- unrefined cereal products, e.g.
  - unsifted wheat and maize meal
  - rolled oats
- biscuits
- jam

76 % and more

- rice
  - white
  - brown
- refined cereal products, e.g.
  - baker's cones
  - cake flour
  - cornstarch
  - maize rice
  - macaroni
- golden syrup
- honey
- sugar
- sweets

From: *Scientific Nutrition and You* issued by Department of Health Services and Welfare. Administration: House of Assembly.

Fats (triglycerides)

The elements forming fats are C, H and O. Fats and oils are combinations of fatty acids and glycerol.

Source

Animal fats: Cream, butter, meat and fish.
Vegetable oils: Sunflower seed, maize, wheat, soy beans, nuts, olives and avocado pears.

Functions

(1) Provide fuel for energy;
(2) carry fat-soluble vitamins;
(3) protect nerves and delicate organs by fat deposited in the body;
(4) building substances, for example, brain tissue, steroids.

Note: Liquid paraffin, a mineral oil, is not a food element and may hinder the absorption of fat-soluble vitamins if taken to excess. Acts as faecal lubricant as it is not digested and absorbed.

A fatty acid is an organic acid which may be either saturated or unsaturated, saturation implying that it cannot absorb any more hydrogen atoms. Unsaturated fatty acids can be rendered saturated by processing, e.g. heating, solidifying.

Examples of fatty acids

Saturated: stearic acid, palmitic acid, butyric acid (in butter). Butterfat is almost wholly saturated and raises the serum cholesterol (TC).
Unsaturated: linolenic acid, linoleic acid. They occur widely in plants. They are termed 'essential' in nutrition as they cannot be synthesised in the body. They are the essential fatty acids which form part of all lipoproteins in the body. Modern studies[4] suggest that a deficiency of essential fatty acids in the diet may contribute to atherosclerosis. The unsaturated fatty acids are thought to keep the level of the blood cholesterol low, as the process of cholesterol catabolism is accelerated by the unsaturated fatty acids in the blood. A low dietary intake for a period of at least a year manifests as a low level of linoleic acid in adipose tissue (body fat). This is a risk factor indicator for ischaemic heart disease.

The kinds of fats found in most plants and fish (oils) are unsaturated. Margarine, a vegetable fat, contains both saturated and unsaturated fats, the amounts being printed on the container. Peanut butter contains about 50 % oil, of which 30 % is polyunsaturated. It has been found that active people metabolise saturated fat better than sedentary ones.

Note: The 'poly-' refers to more than two double bonds in the fatty acid molecule. Hardening of a liquid oil turns it into a solid fat (e.g. margarine). It makes an unsaturated fat partly or completely saturated. When completely saturated it is no longer able to reduce the cholesterol level of the blood.

Cholesterol (closely associated with animal fats)

Cholesterol content of common foods of animal origin (mg/100 g):

Fresh egg yolk	2 000
Beef kidney	405
Beef liver	260
Sardines	70
Whole egg	495
Calf liver	360
Cheese (processed)	135–155
Milk	11
Lamb liver	610

Butter 280
Chicken 90
Fish 50–60

Lean meats and fish, skim milk, all fruits and most vegetables and their oils are low in cholesterol. Cocoa and chocolate are high in cholesterol. All South African margarines are made from sunflower oil and contain no cholesterol.

Cholesterol is a kind of alcohol which is a normal substance in the body of an animal, being found in the human body mainly in the bile (chol. = bile) and in nerve tissue. It forms the basis of all steroids (e.g. hormones of the suprarenal cortex, sex glands) and is tied to fatty acids in the blood. Cholesterol is one of the blood lipids (fat and fat-like substances), the other lipids being fatty acids, triglycerides (true fats), phospholipids (e.g. lecithin, cephalin) and lipoproteins. Cholesterol is necessary for the synthesis of all body cells, especially those of the liver. It is catabolised to cholic (bile) acids and excreted in bile and faeces.

The normal serum cholesterol level is below 200 mg per 100 mg (mg %) (5,2 mmol/ℓ). Normally the cholesterol level of the blood is not affected by dietary intake unless the latter is excessive. Exercise seems to play a role in keeping serum cholesterol levels normal.

Researchers have found that where prudent dietary principles (see p. 269)[5] are followed, one egg once daily (not fried) does not increase total serum cholesterol.

Proteins

The elements forming proteins are C, H, O, N, S and P. Proteins are composed of organic acids called amino acids.

Source

Animal (1st class): Milk, eggs, meat and fish.
Animal (2nd class): Gelatine.
Vegetable (2nd class): Legumes and whole grain.

Functions

(1) Building substances for growth and repair;
(2) fuel for energy;
(3) regulation of body functions.

About 20 % of the mass of the adult body is protein — the second greatest ingredient of the body after water (except in the obese person). Approximately 3,5 % of the total body protein is lost to wear and tear daily and must be replaced as the body does not store protein. The protein from broken-down body cells can, however, be reused to make new protein.

Second-class vegetable protein is body-building only if a variety is eaten or if it is supplemented by the addition of first-class proteins. Gelatine acts as a fuel only.

The quality of a protein depends upon the number of different amino acids it contains, 20 amino acids being required for building a protein. Plants can synthesise these amino acids but humans and animals cannot do this; human beings must obtain at least nine essential amino acids from plants, directly or via animals, in order to build their own protein. First-class proteins are those that contain all the essential amino acids. Second-class proteins are lacking in essential amino acids but in combination provide the body with a first-class source of protein. Each meal should, therefore, consist of a combination of foods which contain all the essential amino acids. Amino acids are not stored in the body if they cannot be used immediately — they are simply used for energy purposes.

The recommendations of the Food and Nutrition Board of the USA for daily protein intake per kilogram ideal body mass for the various age groups are as follows:

- Infancy: 2,2 g
- Childhood: 2–1,8 g
- Adolescence: 1–0,9 g
- Adulthood: 0,8 g
- Pregnancy and breast-feeding: Additional 30–20 g per day (total)

Stress and tension due to injury, fear, anxiety and anger stimulate the breakdown of body protein, as does a starvation diet; if the intake of fats and carbohydrates is insufficient, dietary protein will be used as body fuel; if this is insufficient, body tissue will be broken down to supply kilojoules. This happens in fasting and in undernourished people.

Strenuous activity does not require increased protein intake, except if the activity is aimed at increased muscle mass. Confinement to bed does, however, require increased protein intake, as the bedridden patient excretes more protein than he normally takes in.

Minerals

Minerals are inorganic salts and are obtained from the diet. The major minerals (RDA more than 100 mg/day) include: calcium, phosphorus, magnesium, sodium, potassium, chloride, sulphur.

Trace elements (RDA less than 100 mg/day) are present in small quantities in the diet and include: iron, iodine, zinc, copper, manganese, chromium, cobalt, selenium, molybdenum, fluorine.

Other elements which may act as trace elements include: silicon, vanadium, nickel, tin, cadmium, arsenic, aluminium, boron.

Note: RDA — recommended daily allowance.

Calcium (Ca), Phosphorus (P), Magnesium (Mg)

In: milk, cheese, beans, lettuce, cabbage, celery, almonds, carrots, beet leaves, dried figs, peanuts, sesame seeds, molasses, drinking water.

Functions

(1) Form part of bones, teeth and blood;
(2) regulate the irritability of muscles and nerves;
(3) calcium and magnesium are essential for enzyme activities, clotting of blood and the heart beat;
(4) 99 % of total body magnesium is present in intracellular fluids and bone.

Iron (Fe), Copper (Cu)

Good sources: Kidneys, heart, liver, egg-yolk, lean beef and brown sugar.
Moderate sources: Dried legumes, oats, apricots, prunes and raisins. The iron in spinach cannot be utilised by the human body.
Poor sources: Nearly all fruits and vegetables, maize and milk. Maize inhibits iron absorption from other foods in the diet.

Functions

(1) Iron forms the oxygen-carrying component of haemoglobin;
(2) copper is essential for the utilisation of iron.

Zinc

Good sources: dry legumes, peanuts.

Functions

An important trace element.

Iodine (I)

In: sea foods and water. Iodised salt.

Functions

Iodine forms part of the hormone thyroxin.

Potassium (K), Sodium (Na)

In: all natural foodstuffs, especially meat, cheese and eggs; orange juice and bananas are rich in potassium; extra Na is ingested in the form of table salt (NaCl) and sodium bicarbonate.

Functions

Na and K are the chief electrolytes of the body, whereby body functions are regulated. K is found chiefly intracellularly and keeps the cells alive. Na is found in the blood and tissue fluids (extracellularly), and maintains the fluid balance. A link has been found between high salt (NaCl) intake and: hypertension, stroke, coronary heart disease and gastric cancer.

A reduction in dietary salt is linked to a reduction in hypertension. No one knows what the optimum level of salt in the diet should be, but it is suggested that the average salt intake in a westernised diet should be cut by almost half.

It is a wise precaution in those with developing hypertension not to add salt (NaCl) to food at the table if salt has been used in the preparation of the food.

Vitamins

The water-soluble vitamins are: B complex, C and P. The fat-soluble vitamins are: A, D, E and K. The latter are absorbed only in the presence of bile salts in the small intestine.

Antixerophthalmic vitamin A (Retinol)

Fat-soluble vit. A in: fish-liver oils, dairy products, mammalian liver, egg-yolk and enriched margarine.
Provitamin A (beta-carotene) in: yellow vegetables and fruit, e.g. carrots, pumpkin, paw-

paws, yellow mealies, yellow peaches, mangoes.

Dark green vegetables, e.g. green beans and peas, cabbage, broccoli and spinach.

Functions

(1) Promotion of the natural resistance of the skin and mucous membranes;
(2) essential for the formation of visual purple of the retina, and tears;
(3) normal growth and development of the skeleton, teeth and soft tissues.

Vitamin A is destroyed by ultraviolet radiation and by oxidation. It is resistant to heat in the absence of air.

Vitamin A in every gram of fish-liver oil (LO), measured in international units (IU) —

- Hake (stockfish) LO: 10 000–12 000 IU
- Kingklip LO: 10 000–40 000 IU
- Halibut LO: Up to 50 000 IU
- Cod LO: 1 000 IU

used as a prescribed medicine.

Note: Amount is measured today in microgram retinol equivalents (RE) (see p. 264).

Vitamin A is stored in the liver and the body retains enough of this vitamin to last two years (in the event of protein, vitamin A and carotene starvation). When there is sufficient vitamin A stored in the body, the conversion of beta-carotene to retinol decreases. This is a protective mechanism.

Note: Retinol poisoning may occur from taking in too much retinol, e.g. from self-medication with fish liver oil preparations. These are such concentrated sources of retinol that 10–20 times the recommended daily intake (see p. 264) is consumed.

Vitamin B complex

Antineuritic vit. B_1 (thiamin or aneurine) in: meat, especially pork and liver; most fruits and vegetables, especially legumes; all cereal kernels and, therefore, whole-wheat bread; dried yeast and Marmite.

Functions

(1) Maintains the health of cardiac muscle and nervous tissue;
(2) essential for the oxidation of carbohydrate in the cells;
(3) promotes growth;
(4) prevents beriberi.

In an acid medium, vit. B_1 is resistant to heat, except the high temperatures of superheated steam. It is destroyed by alkalis.

Riboflavin (vit. B_2)

Good sources: Beef and sheep liver, heart and kidneys; legumes and dried yeast: milk and eggs.

Poor sources: Fruit and vegetables with the exception of dried legumes.

Functions

(1) Essential for growth;
(2) important for the metabolism of carbohydrate and protein.

Vit. B_2 is heat stable but is destroyed by light.

Pyridoxine (vit. B_6) and co-enzymes (vitamers)

Endogenous synthesis in gut.

Good source: Vegetable foods such as beans, peas, cabbage, nuts, cereals and bananas.

Poor sources: Meat, eggs and milk.

Functions

Plays a vital role in physiological processes such as amino acid and lipid metabolism and immunity.

Nicotinic acid (niacin)

Good sources: Lean meat, liver, kidneys and fish; legumes, dried yeast and whole wheat; coffee.

Poor sources: Milk, eggs, vegetables and fruit.

Functions

(1) Same as riboflavin;
(2) prevents pellagra.

Niacin causes peripheral vasodilatation.

Note: Niacin can be made from tryptophan in the presence of pyridoxin and riboflavin. The niacin in maize is bound and unusable. It can withstand damp heat. Both maize and millet are pellagragenic (see p. 212 for new maize hybrids).

Anti-anaemic factor (vit. B_{12})

Only in animal foods, especially mammalian liver.

Enriched soya milk.

Functions

Maturation of erythrocytes.

Antiscorbutic vitamins

Ascorbic acid (Vit. C) and rutin (permeability vit. P) in: guavas, citrus fruits, pawpaws, mangoes, berries, raw cabbage, potatoes, turnips, tomatoes and green chillies.
Poor sources: Cow's milk and meat. Eggs contain nil.

Functions

(1) Collagen synthesis.
(2) Vit. C and P maintain health of capillaries and prevent scurvy.
(3) Vit. C stimulates the formation of erythrocytes, bones and teeth, and raises the resistance of the body, as it is essential for the function of the suprarenal cortex.
(4) Improves the absorption of iron if eaten with iron-rich vegetables.

Ascorbic acid content of the fresh mass of the following fruit and vegetables (measured in milligrams per 100 grams — mg %):

- guava: 120–1 000, average 350;
- orange (Valencia): 33;
- pineapple: 23;
- prickly pear: 17–22;
- naartjie: 37;
- avocado pear: 21;
- pawpaw: 73;
- peach: 21;
- potato: 19,2;
- sweet potato: 20;
- turnip: 24;
- pumpkin: 4,41;
- cabbage: 60–87;
- lettuce: 5–35;
- green peas: 30–50;
- tomato: 25;
- green chillies: 111.

Note: Ascorbic acid is destroyed by heat, light and oxidation (see Preparation of Food, p. 272).

Antirachitic vitamin D

Calciferol (vit. D_2) in: irradiated ergosterol of yeast, egg-yolk and dairy products (if cows fed on irradiated ergosterol).
Vit. D_3: Irradiation of the skin with ultraviolet rays, causes the provitamin, 7-dehydro-cholesterol to be converted to vit. D.
Natural sources: Cod-liver and halibut liver oils, egg-yolk and dairy products, if animals are exposed to sunlight.
Poor sources: Mammalian liver, vegetables.

Functions

(1) Absorption of calcium;
(2) calcification of bone.

Vit. D_3 is resistant to heat and oxidation.
Vitamin D in every gram of fish liver oil (LO), measured in international units (IU) —

- Hake (stockfish) LO: 200–300 IU
- Kingklip LO: 200–600 IU
- Halibut LO: 1 000–2 000 IU
- Cod LO: 100 IU

Vitamin E (tocopherol)

In: green vegetables, especially beans and peas, nearly all vegetable oils; egg-yolk; grain kernels, beef liver, fish.

Function

Essential for the prevention of degenerative changes in tissues. It was formerly thought to be an anti-sterility vitamin.

Vitamin K (the anti-haemorrhagic vitamin)

In: vit. K_1 — Green leaves and tomatoes; vit. K_2 — manufactured by intestinal flora.

Function

Used by the liver for the manufacture of the blood-clotting agent, prothrombin.

Water

The elements forming water are H and O (H_2O).

Sources

Drinks, fruit and vegetables.

Functions

(1) Building material — 60 % of the adult body consists of water;
(2) solvent for the transport of solids in the body;
(3) as perspiration, water regulates the body temperature;
(4) essential for taste, peristalsis, digestion and absorption;
(5) essential for the excretion of waste products.

Dietary fibre

Dietary fibre consists of non-starch polysaccha-rides (cellulose and hemicellulose), lignin (a polymer of a certain alcohol) and certain gums. Fibre is the skeleton of all plant cell walls. It is the indigestible part of vegetable foods (rough-age) which provides little energy to humans but increases the bulk (solid matter and water) of stools. The bulk-forming capacity of fruit and vegetables does not equal that of lightly milled cereal products. It is the fibre in cereals that forms the main regulatory factor in transit times and volume of bowel contents, frequency of defaecation and of the chemical and microbio-logical make-up of faeces.

Fibre has been deliberately removed from food in modern countries as in the polishing of rice in the East, the making of white flour in the West and fine maize (mealie) meal in Africa, to make the carbohydrate (meal, flour or rice) more digestible and palatable. The westernised diet is inclined to be low in fibre.

The traditional diet of blacks, consisting mainly of lightly milled maize, supplemented with sorghum, millet, wheat, dried peas and beans, groundnuts, pumpkin and wild greens, has a high fibre content. This pattern of diet is common to that of most of the world's popula-tion.

With urbanisation in an industrial society, blacks in the RSA may follow this diet in part, but usually switch over to refined (white) bread and maize products; they also increase their meat and sugar intake, i.e. their diet becomes westernised.

The diet of urban westernised nations con-tains much less fibre (about 2 to 10 g/day) although people are becoming more conscious of the beneficial properties of whole-wheat bread. The addition to the diet of high fibre 'health' foods, e.g. bran, is now a common and growing practice to raise the low fibre diet's bulk-forming capacity.

Dietary fibre plays an important role in serum total cholesterol (TC) levels. Fibre in oats, legumes, vegetables and fruit lowers se-rum TC levels, but wheat-bran has a negligble effect.

FOOD LABELLING

The labelling of food in containers is required by regulation. This is necessary to protect the consumer and to enlighten the purchaser.

Information displayed on labels includes:

- The name of the product, the manufacturer and the net contents indicated in weight or volume. In containers with mixed products the list of ingredients is placed in descend-ing order of mass.
- All food additives must be indicated. This is especially important for people with certain allergies of which they are aware.

Sometimes the following are indicated on the labels:

- Enriched, fortified (see p. 441).
- Artificial (synthetic). This means that the food resembles a genuine foodstuff, but is nutritionally inferior, e.g. fruit juices.
- Expiry date may be mentioned on the label in the case of high quality perishable food-stuffs. After the expiry date the foodstuff may still be edible but the quality has dete-riorated.
- Nutrition information may be included, for example: a suggested portion, the energy value of the portion in kilojoules and its protein, carbohydrate and fat content in grams. Vitamins and minerals are indicated as a percentage of the RDA.

Recently (1992) there has been a call for stricter food labelling by NGOs concerned with dis-eases caused by nutrition-related diets: heart disease, stroke, obesity and cancer. They advo-cate enforced labelling of the kilojoule, fat, salt and fibre content of all processed foods. The amount of caffeine and lactose (to which people may be intolerant) as well as the egg and wheat content (associated with allergies) should also appear on the label.

Real milk and milk substitutes

The nurse must be aware that there are milk substitutes on the market. Real milk products bear the label 'Real Dairy'.

The following 'real milk' preparations are available:

- Fresh milk (full-cream, low-fat and fat-free)

- Buttermilk (sour, low-fat)
- Long-life milk (sterilised)
- Milk powders (full-cream and fat-free); (vit. A and D added))
- Evaporated and condensed (sugar-added) milk
- Real milk powder blends consisting of fat-free milk powder and milk solids (whey powder)

Milk substitutes contain non-dairy products (sometimes called 'farm products'). These products are not suitable for infants, children and the elderly. There are two kinds:

(1) Non-dairy creamers made from corn syrup, palm kernel oil and coconut oil. This high energy product has a high saturated fatty acid and low calcium content, and should, therefore, not be used by overweight persons and by those with a high blood cholesterol level.

(2) Blends consisting of a mixture of fat-free milk powder, corn syrup, palm kernel oil and coconut oil. The nutritive values of the various proprietary blends differ.[3]

Note: In November 1987, the Minister of Agricultural Economics and Marketing issued regulations with regard to the labelling of real dairy products and milk substitutes. The details to be printed on packaging include the information given above. Milk-powder blends and milk substitutes must display the warning, 'Not for infant feeding'. The regulations also forbid the use of terms which misrepresent the product to give it special merit, or any statement which is not approved of by the Dairy Board.

The purpose of these new labelling prescriptions is to enlighten the public, thereby enabling people to distinguish between real dairy products and nutritionally inferior milk substitutes.

THE BALANCED DIET

The aim of good nutrition is a balanced diet which must comply with the following requirements.

Kilojoules

It should supply an adequate number of kilojoules to satisfy the energy needs of the body, without causing a loss or gain in the normal weight of the adult.

In the normal diet of the westernised South African, kilojoules are supplied as follows:

Carbohydrates: approximately 40 % to 45 % of the total kilojoules.

Fats: approximately 35 % to 45 % of the total kilojoules.

Proteins: approximately 15 % to 18 % of the total kilojoules.

Note: See the composition of the 'prudent' diet, p. 269.

The requirements for protein are related to growth, pregnancy and lactation, these factors increasing protein requirements, as well as to sex and body size, but not to physical work.

Protective and growth foods

Proteins, mineral salts and vitamins.

See table 1 on p. 264 for the Department of Health Services and Welfare's RDAs for proteins, mineral salts and vitamins.

There is a considerable range of values, the lowest applying to women and the highest to adolescents and pregnant and lactating women. Late adolescent boys require very high protein (for rapid growth) and lactating women very high vit. A allowance (to make up for losses in the milk). Men generally need less iron than women because women lose iron every month in the menstrual blood.

Food constituents (nutrients)

The balanced diet must contain the essential nutritive elements in the correct proportions, so that the individual may develop normally, enjoy health and abundance of vitality and develop a high resistance to disease. Whereas the percentage of kilojoules from fats in the diets of underprivileged people may be no more than 10 to 12, that of privileged people may be more than three times as much, an average of 50 to 100 grams of fat being eaten per day.

Balanced diets are of two main kinds: (1) the mixed omnivorous diet, and (2) the vegetarian diet:

(1) *The mixed omnivorous diet* consists of animal (and animal-derived) and vegetable (plant) foods. Proteins come from both sources. At least one third of the protein should be first class. Fat also comes from

TABLE 1
Recommended daily dietary allowances (RDA) of above (the Department of Health Services and Welfare)

	Unit	Infants 0,0–1,0 years	Children 1–3 years	Persons 4 years & older	Pregnant and lactating women
Energy	kJ	460/kg body mass	5 500	10 000	11 000
Protein	g	2,2/kg body mass	23	56	76
Vitamin A activity:					
(1) Vitamin A (retinol)	IU	2 000	2 000	5 000	6 000 (old measure)
(2) Retinol equivalents	µg	400	400	1 000	1 200 (present measure)
Vitamin D	IU	400	400	400	400
Vitamin E activity	IU	5	7	15	15
Ascorbic acid (vit. C)	mg	35	40	45	80
Biotin	mg	0,15	0,15	0,30	0,30
Folic acid	µg	50	100	400	800
Pantothenic acid	mg	3	5	10	10
Thiamine (vit. B_1)	mg	0,5	0,7	1,5	1,5
Nicotinamide	mg	8	9	20	20
Riboflavin (vit. B_2)	mg	0,6	0,8	1,8	2,0
Vitamin B_6	mg	0,4	0,6	2,0	2,5
Vitamin B_{12}	µg	0,3	1,0	3,0	4,0
Calcium	mg	540	800	800	1 200
Phosphorus	mg	400	800	800	1 200
Iodine	µg	45	60	150	150
Iron	mg	15	15	18	18
Magnesium	mg	70	150	400	450
Copper	mg	0,6	1,0	2,0	2,0
Zinc	mg	5	10	15	25

TABLE 2
The most important sources of protein in the mixed, milk-egg–(lacto-ovo-) vegetarian and the strict vegetarian diets

Foods and their protein content in percentages	Dietary types, amounts, (amts) of food and protein (pr.) in grams (g)					
	mixed		lacto-ovo-vegetarian		strict vegetarian (vegan)	
	amt food	pr.	amt food	pr.	amt food	pr.
Milk 3,5 %	400 ml	14	400 ml	14	—	—
Cheddar cheese 25 %	15 g	3	30 g	7	—	—
Egg 12,8 %	1 egg	7	1 egg	7	—	—
Meat—without bone, lean 19 %	100 g (small portion)	19	—	—	—	—
Whole-wheat bread 7,9 %	80 g (2 slices)	6	120 g (3 slices)	9	160 g (4 slices)	12
Cereal for porridge, etc. 10 %	30 g	3	30 g	3	80 g	8
Potato 2 %	100 g	2	200 g	4	200 g	4
Vegetables 1,5 %	100 g	1	300 g	4	300 g	4
Fruit 0,7 %	100 g	1	200 g	1	300 g	2
Dry legumes 23 %	—	—	30 g	7	70 g	16
Nuts 20 %	—	—	—	—	50 g	10
Total amt protein (pr)		56		56		56

both sources. The mixed diet is generally high in cholesterol and saturated fatty acids, especially in affluent, privileged, Western communities. This westernised diet is considered to be atherogenic, i.e. inclined to cause atherosclerosis, the forerunner of coronary heart disease (CHD). Atherosclerosis is very prevalent amongst adult westernised South Africans (see Chapter 17).

(2) *The prudent diet* (see p. 269). The modern trend is to modify the above diet to reduce its atherogenicity. The so-called 'prudent' diet advocates less fat (i.e. not more than 30 % of total kilojoules), an increased ratio of unsaturated to saturated fatty acids, cholesterol intake of less than 300 mg/day, and high fibre content. Saturated, mono-unsaturated and polyunsaturated fat should each provide 10 % of the total energy intake. To make up for fat reduction, complex carbohydrates are increased to 55 %.

Vegetarian diets purport to be non-atherogenic. There are four kinds:

(1) Strict vegetarian, consisting only of foods of plant origin.
(2) Lactovegetarian, including milk and milk products in the above.
(3) Lacto-ovo-vegetarian, including eggs in the above. This diet does not necessarily fulfil the goals of the 'prudent' diet.
(4) Fruitarian, consisting mainly of fruits, green foliage and nuts, with or without the additions of cereals and dry legumes.

Vegetarianism is no longer considered a food fad as it has many advantages in ensuring a healthy life-style when compared with the atherogenic mixed diet of affluent Western societies.

The staple diet of most inhabitants of this planet is vegetarian, because it is the cheapest means of feeding the hungry masses of meat-starved countries, especially those of the Third World. Vegetarianism is, however, also practised in its various forms in First-World countries, for the following reasons:

(1) *Ethical and religious reasons.* Some people avoid meat because it involves the killing of animals. Some religious meat abstainers will, however, use either a lactovegetarian (e.g. Yogi groups), or a lacto-ovo-vegetarian (e.g. Seventh Day Adventists) diet. Both these diets are easier to balance than the strict vegetarian diet.

(2) *Health reasons.* Vegetarian diets purport to be anti-atherogenic, and to ensure adequate nutrition without promoting atherosclerosis.

Note: Faber *et al.*[2] found that a group of lacto-ovo-vegetarians had a lower intake of Vit. B_{12}, ferritin and zinc compared with a group on a mixed diet, and that their blood lipid levels (see p. 289) were on a par with those of the control group.
Full- cream milk and eggs contribute to the atherogenic blood lipid levels, therefore the strict vegetarian diet ensures a lower blood lipid level.

(3) *Economic reasons.* Some people are vegetarians because they cannot afford the expensive meat and/or other animal proteins.

SOURCES OF PROTEIN IN THE VARIOUS BALANCED DIETS

See table 2 on p. 264.

CHEMICAL COMPOSITION OF VEGETABLES AND FRUIT[7]

See table 3 on p. 266.

It is easier to plan a balanced diet if both plant and animal foods are used, but a strict vegetarian diet can conform to the requirement of a healthy diet, provided a great variety of plant foods (including vegetables, cereals, pulses, nuts and fruit) are used.

SOME FOOD SUPPLEMENTS

Ethanol alcohol

Alcohol is formed when fruit and grains ferment. A moderate amount of alcohol will stimulate the secretion of gastric juice. It has good energy value, and requires no digestion before absorption by the stomach and small intestine. Alcohol is broken down in the liver at a constant rate of 1 unit per hour (*note:* NOT in the muscles).

TABLE 3
Chemical composition of common vegetables and fruit (uncooked)

	Cal/100 g	kJ/100 g	gram/100 g of edible product (g %)				
			Protein	Fat	CHO	Fibre	M. Salts
Green beans	180	756	1,57	0,14	4,45	1,17	0,79
Beetroot	182	764	1,56	tr.	7,78	0,68	1,01
Cabbage	120	504	1,73	0,10	4,70	1,09	0,81
Cucumber	62	260	0,94	0,14	2,15	0,77	0,83
Lettuce	83	349	1,17	tr.	1,80	0,68	1,01
Onion	194	815	0,12	tr.	12,21	0,58	0,38
Green peas	409	1 718	7,24	0,59	13,81	2,43	0,83
Potato	317	1 331	1,82	0,05	17,24	0,53	0,94
Squash	76	319	0,87	0,07	3,18	0,74	0,56
Tomato	91	382	1,00	0,20	3,80	0,62	0,50
Apple	249	1 046	0,40	0,36	12,48	0,83	0,31
Avocado pear	396	1 663	1,17	7,32	3,74	1,32	0,66
Banana	365	1 533	1,51	0,25	18,19	0,61	0,80
Grapes	293	1 230	0,73	0,47	14,33	1,45	0,57
Guava	215	903	1,06	0,64	9,47	6,00	0,58
Pawpaw	123	517	0,39	0,08	6,29	0,71	0,36
Spanspek	84	352	0,50	0,06	4,04	0,55	0,53
Orange	200	840	0,90	0,10	9,90	0,60	—
Watermelon	120	504	0,54	0,11	5,87	0,18	0,30

	Cal/ 100 g	kJ/ 100 g	milligram/100 g of edible product (mg %)			
			Ca	Mg	Fe	Phos.
Green beans	180	756	40	23	1,0	37
Beetroot	182	764	11	16	1,0	42
Cabbage	120	504	39	15	1,0	36
Cucumber	62	260	12	12	tr.	24
Lettuce	83	349	19	9	tr.	37
Onion	194	815	27	16	1,0	37
Green peas	409	1 718	38	34	2,0	94
Potato	317	1 331	13	25	1,0	51
Squash	76	319	11	10	tr.	26
Tomato	91	382	6	11	tr.	19
Apple	249	1 046	7	6	0,5	15
Avocado pear	396	1 663	12	17	0,8	27
Banana	365	1 533	10	22	0,7	18
Grapes	293	1 230	21	9	0,8	19
Guava	215	903	11	13	0,8	27
Pawpaw	123	517	11	8	0,4	90
Spanspek	84	352	12	10	0,3	14
Orange	200	840	26	10	0,1	28
Watermelon	120	504	6	9	0,2	9

The energy value of alcoholic drinks depends upon the strength of the alcohol (degrees of proof spirit) and the sugar content.

Examples:

Tot of brandy (35 ml) . . . . 344 kJ
Glass of sherry (67 ml) . . . . 403 kJ
Glass of dry wine (100 ml) . . . . . . 265 kJ
Pint of beer (600 ml) . . . . 900 kJ

Alcohol units

1 unit alcohol (8g ethanol) =

- 120 ml wine
- 340 ml beer
- 25 ml spirits (brandy, cane spirits, whisky, gin)

An excessive intake of alcohol will cause gastritis and anorexia which are not conducive to the ingestion of the protective foods. As the liver cells are very sensitive to this deficiency and to poisoning by alcohol, they atrophy and are replaced by contracting fibrous tissue. The condition in which the liver is shrunken, hard and fibrotic, is referred to as cirrhosis of the liver.

Alcohol abuse contributes to hypertension.

Caffeine

Caffeine is a commonly used stimulant of the central nervous system, kidneys, myocardium, voluntary muscles. It is found mainly in tea (excluding rooibos), coffee, cocoa (and chocolates) and cola beverages. It has no nutritive value; it stimulates the flow of gastric juices and the excretion of urine. Small amounts promote alertness and wakefulness and increase work performance by muscles. Contrary to popular belief, a cup of black coffee will not sober up a drunk person, but because it promotes wakefulness and diuresis, the alcohol may be metabolised and excreted faster by the lungs and kidneys.

Caffeine is an ingredient of some medicines, e.g. analgesics. It counteracts the soporific (fatigueness) effects of the painkiller.

Some instant coffee powders are decaffeinated and contain a minimal amount of caffeine.

Caffeine should be taken in moderation only, i.e. intake should not exceed 450–500 mg (4–5 cups of coffee) per day.

Caffeine content

Coffee (220 ml) . . . . 92–138 mg
Instant coffee (220 ml) . . . . . . 79–91 mg
Tea (220 ml) . . . . 55–69 mg
Cola beverage (1 can) . . . . 38–57 mg

Infants and children are less able than adults to metabolise and excrete caffeine and should be discouraged from drinking tea, coffee and cola drinks. In the pregnant woman caffeine crosses the placental barrier to enter the circulation of the foetus.

Disadvantages of caffeine

(1) Large doses may have a deleterious effect on an existing gastric ulcer.
(2) In overdosage it causes tachycardia and diuresis.
(3) There may be unpleasant side-effects from caffeine taken medicinally, even in therapeutic doses.

Note: Caffeine is sometimes taken medicinally in large doses by athletes to improve their muscular performance. This is a forbidden practice which can be detected by urinalysis.

(Information about caffeine obtained from the subdirectorate Dietetic Services.)

PLANNING THE MIXED (OMNIVOROUS) BALANCED DIET

The westernised mixed diet consists of foods taken from the following five basic food groups.

Group 1

Body-building proteins, viz. animal (meat, fish, liver, eggs) and vegetable (dried legumes and nuts). The daily requirement includes any two of these proteins.

TABLE 4
Food value of fresh fish (raw)

	Protein (g %)	Oil (g %)	Moisture (g %)
Geelbek	20,11	0,68	76,89
Kabeljou	19,81	1,41	76,92
Kingklip	17,12	0,12	81,70
Snoek	21,91	5,15	70,90
Sole	18,39	0,18	79,78
Stockfish (hake)	16,89	0,79	80,82

TABLE 5
Chemical composition of fish and beef

	g/100 g		µg/ 100 g	IU/g	IU/g	µg/100
	Protein	Fat	Iodine	Vit A	Vit D	Vit B$_{12}$
Pilchards (canned)	20	6	135	20	4,5	4
Beef	18	20	30	0,5	4	4
Stockfish	17	0,8	100	neg.	neg.	1,5
			milligram/100 g			
			Ca	Fe	Thiam.	Ribof.	Niacin
Pilchards (canned)			1	4,0	0,05	0,1	5
Beef			neg.	4,0	0,15	0,04	5
Stockfish			0,06	1,0	0,04	0,04	4

Group 2

Real milk

Milk and milk products, excluding butter and including cheese. This group is body-building and protective and contains, *inter alia*, calcium, phosphorus, vitamins A and D, as well as first-class animal protein.

The nurse must be aware that there are milk substitutes on the market. Real milk products bear the label 'REAL DAIRY' (see p. 262).

Calcium in milk is the cheapest way of providing calcium for the development of bones and teeth and the maintenance of bones and teeth in both children and adults.

Milk requirements daily (as beverage or mixed with food):

Pregnant and lactating women . . . . . 650 ml
Children . . . . 500 ml
Adults . . . . 400 ml

Real milk is such an important food, especially for its calcium content, that its use is mandatory in children and the elderly. Where it is refused on account of its taste, fat-free milk powder can be used, either for preparing flavoured milk drinks or for stirring into solid food. Cheese can take the place of milk as it is a 1:11 concentration of the best nutrients in milk. Cheese is very digestible, 90 % being utilised for growth and repair of tissues as well as for energy. One hundred grams of cheese contains as much first-

class protein as one of the following high protein foods:

- 150 grams of raw lean beef without bones;
- 150 grams of raw fish;
- 8 eggs.

Group 3

Group 3A

Fruit and vegetables with high vitamin C content, viz. guavas, citrus fruits, pawpaws, mangoes, berries, tomatoes and cabbage. These foods must be fresh and raw if possible, as vitamin C is destroyed by exposure to air (quick oxidation during open cooking), light and heat. Wilting of vegetables causes loss of nutrients. The daily requirement is one portion (see page 261 for vitamin C content).

Group 3B

Green and dark yellow vegetables and yellow fruit, the source of carotene (provitamin A). The daily essential requirement is one portion, consisting of a cupful for children. Two portions daily are preferable.

The beta-carotene content of the more important sources of the provitamin A (measured in mg/100 g) is as follows:

banana 0,3
peas 0,3
carrot 7,6
tomato 0,5
maize (yellow) 0,3
pumpkin (red) 0,7
mango 0,14
sweet potato 2,0
orange 0,15
watermelon 0,05

Carrots contain 1 875–5 200 IU of beta-carotene and yellow maize 100 to 600 IU per 100 g.

Group 3C

All other vegetables and fruit, from which are obtained mineral salts, vitamins and fibre. The daily requirement is two to three portions of either potato, squash, beetroot, onion, cauliflower, green mealie, cucumber, green beans, bananas, grapes, apples, white peaches, watermelon or pears.

Group 4

Animal and vegetable fats, including butter, margarine, bacon, dripping and plant oils. In order of value, the plant oils rank downwards as follows: sunflower-seed, maize, soy bean, peanut and olive. The cooking-oils are usually a mixture of sunflower-seed, peanut and maize oils. Peanut butter contains 50 % oil of which 30 % is polyunsaturated. The daily requirement of butter or margarine is ½ to 1 level tablespoon. In addition, plant oils can be used in salads and for cooking. Fats are reduced in slimming diets.

Group 5

Cereals, including cakes and bread, with emphasis on whole grain foods. These fuel foods form the bulk of the diet. The daily requirements are one or more portions of enriched or brown bread or whole grain bread and other cereals, to meet the energy requirements of the body.

TABLE 6
Chemical composition of South African bread and cakes

	kJ/ 100 g	Protein g/ 100 g	Fat g/ 100 g	CHO g/ 100 g	Fibre g/ 100 g	Ca mg/ 100 g	Fe mg/ 100 g
Brown bread	950	7,85	0,41	50,93	0,71	34	1,85
White bread	963	7,40	0,70	53,57	0,14	24	1,19
Whole-meal bread	945	8,26	0,99	48,30	1,35	39	1,93
Fruit cake	1 480	5,92	14,83	55,02	0,35	39	1,86
Biscuits	1 880	6,88	21,70	63,27	0,52	43	2,10

Note: Ration scales (total amount of food recommended for a day), menus and recipes for a low-cost diet can be obtained upon request from Subdirectorate Dietetic Services.

THE PRUDENT DIET

The prudent diet is a balanced, omnivorous diet consisting of foods from the five basic food groups with special emphasis on the inclusion of fibre: fibre from whole grain products to combat constipation and fibre from vegetables, fruits and legumes to lower blood cholesterol levels. The special value of the prudent diet is to lower the alarming high blood cholesterol values of westernised populations.

The prudent diet contains lots of fibre, little fat and maintains a normal body mass.

The visible fats (oil, butter, fat meat) and the invisible fats in milk, ice-cream, cheese and nuts must be curtailed.

Polyunsaturated (sunflower and corn oil, soya beans and fat fish) and mono-unsaturated fatty acids (olives, avocado pears and peanut butter) have a beneficial effect on blood cholesterol levels.

Practical hints in compiling the prudent diet:

(1) Five portions of fruit and vegetables daily.

(2) Whole-wheat bread, oats, porridge and fibre-rich breakfast cereals.

(3) Use small portions of lean meat and remove all visible fat.

(4) Have dry legume dishes, fish and chicken at least twice a week and remove the skin from chicken.

(5) Use low-fat dairy products.

(6) Avoid cream (real or imitation), non-dairy creamers, milk blends and chocolates.

From: The Subdirectorate: Nutrition Services. Department of Health Services and Welfare, No. 19.

PLANNING A STRICT VEGETARIAN BALANCED DIET

Strict vegetarians (vegans) can enjoy a balanced diet, but this needs very careful planning to ensure that it includes the correct amount and variety of amino acids from vegetable sources.

The Department of Health Services and Welfare (Nutrition Services) gives the following good combinations of dry legumes, nuts, seeds and cereal products, one combination to be included in each meal:

- Rice and dry legumes such as dry beans, dry peas and lentils
- Rice and sesame seeds
- Rice, wheat and soya beans
- Rice, wheat and peanuts
- Wheat and dry legumes
- Wheat, sesame seeds and soya beans
- Maize and dry legumes
- Sesame seeds and dry beans
- Sesame seeds and peanuts

The strict vegetarian diet consists of foods taken from the following five food groups:[1]

Group 1: Cereals and cereal products

This group includes all dry grains and their products such as bread, porridge, pasta, breakfast cereals, samp, etc. Unrefined cereals are preferable to ensure adequate mineral and vitamin intake.

Nutrients present: complex carbohydrates, proteins, vitamins, minerals and fibre.

Group 2: Legumes

The dried seeds (pulses) of leguminous plants, e.g. peas, beans, lentils and their protein-rich products (e.g. Toppers, SOMOS).

Nutrients present: protein, iron and other trace elements, e.g. zinc, B vitamins, fibre, carbohydrate.

Protein value of South African dried pulses (seeds of legumes), measured in grams per 100 grams:

Field beans: 24,9
Soy beans: 43,2
Lentils: 25,1
Black-eyed peas: 24,6
Cowpea (dehusked): 24,6

Note: Soy beans are closer to animal protein in nutritional value than any other dried pulses.

Group 3: Vegetables and fruit

Dark green leafy vegetables must be eaten daily for calcium and riboflavin, and yellow vegetables (and fruit) for carotene (vit. A precursor). Dried fruit is a good source of energy, minerals and vitamins.

Nutrients present: vitamins, minerals, fibre, carbohydrate.

Group 4: Fatty foods

Nuts and nut-like seeds (sunflower, sesame), olives, avocado, coconut. Peanuts are a source of zinc.

Nutrients present: the essential fatty acid (linoleic acid), protein, energy, saturated and unsaturated fatty acids.

Note: Their use must be restricted to 2 portions per day as they could be fattening.

Group 5: Other foods and supplements

Sugar, oils and vegetable spreads. As they are concentrated 'empty' sources of energy, they must be used sparingly.

Vegetarian recipes are obtainable free of charge from:

PDG-Boards*
Private Bag X135
PRETORIA
0001

*PDG = Potato, Dry beans, Grain sorghum

Note:

- For lacto-vegetarians and lacto-ovo-vegetarians a separate milk and egg group should be included.
- Iodine deficiency is prevented by the use of iodised salt.
- As vit. B_{12} (cyanocobalamin) does not occur in the vegetarian diet, vegans must use either vit. B_{12} enriched soya milk, or meat substitutes (e.g. Toppers), or use medically prescribed supplements.
- Vegans may have to consume a larger quantity of food (only from Groups 1, 2 and 3) than persons on a mixed diet, in order to meet all the nutritional requirements of the body.
- Exposure to sunlight must be adequate for vit. D manufacture.

The following vegetarian diet plan of ± 8 400 kJ for an adult woman is recommended by the Subdirectorate: Nutrition, Department of Health Services and Welfare:

Breakfast

125 ml stewed dried fruit
125 ml maize meal porridge
30 g molasses
50 ml soya milk
35 g whole-wheat bread (1 slice)
5 ml margarine (1 teaspoon)
20 g peanut butter (4 teaspoons)
200 ml soya milk

Snack

1 orange

Lunch

250 ml soya bean stew
125 ml brown rice

125 ml spinach
125 ml carrot, pineapple and orange salad
125 ml canned guavas

Supper

125 ml cabbage salad with
30 g almonds and
15 g sunflower seeds
70 g whole-wheat bread (2 slices)
10 g margarine (2 teaspoons) and
10 g sesame seeds (on the bread)
1 banana
250 ml soya milk
8 g dry yeast (1 dessertspoon)

Taken from: *Facts about Vegetarianism* No. 8

The advantages of a vegetarian diet

Strict vegetarian diet

- It is relatively cheap. It is much more expensive to produce animal protein than vegetable protein and the poor Third-World countries will have to rely almost wholly on plant foods.
- Obesity is not a problem as plant foods (except nuts and avocado pears) have a low energy value.
- Vegans have comparatively low blood lipids and are less likely to suffer from the atherogenic diseases: coronary artery disease and cerebrovascular disease. It is the ideal diet for patients with atherosclerosis.
- The high fibre content prevents constipation and its sequelae, chronic diseases of the colon, e.g. diverticulitis.
- It contains sufficient water-soluble vitamins (except B_{12}).

Lacto-vegetarian diet

- If milk is used in moderation, especially if the milk and milk products are fat-free, advantages are as for the strict vegetarian diet.
- It fully supports growth in children.

Lacto-ovo-vegetarian diet

- If eggs are used in moderation (one per day), the advantages are as for the lacto-vegetarian dict.

Fruitarian diet

- If combined with cereals and dry legumes, advantages are as for the strict vegetarian diet.

Disadvantages of a vegetarian diet

Strict vegetarian diet

- Deficiencies of minerals such as calcium, iron, zinc and iodine, as well as vitamins B_{12} and D can occur in a poorly planned vegetarian diet.
- A strict vegetarian diet is not recommended for children, as proteins, calcium and zinc are insufficient for growth purposes. Mental development is normal, however.[2]

    As the vegetarian diet is bulky, children may be incapable of eating enough food to meet their energy needs. Children also find it difficult to digest dry legumes and a large amount of dried fruit.

Lacto-vegetarian diet

- Some of the disadvantages of the mixed diet (high blood lipids, obesity) will be present if too much full-cream milk and milk products are consumed.

Lacto-ovo-vegetarian diet

- Same as for lacto-vegetarian. Eggs used in excess add to the dangers of high blood cholesterol.

Fruitarian diet

- It may be too high in fat content if an excess of nuts, olives and avocado pears is eaten.
- If not combined with cereals and dry legumes, the fruit and nut diet is nutritionally deficient.

SIMPLE COOKING METHODS AND THEIR EFFECTS ON FOOD

A further aim of good nutrition is the preparation of the balanced diet in such a way that —

(1) the essential nutrients are preserved;
(2) the limitations of body functions are met in health and ill-health.

Meat may be cooked by dry heat (grilling, roasting), water (boiling, stewing or pressure cook ing), or fat (frying). In cooking, the elastin shrinks, the collagen fibres are converted to gelatin, the meat becomes tender, firm and shrunken, and juices are extruded. In moderate cooking, little change takes place in the fat and protein content of the meat, but in prolonged cooking — for instance of stews — the proteins may become denatured, i.e. lose their nutritive value.

The meat fat retains its vitamin A content, but the vitamin B, being water-soluble and sensitive to heat, is reduced according to the amount of cooking.

Overheating fats and oils to smoking temperature causes them to deteriorate rapidly; this and repeated heating cause fats and oils to become rancid, thereby causing vitamin E to be destroyed. If rancid oil is eaten, it destroys the vitamin E of other foods.

Soups have very little nutritional value except if they have been fortified by the addition of starch, protein powders or fat.

In cooking eggs, the coagulated white is rendered more digestible. Hard-boiled eggs are slightly less digestible than those lightly boiled. In cooking eggs, there is some loss of vitamin B.

The cooking of cereals is essential for proper digestion and absorption of starch.

Vegetables can be cooked in the same way as meat (except grilling). Cooking renders the starch more digestible and causes some loss of minerals and vitamins B and C, the greater the volume of water in which vegetables are boiled, the greater the loss.

Large amounts of vitamin C are lost: in cooking green vegetables; in keeping cooked vegetables hot for some time before serving; during the exposure of orange juice to the air. The canning of vegetables destroys a considerable portion of their ascorbic acid content. Tomatoes contain approximately 25 mg/100 g ascorbic acid; 45 % of this vitamin is lost in the canning process; green peas lose 66 % of their ascorbic acid during canning. The cutting up of raw vegetables so that their cut surfaces are exposed to the oxygen in the air also destroys their vit. C content. Approximately 80 % ascorbic acid is destroyed when lettuce is shredded and allowed to stand for 3 minutes.

Vegetables cooked in a pressure cooker, waterless cooker and in a saucepan with cup of water retain more nutrients (Ca, Fe, P, carotene, vit. C, vit. B complex) than if cooked in a saucepan with enough water to cover them.

Boiling vegetables leaches some of their minerals, but if they are cooked in hard water, calcium is added. Cooking also increases the availability of iron in the food. If the mineral-laden cooking water is used for soups and gravies, the minerals are fully utilised.

Vitamins can be preserved by the following practices:

(1) Orange juice should be used for its vitamin C content only when fresh. A corked bottle of juice can, however, be kept under refrigeration for some time without any ill effects.

(2) Vegetables should be prepared immediately before cooking, lest the water-soluble vitamins and minerals are leached in water in which they are kept.

(3) Green vegetables are placed in strongly boiling water (and cooked until just done) in order to destroy the plant enzymes which destroy vitamin C. Vegetables are boiled quickly in a closed container and no soda is added to keep green vegetables green. As little water as possible is used. A pressure cooker and a waterless cooker take second place to the ordinary saucepan, provided the above rules are observed. Cooking in a lot of water results in the greatest loss of vit. C.

(4) Food should not be left standing in the oven and should be served as soon as it is cooked.

Most protein foods are cooked to improve their tenderness and flavour. Moderate cooking improves digestibility but over-cooking at high temperatures cause changes which results in indigestibility.

Such indigestible compounds are found in toast and in the brown crust of baked and fried products that have been toasted, fried, grilled or roasted for too long or at too high temperatures. The proteins of nuts roasted to a dark brown colour become denatured.

The modern trend in hospitals is the preparation of 'convenience foods' to beat the shortage of skilled labour. In the 'convenience system', meals are fully prepared at a convenient time, then frozen and stored and finally heated when required for consumption.

A start has been made at several South African hospitals where the meals are served in this fashion. Meals are either cooked in microwave ovens in their own juices, or they are prepared in the conventional way. Microwave cooked food does not undergo the colour changes of normally cooked food, but special food-browning ovens can be used to make the colour of the food more appetising. The food must be frozen within an hour of preparation.

Flash freezing is done by feeding prepared foods packed in individual portions into a food freezing tunnel in which they are frozen instantaneously by intensely cold liquid nitrogen. The freezing does not affect the taste or nutritional value of the food. The process takes only minutes; the food is then stored indefinitely in cold storage. Reheating of the meal is done in a microwave oven which can reconstitute a frozen meal in 40 seconds.

Freezing and storage of food eliminate peak periods of kitchen activity and allow a wide variety of meals, packed in individual portions, to be kept on hand, thereby preventing food wastage. An à la carte food service for patients is envisaged for the future.

Solar cooking

This means cooking which makes use of the heat of the sun. It is an ideal way of cooking for fuel-starved South Africans who often spend hours of each day gathering firewood. The only expense with this method is the investment in a cooker box and painting the cooking pots black where aluminium pots are used. The usual articles of diet can be solar cooked: maize meal, vegetables, meat, pasta and even cakes and cookies. Even water and the baby's bottle can be pasteurised as the contents of the cooker box can be heated to 95 and even 135 °C, depending upon the heat of the sun. Several pots of food are cooked in 2–4 hours and there is never any danger of the food being overcooked.

A solar cooker box is an insulated box within a box big enough to capture $\frac{1}{3}$ square metre of sunshine. Reflectors inside the box direct the sunlight through a snug-fitting lid on to the cooking pots.

These solar cooking boxes are *inter alia* distributed by the Girl Guides Association of South Africa.

New users of the box must be taught the technique of using the box.

THE PROCESSING AND PRESERVATION OF FOOD

Food shortages can be overcome either by curbing population growth, increasing food production or by processing and preserving food for use in times of crop failure and for distribution to areas where food production is inadequate for local needs. In Africa, half the food produced is either destroyed by rodents and insects, or is spoiled because of storage problems.

Methods of food preservation which facilitate the stockpiling of food for use during lean agricultural periods and distribution to poorly fed communities are:

(1) Canning of fruit, fruit juices, vegetables, meat, condensed milks and soups, fish. The length of time tinned foods can be kept (the so-called 'shelf life' of the can) will depend on the temperature and humidity of the environment, the kind of food and whether or not the tin is damaged. If tins are kept in a cool, dry place, their shelf life will be as follows:
Fish (in tomato sauce) and milk: 1 year
Fruit and fruit juices: 1 to 2 years
Soup, fish (in oil), meat, vegetables:2 years

Note: Any tin that becomes 'blown', i.e. bulges due to the pressure of gas usually produced by bacterial activity, should be discarded.

(2) Dehydration of fruit, vegetables, milk, soups, meat and fish by spray-drying, air-drying, freeze-drying and roller-drying.
(3) Pasteurisation and sterilisation of liquid milk. Sterilisation by microwaves of food in glass jars and flexible pouches.
(4) Freezing of meat, fish and vegetables. Refrigerated transport containers and cold storage facilities have made it possible to transport perishables from one area or country to another, e.g. fish and meat. Fresh fruit can also be exported and imported.
(5) Irradiation with cobalt[60] gamma rays of:
    (*a*) subtropical fruits and potatoes; ripening of fruit is delayed and microbes and

insects are destroyed; the gamma rays can penetrate packaged products;

(b) Chickens; after irradiation, unfrozen chickens can be kept on a shelf for three weeks, as opposed to four days for untreated chickens.

Note: A start has been made in South Africa with food irradiation. In a regulation (of March, 1983) of the Foodstuffs, Cosmetics and Disinfectants Act 54 of 1972, it was proposed that no foodstuff which has been irradiated shall be sold unless the minister or director-general has in writing approved the sale of such irradiated foodstuff.

HEALTH EDUCATION IN NUTRITION

Health education is aimed at the total health needs of a community and one of its major concerns is nutrition. South Africa is a country of contrasts — on the one hand there is poverty and diseases of deficiency and on the other hand there is affluence, often accompanied by dietary excesses. Both nutritional deficiency and nutritional excess are forms of malnutrition; they stem not only from the economic status of the victim but also from ignorance, apathy and cultural factors such as customs, food taboos and preferences.

Poor nutrition may have a number of causes amongst which poverty and ignorance rank first in importance. For example: urban black babies are sometimes reared on a diet of mealie meal gruel mixed with water if their mothers are forced by economic necessity to go to work before they are weaned off milk. Ignorance and poverty are the causes of the protein deficiency disease — kwashiorkor — which may result from this practice. Although malnutrition is not confined to the lower socio-economic classes, the poor man's diet is likely to contain a preponderance of the cheaper carbohydrate foods. The expensive animal protein foods, vegetables and fruit may be beyond the means of the lower income groups. Food fads amongst the higher income groups may, however, also give rise to poor nutrition. Vegetarians generally derive their proteins from vegetable sources and unless they make a thorough study of food values and ensure that they consume a variety of second-class proteins, as well as milk and cheese, they may suffer from protein deficiency. Some faddy children grow up without acquiring the taste for

fruit and vegetables and may suffer from vitamin deficiencies in the midst of plenty.

Nutritional excess may be another cause of malnutrition. Obesity is a disease of affluent populations. Overprotective parents may overfeed their children and children who feel emotionally deprived may overindulge themselves with sweet foods in an effort to obtain some gratification. In this way habits of overeating, especially with non-essential foods, can be established in societies which have the technical skills to produce an abundance of food and which emphasise the importance of rich food and drink on festive and social occasions.

Self-medication with vitamin A (fish liver oils) may lead to vitamin A poisoning as 10–20 times the recommended daily intake may be consumed (see p. 264).

NUTRITION CULTISM (FOOD FADS)

Many affluent people subscribe to the so-called 'health foods' and make a cult of following diets or taking naturopathic medicines which have no nutritional advantages and may, in fact, harm the body if adopted long enough.

Certain 'health foods' are sold as food supplements in health food stores, e.g. vitamin B_{17}, also known as Laetrile and Bee-17. Vit. B_{17} is not a vitamin at all; these preparations are the trade names for a substance derived from berries, seeds and fruit kernels. It contains cyanide (group 1 hazardous substance) and is purported to prevent or cure cancer. Its sale was recently banned in the RSA. Nutrition cultists get around the ban by eating foodstuffs purported to be rich in 'vitamin B_{17}'. Health food stores even sell a recipe book called 'The little cyanide cookbook'.

Other substances sold as food supplements are vitamin B_{15} and Green-Lipped Mussel Extract (Seatone). There is no nutritional value in vitamin B_{15}. The purveyors of this substance get around the problem of false advertising by calling the substance pangamic acid (Pangam) and inserting a notice on the container: 'The B group vitamins are water soluble and must be replaced daily'; moreover, they stock overseas books on nutrition in which pangamic acid and vitamin B_{15} are equated. In this way the undiscriminating buyer is duped into believing that he is buying a valuable food substance.

Reliance must be placed on health education of the public to make them aware of propagated fallacies of 'miracle cures' so often insinuated by the purveyors of so-called 'health foods', or 'food supplements'.

Health food faddists who run health hydros sometimes make amazing nutritional claims e.g. that certain foods 'pollute' the system, that fresh fruit and raw vegetables are the only nontoxic foods, that certain diets get rid of 'toxins' in the body, and many more. Lack of knowledge of nutrition and the requirements of a well-balanced diet cause gullibility and food faddism. The basic rules of good nutrition are: moderation and variety, with an adequate amount of fibre.

Vitamins

Many people in our medicine-oriented society have become addicted to vitamin and mineral supplements. The nurse must be aware that healthy people who are eating a well-balanced diet do not need food supplements, in fact, extra vitamins can be dangerous, causing:

(1) Vitamin A overdosage (hypervitaminosis A). This is characterised by poor appetite, headaches, irritability, dry, itchy skin, swollen legs and liver damage. The patient may also develop alopecia. There is a danger of vitamin A toxicity in babies and people with skin problems (acne) after long-continued treatment with the vitamin. In pregnant women vitamin A poisoning may adversely affect the foetus. Beta-carotine, the precursor of vit. A, does not lead to vit. A toxicity.

(2) Vitamin D overdosage. This vitamin stimulates the absorption of calcium, causing hypercalcaemia and storage of calcium in the heart, lungs, kidneys and other soft tissues. Toxic effects include: muscle weakness, headaches, nausea and vomiting, bone pain, hypertension.

(3) Excessive doses of vitamin C may cause diarrhoea. Excessive secretion of the vitamin by the kidneys causes the urine to become so acid that salts precipitate to form oxalate kidney stones. Excessive intake may interfere with the action of Warfarin and aspirin. Extra vitamin C intake will not prevent periodontal disease with bleeding gums.

A commonly held belief that vitamin C prevents or cures the common cold has never been proved in scientific studies. One portion of fresh vegetables or fruit daily in the well-balanced diet will supply the required amount of vitamin C for normal dietary needs.[8]

Specially grown foods

A commonly used food-related term which may impress members of the public is 'organically grown food'. This term is meant to imply that these foods have superior nutritive value as they are grown in humus-rich soils which have not been contaminated with pesticides and artificial fertilisers.

The US Federal Trade Commission (quoted by Venter[9]) which investigated 'natural', 'health' and 'organic' food claims, came to the conclusion that 'organically grown' foods are not nutritionally superior and that there is no danger of harmful substances accumulating in the foodstuffs due to the regular use of pesticides[9], and that 'natural' foods (minimally processed) are superior on nutritional and/or safety grounds.

'Slimming diets'

The need or perceived need for slimming has given rise to a multitude of fad diets purported to induce weight loss. The common characteristics of fad diets is their imbalance with regard to carbohydrates, proteins and fats to reduce the energy value of the diet. Unfortunately the quick loss of weight which is their main attraction cannot be maintained as the dietary restrictions impose too great a sacrifice on basic food needs.

These diets fail to alter lifetime eating habits and backsliding with weight gain occurs.

The Drinking Man's Diet (high protein and fat), The Complete Scarsdale Medical Diet, 'Calories Don't Count' are examples of low CHO diets. Rapid weight loss on the low carbohydrate diet is accompanied by loss of water and sodium as the kidneys are stimulated by the protein ash to increased excretion. The imbalance (lack of CHO) causes ketosis and uricaemia, and results in fatigue and dehydration. These diets are dangerous in patients with metabolic diseases and in pregnant women.

Very low kilojoule diets (less than 2 500 kJ) cause a rapid loss in weight. They contain high quality protein and mineral supplements, (e.g. the Cambridge diet powder). This type of diet eventually decreases the metabolic rate, making it difficult for the patient to maintain the weight-loss.

The student is referred to the *Manual of Nursing*, Volume I (Vlok) for the principles of the healthy reducing diet.

Apart from its nutritional unsuitability, food may harm people through introducing harmful substances into the body. pathogenic microganisms are ingested in unhygienically handled foods, e.g. cholera, enteric fever and food poisoning. Poor soil conditions in Transkei cause the production of nitrosamines in green plants with deficiency diseases. Nitrosamines have recently been implicated (but not proved) as an aetiological factor in carcinoma of the oesophagus which is extremely prevalent in Transkei. Aflatoxin, a mycotoxin found in mouldy grain, is the product of a fungus which flourishes in the damp conditions of underground grain storage pits favoured by Africans. Aflatoxin is also a carcinogenic agent which is suspected of being the cause of the high incidence of primary liver cancer in the black person whose liver has been damaged by virus infection and malnutrition. See pp. 284 and 800 for the link between cancer and diet.

KNOWLEDGE ESSENTIAL FOR THE NUTRITION HEALTH EDUCATOR

The health educational aids which the health educator uses will depend upon the level of literacy of the people. The health educator must be knowledgeable about the following matters.

(1) The nutritional habits and food preferences of the people and the foods that are locally available:
   (a) at the stores;
   (b) in the home gardens and in the home storage places;
   (c) the special foods (wild fruits, wild spinaches and insects) which are indigenous to the area and are traditionally used to supplement the diet.

(2) The influence of the values and beliefs of the people on diet.

(3) Life-style and its role in diet-related diseases.

(4) Observation as to whether the diet is sufficient to ensure:
   (a) adequate growth of the young (as indicated on the paediatric growth chart);
   (b) high resistance to infection (e.g. tuberculosis);
   (c) the absence of nutritional disease, especially deficiency diseases;
   (d) strong and vigorous children and workers;
   (e) healthy teeth.

(5) The principles of good nutrition and the composition and nutritional value of the common basic foods.

(6) The effects of cooking on the nutritional value of foods; methods of cooking which are least destructive to the nutrients; methods of food preservation.

(7) The balanced diet and diet planning with available foods. In planning a suitable diet for a community, many factors must be taken into consideration to make the diet a practical possibility and acceptable to the people to be helped. The following questions must be considered:
   (a) Can the people afford expensive processed foods, e.g. condensed milk and cheese or expensive natural foods such as eggs and meat?
   (b) Will the people accept the food, i.e. will it be palatable to them?
   (c) Is the food available in the community (shops, home gardens and stores), e.g. fresh milk, fresh fish?
   (d) Is the item of food recommended likely to be a taboo food, e.g. fish and eggs among certain black ethnic groups?

(8) Nutritional diseases, their stigmata, causes, prevention and cure.

(9) Food fortification and supplementation.

(10) Methods of raising the nutritional standards by encouraging self-help with regard to food production.

(11) The signs and causes of soil infertility and erosion; principles of soil and water conservation.

Nutritional habits of people

The two main influences on peoples' nutritional habits are: (1) food preferences, and (2) food availability.

Food preferences

The different cultural groups in South Africa have definite food preferences; if these preferences ensure the ingestion of a well-balanced diet, there is no reason why they should be dropped for the sake of conformity with some idealised version of a well-balanced diet. Each cultural group has its own distinctive ways of preparing food. The Afrikaners are famous for bobotie and koeksisters, the Indians favour curry and highly spiced foods, and the Jews have many distinctive dishes which originated in Europe. The drying of bread and meat to preserve them for long journeys led to the development of boerbeskuit and biltong. Some cultural groups like vegetables prepared with sugar and butter while others like plenty of vegetable oil and pasta. All cultural groups eat bread, although different grains may be favoured, e.g. rye bread by the Jews. Blacks will take bread as a substitute for mealie meal porridge and the majority will consume both white and brown bread.

South Africans are not very partial to fish, although modern quick-freezing methods have made plenty of fish available to all. Rural blacks do not care for fish very much (except those who live near large rivers and lakes), but the urbanised Africans are beginning to eat it, especially 'fish and chips' and canned fish. Some traditional blacks have taboos against fish, thus the Zulu and the Swazi consider the fish a reptile and the Pedi forbid its consumption. Indians like dried fish (Bombay duck).

Soups are generally favoured by white South Africans, but not by the blacks; this is the reason why fortified soups used for black feeding schemes are not very acceptable. The energy value of soups may vary from high to low and depends upon the ingredients. The addition of beans, peas and beef to soups makes them very nutritious because of the high protein, fat and carbohydrate content of these foods. Soups also contain mineral salts, carotene, vitamin A and vitamin B complex.

Sorghum beer, made from sprouting mealies and sorghum, has a low alcoholic content (below 4 %), but *amahewu* (*amarewu, maheu* or *mogou*) — fermented maize gruel — is a non-alcoholic beverage which is adored by blacks. *Mogou* is made either from finely ground mealies or from mealie meal cooked before fermentation, the latter being hastened by the addition of flour or sorghum. Soy beans may also be used as an ingredient. Blacks generally prefer sour milk to sweet milk.

Black migrant labourers working in the gold mines in South Africa are provided with pre-cooked meals, the quantity and quality of the foodstuffs being prescribed by law to ensure the adequacy of the food rations. According to A M Coetzee *et al.*[10] the diet provides roughly the following per man per day:

Mealie meal and maize products . . . . 596 g
Meat and fish . . . . 223 g
Vegetables (cauliflower, spinach, carrot, cabbage, leek, beetroot, pumpkin, turnip and parsnip) . . . . 170 g
Bread . . . . 170 g
Beans . . . . 56 g
Dripping . . . . 8 g
Sugar . . . . 40 g
Milk is not normally provided.

These labourers represent a large number of black ethnic groups from South African and neighbouring territories. Research is constantly being conducted to ensure that the mine worker receives optimal nutrition so that he has sufficient stamina for his arduous task and so that his eyes can adapt to the dark conditions underground. It would seem, therefore, that the foods listed and their proportions (e.g. preponderance of maize products), reflect the cultural preferences of unsophisticated black populations.

Preference for refined cereals may cause vitamin B complex deficiencies even amongst the wealthy classes. With the removal of the grain husks the vitamin content of the grain product is much reduced and if grain foods form the bulk of the diet, the population concerned may be in indifferent health. Many blacks who live on a restricted diet favour the smooth porridge made of refined maize flour and may even prefer white bread to whole-meal bread. The palatability and easy procurability of refined carbohydrate foods at the local stores are apt to remove the incentive for producing home-grown vegetables, fruit and grains.

Some of the dietary preferences of our cultural groups, e.g. caterpillars and wild spinaches, are compatible with a good standard of health and should, therefore, be encouraged. Other preferences, again, cause the diet to be poorly balanced, e.g. too much carbohydrate (causing obesity) and too little protective foods (lowering resistance to infection). In this case

the dietary preferences, whether idiosyncratic or culturally determined, should be discouraged by health education. Where dietary deficiencies result from poor soil husbandry and poor methods of food storage, a programme of practical education is required.

Food availability

The availability of food plays an important role in diet planning. There are always seasonal variations in fruits and vegetables. In the former black homelands milk is not readily available due to overstocking of pastures and poor condition of the cattle. In arid areas vegetables are

TABLE 7
Chemical composition of maize and maize products (Wehmeyer *et al.* 1957)[7]

| | grams/100 grams | | | milligrams/100 grams | | | | |
	Protein	Fat	CHO	Ca	Fe	Thiam.	Ribof.	Niacin
Whole maize								
Yellow dent	10,1	4,3	71,1	5,5	2,6	0,51	0,11	1,39
White dent	9,4	4,0	72,5	4,4	2,0	0,42	0,09	1,42
Maize products								
Unsifted granulated meal	9,1	3,7	73,1	5,3	2,6	0,34	0,09	1,33
Sifted granulated meal	8,4	3,0	75,6	3,3	2,2	0,32	0,09	1,17
Maize rice	8,4	0,7	78,9	1,9	1,1	0,19	0,03	1,07
Stamped maize (samp)	8,5	0,6	78,9	1,4	0,4	0,17	0,04	0,60
Maize flour	6,6	2,3	79,1	2,6	1,6	0,19	0,05	0,80

TABLE 8
Chemical composition of edible insects and special flesh foods[7]

| | grams/100 grams | | | milligrams/100 grams | | | | |
	Protein	Fat	CHO	Ca	Phos.	Fe	Thiam.	Ribof.	Niacin
Red ants with eggs	13	5	9	104	107	—	—	—	—
Caterpillars, dried	55	13,8	7	270	—	20	0,35	2,0	11,2
Locusts, mature, fresh	20	6	—	30	—	1	—	0,5	2,2
Locusts, fried	30,5	10,7	—	149	760	5,2	—	—	—
Termites, mature, fresh	10	12	—	12	—	1,0	—	—	—
Bombay duck (dried fish)	61,7	4,0	2,5	1 389	240	19,1	—	—	—
Goat meat	21,4	3,6	—	12	193	—	—	—	—
Rat (field) meat	23,6	1,0	—	30	242	—	—	—	—
Shrimp, dried	68,1	8,5	—	4 384	1 160	—	—	—	—
Venison	21,0	0,6	1,9	3	233	—	—	—	—

scarce as they cannot be grown without an adequate and reliable supply of water. Natal Indians have access to fish which they preserve by drying. In the Transvaal black rural areas, where meat is usually scarce, some insects and caterpillars are a source of protein and fat. Roasted locusts, roasted or dehydrated flying ants, dried 'mopani' worms (dehydrated caterpillars) are traditional delicacies and rats and field mice are also eaten.

Meat, when available, is a great favourite amongst Africans and comes second only to mealie meal porridge. Grilled meat is usually consumed underdone but meat stews are often cooked for such long periods that the proteins become denatured and the vitamins are de-

stroyed. Pulses are used as a substitute for meat and, although they are excellent as a source of protein, they cannot wholly replace meat (for protein value of pulses, see page 272). Nuts and seeds also have a high protein content and are used as a meat substitute by Africans and Indians who cannot afford meat.

A tour around South Africa through the developing black areas will give some idea of what people are eating.

In the northern Transvaal, among the Tswana-Sotho ethnic group, mealie meal is the most important article of diet because it fills and because it can be used for such a large variety of dishes. According to H C Franz,[11] maize was adopted as the staple cereal food only since the

TABLE 9

	grams/100 grams			IU	milligrams/100 grams							
	Pro-tein	Fat	CHO	Vit. A	Ca	Fe	Phos.	Thiam.	Ribo.	Niac.	Vit. C
Cashew nut	21,2	46,9	22,3	100	50	5,0	450	0,63	0,19	2,1	0
Gingelly seeds	25,3	24,5	33,0	100	1 450	10,5	570	1,01	0,06	4,4	0
Oyster nut	29,7	63,3	—	—	10	4,1	570	—	—	—	—
Pigweed seeds	16,3	2,1	60,1	0	490	11,3	470	0,14	0,34	0,5	1
Pistachio nut	19,8	53,5	16,2	240	140	13,7	430	0,67	0,03	5,0	0
Pumpkin seed kernels	24,3	47,2	15,6	76	50	5,5	830	0,33	0,16	3,1	1
Sunflower seeds	19,8	52,1	17,9	0	280	5,0	670	0,86	0,03	5	1
Kaffir melon seed meal	22,1	31,5	10,7	—	180	18	480	—	—	—	—
Macadamia nut	7,8	71,6	13,4	0	48	2,0	161	0,34	0,11	1,3	0
Marula kernel	23,9	60,7	7,7	—	140	8	690	—	—	—	—
Watermelon seeds	6,0	12,2	7,5	—	68	2,5	—	0,13	—	—	—

TABLE 10
Chemical composition of cereals and pulses used mainly by Africans[7]

	grams/100 grams			IU	milligrams/100 grams							
	Pro-tein	Fat	CHO	Vit. A	Ca	Fe	Phos.	Thiam.	Ribo.	Niac.	Vit. C
Sorghum	10,4	1,9	72,6	79	25	5,8	222	0,37	0,28	1,8	0
Pearl millet	11,6	5,0	67,5	220	42	14,3	269	0,33	0,16	3,2	0
Field bean	24,9	0,8	60,1	0	60	2,7	248	0,52	0,16	1,8	0
Soya bean	43,2	9,5	20,9	710	240	11,5	690	0,73	0,76	2,4	0
Cowpea	24,6	0,7	57,1	0	70	3,8	384	0,41	0,85	—	0

last war, i.e. in the 1940s. The traditional diet prior to this time consisted of three main kinds of food: porridge, relish and vegetables (*morôgô*). Fish and eggs were never eaten. Stiff porridge and its modifications were made either of sorghum or of millet, the cereal being ground by the women and cooked in an earthenware pot. A popular modification was sour porridge cooked with or without whey. The porridge was eaten by hand with a side dish of either relish or *morôgô* or both. A substitute porridge was also made of beans.

As in the past, so today, the relish may be made of meat, locusts, caterpillars, sour milk or beans and adds flavour to the porridge (traditional or mealie meal). *Morôgô* (vegetables) are generally eaten, although vegetables have never been as important as in the westernised diet. Favourite vegetables are: marrakas, watermelon, makataan, sugar reed, leaves of plants (e.g. beans) and wild spinaches and other weeds. Unfortunately the green leaves are often overcooked for the sake of smoothness and lose much of their ascorbic acid content. Some vegetables are cultivated but the majority are collected from the veld. Vegetables are preserved

for the winter by cooking, mashing and drying them, the dried pellets being boiled before use.

The traditional black diet of the northern Transvaal is nutritious and health-promoting, but this kind of diet is seldom available to the rural black because of poor soil husbandry and the absence of the men gardeners in the cities where they work for wages which, in turn, are used by the women to buy refined foods. Because the nutritional value of maize, especially the refined products, is such that it does not supply a well-balanced diet, pellagra due to niacin deficiency and kwashiorkor due to protein deficiency, have become prevalent in these areas.

Maize is the most important staple food of Transkei, being cooked to form a wide variety of dishes, from stiff porridge to thin gruels (*amarewu*). Sour porridge is a great favourite. The second important staple food is dried beans and the third sorghum. Bread is eaten by some people, but millet appears to be unknown. Sorghum is especially important for beer-brewing, but maize can also be used for this purpose.

Traditional stone-on-stone grinding of home-grown grains by the women disseminates

TABLE 11
Leaves and tender stalks eaten by Indians and Africans[7]

	grams/100 grams			IU	milligrams/100 grams						
	Pro-tein	Fat	CHO	Vit. A	Ca	Fe	Phos.	Thiam.	Ribo.	Niac.	Vit. C
Bamboo shoots	3,9	0,5	5,7	0	210	0,1	65	0,08	0,19	0,2	5
Field beans	3,8	0,7	6,7	312	210	1,7	68	0,10	tr.	tr.	9
Madumbe leaves and stems	4	1,2	4,2	—	163	5,6	68	—	—	—	—
Wild mustard	4	0,6	3,2	—	155	16,3	26	—	—	—	—
Indian pea	6,1	1,0	5,5	6 000	160	7,3	100	0,01	0,03	—	41
Spiny pigweed	3	0,3	7,0	5 940	800	22,98	50	0	0,01	0,2	33
Dandelion	2,0	0,6	5,1	11 700	140	1,8	42	0,13	0,16	—	18
Potato leaves	4,4	0,9	3,6	—	120	—	50	—	—	—	—
S. potato leaves	4,2	0,8	10,7	1 250	360	10	60	0,18	0,24	1,7	27
Pumpkin leaves	4,6	0,8	7,7	—	392	—	112	—	—	—	—
Pumpkin flowers	2,2	0,8	5,7	—	120	—	60	—	—	—	—
Tamarind leaves	5,8	2,1	18,2	418	101	5,2	140	0,24	0,17	4,1	106
Turnip leaves	4,0	1,5	9,4	15 660	710	28,4	60	0,31	0,57	5,4	180

silica dust which, when inhaled over a long period, may cause Transkei silicosis — a condition of lung fibrosis which predisposes to pulmonary tuberculosis. Recently Transkeians have developed a preference for refined cereals, buying mealie meal and flour at stores. Efficient milling techniques to produce the refined products unfortunately remove most of the husks and with it the B vitamins. Methods of machine and hand milling which steer a middle course between the two dangers of silicosis and avitaminosis are available at some of the local stores and co-operatives where people are encouraged to take their grain for self-milling. Samp is a great favourite with the Xhosa and Fingo and is made by stamping mealies with a pestle in a mortar. The husks and some of the maize germ is blown away, thus robbing the maize of protein and B vitamins. Samp is, however, sometimes cooked with dried beans to make a nutritious dish. The leaves of wild plants (*imifino*) are eaten as a smooth spinach with thick crumbly maize porridge.

Transkeian blacks eat vegetables: pumpkin, watermelon, spinach, cabbage and beans; they relish the cooked tendrils of creeping vegetables (e.g. pumpkin) and use edible wild plants (spinaches) and wild fruits. Some grow their own vegetables and fruit, especially oranges, guavas and bananas. Some other vegetables are coming into use: green peas, carrots, tomatoes, turnips and cauliflower. Vegetables are cooked with or without the addition of maize meal, fat, curry and onions. Groundnuts are hardly known to Transkeians.

The people of Transkei have herds of cattle, and flocks of sheep and goats and even keep chickens and pigs. The animals are, however, kept mainly for *lobola* purposes and are slaughtered only for ritual sacrifices to propitiate the ancestor spirits or on festive occasions when all the participants get a share of the meat. Wild birds and animals are hunted for food but they are scarce. Few people eat meat regularly, the pattern being once every 1 to 3 months. Milk, especially when soured in calabashes, is an important food in Transkei, but is not in abundant supply because of the poor quality of the cows. Eggs are seldom eaten and not at all by women.

Transkeians favour bitter foods, e.g. bitter wild plants, bitter leaves of peach and potato and animal bile, but they have also developed a preference for sugar, sweets, tea and coffee. The diet is monotonous because the people are very conservative as regards their feeding habits. It would seem that custom rather than poverty dictates the foods eaten. The sign of impinging acculturation with Western food preferences is the inclusion of sugar, tea and coffee in the diet.

TABLE 12
Chemical composition of common vegetables and fruit[7]

	per 100 g		grams/100 grams			IU	milligrams per 100 grams						
	Cal.	kJ	Protein	Fat	CHO	Vit. A	Ca	Phos.	Thia.	Ribo.	Niac.	Vit. C	Fe
Prickly pear	279	1 172	1,00	0,58	13,9	—	26	29	—	—	—	—	0,3
Melon, kaffir	21	88	1,4	0,2	3,4	23	25	24	0,04	0,08	0,3	18	0,9
Gourd, bitter	25	105	1,6	0,2	4,2	210	20	70	0,07	0,09	0,5	88	1,8
Madumbe, tuber	97	401	3,0	0,1	21,1	40	40	140	0,09	0,03	0,4	1	1,7
Sweet potato	422	1 772	1,61	0,12	21,43	—	24	42	—	—	—	—	1
Cassava tuber	132	554	1,0	0,4	32,8	tr.	40	34	0,05	0,04	0,6	19	1,4
Pumpkin	114	479	1,11	0,08	4,97	—	18	29	—	—	—	—	1
Sugar cane juice	39	163	0,1	0,2	9,1	10	10	10	—	0,04	—	—	1,1
Chillis, green	—	—	2,9	0,6	3,0	292	30	80	0,19	0,39	1	111	1,2
Pepper, green	—	—	4,8	2,7	13,7	900	270	70	0,05	0,04	—	1	2,4

The Zulu of northern Natal also have maize as their most important staple food, using it either as samp (cooked with cowpeas), or as thick or thin porridge. Amongst the rural Zulu the diet is not westernised, the people either growing their own food or obtaining wild leaves, fruit and animals from the veld. Those few people who can afford to do so buy the following foods from the trading stores: bread flour, mealie meal, samp, sweets, cold drinks, coffee, tea, condensed and powdered milk, sugar, tinned fish, fat and oil.

Women are the cultivators and the food gatherers and they brew the Bantu beer from sorghum or millet. The men who stay at home are chiefly occupied with tapping the juice of palms to make palm wine for own consumption or for barter. Their traditional role as hunters and stock keepers is almost redundant due to the scarcity of game (cane rats, rabbits, insects, birds) and domestic animals. Cattle and goats are not regarded as a source of food, being used for barter and ritual purposes; some chickens are kept for consumption. Fish is eaten by those people who live near the rivers and lakes. The Zulu, therefore, eat very little animal protein, their main source of protein being peanuts (groundnuts).

Maize, sorghum, groundnuts and millet are grown, maize forming the bulk of the crop. The vegetables cultivated are: madumbe, cassava, sweet potato, cowpeas, peanuts, beans, melon, pumpkin, calabashes, gourds and chillies. Thick peanut gruel is added to all maize and vegetable dishes and chillies are cooked with vegetables. Cane is also grown and the people use this for chewing and for brewing an intoxicating beverage.

Milk is consumed when available but eggs are usually taboo as a source of food, except to men and old women. Supplementary sources of food (sometimes almost the sole source) are wild mushrooms, green leaves (*imifino*) and fruits which are available in many varieties, some throughout the year. Home-made alcoholic beverages, *amahewu* (fermented cereal gruel), *amasi* (sour milk) are traditional beverages.

Usually only one main meal is consumed daily in the late afternoon. It consists of a maize course and a vegetable course. A portion of this meal is left for consumption during the first half of the next day. Wild fruit and beverages, including tea and coffee, may be consumed during the course of a day.

The influence of values and beliefs on diet

The traditional blacks are rigidly conservative because the traditional customs are strongly enforced by religious beliefs which in turn are an expression of the value systems of people who believe in the magical control of their environment; these people are unable to grasp the principles of Western scientific thought which attempts to find a natural cause for all the calamities which befall man. Traditional black medical lore appears to the Western mind to be superstition and black medical practice is regarded as magical hocus-pocus; but these beliefs and practices are the 'truth' for all blacks who share the traditional culture. The traditional blacks believe that everything that happens to them — good or bad — is due to the working out of forces in nature or magical powers residing in important people, like chiefs, to whom only good things happen as their magical powers ward off the evil. If a person is healthy or successful, it is because the ancestor spirits have blessed him for not neglecting them or because of good fortune. Evil forces are always about, however, and need to be warded off or driven out by magical cures. The traditional black cannot see any connection between laziness and poor crops, malnutrition and disease, poor hygiene and disease. To his mind the main causes of disease are:

(1) defilement of the body by breaking a taboo;
(2) anger of neglected ancestor spirits;
(3) bewitchment by a witch or sorcerer — a malicious person who has cast a spell.

Sickness evokes tremendous fear in the sufferer — fear of the unknown malevolent force bent on destroying him. He will seek help from the specialists in his culture — the diviners and the herbalists. Magical causes of disease merit magical cures and if the cure fails he accepts the hopelessness of his fate and exhibits fatalistic and helpless attitudes.

Because of the strong magico-religious beliefs held by the traditional blacks, it is very difficult to establish in the mind of malnourished people a connection between food (or the lack of protective foods) and ill-health. These beliefs are so firmly entrenched that even urbanised blacks who came into daily contact with Western thought cannot abandon them entirely.

Belief in sorcery and witchcraft practised by the living, or in evil forces like the Thikoloshe which is believed to harm people unless they are protected by magical spells, causes much terror and mental and physical ill-health among people who find it difficult to exchange the emotionally charged magico-religious beliefs for the rational, objective, scientific attitudes of Western thinking simply because the latter does not make sense to them. The deeply ingrained magical beliefs regarding the aetiology of disease are rooted in the social structure and are a great hindrance to effective health education. Galli (1972)[12] feels that resistance to change exhibited by developing people is due to an unbridgeable gap between the health educators and those to be educated because of the following faults in the educators: lack of understanding and insensitivity towards the cultural norms of the people, which give rise to judgemental attitudes (i.e. rejection and contempt); basic differences in belief systems and in the status of educator and those to be educated.

The skills of many dedicated health educators are needed in order to establish a firm connection between food and health in people who see ill-health in terms of bewitchment by envious adversaries or as punishment by angered spirits. To quote an example:

'. . . a well-dressed mother presented to our mobile clinic with a month-old marasmic baby that died before it got to hospital. She had the means to buy milk and the knowledge that milk would have saved her baby. She also had healthy breasts. However, she believed the child had *iplate* and fed it on water and thin porridge. Her question is, who murdered the child?'[13]

Note: Iplate is a Xhosa disease of premature infants, believed to start in utero, by transplacental poisoning. The infant is sickly and if it survives for more than a month it becomes marasmic. Xhosa mothers see no connection between poor feeding and *iplate*. Kwashiorkor is believed to be caused by ancestral anger resulting in 'burning' of the child — the Xhosa explanation for the skin lesions.

Religious and cultural beliefs impose taboos on certain foods and must be taken into consideration when planning diets. Examples: meat is generally an accepted article of diet in all South African cultural groups, but is subject to many restrictions on religious grounds. Jews and most African tribes do not eat pork, Hindus do not eat beef, while some religious sects advocate a vegetarian diet. The orthodox Jews observe intricate ritual in order to prepare kosher food.

Cattle, sheep and goats are not readily slaughtered in the black rural areas because cattle denote wealth and play an important role in *lobola*; slaughtering is done for feasts and for sacrifices to the ancestors, after which the beast is eaten by all the participants.

Africans are not keen on eating eggs; tribal blacks believe that eggs increase the man's virility and make women and children sexy. Among the traditional Zulu there is a loosely imposed taboo on certain meats, eggs and milk for women and young girls, men being allowed to eat and drink as they like. As these taboos have a deleterious effect on health, especially that of pregnant and lactating women, one may presume that the rural blacks see no connection between food and health.

THE WESTERN LIFE-STYLE AND ITS ROLE IN DIET-RELATED DISEASES

Many 'Western' diseases are diet-related and are associated with 'progress', especially the rapid cultural changes in industrial society since the industrial revolution in Europe and World War II. These Western diseases include diabetes type II, appendicitis, obesity, hypertension, gallstones, ischaemic heart disease, varicose veins and venous thrombosis, hiatus hernia, diverticular disease of the colon, and cancers (colorectal, breast, prostate, pancreas). These diseases were relatively rare approximately 100 years ago. They are still rare in simple rural societies. It has been found, however, that when communities emigrate from low to high prevalence (of Western diseases) areas, the next and subsequent generations (e.g. where there was large-scale immigration to Hawaii and Israel after World War II) have disease prevalences similar to those of the host countries (Burkitt). These so-called Western diseases are, therefore, apparently environmentally caused.

The 'environment' includes a number of risk factors, viz. tension and stress, sedentary lifestyle due to private transport and sedentary occupations, smoking, obesity and a low-fibre, rich diet. Diet has been implicated as an important risk factor.

The main dietary changes with westernisation that may play a role in Western diseases are:

(1) Protein: the source has become animal rather than vegetable.
(2) Carbohydrate: total energy from CHO has been halved. Half of the CHO is provided by sugar.
(3) Fat: at present three times as much energy comes from fats as before. Its source has changed from vegetable to animal.
(4) Fibre intake has been reduced 3–5 times because of the modern preference for refined foods. Whereas fibre used to come from starchy staple foods, it now comes mainly from fruits and vegetables.
(5) Salt (NaCl): Western man consumes much more salt than man in simple societies.

These dietary changes have taken place over a comparatively short period (i.e. some 200 years) in comparison with the long period (approximately 10 000 years) in which man was a peasant agriculturalist and was, presumably, mainly vegetarian.

Role of fibre in the diet

(See p. 206.)

Burkitt[14] postulates the following role of fibre (roughage) in the prevention of Western diseases.

(1) Fibre increases bacterial mass and retains water in the colon thus ensuring a bulky (large volume) soft stool. Reduction of faecal volume causes the following:
   (a) Constipation; hard constipated stools are difficult to evacuate; straining at stool raises intra-abdominal pressure, a possible cause of hiatus hernia, haemorrhoids and varicose veins.
   (b) Diverticular disease (diverticulosis and diverticulitis). This is the commonest colonic disease, being found in a third of westernised people over the age of 60 years. The diverticula (pouches) caused by high intra-colonic pressure and weaknesses in the wall of the colon are acquired. When they cause no symptoms the condition is called diverticulosis and when they cause symptoms (intermittent functional colonic obstruction, excessive segmentation, abdominal discomfort and severe colicky pain) the condition is called diverticulitis.[15]
   (c) Appendicitis due to obstruction of the lumen of the appendix by faecal impaction.

(2) The fibre content of food affects the nature and amount of intestinal bacteria and consequently the faecal pH. Fibre reduces bacterial degradation of cholesterol and bile acids. The degradation substances are potential carcinogens.
A small amount of hard faeces in the bowel causes prolonged transit time; this increases the concentration of faecal carcinogens or pre-carcinogens and their time of contact with the intestinal mucosa. The presence of increased amounts of potential carcinogens plays an important role in colorectal carcinogenesis.

(3) Reduced bulk in the diet may increase hunger and encourage the intake of empty kilojoules with resultant obesity and diabetes mellitus.

(4) Fibre in diet affects the metabolism of both bile acids and cholesterol and prevents the formation of gallstones.

(5) Dietary fibre plays a role in the prevention of atherosclerosis (see p. 296).

Note: According to the British Agricultural and Food Research Council,[16] tinned baked beans in tomato sauce cause a lowering in blood cholesterol.

The link of a fatty diet with cancer

People on a high-fat diet (40 % kilojoules from fat) run a far greater risk of getting cancer than those on a low-fat diet (20 % kilojoules from fat) (Prof E L Wynder, president of the American Health Foundation, *Rand Daily Mail*, 14.04.1983).

The important cancers related to a high-fat diet are: cancers of breast, colon, prostate, pancreas, body of the uterus and the ovary. Dietary fat increases the bile acids in the stool and also affects the production of certain hormones late in life.

The following are ways of cutting down on the fats in a Western diet:

(1) foods are boiled, poached or grilled instead of fried;

(2) red meat (containing 40 % fat) intake is reduced in favour of chicken and fish;

(3) butter and margarine consumption is reduced;

(4) low-fat milk is used.

REFERENCES

(1) Vorster HH. Vegetarianism. *S Afr J Cont Med Ed* 1987; **5**: 35.

(2) Faber M, Gouws E, Spinnler-Benade AJ, Labadorios D. Anthropometric measurements, dietary intake and biochemical data of South African lacto-ovovegetarians. *S Afr Med J* 1986; **69**: 733.

(3) Facts about Milk and Milk Products No. 5. Subdirectorate: Nutrition, Department of Health Services and Welfare.

(4) Wood, DA, *et al. Lancet* 1987; 179–182.

(5) Edington D, *et al. Br Med J* 1987; **294**: 333–336.

(6) Department of Health Services and Welfare. *Scientific Nutrition and You.*

(7) Fox FW. Studies on the chemical composition of foods commonly used in Southern Africa. *SAIMR* 1966.

(8) SAMJ News. *S Afr Med J* 1986; **70**: xi.

(9) Venter CS. Food Fads. *S Afr J Cont Med Educ* 1987; **5**: 22.

(10) Coetzee AM, *et al. S Afr Med J* 1973; **47**: 739.

(11) Franz HC. *S Afr Med J* 1971; **45**: 1232.

(12) Galli E. *S Afr Med J* 1972; **46**: 1855.

(13) Fehrson GS, Ingle RF. *S Afr Med J* 1973; **47**: 298.

(14) Burkitt DP. Western diseases and their emergence related to diet. *S Afr Med J* 1982; **61**: 1013.

(15) Painter NS. Diverticular disease of the colon. *S Afr Med J* 1982; **61**: 1016.

(16) SAMJ News. *S Afr Med J* 1988; **74**: xxi.

(17) Meyer,B.J.*Die Fisiologiese Basis van Geneeskunde.* Derde Uitgawe. 1983; Opvocdkundigc Uitgcwcrs. Prctoria.

TEST OF KNOWLEDGE

The student has benefited from studying this chapter if he/she can answer the following questions:

(1) 'The overconsumption of fat, generally, and saturated fat in particular, as well as cholesterol, sugar and salt has been related to 5 leading causes of death: ischaemic heart disease, cancer, cerebro-vascular disease, diabetes mellitus and atherosclerosis.' In the light of the above statement, what practical dietary advice would you give a group of affluent young adult South Africans who are desirous of adopting a healthy life-style?

(2) Discuss milk as a food for all age groups and explain why the packaging of milk powder blends and milk substitutes must display the warning, 'Not for infant feeding'.

(3) Discuss the health advantages of a balanced strict vegetarian diet and the health dangers of a vegetarian diet which is used haphazardly without strict attention to dietary requirements.

(4) Write notes on:
    (a) Saturated and unsaturated fatty acids.
    (b) Essential amino acids and their importance in the diet.
    (c) The dietary role of caffeine and the need to limit its intake.
    (d) Cholesterol in the diet.
    (e) Potassium and sodium in the diet.
    (f) Water-soluble vitamins and their functions in the body.
    (g) Fat-soluble vitamins, their sources and functions.

(5) (a) Discuss the difference in fibre content of the westernised diet and the traditional black diet.
    (b) What prophylactic role does an adequate amount of plant fibre in the diet play?

(6) What are the advantages and disadvantages of a lacto-ovo-vegetarian diet?

(7) Enumerate cooking hints calculated to preserve the nutrients in food.

(8) What are the disadvantages of diets which causc rapid wcight loss? What dictary ad-

vice would you give an overweight person who wishes to shed 20 kg of mass?

(9) Prepare a well-balanced menu for a day, for a black rural family of your choice, from articles of food freely available in the community.

17

Hyperlipidaemia and Atherogenesis

GENERAL OBJECTIVES

To give the student an understanding of the aetiology of the commonest cause of morbidity and mortality of the westernised population groups in South Africa — atherosclerosis. This disease is closely asso- ciated with the life-style of these population groups. The community nurse has an important role to play in health education which purports to modify destructive life-styles.

STUDY OBJECTIVES

The student is introduced to:

(1) The condition, hyperlipidaemia, its antecedents and its association with atheroma and atherosclerosis.

(2) The familial hyperlipidaemias (FHLPs) with special emphasis on the monogenically inherited familial hypercholesterolaemia (FH) which has its highest global incidence amongst Afrikaners.

(3) The concept of an interaction between diet, serum total cholesterol (TC) and atherosclerosis and the relationship between a high incidence of hypercholesterolaemia and a high incidence of coronary heart disease.

(4) The primary prevention of hypercholesterolaemia and CHD on both a community level (by education for a healthy life-style and by screening for serum TC levels) and on an individualised level of those persons who are at moderate or high risk of developing CHD.

IN THIS CHAPTER

INTRODUCTION

A large number of disorders of metabolism are expressed only under the influence of unfavourable or inappropriate environmental factors, or when middle age is reached. They have a genetic basis and a multifactorial aetiology. The commonest constitutional metabolic disorders are: glucose intolerance and diabetes mellitus, gout and hyperuricaemia, some types of familial hyperlipoproteinaemia (HLP) and obesity.

The inborn errors of metabolism (see p. 119) merely increase the risk of developing these constitutional disorders of middle age. Thus it is that some people in our affluent society can indulge in smoking, or in a high-fat, high cholesterol diet, or a rich diet with plenty of meat and wine, with impunity, whilst others develop carcinoma of the lung, coronary heart disease, diabetes mellitus or gout under similar conditions of indulgence.

In multifactorial aetiology, the genetic predisposition is strongly affected by the environment, especially by diet, drugs, lack of exercise and stress. Smoking is an important aetiological factor in many constitutional disorders. It would appear that the genetic component of multifactorial aetiology is the inherited inability of the body to handle extra metabolic loads because of the deviation in function of one or more enzymes. It has been found, for example, that only a small percentage of persons with hyperuricaemia develop clinical gouty arthritis. Persons with gout are unable to handle the high purine loads imposed by the diet in Western countries, probably because their kidneys are unable to excrete the additional loads of purine caused by dietary excess or by stress. The same type of aetiological factors probably operate in some types of hyperlipoproteinaemia and coronary heart disease, and hyperglycaemia and diabetes mellitus.

Cardio-vascular diseases are a major cause of morbidity and mortality in South Africa, coronary heart disease occurring very commonly in whites and rarely in rural blacks, and hypertension occurring mainly in urban blacks but also in urban whites. Because of the heterogeneous distribution of these cardio-vascular diseases, epidemiological studies have brought to light the major risk factors involved; an attempt can be made to control these diseases by applying community health measures. The urban/rural variation in incidence offers an opportunity to study the effects of urbanisation/industrialisation/westernisation on health, especially with respect to diet and socio-economic stresses.

Because of its uniquely high prevalence amongst the white, coloured and Asian population groups in South Africa, and its growing incidence amongst urban blacks, hyperlipidaemia (hyperlipoproteinaemia) has been included in this manual as a community health problem.

DEFINITIONS

Atherogenesis means the formation of atheroma (atherosis) — a mass of lipid in the intima of large and medium arteries.

A *lipid* is a fatty substance, the important blood lipids being triglycerides (neutral fats), cholesterol and phospholipids.

Atherosclerosis is an arteriosclerosis caused by atherosis. The irregularly distributed lipid deposits are associated with fibrosis and calcification of the arteries. Severe atherosclerosis leads to reduction of the arterial lumen and predisposes to thrombosis — *atherothrombosis*. The resultant stenosis causes ischaemia of the organ supplied by the artery. Ischaemia commonly manifests as: coronary artery disease (angina pectoris and myocardial infarction), brain infarcts (strokes), intermittent claudication and gangrene of the lower extremities.

The following risk factors are known precursors of atherosclerosis: hypertension, raised serum cholesterol and triglycerides levels, cigarette smoking, glucose intolerance (diabetes mellitus) and a family history of myocardial infarction, i.e. a genetic predisposition.

The *hyperlipidaemias* are a group of metabolic diseases which are characterised by raised serum (plasma) lipid levels, viz. serum cholesterol (hypercholesterolaemia) and/or serum triglycerides (hypertriglyceridaemia).

Hyperlipidaemia may be primary (due to a number of different genetic factors) or secondary due to underlying causes, viz. diabetes mellitus, alcohol excess, cigarette smoking, hypertension, hypothyroidism.

THE LIPIDS

A lipid is a fatty substance. Fat is a lipid but all lipids are not fats. The most important lipids in the blood are: triglycerides (neutral fats), cholesterol esters and phospholipids. The plasma also carries free fatty acids (from adipose tissue triglycerides) which are transported by albumin and are used as a source of energy, especially in starvation.

Triglycerides (Tg) are the energy carriers and can be stored in the body as adipose tissue. They are of exogenous (dietary) and endogenous origin (from the liver). Fasting plasma Tg levels are: 0,4–1,7 mmol/ℓ. A Tg value of greater than 2,3 mmol/ℓ is regarded as abnormally high.

Cholesterol is a sterol which occurs in plasma in the free (alcohol) form (30 %) and esterified form (70 %). The free form is a component of all cell walls; it is required for the formation of new cell walls and for their maintenance. Free cholesterol is also essential for the synthesis of steroids and bile acids. (For serum total cholesterol (TC) levels, see p. 296.)

Note: Dietary cholesterol constantly enters liver cells in chylomicran remnants. The liver cells monitor the cholesterol levels in the body and accordingly synthesise varying additional quantities, chiefly from *saturated* fatty acids. Most of the body's cholesterol is derived from endogenous synthesis, rather than from the diet. Reduction in dietary cholesterol tends to cause a negative feedback stimulation of synthesis. As most endogenous cholesterol is synthesised from *saturated* fats, a diet which is high in saturated fats may stimulate cholesterol production and raise plasma cholesterol levels to a greater extent than a high cholesterol diet. A low cholesterol diet, combined with a low-fat diet which contains a high proportion of *unsaturated* fats, effectively reduces plasma cholesterol levels.

Phospholipids are necessary for the formation of the cell wall. They also play an important role in blood clotting. The normal plasma phospholipid level is: 2,5–3,0 mmol/ℓ.

Lipids are insoluble in plasma. In order to make their transport in blood possible they have to be bound to plasma protein, usually the alpha and beta globulins. They are then called lipoproteins.

Approximate measurement conversions:

Cholesterol: mg/dl ÷ 40 = mmol/ℓ
Triglyceride: mg/dl ÷ 88 = mmol/ℓ

LIPOPROTEINS

A lipoprotein consists of lipids (cholesterol, triglyceride and phospholipid) bound to a protein (globulin). Some proteins bind more lipids than others. The relative density of lipoproteins, therefore, differs; the more lipid bound to the protein, the lower its relative density and vice versa.

The main function of lipoproteins is to transport lipids from sites of absorption or synthesis to sites of use. There are several different proteins to which lipids bind.

The four main lipoproteins, in order of decreasing density, are the following.

HDL — high density lipoprotein

This is the anti-atherogenic protective factor. HDL-C (cholesterol) transports excess cholesterol from the peripheral tissues, e.g. the artery walls, to the liver where it is broken down and excreted in the bile as bile acids and steroids. This is the only way in which excess cholesterol

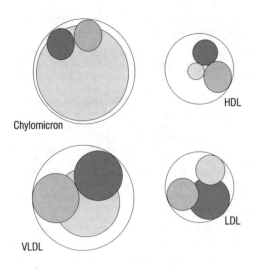

Chylomicron

HDL

VLDL

LDL

Figure 17.1

	Chylo-micron	VLDL	LDL	HDL
Protein	2 %	7 %	21 %	47 %
Cholesterol	7 %	20 %	47 %	18 %
Triglycerides	85 %	55 %	98 %	7 %
Phospholipids	6 %	18 %	23 %	28 %

is excreted. A deficiency in HDL-C could lead to the deposition of cholesterol in the intima of arteries. This pathological condition is called atheroma. High HDL-C levels offer physiological protection from cardio-vascular atheroma and the risk of myocardial infarction.

HDL-C not only inhibits the take-up of cholesterol by the cells but at the same time accelerates the transport of cholesterol away from the cells. In cases of increased risks of myocardial infarction, the concentration of HDL-C in the blood is found to be lowered. The ratio of HDL-C to total cholesterol (TC) is a useful summary of lipoprotein-related risk of developing coronary heart disease (CHD). A 20 % (1:5) HDL-C/TC and higher ratio is 'protective'. HDL-C below 1,0 mmol/ℓ is an indication of increased risk of CHD.

Mean HDL-cholesterol levels in mmol/ℓ:

Males

Age in years	Mean value
6–13	1,45
14–54	1,20
older than 55	1,30*

*Range 0,75–1,95

Females

6–19	1,35
20–70	1,55*

*Range 0,90–2,34

HDL-C values of greater than 1,7 mmol/ℓ in men and 2,2 mmol/ℓ in women are indicative of good health.

Regular strenuous exercise and physical fitness are associated with high levels of HDL-C; obesity and smoking with low HDL-C and high LDL-C. Exercise appears to keep arteries healthy. Oestrogens raise the HDL-C level thus protecting the premenopausal woman from CHD.

LDL — low density lipoprotein

LDL-C is the largest fraction of the lipoproteins and is the main cholesterol transporter. LDL-C becomes bound to specific receptors on cell surfactes; in so doing, it enters the cell and is broken down by lysozyme thus freeing the cholesterol for its anabolic function. Cholesterol will accumulate if the receptors are defective and unable to clear the LDL-cholesterol from the blood, so that the plasma level rises, or if HDL-C is low and therefore not available for the removal of excess cholesterol from the peripheral cells to the liver. This condition is called hyperlipidaemia, or more specifically, hypercholesterolaemia. A high LDL-C plasma level carries a high atherogenic risk.

Its value is approximately two thirds that of serum TC (total cholesterol). Its level can be calculated accurately, however, by doing a fasting lipogram (lipoprotein profile).

Suggested cut-off points (mmol/ℓ) for serum TC (total cholesterol) levels in hypercholesterolaemia (moderate risk):[3]

Note: LDL-C plasma value is approximately 2/3 of the values quoted below.

Age in years	15–24	25–34	35–44	45–54	55–64
Males	4,10	5,00	5,52	5,68	5,75
Females	4,51	4,94	5,31	5,93	6,56

(Established from the findings of the CORIS survey, see p. 294.)

VLDL — very low density lipoprotein

This carries a high atherogenic risk. VLDL contains mostly triglycerides, formed in the liver from alcohol, carbohydrate and free fatty acids, as well as some cholesterol. It is the transporter of endogenous triglycerides.

Chylomicrons

These consist mainly of triglycerides absorbed from the intestines. They are the transporters of exogenous triglycerides, via lymphatics, into the systemic circulation. A chylomicron molecule is too large to enter peripheral cells and it carries only a slight atherogenic risk due to its small cholesterol component.

Note: An additional lipoprotein has recently been identified. It is called Lipoprotein(a) (Lp(a)) and is an apolipoprotein. Only genetically predisposed individuals form apolipoproteins. Lp(a) is strongly associated with atherogenesis. Plasma levels of Lp(a) are measured in order to identify very high-risk persons.

THE HYPERLIPOPROTEINAEMIAS (HLPs)

The term hyperlipidaemia can be used synonymously with hyperlipoproteinaemia, as the lipids are always transported in the plasma bound to proteins.

The hyperlipidaemias are a group of metabolic diseases which are characterised by *raised serum (plasma) lipid levels*. One or more of the plasma lipid fractions may be raised above the desirable level for good health of the relevant population group. Most, but not all, hyperlipidaemias are *atherogenic (atheroma-generating)*.

Although atherosclerosis is caused mainly by hyperlipidaemia, many other risk factors contribute to its genesis. Stress is thought to play an important role as well as cigarette smoking, excessive fat, energy and alcohol intake, hypertension, diuretics, beta-blockers, steroids, and lack of exercise.

Note:
(1) The role of occupational stress as a risk factor is a somewhat controversial subject. Meyers[8] states that CHD (coronary heart disease) is beginning to appear in urban blacks of the upper social strata as well as in some black workers subject to high levels of work-related stress. Contrary to what was formerly assumed, that CHD is a disease of affluent, high-powered executives, work-related stress is more common lower down in the labour hierarchy than in men in management positions. Lewis[9] agrees with him; CHD has been a commoner cause of death in social classes IV–V than in social classes 1–11 in the UK since 1950.
(2) Seedat *et al.*[10] postulate a hereditary factor in hypertension, the genes controlling blood pressure interacting with the genes controlling serum lipids. As blood pressure rises, arteriosclerosis increases.

Hyperlipidaemia may be either a *primary, hereditary, familial disease* (FHLP) or it may be *secondary to other diseases* such as diabetes mellitus, chronic renal failure, hepatobiliary disease, multiple myeloma, SLE, Cushing's disease, obesity and thyroid deficiency.

The separation of the primary from the secondary disorder is not easy; moreover, both types may coexist in the same patient. In this case the secondary cause may potentiate the primary disorder.

The familial hyperlipidaemias (FHLP)

FHLPs are prevalent in South Africa. As most of them are inherited as an autosomal dominant condition, a positive family history is usually obtainable.

FHLPs may be either monogenically or polygenically inherited, the latter often being exacerbated by adverse environmental factors, viz. the risk factors mentioned above.

In a polygenically inherited FHLP many genes interact with environmental factors, especially diet, to produce hypercholesterolaemia. Polygenic disorders are the most common cause of hypercholesterolaemia.[4] The most common environmental factors also affect the clinical expression of single-gene disorders.

Most, though not all, FHLPs are atherogenic, atherogenicity depending on the cholesterol content of their raised lipoprotein. All liproprotein fractions contain cholesterol to a greater or lesser extent (see fig. 17.1), hence their potential for atherogenesis. An accumulation of HDL is, however, entirely benign.

FHLPs must, if possible, be distinguished from the secondary IILDs. In the latter case the hyperlipidaemia may respond to treatment of the primary condition. Effective management of the hyperlipidaemia is, however, not based on the diagnostic label, but on objective laboratory and clinical data.

Classification of FHLP
Frederickson NIH (National Institutes of Health) types

- *Type II(a):* Pure hypercholesterolaemia (LDL-C). There are 3 subtypes, including the Familial Hypercholesterolaemia (FH). They may be either hetero- or homozygous, the latter being rare.
- *Type II(b):* Mixed — i.e. increased cholesterol and triglyceride.
- *Type III:* Mixed VLDL-C and chylomicrons — a rare condition.
- *Type IV:* Pure VLDL, i.e. predominantly hypertriglyceridaemia.
- *Type I:* Pure chylomicrons — hyperchylomicronaemia. This is a recessive, non-atherogenic disorder which may cause much ill-health (see below).
- *Type V:* Increased VLDL and chylomicrons causing hypertriglyceridaemia.

Type II(a): The *hypercholesterolaemias* — and the mixed FHLPs (Types II(*b*) and III) are a common group of disorders which generally cause premature atherosclerosis, especially involving the coronary arteries. Premature atherosclerosis is especially common in FH (Type II(*a*)).

The *hypertriglyceridaemias* are potentially atherogenic, especially if accompanied by elevated cholesterol levels. They are often associated with obesity, hyperuricaemia (gout), hypertension, impaired glucose tolerance (diabetes mellitus) and low HDL-cholesterol levels, the latter predisposing to CHD. They are markedly susceptible to environmental influences, notably diet, but also alcohol and exogenous steroids.

The *chylomicronaemic* syndrome (Type I in children and Type V in adults) may be accompanied by an xanthomatous rash, lipaemia retinalis (creamy appearance of retinal blood vessels), enlarged spleen and/or liver, abdominal pain (colic), acute pancreatitis and neurological deficits.

Familial hypercholesterolaemia (FH)

FH is characterised by a raised plasma LDL-C level and by the deposit of LDL-derived cholesterol in tendons and skin (xanthomas) and in arteries (atheromas). (See p. 293.)

This severe form of atherogenic (for coronary arteries) familial hypercholesterolaemia is of special interest to Afrikaners, with the highest incidence in the world, between 1:50 and 1:100 having heterozygous FH.[4] It is inherited as a monogenic, autosomal, dominant trait (see p. 124).

FH is also known as hypercholesterolaemic xanthomatosis because of the high serum total cholesterol (TC) (7,5–12,5 mmol/ℓ) and the deposit of excess cholesterol (xanthomas) especially in tendons, but also over the knees, elbows and heels and in the soft tissue around the eyes (xanthelosmas). On the other hand, xanthomas may be absent, diagnosis then depending on a serum (plasma) TC level of at least 8,5 mmol/ℓ and signs of FH in close relatives. There may be Achilles tendon thickening. Familial hypercholesterolaemia accounts for early occurrences of coronary heart disease (CHD) and xanthomatosis, usually even in the absence of other risk factors. Affected persons often develop occlusive myocardial atherosclerosis in the early thirties and are then at risk of dying prematurely from myocardial infarction (MI).

Fifty-one per cent of men with FH have MI before the age of 50 and 85 % by age 60. Twelve per cent of women with FH have MI before the age of 50 and 58 % by age 60.[5] If the disease strikes early — being known to occur in children as young as 5 years — the faulty gene has probably been inherited from both heterozygous parents. The homozygous disease occurring in double dose is very severe with plasma TC levels from 14–30 mmol/ℓ and xanthomas within the first decade of life. Cholesterol is even deposited around the aortic valve to produce aortic stenosis. Two heterozygous parents have a 1:4 chance of producing a homozygous child. There is a 1:2 chance of heterozygous parents producing a heterozygous child.

The faulty gene of FH causes a quantitative or qualitative deficiency of LDL-C receptors on cells. This causes a reduced rate of clearance of LDL-C and its subsequent accumulation in the plasma. The excess cholesterol is taken up by macrophages and deposited in tendon and skin xanthomas, in the spleen and in atheromas in the intima of arteries, especially those of the myocardium (coronary arteries). Peripheral and cerebral atheroscleroses are relatively uncommon. Seftel[6] states that the platelets of FH are hyperaggregable thus contributing to atherothrombosis.

Note: Although familial hyperlipidaemia (FHLP) is common amongst Afrikaners, only 1:10 Afrikaners under the age of 50 with acute myocardial infarction suffers from FH.[3] The high prevalence of FH amongst Afrikaners is due to the 'founder effect'. Seftel[6] estimates that approximately 30 000 Afrikaners suffer from FH. FH is also fairly common amongst South African Jews. Its prevalence amongst South African whites of British descent is much lower. The familial hyperlipidaemias are a community health problem amongst the whites in South Africa.

Treatment of the heterozygous FH

(1) Dietary as for all hyperlipidaemias. This treatment should start in infancy if FH is diagnosed as early as that.

(2) Correction of other risk factors.

(3) Lipid-lowering drugs (see p. 298).

(4) If the heterozygous FH is resistant to drug therapy, a partial ileal bypass operation (ileocaecostomy) can be performed. This interferes with bile acid absorption and has a strong hypocholesterolaemic effect. A by-pass operation may, however, cause malabsorption of other nutrients, especially vit. B_{12} and may cause diarrhoea.

(5) Plasmapheresis.

Treatment of the homozygous FH

Diet and drugs as for the heterozygous FH.

Surgery includes a portacaval shunt in which the portal vein is anastomosed to the inferior vena cava.

Plasmapheresis is effective in lowering LDL-C and in ameliorating xanthomas and atherosclerosis. Plasmapheresis is a difficult, time-consuming and expensive procedure done in special units of academic hospitals (see Vlok, ME, *Manual of Nursing*, Volume 2).

The majority of homozygous FH sufferers die before the age of 30. Their response to medical treatment is uncertain.

ATHEROMA (ATHEROSIS) AND ATHEROSCLEROSIS

Atherosclerosis is an arteriosclerosis caused by atherosis. It is sometimes called nodular arteriosclerosis.

An atheroma (atherosis) is a mass of lipid in the intima of large and medium arteries. This atheromatous plaque causes a yellow swelling on the endothelial surfaces. The atheroma contains cholesterol crystals, calcium precipitates, proteoglycans, soluble and insoluble proteins, as well as dead and dying cells. The plaque is separated from the arterial lumen by a cap of fibrous tissue. Atheroma leads to the reduction of the size of the lumen and predisposes to thrombosis (atherothrombosis). Thrombosis follows the exposure of the lipid to the blood but in some cases there is no such exposure. Thrombosis usually develops on plaques undergoing the process known as fissuring, rupture or cracking of the fibrous cap of the plaque for reasons that are not quite clear. Narrowing (occlusion) of the atheromatous arteries, with or without thrombosis, causes ischaemia which may manifest as: angina pectoris and myocardial infarction (heart), cerebro-vascular accident (brain), intermittent claudication and gangrene (lower extremities).

Grades of atherosclerotic narrowing:

- Grade I — up to 25 %
- Grade II — 25–50 %
- Grade III — 50–75 %
- Grade IV — 75–100 %

A collateral circulation may become established if the occlusion is gradual. In cases of coronary thrombosis, the thrombus either resolves rapidly, thus preventing death of tissue (myocordial infarction), or it may grow and propagate distally occluding a centimetre or more of the artery. Death of tissue is not inevitable if a collateral blood flow was previously established due to a partial occlusion of the artery.

The atheromatous lesion is a degenerative condition which is the major but not exclusive consequence of hyperlipidaemia. Atherosclerosis is provoked by a variety of stimuli acting alone or synergistically: imprudent food consumption and stress,[7] cigarette smoking, hypertension, lack of exercise, excessive alcohol intake, diabetes mellitus. There seems to be a definite interaction between diet, serum total cholesterol and atherosclerosis.

In South Africans the risk of CHD is present when the serum TC level exceeds 5,68 mmol/ℓ in men and 5,93 mmol/ℓ in women aged 45–54 years.[3] This was established by the CORIS survey.

THE CORIS SURVEY[3]

CORIS is the acronym for Coronary Risk Factor Study. This survey was a joint undertaking of the S.A. Medical Research Council, the Department of National Health and Population Development, and the Human Sciences Research Council. It is the largest and best-documented population survey in the RSA to date.

CORIS was a dietary survey, done in 1979 on a substrate of 1 113 males and females, 15–64 years of age. It was done in the mainly Afrikaans-speaking districts of Robertson, Swellendam and Riversdale, to determine the prevalence of risk factors associated with the development of coronary heart disease. A cross-sectional survey was done on the eating habits of the test subjects and their blood was tested for serum TC and HDL-C. (LDL-C can be calculated from TC.)

The results of the CORIS survey are used as reference values of serum TC (action limits) which indicate the risk of developing coronary heart disease. Results are often compared with the American MRFIT (multiple risk factor intervention trial) of 1982. It was found that the 80th USA percentile for serum TC equals the 50th South African (CORIS) percentile. The median serum total cholesterol (TC) of South Africans is, therefore, much higher than the median USA serum TC. The age-specific values of serum TC found in the CORIS survey are typical of a high-risk westernised population. If the CORIS findings correspond to those of the rest of South Africa, it means that South Africans are at much higher risk of developing coronary heart disease than Americans. This is, in fact, the case.

In 1984, 12 059 South Africans died from coronary heart disease; 75 % of the deaths were due to acute myocardial infarction. These deaths accounted for 7 % of all deaths in South Africa. Ninety three per cent of these deaths, however, occurred in whites, Asians and col-

oureds, who, together, make up 27 % of the South African population. In blacks, CHD accounted for only 1 % of all deaths.

Asians had the highest mortality rate from CHD in South Africa in 1978–1982, 34 % higher than that of white males and 84 % higher than that of white females. Rossouw places South African white and Asian CHD mortality rates in the highest global bracket. It would appear that the high prevalence of diabetes mellitus in Asians contributes heavily to the high Asian CHD mortality rate, as the prevalence of hypercholesterolaemia and hypertension is moderate.

In blacks and coloureds the urban CHD mortality rates are higher than the rural, probably because the relative affluence of the urban citizens causes them to buy more high-fat animal protein foods and cigarettes and urbanisation exposes them to the stress of acculturation with subsequent rise in the prevalence in hypertension.[11]

COMMUNITY PRIMARY PREVENTION OF HYPERCHOLESTEROLAEMIA AND CHD IN SOUTH AFRICA

A high rate of coronary heart disease (CHD) in a community is a mass phenomenon determined by the lifestyle of the CHD-prone community. Communities which have a saturated-fat intake accounting for more than 15 % of their daily energy intake have high serum total cholesterol (TC) levels and high death-rates from CHD,[3] while in those with a saturated-fat intake of less than 10 % the reverse holds. A great number of westernised South Africans are at risk from CHD. Primary prevention strategies are possible but there must be clarity about how this can be achieved. CHD has a multifactorial aetiology, the most important predictive factor being serum TC. Individual risk of developing CHD increases as the serum TC level rises (hypercholesterolaemia). Most cases of CHD do not, however, occur in the relatively few people at high risk, but in the large number of people at moderate risk in the community. The only approach likely to be effective for the primary prevention of CHD on a national basis is, therefore, a population or community approach.

The community approach includes the following strategies: health education; screening the at-risk population for raised serum TC values.

Health education

The most important primary prevention strategy is education for a healthy life-style and the consumption of a diet which is non-atherogenic, i.e. one which does not raise the serum TC levels to CHD risk levels.

If the serum TC levels of a community at high risk of CHD can be lowered (as has been done in the USA and elsewhere) the incidence of CHD in the community will fall. TC levels can be lowered by persuading people with raised TC levels to take action (see p. 296).

While unique constitutional factors determine the serum TC response of a particular individual to a given environment (e.g. diet, smoking, sloth, stress, alcohol abuse), in a group or community it is mainly the environment which will determine whether the mean serum TC level of the community is high or low.

The important goal of primary prevention is to change the life-style of whole communities with regard to the excesses and indulgences of rich food, drink and cigarette smoking. It involves people at all ages, starting in childhood. Atherosclerosis starts in early life; moreover, behaviour patterns, including those of eating and smoking, are usually established in childhood. Community prevention programmes aim at risk-factor reduction by the adoption of a healthier life-style.

The following action programmes are purported to reach the whole community as well as targeted subgroups:

(1) Professional education, i.e. professional health workers from the medical and allied fields must be trained in the correct orientation towards prevention. As they must set the example it is important that their personal and family health behaviour is health promotive.

(2) Community leader education involves education of leaders of public opinion, e.g. ministers of religion, university professors, members of parliament, etc.

(3) Public education through risk-factor measurements at primary health care facilities. This makes people aware of possible weakness in their health status. Adult education classes, including classes for senior citizens, on risk factors and prevention and school health programmes in effective social behaviour are important vehicles of public education. Education through the mass media can also be very effective.

(4) Environmental change on the part of voluntary and governmental bodies, e.g. the provision of recreational facilities and 'trim parks' encourage increased physical activity; prohibition of smoking in public places makes smokers aware of the health hazards of their addiction.

Statistics show that in countries in which people have responded to health education (USA, Finland), the incidence of CHD has abated. In these countries much publicity has been given to the dangers of smoking, cholesterol-rich foods and saturated fats. However, response is likely to come only if the community becomes health conscious instead of sickness conscious. The nurse or doctor who feels that his/her professional role concerns only the care of sick people is unlikely to be able to impart health education principles by example and inspiration — witness the fact that many members of these professions still smoke! Cigarette smokers must be encouraged and helped by non-smokers to give up the smoking habit.

Affluent communities living on rich diets should be made conscious of the dangers of dining and wining too sumptuously on daily, non-festive occasions.

The health educator will find that this is a formidable task as people in good health, especially hungry growing adolescents, are loath to curb their appetites when they are surrounded by plenty and when they find gratification in the palatability of a rich refined diet. Food occupies a central role in many people's enjoyment of life and unless these people understand and accept that their eating habits may be dangerous to their health — which may or may not be precious to them — they are not likely to make sacrifices.

In order to make the typical diet of affluence more anti-hyperlipidaemic, the following food constituents must be cut down: fat, especially saturated fats in meat, butter and cream; cholesterol which abounds in eggs; red meat; salt and sugar. The amount of cholesterol in one egg approaches the upper limit of the recommended daily intake. The intake of the following foods is to be encouraged: fruit and vegetables, poultry and fish and fibre-containing foods such as unrefined breakfast cereals and pulses. Certain types of dietary fibre (excluding wheat bran which is good for constipated persons) bind intestinal bile acids, keeping them in the faeces and promoting excretion. Cholesterol is broken down by the liver as a substrate for the synthesis and replacement of bile acids. Dietary fibre thus modestly reduces cholesterol levels. Saturated fat should be replaced by polyunsaturated fats and oils which are freely available. These anti-lipidaemic foods can be made palatable enough to suit the most discriminating tastes. Mothers should encourage their children to eat healthy foods, inculcating sound dietary habits from the age of 1 year. Breast-feeding has been found to be anti-hyperlipidaemic.

Diet modifications according to the principles expounded above are especially important for adolescents in privileged homes. A Johannesburg study showed that this age group has disturbingly high serum cholesterol patterns. In this study 40 % of the boys had serum cholesterol levels above 5 mmol/ℓ (200 mg/dl).[12]

Screening

Raised serum TC levels are detected by population screening. As mass screening programmes will be too costly, screening for raised TC in the non-fasting person should be confined to those possibly at risk: those with a personal or family history of hyperlipidaemia, those with xanthomatosis, sufferers from diabetes mellitus, hypertension, obesity and gout, as well as smokers.

Serum TC assessment (screening) should also be included in conventional health examinations, e.g. executive health checks, army induction, insurance examinations, employment medical examinations, etc. This type of case-finding is a useful way of identifying a large number of hypercholesterolaemic individuals in the work-force. Selective screening or 'case-finding' is a very important function of the primary health care nurse.

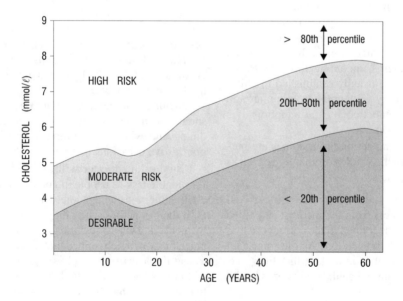

Figure 17.2

Action limits for total cholesterol

Graph of age-specific action limits for serum TC derived from the CORIS 20th and 80th percentiles for both sexes combined.

Clarity about how CHD in a specific community can be prevented rests on the epidemiologically determined serum TC values for that community. The results of the CORIS survey were used by an *ad hoc* committee of the Heart Foundation of Southern Africa to identify serum TC values which require action to be taken. These values, referred to as 'Action Limits for serum TC' were published in the *SA Medical Journal*, June 1988[4] (see fig. 17.2). The Committee agreed that the South African action limits should be age-specific. LDL-cholesterol levels follow the same trend with age as serum TC and are approximately 2/3 of the TC value. They should, therefore, also be age-specific. HDL-cholesterol, on the other hand, has an independent and inverse influence on CHD risk and does not change much with age. Therefore a single cut-point for HDL-C can be used.

It will be noted that age-specific levels of a given serum TC and LDL-C carry less relative risk for an older than for a younger patient.

Note:

(1) A serum TC level indicating moderate risk, in the absence of any other risk factor, may denote high risk in the presence of one or more additional risk factors. These are: low HDL-C level, hypertension, smoking, diabetes mellitus, a family history of early CHD or evidence of CHD. Therefore serum TC measurements should always be accompanied by screening for other risk factors.

(2) For any given level of serum TC, the absolute risk for men is greater than for women, especially before the menopause, because of the higher serum HDL-C in women.

(3) Twenty per cent of whites, Asians and urban coloured people have serum TC levels which put them at high risk and another 60 % have levels which put them at moderate risk.

(4) It is important to screen children regularly for high blood lipid levels in all families in which adults develop CHD prematurely. Where hyperlipidaemia is found to exist in a familial form, diet and body mass control become a lifelong routine for all family members at risk.

(5) The risk of death from CHD rises dramatically as serum cholesterol rises above 5,2 mmol/ℓ. A rise from 5,2 to 6,4 mmol/ℓ doubles the risk, and a rise to 7,6 mmol/ℓ quadruples the risk.[13]

In calculating TC values for South African populations from the CORIS survey, male and female data have been combined. The CORIS data have been expanded by using data from studies on children.[4]

Percentage decline in mortality rates (per 100 000) from 1985 to 1989 from ischaemic heart disease in South Africa[14]

Group	1985	1986	1987	1988	1989	% decline
Asian						
Male	151	147	159	137	128	15,2
Female	71	69	82	69	65	8,4
Black						
Male	5	5	6	7	5	0,0
Female	3	3	4	4	3	0,0
Coloured						
Male	71	70	74	65	57	19,7
Female	49	49	58	48	44	10,3
White						
Male	230	219	209	198	159	30,9
Female	127	123	125	120	102	19,7

INDIVIDUALISED PRIMARY PREVENTION OF CHD IN AT-RISK PATIENTS[4]

The *ad hoc* committee of the Heart Foundation of Southern Africa decided on the following action limits to place individuals into high, moderate and ideal (desirable) serum TC ranges for individualised primary prevention of CHD. Those in the high and moderate ranges are at high and moderate risk, respectively, of developing CHD. The high-risk action limit is also used for screening for familial hypercholesterolaemia (FH).

The high-risk action limit operates for all those with a serum TC level above the 80th percentile; the medium-risk category lies between the 20th and 80th percentile. The ideal serum TC levels fall below the 20th percentile. (See fig. 17.2.) Patients at high and moderate risk of developing myocardial infarction should be under medical care, either at a lipid clinic, from a private physician or a cardiologist, in order to reduce risk factors.

The following advice is given:

Moderate risk group with a serum TC action limit of 5,2 mmol/ℓ in middle-aged adults:

Healthy lifestyle: no smoking, moderate alcohol and salt consumption, daily exercise; maintenance of ideal body weight, regular and balanced meals.

Hypertension and diabetes mellitus must be controlled.

Step 1 lipid-lowering diet according to the following dietetic principles:

The diet must be high in fibre and low in kilojoules if the subject is overweight.

Reduction of saturated fats and cholesterol contained in red meat, full-cream dairy products, eggs and many convenient foods, to reduce fats to less than 30 % of energy intake, saturated fats to less than 10 % (i.e. polyunsaturated (P): saturated (S) ratio 2:1) and cholesterol intake to less than 300 mg/day. The diet is high in fibre (from cereals, fruit and vegetables) and in complex CHO (starches).

This advice regarding a healthy lifestyle and a prudent diet is applicable to the entire population, including high-risk cases during the first three months of treatment.

High-risk group with TC action limit (80th percentile) of 7,1 mmol/ℓ in 45 year old males. Patients with FH often fall in this category. Such individuals need more vigorous dietetic treatment if they have not responded to Step 1 diet and a healthy life-style.

In the Step 2 lipid-lowering diet total fats are reduced to 25 % or less of dietary energy, saturated fats to 7 % and dietary cholesterol to 200 mg/day. These dietetic requirements are met by the strict vegetarian diet (see p. 269).

Note: The 80th American percentile equals the 50th South African (CORIS) percentile. If the MRFIT (American) standards were to be used in the RSA, half the South African westernised population would have to be considered for lipid-lowering drug therapy.

The following cases of hyperlipidaemia are referred to a specialist physician or a lipid clinic:

(1) non-responding high-risk patients after a Step 2 dietetic trial of at least 3 months;

(2) adults with TC or Tg values more than 15 mmol/ℓ especially those with xanthomatosis and serious risk factors, e.g. hypertension and diabetes mellitus;

(3) adults with very low or absent HDL-C;

(4) all children with xanthomas or uncontrolled insulin-dependent diabetes mellitus.[4]

For these serious and intractable hyperlipidaemic cases, the following more drastic lipid-lowering treatments are available.

Pharmacological therapy with lipid-lowering drugs:

(1) Resins which bind bile acids in the gut and therefore prevent their absorption. Example: cholestyramine. It is not absorbed and is therefore safe, but it may cause constipation and other G.I. symptoms, and interfere with the absorption of other medicines and fat-soluble vitamins. Patient compliance is obtained by starting with low doses, mixing the powder thoroughly with water and taking other prescribed drugs half an hour before the cholestyramine. G.I. side-effects are treated symptomatically. The concurrent administration of small amounts of fat-soluble vitamins and folic acid may be advisable.

(2) The fibrates, e.g. clofibrate, fenofibrate and bezafibrate, are useful in the mixed hyperlipidaemias but are also used in the uncomplicated hypercholesterolaemias. They lower triglycerides. They are absorbed and may affect the kidneys and liver. Other side-effects include impotence, alopecia and more. If used with caution, the fibrates are generally safe and effective.

(3) Probucol has variable LDL-C and HDL-C lowering effects. It may cause diarrhoea, nausea and a skin rash. It can be used only if the basal HDL-C is high and can be combined with resins.

(4) Nicotinic acid is effective in lowering both TC and Tg values. Its unpleasant side-effects are flushing, pruritus, nausea, heartburn and diarrhoea. It may be combined with resins or probucol.

(5) HMG CoA reductase inhibitors, e.g. Ravastatin (Prava), Simvastatin (Zocor). These are very good modern drugs for reducing LDL-C. They have been proven to 'regress' and slow the progression of CHD. They have few side-effects but are very expensive.

Lipid-lowering drugs have been shown to reduce CHD mortality in large-scale trials of high-risk patients[4] in the long run.

Note:
(1) Drug therapy should not be started before the serum TC and LDL-C status has been confirmed by a repeat fasting lipogram and other risk factors have been treated.
(2) Non-pharmacological therapy (diet, healthy life-style) to lower serum TC levels is an essential adjunct to the use of lipid-lowering drugs.

(3) In secondary hyperlipidaemia, the treatment of the underlying disorder is the first priority; only then can lipid-lowering medication be helpful.

For plasmapheresis and surgery for intractable hypercholesterolaemia in familial hypercholesterolaemia (FH), see p. 293.

REFERENCES

(1) Tobias PV. *S Afr Med J* 1972; **46**: 552.

(2) Esterhuizen AJ, Berger GMB. Die laboratorium diagnose van hiperlipidemie. *S Afr J Cont Med Educ* 1984; **2**: 86.

(3) Rossouw JE. The extent and significance of hypercholesterolaemia in South Africa. *S Afr J Cont Med Educ* 1984; **2**: 17–23.

(4) Rossouw JE, Steyn K, Berger, GMB *et al.* Action limits for serum total cholesterol. *S Afr Med J* 1988. **73**: 693–700.

(5) Berger GMB, Watermeyer G. The common familial hyperlipidaemias — a clinical approach to diagnosis and management. *S Afr J Cont Med Educ* 1984; **2**: 25–35.

(6) Seftel HC. What the clinician wants to know about familial hypercholesterolaemia in South Africa — 20 questions and answers. *S Afr J Cont Med Educ* 1984; **2**: 39–46.

(7) Walker ARP. Risk factors in the development of coronary heart disease — nutrition and stress. *S Afr J Cont Med Educ* 1984; **2**: 99–102.

(8) Meyers JE. Correspondence to the *S Afr Med J* 1984; **66**: 545.

(9) Lewis B. Correspondence to the *S Afr Med J* 1984; **66**: 545.

(10) Seedat YK, *et al. S Afr Med J* 1978; **53**: 923.

(11) Rossouw JE. Local epidemiology of acute myocardial infarction. *S Afr J Cont Med Educ* 1988; **6**: 27–31.

(12) Quoted by Hansen JDL. Editorial. *S Afr Med J* 1978. **53**: 153.

(13) DiBianco Robert. Focus on hyperlipidaemia. *S Afr Med J* 1992; February supplement.

(14) Department of National Health and Population Development. *Epidemiological Comments* **19**(9). *Ischaemic heart disease mortality in South Africa, 1985–1989.* Sept. 1992.

TEST OF KNOWLEDGE

The student has benefited from studying this chapter is he/she can answer the following questions:

(1) Define the following terms:
 – atherosclerosis
 – lipoproteins
 – homozygous FH
 – plasmapheresis
 – action limits for serum TC
 – cholesterol
 – VLDL
 – triglycerides
 – xanthoma
 – hyperlipoproteinaemia

(2) Discuss the purpose and findings of the CORIS study.

(3) Discuss the significance and extent of hypercholesterolaemia in atherogenesis in the RSA.

(4) Discuss the risk factors for developing atherosclerosis with special reference to the Western life-style.

(5) Discuss the community primary preventive measures against hypercholesterolaemia and coronary heart disease in the RSA.

(6) Write notes on:
 (a) The significance and function of HDL-C in the blood.
 (b) The prudent diet (refer to Chapter 16).
 (c) The significance of a high LDL-C plasma level.
 (d) Familial hypercholesterolaemia (FH).
 (e) The difference in the mortality rates from CHD between black and other South African population groups.

(7) Discuss:
 (a) the advice with regard to life-style modification you would give a patient who is at moderate risk of developing coronary heart disease;
 (b) the principles of Step 1 lipid-lowering diet;
 (c) the principles of Step 2 lipid-lowering diet;
 (d) pharmacotherapy for patients with serious, intractable hyperlipidaemia.

(8) Distinguish between primary and secondary hyperlipidaemias.

18

Preventive Dentistry

OBJECTIVES

The objective of this chapter is to spell out in no uncertain terms the important role prevention plays in the dental health of a community. The two main prophylactic measures to prevent dental caries and premature loss of teeth are good oral hygiene and induced hardening of tooth enamel by means of fluoride. The latter is especially important from birth to the age of 12 years, the time during which calcification of permanent teeth embedded in the alveolar bone takes place. This is the time span when fluoride should be continuously available for maximum benefit in preventing dental caries.

IN THIS CHAPTER

DISEASES AFFECTING THE TEETH

Dental caries

Tooth decay (dental caries) is the most prevalent disease in the world, approximately 98 % of people being affected. It is one of our major community health problems which can be prevented by fairly simple preventive and health-promotive measures.

Information obtained from examining the skulls of ancient man has revealed that the problem of tooth decay is not a recent one; it was found in Egyptian mummies. Dental caries is prevalent in both developed and underdeveloped countries; it is found in people who live on an unrefined as well as in people who eat a refined diet, although the prevalence in the latter group is higher than in the former. Blacks generally have a lower caries prevalence than whites, irrespective of whether they live in rural areas or in the cities. Staz[1] in 1938 found the following average numbers of carious teeth per mouth in young adult South Africans: rural blacks, 0,71; urban blacks, 4,39; whites, 14,97. The whites, therefore, had 21 times as many carious teeth as the rural blacks. Today much the same picture exists.

Caries may begin the moment a tooth appears in the mouth.

Caries, particularly of the front teeth, is common in infants and toddlers whose bottled feeds contain sweetened fluids, and whose dummies are dipped in honey, vitamin syrup and other sticky solutions.[2] Even milk, human and bovine, is cariogenic, if allowed to be in contact with tooth surfaces long enough, e.g. by prolonged suckling at the breast, or sucking a bottle of milk as an inducement to fall asleep.[2] Peters suggests that after the age of 1 year, the child's bedtime bottle should be gradually diluted until the child receives pure water, if the bottle habit persists at that age. If milk teeth are lost prematurely, the child may never learn to chew properly and permanent teeth may be placed unevenly.

Healthy milk teeth which remain in the mouth until the permanent teeth are ready to erupt are the best way of ensuring that the permanent teeth grow out straight and in their proper position, and of preventing malocclusions, i.e. 'bad bite' or uneven contact between the upper and lower teeth. Malocclusions can interfere with the sound development of teeth and can give rise to periodontal problems, speech defects and jaw deformities.

By the time adulthood is reached, many young people are edentulous. In edentulous people artificial dentures cannot effectively replace the natural dentition. Artificial dentures may be cosmetically unattractive and loss of teeth causes an alteration in the shape of the jaw with the appearance of premature ageing. A person with a full set of artificial dentures can never masticate food as well as a person with natural teeth.

Dental caries is known to be due to the interaction of three factors: cariogenic (decay generating) diet which is the substrate, the teeth after they have erupted, which are the target organs, and the oral microflora which contain the enzymes to break down both the substrate and the target organ. One of the common groups of organisms involved in dental decay is the streptococcus groups, especially *Strep. mutans*. In the absence of one of these three factors, teeth will not decay; for example, teeth embedded in the jaw before eruption cannot be carious. A vaccine made from oral microflora to stop tooth decay in children, has been developed in the UK but is not yet ready for commercial production.

The cariogenic diet is a rather controversial topic in that the role of the implicated carbohydrates in dental caries is not always well understood.

Cariogenic organisms break down carbohydrates into acids which decalcify the enamel of the teeth: this applies to any carbohydrate which adheres to the teeth long enough to form the substrate for the organisms. Refined carbohydrates such as sugar (glucose, sucrose and lactose), honey, toffees, sweets, chocolates, cakes, biscuits and candy floss are harmful as they are sticky and adhere to the teeth, but bread and other foods containing carbohydrates are also dangerous if they remain behind on the teeth and on the gums. All sticky foods are dangerous as far as dental caries is concerned. What is important to understand is that it is not the amount of carbohydrate consumed that is dangerous, but the frequency with which it is consumed and whether or not food particles remain in the mouth on teeth and gums. Sucking a tiny sweet every hour is much more cariogenic than eating 250 g sweets at one sitting; if the teeth are thoroughly cleaned after the latter, no damage should ensue. Fermentable carbohydrate food causes the pH of the mouth to drop from 7,4 to below 5,5 within 2 minutes of placing it in the mouth, due to the fermenting action of the mouth bacteria which cause the formation of acid. Normally the pH is restored to 7,4 approximately 30 minutes after eating a meal, a snack or sweet. In people who eat many snacks between meals, the material covering the teeth therefore remains acid. A non-fermentable sugar made from wood pulp, called xylitol, has recently been suggested to be a valuable anti-decay agent as it does not cause acids to be formed and is, therefore, not cariogenic; it is unfortunately too expensive for everyday use.

Acids decalcify the enamel of the teeth and cause cavities to form. Although enamel is the hardest substance in the body, being composed of calcium salts in crystalline form (98 %) and organic matrix (2 %), it can only be remineralised once it has been damaged in the early stages of decay. Any acids, not only those formed by food break-down, which remain in contact with teeth for some time, decalcify the enamel, there-fore sucking lemons frequently will also cause enamel loss.

Certain acid foods such as cheese will not have this effect because the acidity of the cheese stimulates the flow of saliva which neutralises the acid and protects the enamel.

The areas of the tooth where cavities are likely to form are the pits or fissures on the biting surfaces of the molars and the area of contact of two adjacent teeth and alongside the gum margin. These are the areas where dental plaque is found. **Plaque** is a sticky film which adheres to the surface of teeth, collects under and on the edges of the gums (gingivae), and prevents fluid saliva from getting to debris to wash it away. It consists of bacteria and sticky food debris in a film of adherent saliva. It is in the micro-environment within this plaque that tooth decay begins. Plaque starts reforming the moment it has been removed but it takes 24 hours before it is mature enough to cause damage. Once the enamel surface has been eroded by the acid formed by the bacteria in the plaque, food debris and bacteria accumulate in the resultant opening; the dentine is eventually digested by the bacteria and a spreading cavity undermines the enamel. Eventually the carious

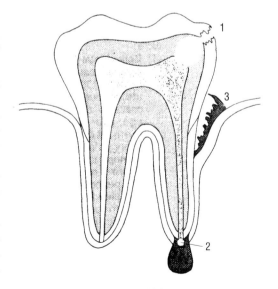

Figure 18.1

Dental and periodontal disease

1. Cavity in tooth enamel
2. Abscess at the root tip
3. Periodontal disease

cavity breaks through into the pulp space and causes excruciating pain. An abscess may form and track down to the apex of the tooth root — an apical abscess. Plaque remains adherent to the tooth unless it is removed by floss or brush. Some plaque left on the teeth will eventually harden into a substance called calculus (tartar). This deposit at or below the gum margin of teeth consists chiefly of hydroxyapatite. It forms a rough surface to which fresh plaque adheres — a vicious cycle which causes tooth, gum and bone disease.

The periodontal diseases (pyorrhoea)

(Periodontal/peridental = around the tooth)
These diseases affect the tissues that surround, support and are attached to the teeth. These tissues include the gingivae (gums), periodontal membrane, the cementum and the alveolar bone. As in the case of dental caries, most periodontal diseases are caused by poor oral hygiene, i.e. failure to completely remove daily plaque from all tooth surfaces and from under the gums. The signs of periodontal diseases are red, swollen, bleeding gums. (*Note:* Healthy gums never bleed; they are pink and firm.) Periodontal diseases may become chronic; then they destroy tissues around the tooth; this leads to

loss of sound teeth usually in adulthood, although the periodontal disease may start in childhood. They can be prevented or stopped through early dental treatment and effective daily oral hygiene.

Periodontal disease usually starts with chronic gingivitis (inflammation of gums). Gum margins begin to recede alongside the teeth, forming pockets in which plaque accumulates, the periodontal membrane surrounding the root of the tooth becomes inflamed and the adjacent alveolar bone destroyed. Periodontal abscesses may also form eventually, causing pus to ooze from the pockets. The teeth become loose and are eventually lost.

Note:
(1) Both dental caries and periodontal disease are caused by plaque and poor oral hygiene. Other factors may also contribute to periodontal disease, e.g. progressive degeneration of tissues with age, poor alignment (biting relation) of teeth, emotional stress, hormonal changes in women during pregnancy and menopause and tartar (calculus).
(2) There is no relationship between scurvy and periodontal disease, despite the fact that bleeding gums may be encountered in both conditions. Vitamin C therapy is of no value in the prevention or treatment of periodontal disease.[3]

Dental trauma during contact sport, e.g. rugby, boxing

Apart from damage to facial bones and soft tissue, front teeth may be fractured or knocked out.

Prevention of damage to front teeth is by the wearing during play of a dental shield specially moulded for the sportsman's upper teeth.

A fractured tooth can be saved by the dentist.

The following first-aid treatment may salvage a knocked out tooth:[6]

- The tooth is held by its crown; on no account must the root be damaged by rubbing off dirt or handling.
- If soiled it is rinsed under a running tap.
- The tooth is then placed back in its socket and held firmly in its correct position for 2 minutes.
- If replacement is impossible, the tooth is protected either in the subject's mouth (between lip and bottom teeth), or wrapped in a clean damp cloth or placed in a glass of milk.

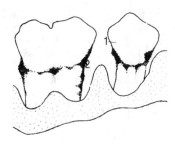

Figure 18.2

Periodontal disease

1. Plaque
2. Soft tissue and bone surrounding tooth destroyed

■ The subject with replaced or non-replaced tooth is taken to a dentist immediately for splinting of the tooth to the two adjacent teeth.

DENTAL HEALTH EDUCATION FOR PREVENTION OF DENTAL CARIES

Health education is needed to prevent tooth decay, especially during the years of childhood when loss of teeth causes malocclusions and interferes with the mastication of food. Where professional dental treatment is available, children should be taught the practical advantages of six-monthly visits to the dentist, even from the third year of life.

All children, black, brown or white, rich or poor, can be taught the importance of preventive dentistry practices: this does not mean that they must forgo the satisfaction of eating certain foods such as sweets and biscuits. It must be remembered that it is not the amount of these satisfiers which causes tooth decay, but the fact that they are eaten between meals and at bedtime — times at which it is unlikely that the teeth will be brushed to rid them of all traces of fermentable carbohydrates. It is also important for the nurse to remember that her bedridden patients are exposed to greater risks of tooth decay during their period of hospitalisation, unless she sees to it that they have the facilities to clean their teeth effectively.

Prevention of dental caries involves good oral hygiene, sensible and sound eating habits, the early and regular visiting of the dentist (for examination and cleaning) and the use of preventive agents such as fluoride and pit and fissure sealants.

Good oral hygiene to prevent dental problems

Instructing children in oral hygiene is the duty of every adult who supervises children, i.e. dentists, nurses, especially school nurses, teachers and parents. The example of parents has the strongest influence on a child's dental health. Parents should be taught to clean their infants' teeth as soon as they erupt. This can be done with a gauze-covered finger at first, and later with a soft child-size toothbrush.[2] Peters quotes evidence that the younger the child when tooth

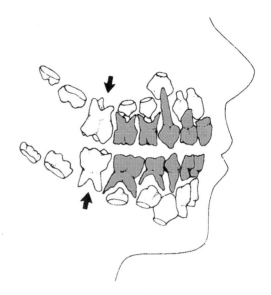

Figure 18.3

Teeth of the six-year-old

The temporary teeth are shaded; the permanent teeth are unshaded. First molars have erupted.

brushing begins, the lower the prevalence of caries.

Every child should be taught to follow a definite routine for life. This daily dental health pattern is aimed at preventing dental caries and periodontal disease by eliminating plaque. Oral hygiene can be made the personal responsibility of every human being and should, therefore, take priority in the fight against dental caries. The Dental Association of South Africa launches a National Dental Health Week every year. To educate pre-primary and primary schoolchildren in oral hygiene or preventive dentistry practices, they recommend the following daily dental care:

(1) Teeth are brushed twice a day for at least one minute at a time, i.e. after breakfast and at bedtime. The thoroughness of brushing must be such that all plaque is removed. This is tested for by running the tip of the tongue over the teeth, which should feel as smooth as glass. Red 'disclosing' tablets can be used to check that plaque is completely removed. After cleaning the teeth, the tablet is chewed and moved about in the mouth for 30 seconds; the mouth is then rinsed. Any area of plaque will be stained red and retain this

colour for an hour unless it is removed by renewed brushing.

Brushing should be systematic, e.g. starting with the outer surface of the upper teeth, two teeth at a time and brushing from the gum downwards to the tips of the teeth. Small circular movements are used and horizontal movements are avoided to prevent the horizontal hollowing out of the surface enamel. The chewing surfaces of the molars are scrubbed clean, using very short horizontal back and forth movements in order to clean the fissures. The inner surfaces of the teeth must always be cleaned. The mouth is rinsed well.

Dentifrices (toothpastes and powders) may be used to assist in the effective cleaning of the teeth but are not essential for oral hygiene. Some toothpastes contain fluorides and are to be recommended for their enamel-hardening properties. For this purpose, fluoride mouth-rinses are also available. Toothbrushes should be procurable by everyone in South Africa; there is, however, the possibility that some people may plead poverty for their lack of this essential instrument of dental hygiene. In this case, the index finger can be used with plain water, salt or soda-bic. to rub the tooth surfaces and the mouth can be rinsed very thoroughly.

(2) The mouth should be rinsed with cold water on rising, after lunch, whenever sticky food has been eaten between meals and immediately after supper. This will help get rid of some food particles and bacteria and will dilute the acid that they form.

(3) The teeth should be flossed after supper, before the final brushing of the day. Flossing, i.e. the pulling through of dental floss (nylon thread obtainable from the chemist) between each two adjacent teeth, should be done gently so as not to damage the gums — as evidenced by bleeding. Flossing is done to remove plaque from between the teeth where the bristles of the toothbrush cannot penetrate because teeth are usually set too close together.

Sound eating habits

A good diet in the pregnant woman and in the growing child strengthens children's teeth. A child whose food (or whose mother's food in the case of breast-feeding) is prepared with fluoridated water from birth has more chance of having strong permanent teeth. If snacks are eaten between main meals, e.g. by schoolchildren, they should consist of low-fermentable foods such as cheese, fruit juices, milk, potato chips, biltong, fruit and raw vegetables. All sticky foods should be avoided between meals and at bedtime unless the mouth can be cleaned immediately afterwards.

Note: Certain medicines stain and damage the teeth and should be taken through a straw, e.g. iron mixtures which stain and diluted hydrochloric acid which erodes the teeth. Tetracyclines given to pregnant women and young children (while the dentition is forming) cause hypoplasia of enamel of the primary teeth and may cause pigmentation (yellow or brown discoloration) of teeth. The damage may predispose to dental caries. Tetracyclines are deposited in calcifying areas in bone and in teeth, both erupted and unerupted. Unerupted teeth may have the material deposited throughout their structure, while erupted teeth have the tetracycline deposited in their roots.

Visits to a dentist

The dentist should be visited at least every six months (where his services are available) for:

(1) dental inspection for early detection and filling of small cavities;
(2) orthodontic treatment of malaligned teeth;
(3) professional oral hygiene for the removal of all deposits on teeth, around the gums, particularly calculus (tartar);
(4) the treatment of periodontal disease;
(5) fluoride dental treatment and the application of pit and fissure sealants.

The preventive agent, fluoride

Although counselling with regard to oral hygiene must always come first in any preventive dental health programme, the counsel of perfection with regard to mouth care is difficult to attain. For this reason the most effective global way of preventing dental caries is to make the teeth more resistant to the onslaughts of dental plaque. This can be done with **fluorides** which have a direct hardening effect on the enamel of the teeth. When contact is made with tooth enamel, soluble calcium hydroxyapatite is converted to insoluble calcium fluoroapatite in the enamel, making it hard and acid-resistant.

It also remineralises eroded enamel. Whereas the untreated tooth may become eroded at a salivary pH of 6, a fluoridised tooth could resist a pH of 5,5 before damage is done. Fluorides do not give absolute protection against dental decay — they merely strengthen the teeth.

The essential trace element fluorine is found abundantly (in nature in rocks and soil and, therefore, in most waters) in combination with other elements as fluorides. In the body it is stored in bones and teeth, the more fluoride found in water, the greater the uptake by teeth (enamel and dentine) and bones. Once a tooth is fully formed (aged 12), fluoride uptake is superficial.

Note: In some areas on earth the natural water contains high concentrations of fluorides. This may cause dental fluorosis characterised by a mottling of the teeth.

Contact of the teeth with *soluble fluorides* can be brought about by:

(1) the fluoridation of water supplies of a community; the fluorides are absorbed and make contact with the teeth via the tooth pulp as well as saliva (in which fluoride is secreted);
(2) the systemic administration of fluorides; and
(3) topical fluoride therapy for those without access to fluoridated water.

Methods (2) and (3) play an important role in preventive dentistry in South Africa. Unfortunately at present due to high cost it can be afforded by the privileged classes only.

Fluoridation of water supplies

Many studies have shown that a low incidence of caries in the permanent dentition is associated with a high fluoride water level (and a low intake of sucrose between meals). People who use artificially fluoridated water are 50 % less likely to develop dental caries without taking any other preventive measures.[4]

Fluorides occur naturally in water but usually in insufficient amounts. Fluoridation of drinking water supplies of a community is generally considered the best method of preventing dental caries, as no one is excluded from preventive care through poverty and lack of privi-

lege. This statement is qualified, however, by the fact that in our rural areas, all sections of the population do not receive tapped water from a communal supply which can be subjected to a fluoridation scheme.

Fluorides are enzymatic poisons but the strength used for the fluoridation of public water supplies (1 part per million — 1 p.p.m.) is not toxic. Fluoridation schemes are used extensively in the United States of America and are endorsed by the WHO (World Health Organization). Fluoridation schemes function in thirty countries and serve a population of 150 million people. Fluoridation of water supplies is not currently in operation in South Africa.

The government is interested in legalising this preventive measure and in 1967 appointed a Commission of Enquiry into fluoridation in order to examine the arguments for and against the process. The commission reported overwhelmingly in favour of fluoridation and recommended that 'Steps should be taken to encourage, advise and assist local authorities to fluoridate the water supplies of their communities as soon as possible.'

In the concentration recommended of 1 part per million (even less in the RSA), the procedure is completely safe for health. This concept is supported by world-wide research and by such influential bodies as the American Dental Association, the Royal College of Physicians of London and the Dental Association of South Africa as well as many other organisations. The 'antifluoridationists' would argue that the continuous ingestion of fluorides could cause systemic fluorosis, a condition of chronic fluoride intoxication with renal damage and even cancer. They fear poisoning, and postulate that the benefits of fluoridation are uncertain. Echoing the sentiments of the conscientious objectors against compulsory smallpox vaccination, they offer the argument that fluoridation of the public water supplies is a violation of the individual's freedom to choose whether he will submit to public health measures or not. The 'antifluoridationists' are a formidable group as they can influence the legislation which is required for compulsory fluoridation of public water supplies. As their arguments are based on emotional premises, education propaganda may sway public opinion in favour of fluoridation of water supplies for domestic use.

Fluoridation follow-up

A committee which reviewed ongoing research in the RSA on fluoride, recommended recently (1990) to the MRC and to researchers what the priorities in fluoride research should be.

A summary of their findings follows:

Extensive research data about the advantages and disadvantages of fluoride on teeth are available. Present knowledge indicates that water fluoridation is the cheapest, safest and most effective way of preventing tooth decay. But, as country-wide fluoridation of water supplies may take many years, differentiated, monitored and structured preventive fluoride programmes should be implemented. This should take place with the co-operation of the DOH and the private sector, with the MRC as a central co-ordinating body.

Fundamental research, apart from applied research, is important to discover: the systemic effects of fluorosis; mechanism and cellular action of fluoride in man and animals; and the therapeutic use of fluoride e.g. in osteoporosis.

Systemic administration of fluoride-containing tablets

The daily intake of fluorides in tablet form, from birth to the age of 12 years, is as valuable a method of preventing dental caries as fluoridation of the water supplies.

In infants, 0,25mg sodium fluoride (e.g. 1 tablet Zymofluor) is crushed and dissolved in the feed. The dose is increased to 4 tablets (i.e. 1 mg per day) in older children who must be persuaded to chew or suck the tablets for their additional topical effect. Regular and continuous use is essential for maximal benefit.

Note:
(1) Gross overdosage (100 mg fluoride for a toddler) may be lethal. This is equivalent to 400 of the 0,25 mg tablets. Fluoride tablets must be kept out of reach of children.
(2) Supplemental fluorides should not be given if the natural fluoride level of the drinking water available exceeds 0,7 p.p.m. The Department of National Health and Population Development will, on request, assist in the determination of the fluoride content of drinking water.[5]

Topical administration of fluoride

(Topical administration of fluorides by dentists or oral hygienists, after the teeth have been cleaned)

Professional administration. This is done with the greatest advantage to teeth as soon as they have erupted because at this stage the enamel incorporates minerals from the mouth with great ease. The preparations used are flavoured gels, solutions, varnishes and pastes.

Gels and solutions are applied to the teeth either with cotton pellets or in dental trays (either preformed or individually moulded), either filled with the gel or lined with filter paper saturated with the fluoride solution. Fluoride can thus be applied to the upper or lower dental arch by allowing the child to bite into the tray, thereby getting close contact of the teeth with the fluoride preparation.

Self-administration

(1) Fluoridated toothpastes used regularly reduce dental caries considerably. Because of their low content of fluoride ions they are safe for children to use.
(2) Mouthwashes with fluoride, if used regularly, i.e. daily, also reduce tooth decay.
(3) Kits for the self-administration of fluoride gel are available for use by responsible persons. The gel is applied in preformed trays in the same way as the professionally administered gel.

The preventive agents: pit and fissure sealants

Pit and fissure sealants are materials painted on to the surface of teeth every 6–18 months by a dentist or oral hygienist to prevent debris (food and *Strep. mutans*) from getting into the crevices of teeth and causing fissure caries.

DENTAL CLINICS

Dental clinics cater mainly for children, being geared to primary and secondary preventive work for the indigent sections of the community, who cannot afford to go to private dentists. Community dental clinics are not administered uniformly in the RSA.

Generally it can be stated that dental clinics operate to implement the Health Act 63 of 1977 which aims at bringing comprehensive medical (including dental) care to all sections of the community, rich or indigent, black, brown or white. Unfortunately there are not enough dentists available to put official policy fully into operation. In order to assist the country's dentists in their task, the following classes of assistants are being trained:

The dental therapist

The dental therapist is a new category of dental worker. At present blacks are given an in-service training lasting three years, only at Ga-Rankuwa Hospital in the northern Transvaal, to work amongst blacks. The dental therapist is allowed to do the work of the dental oral hygienist and may also do simple fillings and extractions.

Dental oral hygienists

Dental oral hygienists who train for 1,5 to 2 years at the dental schools of the Universities of the Witwatersrand, Pretoria and Stellenbosch.

Oral hygienists play an important role in preventing dental caries and periodontal diseases. Trained oral hygienists are registered with the South African Medical and Dental Council and rank as paradental health personnel.

The law requires that a registered oral hygienist shall not:

(1) undertake any work in oral hygiene except under the direction and control of a registered dentist;

(2) advertise himself to obtain work to promote his own professional interests.

The role of the oral hygienist was created to assist dentists to meet the dental health needs of all citizens. Better dental care can be given to more people by using dental auxiliaries to carry out certain clinical functions, e.g.:

(1) cleaning teeth by removing stains, plaque and calculus;

(2) applying fluorides and fissure sealants to prevent dental caries;

(3) teaching people how to prevent caries and periodontal diseases.

By assisting the dentist in this way, the latter is freed to meet the more specialised dental needs of his patients.

N.B.: Dental services for blacks are still inadequate due to manpower shortage. Non-white dentists are being trained at the Universities of the Witwatersrand and Western Cape, and lately, at MEDUNSA.

School dental clinic services

Operating from dental clinics, the dental staff, dentists and oral hygienists visit schools to do dental inspections. After inspecting the teeth of schoolchildren to see what requires to be done, the dental team informs the parents of the dental needs of their children. The responsibility rests with the school principal to decide whether parents can afford to go to private dentists or whether the free services of clinics are indicated. The principal will issue the authority for free dental treatment to the parents and will send the clinic a list of the names of children eligible for free treatment. The clinic then books appointments for the year. The dental clinic often transports children *en masse* from the school to the clinic during school hours. Children from institutions always qualify for free dental care and get regular appointments for 'check-ups'.

Treatment at the dental clinic is comprehensive; fillings, extractions, restorative work, cleaning of teeth, application of fluorides and fissure sealants, as well as education in the prevention of dental caries and periodontal disease. Orthodontic treatment is available on a limited basis as it is very time-consuming.

The Department of Community Dentistry of the University of the Witwatersrand recently (1985) launched a unique mobile dental unit. It visits hospitals and schools in the Witwatersrand area and in rural areas of southern Africa.

ORAL HEALTH

A National Oral Health Survey (NOHS) was carried out in 1988/1989 in the five metropolitan regions of the RSA by the government departments of health and the departments of community dentistry in order to devise 'The Population Strategy' for improving dental health.[7]

A steering committee was formed to formulate a national health plan and in 1993 the interim report for such a plan was completed.

Some of the results of the survey are compared with WHO goals for HFA 2000:

(1) WHO goal: 50 % of 6-year-olds must be caries-free. RSA: 30 %
(2) In South African 12-year-olds the DMFT (Decayed, Missing, Filled Teeth) was within the WHO goal. In the RSA by the age of 15 years there is a doubling of the 12-year-old caries rate – so there is no room for complacency.
(3) WHO goal: 75 % of the population should retain a minimum of 20 functional teeth at the age of 35–44 years. The finding in the RSA was favourable, except amongst the coloured population group where there is a high level of edentulousness.
(4) The survey showed that gingivitis and calculus are widespread in the RSA. It also found a backlog of treatment needs but realised that the top priority for the RSA is oral health promotion, disease prevention and the conservation of tooth structure – subjects that fall within the Primary Health Care approach.

Preventive strategy means targeting specific, high-risk populations and instituting oral hygiene: effective brushing, fluoride applications and the use of toothpastes containing anti-plaque, anti-tartar and anti-gingival agents.

To implement this strategy requires a PHC team led by dental personnel with community health workers, PHC nurses, health educators and school teachers. The main target group are the primary school children.

Primary oral health care in a rural black community

In a South African study on blacks in KaNgwane[8] it was found that, although the dental caries prevalence rate is low, urbanisation causes an increased rate. The prevalence of periodontal disease is high as is the percentage of 12-year-old children with calculus.

In Third-World sections of the population, traditionally curatively oriented, expensive modern dentistry cannot cope with the oral health problems. Except for the need for dentures, the demand for sophisticated dental treatment is low, although it is available by private dentists in nearby 'white towns'.

Du Plessis[8] suggests and is implementing primary oral health care in KaNgwane and suggests that this care be extended on a national scale.

The PHC principles of oral care are:

(1) The full co-operation and participation of the community must be obtained. This entails discussing every step taken with the leaders in order to obtain their consent.
(2) A community diagnosis of the dental health of the community must be made to determine oral health hazards, what the people can do to prevent them and what they can afford to pay towards the implementation of a practical treatment programme (e.g. toothbrushes and dental paste).
(3) Relief of pain and control of sepsis are the highest priority demands of a developing community and can be addressed by the extraction of carious teeth as an emergency manoeuvre. Where there is a shortage of dentists or dental therapists, clinic nurses can be trained and utilised for emergency extractions in their own working environment. The SA Nursing Council rules that a nurse may perform any task for which she has been trained and, as a result of the KaNgwane experience, a training programme has been prepared.

The SA Medical and Dental Council conditionally granted permission to a request by the KaNgwane government for nurses to do emergency extractions.
(4) Primary prevention must be the first priority of dental services, especially the prevention of periodontal disease. Teachers trained in oral preventive work at their Colleges of Education are requested to teach oral hygiene to primary school children. This entails the brushing of teeth with fluoridated toothpaste during school hours.

Note: The thorny issue of the fluoridation of the water supplies of the community must be raised repeatedly with the authorities.

(5) The secondary preventive measures (filling of cavities and the removal of calculus) by the dental personnel of school dental services, usually based in regional hospitals,

must be included in Primary Oral Health Care Programmes.

(6) Health Education must be given, especially to parents, to resist the persuasive arguments of the advertisement media about the energy-providing advantages of sweets and sugar.

REFERENCES

(1) Staz J. (1938) *S Afr Med Sci*; **3**: Suppl. 1.

(2) Peters R. Dental health for the preschool child. *S Afr J CME*. 1986; **3**: 55–60.

(3) Touyz LZG. Vitamin C, oral scurvy and periodontal disease. *S Afr Med J* 1984; **65**: 838–842.

(4) Quoted from Bischoff J, *et al. J Dent Ass S Afr;* **30**: 333.

(5) The Dental Association of South Africa. *Fluoride facts for the health professions in South Africa.* Ciba-Geigy.

(6) Joubert J J de V. Die noodbehandeling en voorkoming van tand- en kaakbeserings tydens sportdeelname. *S Afr J C M E* 1985; **3**: 55–59.

(7) Rudolph, MJ. Oral Health: A model for approaching health promotion and disease control. *S Afr J Epidemiol Infect* 1993; **8**(2)

(8) Du Plessis, JB. The problems of providing dental services – in the rural areas of South Africa. *CHASA* 1990; 61–65.

TEST OF KNOWLEDGE

The student has benefited from studying this chapter if he/she can answer the following questions:

(1) State the main points of a didactic lecture you would give to a group of young mothers on how to prevent dental caries and periodontal disease in their children.

(2) Discuss the role of fermentable (refined) carbohydrates in the aetiology of dental caries. How can caries be prevented in a year-old child?

(3) Distinguish between the following paired words:
   – plaque/calculus (tartar)
   – enamel/dentine
   – calcium hydroxyapatite/calcium fluoroapatite
   – dental fluorosis/systemic fluorosis

(4) Name the main points you would stress in teaching a child a tooth-cleaning routine and general dental hygiene.

(5) (*a*) What is fluorine, how and where is it found in nature and why is it essential in human nutrition?
   (*b*) Discuss the fluoridation of public water supplies with regard to its reputed dangers and its benefits.

(6) How are dental assistants (auxiliaries) used in the RSA as the extended arm of the dentist?

(7) How would you, as a clinic sister, run a primary, oral, health care service for primary school children in a rural area?

19

School Nursing
Some Problems of Adolescence

OBJECTIVES

School health (medical and nursing) services in South Africa are aimed at health surveillance of all scholars in government schools from the age of 5 to 18 years, to ensure that every child shall benefit from education through health. Some school problems of the primary school child are discussed briefly to give the student nurse some idea of the common problems with which teachers have to contend, viz. the attention deficit disorder, school phobia and learning problems.

A large part of this chapter is devoted to teenage pregnancy, the tragedy this causes in the life of a schoolgirl, and the attempts being made by family planning clinics to curb this social evil which is still growing in intensity.

Drug abuse, including smoking and drinking, is another problem among teenagers which is on the increase but which is poorly researched in our schools. The school nurse must be aware of these two great evils in our schools, which ruin the lives of many adolescents. These problems have their inception in the primary schools. Health education should be vigorously aimed at this vulnerable group.

Suicide and parasuicide, anorexia nervosa and bulimia are psychiatric disturbances which occur in apparently normal children and adolescents.

THE OBJECTIVES OF SCHOOL HEALTH SERVICES

(1) To promote health and prevent physical and psychological problems which may lead to antisocial behaviour, by the early identification of problems and referral for treatment at specialised clinics of provincial hospitals, dental clinics, and to social workers, ministers of religion, physiotherapists and occupational therapists.

(2) To create a health climate in schools so that the child may benefit maximally from the teaching programme.

(3) By health guidance in co-operation with the educationists, to support and guide scholars and their parents, so that each child may develop into a healthy, happy and balanced individual.

(4) Inspection of schools and hostels and their environs for health risks, amongst others, ventilation and lighting, toilet facilities, method of water supply, garbage disposal and first-aid equipment.

Note: School nursing is a subdivision of community nursing and the school nurse needs the following professional qualifications:

- General nursing diploma;
- Midwifery and psychiatric nursing diploma;
- The integrated nursing diploma.

A diploma in community nursing is a recommendation.

School nurses should attend in-service training programmes directed at maintaining an acceptable standard of practice in health screening, counselling and health education in particular.

Modern family life with both parents working and single parent families create problems when children's needs for supervision and the profitable spending of free time are not catered for. Parents often have to rely on community services to supplement their basic functions. These services are not always available, or are not used by the older child with resultant child neglect.

SCHOOL HEALTH SERVICES

The aim of the health surveillance function is to ensure that every child shall benefit from education through health. This aim is achieved through the physical examination of children and through recommendations for treatment made to school principals, the child's parents or guardians and family doctors. Physical examination in government schools is compulsory but involves neither treatment nor anything of a nature likely to cause pain or inconvenience to the child. The parent or guardian is notified of the date of the examination and is invited to be present if he is concerned about some aspect of his child's health.

Each school nurse is responsible for approximately 7 000 scholars in pre-primary, primary, high, special and clinic schools. These scholars generate many health statistics which are communicated stepwise to Head Office every three months. Organisational control by inspection of work and receipt of reports, work itineraries and programmes is exerted by the nursing service manager/chief nursing officer: School Health Services.

It is important for the school nurse to maintain a relationship of co-operation and consultative communication with the teaching staff and education support and other welfare services. She assists at the medical examination of students for teacher's training colleges.

All children in schools which qualify for school medical services are subjected to a medical examination by a doctor and/or a school nurse. In primary schools this is done in Grade 1 and Standard 5.

Apart from the regular examination of target groups, teachers are required to identify children with health problems in other classes and refer them for medical examination.

Physical examination and the school nurse

The school nurse helps the doctor with medical examinations or screens for physical and behavioural disorders and refers for medical attention. Abnormal findings and recommendations for treatment are communicated personally by the school nurse to the parent(s). Between medical examinations, the school nurse pays health visits once a year to the schools for which she is responsible. She keeps a health report card on every child on which is recorded his mass, height, any visible orthopaedic defects and their treatment, poor posture. The school nurse examines ears, skin, throat, teeth and notes discharges from any orifices. The types of physical problems which merit priority are those of the special senses. From the time the child enters school, sight and hearing are tested at intervals, sight by means of Snellen's eye-test cards and hearing with an audiometer.

The school nurse must be aware of the signs of malnutrition (both overmass and undermass) and poor personal hygiene. If any infestations such as scabies or head lice are detected during a health visit to a school, the parents are notified and the child excluded from school until treated and pronounced free from infestation. The child can attend the school clinic, accompanied by an adult, for treatment by the school nurse for these conditions. In the areas where doctors are not freely available, medical tasks of a primary health care nature are delegated to the school nurse who works under the long-distance direction of a doctor. Primary health care school nurses should be trained in the use of the stethoscope (for examining the heart and lungs), the ophthalmoscope and the auroscope so that some children are not deprived of expert health surveillance.

The suitably trained primary health care nurse should be able to detect heart murmurs, asthma, diabetes mellitus (by urine tests), epilepsy and recommend referral to appropriate medical services.

Eyes are examined for strabismus, conjunctivitis, nystagmus, corneal scarring, blepharitis and vitamin A deficiency (see p. 213). The adequacy of speech and neurological development is assessed.

The headmaster is held responsible for ensuring that all the children in his school have been immunised against poliomyelitis, diphtheria and tuberculosis. At the instigation of the school medical team, the principal warns parents that their children will be excluded from school unless they are vaccinated against polio before a fixed time, or unless they have a certificate of exemption.

Follow-up checks by the school nurse

When the school nurse does follow-up checks three months after the doctor's examination and recommendations for treatment and finds untreated cases, she will do home visits in order to initiate positive action.

If parents are unable to afford private medical and dental services, they are advised to take their children to one of the following:

- Provincial hospitals
- Municipal clinics
- Welfare services
- Dental services
- District Surgeons
- Community health centres and clinics
- Genetic services.

Where parents cannot pay for glasses or hearing aids, children can be referred by a school clinic (which has the authority to authorise the supply of glasses and hearing aids) to specialist departments in provincial hospitals.

Health education and the school nurse

The school nurse can talk to groups of children during her health examinations on the topic of personal hygiene. She consults with and co-operates with the teaching personnel.

Health education talks can be presented to parents during home visits and at parent-teacher meetings in which school nurses and doctors should be closely involved.

Sex education and the scholar

Selected teachers, both men and women, receive intensive training to enable them to plan the subject of sex education with great caution and circumspection and to present it in accordance with the developmental level of the scholars. If any specific needs with regard to sex education, birth control and teenage pregnancy are identified, health education is given informally to individuals or groups of scholars. For 'AIDS education for children', see Chapter 34.

Whether the school nurse is utilised to her full potential as a community nurse is a moot point. Health education and health promotion, both in the classroom and in the home, should be of the same importance in the role of the school nurse as the physical health surveillance tasks aimed at prevention of physical ill-health.

Smoking, especially in the primary school child, drug abuse and other problems of adolescence are important health concerns which merit attention by school doctors and nurses.

PHC and the black school nurse

Social conditions amongst the South African population groups are different and school nursing procedures require modification to the basic pattern. Wagstaff *et al.*[18] found (in a Soweto study) that only a small percentage of children referred for further medical attention, received further care. What is more, except for dental and learning problems, most of the health problems can be managed by the nurse at a school-based primary health care level. The role and functions of the black school nurse can and are being extended to include the curative care of common medical problems, e.g. sore throat. This meets the special needs of black schoolchildren whose parents seldom have the time or money to take them to a doctor, clinic or hospital for minor indispositions which could be managed by a primary health care nurse.

Note: PHC nurses at the Soweto clinics manage 80 % of sick children who attend their clinics.

Endeavours to promote the total well-being of black scholars need a large number of specially trained primary health care nurses. This kind of training is the answer to many health problems encountered in developing populations.

SCHOOLING PROBLEMS AND THE SCHOOL NURSE
Learning problems

Counselling and psychiatric services for children are available in the larger centres in South Africa. The school nurse can make use of the services by recommending referral of children in her care who present with emotional and persistent learning problems.

Learning problems with emotional sequelae

In the primary school child, early recognition of learning problems and remedial education to overcome these problems in an atmosphere of understanding and support will help to prevent the anger, discouragement, antisocial behaviour and depression of children with learning problems. Concomitant efforts by child guidance clinics and family therapists to help parents to lower their expectations of their learning-handicapped child will prevent poor parent-child relationships and family pathology.

Emotional problems causing under-achievement

The primary school child is emotionally vulnerable and may find it difficult to separate emotionally from his parents (i.e. become relatively independent) in order to form satisfying peer group relationships. Separation anxiety (precipitated when he is forced to leave the home physically in order to go to school), psychosomatic problems (due to his inability to express his fears and angers) and depression due to feelings of inadequacy and rejection by peers, prevent children from learning and achieving according to their potential intelligence. Under-achieving by a child causes much frustration and anxiety to child, teacher and parents.

In urban areas the following community child and family psychiatric services, as defined by the Mental Health Act of 1973, are generally available: child guidance clinics; child psychiatric units.

Note: The Departments of Education and Culture run school psychological services which do not fall under the jurisdiction of the Mental Health Act of 1973. The staff of this service investigates and handles learning problems, as well as behaviour problems which disrupt instruction in the classroom.

School phobia — school refusal

School phobia is the failure to attend school despite the scholastic and physical capacity to do so. The school phobic child does good school work and is worried about missing school but the fear related to some aspect of school is so overwhelming that he has little control over his school refusal. He feels safe at home.

The school phobic child often develops psychosomatic symptoms which are offered as an excuse for missing school but which disappear if he is allowed to stay at home.

The phobic child may develop panic attacks when it is time to leave for school or he may reach school and rush home in a state of anxiety.

In younger children the onset is usually acute but in older children and adolescents the phobia may develop more gradually; it may occur at any age.

School phobia is a neurotic phenomenon with conflicts about separation from the mother and individuation (independence). The child usually feels ambivalent towards his mother and fears something will happen to her or that she may abandon him in his absence. The fears are unconsciously displaced on to the school. The problem has its roots in family relationships, of special importance being the parental relationships. Acute school phobia is a psychiatric emergency which is handled by immediate return of the child to school before the problem becomes intractable. The child is handled by a therapist (social worker, psychiatric nurse, or psychologist) and the parents are enlightened as to familial origin of the problem. Either the parents or the therapist accompany the child to school in the morning when the problem is at its worst and stay with the child for a while until he settles down. The doctor may prescribe anxiolytics for a limited period to help the child cope with the separation anxiety. Family therapy is commenced as soon as the child is back at school and later the problems between the parents may be sorted out in marital therapy. For

successful outcome, close co-operation between therapist, parents and school is important.

The attention deficit disorder

This is the DSM III name for a syndrome affecting schoolchildren, mostly boys, who cause disruption in the classroom through hyperactive behaviour and an inability to attend and concentrate on a task for any length of time. Other names used for this syndrome in the past are: the hyperkinetic (hyperactivity) syndrome, minimal brain dysfunction. Normal healthy primary school children are active and flit from one activity to another and it may be difficult to decide when the natural exuberance of children and their limited attention span reach the abnormal. Leary[19] suggests that when distractibility and sustained motor activity prevent a child from developing abilities and skills appropriate to his age, then he may be suffering from a pathological condition.

Some *causes of hyperactivity* and inability to concentrate and pay attention:

(1) Anxiety caused by family problems, inability to cope intellectually and peer group bullying.

(2) Hunger in the neglected child.

(3) Inadequately controlled asthma with hypoxia.

(4) Partial hearing loss, the child becoming bored when he cannot follow the lesson.

When these causes of hyperactivity and distractibility have been excluded by successful treatment, we are left with the child who, because of neurological immaturity, has a short attention span, cannot complete given tasks, is given to day-dreaming, reads with difficulty, develops a spidery handwriting and may or may not be hyperactive. This is the child with the true DSM III 'attention deficit disorder' who can be helped with stimulant medication. The stimulant used for this purpose is methylphenidate (Ritalin), a Schedule 7 substance. Ritalin is a central nervous system stimulant and, if it is used for the attention deficit disorder in childhood, has a paradoxical calming effect which helps the child to concentrate and learn.

Conditions for use of methylphenidate (Ritalin):

(1) It is obtainable only on medical prescription.
(2) A dosage of 0,5 mg/kg/d is administered after breakfast on school mornings only and only once a day. Weekends and holidays are medicine-free. If the child is not hyperactive a smaller dose of 0,3 mg/kg/d is given.[19]
(3) Maximum effect lasts for 4–5 hours and should cover the school period.
(4) If the medication does not have a dramatic, almost immediate effect, it should be discontinued as it is then not the appropriate medicine. If a child is on a larger dose than 20 mg/d, medication is ineffective and other causes and treatment for the symptoms must be sought.
(5) The drug is not used in pre-school children and teenagers. Its effects are inclined to be stimulating after the age of twelve years and the danger of developing a dependence on Ritalin must always be borne in mind.
(6) No child should be given Ritalin for longer than six months without a two-week trial period off Ritalin. If the child's teacher reports no deterioration in work and classroom behaviour, it may be assumed that neurological maturation has occurred and the child no longer needs the drug. If the child relapses, Ritalin is continued for another six months.[19]

It is a dangerous practice to keep a child on Ritalin for years.

Side-effects of Ritalin:

(1) Insomnia and poor appetite.
(2) Suppression of growth. This is reversible on discontinuation of the drug.
(3) Addiction to stimulants, especially if therapy continues into adolescence.

These side-effects may be avoided with the cautious approach to Ritalin therapy as outlined above.

CHILD ABUSE AND NEGLECT AND THE SCHOOL NURSE

Teachers may report emotional and behavioural disturbances in children, e.g. excessive masturbation in class in full view of other pupils. The school nurse must then pay a home visit and, if necessary, refer the child and his family for investigation and treatment to a child psychiatric unit. She can also bring to the notice of the psychiatric community nurse and social welfare agencies severe family problems she meets on her home visits. Child abuse is frequently perpetrated on primary schoolchildren. Teachers and school nurses should be aware of the signs of child neglect and abuse (see p. 422) and become involved in this social problem.

The school nurse, as member of the multi-disciplinary health and welfare team and in touch with children at school health clinics and at schools, is likely to detect child abuse and neglect during the physical examination. She is legally obliged to notify the police.

The school nurse will refer the child to a Child Abuse Unit at a provincial hospital and the family to a child and family institute or child welfare society. Whatever the court's decision may be, the continuing support of the family by means of home visits either by the school or the community nurse is needed. Parents who fail their children need to be motivated to co-operate in the child welfare or other treatment programme. They need to be taught the principles involved in establishing good family relationships (see p. 400).

SOME PROBLEMS OF ADOLESCENCE

Teenage pregnancy (TAP)

Van Coeverden de Groot describes TAP as 'the premier social evil of the Third World',[2] and 'a major social evil'.[3] Teenage pregnancy is a socio-economic problem. In 1986 there was an explosion of this problem in Cape Town primarily as a result of the high prevalence of unplanned and unprotected coitus among teenagers.

Consequences of TAP:

(1) The girl drops out of school and becomes educationally and vocationally disadvantaged and poor.
(2) The infants of young TAP mothers have high perinatal and infant mortality rates; some are abandoned and others abused.

In a study done in rural Transkei[4] it was found that adolescence *per se* confers no increased obstetric risks. Unwed motherhood, however, constitutes a most disturbing social trend in black rural society because of its implications for family life and community stability. This should be the focus of concern for health care workers.

Education for sexual responsibility should start in the home and continue throughout the school years. For those teenagers who opt for early coitus, contraception especially geared for teenagers should be provided.

While ignorance regarding sexual functions and irresponsibility are important causes of the rising incidence of teenage pregnancy, some adolescents regard contraceptives as very dangerous and are unable to weigh up the risks of contraception and unprotected coitus. This confusion minimises the value of educational interventions aimed at increasing the rate of protection against pregnancy.

In a study done at a teenage clinic in Cape Town[3] it was found that the earlier the age of menarche, the higher the prevalence of coitus at an early age. Young age at first coitus, i.e. under 12 years, is associated with higher prevalence of multiple sex partners (promiscuity) and smoking, and a longer period of unprotected coitus. Those who start coitus after the age of 19 are more likely to use contraception from first coitus, i.e. they practise responsible sex. Earlier sexual maturity therefore leads to earlier sexual activity; sexual maturity does not imply psychosocial maturity. Early age at first coitus is also associated with single-parent families. These results indicate the need for sex education in junior school to reach the large number of girls who start menstruating before they enter high school.

Teenage contraception and parental consent

Section 39 of the Child Care Act 74 of 1983 reads:

'39(4). Notwithstanding any rule of law to the contrary, any person over the age of 18 years shall be competent to consent without the assistance of his parent or guardian, to the performance of any operation upon or any medical treatment for himself.'

This includes contraception.

The doctor's position with regard to prescribing contraceptives to a minor (below 18) without parental consent is not legally defined. The Medical Association of South Africa advises doctors to adopt the following guidelines in prescribing contraceptives: (*a*) doctors can prescribe contraceptives to sexually active minors, but they must make every effort to obtain the client's permission to inform her parents thereof; and (*b*) in the case of a complaint by parents the doctor must cease the treatment immediately.[5]

Note: It is a criminal offence for any male to have intercourse with a girl below the age of 16. Sixteen is the legal age of consent for sexual intercourse.

National Adolescent Programme of the DOH

The National Adolescent Programme was developed by the DNHPD: Directorate of Family Planning, in 1984. In 1983 it had been discovered that 30 % of all family planning clients requiring a contraceptive service were teenagers. In 1987/88 there were 1,8 million visits by teenagers to the 57 **Youth Health Centres** of Family Planning Clinics. There is some resistance to sexuality education from parents, schools and religious institutions; more teenage males need to become involved in the programme.

Objectives of the National Adolescent Programme

Apart from sexuality and contraception education, the programme teaches teenagers interpersonal and life skills; they are taught how to communicate with adults with regard to sexuality and with the opposite sex and how to say 'No'. The programme is also geared to involve adolescent males so that men will ultimately share an equal responsibility for reproductive health. The teenagers are given all the necessary information so that they may make an informed, responsible decision about their sex lives. The more they know, the less likely they are to experiment.

The **Youth Health Centres** are hoping to lower the rate of unintended pregnancies and raise the age of first coitus. Early coitus often leads to promiscuity, smoking, sexually transmitted diseases (AIDS, HPV and HSV infection) and the subsequent danger of cancer of the cervix. Many children are in conflict about sex because of contradictory misinformation. Sex may be classified as 'bad' together with drugs and alcohol; on the other hand, premarital sex is romanticised in the media and peer pressure makes it the 'in thing' — the answer to loneliness and the way to get love and attention. Pregnancy is, therefore, a great risk in the emotionally deprived teenager or in the girl who feels unattractive to the opposite sex. Unfortunately the romantic soap operas of screen and TV do not make the teenager aware of the need for contraception and avoidance of STDs.

At present, adolescent services are rendered under the auspices of the Provincial Administrations by specially selected and trained professional nurses, liaison officers and advisers at:

(1) Youth health centres, for the use of adolescents only.
(2) Specific clinic sessions at adult family planning clinics for adolescents.
(3) In the community at
    – schools
    – school camps
    – special youth projects

The services offered include:

(1) Individual Counselling with
    – adolescents
    – adolescents and their parents
(2) Group counselling with homogeneous groups like
    – single adolescents
    – married adolescents
(3) Informal group discussions for sexuality education.
(4) Training of:
    – peer counsellors, as it is evident that the greatest source of information to the teenager is his own peers; and
    – parents. In order to reduce the communication gap between parents and their children, a course in systematic training for effective parenting (STEP) is offered. The STEP course is also offered to school guidance personnel and school nurses.
(5) Reproductive Health Care
    – full physical examination
    – pelvic examination
    – PAP smear
    – pregnancy tests
    – contraceptive service to aid in lowering the TFR (total fertility rate) by raising the age at first birth to 20 years and above
    – post-coital contraception as an emergency measure
    Detailed records are kept.
(6) Referral services when situations arise which cannot be handled by the staff in the adolescent programme. Cases may be referred to:
    – sexually transmitted diseases clinics
    – antenatal or postnatal care clinics

Results of TAP

(1) Unwanted children.
(2) Early unstable marriage and family stress.
(3) Teenage suicide and abortion.

Because abortions on demand are illegal in South Africa, backstreet abortions are frequently resorted to. This may end in death, infertility and disease.

The effect of pregnancy on the adolescent

Normally adolescence is a time of emotional turmoil and rapid physical development. Unwanted pregnancy at this age is traumatic and may result in permanent damage to the developing personality. In many cases it is an expression of the adolescent's need to be loved — by her boyfriend and later by her baby. There is general consensus that girls in the immediate post-pubertal period, i.e. at the age of 15 and below, should not be exposed to the stresses of pregnancy and childbirth.[7] For both boys and girls this is the time of transition from childhood to adulthood with its identity crisis (i.e. the child/woman, child/man conflict), with ambivalent feelings about sexuality, a conflictual identification with the mother or father (in the case of boys), strong strivings for independence mixed with feelings of dependency on the home and fear of taking responsibility for own decisions. The teenager is unsure of his/her sexual acceptability and needs to experiment with heterosexual relationships. These conflicts have to be dealt with by normal adolescents for them to reach the relative maturity of the young adult stage. Resolution of these conflicts constitutes the so-called 'tasks' of adolescence common to both sexes. Some disturbed teenagers cannot resolve the conflicts of adolescence in a socially acceptable way and may resort to delinquent behaviour, including alcohol and drug abuse, and irresponsible sexual behaviour with disastrous obstetric and developmental consequences. Pregnancy at this age causes a tremendous emotional shock; a teenage girl may deal with it by denying its presence until pregnancy becomes so obvious that she yields the truth on being confronted. This may precipitate a crisis which needs careful handling, often with the help of the boyfriend. Older adolescents who, under normal circumstances, are psychosocially more mature, can face up to the problem in a more realistic way, seeking help at a much earlier stage of the pregnancy.

Counselling the pregnant teenager

Because of her dominant role in the Family Planning Clinic and its Youth Health Centre, the nurse is the proper person to counsel (note: not advise) the pregnant teenage girl on her future and that of her baby. The nurse must state all the options open to the girl and allow her to discover for herself what is best suited to her life.

Some of the options are:

(1) *Abortion*. This is legal in South Africa only in cases of rape, incest, foetal abnormalities, pregnancy risks to the life of the mother or severe psychological problems. The U.K. will no longer accept South Africans for induced abortions. Illegal abortions are a great risk to health and fertility and may cause severe religious conflicts. Even if the girl is not religious, post-abortion guilt remains a problem. If guilt and depression cannot be worked through they may spoil subsequent relationships with men. Unfortunately some pregnant girls and their families can think of no other option in their need to save the family name or accommodate the boyfriend.

(2) *Adoption*. If the pregnant girl is not coerced into making this decision, it is the best solution. The teenager must be helped to mourn her loss and must be allowed to hold and see her baby. She is comforted by encourage-

ment to think of it as an act of selfless love to ensure a better future for her child.

(3) *Marriage to the child's father*. To be successful this depends on the age, financial status and maturity of the young couple and on whether it is a forced or mutual decision. Early forced marriages are usually unstable and end in divorce.

(4) *Single parent*. The attitude of the boyfriend and family may be in favour of keeping the child. Success depends upon the support of the girl's parents, the arrangements for child care and on her job opportunities. Keeping the child may spoil the girl's marriage opportunities and if the stress of coping with work, social life and child care becomes too great, the scene is set for child abuse.

Support of the pregnant teenage girl

The nurse can play a useful role in psychoprophylaxis of the pregnant teenager. She must neither reject the unwed mother nor become emotionally involved. The teenager needs understanding and skilled handling by a professional nurse who is mindful of the teenager's need to mature into a responsible person.

Substance abuse

Substance abuse is increasing world-wide and peaks in the late adolescence and early adulthood in South Africa. Recently one quarter of the Mandrax confiscated in the world was destined for South Africa. Cannabis grows freely in the RSA and enjoys a good overseas market.

The Narcotics Bureau of the SAP is extremely active in tracing the sources of drugs, but drug syndicates which run lucrative, global trafficking networks are very powerful and ruthless. The use of the psychoactive substances, cannabis, heroin, hallucinogens and cocaine, for whatever purpose, is illegal, whereas other drugs of addiction (e.g. morphine, Wellconal) are dangerous but their use is allowed on medical prescription. Solvents, glue and alcohol are freely available. For a description of these drugs and their control, see Chapter 42. Substance abuse in adolescents is a symptom — a means by which inner turmoil, which is uncomfortable, is deadened and a false sense of security and feelings of happiness are created. In adolescence drugs may be used experimentally on a temporary basis, through peer group pressure which also dictates fashions in clothes and jewellery and in music.

Substance abuse may also start when drugs are used as an aid to cope with the tasks of adolescence (see p. 320). On the other hand, it may be a sign of a conduct (antisocial) disorder or psychiatric illness. Whatever the cause of the substance dependence, it can become an established addiction which is extremely difficult to break as the addict has become integrated into the 'drug culture' and no longer feels at ease in normal society. Addicts become dependent not only on psychoactive substances but also on their families of origin or any institution *in loco parentis*.

Diagnosis of substance abuse

A drug history must be obtained.
Clinical signs:[8]

(1) Change in behaviour, e.g. increased isolation, moodiness or irritableness.
(2) Change in functioning, viz. drop in school performance and loss of interest in sport and hobbies.
(3) Episodes of intoxication.
(4) Specific signs from specific drugs:
    - Cannabis: bloodshot eyes, increased appetite, stains on palms from the bottle neck used for smoking, giggling episodes and a characteristic smell.
    - Stimulants: elation alternating with depression, loss of appetite, insomnia.
    - Sedatives: drowsiness, loss of inhibitions without the smell of alcohol which may cause the same signs.
    - Solvents inhaled: slurred speech, confusion, staggering gait.
    - Hallucinogens: markedly abnormal behaviour with hallucinations and paranoid delusions.

The clinical signs of the addiction may be accompanied by physical and psychological dependence if the addict cannot get his 'fix'. The addict may also suffer from physical side-effects, a conduct disorder or a psychiatric disturbance. The addict often steals or resorts to prostitution to maintain his very expensive habit.

Intravenous drug users (IVDU) who share their bodies and their needles may become the victims of HIV/AIDS.

For the management of substance abuse, see Chapter 42.

Suicide and parasuicide

Suicide is self-murder and parasuicide is an unsuccessful attempt at suicide. In parasuicide the person may or may not have attempted to kill himself.

Stengel's[9] definition of suicide, 'any act of self-damage inflicted with self-destructive intention, however vague and ambiguous; sometimes this intention has to be inferred from the patient's behaviour', accepted in 1970, did not include the word 'parasuicide' which is the modern term for 'attempted suicide'.

Until recently parasuicide and suicide were considered criminal offences. At present society has a more tolerant attitude towards suicide and the act has become the subject of scientific research. Some American medical schools have suicidological units and in South African hospitals the trend is towards offering psychiatric help to the person who has made an unsuccessful attempt at ending his life. Suicide prevention is attempted with the aid of voluntary societies such as Suicides Anonymous and Life Line. The recent suicide of Arthur Koestler, philosopher and writer, and his wife in Britain, has highlighted the controversy about the right of the individual to end his life in a dignified way if he feels its quality no longer warrants its continuance.

Suicide and parasuicide in childhood and adolescence

The impact on society of suicide and parasuicide amongst the youth is much greater than that of suicide in older people. The dependency and relative helplessness of children *vis-à-vis* intolerable living conditions are accepted by adults with feelings of social responsibility. When a child commits or attempts suicide some adult is deemed accountable. Childhood suicide or parasuicide, therefore, evokes social guilts and inspires community efforts to help children 'in need of care'.

Shaffer[10] found two common personality types among child and adolescent suicides:

(1) children of superior intelligence, isolated, depressed and withdrawn or in trouble before death;
(2) impulsive, paranoid children prone to aggressive or violent outbursts.

These personality types are not, however, predictive of suicide. The only factor these disturbed child suicides had in common was their familiarity with the phenomenon of suicide in their family or social environment.

Shaffer lists the following determinants of a child's death by suicide:

(1) degree of conceptual maturity, i.e. understanding the concept that death is permanent;
(2) disturbed family background;
(3) depressed mental state;
(4) a precipitating incident (disciplinary crisis, fight with peers, etc.);
(5) access to the means of suicide and privacy to commit the act without disturbance;
(6) familiarity with the phenomenon of suicide.

Garfinkel[11] found the motivation for suicidal attempts, threats or gestures in children and adolescents to be:

(1) a way out of an intolerable situation in persons with high psychosocial stress;
(2) manipulation of important others to change their behaviour;
(3) a cry for help to draw attention to distress;
(4) self-punishment (i.e. depression) or punishment of others. The attitude of the angry suicidal child seems to be 'I'll die and then you will be sorry'.

The adolescent usually has difficulties with one or both parents or relationship problems with peers. It seems to be an age-related stress response to an insoluble problem which the adolescent cannot discuss with a mature adult; it is an impulsive way of solving a problem. The intent to kill may be there but the act may also be a manipulative one born of despair and hopelessness.

Adopted children who feel sensitive about their adoption because of teasing in the younger age group and who cannot share their feelings of being 'different' with their adoptive parents, are an at-risk group for suicide when they reach adolescence.

Suicide methods

A Durban study[12] found the following range of methods used by parasuicides:

	Number	%
Overdose (O.D.)		
— Benzodiazepines	109	35,2
— Analgesics e.g. paracetamol	76	24,5
— Tricyclic antidepressants	18	5,8
— Phenothiazines	12	3,9
— Barbiturates	6	1,9
— Hypnotics/anticonvulsants	7	2,3
Self-poisoning		
— Insecticides	6	1,9
— Solvents	11	3,5
— Alcohol	13	4,2
— Carbon monoxide		
(car exhaust fumes)	6	1,9
— Gas	6	1,9
Laceration of wrists	23	7,4
Gunshot wounds	9	2,9
Miscellaneous	8	2,6

Garfinkel[11] found that in most cases of unsuccessful suicide in children there is a high likelihood of rescue.

Primary prevention

Primary prevention of suicide aims at the prevention of attempts at suicide by health education of the community to recognise risk factors in suicide and to know where to refer people-in-crisis. The community and psychiatric nurses have a special role to play in this regard. Crisis intervention can be carried out by the following community services:

(1) Crisis clinics.
(2) Life Line (telephonic service).
(3) Suicides Anonymous.
(4) Mental health clinics.

These helping and special emergency agencies are useful in crisis situations. Their services make it possible for potential suicides to be held in an interpersonal relationship until tensions (internal pressures) and irrationality (caused by transient situational disturbances) subside to such an extent that problem-solving behaviour is possible. These disturbances need thus not lead to suicide if the crisis can be treated.

The most important primary preventive measure is to help parents communicate with their children. This applies especially to rigid, punitive, authoritarian parents who alienate their children. While children can voice their grievances to their parents, they are not likely to resort to self-destructive gestures.

Secondary prevention

After an unsuccessful or incomplete suicide attempt, the family or the community will intervene by getting medical help for the self-injured or poisoned patient.

The following secondary preventive measures can be taken:

(1) emergency resuscitative or eliminatory treatment in a casualty department (trauma unit) of a hospital. In some hospitals the seriously affected patient is treated in an intensive care unit;

(2) hospitalisation, if necessary, for further treatment of physical problem(s) caused by the suicide attempt;

(3) hospitalisation, if necessary, in the psychiatric ward of a hospital if the patient suffers from a serious psychiatric problem or if evaluation of risk factors predicts a repeat suicide attempt.

The most important secondary preventive measure after the attempted suicide or parasuicide has been resuscitated in a hospital, is to evaluate the risk of the suicide attempt being repeated, this time successfully.

Hawton[13] recommends that all children and adolescents who attempt suicide should be admitted to a general hospital and that a psychosocial assessment of the patient and the family should be carried out as soon as the patient has recovered from the physical effects of the overdose or self-injury. This should be followed by out-patient care. Hawton found that a third of adolescent attempters were relatively normal youngsters who had experienced an acute crisis. These cases can be handled by counselling of parents or family therapy and supervision by their general practitioners.

Anorexia nervosa and bulimia

Introduction

Anorexia nervosa is a psychophysiological disorder characterised by under-eating due to a morbid fear of becoming fat. The mass loss due to dieting causes a body mass of 20–25 % or more below that which is desirable for age and sex.

Bulimia nervosa (bulimarexia) is a variant of anorexia nervosa. In this case the patient indulges in uncontrollable episodes of gross over-eating ('bingeing'). The accompanying morbid fear of becoming fat is allayed by induced vomiting or abuse of purgatives or both.

Anorexia nervosa is a modern disease. It is the commonest single psychiatric disorder affecting adolescent females of the middle and upper classes in the Western World and has not been encountered amongst blacks in the RSA.[17]

Premorbid personality

The at-risk personality pattern is: perfectionism, introversion, compliancy and emotional dependency.[17]

Anorexia nervosa occurs mainly (95 %) amongst females during pre-adolescence, adolescence and early adulthood. It is a complex condition in which personality conflicts, family attitudes and social problems and pressures interact with one another. The struggle for power within a family may be acted out during mealtimes.

Parents may be over-concerned about diet and subscribe to food fads. Thus food may become a matter of central importance in the family. The potential anorexic may be overmass and consequently become over-concerned with mass and dieting to the point of becoming phobic about food. The stereotype of female beauty in affluent Western societies tends towards slimness. Slimness is equated with self-discipline, 'goodness', sexual power and security in heterosexual relationships. To be fat is to be lazy and unattractive, especially to the opposite sex. The insecure adolescent girl may displace anxieties about emerging sexual and social conflicts on to actual problems regarding body mass; thus mass and the shape of her body become the main focus of her anxieties which express themselves in ruminations about mass and food.

Statistics differ with regard to antecedent mass problems. Thus Crisp[14] reports an incidence of 50 % and Bruch[15] an incidence of 12 %.

Anorexia nervosa is sometimes preceded by some other acting-out behaviour but this is not always the case. Parents often describe their anorexic child as 'good and conforming'. The anorexic may have a perfectionistic, hard-driving compulsive personality disorder but the self-starving symptom may also arise in the schizoid or the histrionic personality types. Anorexia nervosa is most common in families with strict moral and religious standards, in which the mother plays a dominant, central role, being closely enmeshed with her anorexic daughter, and the father a passive, peripheral role.

The family of the anorexic patient

Dally and Gomez[16] found wide variations in the relationships of family members of anorexics. They found one parent to be more dominating and forceful than the other. The family invariably has high achievement expectations from its children. Anorexics are usually above average in looks and intelligence, yet for some reason they are angry and afraid of meeting the maturational challenges of adolescence and young adulthood.

Various psychoanalytic reasons have been advanced for the deliberate self-starvation: symbolic rejection of oral sexual impulses; denial of pregnancy; a subconscious wish to become a boy; avoidance of growing up. Whatever the reason may be, anorexics experience themselves as inadequate to form heterosexual relationships. They express their conflicts, frustrations and angers in a way that punishes the family and focuses attention upon themselves, and that is also self-destructive. Self-starvation is a powerful tool for punishing and controlling other people by threatening to, or actually committing suicide.

It may be difficult to get to know the pathology in the family as the parents may present a harmonious facade to the outside world, despite deep and chronic tensions and conflicts. The illness of the index patient may actually serve to hold a marriage together through the shared involvement and concern of the parents. The incidence of broken homes in cases of anorexia nervosa is fairly low.

Clinical picture of anorexia and bulimia

Eating behaviour

The patient is often untruthful about the amount of food eaten. The nurse must realise that the bending of the truth is a reflection of what the patient feels and perceives when eating. A true picture of eating behaviour can only be obtained by observing the patient during mealtimes.

Anorexic patients are preoccupied with food, thinking about the next meal both with dread and with pleasure since each meal is a test of will power and the ability to resist food.

They study food and the kilojoule values of the various foodstuffs. They enjoy buying and preparing food and like to watch others eat. They compare their eating patterns with those of others. Eating patterns differ and mealtimes may reflect the type of battle fought with parents: open refusal of food or covert refusal (hiding of food or feeding the dog discreetly). The anorexic may bargain with her parents, agreeing to take a certain amount of a certain kind of food. The unwilling eater may spend 5–10 minutes cutting the food into small pieces or chewing a mouthful. Anorexics are often fussy about the times they eat, the way food is served or prepared. The diet is often bizarre with many fads and fancies.

Hunger is intense at first but gradually diminishes. Eventually the anorexic patient fails to recognise hunger. This disinclination to eat is not a mere loss of appetite as the name of the disorder implies. There may be a fluctuation between starving and bingeing (bulimia). Bingeing is followed by tremendous guilt and a feeling of disgust. The binge is usually relieved by induced vomiting.

Overactivity

Patients with anorexia nervosa are usually extremely active. In the early stages this overactivity reflects increasing frustration and anxiety. Starvation causes restlessness and overactivity which also serves to heat the patient who is not burning kilojoules which are normally readily available. Physical exercise may also be used to burn up any food ingested. Fatigue resulting from exercise is denied.

Vomiting

Vomiting may either be mild and induced after binges or it may take place secretly after every meal to remove the danger of getting fat. Vomiting produces a sudden loss of tension after eating, thus serving to reinforce its recurrence. The tension associated with bingeing becomes pleasurable as the anorexic knows that the consequences of indulging her appetite can be avoided. The therapeutic prevention of vomiting causes extreme anxiety.

The patient with bulimia differs from the patient with anorexia in that she is more likely to have had sexual experience or to have abused alcohol, drugs or laxatives.

Constipation

Anorexic patients become obsessed with changes in bowel habits. Constipation is to be expected because of the reduction of faecal mass caused by starvation. They deal with constipation either by taking large doses of laxatives or by sitting on the toilet for hours at a time. There is the danger of developing a prolapsed rectum.

Menstruation

Although amenorrhoea is the rule, menstruation may persist for a long period in bulimic patients; they also resume menstruation at a lower body mass than anorexia patients. Starvation causes endocrinological changes, hence the amenorrhoea. Menstruation usually returns when the anorexic patient reaches 80 % of desired body mass. Patients are usually vague about their menstrual cycle and need reassurance that menstruation will return.

Sexuality

The pre-anorexia libido of most patients is probably normal. Once anorexia nervosa develops, sexual feelings and interest diminish. Some are pleased at the absence of 'periods' and aver that they never want to marry. Many dislike and reject physical contact. On the other hand, there are those who look forward to getting married and having children; they discuss these ideals in a child-like way virtually ignoring the role of the male in their plans for the future. The ideal male partner is seen as gentle, undemanding and considerate. The sexual infantilism experienced by the anorexic patient seems to be a way of dealing with sexual conflicts which cannot be resolved in a mature way. Even after recovery heterosexual adjustment is inadequate.

Circulatory disturbances and hypothermia

Acrocyanosis (blueness of the extremities) is often present. Patients complain of feeling cold and their extremities may be painful in winter.

Pulse and blood pressure

Bradycardia is common but tachycardia occurs during the terminal stages of starvation. Hypotension (with dizziness) occurs with loss of mass. The ECG shows the following abnormalities: inverted T-wave and depression of the S-T segment. This could be mistaken for myocardial ischaemia. The abnormalities disappear with mass gain.

Skin, hair and teeth

The skin is dry, rough and pale; patients try to hide this by putting on excess make-up. Lanugo (fine hairs) grow on the back, arms, legs and face of anorexic patients. Teeth are usually normal but chronic vomiting may cause acid erosion of the enamel.

Hydration

Severe dehydration and electrolyte disturbances can occur in the vomiting or/and purging patient. In severe emaciation, oedema of the legs is common, the retention of water causing mass gain.

Body image

The anorexic patient has a distorted body image, fearing obesity even after treatment. She tends to overestimate her width but not her height. Perceptual distortion increases with increased mass loss. She avoids looking at her body. The fear and shame of being fat even extends to avoidance of swim suits.

Treatment of anorexia nervosa and bulimia

A wide range of treatments has been used. Early therapists advocated that anorexic patients be separated from their families. The value of separation is still recognised today, although mild cases may be successfully treated at home. Control is best achieved by hospitalisation, however. Treatment focuses either on the gaining of mass or on eating.

Regardless of the focus, a **behaviour modification programme** is commonly used. This entails the granting of privileges for either eating or gaining mass.

The prime goal of treatment is the preservation of life as the disease can be lethal.

Pharmacotherapy

The doctor may prescribe one or more of the following:

(1) *Phenothiazines.* Chlorpromazine is the drug of choice as it reduces anxiety and psychomotor restlessness. It also has anti-emetic properties.
(2) *Sedatives.* Benzodiazepines are used as anxiolytics.
(3) *Beta-blockers.* Propranolol is used to reduce anxiety and for its probable stimulant effect on the hypothalamic appetite centre.
(4) *Antidepressants.* The tricyclic antidepressants, e.g. amitriptyline and trimipramine, are the medicines of choice; besides reducing depression, they have anxiolytic and hypnotic effects.
(5) *Hypnotics.* They are useful at night as starvation causes restless sleep.

Psychotherapy and family counselling

Individual psychotherapy and parent counselling are indicated. Psychotherapy is carried out by trained therapists and only when mass gain is satisfactory. Parents must be given a clear understanding of the dynamics of anorexia nervosa within the family and any attempt to 'side' with their daughter against the 'harsh' therapeutic regime must be firmly dealt with.

Nursing anorexia and bulimia

Assessment of the patient's needs and problems

The nurse conducts the initial interview with the patient to establish a therapeutic relationship. The patient needs the reassurance that her fears and behaviour are understood and that her helplessness is recognised.

The nurse therapist then obtains a history of the illness and elicits the eating pattern. This information should be obtained first separately and then jointly from patient and family in order to eliminate bias and false information.

Goals of nursing care

Short-term goals:

(1) The establishment of a trusting relationship with the patient.
(2) The promotion of mass gain.
(3) The development of non-food-related coping mechanisms.
(4) The increase of self-esteem.

Long-term goals:

(1) The establishment of regular, healthy eating patterns.
(2) The development of the ability to express negative feelings (e.g. anger) in socially acceptable ways.
(3) The preparation of the patient for discharge.

Nursing interventions

Nursing interventions should be planned in conjunction with the multiprofessional team and the patient to ensure consistency and co-operation — essential conditions for successful treatment. Anorexic patients can be manipulative and attempt to play team members off against one another. Good teamwork, which gives the patient a feeling of security that she can depend on her therapists, is insured by team meetings in which members report back on their therapeutic experiences with the patient and treatment strategies are reviewed.

The nurse's attitude towards the patient must be characterised by understanding, consistency and objectivity. Bargaining should be avoided.

Feeding. During mealtimes constant and unobtrusive observation is essential; discussions about food and distractions, e.g. magazines and TV, are disallowed. The patient is served her meal and the nurse insists that everything be eaten within a fixed period, say 40 minutes. Any food left after expiry of time is noted. The left-over food is either liquidised and fed by nasogastric tube or replaced by a substitute drink such as Sustagen. The patient is made aware beforehand of the consequences of non-compliance with the requirements of finishing her meal within the time limit.

Personal likes and dislikes should be taken into consideration when planning the meal. The kilojoule value of the diet must, however, not be diminished by substitute items of food.

Patients are not allowed to go to the toilet or bathroom for one hour after meals in case they use this opportunity to induce vomiting.

Mass. The mass is monitored according to the prescribed programme, i.e. either daily or weekly. The patient is weighed in underclothes to prevent cheating by hidden additives. Privileges are granted according to mass gain. Example: on admission the patient is nursed at bed rest and no visitors are allowed. Earned privileges may include the following: up out of bed, initially for ½ hour per day and thereafter for longer periods; visitors; attendance at Occupational Therapy Department; morning leave; weekend leave. The accurate monitoring of mass is, therefore, a very important nursing task.

Psychological care of the patient. The focus in psychological care is on the person and not on the diagnosis. No two patients are the same. The anorexic patient is usually passively aggressive, i.e. she cannot express anger and guilt directly, using self-destroying eating patterns instead. By her attitude of positive regard, acceptance and empathy, the nurse can help the patient express negative emotions of fear, guilt and anger, especially when these feelings concern family members. The patient is gently weaned from her food rituals and emotional associations with food by de-emphasising them in favour of attention to the worth of the suffering human being. Self-esteem is promoted by encouraging independent functioning.

The encouragement of family involvement. The nurse is required to co-operate with the family therapist. The involvement of the family in the treatment programme must be actively promoted by the nurse.

The nursing of a patient suffering from anorexia nervosa is not an easy task. The acquisition of the skills required for successful nursing are contingent upon emotional maturity, the emotionally mature nurse being capable of feeling compassion and empathy for her extremely disturbed patient who is delusionally out of touch with the needs of her body.

The section on anorexia nervosa was contributed by C J du Toit.

REFERENCES

(1) De Barros H. When children have children. *Southern Africa Today* 1990; **7** (2).

(2) Van Coeverden de Groot HA. Teenage pregnancies — the premier social evil of the Third World. *S Afr J Cont Med Educ* 1988; **6**: 67–68.

(3) Van Coeverden de Groot HA, Greathead EE. The Cape Town Teenage Clinic. *S Afr Med J* 1987; **71**: 434–436.

(4) Ncayiyana DJ, Terhaar G. Pregnant adolescents in rural Transkei. *S Afr Med J* 1989; **75**: 231–232.

(5) *S Afr Med J* 1986; **70**: 582.

(6) Greathead E. The dilemma of the pregnant teenager. *Nursing RSA.* 1988; **3**: 20–28.

(7) Gillis LS. Teenager pregnancy. *S Afr Med J* 1990; **77**: 121.

(8) Ziervogel CF. Substance abuse in adolescents. *S Afr J Cont Med Educ* 1986; **4**: 47–51.

(9) Stengel E. *Suicide and Attempted Suicide.* London: Pelican Books, 1970.

(10) Shaffer D. Suicide in childhood and early adolescence. *J Child Psychol Psychiat* 1974; **15**: 275.

(11) Garfinkel BD, Froese A, Hood J. *Am J Psychiat* 1982; **139**: 1257.

(12) Minnaar GK, Schlebusch L, Levin A. A current study of parasuicide in Durban. *S Afr Med J* 1980; **57**: 204.

(13) Hawton K. Attempted suicide in children and adolescents. *J Child Psychol Psychiat* 1982; **23**: 497.

(14) Pillay M, Crisp AA. Psychological characteristics of patients with anorexia nervosa. *Br J Med Psychol* 1977; **50**.

(15) Bruch H. *The Golden Cage.* Harvard University Press, 1978.

(16) Dally P, Gomez J. *Anorexia Nervosa.* London: William Heineman Medical Books Ltd, 1979.

(17) Norris DL. Anorexia nervosa: The adolescent epidemic. *S Afr J Cont Med Educ* 1986; **4**: 39–45.

(18) Wagstaff LA, De Vries G, Mkhasibe C. Whither school health services for lower primary schoolchildren in Soweto? *S Afr Med J* 1988; **73**: 117–119.

(19) Leary PM. Editorial. Hyperactivity and methylphenidate. *S Afr Med J* 1986; **70**: 383–384.

The author wishes to thank the former Department of Health Services and Welfare (House of Assembly), the Department of National Health and Population Development and the Branch Health Services of the Transvaal Provincial Administration for valuable information supplied.

TEST OF KNOWLEDGE

The student has benefited from studying this chapter if he/she can answer the following questions:

(1) (*a*) Name the objectives and aims of a school health service of your choice.

   (*b*) To what extent, in your experience, are these objectives attained in the school system with which you are familiar. Give reasons for your findings.

(2) (*a*) What are the functions of the school nurse at health visits paid once a year to the schools for which she is responsible?

   (*b*) What is the possible scope of a school nurse who, besides having the present basic qualifications required, has been trained as a primary health care nurse?

   (*c*) What role does the school nurse play in the health education of scholars? How, in your opinion, can this role be extended?

(3) Write notes on:

   (*a*) School phobia

   (*b*) Anorexia nervosa and bulimia

   (*c*) Parasuicide

   (*d*) The dangers of methylphenidate (Ritalin) therapy

   (*e*) The dangers of sexual promiscuity

   (*f*) The objectives of the National Adolescent Programme and functions of the Youth Health centres.

(4) (*a*) Discuss the problem of teenage pregnancy in your community.

   (*b*) How would you, as a nurse, counsel a pregnant schoolgirl aged 17?

(5) (*a*) Discuss the detection of substance abuse in an adolescent scholar.

   (*b*) How can substance abuse in a school be handled?

(6) (*a*) What would alert you, as a school nurse, to the possibility of a scholar's impending suicide?

   (*b*) What are the motivating factors for adolescent parasuicide?

Part 4

MATERNAL AND CHILD HEALTH CARE

20

Family Planning (FP)

OBJECTIVES

Family planning has become a very important nursing skill of the community nurse who may be required to dispense primary health care services in health centres and clinics under indirect medical supervision. It is incumbent upon the nurse, therefore, to acquire the basic family planning skills during training, these skills being augmented later by State Health post-basic certification courses.

Family planning is an integral part of the Population Development Programme and Reconstruction and Development Programme which are aimed at social upliftment and prevention of overpopulation. It has been incorporated in the routine primary health care service. Urbanisation and improvement of socio-economic status are the cornerstones of these programmes and are necessary to create the attitudes which will bring about a decline in the fertility rate. Motivated couples will make use of freely available nurse-oriented family planning services — nurse-oriented as 95 % of State Health family planning staff are nurses. When integrated into primary health care, family planning lowers infant and maternal morbidity and reduces illegal abortions and their hazards. Slower population growth is vital to development.

Dr K. E. Sapire expresses the importance to mankind of contraceptive methods in the following words:

'Few medical discoveries have had more impact on the welfare of human beings than those which provide them with the freedom to make choices about their family size. The aspirations of millions to rise from destitution to dignity could never be realised without this contribution to medical science.'[2]

On the other hand, freely available contraceptives (all except the condom) have had a harmful effect on the STD and HIV/AIDS epidemics due to an increase in sexual promiscuity.

STUDY OBJECTIVES

The student must become conversant with:
(1) The reasons for the urgency of curbing population growth.
(2) The national family planning programme as integral part of the Population Development Programme and Reconstruction and Development Programme.
(3) The growing importance of sterilisation as a method of contraception.
(4) The role of abortions in curbing the population of South Africa.
(5) The various non-surgical contraceptive methods, their relative effectiveness and their advantages and disadvantages.

THE INTERNATIONAL STATEMENT ON FAMILY PLANNING

The 'Declaration of Tokyo' was made in November 1986 by the International Planned Parenthood Federation Members Assembly. This declaration is supported by the Planned Parenthood Association of Southern Africa:

'We, the family planning associations of the world, responding to the new and incontrovertible evidence that family planning saves lives, pledge ourselves, as a matter of urgency, to take the following measures to reduce the appalling toll of sickness and death caused by unplanned pregnancies:

1. Spread awareness of optimum conditions for childbearing, which can save up to 5 million child lives a year and avoid 200 000 maternal deaths through complications of unplanned pregnancy;

2. Launch campaigns in each country to ensure that family planning is recognised as an essential component of primary health care;

3. Discourage pregnancy before the age of 18, thus reducing the special hazards which afflict young mothers and their children;

4. Promote spacing of births at least 2 years apart as an essential life-saving measure;

5. Further reduce infant mortality by giving advice and services to mothers and fathers in order to limit family size, this being one among other critical health interventions for child survival;

6. Counsel parents to cease childbearing after a woman has reached the high-risk age of 35 and provide the necessary services;

7. Work within the national legal and cultural framework to reduce the incidence of illegal abortion, which is responsible for up to a quarter of all maternal deaths in some countries;

8. Act, without delay, to help combat the spread of the acquired immune deficiency syndrome (AIDS) through education and appropriate services.

We, the members of the International Planned Parenthood Federation, which has campaigned for family well-being for 35 years, now undertake to intensify our efforts at international, regional and national levels for realisation of our goals.'

SOME POPULATION PROBLEMS

The most pressing problem in the world today, especially in the Third World, is overpopulation. South Africa's population is expected to double by 2010 from a total of approximately 25 million (excluding TBVC countries) in 1981 to a total of 47–50 million. (Population doubling time with population growth rate of 2,31 % is 30 years.) In order to avoid this catastrophe, families should ideally be limited to two children; this will ensure a zero increase in population. This ideal situation has been achieved in some Western countries. South Africa's population growth rate is amongst the highest in the world: 2,6 % a year. In 1985 natural population growth rates per 100 population for the South African groups were the following:

Asian 1,7
Black 3,1
Coloured 1,9
White 0,7
Average 2,6

High population growth has become one of the most obstinate and persistent hindrances to the improvement of life circumstances throughout Africa.

**Population of South Africa from the 1985 census
(TBVC countries excluded)**

	1985	1990 (projected)	1995 (projected)
Asians	861 300	947 923	1 043 000
Blacks	19 051 500	21 361 203	23 950 923
Coloureds	2 862 200	3 221 432	3 625 771
Whites	4 947 100	5 291 100	5 560 000
TOTAL	27 722 100	30 821 658	34 179 694
Central Statistical Service			

In 1988 the total population of greater South Africa was 36,5 million and, in 1994, 40 million. Housing, education, agriculture, health services, economic and manpower development programmes and family planning programmes for the underdeveloped masses of the RSA should receive urgent attention if co-operation in any government population control programme is to be expected. At 2,31 % growth a year South Africa's population is one of the fastest growing in the world. At this rate it doubles every 30 years. Most of the population growth takes place in the impoverished rural areas.

Note: Africa's population is growing at an annual 2,9 %, the fastest for an entire region.

In 1983 the President's Council (PC) proposed measures to curb population growth (see PDP in Chapter 1). In order to reverse the catastrophic demographic trends, these measures should be launched immediately in order to reach a stabilised population of 80 million by the year 2100 with zero growth rate. This is the maximum affordable population for South Af-

rica. This can only be achieved by a gradual limitation of the fertility rate of women to two children per woman by the year 2020. This will lead to a cessation of population growth by the year 2100.

Thus state interference in parenthood may become a reality in the interests of the future generation. In a democratic country the individual retains the right, however, to decide responsibly on the number of children he will procreate.

Communist China is a very good example of a country which is making an all-out effort to curb its population growth. China is a poor country with over 1 billion of the world's population. The objective of the Chinese is to reduce population growth to zero by the year 2000. To achieve this, the population is being persuaded by various incentives and sanctions to have one-child families, at the most two if the first child is a girl. Pregnant women who have exceeded their child-allowance, are persuaded to undergo abortions; due to concealment of pregnancy, this is often performed during the second trimester. Penalties for non-compliers are severe.

The population growth rate of the USA is, at present, approximately 0,8 %. This slow growth rate has also been attained in Western Europe and East Asia.

Recent studies made by the United Nations Population Division predict the world's population is likely to be 6,1 billion in the year 2000. In July 1987 it was 5 billion.

BIRTH CONTROL

Control of the birth-rate is one of the most important obligations of the present generation.

The term 'population explosion' very aptly describes the possibility which confronts populations of human beings driven by hunger and overcrowding, of taking desperate destructive steps against other population groups for the possession of scarce means — food and land — in order to ensure their survival. Increasing the death-rate by killing other people or by allowing them to starve is one way of solving the global population problem. The 'law of the jungle' operates in the hearts of many so-called 'civilised' people and its feasibility cannot be argued away by logical reasoning. People who function on a primitive emotional level cannot feel concern for the welfare, or concede the rights, of other people whom they do not even know and who might not even form part of their own ethnic group. People who do have the welfare of humanity at heart, however, cannot accept that increasing the death-rate is a civilised way of averting the imminent population explosion. A more humane solution appears to be to limit the population growth.

No form of birth control will succeed for long, however, unless the need for it is understood and accepted. In developing countries, the birth-rate is unlikely to be reduced until the infant mortality rate is brought down. It is important to raise the social status of the woman in an underdeveloped country and provide her with equal opportunities for education, self-development and employment outside the home. By decreasing the emphasis on the role of the woman as wife and mother, the birth-rate is more likely to be reduced. This statement is not meant in any way to disparage the woman who chooses as her vocation the role of wife and mother. All women are not suited for the exacting vocation of motherhood.

In a society geared to believe that to reproduce is woman's ultimate destiny in life, the urge in a woman to have a baby or to prove her fertility and femininity by becoming pregnant is very strong. Despite the ready availability of contraceptive knowledge many women, both married and unmarried, who do not want to carry a baby become pregnant — as evidenced by the perennial demand for abortions. Other women, again, find pregnancy a rewarding state but reject the baby once it is born. The battered baby is a prime example of child rejection. Increasing numbers of women share their responsibilities as mothers by delegating the care of their young children to nannies and crèches while they carry on with a career. Modern woman is facing the dilemma: to fulfil her destiny as a woman or to be productive economically.

The dilemma of the modern woman has in part been caused by the changes in the world situation; the old ideas of woman's prime function in life are changing with the realisation that, unless woman's reproductive abilities can be drastically curbed, tragedy in the form of a population explosion awaits the coming generation. When hunger stares a billion people in the face, a woman's productive potential is more highly prized than her reproductive potential. We are experiencing a tremendous change in our basic human values. Many people are unable to accept these changes in our non-material culture — our beliefs, customs and values — and they cling to time-honoured traditions. This cultural lag causes many conflicts between the old ways of life and the changing demands of the present world.

In this world, birth control and family planning have become important concepts. Young couples who do not want children need no longer feel selfish or guilty of a moral sin. The easy availability of contraceptive advice is actually encouraging them to direct their energies in other socially useful directions. The old bogies of the childless state: the fear of a lonely, unwanted, deprived old age and fear of becoming cranks and social misfits, no longer apply in the modern industrial world in which social services are taking over the functions of the extended family. In this world motherhood is a matter of choice and no woman need feel that it is her duty to produce a child for the sake of the society. Marriages held together because of children are precarious indeed and lead to much mental ill-health, especially when the child is used as a pawn in a parental conflict.

Modern women have the right and the opportunity to choose their own destinies. They have been liberated by modern contraceptive methods from the societal obligation to reproduce by the sheer necessity of reducing world population growth. The choice of having children is theirs. The natural urge for motherhood is very strong indeed in many women who want to make the rearing of children their career. These career mothers are not likely to reject their children; their devoted care makes children feel loved and wanted — the essential prerequisites for mental health.

Unwanted children are usually not rewarding children as they sense parental rejection; this leads to much misery and emotional ill-health.

In a study on children born after their mothers were refused pregnancy termination, Forssman & Thuwe[1] report a 21-year follow-up. The study involved 120 children born to Swedish women who had been refused a therapeutic abortion and 120 control children born at the same time. A number of important differences were noted. In particular, more of the unwanted children had an insecure home during childhood and the incidence of mental disturbance requiring psychiatric care and delinquent or criminal behaviour was much greater among unwanted children than among controls.

Willingness to use contraceptives, especially the IUD and Depo-Provera, is increasing among black women working in urban areas. These women are likely to lose their jobs when pregnancy becomes obvious; therefore, economic circumstances are forcing them to take birth control seriously, especially if unmarried. The liberation of women from their serfdom to male domination has had much encouragement from the ANC. Many women's organisations, under the banner of the Women's National Coalition (WNC), have fought effectively for gender equality, especially in RDP structures.

The ANC has promised one third of its political representation will be women.

Women will have six months paid maternity leave and men ten days paternity leave.

The ANC guarantees women equal rights to land.

Educational opportunities for males and females will be equal.

A ministry of rural development will pay particular attention to the status of women and local authority programmes will be scrutinised for gender sensitivity.

Women are playing a leading role in contraceptive practices; there is, therefore, no physical reason for a woman to bear an unwanted child.

FAMILY PLANNING

Family Planning is not quite the same as birth control. The family planning clinics will assist sterile couples by appropriate referral as well as those who wish to limit the size of their families. They aim at helping mothers to space their children so that each child will be able to get the necessary care during the vulnerable years of complete dependence on a stable mothering figure. The clinics will help parents decide on the optimal size of their family and prescribe suit-

able measures to implement the decision. The chief concern of family planning programmes is, therefore, to guard the health of mothers and children and to promote the welfare of the family. The Planned Parenthood Movement stresses the economic, educational and health advantages of well-spaced, limited numbers of children.

Initially there was religious and other opposition to the birth control movement but today family planning clinics have religious support. The social climate is such that birth control information can circulate freely.

The long-term goal of a successful family planning campaign, which has been achieved in the USA and some European countries, is to reduce the population growth rate of a fully populated country to zero. This goal will be achieved when the number of children in a family is reduced to two.

Three important concepts in family planning

(1) *Crude birth-rate*: the number of live births in a calendar year for a particular area divided by the mid-year population of that area, multiplied by 1 000. In 1980 it was as follows in the RSA:
Whites: 16,5
Coloureds: 27,8
Asians: 24,0
Blacks: 39,1

(2) *Total fertility rate* (TFR): the number of live births in a calendar year for a particular area divided by the mid-year population of fertile women (i.e. aged 15–45 years) in the same area, multiplied by 1 000.

(3) The fertility pattern (children per woman in completed families) Memo: the generation replacement of children per woman is 2,1 during her reproductive years; this implies zero population growth rate.

The following fertility pattern statistics are to hand in the RSA: black women in Soweto 2,8 (1988); black rural women 5,7 (1988); white women 2,2 (1988); coloured women 3,8 (1976).

For the planning of birth control programmes in cities experiencing rapid expansion, it is important to know the intra-urban variability of fertility rates at the community

Birth and fertility rates (per 1 000) according to population group in metropolitan Cape Town[3]

Population group	Birth rate	Fertility rate	Live births	Total population	Females (15–44 yrs.)
White	13,6	57,0	6 573	482 240	115 260
Coloured	28,9	106,4	22 917	793 020	215 430
Black	39,8	199,2	7 299	183 360	36 640
TOTAL	25,2	100,2	36 789	1 458 620	367 330

level. In a study done by Rip *et al.*[3] in Cape Town in 1985, the above results were obtained.

It will be noted that even though it is generally known that urbanisation brings down the fertility rate, the intra-urban rates of reproduction (blacks 3,5 times greater than whites) are dependent upon socio-economic status of the three population groups compared.

A decline in the population growth rate is thus dependent on an interaction of the following factors:
(1) Socio-economic development:
    (a) economic development; and
    (b) adult literacy and formal education.
(2) Health and medical as well as family planning services.
(3) Urbanisation.

Family planning, in contradistinction to contraception, is done for two purposes:

(1) To space children to the satisfaction of the parents and in consideration of their coping abilities.
(2) To limit the size of the completed family. In Western countries most parents wish to have no more than two children, whereas some black women in the rural areas desire to have at least five.

For couples who want children, family planning which allows spaced pregnancies is a potent primary preventive measure as it prevents the exhaustion stress and irritability of the mother saddled with frequent and unwanted pregnancies, as well as the malnutrition, poor child health and high infant mortality rate amongst the lower socio-economic classes, especially amongst the blacks in South Africa. Theoretically, family planning should do away with the problem of unwanted children. Planned parenthood enables the parents to cope with their parenting functions and to raise their socio-eco-

nomic status for the general benefit of the family.

In any national family planning programme, the emphasis falls on family planning for the sake of promoting the health of the family. Together with the family planning service, there must be an efficient maternal and child health service. If women are expected to limit the number of children they produce, the birth of a healthy infant and its subsequent protection against malnutrition and disease must be ensured.

It has generally been found that parents are satisfied with fewer children if they are confident that their children will grow up healthy. A good maternal and child health service and improvement in poor socio-economic circumstances are, therefore, the best insurances against failed contraceptive practices.

Summary

The success of a family planning programme is influenced by the socio-economic status of the people, their literacy rate, their infant mortality rate, the degree of urbanisation, sophistication and emancipation of women, the density of the population and the cultural beliefs of the people. As the life circumstances and education of people improve, so their birth-rate becomes reduced. The success of education in family planning will, therefore, depend upon the level of development of the people to be educated. Unwillingness to practise birth control for the sake of spacing or limiting a family may be a reflection of social problems and cultural values.

Note: See also 'Factors which affect fertility rates in populations' (p. 83).

The national family planning programme

In 1974 the government launched a comprehensive National Family Planning Programme which aims at bringing to the notice of every adult in the country the concept of family planning. It has since 1983 become part of the PDP, and since 1994 part of the RDP. (See p. 319 for the National Adolescent Programme.)

The Department of Health ('State Health') carries the financial responsibility for this nation-wide service which is essentially free.

The full-time services of experts in health administration, fertility control, demography, sociology, communication, nursing, training and evaluation are available. The Directors of Hospital Services (provincial) and Regional Directors of State Health are responsible for the local administration of the programme. Local authorities play a very important part in family planning which forms part of their primary health care services. Primary health care nurses in health care clinics and day hospitals are important educators in family planning. Community health nurses doing 'first visits' after confinements are important carriers of information about contraception and refer patients to the clinics.

District surgeons are also important disseminators of family planning information and contraceptives. The State Health Department has appointed hundreds of doctors and nurses on a full-time or part-time basis to carry out family planning duties. In the rural areas, nurses are employed on a part-time sessional basis; they serve, *inter alia*, the farming communities. Occupational health nurses, trained in contraceptive practices, serve the industrial worker.

Private individuals and voluntary organisations, i.e. the Planned Parenthood Association of Southern Africa, also render family planning services.

The Planned Parenthood Association of Southern Africa (PPASA)

The PPASA is a private, non-profit organisation (NGO) committed to improving reproductive health and well-being. It was founded in the 1930s and relies on committed groups of volunteers for assistance.

The functions of the PPASA are:

- contraceptive education and provision;
- birth-spacing; maternal and child health;

- education in PHC, human sexuality and reproductive and women's health; teenage pregnancy;
- AIDS prevention;
- the development of women.

The PPASA is a national organisation based in Johannesburg and has five branch offices (Durban, Johannesburg, Lenasia, Cape Town and Port Elizabeth).

The professional groups involved in the implementation of the programme include not only doctors, nurses, social workers and guidance officers but also schoolteachers. It is envisaged that teachers and scholars undergo a training course in demography in order to understand the socio-economic problems caused by rapid population growth, especially among developing nations, and that they acquire a sound knowledge of reproductive functions. Thus it is hoped that through education attitudes will be changed to make the idea of family planning acceptable to the coming generation. When this happens, family planning will be practised by all citizens for the benefit of the entire nation — black, white, Asian and coloured.

The family planning (FP) nurse and adviser

The national family planning service is a nurse-oriented service as 95 % of State Health family planning staff are nurses. There are nine FP training centres in the RSA (1983), running multiracial certification courses:

- 2 weeks for basic FP clinic sisters;
- 3 weeks for auxiliary nurses who form part of the team and are trained to assist the registered nurses; they learn to take BP, to weigh clients, to test urine, etc.;
- 1-week course for sister tutors from nursing colleges, in the intensive clinical aspects of FP and the content of the course.

Family planning advisers attend a 3-week course in motivation and clinical information. They must have a Std VIII certificate and be over 25 years of age.

Male advisers (male nurses) are being trained and used to change attitudes to family planning among males.

Certification courses are also run on an in-service training basis at local FP clinics where sisters and auxiliary nurses cannot be released to attend full-time training courses. These courses generally take longer than the full-time courses. The in-service training is done by chief professional nurses who are in charge of each of the thirty-seven FP areas of the RSA.

The syllabus of FP clinic sisters covers not only FP practice and theory but also personal development in interpersonal skills and management.

All FP sisters are expected to spend 30 % of their working time giving health education. Their aim should be to improve the socio-economic status of those with low status.

All family planning sisters are also taught to take PAP smears. Every family planning sister must be updated annually and her certificate endorsed to this effect, otherwise she may not practise as a FP sister. Updating and endorsement are done as follows:

(1) By a chief professional nurse or State Health nurse who visits state FP clinics twice a year. All FP nurses in industry, in the private sector and in local authority clinics must likewise be updated and have their certificates endorsed.

(2) By a provincial nursing manager who visits provincial FP clinics twice a year for updating and endorsement of certificates. The nursing managers, of whom seven were subsidised by State Health in 1983, attend FP meetings at headquarters, Pretoria, every six months.

The extent of the FP service

In 1983 there were 26 000 clinic points run by the state, province and local authorities, with a total of approximately 1,18 million clients. This includes 40–50 % of black fertile women in rural and urban areas. There are more clients in urban than in rural areas. Town clinics are being established in shopping centres and near bus termini. Many more white women than black (proportionately) use contraception, but many whites make use of private services.

Increasing numbers of mobile family planning units are being put into use to reach farms and factories. These units have been part of comprehensive (PHC) mobile clinics since August 1991.

Since 1973 all registered nurses trained in family planning techniques who are on the staff of the departments of NHPD, provincial administrations, local authorities, or are employed in industry and are participating in the National Family Planning Programme, have been authorised by the Director-General: NHPD to issue contraceptives to the public. The contraceptives include hormonal pills. It is expected of these nurses that they decide for themselves on the most suitable method of birth control. Only registered nurses who have undergone a special course in family planning are allowed to control steroidal contraceptives from a medical protocol. The medical practitioner is responsible for delegating family planning procedures to nurses, but the nurse is responsible for her own actions.

The running of a family planning clinic offers very exciting opportunities for the registered nurse practitioner who makes it her vocation. She is allowed to give full family planning services to clients, i.e. she does not work in the capacity of a doctor's assistant, although she functions under the direct or indirect supervision of a doctor. Her success will depend on her own efficiency and enthusiasm.

The family planning clinic

When a recognised authority wishes to start a clinic, application is made through a Regional Director of State Health Services to conduct a family planning clinic. Over the years two types of family planning services have developed and both are operative in South Africa. They differ in the 'core' service given.

(1) In the conventional type, generally used throughout the world, family planning is the core unit of the service. It is either integrated with primary health care services or is an independent unit, run by a sister trained in family planning methods.

(2) In the extended type, the core unit is a maternal/child service, family planning being part of the service, e.g. family health centres. This service is purported to reach the woman at a time when she is most receptive to family planning, i.e. during the postpartum period. The family planning unit is run by the community health nurse who is also

specially trained in family planning methods.

The sister in charge of the clinic must use her ingenuity to make her clinic as attractive as possible; the following hints are guidelines to the running of a successful clinic:

(1) The clinic must be conveniently placed to give easy accessibility and privacy to clients.

(2) Clients must not be expected to wait for long periods; to prevent this, consultations can be arranged on a flexible semi-appointment system. The clinic must be open during hours which suit the clients. Queues must be avoided at all costs and comfortable waiting-room space provided.

(3) The people served by the clinic must respect and trust the staff. Respect and trust are earned by a courteous and helpful approach to people when answering their queries and listening to their problems.

The family planning sister must at all times be aware of the importance of health education, warning women against the dangers of smoking, especially when they are on steroidal contraceptives and over the age of 35 years.

Free contraceptive materials are supplied by the Department of Health to the clinic which is required to submit information at regular intervals in respect of each client. The keeping of statistical records is essential in order to guide the department in its future planning of family health services. Statistics allow for a reliable assessment of the effectiveness of the various contraceptive methods.

The nurse must remember that her clients are perfectly healthy people (usually) who are at the peak of their physical strength. They often come to the clinic for a service about which they may feel ambivalent. Satisfied clients will be enthusiastic about contraception and persuade other clients to practise it; in this way the clinic can become a tremendous force for good in the community.

As an extension to the family planning service, most clinics are geared to help in the detection of early breast and female genital tract malignancy. Sisters specially trained to do so do a thorough bimanual gynaecological examination on all new clients.

Mobile clinics no less than static clinics have all the facilities for providing a quality FP service. Apart from FP advice and help, every woman is given an annual health examination.

Some of the clients at family health clinics seldom see a doctor; clients are, therefore, given a physical examination by the clinic sister or doctor once a year. This includes examination of the eyes (e.g. for jaundice), legs for varicose veins, blood pressure, urine, thyroid gland, skin and breast. Mass is checked. The side-effects of contraceptives are noted and treated. Clients with physical abnormalities are referred for further investigation and treatment. Thus the family planning clinic plays a very important primary health care role in the maintenance of health in women of childbearing age.

Education in family planning

People must be educated to appreciate the benefits of family planning. Family planning educators direct their appeals to the health of parents and children. Most people are not moved by the spectre of world overpopulation; they are more likely to respond if they can be convinced that the quality of their home life will be improved.

The nurse and other guidance personnel will come across resistance to the principles of birth control amongst those who apparently stand to gain most from a regime of family planning. Some may have genuine convictions as to the desirability of having a large family, while others may be breeding with complete disregard for the responsibilities of parenthood. The educator who understands global problems of environmental pollution, resources depletion, water and food shortages and the imminence of the 'population explosion', will be able to channel her preventive skills in helping to guide those who through ignorance or misguidedness are breeding indiscriminately, to exercise some control for the sake of the future generations.

A very comprehensive national guidance (adviser) programme has been organised for the purpose of motivating the population to participate in family planning. Guidance (adviser) field workers undergo a training period of three weeks. State Health plans to employ hundreds of these field workers — one for every 30 000

persons in the community they serve — to disseminate knowledge and persuade people to
limit their families. These workers are especially selected for their ability to contact people
and they match the ethnic group they serve.
They work under the supervision of liaison officers and their effectiveness is measured by
weekly reporting and evaluation of the number
of new clients who report at family planning
clinics through their persuasive efforts.

Personal communication of guidance (adviser) personnel is supported by mass-com-
munication media to encourage the idea of
family planning. These media are: the radio
and television, cinema advertisements, exhi-
bitions at shows, films, newspapers, magazines, photo story booklets, brochures and
pamphlets. Professional literature on all aspects of family planning care can be obtained,
free of charge, from Regional Directors of the
Department of Health.

Many black people associate a large family
with wealth and with security for parents in old
age. A country-wide study done by the Human
Sciences Research Council on the fertility behaviour of black women in South Africa revealed that, of women between the ages of 40
and 44 years, approximately 30 % had given
birth to fewer than 5 children, 40 % had between
5 and 7 children and 30 % had 8 or more living
children.

As the services of the National Family
Planning Programme are available to all
women of South Africa, irrespective of the
colour of their skin, the above statistics give
much food for thought. They reflect the level
of socio-economic development of different
sections of the South African peoples. As in
all diseases associated with poverty (i.e. undernutrition and infection), improvement in
the pernicious condition of overbreeding
seems to occur as the socio-economic status
of the people improves; health education in
the absence of such improvement seems to
have very little effect in persuading people to
limit the size of their families for the sake of
self-interest or for the sake of averting a
global population explosion.

Motivating clients to accept family planning: A guide for nurses

Nurses who attend groups of mothers at preventive (family) health centres or at independent
family planning clinics have the opportunity to
motivate them to practise birth control and plan
their families to suit their means and childbearing capacities.

One of the main functions of nurses in
family planning clinics is educative, in the wide
sense of changing attitudes in order to
strengthen personal motivation so that clients
who come for help will not only persist in the
face of difficulties but will also influence others
to come to the clinics. Most of the family planning educative work is being done by means of
lectures, personal talks, films and literature.
Education is geared towards promoting the
health and happiness of the family. An excerpt
from a booklet published by the Transvaal
Planned Parenthood Association of Southern
Africa, intended for distribution to blacks, illustrate these aims:

'It is natural and good that people should fall
in love and get married. It is natural also that
married people should have children. We all
want healthy children and healthy children need
food and clothing and blankets to keep them
healthy. But all these things, so necessary to a
child's health, cost money and the cost of living
is getting higher and higher . . . so that if parents
want healthy children, they can't afford to have
too many children. Our ancestors knew this in
the old days and they spaced their children. It is,
however, natural and good that married people
should make love. But while making love is
good and natural, having too many children as
a result of making love causes problems. So
sensible people find means of making love without having unwanted children. This is where
family planning or birth control comes in. Let
me explain the various methods of birth control.
None of these methods I will explain causes the
child to be killed. They stop the child from being
made in the woman. And none of the methods I
will explain causes any lessening of sex power.
Birth control methods allow people to make
love completely and yet not have children they
do not want.' (Included by kind permission of
the Transvaal Planned Parenthood Association.)

In motivating parents the nurse can use the following arguments.

(1) She can point out the advantages of limiting the size of the family, especially with regard to poverty prevention. Parents with limited incomes cannot do justice to large families. They cannot give a large number of children proper food, clothing, accommodation and education; the parents also suffer privations as they receive no material rewards for their labours in order to gratify their own needs. Ignorance, overcrowding and malnutrition, the inevitable accompaniments of poverty, cause many preventable diseases, such as tuberculosis, parasitic diseases and kwashiorkor.

(2) The nurse can point out that it is possible to prevent pregnancy-related problems and to promote health by family planning.

  (a) Anaemia, gynaecological problems, mental and physical exhaustion.

  (b) If the mother is not overburdened with pregnancy and childbearing, she will have more time for her husband and children and, in the relaxed atmosphere of her home, promote good family relationships. If the fear of unwanted pregnancies is removed, the couple are more likely to develop healthy sexual relationships.

  (c) If all the children are planned and really wanted, the mother is more likely to make a success of her mothering role. A rejected, unwanted child is prone to abuse by his parents. Child abuse and neglect cause physical and mental ill-health.

(3) The nurse can banish the fear in the minds of many women that contraceptive practices will harm them. If the sensitive nurse can elicit the fears of women who are uninformed with regard to modern contraceptive methods, she will be able to set their minds at rest by giving them the correct information. The usual fears encountered are: fear of cancer, thrombosis, infertility and the fear of some husbands that their wives will be unfaithful to them.

(4) The nurse can sketch the extra advantages of attending a family planning clinic, viz.

the detection of diseases. At these clinics clients are examined not only for the purpose of deciding on a suitable family planning method but also to look for early signs of disease, especially cancer. Anaemia, hypertension, diabetes, venereal (sexually transmitted) disease, leprosy, tuberculosis and malnutrition can be spotted and referred for early treatment.

(5) The nurse must remember that many clients are ambivalent about contraception because of culturally inculcated taboos against anything 'unnatural' with regard to procreation — a function considered a sacred duty. Overcoming religious scruples and cultural taboos requires knowledge of the client's beliefs and value system.

For example, some Christian denominations are against birth control because they maintain that it goes against God's Word. It would appear, however, that for every biblical text which appears to condemn contraception there is one to encourage it. Example: Genesis 1:28 versus Isaiah 5:5.

There are still some people who deny that a population problem exists at all. This denial stems either from ignorance or from an inability to face the problem because of the moral issues involved in artificial methods of birth control. On our own continent there is massive prejudice against the concept of birth control. The population of Africa is increasing at the rate of 8 million per year; at present it totals approximately 350 million. A number of African governments have officially recognised the need for family planning and are collaborating with the International Planned Parenthood Federation (IPPF). Some of their people, however, are obeying the dictates of some churches which forbid birth control by artificial methods. Some believe it is part of the white man's scheme to dominate the black man by keeping down his numbers, while others subscribe to the cultural prejudice that the size of the family is a measure of a man's virility. At present the birth-rate of blacks is more than three times that of whites who have used birth control methods for some time. It must be remembered that 'family planning' is a health service and is entirely voluntary.

(6) The nurse can elaborate on the different methods by which pregnancy can be prevented. The three criteria for an effective contraceptive method are:

    (*a*) it must be effective in preventing pregnancy;

    (*b*) it must not harm the health of the client;

    (*c*) it must be acceptable to the client and his/her spouse.

The nurse can state with authority that the following 'folk' contraceptive practices are totally ineffective:

    (*a*) prolonged lactation (contraception should be started not later than 2 months post-partum, but preferably immediately post-partum);

    (*b*) douching after intercourse;

    (*c*) drinking 'lewensessens';

    (*d*) keeping back by the woman of the emotional release which constitutes orgasm during coitus;

    (*e*) placing cotton wool soaked in oil or vinegar in the vagina during intercourse.

The nurse can explain the following relatively effective contraceptive methods:

    (*a*) rhythm methods;

    (*b*) coitus interruptus;

    (*c*) intra-vaginal spermicidal creams with or without the diaphragm.

These methods are not very acceptable to clients because:

    (*a*) in the rhythm method, coitus must be avoided for half the month;

    (*b*) spermicidal chemicals can cause allergic reactions and burn both the male and female;

    (*c*) coitus interruptus may cause frigidity in the female as she is so often robbed of orgasm;

    (*d*) both spermicidal chemicals and the diaphragm need pre-coital preparation.

The following good and effective methods are explained to the clients. They must be warned, however, that there is a slight possibility of pregnancy occurring even if the methods are used correctly:

    (*a*) injection of Depo-Provera;

    (*b*) oral combined hormonal pills;

    (*c*) intra-uterine devices.

(The above 3 are used by the female.)

    (*d*) The condom used by the male. The condom is very effective if the man withdraws his penis immediately after intercourse and if, during a withdrawal, he holds the condom to the shaft of the penis so that no semen leaks into the vagina.

The only 100 % safe methods of preventing conception are sterilisation and total abstention. Even intercourse outside the vagina, i.e. between the thighs of the woman, is unsafe, as spermatozoa deposited on the vulva can swim upwards through the vagina to eventually reach the Fallopian tubes. See p. 350 for the degree of effectiveness of the various contraceptive methods.

Family planning is a very important aspect of preventive health; it forms the cornerstone of a community health programme as it is aimed at effecting a decline in the birth-rate of the community, thereby promoting many advantages as described. This can be achieved only if it is accepted by the community as a public service.

THE IMPLEMENTATION OF BIRTH CONTROL AND FAMILY PLANNING METHODS

There are three main measures to control the growth rate of a population:

- Sterilisation
- Abortion
- Contraception

Surgical sterilisation

Surgical sterilisation may be used for two purposes:

- for permanent contraception; and
- as a PHC measure to limit population growth.

Permanent contraception

Surgical sterilisation is ideal for couples requiring effective, permanent contraception when their families have been completed or where pregnancy is contra-indicated. The choice is between male and female contraception, the male vasectomy being safer and simpler than the female tubal occlusion.

In this case sterilisation is an elective procedure. Female sterilisation is done either through a mini-semilunar transumbilical incision of 3 cm to expose the peritoneal cavity, or by means of a laparoscope (endoscope) introduced into the peritoneal cavity through an abdominal stab wound.

The interruption in tubal continuity is obtained as follows:

(1) by bipolar tubal cauterisation — an irreversible operation;
(2) by clips (Filshie-silicon-vitallium) or rings (Falope) applied 2 cm from the uterus on each Fallopian tube.

Although these methods are intended to bring about permanent sterilisation, they are potentially reversible as very little tubal tissue is sacrificed.

Laparoscopy is done virtually on an out-patient basis as most patients are discharged on the same day, i.e. if there are no complications. Some patients are able to return to work the next day.

Female sterilisation by tubal occlusion does not affect the menstrual pattern or cause menstrual discomforts, nor does it adversely influence libido.

Tubal occlusion is not an infallible form of contraception, as a small percentage of women thus sterilised may become pregnant.

Recently the Medical Council issued the following directive: 'Except where it is done on purely medical grounds, a sterilisation operation shall not be performed unless:

(1) the full implications have been explained to the patient, or to both husband and wife if the patient is married;
(2) the patient, if unmarried, is a major (a married person, irrespective of age, is a major);
(3) written consent has been obtained from the patient, or from both husband and wife if the patient is married.'

The couple should be counselled prior to the operation. The counsellor must ensure: that both partners understand the procedure and its effects, (i.e. no alteration in weight or sex function), that the marriage is stable, that sex function is satisfactory and that there is no stress or coercion. The couple must consider the loss of a partner or children and the option of reversible contraception. There is less likelihood of regret afterwards if the pros and cons are carefully considered. The couple must be told about the small possibility of a failed sterilisation and this information must be included in their sterilisation consent form.

To limit population growth

Where sterilisation forms part of a primary health care programme to limit population growth, the approach is somewhat different.

Sterilisation as a means of controlling population growth is increasing in popularity. There are World Federation of Health Agencies for the Advancement of Voluntary Surgical Contraception (WFHA–AVSC). The RSA is an affiliated member through the Association for Voluntary Sterilisation of South Africa which was formed in 1980.[5] The World Federation is an international voluntary health service and family planning system. It is estimated that between 1975–1980, 100 million people were sterilised throughout the world.

The Association's four immediate aims are:

(1) To concentrate openly and honestly on demographic aims (2-child families) which request a sterilisation after the second child. The mother is psychologically prepared to give consent during antenatal visits to the antenatal clinic.
(2) To involve all medical practitioners in South Africa in creating quality sterilisation services.
(3) To see that all medical aid patients are immediately compensated for sterilisation expenses.
(4) To encourage all medical personnel throughout South Africa to help make sterilisation services available every day, including weekends and public holidays.

Dr de Villiers[6] is of the opinion that 'voluntary surgical contraception should be South Africa's first and foremost weapon in the fight against overpopulation, underdevelopment of people and the lack of opportunities so necessary to develop the potential of each and every child in our country'. At community obstetric centres counselling for acceptance of post-partum sterilisation is part of the comprehensive antenatal care of all booked patients. The patients are informed about the various methods with the help of audio-visual programmes. Patients attend in groups and two motivators lead them in discussion. At this time written consent for operation is obtained, months before delivery and sterilisation.

The ultimate goal of sterilisation for women with two children attending the clinics has been propagated since 1985. Sterilisation is done within 48 hours after the delivery of the child (post-partum sterilisation).

The chief professional nurse of each of the nine health regions of the RSA co-ordinates sterilisation services with provincial hospitals. Female clients are referred by FP clinics and male clients by male advisers. Before being sent to hospital, a PAP smear is taken from a woman, and blood is tested for haemoglobin.

Sterilisation in males

The operation in males is a simple one called vasectomy, in which the vas deferens on both sides of the scrotum is sectioned and ligated. The man is not sterile immediately afterwards, as some mature sperm may remain in the genital tract; the sperm are eventually expelled after approximately 12 ejaculations. It is, therefore, imperative for the couple to practise contraception until the man is 'safe'. It must be remembered that vasectomy is not castration which implies removal of both testes (orchidectomy). Vasectomy does not in any way interfere with sexual potency and the continuity of the vasa can in some cases be re-established by plastic surgery, if the vas has not been destroyed by electrocautery. In some parts of the world (not SA) frozen semen is stored in case the man wants to impregnate a woman at some future time. Vasectomy is becoming increasingly popular as it is a quick, cheap operation which does not affect sexual desire or competence, the man even ejaculating the same amount of seminal fluid (mainly from the seminal vesicles and prostate) as before vasectomy. In India, male sterilisation is very commonly practised, men actually being paid by the government to have the operation and to persuade other men to do likewise.

The circumstances in which a person who is incapable of consenting or incompetent to con-

sent to sterilisation may be sterilised, as defined by the Abortion and Sterilisation Act 2 of 1975, as amended in 1980 and 1982, are:

Sterilisation shall not be performed on any person who for any reason is incapable of consenting or incompetent to consent thereto, unless:

(1) two medical practitioners, of whom one shall be a psychiatrist, have certified in writing that the person concerned
   (a) is suffering from a hereditary condition of such a nature that if he or she were to procreate a child, such child would suffer from a physical or mental defect of such a nature that it would be seriously handicapped; or
   (b) due to a permanent medical handicap or defect is unable to comprehend the consequential implications of or bear the parental responsibility for the fruit of coitus;

(2) the person who may in law consent to an operation beneficial to that person has granted written consent to the sterilisation, or, if there is no such first-mentioned person or such person cannot after reasonable enquiry be found, the magistrate of the district in which the person concerned finds himself or herself has, after such investigation as he may deem fit, granted written authority for the sterilisation and

(3) The Minister, or a medical officer of the Department of Health authorised thereto by him in writing, has granted written authority for the sterilisation.

The Act defines 'sterilisation' as follows:

'Sterilisation means a surgical operation performed for the purpose of making the person on whom it is performed incapable of procreation, but does not include the removal of any gonads.'

Abortions

It is generally believed that abortion, whether officially sanctioned or not, is the most commonly practised method of population control in the world today. In no country in the world is population growth showing signs of becoming controlled except in those permitting abortion on request.[7]

Eberstadt (Harvard University researcher) states (*Rand Daily Mail*, Jan. 1982) that between 40 million and 60 million abortions are performed world-wide each year. Most of them are performed in poor countries, mostly under unsanitary conditions and by unqualified persons. Complications are the leading cause of death for women between the ages of 15 and 35.

Public opinion regarding abortion has changed in recent years. Potts, Diggory and Peel[8] state that one-third of the world's adult female population can legally obtain an abortion on request. Altogether, 60 % can have a pregnancy terminated for non-medical reasons. Only 8 % live in countries where abortion is illegal.

A report in the *Rand Daily Mail* (25.2.1983) states that 9 727 incomplete abortions were dealt with in four Cape hospitals in the past 3 years and 12 patients, of whom 11 were blacks, died. The Minister of Health stated in Parliament that almost 27 000 women were admitted to hospitals in 1992 as a result of complications arising from illegal abortions.

South African attitudes towards 'abortion-on-demand' are conservative. In 1979 Dommisse[9] investigated the attitudes of South African obstetricians and gynaecologists to the South African abortion laws. (Less than half responded to a questionnaire.) He found that whereas only 30 % favoured abortion on request before 12 weeks, 82 % were in favour of a modification of the present law or its application. Eighteen per cent were satisfied with the present laws.

Many South Africans went to England and Wales for legal abortions in these countries. The UK will no longer accept South Africans for induced abortions.

In 1985, 712 legal abortions were done in South Africa and 609 on South African citizens in England and Wales; in 1987 the figure for the latter was 447. It would seem that for women seeking a legal abortion the South African legislation is too restrictive.[10]

Therapeutic abortions are procured preferably before the twelfth week (i.e. during the first trimester) of pregnancy or after the 16th week (i.e. during the second trimester). It is a safe procedure if done by one of the following methods:

(1) Surgical curettage (D & C).

(2) Suction curettage.

(The above two are done if period of gestation is 12 weeks or less.)

(3) Injections of prostaglandins (intra-amniotic) done after the 16th week of gestation.

Note: The prostaglandins, of which PGE_2 and PGF_2-alpha are examples, are a large new group of hormone-like therapeutic substances which probably play a role in cellular metabolism. They are either extracted from natural tissues or they can be chemically synthesised from unsaturated fatty acids. They can be administered by many routes: intravenous, oral, intramuscular, intra-uterine, per vaginam and intra-amniotic sac. They produce, *inter alia*, the following effects on the body; stimulation of uterine contractions, stimulation of smooth muscle causing diarrhoea and vomiting, inhibition of gastric secretion, pro- and anti-inflammatory effects, lowering of blood pressure, dilatation of bronchial tubes and constriction of nasal blood vessels.

The circumstances in which an abortion may be procured are defined by the Abortion and Sterilisation Act 2 of 1975, which states:

'**3.** Abortion may be procured by a medical practitioner only, and then only —

(*a*) where the continued pregnancy endangers the life of the woman concerned or constitutes a serious threat to her physical health, and two other medical practitioners have certified in writing that, in their opinion, the continued pregnancy so endangers the life of the woman or so constitutes a serious threat to her physical health and abortion is necessary to ensure the life or physical health of the woman;

(*b*) where the continued pregnancy constitutes a serious threat to the mental health of the woman concerned, and two other medical practitioners have certified in writing that, in their opinion, the continued pregnancy creates the danger of permanent damage to the woman's mental health and abortion is necessary to ensure the mental health of the woman;

(*c*) where there exists the serious risk that the child to be born will suffer from a physical or mental defect of such a nature that he will be irreparably seriously handicapped, and two other medical practitioners have certified in writing that, in their opinion, there exists, on scientific grounds, such a risk; or (*d*) where the foetus is alleged to have been conceived in consequence of unlawful carnal intercourse, and two other medical practitioners have certified in writing after such interrogation of the woman concerned as they or any of them may have considered necessary that, in their opinion, the pregnancy is due to unlawful carnal intercourse;

(*e*) where the foetus has been conceived in consequence of illegitimate carnal intercourse, and two other medical practitioners have certified in writing that the woman concerned is, due to a permanent mental handicap or defect, unable to comprehend the consequential implications of or bear the potential responsibility for the fruit of coitus.'

The Act defines 'unlawful carnal intercourse' as follows:

'Unlawful carnal intercourse means rape and incest.'

The law lays down which medical practitioners may certify in writing that a woman is eligible for an abortion, for example, if an abortion is necessary to ensure the mental health of a woman, at least one doctor shall be a psychiatrist employed by the state, and if pregnancy is allegedly due to incest or rape, at least one doctor who signs the certificate authorising an abortion, shall be the district surgeon concerned.

'**5.** (1) An abortion may be procured and a sterilisation contemplated in section 4 may be performed only at a State-controlled institution (including a provincial hospital) or an institution designated in writing for the purpose by the Minister in terms of subsection (2).

(2) The Minister may designate any institution for the purposes of subsection (1), and subject to such conditions and requirements as he may consider necessary or expedient for achieving the objects of the Act and may, if in his opinion it is justified, at any time withdraw any such designation.

(3) A decision of the Minister in terms of subsection (2) shall be final.'

The law lays down further conditions for the carrying out of the above operations:

(1) the consent (written authority) of the doctor in charge of an approved institution must be obtained;

(2) the doctor who is to procure the abortion or perform the sterilisation must apply for authority to the doctor-in-charge of the institution on a prescribed form; this is to be accompanied, *inter alia*, by the necessary certificates;

(3) in the case where pregnancy follows unlawful carnal intercourse a certificate must be obtained from a magistrate attached to the court having jurisdiction in respect of the alleged offence in question;

(4) the doctor-in-charge of the institution (who has granted authority to operate) must notify the Director-General: DOH (giving the prescribed information) within 21 days of the operation. The doctor-in-charge must keep, or cause to be kept, a record of the prescribed particulars.

'**9.** A medical practitioner (other than a medical practitioner referred to in section 6(1) (i.e. the doctor-in-charge of an authorised institution), a nurse or any person employed in any other capacity at an institution referred to in section 5(1) (State-controlled institution or institution designated in writing for the purpose by the Minister) shall, notwithstanding any contract or the provisions of any other law, not be obliged to participate in or assist with any abortion contemplated in section 3 or any sterilisation contemplated in section 4.'

In 1977, the Board of the South African Nursing Association, in considering what constitutes the right of withdrawal of nurses from abortion cases as specified in the above paragraph, resolved that:

'The individual nurse who, for moral reasons, has a conflict of conscience and duty, would still be required to care for the aborted patient after the operation in accordance with the South African Nursing Association's pledge of service — "The total health of my patient will be my first consideration."

The Board advises employing authorities that if nurses and midwives wish to object to co-operating in operations, they should make their attitude known, either when seeking employment in a hospital or, if they have not done this, at an appropriate time, e.g. nursing personnel should be able to refuse to perform specific duties when performance would conflict with their religious, moral or ethical convictions (subject to informing their supervisor in good time and being satisfied that nursing care is ensured) without being penalised.'[11]

The law lays down the penalties for persons who are not medical practitioners and who procure abortions, as well as for medical practitioners who procure abortions and do sterilisation operations without the appropriate certificates, or at an unauthorised institution, or who grant written authority for these operations without being in possession of an appropriate certificate. The maximum penalties are R5 000 or 5 years' imprisonment or both such fine and imprisonment.

In most of the larger centres in South Africa, psychiatric factors are cited in the majority of cases as the indication for legal termination of pregnancy.

At the Johannesburg Hospital, the following procedure has been successfully followed in carrying out the requirements of the Abortion and Sterilisation Act 1975:[4] Applicants for legal abortion are seen at a Pregnancy Advisory Clinic by a Pregnancy Advisory Committee who advises the hospital superintendent on whether an application for abortion should be granted or refused. This committee consists of the following members: social worker(s); state psychiatrist(s), gynaecologist(s); hospital superintendent; other medical officers concerned with specific patients, e.g. referring general practitioner and medical officer from the out-patient department. Patients are referred to the clinic by their general practitioners, gynaecologists or hospital out-patient doctors. A full history is first taken from the applicant by a senior social worker who helps the patient resolve the crisis situation posed by the unwanted pregnancy. A gynaecologist is then consulted about the duration of pregnancy; the patient may be referred from here for further specialist opinion, e.g. to a psychiatrist. Within 10 days of the application being made, the Pregnancy Advisory Committee reviews all the available information gathered and takes the decision whether

to advise or refuse termination of pregnancy. The patient is helped to make an informed decision, especially with regard to going through with the pregnancy. (Some of those refused undoubtedly seek illegal help with the termination of their pregnancy.) Patients who are refused termination are given emotional and physical help during their pregnancy and are referred to community resources. Psychiatric and psychological follow-up care is given to all women referred to the clinic; they are counselled with regard to the use of contraceptives and are referred to family planning clinics.

The ANC supports a pro-choice stance on abortion. In a recent survey conducted for *Modern Medicine*, more than half of the medical practitioners believe that women have the right to abortion on request. This belief is hotly debated by the Pro-Life protagonists who champion the rights of the foetus. Unwanted pregnancies in black townships are a great problem where the schoolgirl pregnancy rate is 14 %. It is not yet known how, and to what extent, the abortion laws in South Africa will be adapted to meet modern needs and demands.

Contraception

There are many methods of practising contraception, some being more effective than others, some being used by the man only and others by the woman only. Some methods will be described only briefly, while those likely to be used on the advice of family planning clinics (which are seldom visited by men) will be discussed in greater detail. There is no one ideal method of contraception; each method has advantages and disadvantages. These and client reliability and personal preferences are taken into consideration when giving contraceptive counselling.

Post-coital contraception (PCC)

Post-coital contraception may be necessary as an emergency measure to protect a woman against a possible pregnancy which is undesired. Unprotected coitus may be due to unlawful carnal intercourse, failed contraception, ignorance of contraceptive methods, unexpected coitus or failure to take the pill for 2 days. The woman who fears she may become pregnant must approach her doctor or family planning clinic within 72 hours after coitus. She is given 2 Ovral tablets stat. and 2, 12 hours later. If she vomits any of these tablets within 3 hours, the dose is repeated after administration of an anti-emetic.

The insertion of a copper IUCD within 120 hours (5 days) of mid-cycle coitus, can also be very effective, although not infallible.

Note: PCC is only recommended as an emergency method in the event of unprotected coitus.

The effectiveness of a contraceptive method

The effectiveness of a contraceptive method is expressed as the pregnancy rate per 100 women years. The more successful the method, the lower will be the pregnancy rate, consequently, the lower the failure rate.

100 woman years = 100 women × 12 ovulations (year)

Only total abstention and hysterectomy will prevent conception. The failure rate varies from less than 1 (pregnancies per 100 woman years) in the case of steroidal and surgical contraception to over 30 in the case of natural family planning. The following methods of contraception are placed in order of effectiveness, from most to least effective:

Surgical

- Vasectomy
- Tubal occlusion

Injectable progestogens

- Depo-Provera
  150 mg 12-weekly
  450 mg 24-weekly
  Nur-Isterate 200 mg 8-weekly

Oral

- Combined steroids
- Progestogen only (mini-pill)

Intra-uterine

- Copper IUCD, 3-yearly

Mechanical

- Diaphragm, prior to/during coitus
- Condom during coitus

Spermicidal

- Jelly, Cream, Foam, Pessaries

Coitus interruptus, withdrawal during coitus

Natural family planning

- Temperature method
- Calendar rhythm
- Cervical mucus method

Many adolescents experiment with coitus and some even indulge in regular sex. In these cases it is a much wiser policy to supply contraceptive information and contraceptives to the adolescent than to expose her to the risk of pregnancy. It is wise to get the consent of the parents, however, and if necessary to counsel them with regard to their relationship with their child. Although the parents of a minor may forbid a doctor or family planning clinic to supply contraceptives to their child, contraceptive advice may be given on request of such minor without obtaining the consent of the parent, guardian or spouse (in the case of an adolescent wife). Sex and contraceptive education can, therefore, be given without fear of parental recrimination, provided the client (adolescent) gives consent (verbal or by voluntary presence) for such education. The following contraceptive advice can be given to an adolescent:

- If coitus is irregular: condom plus spermicidal agent.
- If coitus takes place on a regular basis: combined steroidal pill or an intra-uterine device.

Contraceptives may never be supplied or administered without informed verbal consent. No woman may, therefore, be given an injection of Depo-Provera against her will and without knowing the reason for its administration.

The selection of the best method of contraception for the individual client is essential in family planning. The woman should be followed up by regular appointments so that contraception may be supervised. Supervision includes verbal and written instructions to ensure that clients know what adverse side-effects (if any) to expect and when to report them.

The various contraceptive methods will be discussed below.

Natural family planning

This is essentially a method of periodic sexual abstention. It is the least reliable of the relatively effective methods, as its efficiency depends on knowledge of ovulation times which may be very variable indeed.

Ovulation takes place on the 14th day before menstruation, but it is very dependent on regularity of the menses and on psychological influences. It is a physiological fact that conception can take place only while the ovum is alive in the oviduct, for approximately 1–3 days somewhere during the middle of the menstrual cycle. The spermatozoa can, however, remain alive in the Fallopian tubes for several days, thus prolonging the 'danger' period to approximately 9 days. If coitus takes place during this period or shortly before, conception is likely to take place. The peri-ovulation period is, therefore, the danger period and the rest of the month is the safe period. The problem is to know when ovulation actually takes place. Some women suffer from 'Mittelschmerz' and can therefore fix the time of ovulation accurately. Others use temperature checks, taking their own rectal temperature at exactly the same time every morning before rising. Ovulation causes a slight drop in temperature, followed a day or two later by a rise of 0,5 °C above the normal temperature for the previous 14 days. She will be 'safe' if she avoids unguarded coitus until three days after the temperature has gone up and stayed up. It remains at this level until menstruation starts, when it once more drops to the 'normal' level. By repeating temperature checks for many months, a woman is able to fix her time of ovulation, if her temperature variations have remained constant. Danger periods can be worked out (usually from the 10th to the 19th day after the start of menstruation) and the couple can either abstain from coitus during this period or make use of a condom or a diaphragm.

The mucus secreted by the cervix changes during the menstrual cycle, becoming noticeably copious for a few days before ovulation. This mucus enables the sperm to swim up through the vagina, uterus and into the Fallopian tubes to await the arrival of the ovum. The Billings method of natural family planning teaches women to recognise this change in mucus secretion and to abstain from coitus during this time.

Natural family planning methods cause the highest failure rate. They make use of natural (physiological) anti-pregnancy forces, i.e. thick cervical mucus, periods when the ovum is not present in the tube. These are physiological safe periods. However, spermatozoa may survive up to 7 days and there is no sure way of predicting ovulation except in the case of Mittelschmerz. If coitus is restricted to the pre- and post-ovulation period (determined by temperature and cervical mucus) the risk of pregnancy is decreased.

Clients must be counselled about the relatively high failure rates.

The condom method

The condom is a thin rubber or synthetic rubber sheath worn over the penis by men during sexual intercourse. It is one of the oldest, cheapest, safest and most widely used contraceptive devices. It is the only method which protects the healthy partner against venereal disease — should the other partner be infected. It was, therefore, issued to soldiers in the Middle East during World War II. It is rolled-up when packed and is unrolled on to the erect penis just before coitus. The man must withdraw the penis immediately after coitus and hold the condom to the shaft of the penis.

The condom should be lubricated before use, if it is not self-lubricating. It is wise to use some spermicidal cream or jelly in case some of the semen is spilled in the vagina.

Apart from preventing the spread of sexually transmitted diseases (STDs), including AIDS, it also provides some protection against pelvic infection in the woman, human papillomavirus infection and carcinoma of the cervix. The use of spermicides which are viricidal, in conjunction with a condom, affords double protection against the spread of virus STD infections.

Femshield, the vaginal shield or female condom, is one of the most promising developments in recent years, especially as it offers a protective barrier in the vagina against STDs and AIDS. It is used once only. Femshield is a blind-ending hollow tube, 15 cm long and 7 cm in diameter. It is made of a strong thin plastic material as used in ostomy bags. Attached to the open end of the tube is a soft plastic ring which holds the tube in place against the vulva. The Femshield thus covers part of the vulva, the vagina and the cervix. A separate ring is provided to aid insertion and to retain the tube within the vagina during coitus. It is inserted before coitus.

Coitus interruptus

Coitus interruptus or withdrawal of the penis before male orgasm and ejaculation is a very ancient contraceptive practice which is still widely used, some couples using it intermittently as an emergency measure whilst for others it is standard practice. For the expert it can be a safe method but the danger is that even if one drop of semen leaks into the vagina or if the ejaculate is deposited on the vulva near the introitus, pregnancy can occur. Coitus interruptus can also disturb the sexual relationship as the need for prompt withdrawal may cause anxiety, tension and non-satisfaction of the woman.

Coitus interruptus is a potential cause of sexual dysfunction. Post-coital contraception should be available in case ejaculation took place in the vagina.

Spermicidal chemicals

Spermicidal chemical barrier creams, jellies and foams introduced into the vagina by special applicator spread a protective coating over the vagina and the mouth of the cervix. Pessaries (suppositories) placed in the posterior fornix serve the same purpose and must be inserted at least 15 minutes before coitus to give them time to melt. The contraceptive foams appear to be the most effective and least messy preparations and are the most commonly used.

Their effectiveness depends on the use of sufficient foam before each act of coitus, which is inserted not more than one hour beforehand. All the chemical barriers can be obtained from a chemist without prescription, or from a family planning clinic.

Note:
(1) Directions on the package for the filling of the applicator, timing and method of application must be followed.
(2) The recumbent position is necessary for instillation and retention of the chemical barrier cream, as the woman will not be protected if an amount of the recommended dose escapes from the vagina.

(3) Another dose of the contraceptive must be applied if there is further intercourse after an hour.
(4) The woman must not douche within at least 6 hours after intercourse.

The failure rate is high when used alone, therefore they are used as an additional method (adjunct) when starting oral contraceptives, or when using the condom, diaphragm, IUD or withdrawal methods.

The diaphragm cap

Before the use of hormones and intra-uterine devices, the diaphragm cap was the chief method of contraception recommended by family planning clinics. The diaphragm cap is used in the vagina in conjunction with spermicidal jelly, cream or foam. The diaphragm cap is a shallow, bowl-shaped, tough rubber or synthetic rubber cap with a circular rim which contains a flexible metal ring. It ranges in diameter from 50 mm to 105 mm. It must be fitted and taut when in position. Before use the bowl is filled with a teaspoon or more of contraceptive jelly which is also spread around the inside of the rim. In order to insert the diaphragm, the rim is compressed between the fingers and the appliance is slipped into the vagina. The anterior rim is pushed up behind the symphysis pubis and the posterior rim is placed in the posterior fornix behind the cervix. In this way the diaphragm covers the cervix thereby helping to prevent the sperm from entering the uterus. More spermicidal jelly is then introduced into the vagina as the rim never fits so securely against the vaginal walls as to prevent entry of sperm entirely. In any case, the vagina changes its shape during coitus so that even the most carefully fitted diaphragm floats loosely in the vagina during the ejaculation of spermatozoa.

The diaphragm is inserted just before coitus or up to 3 hours before the time and may remain in position for 24 hours. It must remain in position for at least 8 hours after coitus. The woman may walk about and pass urine with the diaphragm in position.

The diaphragm is removed by hooking a finger under the anterior rim and pulling it out. Its removal can be followed by a cleansing douche but this is not necessary, ordinary vulval washing being sufficient. The diaphragm is washed with mild soap and water, then dried, powdered and stored. Sterilisation is unnecessary. The greatest disadvantage of the diaphragm, apart from failure to prevent pregnancy, is the rather lengthy and somewhat laborious preparation required before its use can be considered safe. The woman must either go to bed prepared for coitus every night, or she must interrupt a romantic moment to prepare herself. In this way the diaphragm may obtrude on the sex lives of couples.

Note:

(1) The diaphragm cap should last from 1 to 2 years if properly cared for, i.e. if dried, powdered and safely stored after use and if not stretched, pricked and subjected to strong soaps or detergents. It should be regularly inspected for holes and thin places as an intact diaphragm is essential for effective contraception.

(2) A different sized diaphragm may be required after the birth of a baby, after abortion or vaginal operation or if there has been great mass loss or gain.

(3) Diaphragms are unsuitable until 8 to 12 weeks after the birth of the infant.

(4) Diaphragms are contra-indicated in cases of cystocele, prolaps, poor muscle tone, poor motivation.

Intra-uterine contraceptive device (IUCD)

IUCDs are compressible pieces of moulded 'memory' plastic which are placed inside the uterine cavity to stop implantation of the fertilised ovum.

IUCDs exert their effect by reason of being irritant foreign bodies which elicit an inflammatory reaction with the outpouring of many polymorph leucocytes which phagocytose spermatozoa and any fertilised ovum which may be present. Copper increases this inflammatory reaction.

They are made in different shapes and are approximately 25 mm in diameter. In 1972 the anti-fertility action of copper was discovered; when copper wire is wound round a portion of the IUCD, the extra effectiveness of the IUCD lasts for approximately three years as the copper then becomes spent. The copper IUCD's in use at present are: Copper T, Cu7 (Gravigard) and Multiload CU 250, Cu 375, Nova-T and more. The silver cord in the TCu380 Ag and Nova-T devices prevents fragmentation of the copper wire, thereby extending the life of the IUCD for up to 5 years. Cuprocept is the first South African-made copper-containing IUCD.

Intra-uterine devices have been used in family planning clinics since 1964 and play a very important role in helping to control population growth. They are safe and effective and require little co-operation from the rather unsophisticated section of our population, who may lack strong motivation to practise birth control or who may be unreliable in carrying out other forms of contraception. They are used extensively in population control programmes in underdeveloped countries throughout the world, being most suitable for women over 30 who have completed their families.

Plastic IUCDs are visible on X-rays. The device is inserted into the uterus by a specially trained doctor or nurse through a small tube which is

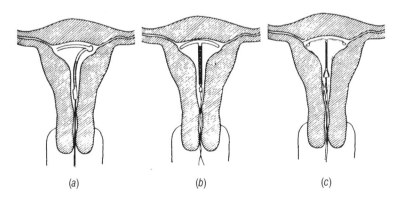

(a)　　　　　　(b)　　　　　　(c)

Figure 20.1

Intra-uterine devices in position

(a) Cu / Gravigard; (b) Copper I; (c) Nova-I

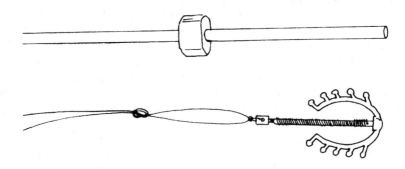

Figure 20.2
IUCD Multiload Cu 250 with inserter (actual size)

introduced through the cervix, by means of a special inserter. When pressure is released after insertion, the device springs back into its original shape. Extrusion is thus prevented.

Multiload CU250 is commonly used in national family planning clinics. Intra-uterine devices and their inserters are supplied either sterile in individual packs or unsterile, in bulk. The unsterile IUCDs are disinfected by immersion in a disinfectant, e.g. Hibicol.

IUCDs are inserted at any time up to the 17th day of the menstrual cycle, but preferably on the last day of the menses or immediately after abortion or birth. They can also be inserted at the post-partum check-up, 6 to 12 weeks after childbirth, when involution is complete. IUCDs can also be used as post-coital contraception. They can be used until the menopause.

Literature supplied by the manufacturers describes the precise method of insertion. Insertion is a sterile procedure and requires a sterile pack with vulsellum forceps, Cusco's vaginal speculum and lubricant and a uterine sound.

Note: The SA Medical and Dental Council considers that a doctor is guilty of improper conduct if he inserts an IUCD without first establishing whether the client is pregnant or not, and if he fails to remove a previously inserted IUCD before commencing to insert a new one. These rules would likewise apply to nurses who are authorised to insert IUCDs.

The nurse and the intra-uterine device

In some clinics suitably trained nurses insert IUCDs, while in others, especially those attached to training hospitals for medical stu-

dents, this task is usually delegated to the latter and their teachers. But even when the nurse does not insert the IUCD, she has many responsibilities as regards its use, viz. deciding who are the suitable clients and motivating these clients to accept the IUCD and to persist in its use despite temporary side-effects. Contrary to earlier teachings, a young nulligravida can be fitted with an IUCD. It should, however, be inserted by an expert, i.e. a doctor with much experience.

An IUCD can be left in position for three years; clinics usually replace them three-yearly as prescribed by the manufacturers. If the client experiences no problems she can continue using her IUCD even after the expiry date. Clients are advised to come for a position check 5–6 weeks after insertion of the IUCD and then annually when they come for a check-up. Clients are advised to consult the clinic sister about any problems with the IUCD.

The clients are warned about the possibility of expulsion of the IUCD and to take other contraceptive action immediately should this happen, as they then have no protection against conception. An IUCD should never be removed at or near ovulation in case a fertilised ovum is proceeding down the Fallopian tube.

The advice to clients on insertion is to do periodic self-examinations for the continued presence in the vagina of the threads attached to the IUCD, especially after menstrual periods. The client must report back to the clinic if: the threads are missing, a hard part is felt in the mouth of the cervix, a period is missed, menor-rhagia or metrorrhagia is present, there is severe pelvic pain, or there is profuse vaginal dis-charge. The client must not wear a tampon for the first six weeks and must examine pads for an expelled IUCD; she must use extra precau-tions mid-cycle if she is worried about preg-nancy.

The woman may wear a vaginal tampon after the first 6 weeks if she can cope with the extra menstrual fluid.

Contra-indications

Pregnancy, pelvic inflammatory disease and uterine growths and anomalies, severe dys-menorrhoea, rheumatic heart disease (risk of S.B.E.), tendency to menorrhagia, cervical pa-thology, e.g. incompetence and infection, small uterus, fixed retroverted uterus.

Relative contra-indications: nulliparae, past history of pelvic inflammatory disease, promis-cuity, immunosuppressive treatment.

Disadvantages of the IUCD

All side-effects are local.

(1) The client is reassuringly warned that the following may occur temporarily:
   (*a*) pain and lower abdominal cramps for 24 to 48 hours after insertion;
   (*b*) vaginal discharge (leucorrhoea) for a month;
   (*c*) spotting, intramenstrual bleeding and heavier periods for 3 months.
(2) The IUCD (copper) has a failure rate of 2 pregnancies per 100 woman years. It is, therefore, a less effective contraceptive than the combined steroidal pill.
(3) Menorrhagia or metrorrhagia.
(4) Persistent pain and dysmenorrhoea.
(5) Displacement of the IUCD, due to expulsion or translocation with perforation of the uterus.
(6) Pelvic inflammatory disease (e.g. salpingi-tis) usually due to reactivation of chronic infection by the IUCD. The risk of infection is greatest during the first 4 months after insertion and in women exposed to STD's.

HANDLING OF TROUBLESOME SIDE-EFFECTS CAUSED BY THE IUCD

(1) Menorrhagia: a large IUCD is changed for a smaller one or the client is given one packet of progestogenic oral pills. An iron tonic is prescribed to combat the anaemia. If menorrhagia persists, IUCD contracep-tion is abandoned.

(2) Persistent pain despite a correctly placed IUCD and the absence of infection: the cli-ent is given mild analgesics and a large IUCD is changed for a smaller one. If the pain does not clear up, IUCD contraception is abandoned.

(3) If menses are delayed, the possibility of pregnancy is excluded by doing a bimanual examination, asking the client about men-struation habits and, if the delay is 10 days or more, doing pregnancy tests. If the client is not pregnant, progesterone is prescribed to produce withdrawal bleeding.

Pregnancy and the IUCD

IUCDs are not as effective as the hormone pills in preventing pregnancy but are safer contracep-tives for the woman over 40 years of age who is at greater risk of developing thrombo-embolism if she takes combined oral contraceptives, espe-cially if she smokes. Not only is there an expul-sion rate and/or discontinuation rate of up to 10 % during the first year of use, but even with the IUCD *in situ*, the failure rate is approxi-mately two pregnancies per 100 woman years, especially during the first 6 months of usage. In these pregnancies, ectopic implantation fre-quently occurs.

Pregnancy with the IUCD *in situ* is not without its dangers; there may be spontaneous abortion in 50 % of cases; there may be ante-partum haemorrhage or premature labour, as well as intra-uterine sepsis. Copper has been found to be teratogenic. It is, therefore, impera-tive for the doctor to remove the IUCD if the woman is pregnant. Removal reduces the abor-tion rate to 25 %. Termination of pregnancy because of the presence of an IUCD is not legally permitted.

Displacement of the IUCD

Failure of an IUCD to remain *in situ* is due either to expulsion, displacement within the uterus or translocation, i.e. displacement of the IUCD to a site other than the cavity of the uterus, usually the peritoneal cavity. Absence of the IUCD is first suspected when either the woman on self-examination or the nurse or doctor on PV examination notices the absence of the threads in the vagina. Sometimes the threads reappear after the next menstrual period and all may be well. If the threads remain missing and the woman is not pregnant, nor the IUCD translocated or expelled (unnoticed), then the IUCD is removed instrumentally.

Translocation is due to perforation of the uterus, either primarily during insertion or secondarily due to erosion of the uterine wall by an imbedded device. Primary perforation can usually be ascribed to a faulty insertion technique, e.g. not sounding the uterine depth and, therefore, inserting the device blindly. Blind insertion is especially dangerous if the depth of the uterus is less than 4,5 cm, a depth which precludes the use of an IUCD. In the case of secondary perforation, the woman may be asymptomatic except for the missing threads, but sometimes lower abdominal pain and menstrual disorders may be present and complications

lead to abscess formation, perforation of hollow organs, adhesions and bowel obstruction.

Diagnosis is made by bimanual examination, probing the uterus, ultrasonography and radiography (if pregnancy is not suspected) as well as other complicated diagnostic techniques. After it has been located, the IUCD is removed either by laparotomy or by posterior colpotomy as soon as possible, before complications supervene.

Steroidal contraception

This is generally considered the best contraception ever invented: if it is used correctly it gives full protection against pregnancy as it prevents ovulation by inhibiting the gonadotrophic hormones of the pituitary gland. The 'pill' also corrects menstrual disorders (polymenorrhoea, hypermenorrhoea and dysmenorrhoea) and by its proper use will establish a regular 28-day menstrual cycle; it is the ideal contraceptive for the young healthy woman.

The menstrual cycle is intimately concerned with the implantation of the fertilised ovum and is controlled by two sets of hormones, those of the pituitary gland stimulating the hormonal secretion of the ovaries as well as the changes that take place in the Graafian follicle which

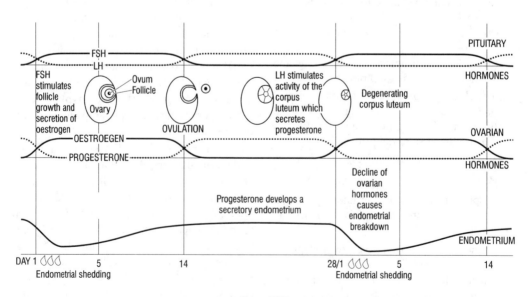

Figure 20.3

The normal menstrual cycle

houses the ovum. The anterior pituitary gland secretes two gonadotrophic hormones:

(1) the **follicle stimulating hormone (FSH)** causes the maturation of the follicle and promotes oestrogen secretion;

(2) the **luteinising hormone (LH)** causes the formation of the *corpus luteum* in the follicle after extrusion of the ovum (ovulation). It promotes the secretion of progesterone by the lutein cells.

The ovaries secrete two ovarian hormones:

(1) Increasing amounts of **oestrogen** during the first half of the menstrual cycle, by the developing Graafian follicle. After ovulation only a little oestrogen is secreted, the amount increasing again with the ripening of the next Graafian follicle once menstruation has started.

Note: A number of follicles start developing each month but usually only one, from alternate ovaries, ripens and is extruded into the abdominal cavity (on the 14th day of the cycle) and sucked up by the fimbriated end of the oviduct.

(2) **Progesterone** by the *corpus luteum*. Progesterone secretion begins after ovulation and rises until just before menstruation when it stops completely. The corpus luteum shrinks to a fibrous body called the *corpus albicans*.

Menstruation is brought about by the withdrawal of progesterone; the endometrium becomes ischaemic and breaks down; the torn blood vessels bleed and the blood carries the endometrial debris away with it.

The purpose of this cyclical activity is to prepare the endometrium for implantation of a fertilised ovum, month after month. The ovarian hormones therefore bring about important changes in the endometrium every month.

(1) *Oestrogens* cause growth of the endometrium from a thickness of 1 mm at the beginning of the cycle to a thickness of 5 mm at the end of the cycle, just before menstruation takes place. It also stimulates duct development in the breasts.

(2) *Progesterone* causes secretion of the coiled, tubular glands of the endometrium. It also stimulates alveolar development in the breasts. It is the important hormone for the maintenance of pregnancy.

Oral steroidal contraception with the 'pill'[12]

Note: A progestogen is any substance which produces biological effects similar to those of progesterone. Progestogens are steroids, like progesterone. A progestin is the generic term for a natural or synthetic progestogen.

The 'pill' consists of synthetic ovarian hormones (steroids), either a progestogen only or a

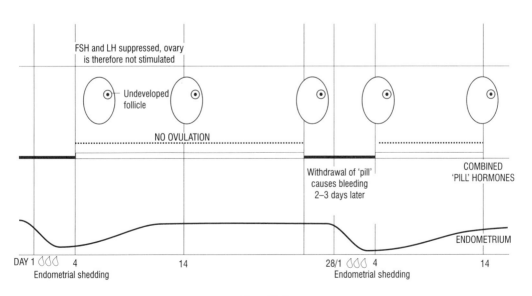

Figure 20.4

Effects of combined formulations on ovulation and hormone secretion

(Compare with 'The normal menstrual cycle', figure 20.3, page 356.)

combination of progestogen and oestrogen. The pill prevents pregnancy in the following ways:

(1) It suppresses the secretion of FSH and LH, thereby preventing the occurrence of ovulation (oestrogen and high dosage progestogen). Inhibition of ovulation is essentially due to oestrogenic action.

(2) It changes the endometrium so that implantation (nidation) cannot occur. This effect is due to the progestogenic component of the pill.

(3) By increasing the viscosity of the cervical mucus, progestogen inhibits the penetration of spermatozoa.

There are several varieties of pills.

The pure progestogen pill

This pill — commonly called the mini-pill — is used continuously, i.e. on a daily basis, even during menstruation. This pill does not depend on suppression of ovulation to prevent pregnancy.

For indications, see p. 363. The progestogen-only pills contain minute doses of progestogens, e.g. norethisterone 0,35 mg (Micro-Novum); lynestrenol 0,5 mg (Exluton); ethynodiol 0,5 mg (Femulen); levonorgestrel 0,03 mg (Microval).

The mini-pill is the safest contraceptive pill, as far as the health of the woman is concerned, but it is not as reliable in preventing pregnancy as the other preparations. It can be started on the third day after delivery (as it does not suppress lactation) and will not do any harm if given inadvertently to a pregnant woman. It is inclined to cause irregular menstrual cycles; the woman may develop short cycles or amenorrhoea, in which case the addition of oestrogen pills will usually start the onset of menstruation.

Note: The mini-pill can be given as the initial contraceptive pill in the middle of a menstrual cycle and will ensure safety from pregnancy (within the limitations of its reliability) six hours after the ingestion of the first pill. The combined pill can replace the mini-pill on the first day of menstruation, i.e. the mini-pill is then discontinued in favour of a combined preparation.

Side-effects with the mini-pill are minimal and lactation is not affected.

Contra-indications:

▪ Impaired liver function.
▪ Previous ectopic pregnancy.
▪ Undiagnosed abnormal vaginal bleeding.
▪ Porphyria.
▪ Pregnancy.
▪ Hormone dependent malignant tumour.

The combined pill

The combined pill contains both hormones and is the commonly used contraceptive pill which suits most women as the hormones are balanced. The active hormonal pills are used for 21 days to be followed by 7 daily inactive pills, thus completing a cycle of 28 days. Most women are started on a low dosage preparation; after three cycles the strength of the hormones is adjusted if the woman develops either oestrogenic or progestogenic side-effects.

For method of prescribing pills, see p. 362. The combined pill is often referred to as OC (oral contraceptive).

Types of combined pills: (*a*) balanced; (*b*) predominantly progestogenic; (*c*) predominantly oestrogenic, see p. 359.

The following synthetic hormones are used in contraceptive pills:

Oestrogenic substances

▪ Mestranol 0,05, 0,075, 0,08, 0,1 mg
▪ Ethinyl-oestradiol 0,02, 0,03, 0,035, 0,05 mg
▪ Mass for mass, ethinyl-oestradiol is more potent than mestranol

Progestogenic substances

▪ Norethisterone 0,35, 0,5, 1, 2, 3, 4 mg
▪ Ethynodiol 0,5, 1 and 2 mg
▪ Megestrol 1 and 4 mg
▪ Lynestrenol 0,5, 1 and 2,5 mg
▪ Norgestrel 0,03, 0,05, 0,125, 0,15, 0,25 mg
▪ Desogestrel 0,15 mg
▪ Norgestrel 0,15, 0,5 mg
▪ Gestodene 0,075 mg
To change mg to microgram (μg) x 1000.

Variations of the combined pill

The triphasic pill (e.g. Triphasil; Logynon, Triminulet, Trinovum, Triodene) was developed in 1979. It has a lower total-steroid content than previously used combined pills. The three dif-

Combined hormones	First phase	Second phase	Third phase	Free period
ethinyl-oestradiol levonorgestrel	6 days 30 μg 50 μg Early, approx 4th day of menstruation to mid-follicular phase	5 days 40 μg 75 μg Higher dosage before normal ovulation to suppress hypothalamic–pituitary–ovarian system, thereby preventing ovulation	10 days 3 μg 125 μg This dosage mimics the luteal phase	7 days placebo placebo Exogenous steroid levels decline — withdrawal menstruation on 3rd day after last hormone pill

ferent dosages mimic the natural 3-phase hormonal fluctuation of a woman's menstrual cycle.

Note: The triphasic pill comes close to being the ideal steroidal contraceptive: low dose of both oestrogen and progestogen and complete reliability of ovulation inhibition by gentle pituitary suppression. There is also rapid return to fertility on stopping the triphasic pills, i.e. full pituitary responsiveness within 10 days. Because of lower dosage of both oestrogens and progestogens, the triphasic pill is suitable for the older woman who is in good health and does not smoke and is, therefore, not at special risk of developing cardio-vascular and thrombo-embolic diseases. It is also safe for the teenager as it does not have a heavy impact on the hypothalamus. Other advantages are: reduction of acne, dysmenorrhoea and breast discomfort during menstruation; neither blood pressure nor mass are adversely affected.

Combined pills are made up in serial packs containing 28 tablets. The pack is started on the first day of the menses and only 21 pills are active, the rest being inactive placebo. Withdrawal bleeding (menstruation) occurs during the week of taking the inactive pills.

Menstruation should start approximately 3 days after the last hormone pill has been taken. It may be very scanty or completely absent for some months, but amenorrhoea does not mean pregnancy if pills have been taken regularly. Whether menstruation has taken place or not, a new package of pills must be started exactly 28 days after the previous package was started and not a single scheduled pill must be missed. The first day of menstruation is always designated Day 1; therefore, if instructions read: start the pill on Day 5, it means the 5th day after menstruation started or should have started.

Each pharmaceutical package contains explicit instructions for the use of its own preparation and these instructions must be strictly adhered to. In some packages the pills are even numbered for the very reason that they are not

all the same and the correct sequencing is important. All the pills supplied by the Department of Health are started on the first day.

A new packet is always started on the same day of the week, e.g. a Sunday. If vaginal bleeding occurs before the time of expected menstruation, the doctor or clinic sister must be consulted. They may double the dose in an effort to stop the so-called 'breakthrough' bleeding. They may decide that it is a true menstruation period and restart the cycle of 28 days with a fresh package of pills. On the other hand, bleeding may be due to gynaecological complaints unrelated to the pill.

The combined oral contraceptive pill is safe to use below the age of 40 years, provided the woman is in perfect health. If middle-aged women wish to continue using the combined pill, their physical health must be carefully monitored and their mass controlled. Some women experience very uncomfortable side-effects from the pill.

The use of the pill does not greatly interfere with a woman's fertility and if a woman 'on the pill' wants to conceive she simply stops using the 'pill' in order to recover her natural fertility. There may, however, be a period of infertility of 6 months and longer due to anovulation.

On the whole, the pill is more suitable than the injection for the younger woman who wants to postpone starting her family or who wants to space her family.

Decrease in dosage has made the pill much safer. One month's supply of oral contraceptives today contains approximately the same amount of steroids as in one pill 25 years ago. Serious complications are now extremely rare due to the policy of prescribing 'low-dose pills for low-risk' women.[13]

Note: There is a difference between oral oestrogen-progestogen combinations used as contraceptives, e.g. Triphasil (Wyeth) and oral oestrogen-progestogen combinations used for oestrogen replacement therapy, e.g. Trisequens (Novo) and Prempack (Ayerst), the oestrogen content of the latter being much higher. The oestrogen replacement preparation does not prevent conception.

Contra-indications

(1) There is a definite link between the pill and thrombo-embolic diseases. Women with varicose veins or those with a history of superficial or deep vein thrombosis should not take the pill. Myocardial, cerebro-vascular and blood diseases are also contra-indications. For the same reason, the pill should be discontinued 6 weeks before elective major surgery and during the post-operative recovery period. Heparin is usually given pre-operatively.

(2) Abnormal vaginal bleeding.

(3) The pill may exacerbate existing liver disease, especially in a woman who has a history of jaundice during pregnancy. A previous attack of infective hepatitis does not exclude the use of the pill, providing there is no residual infection.

(4) A woman should not take the combined oral contraceptive for a period immediately after the birth of a child if she wants to breast-feed the child. The mini-pill will not affect lactation.

(5) Women with the familial disease, porphyria, should not use the pill.

(6) Women who are smokers or who suffer from hypercholesterolaemia or hypertension and are, therefore, at risk of developing myocardial infarction, should not use the combined pill, especially not after the age of 35 years and not if they have been on the pill for over 5 years.

(7) Combined oestrogen and progestogen must not be used during pregnancy or suspected pregnancy. They are, therefore, contra-indicated for pregnancy testing.

(8) No women over the age of 45 should use the pill.

(9) Tumour of breast or genital tract, malignant melanoma, leukaemia.

(10) Psychosis, depression.

Relative contra-indications are: diabetes, renal disease, use of antibiotics, anticoagulants and anticonvulsants, smoking, lactation, epilepsy and tuberculosis.

Side-effects of the pill

(1) Nausea, mass gain, bloating and breast tenderness.

(2) Intermenstrual 'spotting', i.e. slight bleeding between periods.

(3) Anxiety and depression; headaches; loss of libido (sexual desire).

(4) Thinning or loss of hair only with some preparations.

(5) The skin can become affected in several ways: brown discoloration (chloasma, nipples and areola, line stretching from the umbilicus to the symphysis pubis); dryness and itching.

(6) Amenorrhoea due to endometrial atrophy. It is reversible.

If these side-effects do not clear up after a few months, and the use of a different preparation has no effect either, the use of the pill must be discontinued. This happens in about 5 % of women. It is for these reasons that every woman on the pill should have an annual medical examination to assess its effects on her body and on her psyche. On the other hand, some women are inclined to blame all untoward signs on the pill. It must be remembered that there are other causes of indisposition and the pill should not be incriminated unnecessarily.

There are certain advantages of the combined pills, apart from contraception:

(1) Sexual desire and libido may increase.

(2) Acne may improve.

(3) Dysmenorrhoea and menorrhagia may improve.

(4) In the hirsute woman, facial hairs may decrease.

(5) Mittelschmerz will disappear due to the cessation of ovulation.

(6) In some small-breasted women, the slight swelling of the breasts caused by the pill may be welcomed.

(7) A reduction in endometrial and ovarian cancer, rheumatoid arthritis, iron deficiency anaemia, duodenal ulceration, benign breast lesions, ovarian cysts, pelvic inflammatory disease, ectopic pregnancy and endometriosis.

Note: The light, pain free, regular periods which a woman on the pill generally experiences will revert to her former pattern of menstruating when the woman comes off the pill.

The rules, which apply to the pill and/or the 'injection', are:

(1) Regularity in the taking of the pill is the first essential. One pill only is taken daily at the same time every day for as long as contraception is required. This rule applies even if coitus is not contemplated for a period, in order to ensure protection when coitus is resumed. If a pill is forgotten, protection is still assured if it is taken within 12 hours of the usual time. Regularity can be further assured if an extra packet of pills is kept ready to begin with as soon as the old packet is finished.

(2) Extra precautions, e.g. condom or contraceptive creams and foams, are taken until the next normal period starts:
   (*a*) during the first month of starting on an oral contraceptive regime;
   (*b*) if the first 'injection' has been given after the fifth day of the cycle;
   (*c*) if one or more pills have been left out completely;
   (*d*) if there is any diarrhoea or vomiting in pill users.
   During this time the woman must continue taking the pills regularly. She will be completely safe only during the next cycle of regular pill-taking.

(3) The woman must watch her mass and cut down on carbohydrates if she starts gaining weight.

(4) The woman must inform the doctor concerned that she is on a contraceptive 'injection' or pill if she is ill or if surgery is contemplated. For 6 weeks before elective surgery all oestrogen-containing formulations should be stopped to prevent post-operative thrombosis and the woman either put on a mini-pill or advised to use other precautions.

(5) The woman is warned that she might suffer the following side-effects for a few months and encouraged to persevere: irregular bleeding, spotting, amenorrhoea, tenderness of the breasts, tiredness, loss of libido, mood changes (including depression), headache. These side-effects are often due to anxiety if the woman fears that the pill may be harming her; or they may be due to individual sensitivity to either oestrogens or progestogens. If they continue, their cause must be investigated and measures taken to eliminate them. In women on combined formulations, menstrual periods are usually regular and light, but in women on progestogen-only formulations, there may be several short and several long cycles, the woman never knowing when to expect her periods. If she knows what to expect by careful preparation, anxiety is less likely to cause her to abandon oral contraception.

(6) The pills must be kept in a safe place away from children.

(7) There is no justification for stopping the pill at intervals.

(8) The woman must report to the clinic if she has continuous 'breakthrough' bleeding, a missed period or if side-effects continue for more than 3 months.

(9) There is evidence of oral contraceptive failure due to drug interaction. The drugs specially implicated are rifampicin, barbiturates and antihistaminics. While on these drugs, extra precautions must be taken or another contraceptive method practised.

(10) There are certain **absolute contra-indications** for the use of any sort of oral hormonal contraceptive. The pill is not a safe contraceptive in the hands of careless, forgetful, or mentally defective women or any woman who fails to appreciate the necessity for strict adherence to rules of administration.

Suitably trained nurses running family planning clinics, who work under the indirect guidance of a doctor, are allowed to prescribe the pill for clients, provided the latter are perfectly healthy. It is important that systemic diseases be excluded when the woman attends the clinic for the first time and that she has a check-up at least once a year. If there are any complicating factors such as thrombophlebitis, varicose veins, diabetes mellitus, porphyria, liver disease, tuberculosis, heart disease, hypertension, the nurse must consult with the clinic doctor as to the advisability of using oral contraception or as to the nature of oral contraception. The clinical examination includes blood pressure recording, urinalysis, cervical smears (Papanicolaou if facilities are available) and breast palpation to exclude breast cancer.

In prescribing a pill, the nurse must be guided by the suitability of the oral contraceptive for a particular client. The combined formulation is usually used, the triphasic formulation being popular.

In using the combined pill, there are many formulations to choose from. These formulations are prepared from two kinds of synthetic oestrogens and 8 kinds of synthetic progestogens, in different strengths (see p. 360). When a combined pill is to be used, the general rule is to begin with the lowest effective dose, e.g.:

(1) Norethisterone 0,5 mg, ethinyl-oestradiol 0,035 mg (e.g. Brevinor); or

(2) Levonorgestrel 0,15 mg, ethinyl-oestradiol 0,03 mg (e.g. Nordette); or

(3) Desogestrel 0,15 mg, ethinyl-oestradiol 0,03 mg (e.g. Marvelon).

If there is breakthrough bleeding on this dose, a stronger combination in the same range can be tried. If side-effects persist on this formulation, different oestrogens and different progestogens can be tried, e.g. mestranol instead of ethinyl-oestradiol and norethisterone instead of norgestrel. If the side-effects denote oestrogen deficiency and progestogen excess, either the amount of progestogen can be decreased or the amount of oestrogen increased. Conversely, if the side-effects denote that there is oestrogen excess and progestogen deficiency, either the oestrogen content of the pill is decreased or the progestogen dose increased, or a more potent progestogen (e.g. d-norgestrel) is used.

Signs and symptoms of —

(1) Oestrogen deficiency: irritability and nervousness, hot flushes, hypomenorrhoea, breakthrough bleeding during the first half of the cycle.

(2) Oestrogen excess: nausea, vertigo, oedema of legs, headaches, thrombo-embolism, cramps in legs, hypermenorrhoea, breast enlargement, enlargement of myomata.

(3) Progestogen deficiency: late breakthrough bleeding, hypermenorrhoea with clots, delayed menstruation.

(4) Progestogen excess: depression, loss of libido, greasy scalp, acne, increased appetite and mass gain, hypomenorrhoea, dyspareunia.

Note: 'Low oestrogen dosage' preparations contain 0,03 or 0,035 mg ethinyl-oestradiol.[13] Pills containing 0,05 mg ethinyl-oestradiol should only be used as contraceptive by women on treatment for epilepsy, for the treatment of gynaecological conditions, or as contraceptive where breakthrough bleeding persists for more than 3 months.

Oral Contraceptive Prescribing Guide[13]

Initial choice of oral contraceptive

Individual client response is variable; in general, therefore, initiate therapy with a relatively weak progestogenic and oestrogenic preparation, unless a more progestogenic or a more oestrogenic preparation is obviously indicated on initial assessment.

Reassess the response after 8 to 12 weeks and change if necessary.

Group 1: 'Relatively low progestogenic and low oestrogenic (balanced) pills'

Indications:

◼ Initiation of therapy

Preparations:

(1) Triphasic: Logynon; Triphasil.

(2) Other: Brevinor, Marvelon.

Group 2: 'Relatively more progestogenic pills'

Indications:

◼ Breakthrough bleeding
◼ Breast tenderness
◼ Cervical erosion
◼ Heavy menstruation
◼ Mucorrhoea
◼ Persistent nausea

Preparations:

◼ Moderate: Minovlar, Nordette, Norinyl, Ortho-Novum
◼ Strong: Demulen, Nordiol, Ovral.

Group 3: 'Relatively more oestrogenic pills'

Indications:

◼ Acne
◼ Dry vagina

- Lack of libido
- Scanty menstruation

Preparations:

- Biphasil, Normovlar
- Ovostat

Group 4: 'Progestogen-only pills' (Mini-pills)
Indications:

- Lactating patients
- Oestrogen intolerance or contra-indication
- Relative contra-indications to combined pill in a patient prepared to accept the slightly higher pregnancy failure rate
- All women over the age of 45 years (if oral contraception desired). Women who must stop the combined pill 4–6 weeks before and 2 weeks after major surgery.

Preparations:

- Exluton, Femulen, Micro-Novum

Group 5: Cyproterone acetate, ethinyl-oestradiol pills
Indications:

- Severe acne and hirsutism. Diane is also a contraceptive.

Preparation:

- Diane

The State Health Department provides a limited selection of oral contraceptives, free of charge, at family planning clinics. The selection available should be ascertained for prescribing in clinics.

The injectables[12] — pure progestogen given intramuscularly

There are two main kinds of progestogens used for parenteral steroidal contraception.

(1) Medroxyprogesterone acetate (e.g. Depo-Provera).
(2) Norethisterone enanthate (e.g. Nur-isterate).

Indications

(1) For the older woman who has completed her family and for whom oestrogens are in any case contra-indicated. It can be continued till the menopause.
(2) For the woman who wants no children and requests the injection.

(3) For women with 'problem' families, who are too poorly motivated to practise birth control conscientiously.
(4) For women who should not have children: mental defectives (at risk), chronic alcoholics and psychotics.
(5) For women with chronic illnesses where no further pregnancies are considered desirable and in whom, for some reason, sterilisation has not been done.
(6) Depo-Provera is often given to a woman shortly after the birth of a baby, before she leaves the hospital or nursing-home. This will prevent pregnancy for at least 3–6 months, or until she is able to attend a family planning clinic. The client is warned that she may stop menstruating for a prolonged time.
(7) For women who cannot attend family planning clinics regularly.

Contra-indications

(1) Known or suspected malignancy of breast or genital organs.
(2) Undiagnosed vaginal bleeding.
(3) Liver dysfunction or disease.
(4) Hypertension, migraine (relative contra-indication).
(5) Uncontrolled diabetes mellitus (relative contra-indication).
(6) Porphyria.
(7) Pregnancy.
(8) Thrombo-embolism (relative contra-indication).
(9) Depression (relative contra-indication).

Depo-Provera is an aqueous suspension of medroxyprogesterone acetate. One deep intramuscular injection of 1 ml (150 mg) is given every three months, preferably during the first 5 days of the menstrual cycle. This gives protection for a variable period (4 to 11 months), the length of this period not negating the necessity for the regular 3-monthly injection. One injection of Depo-Provera 3 ml (450 mg), given every 6 months, is an effective contraceptive.

Depo-Provera acts as follows:

(1) Ovulation is prevented by inhibition of hypothalamo-pituitary-ovarian function.
(2) Implantation of the ovum is prevented by maintenance of the endometrium in a state unsuitable for nidation (embedding).

(3) Passage of spermatozoa is prevented by the formation of a cervical mucus barrier.

Although Depo-Provera is a most effective contraceptive, its use-effectiveness being 0,24 pregnancies per 100 woman years, it is not suitable for young women who have not yet completed their families and wish to space their children, because a woman finds difficulty in falling pregnant after she has used it for some time.

Complications and side-effects of Depo-Provera

The side-effects are mostly due to oestrogen insufficiency. Depo-Provera has an unpredictable effect and may markedly depress hypothalamopituitary-ovarian function, recovery taking up to two years.

The most important side-effect is alteration of the menstrual cycle. This is its major problem and reason for discontinuation. For one to five weeks after the injection, there may be 'spotting' and even menorrhagia for 12 days, frequently followed by amenorrhoea. Although the amenorrhoea is not harmful, it upsets some women who firmly believe that the 'bad' blood collects in the head and causes headaches. Menorrhagia, in the absence of pelvic inflammation, can be treated by oral or parenteral oestrogen therapy, e.g. ethinyl-oestradiol 0,1 mg daily for 5 to 7 days. Management is not entirely satisfactory, however.

Other side-effects and complications are: headache, bloating, mass gain, depression, loss of libido and hypertension.

Nur-isterate (norethisterone enanthate) is a derivative of norethisterone; it is a long-acting contraceptive which is given by intramuscular injection every 11–12 weeks, in the dosage of 1 ml (200 mg). The first injection is given within the first 5 days of the cycle and protection begins on that day. The indications for use are practically the same as for Depo-Provera. It is not as effective, however, but recovery of fertility takes place within 6 months. For this reason it can be used in women who have not completed their families and who cannot tolerate combined oral contraceptives.

In diabetes mellitus Nur-isterate is preferred to Depo-Provera. The most important side-effects and complications, which do not occur as frequently as with Depo-Provera, are irregular menses, intermenstrual bleeding and amenorrhoea. Headaches, dizziness, temporary nausea may occur, but mass gain is not a problem.

Pure progestogen contraceptives provide health benefits similar to those afforded by the combined oral contraceptives.

Correctly used, parenteral progestogens give extremely reliable protection against pregnancy. It is the contraceptive of choice for long-term use.

Regular monitoring for complications must be done, especially if the injectables are used in cases of cardio-vascular disease and diabetes mellitus.

REFERENCES

(1) Forssman H, Thuwe L. One hundred and twenty children born after application for therapeutic abortion refused. Their mental health, social adjustment and educational level up to age 21. In: *Recent Advances in Clinical Psychiatry*. Granville-Grossman, 1971.

(2) Sapire KE. *Contraception and Sexuality in Health and Disease*. Johannesburg: McGraw-Hill, 1986.

(3) Rip MR, Roux AJ, Roberts MM. Birth and fertility rate variations in metropolitan Cape Town. *SA J Epidemiology & Infection* 1986; **1**: 70–73.

(4) Bloch B, *et al. S Afr Med J* 1978; **53**: 861.

(5) SAMJ News. *S Afr Med J* 1989; **76**: xx.

(6) De Villiers VP. Post-partum sterilization and demographic progress at Paarl Hospital. *S Afr Med J* 1988; **74**: 114–116.

(7) Spilhaus M. (1974) *S Afr Med J* 1974; **48**: 1305.

(8) Potts M, Diggory P, Peel J. *Abortion*. Cambridge University Press, 1977.

(9) Dommisse J. The South African gynaecologists' attitude to the present abortion law. *S Afr Med J* 1980; **57**: 1044.

(10) Bourne DE. Abortions in England and Wales on South African residents. *S Afr Med J* 1988; **74**: 87–88.

(11) Letter to the editor. *S Afr Med J* March 1977.

(12) Sapire KE. Family planning. *S Afr J Cont Med Educ* 1984; **2**: 99–103.

(13) Dommisse J, Sapire KE. Oral contraception — a guide to prescription. *S Afr J Cont Med Educ* 1984; **2**: 105–106.

TEST OF KNOWLEDGE

The student has benefited from studying this chapter if he/she can answer the following questions:

(1) (*a*) Comment on the 'Declaration of Tokyo' with regard to family planning as an essential component of primary health care.

(*b*) Comment on the concern of nations to reduce the population growth rate to zero in order to avert the imminent global population explosion when the 6 billion people predicted for the year 2000 start increasing by geometrical progression (constant ratios between successive quantities).

(2) Explain the difference between:
   - Family planning and birth control (contraception)
   - Crude birth-rate and total fertility rate
   - The mini-pill and the combined pill
   - Oestrogen and progestogen
   - Triphasil and Trisequens

(3) Describe the functioning of the State Health family planning (FP) clinic as an integral part of primary health care and the role of the FP nurse in motivating prospective clients to accept family planning in order to limit population growth.

(4) (*a*) Discuss the health advantages for clients of steroidal contraception.

(*b*) Give the untoward side-effects and complications that may be encountered with the use of: (i) IUCD; (ii) Depo-Provera; (iii) the combined pill.

(5) (*a*) State the change in oral contraceptive prescription that may be recommended for the following side-effects of oral contraceptives:
   — weight gain
   — dry vagina
   — breast tenderness
   — scanty menstruation
   — acne and hirsutism
   — breakthrough bleeding
   — heavy menstruation
   — persistent nausea

(*b*) What are the guiding principles in the initiation of oral contraception?

(*c*) State the absolute contra-indications to the following methods of contraception:
   I Injectable progestogens
   II Oral combined pills
   III Progestogen-only pill (mini-pill)
   IV IUCD

21

Community Antenatal Services

OBJECTIVES

The main objectives of this chapter are to introduce the student to community obstetric services which precede the birth of a child (parturition)—the antenatal services. In order to make antenatal care meaningful, some of the important avoidable causes of perinatal (foetal/neonatal) and maternal deaths are discussed. The epidemiology of perinatal and maternal mortality is highlighted to bring to the attention of the student the effects of unfavourable socio-economic conditions on the perinatal health and mortality of the mother and her child.

DEFINITIONS

Obstetrics is the branch of medicine that deals with the care of the woman during pregnancy (period of gestation), parturition (birth) and the puerperium (period of 6 weeks from termination of labour to complete involution (return to normal size) of the uterus).

An *obstetric service* includes antenatal, perinatal and postnatal care.

An obstetric service in any community needs to be an integral part of a maternal and child health service which includes family planning, immunisation and child welfare facilities. The usual measure of the success of a community obstetric service is the perinatal mortality rate (PMR) (see p. 370).

Divisions of the gestation period:
First trimester: the first 13 weeks
Second (mid-) trimester: 14 to 26 weeks
Third trimester: 27 weeks to birth

The antenatal or prenatal period is the period of pregnancy from conception to the beginning of labour (*ante* = before, *natus* = birth).

The emphasis in this chapter is on antenatal care.

Antenatal care means caring for the pregnant woman to ensure the normal birth of a normal child; where normal pregnancy and birth are not possible because of obstetric problems, it aims to ensure the birth of a live child with the least possible damage to the mother.

Note: Antepartum (*partus* = labour) (before birth) differs from antenatal in that it is contrasted with intrapartum (during labour, birth or delivery) and postpartum (after delivery).

The postnatal period extends from birth to 6 weeks after birth when obstetric care comes to an end with the postnatal 'check-up' visit to the obstetrician or obstetric clinic.

The perinatal period extends from the 28th week of gestation to the 7th day after birth. Perinatal care refers to obstetric and neonatal care.

Note: The antenatal and postnatal periods overlap with the perinatal period. The neonatal period extends from the time of birth up to the moment the infant becomes 28 days of age.

Community obstetric care is the care of all pregnant women and their newborn infants in a community, excluding those who make use of private medical services. It is rendered on three levels: primary, secondary and tertiary. In South Africa primary community obstetric care is given at peripheral clinics, while secondary and tertiary care is given in district (regional) and academic (teaching) hospitals respectively. These hospitals serve as referral centres for the clinics which deal mainly with normal pregnancies, births and infants. In South Africa the peripheral clinics are commonly known as *'mid-wife obstetric units' (MOUs)*, a name which originated from the PMNS in Cape Town.

PERINATAL MORTALITY (INFANT DEATHS)

Perinatal deaths (PND) refer to foetal/neonatal deaths shortly before, during and in the first week after labour. If the infant is born dead after 28 weeks of pregnancy, it is referred to as 'still-born'.

Causes of perinatal deaths[4]

(1) Prematurity.
(2) *Infection*, either infection of the amniotic fluid, infection during vaginal delivery, or congenital syphilis.
(3) Congenital anomaly.
(4) Asphyxia due to:
    (*a*) placental insufficiency (including *abruptio placentae*);
    (*b*) cord accidents;
    (*c*) difficult delivery, birth trauma, meconium aspiration.
(5) Other. The low birth weight infant is at risk.

A 'low birth weight' (LBW) infant is one who weighs 2 500 g or less at birth. LBW infants include not only the majority of preterm (premature) infants but also term (mature) infants who are growth-retarded. (See Perinatal Care Index, p. 370.)

Infection

Amniotic fluid infection syndrome

Ross *et al.*[8] reporting on 200 perinatal post-mortems done on stillbirths and neonatal deaths at King Edward VIII Hospital, Durban, from October 1976 to March 1977, found the perinatal mortality rate (PMR) from the amniotic fluid infection syndrome (congenital pneumonia) to be 15,9/1 000.

The phenomenon of intra-uterine (antenatal) infection of the foetus had not been recognised for very long. It is hypothesised that this so-called 'amniotic fluid infection syndrome' is due to infection ascending through the cervix and membranes (ruptured or intact) and causing a membranitis. It is an important cause of perinatal mortality and morbidity and is associated with unexplained preterm labour.[10] In preterm deliveries, microbes can often be cultured from

placental tissue, blood and gastric aspirate (from liquor swallowed by the infant during the birth process). At present the syndrome cannot be diagnosed by antenatal tests. It is diagnosed on clinical grounds, i.e. offensive smell of liquor, maternal pyrexia.

Possible causes of amniotic fluid infection may be:

(1) deficient antibacterial properties of the amniotic fluid;
(2) poor hygiene;
(3) poverty.[10]

Ross *et al.*[8] found that a high proportion of liquors taken from black patients have little antimicrobial activity. The authors postulate that this may be due to dietary deficiencies, e.g. of zinc. They found the percentage of inhibitory, antibacterial activity of liquor amnii to be as follows:

▨ Blacks: 33
▨ Whites: 76
▨ Indians: 52

Infection during vaginal delivery

Maternal genital infection (herpes simplex, gonococcal, chlamydial) may infect the neonate during vaginal delivery and cause either localised (eye, skin, mouth) or disseminated disease.

Congenital syphilis

Congenital syphilis as a cause of perinatal deaths ranked fourth in the Ross *et al.* study[8] with a PMR of 3,2/1 000. This usually occurred when the expectant woman did not attend antenatal clinics. Naicker *et al.*[11] found syphilis to be an important cause of PMR in developing countries amongst unbooked mothers.

Abruptio placentae

In the study of Ross *et al.*,[8] abruptio placentae, as a cause of perinatal death, came second at a PMR of 9,5/1 000.

Abruptio placentae (AP) means the premature separation of the placenta. It is the single factor causing the majority of stillbirths.

AP was found to cause 25–34 % of intra-uterine deaths during labour among patients in the lower socio-economic groups of South Africa.[2]

Risk factors for abruptio placentae

The possible AP risk factors are smoking, lack of antenatal care, coitus within 48 hours of admission, intrapartum hypertension (rise in blood pressure during delivery).

Early signs and symptoms are pain and bleeding. When intra-uterine death occurs, abruptio involves at least 66 % of the placental surface. Delivery by caesarean section may save the infant's life if the abruptio is smaller.

PMR

The perinatal mortality rate (PMR) is defined as:

$$\frac{\text{The number of perinatal deaths in a calendar year}}{\text{Total births (live and still) during the same period}} \times 1\ 000$$

NMR

The neonatal mortality rate (NMR) is defined as:

$$\frac{\text{Number of deaths in one calendar year of infants under 28 days}}{\text{Total live births during the same calendar year}} \times 1\ 000$$

PCI

Perinatal care index (PCI) is defined as the ratio of the percentage of low birth weight (1 000g–2 499 g) infants to the perinatal mortality rate (PMR).

The ideal ratio is $\dfrac{\text{PMR}}{\%\,\text{LBW}} = \dfrac{25}{25} = 1$

The percentage LBW infants in a community reflects the level of health of the community and is largely independent of hospital or clinic perinatal care. A high PMR can be expected in areas with a high percentage of LBW infants. Hospitals with a high PMR but low percentage of LBW are suspected of giving poor perinatal care.[15]

In a survey of births and perinatal deaths in Mitchell's Plain, Rip et al.[1] found a high LBW (low birth weight) rate (14,9 %) in the PMNS group; more than half these infants were born at term. This suggests a high incidence of infants with growth retardation. They also found that the higher PMR (than amongst the privately delivered infants) is accounted for by the extremely high stillbirth rate.

The high PMR in the lower socio-economic groups in the RSA is a matter of concern; the intra-uterine death-rate (after 28 weeks gestation, i.e. stillbirths) was far in excess of the NMR in a study done by De Jong et al.[3]

BORN BEFORE ARRIVAL (BBA)

A delivery before arrival (at an obstetric unit) is obstetrically undesirable because of the danger that the mother and infant will not receive expert care while they are in a very vulnerable state.

In the PMNS (MOUs) the situation is becoming steadily worse,[17] the rate increasing from 8 % in 1980 to 11 % in 1984.

Causes of BBA in a PMNS study:[17]

(1) Patient default in not arranging for transport to the booked obstetric unit (MOU) timeously.

(2) Short labour, i.e. one less than 2 hours. This may be the cause of transport failure.

(3) Ambulance default, sometimes caused by heavy demands on ambulance services.

(4) Delivery occurring in the obstetric unit without attendance.

Prevention of BBA's is mainly through education and through improved transport and telephone facilities.

Problems associated with BBA:

(1) More preterm and more low birth weight deliveries than under normal conditions of delivery.

(2) Higher perinatal mortality rates.

The PMNS study[17] showed that more unfavourable socio-economic features were present in the BBA mothers than in their peers in the PMNS. These features were:

▪ poor education,
▪ unmarried status, and
▪ unplanned pregnancies.

MATERNAL MORTALITY (OBSTETRIC DEATHS)

Maternal death is defined as 'the death of a woman while pregnant or within 42 completed days of termination of pregnancy, irrespective of the duration or the site of the pregnancy' (WHO).

Direct obstetric death is defined as 'death resulting from complications of the pregnancy itself, from intervention selected or required by the pregnancy or resulting from the chain of events initiated by the complications or the interventions' (WHO).

Indirect obstetric death is defined as 'death resulting from disease before or developing during pregnancy, not a direct effect of the pregnancy, which was obviously aggravated by the physiological effect of the pregnancy and caused the death' (WHO).

At-risk pregnancies. The following pregnant women are at risk and should be monitored every 2 weeks after the 24th week of pregnancy:

(1) those with a history of hypertension;
(2) those with a multiple pregnancy;
(3) those with diabetes mellitus, hydramnios, renal disease (including infection) and hydatidiform mole;
(4) adolescents and primigravida over the age of 40.

The following avoidable factors are associated with maternal deaths:

(1) Delayed admission to hospital where obstetric complications are dealt with. This may be due to transport failure.
(2) Failure of the midwife or doctor attending the patient during antenatal care to recognise warning signs and symptoms of complications.
(3) Delay in giving adequate treatment and neglect of the basic principles of intra-partum care.
(4) Non-attendance for antenatal care.

Direct causes of maternal deaths[18]

Most frequent causes of death:

(1) Hypertensive disorders of pregnancy. This will be discussed in some detail below.
(2) Sepsis of genital tract from abortion, puerperal sepsis, after emergency caesarean section, spontaneous delivery, prolonged labour and BBA.
(3) Haemorrhage from abortion, ectopic pregnancy, abruptio placentae, placenta praevia, ruptured uterus, post-partum haemorrhage, disseminated intravascular coagulopathy (DIC), cervical tears, episiotomy.
(4) Embolism — air, amniotic fluid and pulmonary.
(5) Anaesthetic complications after caesarean section and after epidural anaesthesia.

Hypertensive disorders of pregnancy (including pre-eclampsia)

Definitions

Hypertension in pregnancy is a persistent diastolic pressure of 90 mm Hg or more.

Pre-eclampsia is defined by Moodley[19] as a blood pressure of 140/90 Hg or more or a mean arterial pressure of 105 mm Hg on two occasions 6 hours apart after the 24th week of pregnancy. It may be either proteinuric or aproteinuric. Hypertension in pregnancy with proteinuria and oedema (the triad of symptoms) is, however, not one disease with one aetiology and one pathophysiology, i.e. it is not necessarily pre-eclamptic. Oedema occurs in 80 % of all pregnant women and is frequently found in normal pregnancy (see p. 381 for causes). Hypertension is the end result of a number of different disorders.

Causes of hypertension in pregnancy

(1) Pregnancy-induced hypertension (PIH) (pre-eclampsia). It is often found in primigravidae and in association with hyperuricaemia. The patient is normotensive in early pregnancy and develops the triad of symptoms in the third trimester, sometimes late mid-trimester.

Pre-eclampsia may either present in the previously normotensive woman or be superimposed upon renal disease or essential hypertension. To exclude chronic renal disease in doubtful diagnoses of PIH, urinary microscopy for casts and serum levels of urea, uric acid and creatinine are indicated. Further renal investigations can be done.

In pure pre-eclampsia the renal tract returns to normal and in most patients the elevated blood pressure will have returned to normal within 7 days after delivery.

The aetiology of PIH is uncertain, but there is some indirect evidence for an immunological mechanism.

(2) Hypertension may present in pregnancy due to chronic renal disease or essential hypertension.

(3) Latent or transient hypertension may occur for the first time during labour (intrapartum hypertension) or in the puerperium.

Potential dangers of hypertension in pregnancy, whatever its cause

Maternal: sudden exacerbation with end organ damage

(1) Eclampsia with increasing proteinuria, severe headache, severe nausea, vomiting, epigastric pain and mental confusion. This may lead to hypertensive convulsions and cerebral haemorrhage.

(2) Renal, hepatic and cardiac failure.

(3) Abruptio placentae and DIC leading to generalised bleeding.

A hypertensive crisis has a high maternal and foetal mortality, especially if delivery is delayed for 12–24 hours and longer.

Foetal: loss can occur at all stages of gestation. Foetal loss may be due to early surgical termination of pregnancy or to complications such as uterine growth retardation and abruptio placentae.

Early signs of developing pre-eclampsia

(1) Abnormal mass gain;

(2) oedema of the lower extremities and elsewhere;

(3) elevation of arterial blood pressure.

Note: Oliguria, proteinuria and a rising serum creatinine, urea or urate level are late and serious signs.

The management of pre-eclampsia

The only cure for pre-eclampsia is termination of pregnancy, but this solution is not always acceptable as most parents do not want to sacrifice their child if there is a chance that conservative management in a hospital may bring both mother and child through the crisis. Any blood pressure of 140/90 mm Hg and above in a pre-

viously normotensive pregnant patient is an indication for hospitalisation.

Pregnancy-induced hypertension should always be treated by bed-rest in hospital as the disease process only stops when pregnancy ends. Mother and foetus are monitored for BP, foetal growth and renal function, until the foetus is mature enough for normal birth or until it is viable and can be delivered prematurely, either by means of caesarean section or induction and a closely monitored labour.

Premature delivery is indicated when the risk (to the mother) from hypertension is greater than the risk (to the foetus) from prematurity.

The bed-fast patient is sedated (with Valium) and given antihypertensive agents (methyldopa) if the diastolic blood pressure remains above 100 mm Hg.

Bed-rest must be in the lateral position. This will promote a fall in blood pressure and reduce the risk of premature labour. Bed-rest promotes physiological diuresis.

Diuretics and low salt diet are not recommended.[19]

The management of eclampsia[19]

The woman presents in a hypertensive crisis. In hospital the three immediate objectives are:

(1) To control and prevent further convulsions by means of magnesium sulphate. Post-convulsion restlessness is controlled with intravenous diazepam (Valium).

(2) To reduce hypertension with IV dihydrallazine.

(3) To expedite delivery either by oxytocic induction and forceps under epidural anaesthesia, or by caesarean section under general anaesthesia.

(4) Intubation for adequate ventilation, furosemide diuresis, mannitol and steroids to reduce cerebral oedema.

MATERNAL MORTALITY RATE (MMR)

The MMR is defined as:

$$\frac{\text{Number of deaths (direct or indirect) due to pregnancy, childbirth or puerperium in a calendar year}}{\text{Total number of deliveries (births) during the same period}} \times \begin{matrix} 1\,000 \\ or \\ 10\,000 \\ or \\ 100\,000 \end{matrix}$$

Births (deliveries) are defined as births of babies, dead or alive, with a birth weight of 1 000 g or more.

The maternal mortality rate (MMR) is high in developing communities. Because prevention is possible by community perinatal services, the maternal mortality rate is a sensitive socio-economic index of health care in a community. For this reason the MMR of developed communities in South Africa does not bear comparison with the MMR in developing countries — the so-called Third-World communities.[14] The MMR in developed communities varies between 0,10 and 0,50/1 000 deliveries.[14]

In Cape Town maternal mortality rates (MMR) for 1975–1977 were as follows:[13]

- Blacks: 0,69/1 000
- Coloureds: 0,4/1 000
- Whites: 0,27/1 000

There is a remarkable drop in the black MMR from 1/1 000 deliveries in 1956, due largely to the introduction of the obstetric 'flying squad'.

Nearly half the patients who died were unbooked.

In a South African country-wide survey of maternal deaths in 267 hospitals during the 3-year period 1980–1982, Boes[18] found the following: MMR of 83/100 000 (0,83/1 000). Of these 89,6 % were classified as direct obstetric deaths and 55 % deaths were avoidable. Only 37 % of the infants survived. The MMR may have been artificially increased as many patients do not seek care until complications set in. This is evident from the following study.

Cooreman et al.[14] analysed 81 maternal deaths which occurred at the Pelonomi Hospital, Bloemfontein, for the 6 years preceding December 1985. The overall MMR was 2,87/1 000 deliveries, including deaths related to abortion and ectopic pregnancy. Among booked patients the MMR was 0,32 and among unbooked patients 11,13 per 1 000 deliveries. The MMR for patients from the Bloemfontein area was 0,72/1 000 deliveries. The extremely high MMR of unbooked patients (35 times higher than that of booked patients in this study) is due to cultural factors in black rural women who seek the help of traditional practitioners and come to hospital as a last resort.

THE LAWS THAT PROTECT THE PREGNANT WOMAN AND HER UNBORN CHILD

(1) The Abortion and Sterilisation Act 1975 makes it a criminal offence for a woman to have an abortion procured upon her, except in special circumstances, when it is called a therapeutic abortion. An abortion may be procured only by a medical practitioner. Indications for a therapeutic abortion are discussed on p. 347. Legal control over abortions prevents the indiscriminate termination of pregnancy with its high mortality risks when done by persons who are not qualified to do so.

(2) Compulsory treatment of mothers attending antenatal clinics with venereal (sexually transmitted) diseases to prevent abortion or congenital syphilis in the newborn (if the mother has syphilis) and ophthalmia neonatorum (if the mother has gonorrhoea).

The law also requires the midwife to cleanse and instil antiseptic drops into the eyes of every infant at birth in order to prevent eye infection.

(3) Unemployment benefits.

Maternity benefits are payable to women who are employed in commerce and industry and who, therefore, contributed to the Unemployment Insurance Fund. Even women who do not earn enough to contribute to this fund are eligible for maternity benefits. The woman must apply in person, after she has registered as unemployed with the Department of Labour or nearest magistrate's office showing her record card. Maternity benefits are paid only from the day of registration.

Conditions for qualifying for maternity benefits: the woman must have been in employment for at least 18 weeks during the year immediately before her expected date of confinement. Maternity benefits operate from 18 weeks before expected date of confinement until 8 weeks after the birth of a live child and 4 weeks after the birth of a stillborn child.

(4) Regulations made by the SA Nursing Council in terms of the Nursing Act 50 of 1978 define the scope of practice of a registered midwife. These regulations control midwifery practice to the benefit of mother and

child (including the pregnant woman and her unborn child). Transgression of the regulations is subject to disciplinary action by the South African Nursing Council.

Regulation No. R. 1469 to the Nursing Act 50 of 1978, promulgated in July 1987, is an amendment of Regulation No. R. 2598 of 30 November 1984. It reads as follows:

'2. Regulation I is hereby amended by —

(a) the insertion of the following definition before the definition of 'co-ordination':
   "a 'child' shall include the unborn child".

(b) the insertion of the following definition after the definition of 'health needs':
   " 'midwifery regimen' shall mean the regulation and implementation of those matters, which through midwifery intervention, have an influence on the course and management of pregnancy, all stages of labour and the puerperium and includes the provision of care plans, their implementation and evaluation and the recording of the course of pregnancy, labour and puerperium and of any health problem and the care received by the mother and child whilst in the charge of the midwife".

3. Add the following regulations to the regulations (R. 2598).

CHAPTER 3 — THE SCOPE OF PRACTICE OF A REGISTERED MIDWIFE

3. The scope of practice of a registered midwife shall entail the following scientifically based acts or procedures which apply to the practice of midwifery and which relate to the mother and child in the course of pregnancy, labour and the puerperium:

(a) the diagnosing of a health need and the facilitation of the attainment of optimum physical and mental health for the mother and child by the prescribing, provision and execution of a midwifery regimen or, where necessary, referral to a registered person or by obtaining the assistance of a registered person, as the case may be;

(b) the execution of a programme of treatment or medication prescribed by a registered person;

(c) the prevention of disease relating to pregnancy, labour and the puerperium and the promotion of health and family planning by teaching and counselling individuals, families and groups of persons, by implementation of family planning skills and by monitoring the health status of the mother and child;

(d) the monitoring of —
   (i) the progress of pregnancy, labour and the puerperium;
   (ii) the vital signs of the mother and child;
   (iii) the reaction of the mother and child to disease conditions, trauma, stress, anxiety, medication and treatment;

(e) the prevention of complications relating to pregnancy, labour and the puerperium including:
   (i) the performance of an episiotomy;
   (ii) the suturing of first and second degree tears or an episiotomy;
   (iii) the administration of a local anaesthetic;

(f) the administration of medicine to the mother or child;

(g) the prescribing, promotion or maintenance of hygiene, physical comfort and reassurance of the mother and child;

(h) the promotion of exercise, including antenatal and postnatal exercises, rest and sleep;

(i) the facilitation of body mechanics and the prevention of bodily deformities in the execution of the midwifery regimen;

(j) the supervision over and maintenance of a supply of oxygen to the mother and child;

(k) the supervision over and maintenance of fluid, electrolyte and acid base balance of the mother and child;

(l) the facilitation of the healing of wounds, the protection of the skin and the maintenance of sensory functions in the mother and child;

(m) the facilitation of the maintenance of bodily regulatory mechanisms and functions in the mother and child;

(n) the facilitation, maintenance and, where necessary, the improvement of the nutritional status of the mother and child;

(o) the promotion of breast-feeding;

(p) the supervision over and maintenance of elimination by the mother and child;

(q) the facilitation of communication by and with the mother and father or family in the execution of the midwifery regimen;

(r) the establishment and maintenance, in the execution of the midwifery regimen, of an environment in which the physical and mental health of mother and child is promoted;

(s) preparation for and assistance with operative, diagnostic and therapeutic acts for the mother and child;

(t) the co-ordination of the health care regimens provided for the mother and child by other categories of health personnel;

(u) the provision of effective advocacy to enable the mother and child to obtain the health care they need;

(v) care of the dying patient and a recently deceased patient within the execution of the midwifery regimen.'

Note: Since 1994 every pregnant woman is entitled to free medical care at state hospitals.

PRIMARY OBSTETRIC CARE BY THE MIDWIFE

It is important for every pregnant woman to have effective antenatal and perinatal care either by a general practitioner or obstetrician. In developing countries this is not possible because of the low ratio of medical personnel to pregnant women. The trend, therefore, is to use midwives to give primary obstetric care.

Larsen *et al.*[16] describe the training of midwifery nursing associates (practitioners) in a hospital in KwaZulu serving a population of 110 000. Midwives follow a 3-month post-basic midwives' course which equips them for more responsible work in the hospital and in the community. The midwifery nursing associate is trained to assess the antenatal patient adequately, including pelvimetry and cardio-vascular and respiratory systems.

She is trained to detect risk factors and to refer to the doctors only those patients-at-risk who need specialised care. She is taught to do vacuum extractions and even lumbar punctures on neonates. She also takes major responsibility for teaching pupil midwives. The authors of this experiment claim that the antenatal screening of patients by the midwifery nursing associate has been a great success, relieving the overworked doctor of routine duties and enabling him to give more time to sick patients. These midwives have contributed to a lowering in the perinatal mortality rate of the hospital.

The University of Natal offers an Advanced Diploma in Midwifery and Neonatal Science course (at the King Edward VIII Hospital), the content of which is approved by the SA Nursing Council. The course is available from several universities and its aim is to train midwives for an extended role in smaller peripheral hospitals and community obstetric services where medical staff may be unavailable or overtaxed. Midwifery practitioners may not perform surgical operations such as caesarean sections or sterilisations.

A domiciliary, community-based midwifery service, in which pregnant women attend an antenatal clinic but are delivered at home by a midwife belonging to the service, has long been standard practice in South Africa. Patient delivery in the home is far from ideal, however, as slum conditions frequently prevail. Ideally all women should be delivered in an obstetric hospital in which facilities for coping with emergencies are readily available.

In developing countries, including parts of South Africa, sufficient hospital maternity beds are seldom available and, therefore, alternative measures have been developed in the form of satellite clinics. These midwife obstetric units (MOUs) serve as adjuncts or outlying wards to base hospitals. The MOUs are staffed by resident midwives and visiting medical practitioners. They are used for screening pregnant women and for the antenatal care and delivery of low-risk pregnancies while the base hospitals are used for all high-risk pregnancies. Each hospital has strict criteria for the acceptance of referrals from the MOU. General practitioners visit the MOUs daily and obstetricians once weekly for consultation with and instruction of the midwives. The obstetrician lays down the criteria for referral of patients to the visiting doctors and to the base hospital at the booking visit, antenatally, during labour, in the puerperium and for the neonate. He decides which medical problems (e.g. anaemia, gastro-intestinal and urinary symptoms, vaginal discharge, etc.) can be diagnosed and treated by midwives; he is also responsible for preparing midwives to fulfil their extended role and gives them technical and moral support.

MOUs are situated in the community, within 5 km of the people they serve. They book prospective clients, are responsible for their ante-natal care, refer 'at-risk' women to second or third level care obstetric hospitals and deliver all normal pregnant women on their premises. No home deliveries should be undertaken by MOU staff. The MOUs have replaced the need for domiciliary (home) deliveries.

Selection of patients for delivery in a MOU is controlled by a comprehensive list of referral criteria which are applied at these stages: the booking visit, throughout the antenatal period, and in the first and second stages of labour. At any stage a patient booked for delivery at a 'low-risk' MOU can be transferred to a 'high-risk' hospital.

The usual criteria for referral or for initial hospital booking are:

(1) bad obstetric history; cephalopelvic dispro-portion; antepartum bleeding; previous cae-sarean delivery; two or more consecutive, 1st trimester spontaneous abortions; third stage complications and more;

(2) hypertensive disease including pre-eclamp-sia; diabetes mellitus; heart disease; chronic renal disease; epilepsy; poorly controlled asthma; low haemoglobin level not re-sponding to haematinics;

(3) Rh negative blood with antibodies;

(4) postmaturity; very low birth mass;

(5) foetal distress during labour and after birth;

(6) postpartum haemorrhage;

(7) unbooked mothers.

MOUs in areas with high population density should be placed within reach of all the women in the area, preferably on a bus route and near a shopping centre, to make the trip to the antenatal clinic financially worthwhile for the pregnant woman. Each MOU has a number of beds (e.g. from 1 to 10) and midwives are always in atten-dance. After delivery, the mother and child are kept in for 6 to 12 hours, until there is no longer any danger of complications. If necessary, domiciliary postnatal care is given by midwives or pupil midwives from the clinic.

Although MOUs generally deal with normal deliveries, their doors are open to obstetrical emergencies, for example, preterm deliveries.

MOUs are administered and controlled by the base hospital to which obstetric problems are referred from the MOU during antenatal

care and even during and after delivery. An efficient telephone or radio and ambulance serv-ice is, therefore, essential between the obstetric unit and base hospital.

Where clinic midwifery services have been run according to the above-mentioned princi-ples, perinatal and maternal mortality rates have been reduced and the overcrowding in base hospitals has been relieved. Good, comprehen-sive obstetric care for all pregnant women in developing communities, despite few doctors and insufficient hospital facilities, can become a reality.

In the expanded obstetric units of *rural ar-eas* midwives have a high degree of autonomy. The semi-autonomous MOUs are operating in Ciskei, KwaZulu, Bophuthatswana and else-where.

In *black rural* areas the maternal mortality rate (MMR), apart from the PMR, is still unac-ceptably high, avoidable deaths occurring from obstructed labour, ruptured uterus, postpartum haemorrhage, eclampsia, severe hypertension and cardiac failure. In rural areas with insuper-able communications and transport problems, a 'waiting mothers' area' or maternity village for expected 'high-risk' patients where they can stay from 38 weeks onwards, is very necessary to reduce perinatal and maternal mortality.[6] Timely treatment of medical conditions, good antenatal care, delivery of all women in hospi-tals or clinics with ready access to hospital facilities and early admission of women 'at risk' to a 'waiting mothers' area' if they live far from hospital, are ways of reducing MMR and PMR.

In the black rural areas clinic midwifery services are not available, however, to all women. In these areas home deliveries and per-inatal care are often practised by traditional birth attendants (TBA). In some parts of the Cape and Natal TBAs have been integrated into a regional perinatal care service with gratifying results.[7]

THE PENINSULA MATERNITY AND NEONATAL SERVICE (PMNS)

As an example of a regionalised urban commu-nity perinatal service (CPS) the Peninsula (Cape) Maternity and Neonatal Service (PMNS) will be described.[5]

The PMNS accepts sole responsibility for PNC (perinatal care) in the PMNS region other than that provided by the private sector.[4] It also promotes family planning in the perinatal region (PNR).

PMNS comprises all maternal and neonatal services in the Cape Peninsula and was officially designated as the obstetric authority by the Director of Hospital Services in January 1980. The PMNS comprises 5 maternity hospitals (high-risk institutions) and 4 midwife obstetric units (MOUs) (low-risk institutions); it has close contact with the Day Hospitals Organisation. In 1980 its turnover of deliveries was 20 694 with an ethnic distribution of: blacks 27 %, coloureds 69 %, whites 4 %, and an overall PMR of 29,2 per 1 000 births. The PMNS is administered by the PMNS Executive Committee (EC), (matrons, medical superintendent, medical officers, under chairmanship of the senior lecturer in community obstetrics UCT) and the PMNS Co-ordinating Committee consisting of members of the EC, Director of Newborn Services, as well as the medical superintendent and the principal matron of the Day Hospital Organisation. Clearly defined lines of communication are provided between the hospitals and the MOUs, any problem which the latter cannot or should not handle, being discussed with the hospital staff as soon as it occurs; transfers are effected only after consultation. An adequate transportation service is provided between low- and high-risk institutions.

The staff of the midwife obstetric units (MOUs) consists of midwives and doctors of first contact (primary care). PMNS midwives are less autonomous than those operating in the black rural areas in MOUs. They are part of an urban programme and have easy access to base hospitals. Moreover, PMNS MOUs are widely used for the training of student midwives and medical students, and to provide experience in community obstetric practice for post-registration students (doctors and nurses). Medical supervision of the PMNS MOUs is, therefore, more comprehensive than that of the MOUs in the black rural areas. The urban MOUs even include perineonatologists on their staff to obviate referrals to hospitals. The PMNS MOU midwives deliver almost one-third of all women in the PMNS (1982), detect and refer high-risk

cases to hospital, staff outlying antenatal clinics and make a large number of domiciliary postnatal visits to mothers and babies discharged from both the obstetric hospitals and the MOUs. In 1980, 67 000 postnatal visits were made.

Most black and coloured pregnant women of the Cape Peninsula go to their local MOU for booking. They are delivered either at a MOU or at a PMNS hospital.

The PMNS MOU staff are subjected to a vigorous programme of continuing education in the form of practical teaching (by doctors and midwives) in the antenatal clinics and by attending meetings conducted by visiting experts at the MOUs, at which perinatal deaths, referrals and other problems are discussed.

Epidemiological and clinical research projects have been started. The PMNS is an important urban community health programme which stresses the importance of perinatology and family planning.

The PMNS caters essentially for the lower socio-economic groups of the community. The mothers in these groups have high illegitimacy and teenage pregnancy rates, are younger than privately delivered mothers, have low levels of education, tend to book late and are more likely to have their third or subsequent baby.[1]

ANTENATAL CARE BY MIDWIVES

Antenatal care is the care of the pregnant woman until the birth of her child. It overlaps with perinatal care. Antenatal care plays an important role in lowering the PMR and MMR and in preventing cerebral palsy through birth damage to the infant's brain. Antenatal care protects the health of the pregnant woman and her unborn child.

Aims of antenatal care

(1) The promotion and maintenance of good physical and mental health during the pregnancy;

(2) the ensuring of a live, mature and healthy infant;

(3) the preparation of the woman for labour;

(4) the early detection and treatment of medical and obstetric conditions that would endan-

ger the life or impair the health of mother or baby.

Booking for antenatal care

All pregnant women are encouraged to attend antenatal clinics from approximately 8 weeks into their first trimester. As soon as the woman comes for her first antenatal visit, she is booked, i.e. placed on the records, and an antenatal regimen is worked out with her so that she knows what is expected of her and the reasons for regular attendance. A booked patient can be defined as one who attended at least two antenatal clinics. An unbooked patient attended one or no antenatal clinics. Unbooked women, i.e. those who do not receive antenatal care, are at greater risk of developing obstetric problems and of losing their babies.

Pattinson and Rossouw[9] discuss the problem of the unbooked mother at Tygerberg Hospital and district clinics: in 1984 unbooked mothers comprised 11,3 % of patients delivered at hospital. These deliveries accounted for 59 % of all stillbirths and 44 % of all early neonatal deaths for the year. All these mothers knew where their nearest antenatal clinic was and 70 % had had previous deliveries, of which half were abnormal ones. The authors came to the conclusion that the unbooked mother tends to be unmarried, of low income and without permanent heterosexual relationships.

In Southern Africa many women, especially black rural women, do not seek antenatal care when it is available and prefer delivery at home. Traditional medicine still has a strong hold and the help of western doctors and hospitals is sought as a last resort when the patient's life can no longer be saved.

Many grand multiparous deliveries amongst black rural women also take place at home because they have no transport or money. They have children at home needing their care and the services of TBAs (traditional birth attendants) are available. Most home deliveries are unintended though, due to transport failure; thus the motivation for waiting mothers' areas is strengthened.

Rip et al.[1] found a low proportion of preterm and LBW infants born to mothers who booked in the first trimester. Early booking is probably an indication of a well-motivated, better educated mother.

Women are generally anxious to attend antenatal clinics, however, to confirm that they are pregnant and to make sure of the expected date of delivery. Even amongst the rural blacks, women are beginning to realise the importance of antenatal care and the necessity for booking a bed at the clinic or base hospital, where obstetric services are free.

Visits to the antenatal clinics

Pregnant women should be seen by the midwife every 4 weeks until the 28th week of pregnancy. Checks should then be made once every fortnight until the 36th week and, thereafter, weekly, until 40 weeks. The patient is advised to be medically examined at least once before and at least once after the 34th week of pregnancy.

Antenatal visits subsequent to the initial visit can be fairly brief. Blood pressure, urinalysis, weighing and an abdominal examination are necessary investigations.

History taking

The purpose of a comprehensive history on initial contact is to assess the health and social circumstances of the pregnant woman and to record facts about her previous obstetric and medical history.

Any problems or defects which would adversely affect childbearing are especially important at this stage in order to alert the midwife or doctor for future treatment of the mother.

A family history should be acquired to ascertain whether a predisposition to certain diseases such as: diabetes mellitus, essential hypertension, psychiatric disorders and cardiac disease, is present. Amniocentesis is offered to women with a known increased risk of having a child with a chromosomal abnormality, e.g. in women over the age of 35 years. Obstetric facts regarding previous pregnancies, labours and puerperia are of vital importance and need to be carefully recorded. This knowledge will enable the nurse/doctor to anticipate problems with the present pregnancy and act accordingly. Previous antepartum and postpartum haemorrhages, caesarean sections, abortions and placenta praevia are among the problems which should alert the nurse/doctor regarding the present pregnancy.

A history of the previous infants and their mass is also important.

Examinations

Urinalysis

The urine must be tested at the initial visit and every visit thereafter.

Inspection, testing for blood, ketones, protein and glucose are the tests which must be carried out on every urine specimen. Proteinuria is of vital significance in the pregnant woman, as it is one of the signs of pre-eclampsia, a condition which must be treated promptly to avert more serious developments. Proteinuria may be caused by such conditions as pyelonephritis and chronic nephritis. On the other hand, albumin could be a contaminant to be confirmed by a midstream specimen of urine.

The Dornfest method[20] of urinalysis can be used as a screening test to detect asymptomatic bacteriuria, if simple laboratory facilities are available in the antenatal clinic.

Method: A midstream urine specimen is centrifuged and within half an hour a smear is made of 1 drop of the resuspended sediment. The smear is heat-dried, fixed with a few drops of 95 % alcohol and stained with a few drops of 1 % aqueous methylene blue. Under a microscope the total number of bacteria present in 5 oil immersion fields is obtained. A positive Dornfest test (i.e. significant bacteriuria) is indicated by a total of more than 35 bacteria. The result can be controlled by a laboratory culture of the same midstream specimen. If there is a delay in despatching the specimen, it should be stored at 4 °C.

If there is a significant bacteriuria, the patient is treated to prevent pyelonephritis.

Glycosuria is fairly common during pregnancy and, if more than a trace of glucose is present on two occasions, further investigations such as random blood sugar, and glucose tolerance tests must be carried out to ascertain whether diabetes mellitus is present or not.

Blood tests

The following blood tests must be carried out:

(1) *Serological tests for syphilis (STS)*
   (*a*) The VDRL and RPR agglutination tests are screening tests for syphilis and reflect disease activity. RPR positive sera are subjected to the

   (*b*) TPHA (T. pallidum haemagglutination) test
   (*c*) The FTA-ABS (fluorescent treponemal antibody absorption) test is used as a confirmatory test, if RPR is positive but TPHA is negative.

Note:
(1) FTA–ABS test should also be used to detect syphilis in mothers with unexplained stillbirths, neonatal deaths and abortions.
(2) STS should be repeated during pregnancy as seroconversion from negative to positive can take place between initial antenatal testing and delivery. This is especially important in population groups with high prevalence of STDs.
Unbooked mothers should be tested on admission.

(2) *Haemoglobin*—which is taken at 28 weeks and 36 weeks; the normal haemoglobin in pregnancy is 12,6 g % or above. If the haemoglobin is below 10 g %, a full blood count must be done to investigate the anaemia.

(3) *Blood ABO grouping and rhesus typing*
Rhesus factor: A woman who has a Rhesus negative blood grouping will need monthly blood tests for antibodies from 20 weeks until term. The blood of the husband is also tested for grouping and Rhesus typing. In the pregnant woman with Rhesus negative blood, the antibody titre is of great significance. If there is a rapid rise in the titre level before 28 weeks, very little can be done. Intra-uterine exchange transfusions have been attempted with relatively little success.

After 28 weeks of pregnancy an amniocentesis may be done to assess the bilirubin level, which will provide a guide to the obstetrician as to whether the foetus can remain *in utero* or whether the pregnancy must be terminated to save the baby.

Note: Neonatal jaundice from Rh incompatibility can be prevented in future offspring by injecting anti-D immunoglobulin into an Rh negative mother within 72 hours after delivery.

(4) *Blood screening test for the alpha-fetoprotein (AFP) level* (see p. 137). This test was recently introduced in South Africa.

(5) *Screening of antenatal blood samples for HIV antibodies.* The SA Blood Transfusion Service recently screened the blood of over 100 000 pregnant women from a wide geographical area in the Transvaal for HIV an-

tibodies. The blood samples had been submitted by private practitioners and antenatal clinics for routine ABO grouping, rhesus typing and irregular blood group antibody screening. Testing was done anonymously, the results being used for population screening to assess the heterosexual spread of AIDS.[27] (For results, refer to chapter 34.)

Cytological examination

Ideally a PAP smear should be taken on every pregnant woman, with special regard to women over 25 years of age and multigravida, e.g. the woman with a parity of 3 or more.

Height and mass

The height and shoe size, especially 3 and smaller, of a woman could be of significance in ascertaining the size of her pelvis with regard to the birth process. This estimation is not to be used as the absolute criterion — it is only a rough guide to consider with other factors. However, a note is made of a woman of short stature.

Early in pregnancy the woman should be weighed to determine her normal mass. She should be weighed on each subsequent antenatal visit. Her mass gain is of significance with regard to diet control, oedema associated with pre-eclampsia, hydramnios. The nurse is alerted if the woman gains more than 1 kg per week.

The maximum mass gain allowed during the pregnancy is approximately 11,5 kg. Two to 2,5 kg is the average mass gain during the first 20 weeks of pregnancy and, thereafter, 9 kg of mass gain is allowed in the second 20 weeks. A loss of more than 2 kg during the pregnancy could be a possible indication of hyperemesis gravidarum or intra-uterine growth retardation, or the mass loss may have sociological or psychological implications which will need investigation.

Abdominal examination

The midwife/doctor should examine the patient abdominally and record her findings. By carrying out this procedure the nurse/doctor will be able to determine whether the dates correspond with the foetal growth. Regular recordings of the midwife's/doctor's examination findings will ascertain whether the foetus is healthy and growth is normal. The lie of the foetus, the presentation and engagement of the presenting part must be assessed. A record of the date of quickening, amount of liquor and the foetal movements must be kept, so that a comparison can be made at further clinic visits. Multiple pregnancies and intra-uterine growth retardation can be determined during the pregnancy by these means.

The foetal heart sounds can be picked up and noted between 24 and 26 weeks, provided there is no excess liquor, anterior placenta or obesity.

Physical examination

On an initial visit to an antenatal clinic a full physical examination should be carried out by an experienced nurse or doctor. Heart, lungs, breasts, liver, upper and lower limbs, spleen and femoral pulses must be examined for abnormalities. The vulva and anal canal must be inspected.

A vaginal examination should be carried out to exclude any pelvic abnormalities. Conditions such as retroversion of the uterus, fibroids, vaginal cysts, double uterus and septate vagina can be recognised and dealt with if necessary at this stage.

Blood pressure

On the initial visit and each subsequent visit the blood pressure must be taken and recorded. In pregnancy the auscultated sound may persist to zero, therefore, muffling of the sound should be taken as an indication of the diastolic blood pressure (DBP). Sometimes the mean arterial pressure (MAP) is used for the diagnosis and management of hypertension.

This is calculated as follows:

$$\frac{SBP + 2DBP}{3} \text{ e.g. if BP} = 140/90, \text{ then:}$$

$$\frac{140 + (2 \times 90)}{3} \frac{180}{} = \text{MAP of 107 mm Hg}$$

In an out-patient antenatal clinic the blood pressure of a patient should be taken more than once, i.e. at intervals during one visit, and the lowest reading recorded, as anxiety may cause a rise in blood pressure.

The blood pressure in normal pregnancy falls by approximately 15/5 mm Hg from the sixth week and remains low until the third trimester when it rises slowly to reach slightly above pre-pregnancy levels towards term.[21]

The upper limits of normal BP (rounded to nearest 5 mm Hg) according to MacGillivray *et al.*[22] are:

	Before 28 weeks	29–34 weeks	From 35th week
DBP	75 mm Hg	80 mm Hg	90 mm Hg
SBP	120 mm Hg	125 mm Hg	130 mm Hg
MAP	95 mm Hg	100 mm Hg	105 mm Hg

BP was measured with the patient in the sitting position.

Note: Any BP equal to or exceeding these values should be regarded as abnormally high and the patient hypertensive for the stage of pregnancy (see p. 371 for hypertension criteria).

Davey and Dommisse[21] stress the following important points in measuring the BP in pregnant women:

(1) The SBP reading may differ more than 10 mm Hg in right and left arms in which case the arm giving the higher reading should be used throughout the rest of the pregnancy.
(2) The cuff must fit comfortably around the upper arm and be applied over the brachial artery.
(3) The BP must always be measured with the patient lying semi-recumbent (half-sitting) tilted at an angle of 45 ° towards the side on which the BP is to be measured.

Oedema

Oedema during pregnancy is common; it can occur for a number of reasons:

(1) physiological oedema in the lower and upper limbs;
(2) oedema associated with pre-eclampsia; it is found on the upper limbs and face (i.e. it is non-dependent);
(3) orthostatic oedema, often found in the lower limbs in pregnancy;
(4) renal pathology which can cause oedema in the upper limbs and face.

Due to the conditions associated with oedema, a careful check must be kept on the patient.

Clinical evidence of foetal growth

Foetal well-being and growth must be monitored by the midwife, especially if there are signs of hypertension. This is done by:

(1) Recording maternal weight. A loss of more than 2 kg during the pregnancy could be a possible indication of foetal growth retardation.
(2) Measuring the fundus height. Normally the fundus rises as follows:
    – at 16 weeks — halfway to umbilicus
    – at 22 weeks — at the umbilicus
    – at 30 weeks — halfway between umbilicus and xiphisternum
    – at 36 and 40 weeks — at the xiphisternum
    – at 36 weeks in primigravida the level of the fundus drops approximately 5 cm as the head engages in the pelvis.

Genetic counselling

If there is a history of a previous abnormal child the mother must have genetic counselling as to the likelihood of her present pregnancy being affected.

Minor disorders of pregnancy

Although the minor disorders do not endanger life, they must not be ignored or treated lightly. The cause should be explained to the expectant mother and advice given on how she can alleviate discomfort. A few of the minor disorders are discussed below.

Morning sickness

About 40 % of pregnant women vomit between the 4th and 14th week of pregnancy. This usually occurs immediately after getting up in the morning.

Advice. The woman should eat small, frequent meals, avoiding fatty foods and an empty stomach. Digestive biscuits or cream crackers are more easily tolerated and should be eaten instead of heavy meals early in the morning. Motion must be avoided while nausea is present. If the nausea and vomiting become extremely bad, medical assistance should be sought before the woman becomes dehydrated.

Heartburn

Because of the enlarged uterus displacing the stomach upwards, when in a recumbent position the expectant mother may experience discomfort. A relaxed cardiac sphincter allows the reflux of gastric juices into the oesophagus, causing a burning sensation.

Advice. The woman should be advised to tilt the head of the bed and avoid fatty foods. An antacid tablet can be sucked to relieve pain and burning.

Backache

Backache associated with other symptoms, e.g. burning on micturition, suprapubic pressure and frequency of micturition, could indicate a urinary tract infection.

A faulty posture can cause severe backache and can be extremely troublesome.

Advice. The posture must be corrected with the aid of antenatal exercises which will strengthen the back muscles. Supportive, low-heeled shoes and a firm mattress or bed board will probably relieve backache. Occasionally, physiotherapy may be required and a special corset may need to be fitted.

Constipation

The pressure of the enlarged uterus and the possible relaxing effect of progesterone on the intestinal muscle diminish peristalsis and may cause constipation during pregnancy.

Advice. The woman must be advised to include plenty of roughage in the form of whole-wheat bread, fresh fruit and vegetables and bran cereals in her daily diet.

Exercise will aid peristalsis and help to relieve uncomfortable constipation.

Varicose veins

Due to the relaxing effect of progesterone on the muscles during pregnancy, varicose veins become worse at this time. This condition may predispose to vein thrombosis, therefore it is advisable to obtain medical advice.

Advice. The pregnant woman is advised to wear elastic stockings which she must put on before she gets out of bed in the mornings. She is advised to raise her legs for ten minutes in every hour.

Haemorrhoids

External haemorrhoids are varicose veins in the anal region and can cause great discomfort to the pregnant woman.

Advice. Treatment with an anaesthetic cream can be administered to relieve the pain of the haemorrhoids.

In order to avoid this condition, the woman should ensure that she does not become constipated.

Fainting and dizziness

Fainting in pregnancy is thought to be due to the irritability of the vasomotor centre in the medulla oblongata which controls arterial tone. If a rapid fall in blood pressure takes place, the woman faints. The pressure of the uterus on the vena cava may also be a cause of fainting in pregnancy.

Muscle cramps

Cramps in the muscles of the legs, thighs and buttocks occur in some pregnant women, usually primigravidas after the 32nd week of pregnancy. Cramps usually occur while the woman is at bed-rest, especially at night and in the early hours of the morning. The aetiology and treatment of muscle cramps are uncertain. Some women are helped by massaging or exercising the muscle, while others ingest a little table salt for relief.

Conditions in pregnancy associated with bleeding

During the discussions the midwife has with her patient in the antenatal clinic, she should forewarn her of any complications that may occur and the signs and symptoms to watch out for and report as soon as possible.

All vaginal bleeding should be reported by the midwife to a doctor and prompt attention must be given to the pregnant woman. This will often save the pregnancy and prevent serious loss of blood.

Causes

(1) An implantation bleed occurs when the trophoblast erodes the endometrium during the process of embedding.
(2) Cervical lesions:
   (*a*) erosions;
   (*b*) mucus polyps;
   (*c*) carcinoma of the cervix.
(3) Threatened abortion or complete abortion.
(4) Ectopic gestation which is an extra-uterine pregnancy, most commonly occurring in the tubes; immediate termination by salpingectomy is necessary.
(5) Hydatidiform or vesicular moles; the evacuation of the uterus will be necessary.

Counselling in family planning

The antenatal midwife should broach the subject of family planning at the first antenatal visit. She should help the young mother plan her future family with due attention to spacing, number of children and contraceptive method of choice.

The teenage primipara should be advised to wait until she is in her twenties before she has her second child. Women who are having their second or third child are persuaded that this may be enough for the sake of the health of the family and that the best kind of contraception would be a surgical sterilisation within 48 hours of the birth of a normal child. The midwife must ensure that the woman's husband forms part of the decision-making process. Unwed mothers are counselled about giving their baby up for adoption if they have no support system in the community. A good education in contraception is vitally important here. (See p. 320 for the counselling of the school-going pregnant adolescent.)

Women of 35 years and older and multipara of 4 and more are advised not to have any more children. The risk factors to themselves and to their unborn children can be pointed out.

Generally the risks with regard to reproduction are greater for the under 18-year-olds, for those over 35 years, for those who have had 3 children and more and for those whose spacing of children has been less than 2 years, than for women in their 20s who have just started having their families.

Women who have been exposed to enlightened counselling can prepare themselves for contraception as soon as their baby has been born, even before they leave the hospital.

The antenatal midwife must support the woman who is unmarried or who does not want her baby as she may be having a problem pregnancy without supportive relationships. She must also be aware of the need for curative treatment of women with sexually transmitted diseases (STDs). She must teach her patients how to avoid STDs with special reference to the use of the condom and the avoidance of promiscuity.

It is also very important to discourage women with health problems such as hypertension, diabetes mellitus, tuberculosis and heart conditions from having any more children.

Note: At community obstetric centres, counselling for acceptance of postpartum sterilisation is part of the comprehensive antenatal care of all booked patients.

Health education of the pregnant woman by the midwife

When the expectant mother attends the antenatal clinic, the midwife should take the opportunity to advise, encourage and answer the many questions she may have on her mind.

Sexual relations during pregnancy

Contrary to the old school of thought, the pregnant woman is today advised that she can enjoy sexual relations throughout the pregnancy. If during the last trimester of her pregnancy she finds deep penetration uncomfortable, she is advised to change positions, thereby facilitating less uncomfortable intercourse.

In the presence of any vaginal bleeding during the pregnancy, the woman is advised to abstain from coitus during the third trimester. Abruptio placentae (AP) is often preceded by coitus within 48 hours of AP.

Alcohol use and the foetal alcohol syndrome

(See p. 117)

Because of the dangers to the infant should the pregnant woman be a heavy drinker, it is important for the nurse to take note of signs of chronic alcoholism. The problem drinker should be enlightened about the dangers of alcohol to her infant and referred for help to SANCA.

Smoking

Pregnant women should not smoke, as smoking harms the child. Not only is smoking a risk factor for abortion, but smoking mothers produce small-for-gestational-age babies with possible brain damage due to chronic anoxia during the pregnancy. Babies of smoking mothers are also inclined to suffer from chest complaints. Perinatal mortality is higher, the excess deaths being due to anoxia, possibly due to high carbon monoxide levels in the pregnant woman and her foetus. The higher perinatal mortality (neonatal deaths) may also be associated with premature delivery.[23]

Breast-feeding

The midwife should endeavour to instil positive feelings towards breast-feeding in her pregnant patient. This is a tremendous contribution she can make towards promoting the health of the mother and her baby. (For advantages of breast-feeding, see p. 398.) In preparation for breast-feeding the woman can be taught how to toughen her nipples to accustom them to friction and to prevent cracked nipples. During the last two months of pregnancy, the nipples can be rolled between finger and thumb and drawn out every day while she is in the bath. The use of spirits for hardening is not recommended as it is too drying; instead lanolin or other cream can be rubbed into the nipples a few times per week.

For breast-feeding in tuberculosis, see p. 535.

Nutrition

A well-balanced diet is essential for every pregnant woman, not only for the sake of her own health but also to prevent impaired growth of the foetus and subsequent stunting. This does not mean that licence is given to the woman to overeat; first-class proteins such as meat, milk, fish and eggs must be taken regularly, the protein requirements of a pregnant woman being somewhat greater than for the non-pregnant woman, i.e. 80 g per day. Fresh fruit and vegetables are essential and also foods that supply roughage, e.g. whole-wheat bread and whole-

grain cereals, as well as plenty of water to prevent constipation. Animal fats are needed to supply vitamins A and D. Sugar, starches and fats must be curtailed so that the woman does not gain more than 11,5 kg–16 kg mass during an entire single pregnancy in a woman of normal weight. In an underweight woman, the recommended weight gain is 12,5 kg–18 kg and in the overweight woman, 7 kg–11,5 kg. Calcium in the form of milk and cheese is needed, especially during the last 12 weeks of pregnancy when the foetus needs large amounts for skeletal ossification. Folic acid, to prevent anaemia, can be taken in fresh, preferably uncooked, vegetables, but for the Indian women in Natal, among whom iron deficiency is endemic, extra iron should be taken in medicine form. This also applies to women whose diets lack iron.

The following risk groups may also require supplementary iron: teenagers, strict vegetarians, smokers and drinkers, and women who are very underweight.

Note:
(i) The excessive intake of iron reduces zinc absorption.
(ii) Caffeine must be taken in moderation.

Walker and Kruger give the following dietary advice to:

- Western pregnant women: eat a varied diet with greater reliance on plant foods (vegetables and fruit). Supplementation with vitamin-mineral mixtures should not be encouraged.
  Iron and folic acid prophylaxis may be advisable, but only when tests indicate the need.
- Third-World pregnant women: eat a mixed diet especially cereals *and* legumes with more vegetables when possible. Iron and folic acid should be given only where a definite deficiency exists.[24] See p.135 for the use of dietary folic acid supplementation for women of childbearing age.

Note: Insufficient nutrition in the mother during pregnancy is a cause of low birth weight (LBW) in full-term infants. The infant mortality rate is higher in such infants than in normal BW infants. Pregnancy and lactation may precipitate deficiency diseases in an underfed mother.

Rest, sleep and recreation

Ideally the woman should have rest periods during the day, especially towards the end when she feels heavy and uncomfortable, and should sleep at least 8 to 9 hours per night, but this may be a counsel of perfection if she is a working woman or has heavy household duties. She must be reminded, however, that her health will suffer if she becomes overtired and allows herself no recreation. In order to prevent exhaustion, no unnecessary work should be done and full use made of all the helping agencies in her community, as well as friends and family.

Prevention of infection

Since the foetus is at risk from virus infections capable of crossing the placental barrier, the avoidance of such infections must be discussed with women early in pregnancy. Should the woman have been exposed to rubella early in pregnancy, she must be referred for antibody screening. For the prevention of the congenital rubella syndrome, see p. 572.

Use of medicines

The pregnant woman must be warned against the *use of medicines*, except those prescribed by her doctor or the clinic, as medicines may have a teratogenic effect and harm her infant.

It must be brought to the notice of the pregnant woman that aspirins can cause bleeding in the neonate and the mother, especially if taken within 5 days before birth. A pregnant woman must not expose herself to radiation hazards, e.g. no woman who is pregnant should work in an X-ray department or nurse patients harbouring a source of radiation.

The anticoagulant, warfarin, crosses the placental barrier and has a teratogenic effect on the embryo and foetus during the first trimester. It can be used from the 13th to the 36th week of pregnancy. If used after the 36th week of pregnancy there is the danger of bleeding in the mother and foetus. Instead of warfarin, intravenous or subcutaneous heparin, which does not cross the placental barrier, can be used throughout pregnancy for thrombo-embolic conditions. Long-term heparin may, however, adversely affect the mother by causing bleeding and demineralisation of bones (heparin-induced osteopenia). It is, therefore, very important for the pregnant woman on antithrombic therapy to be medically supervised.

Conventional anti-asthma medicines are safe during pregnancy, therefore the principles of asthma therapy remain the same during pregnancy.

Antituberculosis therapy is reasonably safe during pregnancy. See p. 535 for TB therapy during lactation.

Clothes and shoes

The clothes and shoes of a pregnant woman must be comfortable and no restricting bands may be worn around the lower limbs or tight brassières or corsets used to bind her in. She should, however, wear an uplifting brassière from the 12th week to support the breasts and a maternity belt, e.g. pull-on maternity pantie girdle, from the 20th week, to give her good posture. High heels and a pendulous abdomen which pulls her forward cause lordosis and backache.

Cleanliness

Body cleanliness is important, a daily bath or shower with water which is neither too cold nor too hot being ideal. Pruritus vulvae can often be cured with meticulous vulval hygiene; the possibility of pubic lice must not be forgotten.

Exercise

The pregnant woman must have exercise, besides housework, but she should stop playing tennis or any other sport which causes jolting. Taking a walk in the fresh air while wearing flat-heeled shoes is the ideal kind of exercise. She must on no account climb on chairs or steps to reach articles in case she overbalances and falls. If she can afford the expense and time, it is a good idea to join 'keep fit' classes and later on in pregnancy to join a physiotherapy class to learn relaxation in preparation for the birth experience. The pregnant woman must not lift heavy weights, nor must she stand for long periods as this may aggravate varicose veins if she tends to have them.

Travel

It is not wise to travel to medically inaccessible places after the 28th week of pregnancy, nor to travel by plane after the 32nd week. After the 28th week of pregnancy the pregnant woman should get a certificate of fitness from her obstetrician should she wish to travel by plane.

Dental care

The teeth of the pregnant woman need care and pregnancy is no reason why she should not continue with routine visits to the dentist. Extractions should be done under local anaesthetic as a general anaesthetic will affect the foetus.

Antenatal psychological care

(With special reference to westernised women.) Whether a woman enjoys her pregnancy and accepts her child, or resents her pregnancy and feels rejecting towards it, depends very much on how supported and secure she feels. Cultural practices and customs are important in defining the role of the husband, mother and mother-in-law during pregnancy, childbirth and the postnatal period, and also in determining the importance a woman attaches to her reproductive functions and the value of the child to the family and the community. Whatever the culturally determined attitudes are, however, the task of pregnancy, labour and mothering is the greatest adaptive task any woman is expected to face. During this time a woman needs a tremendous amount of support, especially if this is her first experience. Although little can be done to change a woman's motherliness, she can be helped to improve her mothering functions and the mother-child relationship by primary preventive psychological care during the antenatal, perinatal and early postnatal period.

If anxious or frustrated and angry by concern about the future, the pregnant woman cannot find gratification in her pregnancy. The most feared complication of the postnatal period is puerperal insanity which, in extreme cases, may give rise to infanticide or attempted infanticide. Puerperal depressions and anxieties are fairly common and do not necessarily pose a threat to the infant; they may, however, cause a subtle rejection of the child by its mother and lead to later family problems and personality distortion in the developing child.

Stresses precipitated by pregnancy

Emotional stresses in the pregnant woman are usually generated in the family. The pregnancy may be accidental and unwanted or extra-maritally conceived; the pregnant woman may experience rejection from her husband or she may be worried because the family cannot afford an additional member. She may feel inadequate or fatigued and unable to cope or she may resent the unborn child for some other reason. The woman may also resent her pregnancy because she resents her femininity and procreative functions; this influences her motherliness.

Stress caused by pregnancy may manifest itself in psychological symptoms such as depression or in psychosomatic symptoms such as hyperemesis gravidarum, cravings and aversions. Some women abort spontaneously while others attempt to procure an abortion and, if unsuccessful, suffer feelings of guilt, fearing that the foetus may have been damaged. Intense anxiety in the mother, especially if she cannot stop smoking, may cause small-for-date babies or hypertonic infants who are difficult to manage.

The highly anxious pregnant woman may develop uterine inertia which causes prolonged labour, hazardous to the child; on the other hand, anxiety can lead to precipitate birth; both extremes may cause anoxia or other brain damage to the child. Abnormal birth, especially if the mother suffers much pain, may prevent the immediate close physical contact between mother and child, which is so important for the initial bonding of a mother with her child; this may cause the mother to resent the child.

Anxiety in the parturient woman, especially in the primipara, may be caused by fear of the unknown. If the woman has not been instructed during the antenatal period on what to expect when she is in labour, or if she is left in isolation during the first stage of labour, she may become extremely anxious and build up resentment against her husband and the child. The anxiety may cause emotional regression and an inability to bond with mother and the child. This resentment may carry over into the postnatal period and affect milk production adversely.

A woman can be prepared psychologically for childbirth in order to help her control her body during the process of labour; knowledge and control are purported to banish fear and tension, the main cause of pain in a normal delivery. If the woman can learn to relax, she is more likely to deliver spontaneously. An international conference of specialists in human and animal behaviour sponsored by the Ciba Foundation found that 'the more medical routines intrude during the immediate postnatal period, the more difficulties are posed for the establishment of the parent-infant relationship and the greater the long-term risks to the stability of the family and to the later health of the child'.[25] The promotion of a spontaneous delivery is, therefore, an important primary preventive task of obstetrical staff.

The preparation of a woman for a tension-free birth is called *psychoprophylaxis*. The advocate of this method in Western countries was Grantly Dick-Read who, in 1933, published the book, *Childbirth without Fear*, in which he described how women could aid childbirth through relaxation. Later Lamaze, a French obstetrician, invented the term psychoprophylaxis, and popularised the idea of relaxed childbirth which he had learned in the USSR.

In the Lamaze method, preparation for childbirth consists of educational sessions with both husband and wife in the physiology of pregnancy, the process of birth and the active role they can play in it. The husband is included so that he can support his wife during pregnancy and labour, being encouraged to be present at the birth. The woman is instructed for 6 weeks during the last trimester of pregnancy in breathing and relaxation techniques which can be synchronised with uterine contractions during the first and second stages of labour. She can, however, request analgesia during labour. In order to assess the advantages of the Lamaze course, Scott & Rose[26] carried out a controlled study on two groups of primiparas: those who underwent the Lamaze course and those who did not. They found that the trained women required less analgesia during labour and were able to deliver spontaneously more frequently than the controls. There was no indication of any harm resulting from the breathing exercises as had been suggested.

In the following aspects of labour, however, there were no significant differences between the two groups: length of labour, number and type of maternal complications, frequency of foetal distress, neonatal problems and mean Apgar score.

Hypnosis and acupuncture have also been used to banish fear and promote relaxation and spontaneous delivery. These methods make use of suggestion to help the woman cope with pain and in some instances even experience 'painless' births. The main emphasis in all psychoprophylactic methods is on the psychological or emotional preparation for childbirth and on spontaneous delivery, thus enabling the mother to make immediate skin contact with her infant, even before the cord is cut. This immediate contact is purported to promote the bonding of the mother with her child.

Note: The advantages of spontaneous delivery will be cancelled if the labour room atmosphere is so cold that the neonate needs immediate covering.

It is believed by many that a newborn is aware of what is going on around it, i.e. that the 'austistic shell' in no way insulates the infant from sensory experiences during the birth process and during its early postnatal life. Some even believe that the infant sees clearly and can use its eyes to signal to its mother. It will cry to be fondled and its sense of smell is sufficiently acute to enable it to distinguish its mother's smell. These beliefs are the basis of the Leboyer technique, called Birth without Violence.

Leboyer is a French obstetrician who goes against the modern stream of medical opinion. He believes the birth process to be painful for the child; that because the infant is exquisitely sensitive to its surroundings immediately after birth and for the first 24 hours of life, it must be treated accordingly to enable it to adapt to its new environment gradually. A *Leboyer delivery* takes place in a quiet, warm room. The lights are dimmed after the delivery of the infant's head and the staff either remain silent or talk in whispers. Before the cord is cut, the infant is placed naked on its mother's abdomen so that it does not lose its sense of continuity with her body and the sound of the heartbeat, and remains warm. Cord cutting is delayed until the blood supply from the placenta closes naturally. During this time the mother is encouraged to massage her baby, thus establishing mutual tactile 'knowing'. Later the infant is immersed in a bath of warm water to simulate its experience of warm weightlessness in the uterus.

Although the Leboyer method has become fashionable in some cultural circles, the theory of birth trauma and acute sensitivity is not generally accepted. Some paediatricians frown on the opportunity this method offers for surface cooling of the neonate whose ability for temperature control is very poor.

REFERENCES

(1) Rip MR, Keen CS, Woods DL. Births and perinatal deaths in Mitchell's Plain. *S Afr Med J* 1986; **70**: 827–830.

(2) Brink AL, Odendaal HJ. Risk factors for abruptio placentae. *S Afr Med J* 1987; **72**: 250–252.

(3) De Jong G, Pattinson RC, Odendaal HJ. Influence of perinatal care on stillbirths in patients of low socio-economic class. *S Afr Med J* 1988; **74**: 53–54.

(4) SAPA–SASOG Joint committee on Perinatal Care. Asphyxia and perinatal mortality. *S Afr Med J* 1986; **69**: 595.

(5) Van Coeverden de Groot HA, Davey DA, Howland RC. The Peninsula Maternity and Perinatal Service. *S Afr Med J* 1982; **61**: 35.

(6) Larsen JF, Muller EJ. *S Afr Med J* 1978; **54**: 1137.

(7) Van Coeverden de Groot HA. Editorial. Community perinatal care. *S Afr Med J* 1982; **61**: 30.

(8) Ross SM, MacPherson T, Wallace J, *et al.* Unsuccessful pregnancies — report on 200 perinatal postmortems. *S Afr Med J* 1978; May: 828–9.

(9) Pattinson RC, Rossouw L. The unbooked mother at Tygerberg Hospital. *S Afr Med J* 1987; **71**: 559–560.

(10) Roos PJ, Malan AF, Woods DL, *et al. S Afr Med J* 1980; **57**: 347.

(11) Naicker SN, Moodley J, *et al.* Serological diagnosis of syphilis in pregnancy. *S Afr Med J* 1983; **63**: 536.

(12) Ross SM, Windsor IM, Robins-Browne RM, *et al.* Microbiological studies of the perinatal period. *S Afr Med J* 1984; **66**: 598–603.

(13) Van Coeverden de Groot HA. Trends in maternal mortality in Cape Town. 1953–1977. *S Afr Med J* 1984; **56**: 547.

(14) Cooreman BF, Cronje HS, Grobler CJF. Maternal deaths at Pelonomi Hospital. Bloemfontein, 1980–1985. *S Afr Med J* 1989; **76**: 24–26.

(15) Theron GB, Pattinson RC, Engelbrecht BHJ. Kaaplandse plattelandse perinatale sterftes, January–December 1985. *S Afr Med J*; **73**: 211–213.

(16) Larsen JV, *et al. SA Nursing Journal.* November 1976, p. 7.

(17) Van Coeverden de Groot HA, Van Coeverden de Groot AA. Born before arrival at the midwife obstetrics unit in Cape Town. *S Afr J of Epidemiology and Infection* 1987; **2**: 19–22.

(18) Boes EGM. Maternal mortality in Southern Africa, Parts I and II. 1980–1982. *S Afr Med J* 1987; **71**: 158–161.

(19) Moodley J. Raised blood pressure in pregnancy. *S Afr J Cont Med Educ* 1987; **5**: 41–51.

(20) De Wet A, Louw NS. Voorkoms van asimptomatiese bakteriurie tydens swangerskap met behulp van die Dornfest-metode as siftingtoets. *S Afr Med J* 1982; **62**: 285.

(21) Davey DA, Dommisse J. The management of hypertension in pregnancy. *S Afr Med J* 1980; **58**: 551.

(22) MacGillivray I, Rose GA, Rowe B. *Clin Sci* 1969; **37**: 395.

(23) Editorial. *S Afr Med J* 1977; **52**: 1107.

(24) Walker ARP, Kruger S. Nutrition in pregnancy. *S Afr J Cont Med Educ* 1987; **5**: 27–34.

(25) Quoted from *The Star*, 20 July 1977.

(26) Scott JR, Rose NB. *New Engl Med J* 1976; **294**: 1205.

(27) Shapiro M, Crookes RL, O'Sullivan E. Screening antenatal blood samples for anti-human immunodeficiency virus antibodies by a large-pool enzyme-linked immunosorbent assay system. *S Afr Med J* 1989; **76**: 245–247.

TEST OF KNOWLEDGE

The student has benefited from studying this chapter if he/she can answer the following questions:

(1) Write notes on:
  – The amniotic fluid infection syndrome
  – Abruptio placentae
  – Pre-eclampsia

- The low birth weight infant
- Born before arrival (BBA)

(2) Define the following terms:
  - Pregnancy-induced hypertension (PIH)
  - Perinatal care index
  - Mid-trimester
  - Intrapartum
  - Maternal mortality rate
  - Perinatal deaths
  - Neonatal mortality rate

(3) Discuss the following features which exacerbate obstetric problems in socio-economically deprived, developing nations:
  - High teenage pregnancy rate
  - High illegitimacy rate
  - Unbooked status
  - Low level of education
  - Multiparity

(4) (a) Name the causes of maternal deaths.
   (b) Define eclampsia.
   (c) What are the potential dangers of hypertension in pregnancy?

(d) Discuss the taking and interpretation of the blood pressure in pregnancy.

(5) Define the aims of antenatal care and give examples of how these aims may be realised.

(6) How can the following be avoided by good antenatal care:
  - Congenital syphilis
  - Congenital rubella syndrome
  - Neonatal jaundice
  - Anencephaly and spina bifida
  - Cerebral palsy
  - Stillbirths

(7) What antenatal advice would you give a group of expectant mothers on the following topics:
  - Diet
  - Morning sickness
  - Family planning
  - Coitus during pregnancy
  - Breast-feeding

22

Child Mortality
Child Health Clinics

OBJECTIVES

The objectives of this chapter are to highlight the great discrepancy between child mortality amongst the privileged and underprivileged children of South Africa and to suggest interim ways in which this discrepancy can be alleviated through the application of WHO GOBI-FFF principles.

The concept of growth monitoring is introduced by explaining the use of Road-to-Health cards. The student is guided in understanding a percentile chart and the correct interpretation of the mass/age charts used by child clinics to monitor satisfactory growth.

GOBI-FFF principles form the basis of primary health care dispensed from the hospital out-patient and community clinics which cater especially for the needs of children and their mothers. The importance of early (pre-school) child education is an important facet of primary health care and to this end the state is subsidising organisations which care for the young child of the working mother.

For Community Health Centres and Clinics, see Chapter 4.

CHILD MORTALITY*

Definitions

Infant mortality rate (IMR)

The number of deaths in children under 1 year per 1 000 live births for a defined community during 1 year. WHO's global aim in 1979 *vis-à-vis* IMR: less than 50/1 000 by the year 2000.[1] All South African population groups, except blacks, have exceeded this target, i.e. their IMRs are below 50.

In the RSA there were close on 40 000 infant deaths in one year (1986) of which 82,5 % were due to three major causes: perinatal 41,6 %, intestinal 27,5 %, respiratory 13,4 %.

One strategy is needed to deal with all three: essential community-based primary health care services.[1]

Factors influencing the IMR:

(1) The general nutritional status of the mother.
(2) Antenatal and maternity services.
(3) The optimal spacing of pregnancies — ideally 3 years, but not less than 24 months.

(4) Age of the mother. The IMR is higher in teenage mothers and mothers over the age of 35 years.

(5) Educational standard of the mother. This is the single most important factor influencing the IMR.[1]

(6) Conditions relating to the infant such as mass at birth, nutrition of infant, regular attendance at clinics for immunisation and growth monitoring and the quality of mothering.

(7) Socio-economic levels with regard to income (in relation to the size of the family), water, sanitation and housing.

Child mortality rate (CMR)

This is the number of deaths at year 1–4 in a given year per 1 000 children in that age group at the midpoint of the year concerned.[2] CMR excludes the IMR. The CMR reflects mainly environmental factors affecting the health of the child such as nutrition, sanitation, water supplies, the communicable diseases of childhood and accidents occurring in and around the house. It is a sensitive indicator of the socio-economic development of the community.

Causes of CMR[2]

The following make up 74,5 % of all known causes:

- Intestinal infections 32,3 %
- Respiratory diseases 18,9 %
- Nutritional diseases 12,2 %
- Viral diseases 11,1 %

These causes of child mortality are typical of a developing country. White and Asian CMRs in the RSA are on a par with those of developed countries.

Under-5 mortality rate (U5MR)

This is the mortality rate of all children under 5 years of age and is a combination of IMR and CMR. When calculating the U5MR an estimate of the midyear population under the age of 5 years is used as the denominator.

___
* See also page 95.

South African mortality rates in 1986[1, 2]

	Blacks (estimated)	Whites (registered)	Coloureds (registered)	Asians (registered)	Mean for RSA (estimated)
IMR	54,6	7,0	31,6	13,6	47,7
CMR	8,01	1,0	4,78	1,39	6,89
U5MR	18,90	2,11	11,38	4,20	16,25

The IMR and CMR vary among the different population groups. The majority of Third-World deaths in children can be prevented by improving their socio-economic circumstances. Communities lacking basic facilities (First Level of Care of the National Health Plan, see p. 17) should be identified and selected for special attention, either the establishment of PHC clinics where none exists, or upgrading of clinics where they are deficient, or mobile PHC clinics for places that are inaccessible. Community primary health care services can greatly reduce the high mortality rate in black and coloured South African children. The important PHC services are community midwifery and health education, especially of the mother; of special importance in death prevention is the application of the WHO GOBI-FFF principles.

WHO GOBI-FFF PRINCIPLES

Medical services concentrating on the principles of GOBI-FFF have been shown to decrease morbidity and mortality in southern Africa, i.e. to promote child survival.

These principles are:[3]

G　growth monitoring from birth to school age

O　oral rehydration given promptly for treatment of diarrhoea and vomiting

B　promotion of breast-feeding as an exclusive form of feeding for the first 4 months of life

I　insistence on total immunisation cover of all infants and children

F　female (and father) education in proper care and feeding of infants and toddlers

F　food supplements for children under the 3rd percentile in weight and height, and for mothers not gaining weight in pregnancy

F　family spacing or fertility control; children are known to thrive better if there are at least 24–36 months between pregnancies.

GOBI-FFF is the best interim measure to bring down high death-rates in children while First Level Care of the National Health Plan is being put into practice by community development measures.

THE CONCEPT OF GROWTH MONITORING[4]

Road-to-Health cards

One of the main strategies for improving the health of young children is the Road to Health card (pre-school record card) initiated by Professor David Morley as a result of his experiences in Third-World countries. The use of the card is advocated by the WHO.

The cards incorporating percentile mass/age charts are extensively used by child preventive and health promotive (well-baby) clinics. Satisfactory mass gain (measured monthly during the first year of life) signifies adequate protein-energy nutrition. Satisfactory mass gain after a wasting illness can be monitored on the chart. Mass loss (dipping of the graph) or stationary mass in the absence of illness is evidence of incipient malnutrition which will respond to timely corrective measures. The community health nurse at the well-baby clinic monitors both immediate and long-term nutrition.

Note:
(1) The nurse must guard against erroneously diagnosing obesity or under-nutrition if the child's mass falls within the 3rd to the 97th percentile. These diagnoses are valid only if the mass falls beyond these limits.
(2) Mothers must be taught to interpret the mass charts correctly so that they may be able to follow the progress of their children.
(3) Apart from the mass charts on health cards issued by well-baby clinics, PHC child clinics use mass, height and skull circumference charts which are attached to the patient records which the clinic retains. PHC nurses use the mass/age chart as a diagnostic tool to recognise poor nutrition (i.e. mass below the 3rd percentile) and the effects of ill-health.

Although the Road-to-Health cards were originally devised to improve child health in Third-World countries, the information carried on the card can be of tremendous benefit to all children, whether cared for by the public or the private sector. Cards are continually being modified to enhance their practical value.

Figure 22.2 on page 395 illustrates both sides of a pre-school health card (age 0–6 years) designed by a working party of the South African Paediatric Association for use throughout the RSA; it has the approval of the Department of Health.

The card should be issued to the mother on the birth of her child, in a strong protective polythene bag to preserve the card. The mother retains the card and is taught to produce it whenever she takes her child to any clinic.

The card is divided into four main areas. The inside of the folded card is designated the A area and has five subdivisions:

A1: Child's age at each visit.

A2: Mass graph for the plotting of mass. The solid lines on this graph represent the 50th percentile (for boys) and the 3rd and 97th percentiles for girls. The lowest, broken line is called 'the marasmus line'. Mass is based on the National Centre for Health Statistics (USA) (NCHS).

A3: Space to record type of feeding.

A4: Space to record the achievement of the developmental milestones and the results of hearing and vision tests.

A5: Space for recording height, head circumference and haemoglobin value.

The outside of the card has the divisions B, C, and D.

B: Personal particulars and perinatal information including the APGAR score and neonatal complications, e.g. jaundice.

C: A record of immunisations and the results of tuberculin testing, etc.

D: Brief medical notes about illnesses and visits to a doctor.

Percentile growth charts[5]

Growth charts (A2 on Road-to-Health cards) are commonly known as 'percentile' charts. They give an indication of whether the child's growth (height, mass and head circumference) are within normal limits. Some clinics use only mass charts as their main concern is undernutrition. Some charts make provision for monthly recording during the first two years of life and two-monthly after that to the age of 6 years, while others extend to the 13th year.

The normal limits presumed by the growth charts lie between the 3rd and the 97th percentile, the 'population' in this case being all the children from birth to the age of 6 years (in the case of a pre-school health card).

Percentiles give an indication of how a measure of an attribute of an individual compares with that of the population of which the

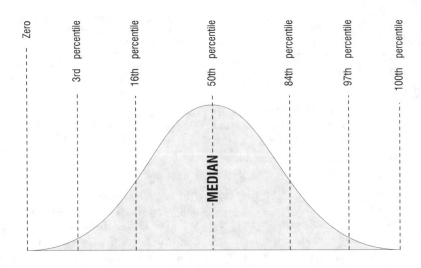

Figure 22.1

Percentiles on normal distribution curve

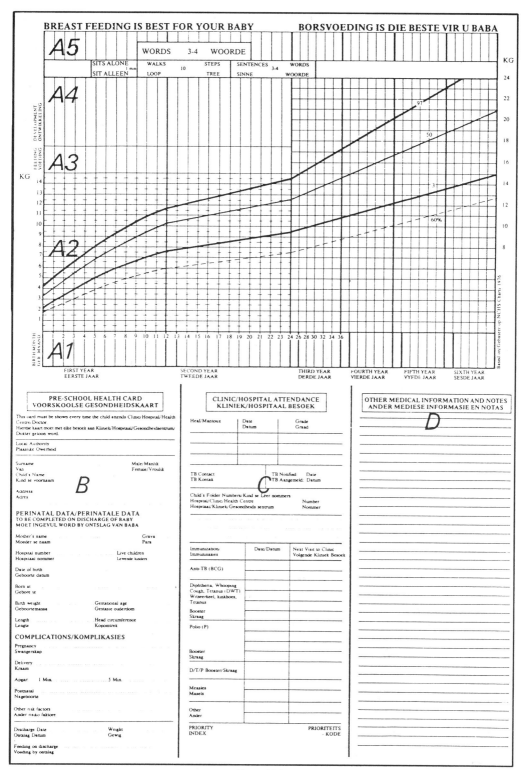

Figure 22.2

Road-to-Health card for use in South Africa

individual is a member. When certain attributes, e.g. head circumference, mass, height, of a population are measured, a large variation is found to exist. This variation is not evenly distributed but clusters around the mean (average) and median values. Thus a bell-shaped curve characterises the 'normal' distribution of a population parameter, with the mean and median values in the middle. Larger and smaller values are equally distributed on either side of the central values.

Note: By the median is meant the score which is so situated that half the scores are higher and half are lower.

Example

If the range of birth mass in a population is 3 kg to 4 kg and birth mass has a normal distribution, then the mean birth mass is 3,5 kg and the median birth mass value is also 3,5 kg. The term *percentile* is related to the median and indicates a percentage of the whole. If the area under the normal distribution curve (i.e. the total population measured — in our example all babies born) is divided by imaginary vertical lines into 100 equal portions, each line demarcates 1/100th of the population — one percentile. The 50th percentile (counting from left to right) is the median. The 3rd percentile means that 2 % of the population weigh less than, and the 97th percentile that 96 % of the population weigh less than (or 3 % weigh more than) the child in question.

A normal distribution of height, mass and head circumference has been established for every month (first two years of life) and every two months up to the 13th year of life. By looking at a growth chart, the nurse will realise that a large range of measures can be considered normal. For example, in the mass chart all masses that fall between the 3rd and 97th percentiles could be normal. If a child's mass lies between the 97th and 100th percentile, a state of obesity due to overnutrition exists; if it falls between the 3rd percentile and zero, failure to thrive — which may be due to undernutrition — is indicated. If the child's mass falls beyond the normal distribution range, a state of malnutrition (either overfeeding or starvation) is suggested. The World Health Organisation considers that if a child's mass is below the 3rd

percentile, he is starving. This statement applies to all races in all parts of the world.

In the normal growth record there should not be a large discrepancy between the height and mass percentiles. If the records show a developing discrepancy, the mother must be advised about feeding and the community health nurse and social worker concerned notified to keep the child under surveillance.

FAMILY HEALTH CENTRES

Family health centres or clinics dispense preventive health services and are staffed by doctors, community health nurses (formerly called health visitors), family planning nurses, social workers and family counsellors. The community health nurse (CHN) provides a health service to families either in the home or in the clinic. Because the CHN is closely involved with families, she assumes special responsibility for the detection of deviations (sight, hearing, intelligence, physical anomalies) and for prompt referral to specialist agencies.

Preventive community health clinics are the responsibility of local authorities who provide health-promotive and ill-health preventive services such as the prevention of communicable diseases by immunisation. One of their most important services is the Child Health (well-baby) clinic.

Child health (well-baby) clinics

Mothers attend these clinics with their babies at regular intervals. Here the progress of the child is monitored, advice and health education are dispensed and the infant screened for abnormalities.

The infant is usually checked by a doctor at the ages of 1 month and 6 months and referred for treatment if necessary.

Audiometric tests are done at 7 months: they are repeated at intervals if the child appears to have a hearing problem. A child with a confirmed positive screening test will require referral to a speech and hearing clinic or the ENT department of a hospital, or a private specialist.

Note: Nearly all deaf-born babies have some degree of hearing which can be amplified by the use of hearing aids which help the infant to acquire normal speech.

In some clinics developmental screening tests are done on all infants and toddlers. The Denver Developmental Screening Test for infants and pre-school children is useful for this purpose. It is designed to identify children with serious development delays in the following areas: gross motor, fine motor-adaptive, language, personal-social. The Denver test can be used by individuals who have no training in administering psychological tests.

Note: This test should pick up gross visual problems. If a developmental delay is observed, the child can be referred to a developmental assessment clinic.

Mothers of children with genetic abnormalities are referred for genetic counselling to counsellors of the Department of Health Genetic Services. The CHN does follow-up work with the parents after the counselling session, which she attends with the parents.

At the well-baby clinic, help and advice with minor ailments will be given, the infant immunised against infectious diseases (see Chapter 28) and mothercraft counselling done.

Mothercraft counselling by the CHN

At the well-baby clinic, babies are regularly weighed and measured; their mothers are counselled with regard to feeding and food supplementation with iron and vitamins. A health card (Road to Health) with appointments and a record of attendances, feeding schedules, immunisation and growth record (percentile charts) is kept for each child.

The mother should be instructed in the use and meaning of the percentile charts, so that she may follow her child's progress intelligently.

Bottle-feeding

An extremely controversial subject in artificial (bottle) infant feeding is the nature of the feed: should the mother use liquid or powdered full cow's milk, or should she resort to modified (humanised) milks? Leary[8] states that the human infant has all the digestive enzymes (except amylase) and can, therefore, digest undiluted cow's milk. Only in the neonate is it necessary to dilute the milk (and add sugar to supply needed kilojoules) because of the high concentration of mineral salts which the kidneys of the neonate cannot excrete satisfactorily. After the

first two weeks of life, the kidneys of an infant are as competent as those of an adult. The only indications for humanised milk are: extreme prematurity, heart failure, renal disease. Leary warns, furthermore, that the use of humanised milk can lead to undernutrition if, because of its high cost, the mother over-dilutes the feed to make one tin go further.

The comparative cost of 100 g of protein in different kinds of cow's milk (1979):

In skim milk . . . . 46 cents
In full cream milk . . . . 84 cents
In dried full cream milk . . . . 88 cents
In humanised milk R2,00

Breast-feeding

Breast-feeding is an emotive subject; modern, sophisticated westernised women generally prefer bottle-feeding and may do so with apparent success; yet for infants born into the lower socio-economic classes, especially in the developing countries of the Third World, artificial bottle-feeding is a tragedy as it invariably leads to under-nutrition and infection. These are frequent causes of infant mortality. Dr David Morley of the University of London, an expert on child health in the developing countries of the world, is of the opinion that in these countries a child should be breast fed for as long as 2 years. He feels strongly that the toddler, fed the traditional diet of maize, does not get enough kilojoules (and protein) due to the bulkiness of the porridge diet. Dr Morley is especially concerned with the deteriorating nutritional standards in developing countries. Among the better-fed middle class, breast-feeding for 6 to 9 months remains the goal.

Modern scientific medicine is constantly finding more proofs for the superiority of breast-feeding over bottle-feeding, and yet the popularity of the latter is growing, especially in the developing countries amongst the more sophisticated urban mothers. It has become almost a matter of status to buy expensive humanised milks for infant feeding, some mothers genuinely believing that they are promoting the health of their child by so doing.

From a survey done in Soweto, Johannesburg, it appeared that although 75 % to 90 % of mothers attended an antenatal clinic, only 72 % of them breast-fed. A quarter of the mothers who bottle-fed their infant believed that breast-feeding would make them ill.[6]

Nurses and doctors are taught the advantages of natural feeding yet seem to be unable to stem the tide of failed lactations in their patients. Can it be that their own scepticism — their lack of enthusiasm and conviction — is transmitted to their patients and that in their health educative efforts they transmit their doubts as to the superiority of natural feeding for the health of both mother and child?

On the other hand, few modern women find complete fulfilment in their traditional role of mother and homemaker and therefore favour bottle-feeding, which does not require total commitment to their infant.

Ransome et al., in a study of urban coloured mothers, found that 97 % began by breast-feeding and 50 % were still doing so at 20 weeks. Some mothers introduced solids very early, the overall feeding and growth pattern being very similar to UK data. It could not be demonstrated in this sample that prolonged breast-feeding protected infants against gastro-enteritis or that the infants were better off nutritionally than those in whom breast-feeding was stopped before 12 weeks.[7]

Leary[8] found that amongst a group of middle-class white women in Cape Town, a mere 5 % to 7 % of mothers were still breast-feeding at the time of their 6-week postnatal check-up visit. Even amongst the coloured mothers of Cape Town, only 10 % of the infants were breast-fed at 4 months.

The main advantages of breast-feeding are:

- Lower incidence of gastro-enteritis and respiratory infections in infancy.
- Greater protection against under- and over-feeding; no obesity.
- Lower incidence of milk allergies; there is no constipation.
- Better protection against infectious diseases to which the mother is immune.
- Lower incidence of crib deaths.
- Promotion of the mother/child relationship; facility in providing demand feeding for the infant; it is economical and time-saving.
- Breast milk has the correct constituents for the development of the child; it has more than a hundred components which differ from those of the milk of other animals. Although breast milk has a low iron content, supplementary iron is not required, as nearly all the iron is absorbed.

Ebrahim[10] states that 'human milk is a substance of great biological potency'. One of its prime functions is to help in the development of the immune system of the infant. Apart from the immunoglobulins (antibodies) in breast milk, it also teems with cells — macrophages, neutrophils and B-cell and T-cell lymphocytes, all well controlled by immunoregulatory proteins to prevent the newborn from overreacting immunologically to the environmental antigens after birth. In this way it helps with the development of the newborn's immune system and enhances the breast-fed infant's survival potential. Breast-fed infants respond better to BCG and DPT vaccines compared to formula-fed ones.

Cow's milk contains approximately three times as much protein and almost four times as much mineral salts as human milk. The protein of human milk is mainly albumin which forms a soft, easily digestible curd.

The casein of cow's milk forms a tough curd in the infant's stomach. The fat of human milk contains more unsaturated fatty acids. This has a favourable effect on blood cholesterol. There can be no suggestion that human milk does not agree with the infant. Leary states that human milk is 'qualitatively the best food which can be provided for the human infant and [that] it may bestow advantages which last into adult life'.[8] These advantages include relative immunity in infancy to gastro-intestinal infection and lowered incidence of atherosclerosis in adult life.

In order to successfully breast-feed her infant the mother must, however, be prepared to make some sacrifices. She must persevere with the establishment of a satisfactory supply of milk. In order to make this possible, motivation aided by paternal involvement and social support is important. The mother must be prepared antenatally and the infant must be allowed to suckle soon after birth — within the first hour — at first only for 5 minutes on each breast to prevent sore nipples. The lactating mother must not take medicines, such as aspirins and antibiotics, because these medicines are excreted in the milk and can harm the infant. The mother must not smoke or drink. If the mother does not have sufficient milk, the infant must be put to the breast 2- to 3-hourly, without resorting to complementary or supplementary feeds. A good well-balanced diet and plenty of fluids are good lactogogues.

Reassurance of the lactating mother is important as the volume of milk secreted will depend very much on the emotional state of the mother. Worry and anxiety will result in a decrease of the supply. Few working mothers successfully breast-feed their infants, but this is by no means impossible as even the working mother can feed her infant at least twice a day, while entrusting the bottle-feeding of her infant to a substitute mother during her absence.

Encouragement and information for the mother who is motivated to feed her infant may be had from organisations of mothers who advocate breast-feeding because of their own gratifying experiences. An example is the la Leche League which has groups in most cities in South Africa. The league publishes literature for lay people, doctors and nurses, amongst which is a manual called *The Womanly Art of Breastfeeding*.

Breast-feeding options for the working woman[11]

Community nurses, especially occupational health nurses, have a very important role to play in promoting breast-feeding by mothers during employment. Early immunisation and breast-feeding play pivotal roles in child survival. Therefore the working mother needs education and counselling to manage lactation. The help of the father can be elicited to help with the other children and the housework, preventing the mother from losing her milk through sheer exhaustion. The nurse can also help the mother secure a suitable caretaker or crèche which will co-operate with the mother's wish to breast-feed. The mother is taught the best way of preserving lactation.

(a) A well-balanced diet and plenty of fluids — the simpler the better, i.e. water.

(b) Vigorous sucking by the infant, i.e. stimulation of the nipple and areola is the best 'lactogogue'.

(c) Avoidance of exhaustion; unhurried feeding at the breast.

The infant must not be bottle-fed between feeds if the mother has to leave it during the day. Breast milk expressed by fingers or a breast pump can be kept cool, preferably in a fridge, and fed by spoon from a cup by the caretaker. In the older infant, solids can be given from the 4th month during the time of mother's absence; baby's thirst can be quenched by feeding water or orange juice by spoon from a cup. Bottle feeding may cause the infant to refuse the breast, as it is easier to suck from a bottle. The nurse must teach the mother the correct hygiene and technique of manual expression with the fingers placed on the areola before pressing towards the nipple. The giving of an expressed milk feed can be started before the mother goes back to work to facilitate this method of feeding by the caretaker.

(d) Some mothers train their babies to sleep during the day and feed them frequently at night on a 'demand' schedule, or the mother may give the infant a large feed early in the morning and a smaller one before she leaves for work.

(e) If the mother leaks milk at work, she is taught either to express milk in a clean receptacle (to be covered and stored in a cool place) or to apply pressure to the breasts (with palms of hands) or nipples (with fingers) or to cross her arms over her breasts and press. She can also wear breast pads.

The occupational health nurse must make employers aware of the special needs of nursing mothers and of the importance of breast-feeding for mother and child. Conditions of employment can sometimes be arranged to suit the breast-feeding mother, e.g. flexitime or half-day work or taking work home, or bringing baby to the workplace for the first few months. The workplace may have a crèche thus affording the mother the opportunity to feed her baby during breaks. Some firms may be persuaded to give maternity leave benefits which enable the mother to work up to the birth and return to work when the baby is 6 months old and able to take solids during the day. Then two or three breast feeds per 24 hours will be sufficient.

Legislation in South Africa allows a woman who has contributed to the Unemployment Insurance Fund to draw 45 % of her normal weekly earnings (provided she receives one third of her normal earnings from her employer) for a maximum of 26 weeks. Some trade unions have been able to negotiate even better benefits for their members.

Because of her close contact with the young family, the CHN can play an important role in promoting mental health by teaching the principles involved in establishing good family relationships.

SOME PRINCIPLES INVOLVED IN ESTABLISHING GOOD FAMILY RELATIONSHIPS

Community nurses, i.e. school nurses, occupational health nurses, community health nurses, district nurses, midwives and psychiatric nurses, who go into the schools, homes, crèches and family health clinics where they deal with children and their parents, are in a favoured position to prevent mental ill-health and promote mental health amongst the youth. This can be done by teaching parents skills which will promote good parent/child relationships, thereby helping children to deal effectively with the frustrations inherent in socialisation.

The essence of good relationships between human beings is the mutual respect of each for the needs of the other. This applies not only in adult to adult relationships but also in child to adult relationships. Good relationships contribute to the psychological growth towards maturity of both children and adults.

It is ironic that, although the mental health of the child depends upon the quality of family life and is essential for the creation of co-operating, contributing citizens, parents are not taught the skills which promote good intra-family relationships; they muddle along as their parents did before them, sometimes raising responsible citizens but at other times thrusting upon society a crop of angry, destructive, fearful and dependent young adults.

Child-rearing skills are based on knowledge and an important task of the community nurse is to teach parents about child development and the needs of children, which vary at different developmental stages. Children need to feel secure, i.e. that their dependency needs will be met while they are legitimately dependent on their parents. They need to separate gradually from their parents, however, to become autonomous human beings who can think for themselves, make choices and decisions and have preferences without constantly feeling the need to ask their parents or others for help and advice.

The infant needs to have a trusting relationship with his parents while he is powerless and helpless. Trust can only be established fully where there is a continuity of the caring, need-satisfying parent/child relationship in order for the child to form an emotional bond and the parent to become a psychological parent. Bonding occurs as a result of the day-to-day physical care of the child, being initiated by early postnatal physical contact between parents and infant.

A child's psychological tie to a parent figure is rooted in the small child's dependence on a caring adult who is preoccupied with the care of the child and becomes emotionally involved with him, in a stimulating, intimate relationship. In an institution where the caretakers do their job efficiently but impersonally and where there are multiple caretakers, psychological bonding does not take place; the child's body, and not the social relationship between infant and adult, becomes the focus of attention.

In order to develop self-esteem, a child must have at least one adult whom he can love and by whom he feels loved and valued. When this mutual loving is absent in infancy, the individual's later capacity to love and care for others is damaged.

As the trusting child develops some ability to move independently (1–3 years), his dependency needs will become less urgent. The child now needs to feel that he has some power and can assert himself, albeit within the protective circle of his family. This stage of development is recognised by the negativism and dawning independence of the toddler who loves playing messily with water and sand, starts communicating with speech and learns to control eliminatory functions.

The normal 'negativism' of the 2–3-year-old can be very trying to parents and, if the natural assertiveness of a child is suppressed at this stage, this can lead to either destructive, angry behaviour or withdrawn, nervous behaviour.

During the pre-school years (3–5 years) the 'oedipal' child needs to form 3-person relationships, i.e. with mother and father at the same time, the relationships being sex-appropriate.

A little girl, therefore, needs to identify with an acceptable feminine model with whose male partner she learns appropriate flirtatious behaviour. A little boy needs to identify with an acceptable male model and displays a protectiveness and possessiveness towards his mother, as he copies his father's role. In order for this stage to be passed successfully, parental harmony is necessary. The 3-person relationships necessarily evoke jealousy and rivalry towards the same-sex parent which the child may find difficult to manage, especially if marital relationships are poor and a parent uses a child for his/her own emotional gratification.

During the juvenile, 'primary school' stage (6–11 years), peer group relationships become very important. The child needs to move away from the home to explore the environment. Parents become less important as satisfiers of emotional needs and their stable presence in the background needs to be taken for granted.

During adolescence the main needs of the emerging adult are the establishment of ego identity, the establishment of roles in the adult world, the establishment of heterosexual relationships and the liberation from adult control. Although the striving for autonomy is very strong during adolescence, the teenager feels ambivalent towards control and needs to feel that parents care enough to set some limits.

These are the main needs of the developing child, the striving for autonomy to become an independent, strong, responsible human being who can relate to other human beings on an equal footing, being a continuous process. The degree of independence should be age-appropriate; both precocious and retarded independence cause emotional and behavioural disturbances in the child.

In our competitive, power-driven society many parents use their power to control their children and many children either resist and rebel, or withdraw and become inhibited, some children becoming saddled with the crippling burden of feelings of inferiority, guilt and low self-esteem. A great problem in child-rearing is caused by parents who feel it their duty to punish in order to produce 'nice' unspoilt children who will be a credit to them; children are often blackmailed to accept their parents' nurturing behaviour and develop a load of guilt if they need to resist the 'good intentions' of their parents. Parents who believe in punitive discipline feel that children must be coerced to accept the cultural values and customs and that they will become selfish unless cultural conformity is punitively induced.

Yet it is possible for children to become socialised without the use of punishment, just as it is possible in a motivated student to acquire an education without punitive coercion. In order to be successful, parents need to understand their children, to make allowances for their faults, to be flexible in handling them and, above all, to set the example they wish their children to follow. Children who relate well to their parents are motivated to co-operate with them in their child-rearing tasks.

COMPREHENSIVE COMMUNITY CHILD CARE — THE UNDER-FIVES' CLINIC

In most warm climate (developing) countries, the mortality from infection in childhood is very high, 40 % to 50 % of children dying before the age of 5 years. The great killers are diarrhoea and pneumonia, these diseases being closely associated with poverty and malnutrition. The under-fives' clinics have been started in many developing countries through the influence of Dr David Morley, Reader in Tropical Child Health, University of London. Dr Morley is well known in South Africa and has greatly influenced paediatric community health care, especially amongst the black people.

The following ideas have been gleaned from his book, *Paediatric Priorities in the Developing World.*

The aims of the people who run the under-fives' clinics for the central hospital or health care centre are:

(1) the early diagnosis and treatment of disease; health education;

(2) to extend low-cost curative and preventive care to as large a proportion of the popula-

tion as possible and to encourage regular visiting of the clinic;

(3) the supervision of the health of all children up to the age of 5 years;

(4) the prevention of malnutrition and all those infectious diseases which are preventable by immunisation;

(5) the provision of simple treatment of diarrhoea, pneumonia and common skin disorders.

Acute 'weaning' diarrhoea is frequent because the protective effects of breast-feeding have ceased. The habit among many black ethnic groups is to send the child away from its mother during weaning; this means that the child does not attend the clinic. The diarrhoea is likely to have a multiple aetiology (see p. 445). In kwashiorkor, pathogenic organisms are not always found, diarrhoea being due to the atrophic small intestine and lactose intolerance. Malnourished children are inclined to get diarrhoea and vice versa.

Under-fives' clinics offer the following curative and preventive services in rural and urban areas (the services should be available at any time of the day, on every day of the week):

(1) Health education of the mother, especially with regard to the nutrition of her family; this is done by means of demonstrations and talks to groups of mothers.

(2) The maintenance of records which are filled in by the staff on health cards which are usually kept and cared for by the mother once she realises how important they are. Dr Morley believes the mother should take the responsibility for the card and be able to read the mass graphs. The information on the cards includes: major illnesses the child has had, his immunity status, reasons for special care (if any), and a growth record which is obtained by regular weighing and measuring of the child. The growth curve gives an indication of the success of the health education of the mother, the effectiveness of immunisation and the adequacy of curative services. When interpreting growth curves, the importance of the direction of the curve, i.e. whether up or down, must be appreciated, not just whether the child is at or below the third NCHS percen-

tile. If a child whose mass normally lies on the 50th percentile starts losing mass, i.e. the direction of the curve is downward, he is considered a 'child at risk' (of developing the sequelae of malnutrition). If a child persistently fails to gain mass despite an adequate diet, chronic infection or psychosocial disorganisation of the family are probable aetiological factors.

(3) Immunisation (see p. 492).

(4) Primary health care (see p. 26) (curative services), in which ample use is made of chemotherapy, hydration of the dehydrated child with diarrhoea (see p. 445), and feeding of the malnourished child. Very often curative services are the only reason why the mother attends the clinic with her child, as many unenlightened mothers do not comprehend the need for prevention. Primary health care is, therefore, an inducement to attend the clinic; thus the child will eventually reap the benefits of promotive and preventive health care. Freely available primary health care, dispensed by specially trained nurses, can cut the under-five mortality by 50 %; further reduction in the mortality rate is contingent on preventive paediatrics, however. Any cases with which the nurse cannot deal because of the limitations of her knowledge and competence, or because the mother insists that her child be seen by a doctor, are referred to the base hospital or to the medical practitioner who works in the clinic on a consultative basis.

(5) Severe malnourished infants are admitted with their mothers, either to the base hospital or to a special unit attached to the clinic. After discharge, the infants are followed up at the clinic and are supplied with free milk until their mass is normal.

Note:
(1) The following services for adults are usually run in conjunction with the under-fives' clinic: antenatal clinic; family planning clinic.
(2) Visits to under-fives' clinics should take place monthly during the first year of life, if the child is healthy, otherwise more often.

PRE-SCHOOL EDUCARE PROGRAMMES AND THE WORKING MOTHER

Pre-school institutions for children up to school-going age are a tremendous boon to working-mothers. In modern urban societies, the children of working mothers attend crèches (and child minders) from some time during the first year of life until the school-going age. Pre-primary (nursery) schools, on the other hand, cater only for the 3- to 6-year-old. Pre-school institutions may be either profit-making and run by private enterprise, or non-profit making and run either by welfare societies, churches, local authorities or hospitals and business concerns for their staff.

The pre-primary school is almost a cultural 'must' in developed countries, even in families in which the mother does not work outside the home. In these countries the family is becoming less and less self-sufficient as specialised external agencies take over the functions of the nuclear family.

Pre-primary schools are open half-day only and close during the school holidays. Trained pre-primary school teachers guide the children in educational and socialising activities, but no formal teaching is allowed by government decree.

Child minders are private women, approved by the Health Department of the local authority who, in their own homes, may care for up to six children for the whole day or part of the day.

Crèches or day nurseries take children either from early babyhood or from 6 months, or from 1 to 3 years, up to school-going age. They are strictly controlled by the local authority and children are not subjected to any formal educational activities. The caretakers are gradually being trained and, in crèches accepting infants, a registered nurse must take charge. Play is supervised and stimulated and children's physical and health needs are catered for. Community health nurses are involved with problem children at crèches and will visit the home of the problem child, counselling the mother in mild cases and referring to a child guidance or child psychiatric clinic when the child and his family are more severely disturbed.

The private sector has played a very active role in providing the facilities for the care of pre-school children and for the training of staff.

Several organisations exist at regional level to co-ordinate ideas and activities at national level. The state has also become increasingly concerned with pre-school education, especially pre-primary education to prepare 5-year-olds in disadvantaged communities for entry into formal education. The state controls and regulates all pre-school institutions, subsidising those that qualify for registration. Health care in the crèches is regulated by legislation.

Crèches not only provide care for children of working mothers but also play an educational role. In underprivileged children, pre-school crèche education is part of preventive medicine in that the play and stimulation to which children are exposed in well-run crèches contribute to the total well-being of the child.

The primary health care nurse must be aware of the extent of the 'educare' programmes for pre-school children in her community as they are part of primary health care services.

Organisations which run places of care for the care of children older than 1 month and younger than 7 years are entitled to a government grant, provided the mother must of necessity work away from the home (see p. 422).

There has been much speculation as to the long-term effects on young children reared in day nurseries and crèches because their mothers are working, the deleterious factor being the multiplicity of mother figures which prevents the infant from bonding with one mother figure. A WHO Expert Committee (1951) came to the conclusion in 1951 that day nurseries and crèches cause permanent damage to the emotional health of a future generation. Rutter[9] found no evidence, however, that young children suffer through having several mother figures, provided the multiple mothers give good care and are stable figures in the child's life. Poor quality maternal care may be the lot of the home-reared child no less than the crèche-reared child — the poor quality of the care will have long-term bad effects on the mental health of the child in both instances.

There can be no doubt, however, that if the infant is separated daily for long periods from his mother during the first year of life, he will have difficulty in bonding with her and in separating from her psychically in order to start individuating and developing towards an autonomous human being. The 'bonding' role of the mother can, however, be taken by any stable mothering figure with whom the child has a one-to-one trusting relationship which endures for a reasonable period of time.

REFERENCES

(1) Department of National Health and Population Development. South African Mortality Rates. *Epidemiological Comments* 1989; **16**(1).

(2) Department of National Health and Population Development. South African Child Mortality Rates. *Epidemiological Comments*. 1989; **16**(4).

(3) Hansen JDC. Nutritional deficiencies in children. *S Afr J CME* 1986; **3**: 17–25.

(4) Wagstaff L, De Vries G. Children's growth charts in theory and practice. *S Afr Med J* 1986; **70**: 426–427.

(5) Vlok ME. *Manual of Nursing* Vol. II. Cape Town: Juta, 1988.

(6) Shuenyane E, *et al*. *S Afr Med J* 1977; **51**: 495.

(7) Ransome OJ, Chalmers B, Herman AAB, *et al*. Infant feeding in an urban community. *S Afr Med J* 1988; **74**: 393–395.

(8) Leary PM. *S Afr Med J* 1976; **50**: 1271.

(9) Rutter M. *Journal of Child Psychology and Psychiatry* 1971; **12**: 233–60.

(10) Ebrahim GJ. Human milk and the child survival revolution. *CHASA* 1993; **4**(i).

(11) Bergh AM. Breast-feeding options for the working woman. *Nursing RSA Verpleging* 1991; **6**(2).

TEST OF KNOWLEDGE

The student has benefited from studying this chapter if he/she can answer the following questions:

(1) Define the following mortality rates: infant, child, under-fives. Discuss the predisposing and precipitating causes of the high mortality rates amongst the coloured and black communities in South Africa.

(2) Explain the principles on which health cards issued by child clinics are based and state their usefulness in primary health care.

(3) Define the relationship between the WHO GOBI-FFF health principles and First Level Care of the National Health Plan.

(4) Compare the 'under-fives' clinics as advocated by Dr David Morley with the 'well-baby' clinics of family health centres run by some large urban local authorities.

(5) Discuss the importance of pre-school education in underprivileged communities and the role of 'educare' in primary health care.

23

Child Welfare in the RSA
Child Care Act
Child Abuse
Social Assistance Act

OBJECTIVES

To introduce the student to the plight of the disadvantaged child in need of care in our society and the socio-legal measures taken to salvage from young wrecked lives the remnants of a healthy personality, or to prevent damage to the personality by instituting early adoption or foster care. Although the implementation of the Child Care Act 74 of 1983 lies largely within the ambit of the social worker, the community nurse is involved because of her close contact with problem families in the community.

The attention of the nurse is drawn to the fact that it is legally incumbent upon the community nurse, and especially the CHN and school nurse, to report cases of suspected physical and sexual abuse, as well as neglect in the form of deliberate undernourishment, to a regional director of health or the police. This may lead to the removal of the child concerned to a place of safety or a hospital.

Midwives, school nurses and CHNs are also in a position to apply primary and secondary preventive measures in cases of child abuse.

The Social Assistance Act 59 of 1992 provides for the financial needs (through grants) of: the aged, the disabled (physically, mentally or psychiatrically), war veterans, foster children; gives maintenance grants to the indigent parent for the maintenance of a child in his custody, capitation (individual) grants to prescribed institutions, including places of safety for the care of persons committed by the court.

The Act also makes financial awards to national councils and welfare organisations which co-ordinate organised activities or social welfare programmes for some of the disadvantaged people in our society.

With the promulgation of this Act in 1992, parts of or entire social welfare Acts became obsolete and were repealed.

INTRODUCTION

Children develop best in the warm, intimate setting of the elementary family; where this nuclear family fails them, either through sickness, death or divorce of the parents, or through alcoholism, pauperism or criminality, or because they abuse them, they must be cared for by others. In most cases where the parents are unable to look after their children, foster caring is done by relatives or carefully selected unrelated families who act as surrogate parents and give the children the warmth, interest and intimacy of primary group relationships. These primary human relationships are essential for the inculcation of feelings of being wanted and loved and of belonging somewhere. Children who are sent to institutions in infancy are usu-

ally deprived of these primary group relationships and may thus be permanently handicapped as they feel rootless, unloved and unlovable and are in turn unable to love in the mature sense of the word. These are our deprived children who develop psychiatric disorders because they feel rootless and unwanted and bear a grudge against society. Depriving children at an early age of loving parents or parent surrogates, and parental failure to make a child feel loved and wanted, are the most serious forms of social pathology. The prevalence of child neglect and its consequences — juvenile and adult delinquency — is therefore an accurate indication of the social health of a society.

The Bill on Human Rights of the United Nations, states:

> 'There is no human right more basic to humanity or more imperative for the individual, than the right to be brought into this world as a wanted human being who will be fed, cared for, loved, educated and given the opportunity for a constructive life.'

In 1985 there were 20 000 children (all races) in all types of institutions in the RSA — only 2 % of them were orphans. An additional 17 000 places were still required for black children in need of care.[1]

COMMUNITY CARE OF THE DISADVANTAGED CHILD

Care of the emotionally and socially damaged child who has been subjected to parental cruelty and neglect and to social rejection is aimed at preventing adult delinquency and criminality, vagrancy, child abuse as well as addiction to alcohol and drugs. Child welfare work in these cases can be termed tertiary preventive work as it is concerned with reducing the sequelae of psychological damage through rehabilitation. The main focus of tertiary preventive measures is on the disadvantaged, deprived child, the 'child in need of care' who often exhibits antisocial behaviour when he comes within the ambit of child welfare services. Johannesburg shelters for street children estimate that between 14 000 and 20 000 children live on city streets (*The Star*, 23.06.1994). Without food and education, these children will turn to crime. Attempts are made by family and child welfare agencies to do reconstruction work with the families that fail their children in order to restore the child to a reasonably functioning family. Aiding the state in its family welfare activities are a number of voluntary welfare organisations.

Voluntary family welfare organisations (NGOs)

A welfare organisation must be registered in terms of section 13 of the National Welfare Act. A family welfare organisation is subsidised by the state in that the state provides a subsidy for every approved social worker's post.

The following family welfare organisations or child welfare agencies assist the state in caring for children in need of care:

- Child and Family Welfare societies; they deal with all racial groups
- Indian Welfare associations deal with Indian children and families only
- Christelike Maatskaplike Raad (CMR) of the Dutch Reformed Church (NDGK)
- Catholic Family Welfare of the Roman Catholic Church
- Ondersteuningsraad of the Hervormde Kerk
- Apostolic Faith Mission of SA, Welfare Council
- Jewish Welfare

The most frequent type of care of children in need of care is by placement with foster parents. In 1985 there were 37 000–38 000 children in foster care in the RSA.[1]

PLACEMENT WITH FOSTER PARENTS

A foster parent is an adult who receives a child on a temporary basis for board and care. The placement is made either by the Social Welfare Department or by a family welfare agency under the direction of the Commissioner of Child Welfare. The placement is either short-term on a retention order or long-term on a committal order. The supervising department or agency can remove the child at any time, either because the placement is not suitable, or because the child is to be adopted or returned to his own parents.

The legal rights of foster parents

Although social workers employed by a child care agency make recommendations to the Commissioner of Child Welfare for the removal of a child from his own parents' home, the final decision rests with the Children's Court (see p. 411). With regard to placement in a foster home, the Commissioner of Child Welfare may order the following:

(1) Where the child's life is deemed to be in danger, the child can be placed with temporary foster parents on a retention order.
(2) At a subsequent Children's Court enquiry, the child can be placed on a committal order in long-term custody of foster parents, under supervision of a social worker.

The state pays a foster care grant to the foster parents for every child thus committed. This grant is not taxable.

Certain parental powers are transferred to the foster parents, viz. the right to punish the foster child and to exercise discipline. The child is legally placed in the care of the foster parents. In the case of an application for the adoption of a foster child by a person other than his foster parent, the foster parent must consent in writing to the adoption of the child. The foster parent cannot withhold consent but has adoption priority.

The legal position of the foster parents also ensures that the child cannot be returned to his natural parents or be placed in the care of anyone without the reversal of the custody order by a Children's Court.

Although the natural parents have lost the custody of their child, they have not lost access to the child. The natural parents are allowed to see their child at times agreed upon by the foster parents.

Both natural parents retain the following guardianship rights over their minor child:

(1) the legal authority to sign consent to operation or to adoption;
(2) the legal authority to sign consent for a minor child to marry;
(3) the legal authority to deal with any property the child may have (section 53 of the Child Care Act 1983);
(4) when a passport is applied for (Guardianship Act, 1993).

If the child dies while in the care of foster parents, the natural parents are responsible for funeral expenses. A foster child can be taken out of the country temporarily, provided the consent of the natural parents (if contactable) and the chief social welfare officer is obtained. The social worker in charge of the fostered child will arrange for consent to be obtained.

Although theoretically foster care is a good solution to the problems of the child whose own parents cannot care for him, in practice this is not always so. In the first place, it is difficult to recruit suitable foster parents, i.e. mature adults who foster children because of their compassion and love for children, and who will not become over-involved emotionally with the foster child if the placement is temporary. In the second place, some foster parents are inclined not to become emotionally involved at all with the child for fear of being hurt when the child is removed from the foster home.

The role assigned to foster parents is to establish a limited parent/child attachment and to give adequate physical, religious, medical and educational care. The child must be treated like the natural children of the family, e.g. in so far as privileges and pocket money are concerned. The child may not be exploited as a source of labour. Biological parents are to be allowed to visit the child and to maintain their emotional bond with him.

The fact that the placement is supervised by an outside agency may prevent the foster parents from feeling that they 'own' the child and, conversely, the child from feeling that he 'belongs' to the family. Thus the child's emotional need for feeling wanted and for belonging is not satisfied. The older fostered child will become aware that he is merely a sojourner in the home and that the state pays for his board. The child/foster parent relationship has little chance of developing the parent/wanted-child quality. The child feels insecure and may become very troublesome, thereby further compromising the parent/child relationship. Foster parents are, therefore, encouraged to adopt 'adoptable' children.

If adults take on foster children for the sake of the money the state pays them and if the parents feel free to return the child whenever it is no longer convenient to keep him, the chances of a limited emotional bond developing are slim indeed and foster care placement is as conducive to emotional deprivation as placement in a children's home.

Because the successful fostering of children is such an exacting task, child welfare societies have recently started foster parent training programmes.

Parents who wish to take children into foster care are advised to join a foster parent association operating in some of the larger centres. Child welfare agencies which are constantly searching for suitable foster parents to place their children in need of care can be contacted for information of foster parent groups.

Prospective foster parents are screened by child welfare agencies, the following issues being considered and discussed with them:

(1) Do they have physical and emotional room for a child, i.e. is the whole family willing to adapt to the needs of a child, often very difficult, who has just lost his own family and is therefore in a state of mourning?

(2) Can they accept more disorder in the home in view of the fact that the foster child may take some time to learn the rules of the home?

(3) Can the physical health of the family stand up to the extra work involved?

(4) How stable are family relationships? Can problems be openly discussed and acted upon? Is there the danger that all existing family problems are going to be projected on to the new child?

(5) Is the husband-wife relationship good enough to withstand extra stress and are both in agreement about taking on a foster child?

(6) How successful are the parents in the rearing of their own children?

(7) How do the children feel about having a foster child in their midst? Will they help the parents with meeting the needs of a child who has just lost his family?

(8) The kind of child and his age are important for successful foster care and care should be taken to match the prospective client's

choice. Some foster parents want to give short-term care while others prefer long-term placements.

(9) The attitude of prospective foster parents to the child's natural parents is important. A friendly relationship between the adult parental figures is essential. The child's parents should be boosted so that the important parent-child bond may be preserved. Foster parents should not try to usurp the role of the natural parents. Their role should be that of good, trustworthy adult friends whose friendship will stand the disadvantaged child in good stead for a lifetime.

THE CHILD CARE ACT 74 OF 1983 AND CHILD CARE AMENDMENT ACT 1991

The following sections are extracts from the Child Care Act 74 of 1983 and its amendment which has replaced the Children's Act 33 of 1960 and all its amendments. The appointment of probation officers and the establishment, maintenance and management of schools of industries and reform schools of Act 33 of 1960 remain in force.

'**Child** means any person under the age of 18 years;

Pupil means any child who has been sent to or transferred to an institution in this Act and in terms of the Criminal Procedure Act of 1977.'

Children's courts

'**5.** (1) Every magistrate's court shall be a children's court for the area of its jurisdiction.

(2) Every Commissioner's court is a children's court for the area for which it has been established . . .

Procedure in children's courts

7. (1) A Commissioner or assistant commissioner of child welfare shall preside over a children's court . . .

8. (1) A children's court shall sit in a room other than that in which any other court ordinarily sits.

(2) At any sitting of a children's court no person shall be present unless his presence is necessary or he is the legal representative of any person whose presence is necessary unless the Com-

missioner presiding at that sitting has granted him permission to be present.

(3) No person shall publish in any manner whatever any information relating to proceedings in a children's court which reveals or may reveal the identity of any child who is or was concerned in those proceedings.'

Juvenile court

A juvenile court, in contradistinction to the children's court, is an informal criminal court in which juvenile delinquents, under the age of 18 years, are brought to trial and are sentenced, leniently, by a magistrate. Only the juvenile, his parents and a probation officer who has 'screened' the case are allowed to be present, i.e. the proceedings are held *in camera*. Psychiatrists have been appointed since 1927 to assist the juvenile courts at Pretoria, Johannesburg, Cape Town, Durban, Pietermaritzburg and Port Elizabeth.

The juvenile may be sentenced to cuts (abolished in 1995) and is either:

(1) placed with his parents under the supervision of a probation officer;

such a child is then deemed to be placed on probation. The court requires that such a child shall:
  (*a*) abstain from the use of dependence-producing substances;
  (*b*) submit himself to medical, psychiatric or psychological examination or treatment determined by the court;
  (*c*) make good loss or damage caused by him, or render some suitable community service;
  (*d*) at all times co-operate with the social worker;
  (*e*) join and become an active member of a specific club or movement.

In the case of a scholar, he shall attend a specific school and not absent himself from school without good reason.

In the case of a child who has already left school, he must remain in the employment of a specified undertaking and remain in regular employment.

The parent or guardian shall to the satisfaction of the social worker provide the child with the necessary material means.

(2) sent to a school of industries; or

(3) sent to reform school if he has had previous serious convictions.

A *school of industries* means a school maintained for the reception, care, education and training of children sent or transferred thereto under the Child Care Act.

A *reform school* means a school maintained for the reception, care and training of children sent thereto in terms of the Criminal Procedure Act 51 of 1977 or transferred thereto under this Act.

For the functions of a children's court, see p. 413.

The protection of children

'Maintenance of certain children apart from parents

10. (1) No person other than the managers of a maternity home, a hospital, a place of safety or a children's home shall receive —

(*a*) any illegitimate children under the age of seven years; or

(*b*) any child for the purpose of adopting him or causing him to be adopted,
and maintain him apart from his parents for a longer period than 14 days, unless such person —

 (i) has applied in terms of section 18 for the adoption of the child; or

 (ii) has obtained the consent in writing of the Commissioner of the district in which the child was residing immediately before he was received.'

Investigation of allegations that a child is in need of care

A case of child neglect, ill-treatment, abandonment or exploitation is usually reported by a member of the community to the police, a Social Welfare Department, regional director or a child welfare agency. The person who reports need not reveal his name. Cases are referred by these authorities to the family welfare organisation which is best able to deal with the case, e.g.:

(1) an appropriate religious welfare agency;

(2) if the parents have no strong attachment to a church, then to a child welfare society;

(3) juvenile delinquents or drug dependants to a social welfare officer;

(4) if the parents of children in need of care are alcoholics, they are referred to family welfare organisations to institute the legal action required to commit the parent(s) to rehabilitation centres.

'Removal of child to place of safety on order of court or on sworn information

11. (1) If it appears to any court in the course of any proceedings before that court that any child has no parent or guardian or that it is in the interest of the safety and welfare of any child that he be taken to a place of safety, that court may order that the child be taken to a place of safety and be brought as soon as may be thereafter before a children's court . . .

(3) Any policeman or social worker or other person authorised by the said warrant to search for and remove a child may enter (by force if necessary) any house or other premises mentioned in the warrant and may remove the child therefrom.

Removal of child to place of safety pending inquiry

12. (1) Any policeman, social worker or authorised officer may remove a child from any place to a place of safety without a warrant if that policeman, social worker or authorised officer has reason to believe that the child is a child referred to in section 14(4) and that the delay in obtaining a warrant will be prejudicial to the safety and welfare of that child.

(2) The policeman, social worker or authorised officer who has so removed a child shall as soon thereafter as may be —

(*a*) inform the parent or guardian of the said child of his removal if such parent or guardian can be traced without due delay;

(*b*) inform a children's court assistant concerned of the reasons for the child's removal; and

(*c*) bring the child before the children's court.'

The functions of a children's court

'Bringing children before children's court

13. (1) Any child referred to in section 11(1) or (2) or 12(1) shall be brought before the children's court.

(2) Any child in regard to whom a children's court assistant is of opinion that he has no parent or guardian, or has a parent or guardian who cannot be traced, or has a parent or guardian or is in the custody of a person unable or unfit in terms of section 14(4) to have the custody of him, may be brought before the children's court of the district in which the child resides or happens to be by any policeman, social worker or authorised officer or by a parent, guardian or other person having the custody of the child.

(3) The children's court before which a child is brought in terms of subsection (1) or (2) shall hold an inquiry in the prescribed manner and determine whether the child has no parent or guardian, or has a parent or guardian who cannot be traced, or has a parent or guardian or is in the custody of a person unable or unfit to have the custody of that child. Provided that if the child ordinarily resides in the district of another children's court the first-mentioned court may refer the inquiry to the children's court of that other district.

(4) If it appears to a children's court that a child referred to in subsection (1) or (2) who is subject to the court's jurisdiction, should by reason of his infancy, ill-health or other sufficient cause not be brought before the court, the court may hold the inquiry in the absence of the child.

Holding of inquiries

14. (1) Any children's court holding an inquiry in terms of section 13(3) may at any time during the inquiry order any medical officer to examine the child concerned and to report to the court.

(2) The commissioner presiding over a children's court may request any social worker to furnish a report on any matter affecting the child concerned or his parents. . . .

(4) At such enquiry the children's court shall determine whether —

(*a*) the child has no parent or guardian, the child has a parent or guardian who cannot be traced, or

(*b*) the child has a parent or a guardian or is in the custody of a person who is unable or unfit to have the custody of the child, in that he —

   (i) is mentally ill to such a degree that he is unable to provide for the physical, mental or social well-being of the child;

   (ii) has assaulted or ill-treated the child or allowed him to be assaulted or ill-treated;

   (iii) has caused or conduced to the seduction, abduction or prostitution of the child or the commission by the child of immoral acts;

   (iv) displays habits and behaviour which may seriously injure the physical, mental or social well-being of the child;

   (v) fails to maintain the child adequately;

   (vi) maintains the child in contravention of section 10;

   (vii) neglects the child or allows him to be neglected;

   (viii) cannot control the child properly so as to ensure proper behaviour such as regular school attendance;

   (ix) has abandoned the child; or

   (x) has no visible means of support.

Powers of children's courts after inquiry

15. (1) A children's court which, after holding an inquiry in terms of section 13, is satisfied that the child has no parent or guardian, or has a parent or guardian who cannot be traced, or has a parent or guardian or is in the custody of a person unable or unfit to have the custody of the child, may —

(*a*) order that the child be returned to or remain in the custody of his parents or, if the parents live apart or are divorced, the parent designated by the court or of his guardian or of the person in whose custody he was immediately before the commencement of the proceedings, under the supervision of a social worker; on condition that the child or his parents or guardian or such person complies, or the parents of the child comply with such of the prescribed requirements as the court may determine; or

(*b*) order that the child be placed in the custody of a suitable foster parent designated by the court under the supervision of a social worker; or

(c) order that the child be sent to a children's home designated by the Director-General; or

(d) order that the child be sent to a school of industries designated by the Director-General . . .

(3) A children's court which has made an order under subsection (1)(b), (c) or (d) may also order that the child be kept in a place of safety until such time as effect can be given to the order which the court has made. . . .

(5) (a) If the Director-General cannot designate a children's home in terms of subsection (1)(c) or a school of industries in terms of subsection (1)(d), he shall without delay furnish the Minister with a report in connection with the child concerned.

(b) The Minister may, after consideration of the Director-General's report referred to in paragraph (a), deal with the child concerned in terms of section 34 or 37 as if the child has been admitted to a children's home or a school of industries, as the case may be.

Duration of orders under section 15

16. (1) Subject to the provisions of this section and of section 34 (transfer of children and pupils from one custody or institution to another) any order made under section 15 shall lapse after the expiration of a period of two years after the day on which the order was made or after the expiration of such shorter period as the children's court may have determined at the time of making.

(2) The Minister may extend the validity of an order referred to in subsection (1) for a further period not exceeding two years at a time.'

During a children's court hearing, the Commissioner of Child Welfare does not pass sentence on a child or his parents but decides what steps are to be taken to help the child (and his family). He is assisted in his decisions by the recommendations of the social worker concerned with the investigation of the case.

The types of problems dealt with by the Commissioner of Child Welfare and the children's court include:

(1) Adoption and the supervision of a protected infant.

(2) The issue of a temporary retention order in an emergency where a child's life is deemed to be in danger. On a retention order, the child is retained either in a hospital, in a place of safety, in a children's home or with temporary foster parents. A retention order marks the opening of a Children's Court Inquiry. After this, a full investigation by a social worker is made and a complete report of findings and recommendations drawn up. This is presented at the subsequent full court inquiry.

(3) The issue of a more permanent committal order at a children's court hearing. A committal order places a child in the long-term custody of a children's home, foster parents or his own parents, under supervision of a social worker.

The proceedings of the children's court (i.e. court inquiry or hearing) are as follows. The social worker reads the report on the circumstances of the family and deals with the special needs of the child (children). The social worker gives an assessment of the case and may make recommendations.

The parents are asked if they agree with the recommendations of the social worker and the contents of the report. If they wish to dispute the social worker's recommendations, they have their own lawyer. Every effort is made, however, for the decision to be a joint one between parents, social worker and children's court. Once all the evidence is heard, the Commissioner of Child Welfare will declare that he finds the child (children) to be 'in need of care' and he will order that the child (children) be placed as recommended by the social worker. (See section 15, Child Care Act.)

A child can be discharged from the provisions of the Children's Act at any age if the family has solved its problems and is coping well on its own; the social worker then recommends that the child be discharged from the provisions of the Act.

If a committed child is not discharged, he remains the responsibility of the state and/or a welfare organisation until the age of 18 years or, in certain cases (if found to be 'in need of care' at the age of 17 years), until the age of 21 years. Even if the committed child works from the age of 16 years, he is still supervised until the age of 18, unless he is discharged from supervision by the children's court.

Note: In section 16: any order made by a children's court lapses after 2 years. This requires that the case be reviewed at least every 2 years.

The legal process of adopting a child

In South Africa children are frequently adopted through family welfare agencies. Each adoption is carefully arranged by the social worker dealing with the case. Private adoption is, however, not prohibited by law; it is, therefore, still possible for individual persons and organisations to place children in adoption without the necessary precautions.

'Qualifications for adoption of children

17. A child may be adopted —

(*a*) by a husband and his wife jointly;

(*b*) by a widower or widow or unmarried or divorced person;

(*c*) by a married person whose spouse is the parent of the child.

'The adoption of children

18. (1) The adoption of a child shall be effected by an order of the children's court . . .

(4) A children's court shall not grant the application unless it is satisfied —

(*a*) that the applicant is or that both applicants are qualified to adopt the child;

(*b*) that the applicant is or that both applicants are of good repute and a person or persons fit and proper to be entrusted with the custody of the child; and

(*c*) that the proposed adoption will serve the interests and conduce to the welfare of the child; and

(*d*) that consent to the adoption has been given by both parents of the child, or, if the child is illegitimate, by the mother of the child;

(*e*) that the child, if over the age of ten years, consents to the adoption and understands the nature and import of such consent;

(*f*) in the case of a child born of any person who is a South African citizen, that the applicant, except an applicant referred to in section 17(*c*), or one of the applicants is a South African citizen resident in the Republic, or the applicant has or the applicants have otherwise the necessary residential qualifications for the grant to him or them under the South African Citizenship Act, 1949 (Act 44 of 1949) of a certificate or certificates of naturalisation as a South African citizen;

(*g*) in the case of an application for the adoption of a foster child by a person other than his foster parent, that the foster parent consented in writing to the adoption of the child: Provided that such consent shall not be necessary if the foster parent refuses or fails, within one month after being called upon in writing by an assistant of the children's court to do so, to indicate to him in writing whether he so consents or not. . . .

(6) The said consent shall set out the names of the proposed adoptive parents, but the children's court may admit, as satisfying the requirements of subsection (4)(*d*), a consent by the child's parents or guardian which does not set out the names or any other particulars of the proposed adoptive parents, if it is satisfied that the interest of the child will be served thereby.

Circumstances in which consent to adoption may be dispensed with

19. No consent in terms of section 18(4)(*d*) shall be required —

(*a*) in the case of any child whose parents are dead and for whom no guardian has been appointed;

(*b*) from any parent —
   (i) who is as a result of mental illness incompetent to give any consent; or
   (ii) who deserted the child and whose whereabouts are unknown; or
   (iii) who has assaulted or ill-treated the child or allowed him to be assaulted or ill-treated; or
   (iv) who has caused or conduced to the seduction, abduction or prostitution of the

child or the commission by the child of immoral acts; or

(v) whose child is by virtue of the provisions of section 16(2) in the custody of a foster parent or is a pupil in a children's home or a school of industries; or

(vi) who is withholding his consent unreasonably.

Effect of adoption

20. (1) An order of adoption shall terminate all the rights and obligations existing between the child and any person who was his parent (other than a spouse contemplated in section 17(*c*)) immediately prior to such adoption, and that parent's relatives.

(2) An adopted child shall for all purposes whatever be deemed in law to be the legitimate child of the adoptive parent, as if he was born of that parent during the existence of a lawful marriage.

(3) An order of adoption shall, unless otherwise thereby provided, confer the surname of the adoptive parent on the adopted child.

(4) An order of adoption shall not have the effect of permitting or prohibiting any marriage or carnal intercourse (other than a marriage or carnal intercourse between the adoptive parents and the adopted child) which, but for the adoption, would have been prohibited or permitted.

Rescission of order of adoption

21. (1) A parent of a child or the adoptive parent or parents of the child, the children's court assistant may apply to the children's court by which the order was made for the rescission thereof on one or more of the following grounds, namely —

(*a*) if the applicant is the parent of the child, that he did not consent to the adoption and that the order of adoption should not have been made without his consent; or

(*b*) if the applicant is an adoptive parent, that his adoption of the child was induced by fraud, misrepresentation or that the child is mentally ill, and that the mental illness existed at the time of the making of the order of adoption, or that the child suffered from a congenital disorder or injury of a serious nature at the

time of the making of the order of adoption;

(*c*) that for reasons set out in the application the adoption is to the detriment of the child;

(*d*) that at the time of the order of adoption the adoptive parent or parents did not qualify in terms of section 17 for obtaining the order of adoption.

(2) If the application is made —

(*a*) it shall be made within a period of six months but not later than two years as from the date upon which that order was made . . .

(3) (*a*) An application on the ground that the child is mentally ill may only be made if the applicant was, or if husband and wife jointly adopted the child concerned, they both were, at the time of the making of the order of adoption, ignorant of the mental illness of the child and that ignorance was not due to failure of the adoptive parent or parents to exercise reasonable care in examining the child or causing it to be examined.

(*b*) An application on the ground that the child suffered from a congenital disorder or injury of a serious nature, they both were, at the time of the making of the order of adoption, ignorant of that genetic disorder or injury, and this ignorance was not due to failure of the adoptive parent or parents to exercise reasonable care in examining the child or causing it to be examined . . .

(8) On the rescission of an order of adoption in terms of subsection (7), the child concerned shall for all purposes be restored to the position in which it would have been if no order of adoption had been made: Provided that the rescission of the order shall not affect anything lawfully done while the order of adoption was in force. . . .

Adoption of adopted child

23. (1) An adopted child shall be capable of adoption, and upon the making of an order for the adoption of a previously adopted child all the legal consequences of the earlier adoption shall terminate, save in so far as the adopted child has acquired any property by virtue of the earlier adoption . . .

Prohibition of consideration in respect of adoptions

24. (1) No person shall, save with the consent of the Minister, give, undertake to give, receive or contract to receive any consideration, in cash or kind, in respect of the adoption of a child.

(2) Any person who contravenes any provision of subsection (1) shall be guilty of an offence and on conviction liable to a fine not exceeding R8 000 or to imprisonment for a period not exceeding two years or to both such fine and such imprisonment.

Alteration of births register as a result of adoption

25. (1) When an order has been made for the adoption of a child the appropriate Director-General shall on the application of the adoptive parent and on production of the order of adoption and on payment of the prescribed fee, cause the fact of adoption and a statement whether the surname of the adoptive parent was or was not conferred upon the child by virtue of the adoption, to be recorded on the birth register.

(2) If the surname of an adoptive parent has been conferred upon an adopted child and that fact has been recorded on the original birth information form, a birth certificate in the surname of the adoptive parent may be issued in respect of the child.'

Adoption practice of family welfare organisations

In all adoption casework, the welfare of the child is of paramount importance, but the well-being of the child's natural parents and of the adopters is also considered. Placement agencies must work within the framework of the law (Child Care Act) which regulates and controls the adoption of children. Placement agencies are attached to Family Welfare Agencies and placement is done by social workers with special placement skills who are employed by the agency.

Some of the agencies with adoption services are: Apostolic Faith Mission of SA Welfare Council; CMR of the Dutch Reformed Church; Catholic Women's League Adoption Society; Cotland's Babies' Sanctuary, Johannesburg; Child Welfare Societies (black, coloured and white); Princess Alice Adoption Home of the Johannesburg Child Welfare Society; Ondersteuningsraad, Hervormde Kerk; Indian Social Welfare Association.

Casework with the child's natural parent(s)

Parent(s) are helped to arrive at a decision when contemplating giving up their child for adoption; indecision is the result of emotional conflicts which cause ambivalence. They are also helped to understand the implications and desirability of adoption, viz.:

(1) (*a*) In a non-disclosure adoption, they will have no access to their child and no legal rights and responsibilities, as the adopters will become the legal parents;

    (*b*) the fact of adoption is entered in the births' register and a new birth certificate will be issued to their child with his new surname and sometimes even with new forenames.

(2) The agency will do its best to give the child a secure and permanent home.

(3) Their own capacity to meet their child's needs. A discussion of this point is especially important in the case of a teenage, unmarried mother who is totally unable to care for an infant, especially if she does not have the support of her family and does not understand the implications of parental responsibility, yet needs her baby to satisfy her own need for love.

When the parent(s) have given verbal consent to adoption, the caseworker must elicit as much background information about the child and his parents as possible in order to facilitate the selection of the most suitable home for the child. Information includes:

(1) health and medical history of the parents, especially with regard to hereditary disorders;

(2) social, cultural, religious and educational status;

(3) an older child's experiences within the family and when two or more children from a family are to be placed, their interpersonal

relationships to judge whether separation would be traumatic or not;

(4) the nature of the pregnancy and birth and the child's medical, developmental and psychiatric history, especially with regard to frequent separations which will hamper bonding with the adoptive parents;

(5) psychometric examination of the mother if she appears to be psychiatrically disturbed or intellectually subnormal.

In the case of an unmarried pregnant woman whose infant is up for adoption and who has emotional problems and poor resources (mentally and materially), the placement agency has a responsibility for her care and support by direct supportive services or suitable referral. Where the father of a child up for adoption is available and willing to be involved and the mother (in the case of an unmarried woman) consents to it, he is approached to give information about himself and his family and to help in the planning of his child's future.

Parents of the mother are sometimes counselled as well. Casework counselling may bring the family together and provide much-needed support for the unmarried mother.

Parents may need counselling to help their daughter make a social adjustment on her return from the maternity hospital.

The parent(s) of the child to be adopted must sign consent after the birth of the child. Both parents, or the mother alone if she is unmarried, must sign consent in the presence of a Commissioner of Child Welfare; the caseworker should accompany her/them to the children's court for this giving of formal, legal consent to adoption.

The caseworker must help the parent(s) separate from their child as soon as possible after they have decided to give him up for adoption. The question of whether an unmarried mother should see her child depends upon the individual mother, but it is usually advisable for her to see the baby once in the presence of the social worker. It is usually considered unwise for the unmarried mother to breast-feed her child in the maternity hospital and steps should be taken to dry up her milk and to give her contraceptive counselling before she is discharged from hospital. She may need counselling for some time after discharge by the case-worker, to help her adjust to life in the community.

Casework with adoptive parents

Screening

An important function of placement agencies is the investigation of the background of applicants for a child. In South African white society, the demand for babies is always much greater than the supply, therefore there is no excuse for selecting unsuitable adopters just to find a home for a child. The age of the adopters (ideally between 25 and 40 years), the stability of the marriage, the ability of the prospective parents to meet the child's material, educational and emotional needs, the religious and socio-economic background, as well as the nationality of the adopters, are the important criteria to be investigated. Adoption casework is done to obtain a good match between the child and his adoptive parents and to ensure the best interests of the child.

Another important aspect of screening is ascertaining what kind of child parents can accept and what their later expectations of the child are likely to be.

Education

Prospective adoptive parents should receive education about adoption: how and when to tell a child about adoption and how to share effectively with the child the background report concerning his origins that should be given with every placement. It is also important to educate prospective adoptive parents about the legal aspects of adoption, including the rights of adopted persons to information about themselves. It must be pointed out that adoption has not been finalised on placement. Biological parents have the right to withdraw consent until the adoption is finalised (usually about 3 months after placement). Group discussions with a number of prospective adopters have many valuable functions: they reduce feelings of isolation common in infertile couples and they help to build support networks amongst adoptive parents.

The child for adoption

Adoption at birth or within a few months is the ideal situation, as the chances of secure bonding and 'owning' of the child by his adoptive parents are maximal. Sometimes, however, an older child who may have had unfavourable early experiences with mothering figures is adopted and this may cause many problems which may need long-term counselling of the adopters.

It is important to have the child examined by a paediatrician. The prospective adopters are told what the child's future development is likely to be, to prevent later disappointment and rejection of the child.

A Guide to Adoption Practice states that the following children are not suitable for adoption and that alternative plans must be formulated for their future, if necessary by appropriate referral:

(1) children with close family ties whose parents or relatives can meet their needs, helped if necessary by casework services from the appropriate agency;

(2) children so severely mentally or physically handicapped that they need specialised permanent institutional care;

(3) older children whose early life experiences have been such as to have deprived them of the ability to make new personal relationships.

Adapted from: *A Guide to Adoption Practice* prepared for the South African National Council for Child and Family Welfare.

Places of safety

'**28.** (1) The Minister may, with the concurrence of the Minister of Finance, ... establish and maintain places of safety for the reception, custody, observation, examination and treatment of children under this Act, and the detention of children awaiting trial or sentence.'

A *place of safety* means any place established under section 28 and includes any place suitable for the reception of a child, into which the owner, occupier or person in charge thereof is willing to receive a child.

A place of safety also includes a police station, a hospital or other institution which is willing to receive a child in need of care.

Note: Any place of safety or place of detention under the Children's Act of 1960 shall be deemed a place of safety under the Child Care Act of 1983.

Except in an emergency, children are removed from their parents and committed to substitute care only after a great deal of preventive work has been attempted with the family, with no positive results. The general public are under a misapprehension that when a family comes to the attention of a welfare agency, the children will be removed. Child welfare agencies go out of their way to preserve family life. A child is never removed from his home and committed to an institution or foster home until a full investigation has been made and the investigating officer is quite sure there is no other way of dealing with the child. The committal of a child is done in a children's court.

Social workers do reconstruction services by helping the family of the child in need of care to solve their problems. The main problems in families are:

(1) breakdown in relationships, either between parents or between parent(s) and child(ren);

(2) alcoholism;

(3) behaviour problems in children and inability of parents to cope with them and to control the child;

(4) severe rejection of children by parents, presenting as child abuse.

Poverty is not usually an insuperable family problem as it is state policy that no child should ever be removed from his parents just for financial reasons (see maintenance grants p. 429).

Amongst black and coloured families poverty is an important cause of family problems, poverty often giving rise to the abandonment of infants. Amongst coloureds, many children find their way into a children's court because of poverty and alcoholism of parents, factors which cause instability and break-up of the family.

Children's homes and places of care

Children's homes

A children's home means any residence or home maintained for the reception, protection, care and bringing-up of more than six children or pupils apart from their parents, but does not include any school of industries or reform school.

Many children's homes belong to family welfare organisations, but some are independent, and some are run by the state. The state pays an allowance to children's homes for every committed child.

Place of care

A place of care means any building or premises maintained or used, whether for profit or otherwise, for the reception, protection and temporary or partial care of more than six children apart from their parents, but does not include any boarding school, any school hostel or any establishment which is maintained or used mainly for the tuition or training of children and which is controlled by or which has been registered or approved by the state, including a provincial administration; example: day care centre.

Children placed in a children's home at a young age and for a long period are likely to suffer emotional deprivation. The mental health of emotionally deprived children is adversely affected. Residential care cannot quite compensate for the lack of warm, concerned family life which gives a child the feeling of belonging somewhere and security, and helps him develop self-esteem and an identity. It is not impossible for young children to develop normally in an institution, but normal development will depend very much on the quality of the emotional care practised in the institution. An attempt is being made to improve the quality of interpersonal relationship between the caretakers (house parents) and committed children.

Some technikons and universities are offering courses in child development and child management to enable child caretakers to carry out their highly responsible task with confidence and efficiency. Some children's homes are run on the 'cottage system', the home being comprised of a number of cottages, each with a housemother and -father and up to 12 children of varying ages. This is an attempt to provide a 'family' environment for children deprived of their own families.

Another very effective type of residential care for boys 'in need of care' is provided by the Boys' Town organisation under the aegis of the Roman Catholic Church. The first Boys' Town was built in 1958 in Magaliesberg on the pattern of Fr. Flanagan's Boys' Town which was founded in Nebraska, USA in 1917. Boys' Towns have since been established in the Cape and Natal. Homes 'in the community' for boys 'in need of care' but with no behavioural problems were established in Cape Town, Johannesburg and Durban, different from the conventional Boys' Towns in that the boys make use of local schools and community amenities.

Boys' Towns cater for older boys with behavioural problems due to antisocial attitudes. The boys (mostly problem and neglected teenagers) form a self-ruling community with a strong religious bent, under the tutelage and care of housefathers, some religious sisters and schoolteachers.

'29. (1) The Minister may, with the concurrence of the Minister of Finance, out of moneys appropriated by Parliament for the purpose establish and maintain **children's homes** for the reception, care and bringing-up of children in terms of this Act . . .

30. (1) No child may be received in any children's home (other than a children's home maintained and controlled by the State) unless that children's home is managed by an association of persons consisting of not fewer than seven members and has been registered under this section, or otherwise than in accordance with the conditions on which that children's home has been so registered.

(2) No child may be received in any place of care (other than a place of care maintained and controlled by the state) unless that place of care has been registered under this section, or otherwise than in accordance with the conditions on which that place of care has been so registered.

(3) Application for the registration of a children's home or a place of care shall be made to the Director-General in the prescribed manner . . .

(5) Any children's home or place of care which immediately before the commencement of this section was registered and classified under section 42 of the Children's Act, 1960 (Act 33 of 1960), shall as from that commencement be deemed registered under this section of this Act as a children's home or place of care.

31. Subject to the provisions of the Act and these regulations no children's home shall be registered in terms of section 30 of the Act unless the Director-General is satisfied that proper arrangements have been made or will be made —

(a) for the treatment of the children in the children's home by a social worker, medical practitioner, psychiatrist or psychologist when such treatment is necessary;

(b) for the proper feeding and care of the said children; and

(c) to ensure that children who are of school-going age attend school.'

Many of the problem children have severe behavioural problems and have been uncontrollable at home. Some adolescents have become involved in prostitution, drug taking and drinking, while others play truant from school, steal and have violent temper outbursts. All are disturbed children whose families have failed them and who have to be controlled and helped by the community to sort themselves out. Their handling presents many problems for the staff as the children are often aggressive, uncooperative and self-mutilating, absconding when the opportunity presents itself.

'Maintenance of good order and discipline

32. (1) Any pupil in a children's home who —

(a) obstructs any persons in authority over him in the execution of his duties;

(b) refuses or fails to carry out or comply with a lawful order by any person in authority over him;

(c) incites, encourages or advises another pupil to create, cause or participate in any disturbance, dissatisfaction or to commit any act of insubordination;

(d) incites or encourages any other pupil or person to acts of violence or endangers or interferes with the good order or administration of the children's home;

(e) without the consent of the owner thereof appropriates, uses or intentionally or through gross negligence damages or destroys any property not belonging to him;

(f) absconds from the children's home or is absent without leave;

(g) brings into the children's home or possesses any alcoholic drink or habit-forming drugs; or

(h) behaves in an improper manner inside or outside the children's home;

may be punished in accordance with the provisions of these regulations.

(2) Any punishment referred to in subregulation (1) shall be determined by the head of the children's home, with due regard to the nature of the transgression, the age of the child and the instructions which the management of the children's home may give in case of a particular pupil or pupils in general; Provided that isola-

tion, confinement or refusal of leave shall not be used as a form of punishment.

(3) Corporal punishment may not be inflicted on a girl and also not on a boy in respect of whom a social worker, psychologist or medical practitioner has forbidden the infliction of such punishment.

(4) Before any corporal punishment may be inflicted the head of the children's home, or, in his absence, a member of the staff designated by him, shall satisfy himself that the pupil on whom he intends to inflict corporal punishment will not be physically or mentally adversely affected by such punishment.

(5) Corporal punishment shall be inflicted with an instrument approved by the management for that purpose on the buttocks in the presence of a person designated by the management for that purpose.

(6) A boy receiving corporal punishment shall wear a shirt, trousers and underpants.

(7) Immediately after the infliction of punishment the following information shall be entered in a punishment register:

(a) The name of the pupil punished;

(b) the date and the nature of the transgression;

(c) the nature of the punishment inflicted; and

(d) the name of the person who inflicted the punishment and the person in whose presence the punishment was inflicted.'

Note: As corporal punishment is no longer allowed in schools, this prohibition should also apply in children's homes.

'**35.** (3) Any person who directly or indirectly counsels, induces or aids any child or pupil to whom leave of absence has been granted under subsection (1) not to return to the custody of the foster parent or the institution or who prevents him from returning to such custody or institution after the expiration of the period of leave or after the cancellation of such leave, shall be guilty of an offence.

36. (1) The Minister may, if he considers it desirable in the interest of any pupil or foster child who is in an institution to which he has been sent under this Act or any other law or in the custody of a foster parent in which he has been placed under this Act or any other law, by order in writing direct that pupil or foster child be taken to a place of safety and be kept therein for observation or to be examined and treated . . .

39. (4) Notwithstanding any rule of law to the contrary —

(*a*) any person over the age of 18 years shall be competent to consent, without the assistance of his parent or guardian, to the performance of any operation upon himself; and

(*b*) any person over the age of 14 years shall be competent to consent, without the assistance of his parent or guardian, to the performance of any medical treatment of himself or his child.

40. In the application of the provisions of section 15(1)(*b*) or 34 regard shall be had to the religious and cultural background of the child concerned and of his parents as against that of the person in or to whose custody he is to be placed or transferred.

41. (1) No person or children's home shall be obliged to receive or resume the custody of any child, but any person or management of any children's home that has received or admitted any child shall be deemed to have the custody of that child and shall maintain and care for that child. . . . .

42. (1) Every dentist, medical practitioner, nurse or social worker who examines, attends or deals with any child in circumstances giving rise to the suspicion that the child has been ill-treated, or suffers from any injury, single or multiple, the cause of which might probably have been deliberate, or suffers from a nutritional deficiency disease, shall immediately notify the Director-General or any officer designated by him for the purpose of this section, of those circumstances.

(2) On receipt of a notification in terms of subsection (1) the Director-General or the said officer may issue a warrant in the prescribed form and manner for the removal of the child concerned to a place of safety or a hospital.

(3) The Director-General or the said officer shall thereupon arrange that the child and his parents receive such treatment as the Director-General or the said officer may determine.

(4) This section shall not exclude any other action against or treatment of the parent and his child in terms of this Act.

(5) Any dentist, medical practitioner, nurse or social worker who contravenes any provision of this section shall be guilty of an offence.

(6) No legal proceedings shall lie against any dentist, medical practitioner, nurse or social worker in respect of any notification given in good faith in accordance with this section . . .

49. (1) Any summons, subpoena or notice in connection with any proceedings under this Chapter may be served without fee by any policeman in the manner prescribed by the rules framed under the Magistrate's Courts Act, 1944 (Act 32 of 1944), for the service of similar documents in civil proceedings in magistrates' courts, unless any other manner of service has been prescribed.'

Prevention of ill-treatment

'**50.** (1) Any parent or guardian of a child or any person having the custody of a child who —

(*a*) ill-treats that child or allows it to be ill-treated; or

(*b*) abandons that child, or any other person who ill-treats a child, shall be guilty of an offence, and

(2) Any person legally liable to maintain a child, who, while able to do so, fails to provide that child with adequate food, clothing, lodging and medical aid, shall be guilty of an offence.

(3) Any person convicted of any offence under this section shall be liable to a fine not exceeding R20 000 or to imprisonment for a period not exceeding five years or to both such fine and such imprisonment.

51. Any person who abducts or removes any child or pupil, or directly or indirectly counsels, induces or aids any child or pupil to abscond from any institution, place of safety or custody in which the child or pupil was lawfully placed, or knowingly harbours or conceals a child or pupil who has been so abducted or removed or has so absconded, or prevents him from returning to the institution, place of safety or custody from which he was abducted or removed or has absconded, shall be guilty of an offence.

52. Any person who without the approval of the Minister removes a foster child or pupil from the Republic shall be guilty of an offence.'

Prohibition of employment of certain children

'**52A.** (1) Subject to the provision of this Act or any other law, no person may employ or provide work to any child under the age of 15 years.

(2) The Minister may, on the conditions determined by him —

(*a*) by notice in the *Gazette* exclude any employment or work from the provisions of subsection (1); and

(*b*) grant any particular person, or persons generally, exemption from the provisions of subsection (1).

(3) An exemption under subsection (2) *(b)* shall—

(*a*) in the case of the exemption of a particular person be granted by issuing to such person a certificate of exemption in which his name and the conditions of the exemption and the name of the child or a description of the category of children with respect to whom exemption is granted are specified;

(*b*) in the case of the exemption of persons generally, be granted by the publication in the *Gazette* of a notice in which such persons are described and the conditions of the exemption and a description of the category of children with respect to whom exemption is granted are specified.

(4) A certificate of exemption contemplated in subsection (3)*(a)* and a notice contemplated in subsection (3)*(b)* may at any time be amended or withdrawn by the Minister.

(5) Any person who contravenes any provision of this section shall be guilty of an offence.

53. (1) (*a*) a parent or a guardian of any pupil or of any child who has under this Act or under section 290 of the Criminal Procedure Act been placed in any custody other than the custody of the parent or guardian, shall be divested of his right of control over and of his right to the custody of that pupil or child, and those rights, including the right to punish and to exercise discipline, shall be vested —

    (i) in the management of the institution to which the pupil was sent; or

    (ii) in the person in whose custody the child was placed.

(2) If a minor living with his parent or guardian has been placed under the supervision of a social worker, the parent or guardian shall exercise his right of control over the minor in accordance with any directions which he may have received from the said social worker.

(3) The rights transferred shall not include the power to deal with any property of a pupil or child or the power to consent to the marriage of a pupil or child or to the performance upon or the provision to a pupil or child of an operation or medical treatment which is attended with serious danger to life.'

Place of care grants

(From R 2612 of the Child Care Act.)

'**38** (1) The Minister may, with the concurrence of the Minister of Finance, give approval for a grant to be paid to an organisation for the care of children older than one month but younger than 7 years of *bona fide* working mothers who must of necessity work away from home, or *bona fide* work-seeking mothers.'

CHILD ABUSE — PHYSICAL, SEXUAL, EMOTIONAL

Child abuse includes the physical and emotional battering of a child by his parents or guardians. The term commonly refers to physical cruelty, however, because emotional battering is difficult to prove. Recently the sexual abuse of children from infancy to adolescence has been exposed as a frequent cause of child abuse, probably because the public media have made people aware that such things can happen, frequently within the family.

    The attention of the Community Health Nurse is drawn to section 42 of the Child Care Act (see p. 420) which stipulates that the health team, including nurses, is legally liable to report cases of child abuse (physical violence and neglect, emotional abuse and sexual abuse) to the police (Child Protection Unit) or to the relevant regional directors of Departments of Health. The shift in emphasis of the law has been from the welfare of the child to the competence of the parents or guardians to care for the child.

Physical abuse: the battered child syndrome

The fact that parents may violently assault young children was medically recognised only 35 years ago, when descriptions started appearing in the medical literature of young children being seen at casualty departments with multiple fractures and bruises, some healed and some fresh. Many of these children had head injuries leading to permanent brain damage and others had injuries to internal organs, such as ruptured livers. Professor Kempe of the University of Colorado School of Medicine named this phenomenon the **'Battered Child Syndrome'** and in 1967 Simpson[2] defined it as follows:

(1) infants, usually 2–3 years of age, are subjected to:

(2) persistent or repeated violence at the hands of . . .

(3) either or both parents or guardians who . . .

(4) either fail to report — or delay reporting — the injuries they are aware of, and who . . .

(5) affect ignorance or lie; offering a simple explanation for the injuries, and who are usually . . .

(6) inadequate, subnormal or simple, but seldom under medical care.

Child battering occurs in all races, ethnic groups and socio-economic strata of society. In practice, it is sometimes difficult to distinguish between so-called legitimate punishment (e.g. a severe thrashing and hanging up a child in a sack) and child battering. Both kinds of treatment terrify and damage a child emotionally and lead to emotional ill-health in later years, often manifested as antisocial, delinquent behaviour.

Certain high-risk children are more likely to be victims of child abuse than other children, viz. premature infants, especially those nursed in incubators with whom the mother has been unable to bond, unplanned and illegitimate babies, stepchildren, physically and mentally handicapped children, sickly infants who cry a great deal, difficult children who do not sleep well and suffer from colic, and wrong-sex children. The usual age of abuse is under 3 years, although many children of school-going age are victims. Child abuse is usually triggered by a crisis: a move to which the family cannot adapt, a husband or wife losing a job, a crying child, an unwanted pregnancy, criticism from a spouse. The abusing parent's control snaps and the child is viciously attacked.

If the parent feels guilty he may feign amnesia for the event, deny that it occurred or that the injuries are serious and delay seeking medical attention. Parents, however, usually bring the child to hospital for 'investigation'. Sometimes the injuries are not reported and the child recovers without medical attention. In a chronically abused child, multiple healed fractures may be discovered on X-ray examination when the child is eventually brought to hospital. The parent usually tells a discrepant story to account for the child's injuries and his behaviour is not that of a loving parent concerned about the injury to his child. Some children will not look to their parents for reassurance and comfort, while others do; the child may assume a facies of 'frozen watchfulness', alert for future attack yet inhibited by his fear of offending adults and eliciting a fresh attack. The type of history, the nature of the injuries and the behaviour of the child and his parents arouse the suspicion of the doctor who notifies the Child Abuse Unit or an approved agency who will proceed to investigate the matter.

The child may be admitted to hospital for full investigation, including skeletal survey and haematological investigations. This is done to find out if there are any other fresh or old lesions and to rule out any blood or bone disorders, e.g. bleeding diathesis and brittle bones.

The abusing home

Blair and Rita Justice[4] postulate that chronic child abuse is not just the product of pathological relationships between parent and child but is a family problem, the result of interactions and collusions between the spouses and the impact of certain children on the parents. Environmental stresses, alcoholism, unemployment, financial problems, frequent moves and cultural values which uphold the right of parents to own their children and to use physical punishment, also play a part in the battering of children. As all the interactions take place in the family, the Justices speak of the 'abusing family', and of child abuse as a 'family affair'. It does not matter which spouse does the battering, both are implicated as both are immature and share the same basic personality.

Battering parents are dependent people who seek a symbiotic relationship with others from whom they want love, approval and nurturance. They are feeling, i.e. non-thinking people, adult in body only, with poor self-image, mistrustful of others, and with very low stress tolerance and self-control. They are usually isolated persons who have no one to turn to for advice and help. Because of their quest for love, they often marry very young, sometimes being forced to because of pre-marital conception. The spouses may compete with one another for mutual nurturance, each one trying to be spoiled by the other and feeling very angry with the spouse if his/her attempts to obtain nurturance fail.

Abusing parents seek from their child satisfaction of their own need for nurturance which the young child is unable to give. Older children often respond by caring for the parent. Battering parents do not see their young child as a helpless little human being dependent on them for its nurturance, because they are so busy either seeking love and approval from others or attacking others for not meeting their needs. They do not know how to accept responsibility for the life they created and the child may become a source of either irritation through its apparent rejection of parental worth (with its constant crying and whining) or disappointment when it cannot fulfil the parent's needs and expectations, or it may become a rival for the other spouse's love and attention. Due to low frustration tolerance, the parent's frustration easily spills over into physical aggression against the child.

The kind of psychopathology cited above is fairly common in Western societies, the difference between abusing and non-abusing immature parents being the strength of inner controls, stress tolerance and the severity of the stress which precipitates the physical attack on the child.

Abusing parents have usually suffered abuse and certainly emotional deprivation in their own childhoods. Because of their loveless childhood — many grew up in children's homes — they have difficulty in relating to people in an emotionally satisfying, adult way.

Primary prevention of child abuse

Midwives can play a very important role in the primary prevention of parental abuse of unwanted children because, more than any other members of the helping professions, they have the opportunity to be in intimate contact with mothers and to recognise problems in the mothering situation.

Recognition of potential abusers and rejecters of young children

During pregnancy the midwife can elicit the following warning signs of maternal rejection and possible child abuse during her antenatal care of the mother:

(1) an attitude of helplessness: the woman expresses her doubt that she will be able to cope; she expresses her dismay at finding herself pregnant and would like an abortion;

(2) the woman complains of feeling isolated, of having no supporting friends or relatives;

(3) the woman does not feel supported by the child's father and might even be abandoned by him;

(4) the woman expresses hatred for the child's father;

(5) the woman appears to be hypersensitive to criticism and rejects proffered advice.

After the infant's birth, the midwife has the ideal opportunity to observe the attitude of the mother to her child and to assess her potential for bonding with the child:

(1) The rejecting mother is not interested in naming, feeding and holding her baby; she holds the baby clumsily, away from her body. She does not allow the child's body to mould to hers when she feeds it. Breast-feeding is repulsive to her.

(2) She sees her child as ugly, does not support its head, handles it roughly and does not coo or talk to it.

(3) She feels that her husband does not support her and that the baby does not love her.

(4) She cannot comfort her baby and is nauseated by its smells and messes.

(5) She suffers from post-partum depression and feels her husband prefers her baby to her.

(6) She becomes enraged at the infant and is not averse to slapping it, often rationalising this as an attempt to start its training at an early age.

(7) She visits her premature infant (kept at the hospital in an incubator) less and less frequently after her discharge and is averse to handling it when given the opportunity to do so.

Note: The modern trend is to encourage bonding by allowing the mother to care for her premature infant in hospital and by intermittently removing the infant from the incubator for purposes of feeding and tactile stimulation.

Signs of prenatal and postnatal maternal depression can be observed by the midwife who can institute primary preventive measures by summoning psychological help for the mother, either in the maternity hospital or after she has returned home. In this way, harm to the baby (infanticide, early mother/child alienation and failure to bond) may be prevented.

Family planning and spaced parenthood are very important measures to prevent child abuse.

The rejecting mother who does not show signs of increasingly enjoying and accepting her infant and who is not returning to a supportive husband and family, needs follow-up care by the community health nurse in order to prevent child abuse. Ideally, the maternity hospital or clinic should notify the regional community health nurse when a potentially abusing mother has been discharged, in order to ensure prompt and extra attention to this mother in need of care and support.

Secondary prevention of child abuse

Once a case of child abuse comes to the notice of the authorities, attempts are made to prevent further abuse.

In all big centres in South Africa, Child Abuse Units have been established in conjunction with a children's hospital. The unit consists of an interdisciplinary team of members of the helping professions. The unit co-ordinates all the work done with the courts, the police and approved agencies, to protect the child and rehabilitate the family, if this is at all possible.

When medical opinion confirms the suspicion of battering, the child is sometimes removed from his family on a retention order and placed either with foster parents, or in a children's home or place of safety, or is kept in the hospital for a full investigation and to recover from his injuries. The abusing parent is encouraged (sometimes compelled by the court) to visit the child and care for him under the supervision of the temporary caretaker if there is a court order. There will be a court enquiry at some time.

The courts are very lenient to child abusers who show willingness to work at rehabilitation. Abusing parents are often hostile to members of the helping professions because of fear of what will happen to them, should they confess to their crime; they expect to be punished. Punishment does not seem to play a part in deterring child batterers, but the courts do sentence to terms of imprisonment sadistic, psychopathic batterers who treat children with the utmost callousness and cruelty, e.g. burning their genitals with cigarettes or making them sit on a hot electric plate to dry their pants.

Some child abusers can be rehabilitated completely, some can improve with therapy, but 40 % are untreatable. In the latter case, the child is never returned to his parents, being placed permanently with alternative caretakers and becoming a state responsibility.

Rehabilitation therapy ideally consists of the following treatment: the abusing parent may be taken into long-term individual therapy in an effort to compensate for his/her chronic emotional deprivation through an intensive mothering, therapeutic relationship.

This is done only in cases where the abusing parent is motivated to grow emotionally and prospects for growth are good, as it makes great demands on the time of therapists. Any intelligent parent who is afraid of abusing or who has just started abusing and comes to ask for help, is a good prospect for intensive therapy. Sometimes couples are treated in a group with other abusing couples. In the group, members learn to express their anger effectively and in an acceptable way. They are taught to relax and control their impatience and violent outbursts of temper. They learn to communicate with people and in this way they lose their feelings of isolation. Spouses are taught to listen to and talk to one another, to share with and to gratify another's needs in an adult way.

The common way of rehabilitating an abusing mother is for a social worker or community nurse or even a volunteer lay homemaker to visit her at home in order to establish a good relationship, win her confidence and teach her simple housekeeping skills. The mother is taught how to budget, how to run a home and how to care for the baby. The helper provides support, aid and human contact for an isolated person. The helper also teaches parents about child development and the needs of children so that they do not make unrealistic demands on their children. The nurse helper can become a friend to the family and be a link between the family and the agency that serves it. She can follow up the family over long periods, making sure that abuse is not recurring.

Note:
(1) A therapist who cannot shake off her sense of outrage at the heinous crimes committed by abusing parents should not work in this field as she cannot be an effective helper.
(2) Therapists who work with abusing parents should not work with or see the abused child, as they may thus become unable to contain their repugnance and hostility towards the parents.

Conclusions

In order to deliver an effective secondary preventive service, a co-ordinated interdisciplinary team approach is mandatory. The team consists of: social workers (from hospital and approved agency), community health nurse, psychiatrist, psychologist, paediatrician, ward doctor, paediatric nurse and family doctor (if available).

The team functions as follows:

(1) Child abuse is recognised either in a hospital casualty department or by a teacher, school nurse, or neighbour and is reported either to an approved agency, to the police Child Protection Unit or to a Child Abuse Unit. People reporting child abuse need not disclose their names.
(2) The child is examined and treated medically and if necessary admitted to a hospital ward.
(3) A social worker from the agency or Child Abuse Unit sometimes approaches the Commissioner of Child Welfare and obtains a retention order which gives permission to remove the child from the custody of his parents temporarily to a place of safety, i.e. a hospital, foster home, children's home or

baby sanctuary. This is done if the child is deemed to be in danger.
(4) The parents are approached by a team member in an accepting, sympathetic way and an attempt is made to obtain a history of family relationships (present and past), and of the events that led up to the injury to the child. A social worker, community psychiatric nurse, or community health nurse visits the home to assess the family's social and economic circumstances.
(5) The interdisciplinary team meets after a few days to discuss their findings, diagnosis and future plans of action.
  (*a*) The diagnosis of abuse is verified.
  (*b*) The major psychological and social problems of the family are discussed.
  (*c*) A decision is taken as to who will deal with each problem:
    (i) treatment of parents;
    (ii) placement of the child;
    (iii) treatment of the child;
    (iv) housing and employment.
  (*d*) A co-ordinator of action is appointed.
  (*e*) Minutes are taken to be included in the report of the children's court.
(6) The plan is put into action and the team meets regularly to report on the family's progress.
(7) When the team agrees that the reconstruction services with the parents have been successful and the home is safe for the child, the court is petitioned to return legal custody of the child to his parents.
(8) The parents remain in therapy or in counselling for at least one month after return of the child until all problems of readjustment have been overcome.
(9) A person appointed by the team to do so checks periodically to find out if the family is functioning satisfactorily.

Sexual abuse of children

Kempe defines sexual abuse of children as 'the involvement of dependent children and adolescents in sexual activities that they do not fully comprehend and in which they are unable to defend themselves' (quoted by L Cohen).[3]

Although sexual abuse is generally associated with little girls, boys can also be the victims of sodomists (homosexuals who commit anal intercourse).

Rape is a criminal offence and occurs at all ages, its annual incidence in children and adults in the RSA being approximately 150 000.[3] Rape is the unlawful intentional carnal connection with a female without her consent.[3] The latter implies that it is accompanied by violence and genital trauma and occurs outside the family. Although shame may beset the victim, rape is usually reported soon after the incident. It was recently recognised that a husband is capable of raping his wife.

Incest, on the other hand, occurs within the family, is seldom violent and genital trauma is usually absent. It may be psychologically forceful in that the victim is bound to secrecy through threats to self and others in the family, especially where the father is the perpetrator.

Incest is a symptom of disturbed family relationships. Fathers involved with daughters have unsatisfying sexual relationships with women. This may be a mutual feeling between a husband and a wife.

An incest pattern may gradually establish itself in early childhood, the victim only presenting at adolescence after years of ongoing sexual abuse. The mother is often aware of what is going on and colludes to maintain the precarious balance of sick family relationships. She is, therefore, unable or unwilling to protect her daughter. Incest is an expression of a pathological family constellation in which the incest victim is trapped. Incestuous fathers have low self-esteem and may be alcoholic. Incest can also take place between siblings and between a mother and her son. Incest victims carry a load of guilt and distress which they cannot share, being afraid of being blamed, punished or disbelieved.

Children should be taught the basic skills of self-protection by their families and at school. They must learn to say 'NO' to strangers who offer them lifts or gifts. Sex education should be given at school, preferably by school nurses or specially trained sex educators, as so many parents avoid the subject. Victims of incest could thus be helped if they make use of the opportunity to talk about their problem to a sympathetic sex educator.

Types of sexual abuse of children (excluding rape):

(1) Sexual exploitation of children
   (a) Sex syndicates use children for the production of erotic material for pornographic magazines and films.
   (b) Children, both males and females, may be bribed or abducted to join prostitution rings which supply children for their paedophilic clients. The great danger here is the transmission of AIDS and other STDs.
(2) Sexual interference (erotic touching) such as fondling, digital penetration of vagina or anus, oro-genital stimulation, all without actual intercourse (coitus). This is usually an incestuous practice.
(3) Adult type heterosexual or homosexual relationship with full intercourse, either vaginal or anal. When a heterosexual relationship continues into adolescence, there is the possibility of pregnancy.

Apart from the emotional trauma caused by incest, physical harm may present as:

(1) STDs and AIDS in a young child.
(2) Pregnancy in an adolescent.
(3) Genital inflammation and/or lacerations; bruising around the genital area.

The younger child is often seductive towards males, may have a precocious sexual vocabulary, or may present with fearfulness, enuresis and urinary tract infection. The older child may present with truanting (from home and school), underachieving, promiscuity, delinquency or suicidal ideation.[3] The long-term sequelae for the victim are often sexual and social maladjustment, prostitution, drug-abuse, low self-esteem and chronic depression. Sexually abused children make poor parents. Sexual abuse is a criminal offence and the courts impose sentences on the guilty parties, especially if there has been violence. The Child Protection Units of the SAPS play an important role in investigating all cases of abuse reported to them. Direct 'Child Lines' in the major centres are also facilitating the reporting of sexual abuse and all types of abuse by children themselves.

In cases of incest, the most effective psychosocial intervention is family therapy, initially while the family is in crisis. If the guilty father has not been violent, the family can be held together in ongoing family therapy to improve family relationships. If there has been violence, the Child Commissioner will remove the child temporarily or permanently from his/her family, for placement in foster care or a children's home.

Emotional abuse of children

Extreme emotional abuse accompanies physical neglect (deprivation), and physical and sexual abuse, but the emotional abuse of children can also occur in the absence thereof. Emotional abuse on its own is difficult to assess by people outside the family and is, therefore, not a reportable condition to the same extent as those conditions which bear the physical stigmata of abuse. Emotional abuse gives rise, however, to much childhood unhappiness and in some cases may be the cause of learning disabilities and poor school achievement. The emotional abuse of children also gives rise to distortions of personality development. The emotional abuse may not be deliberate and may be perpetrated by inadequate parents who know no better because they were also emotionally deprived ('love starved or love smothered') by inadequate parents. Poor nurturing is usually referred to as poor mothering, but both parents may be inadequate in their parenting role, therefore the term 'poor parenting' is more appropriate.

Some examples will be given of poor parenting which, in their extreme form, could be regarded as constituting emotional abuse.

Non-satisfaction of the early biological needs

(The so-called 'dependency needs'.)

The infant fails to bond with its primary person. These needs are for cuddling (stroking and rocking), food, warmth, a variety of sounds, sights, smells and tastes (with which the immature sensory apparatus can cope without the infant becoming bewildered and anxious), for sleep and for the absence of pain and discomfort. Abuse implies that the infant is deprived of these need-satisfactions because of maternal rejection or neglect due to many reasons, alcohol abuse playing an important role here.

The practice of allowing an infant to cry itself to sleep may have serious repercussions if frustration and anxiety become chronic as the infant may withdraw and find difficulty in forming a secure, trusting, focused relationship with its parents.

Punitiveness

Parents who 'teach' their children by insulting, rejecting or punishing them for mistakes, merely impede their progress and make their children aggressive, negativistic, rebellious and antisocial. Punitive parents become authority figures to be feared and hated as 'enemies'. Toddlers punished for destructive behaviour, for instance, are more likely to view the punishing parent as a 'persecutor' to be feared, than to make the connection between their bad deeds and the punishment. If punished frequently, the young child may become either timid, nervous, inhibited and afraid of people, or angry and wildly aggressive and destructive. If parents are punitive yet loving, the child is likely to internalise a very severe superego which sets rigid standards of conforming behaviour for the self and for others. These children become rigid, obsessional, intolerant adults who drive themselves and others mercilessly.

Punishment instils feelings of badness and inferiority; punished children feel resentful and scheme revenge. Death wishes towards the punishing parent may remain confined to the fantasy level, yet produce feelings of guilt and depressive anxieties. Punitive parents make children feel that they are unworthy and unlovable; these feelings in turn engender inability to love (except in a possessive or dependent way). Feelings of worthlessness and unlovableness may later cause an overwhelming ambition to achieve power, wealth and status in order to make good the deficit in worth. The feeling of unlovableness is a socially inherited trait which often manifests itself as a psychosomatic disease in people who are in a chronic state of anxiety because they cannot satisfy their need for power, wealth, status and social acceptability. Because of their early love deprivation, their greed for security and social acceptance is insatiable. Intense anxiety is, however, not caused only by punishment but also by frustration of needs — in fact by anything which makes young children scream and throw temper tantrums.

Masked parental rejection

A woman who has not had adequate mothering herself cannot (under ordinary circumstances) become a loving wife and mother. She will be inclined to reject her child in the same way that she was rejected. Rejection may be obvious or it may masquerade as maternal (or paternal) love. The following are two examples of masked parental rejection.

(a) The over-protective parent smothers his/her child with 'love' and keeps him dependent upon him/her. These parents have not really separated emotionally from their parents, so are unable to allow their children to separate from them to become autonomous human beings. By keeping their children dependent upon them they are hampering their emotional development.

(b) Appeasing and guilt-ridden parents heap material gifts and cultural privileges on their children — to hide the fact that they cannot give of themselves in the form of real caring, self-sacrificing behaviour towards their children, for example, by speaking to them in the language of acceptance, by sharing their interests and by giving them of their time.

Although adults may be fooled by these displays of 'good parenting', children are sensitive to the underlying rejection and become anxious and insecure.

Conditional love

('I will love you if you are good, or do well at school, or win the race.') This is a form of parental rejection which can do much harm to the developing self-concept of the child. The struggle to appear good and acceptable in the eyes of the parents may cause depression and a lifelong feeling of being a failure. Perfectionistic parents who demand high standards of behaviour and achievement from their children may cause them to become discouraged, anxious and nervous. The high standards demanded by these parents serve to boost their own feelings of pride and worth. Some anxious children become either appeasing (in order to placate their parents by ingratiating behaviour), or exhibitionistic or precocious in an attempt to win the approval or attract the attention of their parents.

Discordant family relationships

Children who grow up in a discordant home will suffer from some manifestations of emotional ill-health, for example, poor relationships with parents, siblings and peer group, learning problems and physical ill-health. Psychosomatic symptoms in a child are a sure sign to the outside world that there is something wrong with family relationships.

It would seem that the most important factors which have an adverse effect on a child's psychological development have to do with the unhappy home life caused by marital discord. The tension caused by disturbed family relationships causes much anger, hostility and guilt.

The double bind home

In some families, children get confusing 'messages' which are contradictory, during interaction with parents. Example: the mother insists that the child voice his honest opinion on a certain matter; when he does so (and she does not like it) she scolds him for being ungrateful, etc. This kind of interaction, called a 'double bind', places a child who is aware of his dependency on the parent in a dilemma: he can neither ignore the mother's request (for fear of rejection), nor can he avoid being rejected by her because of his communication. He is thus rejected no matter whether he accedes to her request or not. If this is the parent's customary way of communicating, the child eventually avoids communicating in any meaningful way.

Double bind communication is especially common in families of schizophrenics, the mother who involves her children in a double bind being known as the schizophrenogenic mother. The child feels entrapped in the double bind and may withdraw from reality into madness. Although the double bind cannot be implicated as the cause of schizophrenia, it will certainly cause poor communication and mental ill-health in families who customarily communicate in this confused manner.

SOCIAL ASSISTANCE ACT 59 OF 1992

This Act provides for social assistance by the state to aged and disadvantaged persons and to national councils and welfare organisations which render organised activities and social welfare programmes for such persons.

'Payment of grants

2. The Minister may . . . with concurrence of the Minister of State Expenditure, out of moneys appropriated by Parliament for that purpose, make —

(*a*) social grants to aged and disabled persons and to war veterans;

(*b*) in addition to a social grant, a grant-in-aid to or on behalf of any person referred to in paragraph (*a*) or a war veteran who is in such a physical or mental condition that he requires regular attendance by any person;

(*c*) in addition to social grants and grants-in-aid, supplementary grants to war veterans;

(*d*) a maintenance grant to a parent for the maintenance of a child in his custody;

(*e*) a foster child grant to a foster parent;

(*f*) to prescribed institutions, including places of safety, capitation grants for the care of persons admitted to such an institution or place of safety in terms of an order of court or with the approval of the Director-General.

Social grants

3. Subject to the provisions of this Act, any person shall be entitled to the appropriate social grant if he satisfies the Director-General that he —

(*a*) is an aged or disabled person or a war veteran;

(*b*) is resident in the Republic at the time of the application in question;

(*c*) is a South African citizen; and

(*d*) complies with the prescribed conditions.

Maintenance grants

4. Subject to the provisions of this Act, any person shall be entitled to a maintenance grant if he satisfies the Director-General that he —

(*a*) is the parent of the child whom he supports;

(*b*) as well as the child concerned is a South African citizen; and

(*c*) as well as the child complies with the prescribed conditions.

Financial rewards to national councils, welfare organisations and persons

5. (1) The Minister may, subject to the provisions of this Act and with the concurrence of the Minister of State Expenditure, out of moneys appropriated by Parliament for that purpose, make financial awards to —

(*a*) national councils or welfare organisations which undertake or take or co-ordinate organised activities, measures or social welfare programmes regarding —

(i) family care;

(ii) care of the aged;

(iii) social security;

(iv) care of the disabled;

(v) alcohol and drug dependency; and

(vi) care of the offender;

(*b*) any organisation contemplated in section 1 of the Fund-raising Act, 1978 (Act 107 of 1978), which in terms of its constitution has the care of mentally or psychiatrically disabled persons as one of its objects.

(2) The Director-General may, subject to the provision of this Act, make a financial award to a person if he is satisfied that such a person is in need of social relief of distress.'

REFERENCES

(1) Danilewitz D, Schreier A. Health care needs in children's homes. *S Afr Med J* 1987; **71**: 346.

(2) Simpson K. *Roy Soc Hlth J* 1967; **87**: 168.

(3) Cohen L. Sexual abuse of children — a review. *S Afr Med J* 1985; **67**: 730–732.

(4) Justice B, Justice R. *The Abusing Family*. New York: Human Sciences Press, 1976.

Schedule to Social Assistance Act of 1992
Acts repealed

Number and year of Act	Short title	Extent of repeal
81 of 1967	Aged Persons Act, 1967	Section 2(b) and (c)
25 of 1968	War Veterans' Pensions Act, 1968	The whole
26 of 1968	Blind Persons Act, 1968	Section 2(a) and (b)
27 of 1968	Disability Grants Act, 1968	In so far as unrepealed
41 of 1971	Abuse of Dependence-producing Substances and Rehabilitation Centres Act, 1971	Section 28
18 of 1973	Mental Health Act, 1973	Section 71
37 of 1973	Social Pensions Act, 1973	The whole
100 of 1978	National Welfare Act, 1978	Section 20
74 of 1983	Child Care Act, 1983	Section 56(1)
96 of 1983	Pension Laws Amendment Act, 1983	Sections 12, 13, 14, 15 and 16
104 of 1987	Community Welfare Act (House of Representatives), 1987	Section 20, except in so far as it relates to hospitals
37 of 1989	Social Aid Act (House of Assembly), 1989	The whole

TEST OF KNOWLEDGE

The student has benefited from studying this chapter if he/she can answer the following questions:

(1) (a) Discuss foster care as a solution to the problem of placement of children in need of care.

    (b) What qualities of a foster home are necessary for the successful long-term fostering of children found to be in need of care?

(2) Discuss the legal requirements for the maintenance of good order and discipline in a children's home. Why should these regulations to the Child Care Act have been necessary?

(3) (a) Discuss the role of the community nurse in the primary and secondary prevention of child abuse.

    (b) What are the legal obligations of a nurse who encounters cases of suspected child neglect or abuse in the course of her duties?

(4) Define the following terms:
- Child and pupil (in terms of the Child Care Act)
- Children's court and Commissioner's court
- School of industries and reform school
- Conditional love and smothering love of parents for children
- The double bind communication in families

(5) Describe the advantages of the adoption practices of placement agencies over private adoption procedures.

(6) What symptoms in a child would make a school nurse suspect that a child may be a victim of an incestuous relationship? What are the sequelae of incest for the victim?

(7) State the difference between:
- A children's court and a juvenile court
- A temporary retention order and a permanent committal order by a commissioner of child welfare
- A place of safety and a place of care in terms of the Child Care Act.

(8) What are the legal determinants for declaring a child in need of care?

(9) Name the circumstances in which parental consent to adoption may be dispensed with.

24

Malnutrition in Children
Nutritional Rehabilitation
Acute Infantile Diarrhoea (AID)
Oral Rehydration Therapy

OBJECTIVES

Malnutrition in children is a very important topic of study for the community nurse who must be able to recognise the early signs and symptoms of protein-energy malnutrition (PEM) and make his/her contribution to the development of the community in which he/she lives and works in order to combat this social evil in our midst.

The student is introduced to the RHOSA nutritional survey which has found that 25 % of South African black rural children under the age of 5 suffer from chronic malnutrition. The student must understand the association between stunting (physical and intellectual)

and PEM and that the root causes of PEM are social and economic. Drastic changes to the social structure of a society are needed to wipe out the poverty underlying PEM. Poverty robs children of the opportunity to develop to their full potential. Chronic community deprivation is a pernicious condition which must be tackled from many sides.

The attention of the student is also drawn to the association between malnutrition and low socio-economic status, and the high prevalence of acute diarrhoeal disease which is the biggest killer of children (excluding white and Indian) under five in the RSA.

IN THIS CHAPTER

RHOSA NUTRITIONAL SURVEY[1]

At the end of the 1986, the South African component of RHOSA completed its first anthropometric survey of the present nutritional status
of black rural children under the age of 5 in 5 of
the 7 health regions of the RSA.

RHOSA is the acronym for the Regional
Health Organisation for Southern Africa. It was
inaugurated in 1979 and is an independent or-

ganisation consisting of 11 member states, all of
which administer their own health services.
Their special interests are: health manpower,
health promotion and epidemiology.

This anthropometric nutrition survey is
based on the WHO 'indicators for monitoring
progress towards Health for All by the Year
2000' (WHO Geneva, 1981).

According to the WHO, anthropometric
measurements to assess growth and development in young children are the most widely used
indicators of nutritional status in a community.

The anthropometric measures of nutritional
status used are:

- Height for age percentage H/A %: This
  percentage reflects the cumulative effects of
  undernutrition and infection since birth and
  even before birth. Low H/A % (stunting),
  therefore, indicates poor environmental
  conditions and/or early malnutrition.
- Weight for height percentage W/H %:
  This percentage reflects current effects of
  undernutrition and infection. Low W/H %
  indicates current undernutrition or disease.
- Weight for age percentage W/A %: This
  percentage reflects both the cumulative effects of episodes of undernutrition or
  chronic undernutrition since birth and current undernutrition. Low percentage W/A
  therefore indicates chronic and current undernutrition.

In order to obtain percentage scores of H/A,
W/H and W/A, the respective measurements are
compared with a normal range, either locally
defined or based on international standards.

The WHO has recommended the use of the
United States National Centre for Health Statistics (NCHS) data. Low weight and low height
are defined as less than the value corresponding
to two standard deviations below the median of
the respective frequency distributions for
healthy children. This is generally described as
the third percentile on the Road-to-Health
charts. In order to obtain the percentage of low
scorers of H/A, W/H and W/A in a community
(the target population), a sample of the target
population is tested and a percentage of low
scorers (as defined above) obtained by using the
following formula:

$$\frac{\text{Number of low scorers (on a single measure)}}{\text{Number of subjects in a sample}} \times 100$$

Results of the first RHOSA nutrition study

Anthropometric assessment of nutritional status in black under-fives in rural RSA was as follows:

- Weight for age: 8,4 % were estimated to be underweight.
- Height for age: stunting occurred in 24,5 %, with lower prevalence in Natal and northern Transvaal.
- Weight for height: low W/H % (current undernutrition or disease) occurred in 1,8 % of the population.

The authors of the first anthropometric survey come to the following conclusions: 'Compared to the healthy reference population in which the prevalence of each of the three indicators was 2,3 per cent, the rural black under-five population did not have an acute protein-energy-malnutrition problem as reflected by the weight for height status. However, the relatively high percentages of underweight and stunted children indicate that a chronic malnutrition problem exists.'[1]

Protein-energy-malnutrition (PEM) in children

Food shortages and maldistribution of available food are some of the gravest world problems, leading to undernutrition and PEM (protein-energy-malnutrition), especially amongst the world's children. PEM is defined thus by the WHO: 'a range of pathological conditions arising from coincident lack, in varying proportions of proteins and calories (kilojoules) occurring most frequently in infants and young children and commonly associated with infections'.[2]

Bengoa[3] has estimated the following numbers of children aged from 0 to 4 years, in three regions of the world, suffering from PEM:

Latin-American 9 700 000
Africa 18 700 000
Asia (excluding Japan and China) 70 000 000
TOTAL 98 400 000

PEM comprises, in ascending order of gravity, growth retardation, kwashiorkor, marasmic kwashiorkor and marasmus. The word kwashi

orkor means 'deposed child', i.e. the child who has had to give up the breast for a new sibling. The disease has been known to blacks for a long time; they established a connection between kwashiorkor and weaning. In addition to protein deficiency, the diet may also lack vitamins, especially the A and B vitamins and the stigmata of these deficiencies may be superimposed on PEM. Rickets due to vitamin D deficiency does not occur concomitantly with severe PEM, however, because it occurs only in growing children and growth stops in severe PEM.

PEM has taken the place of earlier epidemic infectious diseases as the most widespread disease and the greatest public health problem in the world. PEM is a disease of poor, underfed, ignorant and overpopulated peoples. There is a positive correlation between malnutrition, low income, large families, lack of education, high sickness and mortality rates and retarded growth. PEM affects all underprivileged and developing communities whose diet consists mainly of carbohydrates and whose staple diet is a cereal or root, e.g. yam and cassava in the tropics, rice in the East and maize in southern Africa. Growth is adversely affected in all South African malnourished children, black, white, Indian and coloured, whatever the nature of their staple diet.

Causes of PEM

(1) The root causes of PEM are social and economic; PEM is a disease of poor and developing communities and it disappears as people become more affluent and educated.

Undernutrition is basically not a medical problem; furthermore, as the standard of living in countries improves, so the incidence of infectious diseases declines. Poverty may be due to unemployment, alcoholism, low wages, large families, illegitimacy and homes with one parent only, e.g. fatherless homes in rural areas due to migrant labour and psychosocial disorganisation of the family. There is a direct relationship between the growth rate of children and their parents' income and social and marital adaptation.

(2) Ignorance of parents with regard to the nutritional needs of their children, especially the importance of breast-feeding. Black in-

fants are often weaned on to a high cereal diet, the maize meal being prepared with water. The feed thus lacks protein.

(3) Working mothers not making adequate provision for their children while they are at work; insufficient crèches for working mothers in the community.

(4) Chronic debilitating diseases such as tuberculosis, worm infestation and schistosomiasis. Gastro-enteritis is considered an important cause of PEM.

Conditions associated with PEM

Increased susceptibility to infection

It has been observed that undernourished children are more prone to infection, especially gastro-enteritis, pneumonia and tuberculosis, than well-nourished children. Malnutrition affects the body's immune system. It has been found in PEM that while the body's humoral immune defences are relatively intact, cell-mediated immunity is adversely affected. Moreover, the inflammatory response is also suppressed. Malnutrition, therefore, has an immunosuppressive effect.

It is a fact that malnourished children get infectious diseases, e.g. measles, in a more severe form than well-nourished children, measles being a 'killer' disease in undernourished, developing communities. Other severe infections which are prone to occur in grossly underfed children are Gram-negative septicaemia, disseminated herpes simplex infections and tuberculosis, the host defences against these infections being cell-mediated.

The relationship between malnutrition and infection (except in cases of extreme nutritional inadequacy) is by no means clear, however, as studies reveal equivocal results. It is commonly believed that nutrition affects resistance to infection, but the objective evidence from scientific studies is lacking. On the other hand, some infections have a direct effect on food intake: measles and herpes cause painful stomatitis; in pertussis food is vomited, febrile infections burn up energy and suppress the appetite, infective diarrhoea is accompanied by vomiting and interferes with food absorption.[4] Malnourished infants may have intestinal mucosal villous atrophy with resultant nutrient malabsorption leading to diarrhoea.[12]

The association between childhood infections and malnutrition may pose an aetiological problem.

Intellectual stunting

Progress in social development in developing countries, including parts of South Africa, is related to standards of education. A prerequisite for social development is the production of healthy and stimulated children who will be enabled to reap full benefit from available educational programmes. If children have been exposed to undernutrition, lack of cultural stimulation and debilitating infections and infestations, they become 'too lazy' to study. The undernourished child is inactive and does not explore the world around him. A stimulating environment is also very important for intellectual development; in fact, the overriding factor in mental development is stimulation by exposure to a culturally rich environment. Thus social development is retarded through lack of privilege and low socio-economic status — a vicious cycle.

There is still much controversy about the extent of the impact of early undernutrition on later intellectual development. Although the child who survives severe malnutrition in infancy suffers long-term intellectual deficit, especially for abstract thinking, there is no proof that the intellectual impairment is directly due to malnutrition.

To repeat: underfed, underweight children are stunted in growth. There is no proof that they suffer brain damage with consequent retarded intelligence. They are, however, educationally disadvantaged due to concentration problems caused by hunger, insufficient energy to cope with the school activities, lack of intellectual stimulation and the prepotency of survival needs. Richter-Strydom et al.[10] found that children malnourished during their first year of life are intellectually disadvantaged during a 10-year follow-up period.

A prospective study of kwashiorkor in Cape Town[5]

A 15-year follow-up study of children who survived at least one episode of kwashiorkor was done by the Institute of Child Health, Red Cross War Memorial Hospital. The kwashiorkor patients were admitted to hospital between 1958 and 1960, aged between 5 months and 4 years, 4 months. One-third of the group died early of malnutrition; some moved away and the remainder (116) were compared with a group of siblings (89) nearest in age to each patient. The comparison group, therefore, shared the same environment as the patient group but had not contracted kwashiorkor. Mass and height of this study group of ex-patients and siblings were measured at 2, 7, 12 and 17 years. Finally, an assessment was made of the social circumstances, attainment in education and adjustment to society of the study groups.

Findings

Comparison of mean values of, for instance, percentage of expected mass for age revealed no difference between the ex-patients and their siblings. All remained close together, near the third percentile, i.e. siblings also suffered from PEM. The girls had a growth spurt after the age of 11–13 years to approach the fiftieth percentile. Mass increase was, however, greater than height increase so that many became obese. It appears that the growth processes of girls are more resistant to stress than those of boys.

The growth of ex-patients and their siblings was, therefore, identical. Their growth potential was equally poor. It would seem that if kwashiorkor develops in one child in a family, the other siblings are also at risk of poor long-term growth.

Economic, intellectual and social assessment at the end of the study revealed that except for housing (which deteriorated due to rapid population growth), socio-economic status, family stability and dietary adequacy had improved, probably due to rapid industrial development in this area.

Achievement in education was similar to that of the population from which the study groups came, i.e. inferior. The scholastic achievement of ex-patients and their siblings was the same. They left school early (some were still at school) and most were employed, but in semi-skilled or unskilled occupations. They were earning fairly adequate wages but capacity for achievement is limited, i.e. they cannot become skilled workers.

The delinquency rate was equal for both groups, the antisocial behaviour amongst boys being a serious problem, especially amongst the unemployed; poor use was made of leisure time, the study groups generally lacking special interests. This is probably typical of the socio-economic group from which the study groups came.

Psychometric assessment of a sample of ex-patients and their siblings showed no significant differences in intelligence scores.

This study was done on children who experienced an underprivileged childhood and, therefore, exhibited many of the stigmata of the pathological life-style of the culture of poverty (chronic community deprivation). The kwashiorkor *per se* did not, however, differentiate non-sufferers from sufferers in terms of scholastic attainment and social adjustment.

The picture that emerged from this study of physical, intellectual and social development of children reveals poor development which is typical of an entire social class in which individual potential is never fully realised, occupational skills are not acquired and earning capacity and social integration are poor. Kwashiorkor is merely the tip of the iceberg.

PRIMARY PREVENTION OF MALNUTRITION (UNDERNUTRITION) IN CHILDREN

Preventive measures need not necessarily be nutritional in nature; thus, raising the socio-economic status of an impoverished subgroup of the population is the most effective way of combating undernutrition (PEM).

In general, malnutrition can be prevented by applying the UNICEF principles contained in the acronym GOBI-FFF (see p. 393).

Besides these principles, the following preventive measures can be applied:

(1) Adequate food production. Long-term health education programmes have as their aim the education of underprivileged people to be independent in their food-producing activities, giving them the necessary financial and technological help while they are in the process of developing. The cultivation of home gardens is important.

(2) Environmental sanitation, deworming of heavily infested children, personal hygiene and promotion of hygienic preparation of food.

(3) Optimal diet for the pregnant woman and adequate antenatal and perinatal care to ensure the birth of a healthy infant.

(4) Promotion of breast-feeding. Amongst people with suboptimal nutrition, breast-feeding can be continued for up to 2 years in the interest of the child.

(5) The establishment of 'under-fives' clinics (see p. 401) and health promotive and preventive (well-baby) clinics and the maintenance of Road-to-Health cards which incorporate mass/age percentile charts to detect incipient malnutrition (see p. 394).

(6) Health education of the public, especially the parents of young children. Mothers can be educated in infant feeding, especially with regard to the giving of a nutritious, easily digestible 'weaning' diet.

Buchanan[6] suggests employing an army of mothers with well-nourished children as basic health educators in areas where undernutrition is rife, e.g. urban black townships. For a small monthly stipend, these part-time educators can be employed to visit and follow up a certain number of homes per week, to serve as models in child-rearing with whom the ordinary woman with low income can identify. The idea is for these ladies from the community to supplement the work of health educators of the Department of Health, in combating ignorance with regard to health matters in order that all those who need enlightenment can be reached. In this way the community can help itself and develop a real interest in health matters.

Nutritional management of underprivileged weanlings in order to prevent PEM

The problem of undernutrition is especially prevalent during the weaning period when the child is no longer receiving adequate nourishment from the breast and the adult-type solid diet is deficient in proteins, kilojoules, vitamins and mineral salts. The diet of some impoverished children consists entirely of mealie meal, sometimes fed only once a day. In order to get sufficient joules (4 000 kJ), a child requires 1,7

kg dry meal; when cooked to a soft porridge, this amount of mealie meal has a mass of 5 kg — too much bulk for a small child to consume. The net result is that the child takes in deficient joules, fats and proteins and eventually suffers from PEM.

The nutritionists of the Department of Health recommend giving an underprivileged 1-year-old child 100 grams of unsifted (No. 2) mealie meal a day to supply half the required amount of proteins. When cooked to the consistency of a soft porridge, this will make 2,5 cups of porridge. To increase the kilojoules, a tablespoon of margarine or oil can be added. Other recommended unrefined cereal products which can be used instead of mealie meal are: unsifted mabela, unsifted wheatmeal, oats, whole-wheat bread. In order to supply the rest of the protein required, the mother can be taught to stir some fresh or sour milk or approximately 4 level tablespoons of skim milk powder per day into the child's porridge. If sufficient milk is not available, use can be made of other protein-rich foods such as eggs, meat (e.g. ground dried caterpillars in black rural areas), fish and cheese. Where animal proteins are not available, plant proteins such as dry legumes (beans, especially soy beans, peas and lentils) and purées made of dark green leaves and yellow fruit and vegetables can be used. For the small child the legumes must be well cooked and put through a sieve to remove the skins and make them smooth and acceptable to the child. One cupful of legumes and one cupful of vegetables should be adequate per day. Roasted or cooked peanuts (mashed) or peanut butter are excellent substitutes for legumes. The food rations for the day should be divided into at least 4 feeds.

Note: Soy beans should be soaked for 24 hours before cooking them in order to remove an enzyme which prevents protein digestion.

SECONDARY PREVENTION OF MALNUTRITION (PEM)

Growth retardation

Growth retardation is the earliest sign of PEM, especially in the pre-school period, but also throughout childhood. The surest way of detecting early signs of PEM is by keeping growth records of children at risk, i.e. those under the age of 5. Child health clinics issue health cards, on which are plotted the child's gain in mass and height, to children who visit them regularly. (See Chapter 22 for 'Health Cards'.)

Any negative deviation from the norm is a warning that the protein and/or energy intake is insufficient. Nutritional stunting of growth can start before birth and continue right throughout the growing period.

Richter-Strydom et al.[10] report that recent studies covering a 10-year follow-up period, have found that children malnourished in their first year of life remain more easily distracted and function at a lower intellectual level than their normal peers.

Recording of the mass curves in the preschool child is important because if malnutrition can be detected and reversed before the age of 5 years there will be no physical after-effects. Other ways of detecting early PEM is by measuring any reduction in total muscle mass. This can be done by measuring the circumference of arm or leg muscles and by biochemical assay of urinary creatinine output, the assumption being that a given mass of muscle produces the same amount of creatinine per day. If the creatinine output remains the same or decreases, the total muscle mass of the body is either stationary or is wasting. Of all the black malnourished children affected by PEM, only 5 % suffer from kwashiorkor and 1 % from marasmus, nutritional growth retardation without the skin stigmata of kwashiorkor being by far the most important component of PEM.

Note: In assessing satisfactory growth, both height and mass must be taken into account. The NCHS (p. 394) mass represents the normal lower limit for well-fed rural black children. When there is increased undernutrition, measurement dips below the NCHS, height responding more slowly than mass to the body's nutritional state.

After the age of 6 years growth normally slows down; because of this slowing down the stigmata of severe clinical PEM will no longer be striking. From now on the effects of chronic protein deficiency will be permanent, however, with physical immaturity and poor school performance being its main crippling effects. The intellectual and physical achievements of a poorly nourished community compare unfavourably with those of a well-nourished one; the resistance of underfed people to tuberculosis is notoriously poor. (For a discussion of these statements, see p. 436.)

Nutritional dwarfing is easily overlooked as the child's appearance may be normal, except for his size. Therefore growth retardation due to a deficit of kilojoules and/or protein in the diet may be masked in the older child, especially if many children in a community are malnourished.

Kwashiorkor

In kwashiorkor, the diet lacks first-class protein, but has a high starch content, so that the child may appear 'chubby'. There is usually a history of some upset: birth of a sibling, psychosocial upset in the family causing anxiety and anorexia or a chronic infection. Kwashiorkor is often precipitated by an attack of diarrhoea.

The peak incidence of kwashiorkor is between the age of 9 months and 2 years, coinciding with the time of weaning. At this age the following *stigmata of kwashiorkor* are present:

(1) The hair becomes thin, straight (if the child has peppercorns), and slightly brown or red (if it has been black).

(2) The child is apathetic, miserable and irritable if disturbed.

(3) Hypoproteinaemia (reduced amount of serum albumin (i.e. less than 3 g/100 ml)).

(4) Oedema of the feet, hands and eyes; anasarca develops as the condition deteriorates. The cause of the oedema has not been established with certainty; it is probably due to an increase of sodium in the extracellular space with hypokalaemia or it may be due to hypoproteinaemia. Apart from the swelling and enlargement of the body, the child may be fat.

(5) Dermatosis is characteristic and appears in the neck region (Casal's necklace), in the groin, on the face and buttocks. There is depigmentation of the skin and drying, accompanied by dark discoloration of exposed areas. The skin may strip off, leaving excoriated areas. The skin lesions may resemble those of pellagra.

(6) The child is small, the abdomen being distended. There is an enlarged, fat-infiltrated liver, the fat comprising from one-third to half of the wet weight of the liver.

(7) The child suffers from anorexia.

(8) Gradually the subcutaneous fatty tissue disappears, and the muscles waste.

(9) There may be accompanying anaemia and signs of vitamin B complex deficiency; sometimes there is a pellagra-like rash; the tongue may be raw and red and there may be angular stomatitis and cheilosis due to ariboflavinosis. Fissuring may occur on the lips and around the eyes and anus.

(10) Diarrhoea may be persistent and due to lactose intolerance. Acid diarrhoea often responds to lactose-free feeds.

Kwashiorkor usually attacks the toddler under 3 years of age while pellagra is found in the child above 4 years.

The body of the child with kwashiorkor has not been able to adapt to low protein intake and blood levels of albumin are reduced. In marasmus (infantile atrophy), on the other hand, growth stops as protein is diverted from the muscles to the blood to maintain the normal blood level of albumin. There is no nutritional oedema and no energy is needed for growth. Therefore the body is able to cope with the energy-food starvation, literally by a state of suspended growth. Marasmus is caused by chronic starvation in infancy. In marasmus there is an insufficiency of both protein and kilojoules.

Marasmus

Marasmus is characterised by stationary mass or mass loss and decreased food tolerance. The infant fails to thrive even when the food intake is increased to normal. The child is usually under the age of 6 months.

Causes

(1) Chronic starvation in famine conditions.

(2) Neglect on the part of a mother who does not realise that her infant is not getting enough food and whose poor mothering is an expression of her rejection; feeding mismanagement from birth.

(3) Ruminative vomiting in a deprived, unloved, rejected infant may likewise cause chronic starvation.

(4) In older children, marasmus may accompany malabsorption syndromes and chronic infections.

Signs

(1) Gross under-mass with wasting of body tissues. The liver shrinks and the skin becomes inelastic and hangs in folds round the thighs and buttocks.

(2) Muscle hypotonia and wizened small sharp face with prominent suction pads.

(3) There may be food intolerance, vomiting and diarrhoea.

Marasmic kwashiorkor

Marasmic kwashiorkor has features of both kwashiorkor and marasmus, viz. wasting and oedema, with dwarfing. It results from a diet which has been chronically low in both protein and kilojoules.

Hospital treatment of severe forms of PEM

A balanced diet is the only treatment required. For black children who prefer a maize diet, the latter can be fortified with skim milk powder, PVM or Somos. It has been found that large amounts of protein in the diet are unnecessary, the following being sufficient: 4 g protein and 400 kilojoules per kg body mass daily. If the child is anorexic, 3-hourly nasogastric milk feeds are indicated. If the child is hypoglycaemic, IV dextrose is administered. If the child has lost his oedema fluid and is unable to gain mass on a normal diet during the recovery period, he is probably lacking kilojoules because a tremendous amount of energy is required by the body for synthesis of protein and growth (21 kilojoules per gram of mass gain). The skin stigmata clear up and even the fatty liver reverts to normal liver tissue within 30 days on a diet containing a normal amount of protein.

In marasmus, food tolerance is gradually increased after an initial blood transfusion. The infant is fed according to expected weight as soon as the food tolerance is normal. Milk is usually the mainstay of diet in the young child, together with vitamins, potassium and antibiotics. Full-cream acidified powdered milk is the main article of diet to help the infant gain mass.

Milk feeds are supplemented with fruit juices, cereals, vegetables, eggs and meat, as soon as the infant is able to tolerate these foods. Vitamins and blood-forming agents are added to the diet. The dehydrated child is given IV half-strength isotonic Darrow's solution with 5 % dextrose. Emotional neglect in the marasmic child must be counteracted by adequate stimulation in order to get the withdrawn infant to react to its environment. For this purpose, cuddling the baby and allowing it to suck as much as possible are very important measures. Education of the mother in nutrition and follow-up care after discharge of the child are essential to prevent recurrence of PEM.

Treatment of PEM at community clinics

(1) Extra food should be available for older pre-school and primary schoolchildren as for infants (0,5–2 years) attending the various child health clinics (municipal and provincial). School feeding schemes for under-privileged children are to be recommended.

(2) Infants at the clinics between 6 months and 2 years qualify for extra feeding if their mass falls below the third percentile.

(3) Incipient stunting can be discovered before growth stops at adolescence, by recording mass and height for age on Road-to-Health charts which should be kept for all under-nourished children, both pre-school and school.

(4) Once stunting has occurred at adolescence, additional nutrition may lead to obesity, causing short, fat children. This should be avoided.

TERTIARY PREVENTION OF UNDERNUTRITION (NUTRITIONAL REHABILITATION)

There has been much controversy and speculation about the long-term beneficial effects on intellectual and physical growth of intervention programmes for those children who have suffered PEM during the first three years of life.

Richter-Strydom *et al.*[10] found no significant difference, after a period of three years, between the physical growth and intellectual functioning of PEM children whose mothers had received 6 home-based nutrition education sessions and a control group of PEM children whose mothers had not. Both groups of PEM children compared unfavourably with normal children from a similar cultural and income group, but whose parents were better educated and who had a more stable family life in a less crowded environment.

These authors[10] quote two recent overseas reviews of major intervention studies on uni-dimensional programmes such as nutritional supplementation and developmental stimulation. These studies found the developmental effects on impoverished children too small to bring the development of the disadvantaged children into line with that of socio-economically advantaged children.

The authors[10] suggest that small-scale intervention is not really successful in rehabilitating the victims of the malnutrition caused by chronic deprivation. Unidimensional programmes merely satisfy the need 'to do something'. Only a complete change in the socio-economic milieu and life-style (as occurs with adoption or long-term foster care) or multi-dimensional intervention programmes (upgrading housing and income of the family, food supplementation and intensive intellectual stimulation of the affected children) is likely to succeed in combating the malignant effects of chronic community deprivation, social disorganisation and malnutrition.

Tertiary prevention includes the education of adults in a socio-economically deprived rural community in small-scale methods of food production so that they may meet the nutritional needs of their families.

Food supplementation, enrichment and fortification

Community feeding schemes and food fortification and enrichment for underfed people have been launched by local authorities through their clinics, and by voluntary welfare organisations.

Subsidised skim milk powder

The Department of Health has since 1961 subsidised skim milk powder to local authorities for supplementing the diet of pre-school children suffering from PEM. The child with PEM is entitled to 500 g skim milk powder per week until his condition is satisfactory.

Subsidised protein-vitamin-mineral (PVM) mixture

Since 1974, a protein-vitamin-mineral (PVM) mixture has been subsidised by the Department of Health as an alternative to skimmed milk powder, the pre-school child over the age of 6 months with PEM being entitled to 200 g powder per week (6 level teaspoonfuls per day mixed in water and given as a medicine).

PVM mixtures were formulated by the National Nutrition Research Institute of the CSIR and are manufactured by the food industry. The most important user is the Department of Health. (They are, however, also used by the private sector as a cholesterol-lowering food supplement for the 'rushed business executive') Thirty grams supplies 1/6th of the adult's protein, vitamin and mineral needs.

PVM is used primarily for the prevention and treatment of undernutrition resulting from the intake of a predominantly cereal diet, especially in the post-weaning and pre-school age group of children and in adult labourers on farms and in industry. Babies fed breast milk or cow's milk do not require PVM. PVM is always used only to supplement the diet, children requiring 30 grams (6 level teaspoonfuls) daily.

PVM must never be given as the sole diet of a young child as the amount which will supply sufficient joules will contain too much protein and minerals.

PVM contains first-class proteins and all the vitamins and well-balanced minerals needed by the body for health and growth. It is made from: deodorised whole fish flour, full-fat heat-treated soy bean meal, skim milk powder, egg albumin, whole egg powder and wheaten flour as thickener. It therefore has a low lactose content and can be used for children with diarrhoea due to lactose intolerance. Its protein content is higher than that of dried skim milk.

Both skim milk powder and PVM must be supplemented with carbohydrate-rich food such as mealie meal. Skim milk powder is cheaper but requires the addition of vitamins and iron.

Vegetable protein foods to replace animal protein

The production commercially of several valuable *high protein foods* of vegetable origin helps to replace animal proteins which are in short supply. Examples are: ProNutro, Somos (artificial meat from soy beans), Protone soup powder, Complan. See table 1.

TABLE 1
Nutritional values of vegetable protein foods

	grams/100 grams			I.U.
	Protein	Fat	CHO	Vit. A
Complan	31,0	16,0	44,0	1 100
ProNutro	22,0	12,9	54,8	1 500
Protone soup powder	23,5	1,40	48,5	5 000
(Skim milk powder)	35,6	0,80	51,7	—

	milligrams/100 grams					
	Ca	Fe	Phos.	Thiam.	Ribof.	Niacin	Vit. C
Complan	825	8,0	780	1,20	1,10	7,7	10
ProNutro	460	8,9	480	0,86	1,20	7,7	—
Protone soup powder	240	5,4	730	1,50	3,00	13,1	200
(Skim milk powder)	1 301	0,6	1 011	0,35	1,80	0,9	7

Food fortification and enrichment in South Africa

The World Health Organisation considers food fortification a public health measure to improve and maintain the health of the population through the provision of an adequate food intake. Food fortification programmes are designed specifically to meet the needs of population subgroups exposed to malnutrition, e.g. in protein deficiency, the target population are pre-school children and pregnant and lactating women. The relatively small quantity of nutrients added to the staple food which requires fortification may be either extracts of natural foods or synthesised products. In 1977 the Medical Research Council Project Group, who studied all aspects of food fortification in South Africa, made the following food fortification and enrichment proposals for immediate implementation:[9]

(1) The enrichment of maize meal with riboflavin and niacin. The enrichment of maize meal was legally sanctioned and controlled in December 1979.
(2) Maize meal can, and should be, fortified with folic acid.
(3) The restoration of the vitamin A content of skim milk by the addition of 1 500 IU per litre.
(4) The fortification of all processed and evaporated milks with 400 IU vitamin D per litre.
(5) The fluoridation of water supplies in areas of low fluoride intake.

Envisaged for the future, after investigation and testing by the MRC, are included the following:

(1) Fortification of maize meal with soya, other vegetable protein or whey powder.
(2) The development and testing of high lysine maize.
(3) Enrichment of sorghum beer with thiamine, riboflavin and niacin.

Note: Natural food supplements, such as tinned pilchards, skim milk powder, and beans, are the most economical way of enriching maize diets on an individual basis. Somos, a textured vegetable protein food derived from soy beans, is also an excellent supplement.

Enrichment of food means the addition of a nutrient which is present in the foodstuff, but in an undesirably small quantity.

Fortification means the addition of a nutrient which was not originally present, e.g. iodine to table salt, vitamin C to jelly, vitamin A to margarine.

The Nutrition Development Programme

The government has set aside money to help with the feeding of the poor — the Nutrition Development Programme. It is administered by committees headed by a regional director of health, from each of the nine health regions of the Department of Health. Welfare and other service-rendering organisations which already offer a nutrition-related service, can apply to a regional office for assistance. The committee will assess applications and supervise the implementation of the programme. Some of the private feeding schemes which may benefit from the Nutrition Development Programme are discussed.

Feeding schemes

Feeding schemes are subsidised and organised by voluntary welfare organisations, for example: African Children's Feeding Scheme operating in the black townships of the Witwatersrand. Aside from feeding needy children, the scheme employs registered nurses, social workers and domestic science teachers who do health education and community development, involving the community in these activities.

Operation Hunger was started by SAIRR in Johannesburg in 1979 in response to the need felt by many voluntary organisations for co-ordinated action on rural hunger and poverty.

It is now an independent organisation headed by a board of trustees and run by a number of sub-committees, regional directors and an executive director. Fund-raising is on a national scale. Operation Hunger is committed to feeding at least 1 million needy people daily, both black and white, but mostly rural blacks. It sees feeding as 'crisis intervention' only. Its main aim is that of helping people to help themselves by establishing work projects, such as vegetable growing, beadwork and other crafts, brick and fence making and sewing.

Operation Hunger responds to community request and works through community committees, i.e. the community-in-need of help is actively involved in the feeding and distribution of food. The community accepts responsibility for the work that has to be done. For example, the community needing assistance for feeding its members has to accept responsibility for the firewood, water and utensils. The cooking and serving of the food is done by the community and no one is paid for his services.

Operation Hunger thus involves the affluent private sector in giving to the needy in such a way that the needy are enabled to help themselves. Similar organisations operate elsewhere, e.g. the Child Nutrition Education Programme of the UCT Child Health Unit in Cape Town.

Education in food production

Health educators must encourage the underfed people from rural areas to utilise their soil potential to its fullest. People must be encouraged to grow grains and vegetable foods with good nutritional value (e.g. sorghum, soy beans, groundnuts) and to produce small animals (rabbits, pigs), birds (chickens, ducks) and fish for home consumption and for the production of manure to increase the productivity of home gardens. Health education which encourages people to be conscious of the value of their soil is much more important than education in the desirability of consuming high quality foods which can only be bought at stores by the fortunate few who can afford them. Soil conservation is the cornerstone of nutritional health education and its principles should be understood by the health educator. For the principles of soil conservation, see p. 156.

Self-help nutritional projects

When the nurse who works in a malnourished community is familiar with the customs and beliefs, with the methods of horticulture and food storage, with the foods available and the foods preferred, as well as the economic status of the people, she will be able to start her educating programme. She will be able to suggest better methods of food production and introduce variety into the diet to bring it into balance. She will help the people utilise their resources to the utmost, bearing in mind that self-help encourages self-esteem and feelings of adequacy — the most important motivating factors towards industry and independence.

How does one start with the health education of people whose apathy, beliefs and customs cause ill-health and who are ignorant of scientifically gathered medical knowledge? As an example of a way which was found to raise the nutritional standards of an impoverished, underdeveloped rural African community, the Valley Trust experiment will be described.[11]

The Valley Trust, a registered welfare association, conducts an ongoing socio-medical experiment to promote health by raising the nutritional standards among a Zulu community, living in the Valley of a Thousand Hills near Botha's Hill. The people had lost their traditional method of soil husbandry and had replaced their traditional well-balanced diet with a diet consisting largely of refined carbohydrates bought at local stores. Soil erosion and destruction of the covering vegetation were rife, therefore the soil had become lifeless and its productivity was low. Furthermore, poor cooking practices (e.g. prolonged boiling of spinaches) largely destroy the vitamin content of the food. Premature weaning of sick infants because of erroneous beliefs about the cause and treatment of their disease, promoted a high infant mortality rate. Poverty, ignorance and apathy caused malnutrition and a high incidence of disease. The birth-rate was high to compensate for the high infant mortality rate. Because of lack of scientific knowledge, the people did not associate food with health, especially infant health; they ascribed ill-health and premature death to the anger of ancestors or to bewitchment and the malice of enemies. These beliefs gave rise to a search for magical cures — those of their own medicine-men and the medicines and injections at the clinics of health services.

The challenge which faced the educators of the Valley Trust socio-medical experiment was to break through the wall of ignorance and apathy in order to arouse interest in self-help activities. The experiment has been in progress for more than 20 years and the people have responded to the health-promotive education. Doctors and nurses working at the Botha's Hill Health Centre have found that the incidence of malnutrition has diminished amongst the people reached by the Valley Trust experiment.

The health educators in this experiment consist of a doctor and a nurse at the Botha's Hill Centre — a medical service run and financed by the state — a nutritional educator (a registered nurse) to give nutritional advice and practical demonstrations on the preparation of available foods, and an agricultural demonstrator to teach soil rehabilitation and food production. The nutrition education programme is initiated at the health centre where the doctor and/or nurse stimulates the patient's interest in good dietary habits, attempting to establish in the patient's mind a connection between diet and health. The suitably conditioned patient is then sent to the nutrition education unit for advice regarding infant and family feeding and for cooking demonstrations. The emphasis is on the optimal utilisation of available foods, with available equipment. The vegetables used for the demonstration are picked in the demonstration vegetable garden in which the 'cooking' hut is situated. The nutrition educator, therefore, stimulates interest in vegetable gardening which is taught on a return visit (to the agricultural section) by the agricultural demonstrator. Thus, the interest aroused at the health centre and developed at the nutrition education unit is brought to fruition by the agricultural demonstrator who teaches soil management at such a practical level in the demonstration garden, that even the simplest peasants can grasp it.

The home-produce marketers are encouraged to produce surplus vegetables and fruit for sale, to keep poultry in pens by the deep-litter system (later using the deep-litter as a garden fertiliser), to make use of a maize-grinding mill provided by the Valley Trust (in order to preserve the maize nutrients) and to rehabilitate the soil by adding humus to it. Interested persons are also taught water conservation and fish culture. School children are gainfully employed during the holidays. Those people who need special help (i.e. handicapped families with chronic illness or whose breadwinner is absent) are helped to lay out and fence gardens and are given fruit trees, seed and seedlings at a time for planting.

The people have responded to the gardening campaign and all the families producing vegetables are eating them, some producing surplus for sale. The experiment is proving that effective health education, aimed at raising nutritional standards and preventing deficiency diseases, is possible even amongst people who are poor, ignorant and apathetic. Long-term educating programmes which foster active participation in the utilisation of natural resources, as

well as attitudes of self-reliance, are infinitely more satisfactory than temporary, emergency relief measures such as food distribution schemes. The developmental process can never thrive on the sterile principle of 'hand-outs'. People will only absorb change to the extent that they participate in it. In order to accelerate development, we must, therefore, always succeed in moving the initiative into the target group.

The health educators changed the helpless and fatalistic attitudes of the people and imbued them with confidence in their own ability to improve their lot. They achieved the aim of health education, viz. to change attitudes which have a deleterious effect upon health.

ACUTE INFECTIVE DIARRHOEAL DISEASE (AID) IN CHILDREN UNDER FIVE

Loening defines acute infective diarrhoea (AID) as an illness of sudden onset with 4 or more watery stools and recovery within 2 weeks.[13] The child starts to lose essential water and salts from the onset of the illness.

The primary clinical features of AID are: diarrhoea, infection (with or without pyrexia) and dehydration with electrolyte imbalance and metabolic acidosis.

Acute infective diarrhoea (AID) with or without vomiting and with dehydration is due to enteral infection, i.e. gastro-enteritis caused by, *inter alia*, E. coli, rotavirus and other viruses, shigella, salmonella, V. cholerae or the parasites, Giardia lamblia and amoeba. Many infants with diarrhoea, especially those with rotavirus infections, are also severely malnourished.[14]

The enteral infection is transmitted through the oro-anal route, the major source being unsanitary living conditions (flies, fingers, faeces, food) and an inadequate supply of safe drinking water.

Note: Other causes of infantile diarrhoea which cannot be considered AID are: lactose intolerance, maternal medication in breast-fed infants, e.g. certain laxatives and antibiotics, parenteral infections of the ears, lungs, ureter or throat (sometimes accompanied by diarrhoea).

The malnutrition associated with diarrhoea may be caused by: decreased intake, extra losses and malabsorption of nutrients. In a retrospective study, Wittenberg and Loening found an association between diarrhoea and malnutrition: a higher proportion of children with diarrhoea had a mass under the third percentile than children with bronchopneumonia.[12]

Malnourished children take longer to recover from each episode of diarrhoea than well-nourished children.

Repeated attacks of gastro-enteritis play an important role in the pathogenesis of malnutrition in children under the age of 5 in the Third World. The repeated attacks cause small intestinal mucosal injuries (with ineffective repair of the villi), bacterial overgrowth and infection. There is subsequent malabsorption of nutrients, especially proteins. Gastro-enteritis may, therefore, be a nutritional disease because of the oft-infected child's very low nutrient absorption rate.[15]

In the management of AID, therefore, both the short-term problem of dehydration and the long-term risk of a deterioration in the nutritional state of the child must be addressed. Nutritional rehabilitation during and after episodes of diarrhoea is mandatory in malnourished children.

Epidemiology of AID

AID is more common in the rainy season and in hot weather, probably due to an increase in the fly population. Eighty per cent of deaths occur before the age of two years,[4] especially during the period of weaning. The average African child will have 4,9 attacks of diarrhoea annually, each lasting 5 to 6 days.[4] The mortality rate from AID is high in the lowest socio-economic group in which poverty and malnutrition are rife.

It was estimated in 1985 that there were 1 000 million episodes of diarrhoea globally among 300 million children, resulting in 5 million deaths.[4] The commonest cause of death (60–70 %) was dehydration. In the RSA, AID is the leading cause of death in children under the age of 5 years, excluding white children among whom it ranks fourth.

Primary prevention of AID

■ Education of mothers in the promotion of health and breast-feeding for 6 to 12 months.
■ Immunisation against the common childhood diseases and selective immunisation against cholera and rotavirus.

■ Supply of uncontaminated water and food.
■ Attention to environmental health, including fly control.
■ Good personal hygiene of the mother or child-minders, especially with regard to hand-washing.
■ Training of community health care workers in primary health care and the principles of GOBI-FFF.
■ The long-term prevention of diarrhoeal disease is ensured by: social upliftment to improve child health generally, and state commitment to primary health care which is accessible to all those South Africans who cannot afford private medical services.
■ Diarrhoea rehydration rooms should be established at every hospital and clinic.

Secondary prevention of AID

■ Early diagnosis of intestinal infections which require antibiotics. If organisms are isolated from the stools on culture, antibiotics, e.g. gentamycin or/and the antimicrobial, metronidazole, are used. Antimicrobial medicines should be used only for specific infections such as cholera, shigellosis, amoebiasis, salmonellosis with bacteraemia and giardiasis.[4]

In the majority of cases infection is not identified and, as it is in any case self-limiting, it is modern practice not to give antibiotics automatically to every child with diarrhoea.

Note: antidiarrhoeal and anti-emetic preparations must never be used for infective diarrhoeal disease, for example, kaolin-pectin mixtures, diphenoxylate, loperamide, cyclizine.

■ Early home or clinic treatment of diarrhoea by:
  (1) Oral fluid therapy with oral diarrhoeal disease solutions (ODDS). This is the first-line home remedy for diarrhoeal disease.
  (2) Feeding (preferably by breast in the case of infants), which should be maintained throughout the course of the diarrhoeal disease, as diarrhoeal disease is associated with malnutrition.[15] Soft solids can also be continued. Foods rich in potassium, such as bananas and fruit juices,

should be given if available. Unless very severe and persistent, vomiting is not an indication for stopping ORT. The severely vomiting child needs hospital care and the parenteral administration of fluids.

To cope with the mildly vomiting child at home, very small amounts are given very frequently.

- Mothers must be reassured that the diarrhoea will stop and that the ORS is not an antidiarrhoeal medicine, therefore the diarrhoea may continue despite ORT. Thus the mother's co-operation with ORS therapy is gained by careful enlightenment of the mother in its use and its mode of action. An ignorant mother may abandon therapy if her false hopes for ORT are not fulfilled.

Note: Tinned juices are not suitable and may make the diarrhoea worse.

Oral fluid therapy (ORT) for diarrhoeal disease

Definitions

ORT — oral rehydration/replacement therapy
OHT — oral hydration therapy
OFT — oral fluid therapy

(The above three are used synonymously.)

ODDS — oral diarrhoeal disease solution
ORS — oral replacement/rehydration solution

(The above two are used synonymously.)

OHS — oral hydration solution

The oral administration of a hydration solution in the early phase of diarrhoeal disease and subsequently will significantly reduce morbidity and mortality. In areas dependent on community primary health care services this therapy is a major survival strategy for children living in poor and underdeveloped communities as it is home-based and can be initiated by the mother or child-minder at the onset of the illness.[16]

ORT is used mainly in the community, by the family, peripheral health workers and primary health centres.

The use of glucose and sucrose and electrolyte solutions has been encouraged by the WHO through its Diarrhoeal Diseases Control Programme.

Fluid therapy can be considered in 3 phases.

Phase 1
Maintenance of hydration. OFT is commenced at the time of the first loose stool. Treatment is home-based by a mother who has been instructed beforehand and has the necessary equipment (cup or litre bottle and standard teaspoon) and salt and sugar. The key to success is: frequency (after every loose stool), amount (1–2 cupfuls at a time), and immediate use after onset of diarrhoea. All households with susceptible children should be shown how to make the salt, sugar and water solution, viz:

- 8 level teaspoons of sugar, and
- half a teaspoon of salt,
added to one litre of water

or

- two level teaspoons of sugar, and
- one 2-finger pinch of salt,
added to 1 cup of water.

The water must preferably be sterile but, as no time must be wasted initially, the use of clean water is acceptable.

If a litre of solution is mixed but not used within 24 hours, the remaining solution must be discarded in case it has become contaminated.

Phase 2

Rehydration by the replacement of accumulated deficit due to fluid and salt losses in stools and vomitus.

In this case the use of pre-packaged salts and sugar in sachets, as recommended by the SA Paediatric Association (SAPA), must be used under the supervision of a community health worker. The pre-packaged salts are produced commercially and are usually available only at clinics. Although they can be used for any phase of the diarrhoeal disease if they are freely and promptly available, their use for phase 2 is mandatory because, in addition to NaCl and sugar (glucose), they contain potassium, lost in stools and vomitus, and bicarbonate to correct metabolic acidosis.

Phase 3

Maintenance by replacement of ongoing abnormal losses due to continuing diarrhoea and vomiting and replacement of the normal physiological losses due to respiration, sweating and urination.

Formulations of ODDS (ORS)

The home-made salt/sugar recipe advocated by SAPA delivers the same sodium concentration as the sachet-packed salts. The problem here is the differing sizes of household measures for both salt and fluid. The double-ended plastic spoon is the safest measure and is issued to all mothers by some local authorities after the birth of a child.

The sachet contents were formulated by SAPA at the request of the Department of National Health and Population Development.

Rehydration sachet[17] dissolved in 1 000 ml water

- Sodium chloride: 2 g, Na 64 mmol/ℓ, Cl 54 mmol/ℓ
- Sodium bicarbonate: 2,5 g, HCO_3 30 mmol/ℓ
- Potassium chloride: 1,5 g, K 20 mmol/ℓ
- Glucose: 20 g, 2 %

Replacement and maintenance home measures dissolved in 1 000 ml water

- Sodium chloride: 2 g, Na ± 60 mmol/ℓ
- Cane sugar: 20 g, 2 %

The sachet ORS resembles half-strength Darrow's/dextrose solution. The NaCl content of the South African formulation is somewhat lower than that of the WHO formulation, which is Na 90 mmol/ℓ.

Note: Taste as a test of salt content must be avoided as experience shows the resulting solution to contain a dangerously high salt content, especially if the mother is asked to use the saltiness of tears as a comparison.

If the mother has no salt or sugar in the home and sachets are not available, any fluid can be given, e.g. rice water, soup, maize porridge (thin), water.

An extract from the WHO Programme for the Control of Diarrhoeal Diseases[18]

'Remember this about the prevention of *diarrhoea* —

The best ways to prevent diarrhoea are:

- Breast-feeding

- Improved weaning practices
- Use plenty of clean water
- Hand-washing
- Use of latrines
- Proper disposal of babies' stools
- Measles immunisation

■ It is important to assess a community's current practices related to diarrhoea and the reasons for them to know what preventive interventions are needed.

■ Use the step-by-step approach to select the specific preventive practices to emphasise in a health area. Briefly, the steps include:
  - List the practices that need to be improved in the area
  - Select the more important practices to improve
  - Identify the practices that will be more feasible to change
  - Select one or two preventive practices to emphasise

■ Health services should play an important role in bringing about improvements in a community's practices. Some activities that health workers can do to support selected preventive practices include:
  - Use of counselling techniques
  - Set a good example
  - Participate in community projects to improve preventive practices
  - Support breast-feeding
  - Build and maintain a latrine at the health facility
  - Advise community members of the cleaner water sources and ways to improve water sources.'

REFERENCES

(1) Department of National Health and Population Development. First RHOSA nutrition study. Anthropometric assessment of nutritional status in black under-fives in rural RSA. *Epidemiological Comments* 1987; **14**(3).

(2) Food and Nutrition Terminology (Terminology Circular No. 27). Geneva: WHO, 1975.

(3) Bengoa JM. *WHO Chron.* 1974; **23**(3).

(4) Coetzer PWW, Kroukamp LM. Diarrhoeal disease — epidemiology and intervention. *S Afr Med J* 1989; **76**: 465–471.

(5) Bowie MD, Moodie AD, Mann MD, Hansen JDL. A prospective 15-year follow-up study of kwashiorkor patients. *S Afr Med J* 1980; **58**: 671–681.

(6) Buchanan NS. *S Afr Med J* 1975; **48**: 903.

(7) Letter to the Editor, *S Afr Med J* 6 September 1980.

(8) Food Fortification: Protein-Calorie-Malnutrition (Technical Report Series No. 477). Geneva: WHO.

(9) Metz J, *et al.* Food fortification in South Africa. *S Afr Med J* 1978; **53**: 744.

(10) Richter-Strydom, LM, Griesel RD, Glatthaar I. Effects of a nutrition education programme on the psychological performance of malnourished children. *S Afr Med J* 1985; **68**: 659–662.

(11) Stott, HH. *S Afr Med J* 1972; **46**: 1572.

(12) Wittenberg DF, Loening WEK. Diarrhoea is a nutritional disease. *S Afr Med J* 1989; **76**: 476–478.

(13) Loening WEK. Management of acute infective diarrhoea. *S Afr J CME* 1986; **3**: 69–74.

(14) Editorial. *S Afr Med J* 1978; **53**: 777.

(15) Ransome OJ, Roode H. Early introduction of milk feeds in acute infantile gastro-enteritis. *S Afr Med J* 1984; **65**: 127–128.

(16) Ferrinho P, Evian C, Wagstaff L, Pretorius JHO, Gear J. Editorial: Towards consensus on oral fluid therapy in diarrhoeal disease. *S Afr Med J* 1989; **76**: 459–460.

(17) Bowie MD & Hill ID. Oral rehydration therapy — South African Paediatric Association Recommendations. *S Afr Med J* 1989; **76**: 461–462.

(18) The programme for the control of diarrhoeal diseases. WHO *Epidemiological Comments* 1991; **18**(6).

TEST OF KNOWLEDGE

The student has benefited from studying this chapter if he/she can answer the following questions:

(1) Discuss the causes of undernutrition in the rural areas of South Africa, as well as the role of the community nurse working from a primary health care clinic in recognising and relieving undernutrition in the under-five group.

(2) What anthropometric measurements (as defined by the WHO) are used to assess growth and development in young children. What are the conclusions of the first RHOSA nutrition survey based on?

(3) Distinguish between the different forms of protein-energy-malnutrition. What form is likely to cause the greatest harm to the underprivileged youth of South Africa? Give reasons for your choice.

(4) Discuss the following statement: Poor sanitation, personal hygiene, water supply and fly control cause repeated attacks of acute infective diarrhoea (AID) in children under 5 and this leads to malnutrition rather than the opposite: malnutrition underlies the high incidence of AID amongst underprivileged children.

(5) Write an essay on nutrition rehabilitation in a deprived rural community.

(6) How would you educate a group of mothers attending an under-fives' clinic in the prevention, home management and rehabilitation of their under-5 children (various ages) who contract acute infective diarrhoeal disease?

Part 5

COMMUNICABLE DISEASES

25

Elementary Microbiology in Medicine

Microbiology is the biology (life science) of micro-organisms — microscopically visible organisms, mainly vegetable but also animal — which cause communicable diseases.

STUDY OBJECTIVES

The student will be introduced to:

(1) The concepts of the pathogenicity of microbes and host resistance.
(2) A simple classification of the protists (predominantly unicellular organisms) and viruses (subcellular living particles).
(3) The identification of microbes in simple theoretical terms, their living characteristics and the conditions for their growth and multiplication.
(4) The viruses in a classificatory context, while
(5) Three important and common pathogenic bacteria are discussed in some detail.

PATHOGENICITY AND HOST RESISTANCE

Microbiology is a branch of science which deals with living, mainly unicellular organisms (microbes). Microbes (germs) are so called because they are visible only under a microscope which may magnify from 75 to 100 000 times. The greater majority (viz. the non-pathogenic microbes) are of benefit to mankind; only a small percentage (viz. the pathogenic microbes) are harmful to man and beast because they are parasites which cause disease.

Pathogenic microbes are disease-producing microbes which live parasitically on plants, animals and human beings. They use the food intended for the host and secrete toxins which poison the host and cause tissue destruction.

Non-pathogenic microbes include saprophytes which decompose dead organic material and serve to make soil fertile, ripen cheese, acidify milk, make alcohol from carbohydrate fermentation, and manufacture vitamin B complex and antibiotics.

Potential pathogens are harmful only under certain circumstances, i.e.:

(1) The intestinal flora, for example, *E. coli*, are pathogenic only in tissues outside the bowel, e.g. in the urinary tract. These and other indigenous organisms are also called commensals.

(2) The normal flora (microbes) of the respiratory tract affect its mucous membrane only when the latter's resistance has been lowered by rapid cooling, malnutrition, etc.

Potential pathogens which cause infection when the host's immunity is lowered are *opportunists*.

Opportunistic micro-organisms include viruses, mycobacteria, bacteria, fungi and protozoa. They are potential pathogens which normally live either as commensals in the body or are found in the environment and normally do not cause infection. When the resistance of the body (host) is lowered for some reason or another, opportunists become invasive and cause infection.

Lowered resistance is caused either by the natural debilitation of a sick or malnourished patient, by the intake of immunosuppressive drugs or by the use of instruments in body cavities, e.g. urethral and cardiac catheters. Opportunistic infections are especially important in immunocompromised patients, i.e. those patients whose host defences are weakened by the use of immunosuppressive drugs, e.g. in transplant surgery and in patients with leukaemia. Immunocompromised patients are much less resistant to invasion by microbes which, under normal circumstances, are held at bay by the biological defences of the body.

Opportunistic infections may also occur in patients on steroids or those with diabetes mellitus and collagen diseases, and those who suffer from immunological deficiency diseases, e.g. AIDS.

Microbes can be classified in two main classes: (1) Protists; (2) Viruses.

THE PROTISTS

The protists are living organisms which include the lowest orders of animals (protozoa) and plants (e.g. bacteria).

Two main groups of protists are distinguished: the higher and lower protists.

The higher protists: protozoa and fungi

The cells of the higher protists have a true nucleus containing chromosomes; they are capable of cell division by mitosis or meiosis. Reproduction of protozoa can be either sexual or asexual, asexual reproduction being either a simple binary fission or a multiple fission (schizogony).

The following unicellular *protozoa* cause human infections:

(1) *Entamoeba histolytica* (for amoebiasis, see p. 648).
(2) Trypanosoma causes trypanosomiasis (sleeping sickness), a tropical disease transmitted by the tsetse fly (see p. 666).
(3) The plasmodium causes malaria (see p. 653). It is non-motile and needs a biological vector, the anopheles mosquito, for spread.
(4) *Trichomonas vaginalis* is a genito-urinary flagellate which causes trichomonal vaginitis, a sexually transmitted condition (see p. 597).
(5) Toxoplasma causes toxoplasmosis (see p. 683).

Fungi are of two kinds:

(1) Yeasts — unicellular organisms which are either ovoid or spherical in shape. They cause fermentation of starches and sugars and are used for the manufacture of vit. B. Some variants are pathogenic, e.g. *Candida (Monilia) albicans* which infects mucous membranes, causing thrush.
(2) Multicellular moulds — i.e. filamentous branching fungi which consist of hyphae forming a mycelium (mould). They are very common in damp soil and cause rotting of fruit and vegetables, as well as the mould on bottled fruit and old bread. Fungi are used in the manufacture of cheese and antibiotics. The pathogenic variants cause dermatophytoses, a group of diseases commonly known as ringworm (tinea).

The soil fungus, *Histoplasma capsulatum*, causes histoplasmosis which is contracted by the inhalation of spores liberated into the atmosphere. The organism grows well in bird and bat droppings (see p. 455).

Reproduction of fungi:

(1) by special reproductive cells, called spores, on the extremities of the hyphae of branched fungi;
(2) by the budding of nodules which break off and form new cells, in the case of yeasts.

Fungi are important opportunistic microbes, especially in the immunocompromised patient.

Note: The actinomyces (ray fungus), which radiates club-shaped rods which end in the tissues, is not a true fungus, being closely related to the bacteria. *Actinomyces bovis* causes actinomycosis, a disease of cattle that can be transmitted to man.

The lower protists: bacteria, etc.

The cells of the lower protists are primitive and have no true nucleus. In human medicine, bacteria are the most important kind of lower protists.

Bacterial classification

Classification of the important bacteria according to Gram staining

Gram-positive cocci

(1) *Staphyloccus* species:
   Staph. aureus (golden) (*Staph. pyogenes*)
   Staph. albus (white) (*Staph. epidermidis*) (an opportunist)
(2) *Streptococcus* species:
   Strep. pyogenes (pus-forming) or haemolyticus
   Strep. viridans (green)
   Strep. faecalis (in faeces) — (an opportunist)
   Strep. pneumoniae (pneumococci)
   Strep. mutans (in mouth)

Some of the strains of staphylococci and streptococci are aerobic, while others are anaerobic.

Gram-negative cocci

(1) *Neisseria gonorrhoeae:* Gonococcus

(2) *Neisseria meningitidis:* Meningococcus

Gram-positive bacilli

(1) Aerobic
  (a) *Corynebacterium diphtheriae*
  (b) Diphtheroids
  (c) *Bacillus anthracis*
  (d) *Bacillus subtilis*
(2) Anaerobic
  (a) *Clostridium botulinum*, causing food poisoning
  (b) *Clostridium tetani*
  (c) *Clostridia* causing gas gangrene (welchii or perfringens)
  (d) *Bacteroides urealyticus* causing NGU (see p. 588)

Gram-negative bacilli

(1) *Salmonella*
  S. typhi (typhoid bacillus)
  S. paratyphi (paratyphoid bacillus)
  There are many other types, some causing salmonella gastro-enterocolitis (food poisoning).
(2) Escherichia
  E. coli (neonatal meningitis, infantile diarrhoea) (an opportunist)
(3) Klebsiella
  K. pneumoniae (Friendlander bacillus) — an opportunist — urinary tract infection
(4) Shigella
  (a) *Sh. dysenteriae*
    Sh. shiga
    Sh. Schmitzii
  (b) *Sh. paradysenteriae*
    Sh. flexneri
    Sh. boydii
    Sh. sonnei
(5) Proteus (causing urinary tract sepsis — opportunists)
  (a) *P. vulgaris*
  (b) *P. mirabilis*
  (c) *P. morganii*
(6) Pseudomonas
  (a) Ps. *pyocyanea* (causing sepsis)
  (b) Ps. *aeruginosa* (an opportunist)
(7) Haemophilus
  (a) *H. influenzae* (Koch–Weeks bacillus) infection of air passages, meningitis
  (b) *H. ducreyi*, causing a STD

(8) Brucella
  (a) *B. melitensis*, causing brucellosis
  (b) *B. abortus* (Malta fever)
(9) Yersinia
  Y. pestis (causing plague)
(10) Bordetella
  Bordetella pertussis, causing whooping-cough
(11) Legionella
  L. pneumophila (Legionnaires disease)
(12) Enterobacter aerogenes (aerobic)

Other Gram-negative bacteria

(1) Vibrio
  V. cholerae
(2) Spirillum (spirilla), Vincent's spirillum causing mouth and throat infection.
(3) The intracellular *Calymmatobacterium granulomatis* (Granuloma inguinale (donovanosis))

Bacteria resistant to Gram staining

Acid-fast *Mycobacterium tuberculosis* (tubercle bacillus):

(1) Human type
(2) Bovine type
Acid-fast *Mycobacterium leprae* (leprosy bacillus)

Spirochaetes

(1) Borrelia
  (a) *B. duttoni*
  (b) *B. recurrentis* (relapsing fever)
  (c) *B. vincenti* (Vincent's angina)
(2) Treponema
  T. pallidum (syphilis)
(3) Leptospira (causes leptospirosis in man and animals)
  (a) *Lepto. icterohaemorrhagiae*
  (b) *Lepto. canicola*

Mycoplasma

The mycoplasma is a Gram-negative organism which does not possess a true cell wall and is, therefore, resistant to penicillin but not to tetracyclines. Both pathogenic and saprophytic species of mycoplasma occur, e.g. in the normal flora of the oropharynx.

Pathogenic species of mycoplasma, *M. pneumoniae*, causes primary atypical pneumonia and PID. Mycoplasma genitalium causes NGU (see p. 588).

Rickettsiae and Chlamydiae

The rickettsiae and the chlamydiae are obligate intracellular microbes which resemble bacteria. They live inside cells to ensure their own survival, the needs of each genus being different.

Rickettsiae are Gram-negative organisms, coccoid to rod-shaped, which are carried by bloodsucking arthropods (insects), viz. lice, fleas, ticks and mites, from animal to human hosts, causing tick-bite fever and different kinds of typhus. The rickettsiae gain entry through skin lesions (bites or scratches) and live in the endothelial cells of blood vessels.

Chlamydiae fall into two main groups:

(1) *C. psittaci* causes psittacosis, a disease of birds which is transmitted to man when he inhales infected, dried droppings.
(2) *C. trachomatis* causes the trachoma-lymphogranuloma venereum complex. It is a human disease spread either directly (by coitus) or indirectly by flies and fomites, or by the fingers from genitalia or eye to eye. The *C. trachomatis* causes both eye infection (trachoma) and a sexually transmitted disease (genital infection).

IDENTIFICATION OF MICROBES (LOWER PROTISTS)

Microbes are identified either by microscope, or by the effect they have on sugars and blood in culture media, or by the shape and colour of the visible colonies they form when cultured on a solid medium in a shallow Petri dish.

Microscopic identification

Under the microscope the following characteristics can be studied: shape, size, way of clustering together and the way in which they stain with different dyes. The nuclei are invisible.

Shape

- The coccus (cocci) is a spherical, oval, lanceolate or bean-shaped bacterium.
- The bacillus (bacilli) is a rod-shaped organism.

- The vibrio is curved and rod-shaped.
- The spirochaetes and spirilla are delicate, mobile, spiral threads.
- Rickettsiae are small, rod-shaped organisms.

Size

Bacteria have an average diameter of 1 μm (1/1 000 mm) and rickettsiae are smaller.

Method of clustering together

- Streptococci form chains of adjacent cells
- Staphylococci form bunches of adjacent cells
- Diplococci are paired cocci.

Staining characteristics

All bacteria, except spirochaetes which are studied in the live, motile state against a black background on which they appear as contorting silver threads, are stained with different dyes in order to make them visible under the microscope. The most common method of staining is the *Gram method*. It is done in the following manner. The material to be studied (colony of cultured bacteria, pus or sputum), is smeared thinly on a polished glass slide by means of a sterile platinum loop, and is drawn through a flame a few times in order to fix the smear. The dye, methyl violet, is then poured on to the slide and left on for a fixed time. It is poured off, the slide is washed under water and then repeatedly washed with alcohol until there is no further discoloration of the alcohol washings. Then a red counter-stain of dilute carbon fuchsin is poured on to the slide, left for a fixed time before it is washed off under water. The slide is then blotted dry and is ready for inspection. It is viewed under the oil immersion lens of the ordinary microscope and, therefore, a drop of oil is placed on the surface with which the lens will make an oily contact.

Many bacteria will absorb the violet dye and show up as violet specks under the microscope. They are called *Gram-positive*. Others will lose the violet dye to the alcohol washings but will retain the red carbol fuchsin dye. They will show up as red specks under the microscope and are called *Gram negative*.

A few bacteria are resistant to Gram staining and are, therefore, stained by other methods. A common stain used is the acid-fast stain, which means that a red stain is absorbed by the bacteria and is not removed with acid.

LIVING CHARACTERISTICS OF MICROBES (LOWER PROTISTS)

Motility

Motility — ability to move spontaneously. Few microbes are capable of spontaneous motion. Motile organisms are:

(1) Those with *flagella* (whip-like appendages), for instance, *S. typhi*, and the vibrio.
(2) The spirochaetes, because their bodies are *flexible*.

Resistance to destruction

Methods of resistance are:

(1) Highly virulent (poisonous) bacteria are *encapsulated*. This enables them to resist phagocytosis (engulfment by phagocytes).
(2) The formation of *spores* by certain bacilli enables them to resist desiccation (the state of being dried), heat and disinfectants. A spore is the inactive encapsulated part of the organism which survives unfavourable conditions. The active multiplying form is called the *vegetative* form. The common spore-forming organisms are the clostridia and the *Bacillus anthracis*.
(3) Microbes exposed to antibiotics and chemotherapeutic drugs are inclined to develop resistance (i.e. insensitivity) to the drugs by manufacturing counter-enzymes, for instance the staphylococcus produces betalactamase which neutralises the action of penicillin and cephalosporins.

Virulence

The harmfulness of pathogenic bacteria is caused by toxins — poisonous substances secreted by the bacteria. Two kinds of toxins are secreted:

(1) *Exotoxins* which are liberated by live bacteria and disseminated by the blood. Bacteria having this property include the *C. diphtheriae, clostridia, Strep. haemolyticus*, the shigella and certain strains of the staphylococcus.
(2) *Endotoxins* which are enclosed in the bacterial cell and are liberated with the lysis of the dead cell. This is the more common kind of toxin.

N.B. — Poisoning of the body with toxins is known as *toxaemia*.

Secretion of enzymes

Microbes secrete enzymes to break down complex organic compounds for their own use. Some of the enzymes are used therapeutically in human medicine, e.g.:

(1) Streptokinase-streptodornase (Varidase) are bacterial enzymes which liquify fibrinous exudate and fibrin of a blood clot.
(2) The antibiotics are enzymes derived principally from moulds. These enzymes are harmful to the microbes.
(3) Certain bacteria, called haemolytic, secrete enzymes which break up (haemolyse) red blood cells. If cultured on a blood-enriched, solid medium in the laboratory, their colonies are surrounded by a pale area of haemolysis in the blood-red medium.

Multiplication

Multiplication or growth of microbes takes place by asexual splitting of one cell into two daughter cells. This is called binary fission.

CONDITIONS FOR GROWTH AND MULTIPLICATION OF MICROBES (LOWER PROTISTS)

Temperature

The optimum (best) temperature for the growth of pathogenic microbes is 30 °C–37 °C. Higher and lower temperatures inhibit the rate of growth until it ceases altogether at 16,7 °C and 42,2 °C respectively. As the temperature rises above 42,2 °C bacteriolysis takes place gradually. At boiling point all microbes, except spores, are destroyed, provided they are exposed to the heat for a sufficiently long period. Cold does not destroy microbes.

Nutrition

Microbes require the following chemical elements for their existence: O_2, H_2, N, C, S, P, Ca, K, Mg, Na and Fe. They contain no chlorophyll and are, therefore, dependent upon the vegetable and animal kingdoms for their food supplies, as is man. The nutritive elements may be dead or alive in the case of the majority of the microbes; they can, therefore, be grown on or in nutritive media in the laboratory. These media contain protein, sugar, blood, serum, and bile in different combinations. Some media are in the form of a liquid broth, while others are solidified by the addition of agar. For bacterial growth vitamin B complex is especially important. The sulphonamides exert their bacteriostatic action for the very reason that they replace one of the vitamins of the B complex. The strictly parasitic organisms, such as the chlamydia and rickettsiae, however, require live and actively-growing tissues for growth and multiplication. For this purpose hatching eggs and kidney tissue of the Rhesus monkey, cultivated to grow in a special medium, are used.

Reaction of the medium

The majority of pathogenic organisms live best in a slightly alkaline medium, i.e. pH 7,2 to 7,6. An acid medium is unfavourable for most microbes.

Moisture

Water is essential for the growth of the microbes. Multiplication cannot take place on a dry surface, non-sporing bacteria dying after two hours. Dried spores, however, may remain viable for twenty years.

Darkness

All micro-organisms multiply more rapidly in the dark than in the light. Direct sunlight is bacteriolytic on account of the ultraviolet rays.

Oxygen

All microbes require oxygen in order to live, but some cannot utilise the free oxygen in the air. Hence the following kinds of microbes are differentiated:

(1) *Obligate aerobes:* They grow best in atmospheric air and free oxygen is essential for multiplication.
    Examples: *M. tuberculosis*, gonococcus, *B. anthracis*.
(2) *Obligate anaerobes:* They cannot grow in the presence of free oxygen. As example, we can take the clostridia which grow in deep traumatic wounds. Growth of anaerobes is arrested by the presence of oxygen.
(3) *Facultative anaerobes:* A great many aerobic bacteria are facultative anaerobes because they can live in the absence or presence of free oxygen.

The staphylococcus

The staphylococcus is found everywhere — in dust, in the nose, in the air, in sewage, milk and fomites, although it normally lives luxuriantly on the intact skin and the intestinal canal of man and animals.

Only some of the staphylococci are pathogenic and cause the formation of thick, yellow pus. There are two main kinds.

The *Staphylococcus aureus* (forming golden colonies on cultivation) grows in any tissue in the body and causes an acute abscess. On the skin it causes boils, carbuncles and impetigo contagiosa. It can also cause enterocolitis and an intoxication through food poisoning.

The *Staphylococcus albus* (forming white colonies on cultivation) is a normal skin commensal which is sometimes pathogenic, but is never as virulent as the *Staphylococcus aureus*. It causes acne vulgaris and stitch abscesses, as well as gastro-enterocolitis if infected food is ingested, and subacute bacterial endocarditis.

Staphylococci multiply readily outside the body and can resist desiccation. They are destroyed by the usual methods of sterilisation, but in the human body they are inclined to become insensitive to one antibiotic after another. The so-called 'Hospital Staphylococcus' causes much sepsis of wounds because it is resistant to a large number of antibiotics.

The streptococcus

The streptococcus is found everywhere, some strains being pathogens while others are potential pathogens (opportunists). Streptococci are capable of causing haemolysis through the action of enzymes, streptolysin O and S, some strains causing greater destruction to erythrocytes than others, e.g. the beta haemolytic streptococcus. Streptococci can be classified according to Lancefield grouping, each different group being designated by a letter, e.g. A, B, C, etc. Lancefield grouping is based on the specific antigenic structure of the carbohydrate layer of the microbe.

The following kinds of streptococci are important in human medicine:

Streptococcus agalactiae — Beta haemolytic streptococcus, Lancefield Group B. This organism is part of the flora of the female genital tract. Under certain abnormal conditions of labour, the organism may be inhaled by the infant and cause neonatal meningitis or septicaemia.

Streptococcus viridans secretes a pale green substance (haemolysis) when growing on a culture medium. It forms part of the flora of the mouth, nose and throat. After tooth extraction it may gain entry to the bloodstream and cause subacute bacterial endocarditis in a person with damaged heart valves.

Streptococcus pneumoniae causes opportunistic infection of air passages, pneumonia and meningitis. It has recently become a dangerous, multiple resistant organism.

The opportunistic *Streptococcus faecalis* forms part of the intestinal flora.

Streptococcus pyogenes — Beta haemolytic streptococcus, Lancefield Group A. This is a virulent, pathogenic organism which is very sensitive to destruction by penicillin. It may be disseminated by throat carriers. It produces virulent toxins and causes the formation of thin pus and the following pathological conditions:

(1) Erysipelas — a streptococcal infection of the skin.
(2) Cellulitis — a spreading infection of the subcutaneous tissue.
(3) Gastro-enterocolitis caused by food-borne infection.
(4) Scarlet fever — no longer a notifiable disease. The erythrogenic exotoxin of a par-

ticular strain of the haemolytic streptococcus is responsible for the characteristic scarlatiniform rash of scarlet fever (erythema punctata).
(5) Rheumatic fever and acute glomerulonephritis. These delayed sequelae are immune responses of the host to the toxins elaborated by haemolytic streptococci, especially after repeated attacks of acute tonsillitis (see p. 545).

The clostridia

The clostridia may be harmless inhabitants of the intestinal tract. They harm the body when they enter the tissues through a wound and become established in a suitable medium for growth.

The clostridia are found in:

(1) the intestinal tract of man and beast and, therefore, in faecal matter;
(2) in soil and street sweepings which contain manure, especially horse manure.

The clostridia are spore-forming anaerobes and are very resistant to destruction. Spores are killed either by dry heat at 160 °C for one hour and 140 °C for two hours, or by superheated steam under pressure.

The *Clostridium tetani* causes tetanus (see p. 549). Infection takes place after deep inoculation of the tissues with the microbes, i.e. after stab wounds, especially those caused by thorns in the veld where animals graze. Street accidents are also a hazard. The clostridia cause little local damage, but they secrete a powerful exotoxin which affects the anterior horn cells of the spinal cord, thus giving rise to spasmodic contractions of the muscles whenever there is sensory stimulation.

Clostridia causing gas gangrene

There are several kinds of which the *Cl. perfringens* and *Cl. septicum* are the most important. They may cause wound and puerperal sepsis without necessarily giving rise to acute, fulminating gas gangrene which is usually fatal. Tissue trauma is the essential condition for infection by these clostridia. Gas gangrene is prone to occur after street accidents with extensive injuries, or in war casualties. After infection by the clostridia of gas gangrene, a widespread putrefaction of tissues takes place with the formation of gas (H_2 and CO_2). The powerful exotoxin liberated causes haemolysis and liver damage with jaundice.

VIRUSES

Viruses are subcellular particles that pass through the smallest filter and are visible only under an electron microscope. They live parasitically inside the cells of the host. The virus consists of a virion (the parasitic particle) surrounded by a protective protein coat, the capsid. The capsid is lost after the virus enters the host cell. The virion consists of nucleic acid, either DNA or RNA (see p. 110) which may be either single- or doublestranded. The virion has an inner core and an outer envelope, both of which have antigenic properties which elicit antibody (immunoglobulin) production.

Multiplication of the virus is by replication of its nucleic acid after the virus has taken control of its host cell's enzymes to change the host cell into a virus-producing factory. The host cell may either disintegrate ('lyse') or remain in equilibrium with the virus; or it may change its function (e.g. if it is a bacterium) and become capable of producing toxins, e.g. the erythrogenic toxin produced by the *Streptococcus pyogenes* in scarlet fever.

Viruses are shed from the host cell and infect other cells or they can be released into the environment and infect other individuals. After infection they cause a primary and then a secondary viraemia.

Viruses usually have specific target organs, e.g. the nervous system in the case of poliomyelitis. Measles and rubella viruses first affect the respiratory tract and eventually cause skin rashes.

Classification of medically important viruses

- Respiratory
  Influenza virus type A, B, and C.
  Respiratory syncitial virus.
  Adenovirus causing acute respiratory infection.
- Rabdovirus of rabies and Marburg disease.

- Gastro-intestinal: enterovirus, rotavirus, adenovirus.
- Common cold: rhinovirus, echovirus.
- Herpes viruses: Herpes 1 (lip); Herpes 11 (genital); varicella; cytomegalovirus; Epstein-Barr (EBV) of mononucleosis.
- Slow viruses: polio; measles; mumps; rubella; hepatitis A and B.
- Arboviruses (those transmitted by arthropods, e.g. ticks and mosquitos): dengue fever; yellow fever; haemorrhagic diseases, e.g. lassa fever; Congo fever.
- Retroviruses: HIV (of AIDS); sarcoma; T-cell leukaemia.
- Human papillomaviruses: warts; condyloma and papilloma. Several types may be responsible for cancer of the cervix.[1]

In the past viruses were detected by tissue culture which took 7 days to complete, and animal inoculation. Former lengthy virus identification and antibody detection tests are being replaced by tests which ensure rapid viral diagnosis, the tests being completed within one day. Thus it is now possible to establish a quick clinical diagnosis; this is especially important for those virus diseases which can be treated by chemotherapy, e.g. influenza A, herpes and condyloma.

Examples of tests

Antigen

- Direct nucleic acid detection for respiratory viruses.
- Various ELISA (Enzyme-linked Immunosorbo) assays.
- Latex agglutination test.
- Initial tissue culture (for 24 hours) followed by fluorescent antibody stain for genital herpes and other viruses.

Antibodies

- Latex agglutination; IgM ELISA.
- IgM-specific antibody test for recent infection.[1]

REFERENCE

(1) Sever L. Future perspectives in virology — diagnosis, treatment and immunoprophylaxis. *S Afr Med J* 1986; Supplement.

TEST OF KNOWLEDGE

The student has benefited from studying this chapter if he/she can answer the following questions:

(1) Distinguish between bacteria and viruses with regard to the following:
   (a) size;
   (b) structure;
   (c) harmfulness (virulence);
   (d) multiplication.
(2) Define:
   (a) Opportunistic infection.
   (b) Pathogenic microbes.
   (c) Potential pathogens.
   (d) Lower protists.
   (e) The immunocompromised patient.
   (f) Aerobic microbes.
   (g) Protozoa.
(3) Write notes on:
   (a) Fungi and their reproduction.
   (b) The Gram stain and its use in the identification of bacteria.
   (c) Bacterial nutrition for growth.
   (d) The chlamydia.
   (e) Bacterial resistance to destruction.
(4) Distinguish between:
   (a) Exotoxins and endotoxins.
   (b) Mycobacteria and mycoplasma.
   (c) Bacterial spores and fungal spores.
   (d) Obligate and facultative anaerobes.

26

Infection
Immunology and Immunity

GENERAL OBJECTIVE

This chapter introduces the nursing student to the subjects of specific infection and the way in which the body naturally resists infection — immunology.

Immunisation, the cornerstone of the fight against infections, is discussed in Chapter 28.

STUDY OBJECTIVES

These are to get to know the general characteristics of communicable diseases — specific infective diseases — their degree of communicability, their mode of infection, the spread of microbes in and outside the body, their incubation periods and periods of infectivity and some of their specific signs, e.g. the rashes which characterise some diseases.

The subject of immunology and immunity needs careful study to give the student an understanding of the ways in which the body resists and overcomes infection, either naturally or artificially by immunisation.

IN THIS CHAPTER

INFECTION

The pathological effects of the invasion of the body by microbes is called infection. A disease caused by infection is called an infective disease; such a disease is infectious, i.e. it can spread from one person to another; it is, therefore, communicable. The pathological effects of infection become manifest when the multiplication of the microbes cannot be halted and tissues are destroyed and poisoned by the microbial toxins. Infection thus harms the body by causing localised inflammation and tissue destruction, and generalised ill-health when the microbes and/or their toxins are disseminated throughout the body by the bloodstream to cause *septicaemia* or *bacteraemia and toxaemia*.

Infection may be either specific or non-specific. A *specific infection* is caused by one particular organism, e.g. diphtheria is a specific infective disease as it is always caused by the *Corynebacterium diphtheriae*. A *non-specific infection* of a circumscribed area of the body is an infection which can be caused by any one of a number of microbes. Cystitis is a non-specific infection as it may be caused by either *Proteus vulgaris*, *Pseudomonas pyocyanea*, *Staphylococcus* or *Streptococcus*. Likewise, pneumonia is a non-specific condition. The emphasis in this chapter will be on specific infective diseases.

When the signs and symptoms of an indisposition are of sufficient intensity, duration and specificity to be clinically recognisable as those of a specific infective disease, the person thus affected is a '*clinical case*' of the disease. An '*abortive or suspected case*', recognised only because it occurs in association with clinical cases of the disease, is not of sufficient intensity and duration to permit a clinical diagnosis of the specific disease to be made. When the infection is so slight that the symptoms pass unnoticed, but the presence of the infection is shown by laboratory or other diagnostic tests, then the infection is of a *subclinical degree*. For example, if a healthy person has a positive Mantoux reaction, he is a 'subclinical case' of tuberculosis. The specific infective diseases are transmitted (communicated) from person to person or, in rare instances, from animal to person, either directly or indirectly. They can be classified according to their degree of infectiousness (communicability) as follows:

(1) slightly infectious (communicable) diseases;

(2) highly infectious, epidemic diseases;

(3) endemic infective diseases; and

(4) chronic communicable infective diseases.

SLIGHTLY INFECTIOUS (COMMUNICABLE) DISEASES

The slightly infectious diseases do not require strict isolation. Patients suffering from these diseases can be nursed in a general ward, provided reasonable care is taken to disinfect the stools (in the case of infective hepatitis and the dysenteries), the skin discharges (in the case of erysipelas) and the cutlery and crockery (in the case of glandular fever).

Examples:

- Glandular fever (infective mononucleosis)
- Erysipelas
- Herpes zoster (shingles)
- Amoebic dysentery
- Infective hepatitis
- Bacillary dysentery
- Malta fever (brucellosis).

HIGHLY INFECTIOUS (COMMUNICABLE) EPIDEMIC DISEASES

These are the acute infective diseases which can also be called acute febrile (feverish) diseases. While suffering from one of the following febrile diseases, the patient needs to be isolated from the healthy members of the community: enteric fever, cholera, poliomyelitis, whooping cough, influenza, measles, diphtheria, cerebrospinal meningitis, encephalitis, chicken-pox.

The main characteristics of acute infective diseases are:

(1) They are highly infectious and are likely to occur in epidemics.
  Epidemic is the term used to describe the outbreak of an infective disease affecting a large number of people at the same time in a limited specified area, for example, a city, town or district. *Pandemic* is the term used to describe the outbreak of a world-wide epidemic. Influenza and cholera sometimes assume pandemic proportions.
  Epizootic is a disease attacking a large number of animals at the same time, akin to an epidemic in human beings.
(2) One attack usually confers lifelong immunity.
(3) They are characterised by *toxaemia* or by *bacteraemia* and in many cases a rash (erup-

tion), in which case they are called *exanthemata*.
(4) They follow a definite pattern consisting of *five stages*.

Signs and symptoms of toxaemia (and bacteraemia)

Fever

The temperature is raised, i.e. the patient is febrile. This is sometimes initiated by a rigor in adults and convulsions in children. The pulse and respiratory rates are raised in proportion to the temperature.

Nervous system

Symptoms are:

(1) Headache and malaise (general unwell feeling).
(2) Mental dullness and stupor.
(3) Delirium with hallucinations (the patient sees and hears thing that do not exist).
(4) Typhoid state with carphologia (plucking at the bedclothes), low, muttering delirium, noisiness at night and stupor during the day, incontinence, and eventually coma vigil (unconsciousness with staring eyes).

Note: Delirium and typhoid state are indicative of extreme toxaemia. In the modern antibiotic age, these conditions are rare.

Alimentary tract

Symptoms are:

(1) Anorexia, nausea and vomiting.
(2) Dehydration with constipation, dry coated tongue and sordes.
(3) Loss of weight with sunken eyes and dry, wrinkled skin.
(4) Herpes febrilis (fever blisters).

Urinary system

Symptoms are oliguria with high SG and albuminuria.

Characteristic rashes

Note: An external rash is termed an *exanthem*, and a rash on a mucous membrane an *enanthem*.

In chicken-pox (varicella) the rash appears on the second day of the disease and is seldom found on the distal parts of the extremities. This distribution is called centripetal (seeking the centre). The rash appears in the following order: macules, papules, vesicles then pustules which later encrust. Crops come out at different times so that all stages of the rash may be present concurrently. The rash affects the epidermis and in uncomplicated cases should leave no scars.

In *scarlet fever* the exanthem appears on the second day of the disease, and desquamation (shedding of the skin) lasts from the sixth to the twenty-first day. The characteristic exanthem is an *erythema punctata* of the entire body, the face being flushed with circumoral (around the mouth) pallor. The enanthem on the inside of the mouth, tongue and throat is a bright red flush, with puncta on the palate.

In *measles* (morbilli) the prodromal granular eruption (Koplik's spots) and bright red enanthem appear on the buccal mucosa before the exanthem which erupts on the fourth day of the disease. The exanthematous eruption is brick-red and macular, many macules coalescing to form coarse, blotchy, crescentic patches over the face and trunk. The rash starts behind the ears and on the face and spreads over the entire body within twenty-four hours. It starts to disappear on the second day and is followed by a fine branny desquamation of the skin. The patient suffers from photophobia, conjunctivitis and blepharitis (enanthem on the eyelids).

In *German measles* (rubella) the pink, discrete and moderately fine macular exanthem appears on the second day of the disease. It starts on the face, spreads over the entire body within twenty-four hours, and disappears progressively within forty-eight hours. It is accompanied by suboccipital, axillary and inguinal glandular enlargement.

In *typhoid fever* the rash consists of rose-coloured spots (macules) — approximately twelve in number — which appear on the abdomen, a few at a time, from the ninth day onward for a few days.

The five stages of an acute infective disease

Stage 1

The first stage is the *incubation period* which extends from the time of contamination of the

tissues until the first signs of infection appear, during which time the patient is sickening for the disease. This period varies from short to medium or long, for example —

Infection	Incubation period: maximum range
Short incubation periods (less than 7 days)	
Anthrax	2–5 days
Bacillary dysentery	1–7 days
Cholera	Hours–5 days
Diphtheria	2–5 days
Gonorrhoea	2–5 days
Meningococcaemia	2–10 days
Scarlet fever	1–3 days
Intermediate incubation periods (7–21 days)	
Amoebiasis	14–28 days
Brucellosis	7–21 days
Chicken-pox	14–21 days
Lassa fever	7–14 days
Malaria	10–14 days
Measles	7–14 days
Mumps	12–21 days
Whooping cough	7–10 days
Poliomyelitis	3–21 days
Psittacosis	4–14 days
Rubella	14–21 days
Trypanosoma rhodesiense infection	14–21 days
Typhoid fever	7–21 days
Typhus fever	7–14 days
Long incubation periods (more than 21 days)	
Filariasis	3 months or more
Hepatitis A	2–6 weeks
Hepatitis B	6 weeks–6 months
Primary tuberculosis	4–6 weeks
Leprosy	Months–years
Rabies	Variable
Trypanosoma gambiense infection	Weeks–years
Syphilis	10 days–10 weeks Mean: 3 weeks

Stage 2

The *prodromal stage* (or stage of invasion) is the most infectious period and extends from the appearance of the first symptom of the ailment until the first characteristic signs and symptoms of the disease, usually a rash, appear. During this period the temperature rises, the patient feels very ill, and sometimes a prodromal rash appears.

Stage 3

The fastigium (culminating point) is the advanced stage extending from the appearance of the first characteristic signs of the disease, and lasts for as long as the temperature remains elevated and the rash, if present, is visible.

Stage 4

The defervescent stage (or stage of decline) starts from the time when the patient improves; the temperature subsides and the rash disappears. Some infective diseases, for example typhoid fever, were characterised by relapses during this period, before the use of chloramphenicol.

Stage 5

The convalescent stage occurs after the infection has been completely overcome. The patient's general condition is low and requires a diet rich in protein to replace broken-down tissue.

ACUTE ENDEMIC INFECTIVE DISEASES

An endemic infective disease is spread indirectly by means of biological vectors (e.g. mosquitoes, lice), or by carriers and sporadic cases who contaminate the water and food supplies of a community.

Endemic: A disease is said to be endemic when the causative microbes are constantly harboured in a certain area, for example, malaria occurs where the anopheles mosquito breeds, i.e. in a hot and damp climate, e.g. the Transvaal lowveld; and sleeping sickness occurs where the tsetse fly breeds, e.g. Central Africa. Cholera occurs where there is no safe, reticulated supply of water.

Note:
(1) The term endemic can be used to denote the continued presence of any disease, whether infectious or not, in a specific locality.
(2) A disease of animals which is indigenous to an area is called an enzootic.

Patients suffering from vector-borne endemic infective diseases need not be isolated, provided the biological vectors have been eradicated. The insect or animal vector is the intermediate host of the microbe and, therefore, the disease cannot be transmitted directly from man

to man. Pneumonic plague is an exception because it is transmitted by droplet infection.

- *Malaria:* transmitted by the anopheles mosquito.
- *Yellow fever:* transmitted by the *Aedes Aegypti* mosquito.
- *Typhus fever:* transmitted by the rat flea or the louse.
- *Tick-bite fever:* transmitted by the small, red tick.
- *Schistosomiasis:* transmitted by the freshwater snail.
- *Trypanosomiasis:* transmitted by the tsetse fly.
- *Bubonic plague:* transmitted by the rodent flea.

Note: Plague is a disease of rodents. In South Africa the main wild rodent reservoirs of *Yersinia pestis* are gerbilles — wild field mice. There are many inland areas in South Africa where plague is enzootic and occasionally occurs in epizootic form (i.e. assumes epidemic proportions in animals). Human plague is a rare disease but is still found in South Africa, the last outbreak (18 cases) occurring in 1982.

CHRONIC COMMUNICABLE INFECTIVE DISEASES

These diseases can be communicable to a greater or lesser extent. Leprosy and tuberculosis are the most important chronic infections which may require isolation care in isolation hospitals.

AIDS and syphilis are blood-borne diseases and do not require care in isolation hospitals.

TRANSMISSION OF MICROBES

Portals of entry

(1) By ingestion (swallowing) of microbes which affect the tonsils and the gastro-intestinal tract whence they may be absorbed into the bloodstream. Examples: enteric fever, dysentery.

(2) By inhalation of infected dust or droplets of sputum. The microbes gain entry to the body through the Eustachian tubes, tonsils or lungs. Examples: diphtheria, influenza, whooping-cough, measles.

(3) By inoculation through the skin or mucous membrane. This may take place by —

    (*a*) a puncture made by an injection needle or insect bite or sting, or through a wound; examples: tetanus, gas gangrene, insect-borne diseases, AIDS;

(b) direct contact of microbes with susceptible mucous membranes, for example the conjunctiva, bladder and the genital tract, and with soggy skin (in fungous infections).

(4) Through the placenta, e.g. congenital syphilis, rubella.

Spread of microbes in the body

If the local inflammatory reaction of the tissues is not powerful enough to combat the invading microbes, infection may spread in one of the following ways.

Directly from cell to cell

In the skin, direct spread occurs in *erysipelas*, and in the subcutaneous tissues the spreading infection is known as *cellulitis*. Cellulitis is an acute spreading inflammatory process in which there is at first no localising pus-formation. The causative organism of a spreading infection which does not localise is usually the haemolytic streptococcus. Infection may also spread directly from the lungs to the pleura.

Through the natural channels

The infected secretions and excretions flow along the ducts and infect organs *en route*. Infection can therefore spread from, for example:

(1) the kidneys to the bladder via the ureters;
(2) the gall-bladder to the pancreas via the bile and pancreatic ducts;
(3) the nose to the larynx and trachea, via the pharynx.

Through the lymphatic vessels to the regional lymph nodes

A pyogenic infection may cause *lymphangitis* (inflammation of lymphatic vessel). It is characterised by a painful red line under the skin. Resultant inflammation of the lymph node is known as *lymphadenitis*. It is characterised by a painful, swollen gland. Lymphadenitis is a protective mechanism whereby bacteria in the lymph stream are destroyed before they gain entry to the bloodstream. Should the lymph nodes fail to stop the infection, bacteria will gain

entry to the bloodstream through the subclavian vein, via the right lymphatic or the thoracic ducts.

Through the bloodstream

The following conditions are characterised by the presence of bacteria in the blood:

(1) *Bacteraemia.* This means the transient presence of bacteria in the blood during transit from the portal of entry to the susceptible organ, or by intermittent distribution from the primary focus. It is characteristic of many acute infective diseases, for example meningitis and typhoid fever.

(2) *Septicaemia.* This denotes the more permanent presence of bacteria in the blood. In contrast to bacteraemia, bacteria are distributed constantly from the primary focus of infection. It is an extremely dangerous kind of blood poisoning, for example meningococcal and streptococcal septicaemia and septicaemic plague. It is a common cause of death in immunocompromised patients.

(3) *Pyaemia.* This denotes the presence of pus in the blood from septic emboli which have their origin in a pyelophlebitis (purulent inflammation of a vein) adjacent to infections. The pus is carried by the blood to other organs, causing multiple metastatic (secondary) abscesses.

Note: AIDS and syphilis are sexually transmitted diseases which are blood-borne.

Reaction of the body to infection

The body's reaction is either non-specific or specific.

Non-specific

(1) The formation of large numbers of antibodies by the plasma cells (B-lymphocytes) in response to the dissemination of microbes.

(2) Leucocytosis, i.e. the physiological increase in leucocytes. The granulocytes (polymorphs) and monocytes are the phagocytic leucocytes of the blood, i.e. they engulf the bacteria. The degree of leucocytosis is an indication of the resistance of the body. In leucocytosis all the varieties of white cells are not necessarily increased. This relative

increase of particular cells is an important diagnostic tool, viz:

(a) Neutrophilia (increase in neutrophil granulocytes) in pyogenic infections.

(b) Monocytosis (increase in monocytes) in tuberculosis, syphilis, brucellosis and malaria.

(c) Lymphocytosis (increase in lymphocytes) in chronic inflammatory states, i.e. the active stage of tuberculosis and syphilis, and in malaria, mumps and whooping-cough.

(d) Eosinophilia (increase in eosinophils) in allergic conditions and worm infestations of intestines.

(3) Increase in temperature (pyrexia).

Heat production and loss are controlled by the hypothalamus on the base of the brain, the thermoregulatory centre in the hypothalamus being likened to a thermostat. Elevation of the body temperature is called fever or pyrexia. In fever the thermoregulatory centre is set to a higher level; heat production and loss occur in the normal way, but at this higher level.

Substances circulating in the blood which cause the rise in body temperature are called pyrogens. Pyrogens may be either exogenous (e.g. particles introduced into the circulation by intravenous injection), or endogenous, i.e. formed in the body.

Many factors stimulate the release of pyrogens by phagocytes (monocytes and macrophages, but excluding neutrophils), viz. infections (viruses, bacteria, fungi, protozoa), toxins (e.g. endotoxins), immune complexes, as well as lymphokines released by antigen-sensitised lymphocytes. Endogenous pyrogens are small proteins which act on the thermoregulatory centre. Information from here is transmitted to the vasomotor centre in the medulla oblongata to increase heat generation and prevent heat loss. The message is probably conveyed by prostaglandin E_2 which is locally produced.[1]

Note: Certain neoplasms, e.g. lymphomas, and rare diseases, e.g. hypothalamic lesions, may cause pyrexia by directly influencing the hypothalamus.

Specific

Specific reaction entails either a humoral or cell-mediated immunological response. (See p. 473.)

The resistance of the body to infection

Factors promoting resistance

(1) Healthy, unbroken skin and mucous membrane which are impermeable to bacteria. An essential requirement for health is that the skin be dry and the mucous membranes moist.

(2) The hydrochloric acid in the stomach, which destroys many bacteria ingested with the food.

(3) The presence of intestinal flora, consisting principally of *Lactobacillus acidophilus, Streptococcus faecalis* and coliform bacilli. These bacteria are antagonistic to the pathogenic bacteria.

(4) The bile in the duodenum, which destroys many pathogenic bacteria.

(5) The tears, which are slightly antiseptic and mechanically remove particulate matter.

(6) The airway, which reacts to the presence of bacteria and dust by an increased secretion of mucus and movement of the cilia, in order that the foreign bodies and mucus may be expelled by coughing and sneezing.

(7) The acidity of the adult vagina, which inhibits the growth of pathogenic bacteria.

(8) The presence of antibodies and leucocytes in the blood.

(9) Good health ensures good resistance. Good health is achieved not only by attention to the rules of personal hygiene but also by psychological security which ensures the absence of anxiety and tension, emotional states which prevent the normal functioning and health of the body.

(10) Immunity.

Factors lowering resistance

(1) Sudden lowering of body temperature. Cooling causes vasoconstriction and thereby lowers resistance sufficiently for the virus of the common cold, and the pneumococcus to cause infection of the mucous membrane of the airway.

(2) Malnutrition. This is the most important cause of lowered resistance. The food elements especially concerned are contained in the protective foods, viz. the anti-infective vitamins A and C, and proteins which are

essential for the formation of leucocytes and antibodies.

(3) Fatigue. This lowers the resistance by causing an accumulation of waste products in the body, which act as tissue poisons.

(4) Destruction of the intestinal flora by the ingestion of antibiotics, whereby the non-sensitive fungus, *Candida albicans*, gains ascendancy and causes, *inter alia*, inflammation of the intestines.

(5) Drying of the mucous membranes and maceration (sogginess) of the skin.

(6) Anxiety and tension caused by conflict and fear, which influence the autonomic and endocrine functions of the body adversely.

THE SPREAD OF MICROBES OUTSIDE THE BODY

The spread of infection implies the spread of microbes. It is, therefore, important that the nurse should know the sources of microbes, the factors limiting or encouraging their growth, how they can be destroyed and, most important of all, how they are spread, in order to enable her to contribute intelligently to the protection of patients against cross-infection, and to help in the enlightenment of the public.

The precautionary measures taken against the spread of pathogenic microbes are:

(1) Isolation and treatment of the source of the infection.

(2) Protection against, and disinfection of, contaminated media.

(3) Combating the dissemination of the microbes.

The source of infection

Sufferers

Either a clinically recognisable case, or an abortive case, or a subclinical case.

Contacts

Persons who have been in contact with the disease.

A contact may be either:

(1) immune; or
(2) susceptible.

An immune contact means any person who, owing to his having contracted a certain com-

municable disease in the past, or because he has been successfully immunised against it, is not likely to contract the disease again on exposure thereto.

A susceptible contact means a person —

(1) who has not previously contracted a certain communicable disease;

(2) who has not previously been immunised successfully against such communicable disease;

(3) in respect of whom the period of immunity after successful immunisation against such communicable disease has lapsed.

(From Act 63 of 1977.)

Carriers

A carrier means a person who, although not exhibiting clinical symptoms of a communicable disease at the time, is for well-founded reasons and after a laboratory or other tests, suspected of being thus infected and who could therefore spread such a communicable disease (from Act 63 of 1977). Types of diseases which are characterised by the carrier condition are: typhoid (enteric), diphtheria, poliomyelitis, cerebro-spinal meningitis and streptococcal infection of the throat, cholera, amoebiasis, shigellosis and malaria.

Birds and animals

Man is susceptible to the following animal diseases (zoonoses):

■ Psittacosis (of parrots)
■ Hydrophobia (rabies) (of dogs, meerkats)
■ Tapeworm (of pigs, cattle and dogs)
■ Foot-and-mouth disease (of cattle)
■ Leptospirosis (rats and other animals)
■ Plague (of rats)
■ Malta fever (brucellosis) (of cows)
■ Bovine tuberculosis (of cows)
■ Actinomycosis (of cattle)
■ Anthrax (of cattle)

Portals of exit from the body

(1) The anus. Infected stools may contaminate water supplies and food.

(2) The urethra which gives exit to the urine, which may be infected with bilharzia eggs, tuberculosis, common organisms causing cystitis and enteric fever.

(3) Pus and bacteria from mucous membranes and wounds. In sexually transmitted diseases, direct contact between skin and mucous membrane lesions between two people is necessary for infection to take place, but indirect contact through fingers, flies and fomites cause wound infections.

(4) Mouth and nose. Infected sputum may be sneezed out, coughed up or expelled while talking.

(5) Blood leaving the body via needles (e.g. blood transfusions), and blood-sucking insect vectors may infect others.

The contaminated media

The best medium for the growth of parasitic microbes is the body of the host. On being shed from the body in its discharges, the microbes do not necessarily die, as they may land in a medium favourable for their growth and multiplication, for example:

(1) the discharges themselves as long as they remain moist, especially pus and faeces;

(2) water, milk, raw fruit and vegetables, tinned foods, raw meat, and food prepared for public consumption, especially cold meats and meat pies;

(3) manured soil and street dust.

Disseminators of microbes

(1) Passive disseminators include the following:
   (a) dust in the air near an infected person;
   (b) fine droplets (aerosol) of sputum in the air disseminated by coughing, sneezing or talking; this gives rise to *droplet (aerosol) infection*;
   (c) fomites (objects), for example bed linen, cutlery, crockery and surgical dressing equipment.

(2) Active transmitters may be mechanical or biological vectors (carriers):
   (a) mechanical vectors are flies, rats, mice, cockroaches, human hands and contacts; a contact is a person who has been in contact with the disease himself, carries the microbes on his body and thus serves as a temporary source of infection;
   (b) biological vectors which serve as intermediate hosts for the infection. They are: lice, fleas, tsetse flies, ticks, snails and mosquitoes.

(3) The placenta. Fortunately very few diseases are transmitted from the mother to the foetus in this way. Syphilis, rubella and AIDS may affect the foetus *in utero* so that it either dies or is born with the disease (congenital). Toxoplasmosis in its destructive form is also a congenital disease.

The housefly (*Musca domestica*)

The fly is a mechanical vector of a large number of diseases, e.g. those of the alimentary tract (especially AID and bacillary dysentery) and ophthalmia with purulent discharge.

The adult fly feeds upon fluids, the infected fluids being fresh excreta, pus and rotting and fermenting matter. The fluid is sucked up through its proboscis (elongated part of its mouth). It deposits the microbes in the infected fluids on food, mucous membranes, etc. by means of its hairy, sticky feet, its own infected excreta and vomitus, the latter being used to dissolve solids, e.g. sugar.

The female fly lays eggs, 2 000 in a life lasting 6–8 weeks, in a place where the larvae (maggots) will be able to find food, principally decaying matter, either vegetable or animal. The maggots, which look like little white worms, hatch after 12–24 hours and feed voraciously, breaking down organic matter. Maggots have been used to 'clean' sloughing wounds. The maggots, fully grown in a few days, move to a drier place, either sand or a dry shelter, where they pupate. No further growth takes place and after a few days the fully grown, adult fly emerges.

Flies and their larvae are killed by spray insecticides which contain organophosphates and pyrethroids. During spraying the room must be shut and left thus for 15 minutes. Food, food utensils and water must not be contaminated by the insecticide. Sticky fly strips can be positioned to trap the flies. Fine mesh is used to prevent entry of flies into buildings.

Note: The main way of combating the fly menace is to destroy their breeding places, especially if they are in the vicinity of the house.

IMMUNOLOGY

Immunology is the science which deals with immunity, induced sensitivity and allergy (Stedman).

The immune response — the specific biological defence system

Immune is the state of being resistant or relatively resistant to an infective disease.

The immune response occurs in two separate but co-operative ways:

(a) recognition by lymphocytes and the body's histocompatibility (HLA) molecules of foreign antigens;
(b) elimination of antigens by effector mechanisms, i.e. phagocytosis, antibody and killer T-cells (lymphocyte) action and complement activation.

Recognition of antigens

The specific immune reaction depends on the body's ability to recognise the potentially harmful nature of invading microbes and irritants — the so-called antigens of external origin. Foreign substances become antigens after they have been subjected to the body's immune processes on at least one previous occasion. This enables the body to recognise their antigenicity. Recognition is thought to be obtained by macrophage engulfment and processing of the foreign protein, in conjunction with the products of the body's own self-recognition histocompatibility (HLA) system.

The properties of an antigen of external origin are:

(a) It is a foreign substance.
(b) It elicits either mainly a humoral (antibody) or mainly a cellular (T-cell) response.
(c) A reaction between antigen and antibody or between antigen and T-lymphocyte ensues.

If the reaction is successful, the antigen is eliminated; either mainly humoral or mainly cell-mediated immunity has been acquired.

The immune response is, therefore, the interaction of humoral and cellular components with antigen. Depending on the nature of the antigen, the response will be either predominantly humoral or predominantly cellular, but sometimes there is a combination of both.

Elimination of antigens

The immune response makes use of three major immunocompetent cell types (the lymphocytes, the polymorphs and the macrophages) and their secretions, the cytokines. Cytokines (including lymphokines and interleukins) act as signals between leucocytes.

Phagocytosis

This is the process by which a phagocyte ingests and digests a substance.

A phagocyte is a cell which is attracted to a foreign protein (microbe, allergen (particle), donor organ cell) or a harmful body cell by a process called chemotaxis, engulfs the foreign protein or body cell and then digests or destroys it by means of enzymes (e.g. lysozymes). Contact between the foreign protein and the phagocyte is essential before phagocytosis can take place.

Phagocytosis is the most important aspect of the biological defence system of the body. The phagocytes of the body are the polymorphs and the macrophages.

(1) The polymorphs are:
    (a) The neutrophils which move through capillary walls to the site of the threat and play the major phagocytic role. Dying neutrophils release lysozymal enzymes which destroy tissues and contribute to the formation of pus (where applicable).
    (b) The eosinophils which are not as efficient at phagocytosis as the neutrophils and are associated with parasitic infestations and allergic inflammatory reactions.
    (c) The basophils which release vaso-active enzymes, e.g. histamine, serotonin.
        The polymorphs (polymorphonuclear leucocytes) are the main white blood cells (leucocytes) of the blood. They play a very important role in inflammation — the body's immediate non-specific reaction to an irritation which has penetrated its superficial defensive barriers, e.g. the skin.
(2) The macrophages form the reticulo-endothelial system (RES). The cells of the RES are spread throughout the body. This mono-

nuclear scavenger system consists of the monocytes of the blood and their precursor cells in the bone marrow, as well as the structurally heterogenous tissue macrophages. The latter are also made in the bone marrow, and are carried by the blood to the tissues. Macrophages exert phagocytic, secretory and antigen-processing functions. The macrophages are the main link between the non-specific and specific defences of the body and are involved in both the inflammatory (non-specific) and immune reactions.

Macrophages have receptors for IgE antibodies on their surface and can react to parasites and allergens. Antigens are processed by the macrophages after engulfment; they are then presented by the macrophages to the T-lymphocytes. This elicits a specific protective immune response.

Examples of tissue macrophages are: histiocytes in the spleen, peritoneal cavity, lymph nodes and bone marrow. Kuppfer cells in the liver, osteoclasts in bone and alveolar (acinar) macrophages in the lungs. Some of these cells are fixed and some are mobile.

Lymphocytes (T-cells and B-cells)

Lymphocytes are produced by the so-called 'stem' cells of the bone marrow. The specific immune apparatus consists of 'virgin' lymphocytes formed from the precursor cells in the bone marrow. They migrate to the primary lymphoid organs (the thymus and the bone marrow) where they become respectively T-cells (thymus dependent) and B-cells. T-cells and B-cells then migrate to the secondary lymphoid organs (spleen and lymph nodes). Their lives are short if they do not meet up with specific antigens in the secondary lymphoid organs. The specific cellular response is dependent on the ability of the lymphocytes to recognise that the invading protein is different or foreign, i.e. that it has antigenic properties. The macrophage is thought to pass knowledge of the antigenic (foreign) properties of the antigen to the lymphocytes after it has engulfed and processed the antigen (as stated before). The HLA system of the body is also implicated.

(a) Cellular defence — the CMI system

The T-lymphocytes are the cellular components of the specific immune response. They comprise 65–75 % of the recirculating lymphocytes. They play the major role in cell-mediated immunity (CMI). T-cells mature under the influence of the thymus.

T-helper (CD4+) cells release macrophage-activating cytokines, also called lymphokines. They consist of interleukins, chemotatic factors, interferons which assist the body's immune response by, for instance, activating macrophages and stimulating B-cells to divide, differentiate and produce antibodies.

T-suppressor cells have a feedback role in immunosuppression.

Cytotoxic (killer) (CD8+) cells kill antigens to which they have been previously exposed.

Note: CD8+ cells also kill cancer cells and donor organ cells; they protect the body against cancer and are responsible for the rejection of donor organ (graft) in transplant surgery.

Cell-mediated immunity is limited to specific infections, e.g. M. tuberculosis, some viruses, (e.g. herpes), Aspergillus, Candida, Histoplasma, Toxoplasma, Pneumocystis. Tuberculin reactions and contact allergy reactions are also cell-mediated.

(b) Humoral defence — the ACP system

The B-cells give rise to the humoral component of the specific immune response. The B-cells differentiate to form memory B-cells and effector B-cells. The latter further develop into plasma cells which are directly responsible for antibody (immunoglobulin) secretion. The antibodies together with complement and phagocytes form the antibody/complement/phagocyte (ACP) system.

The structure of the antibody

The molecule of an immunoglobulin comprises aliquots of 4 polypeptide chains, two called heavy (large) and two called light (smaller). These basic structural units have areas of constant and areas of variable amino acid sequences. Complement attaches to the areas of constant amino acid sequences and antigen to the areas of variable amino acid sequences, an area being specific for one particular antigen. Antibodies vary in size from 2–5 basic units.

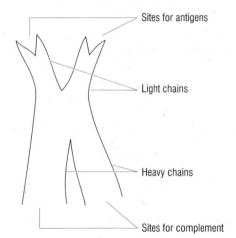

Figure 26.1

The antibody molecule

One theory postulates that macrophage-processed antigen gives the variable sequence area of the freshly made, non-specific immunoglobulin the structure which determines its antigenic specificity.

The important protective immunoglobins are:

(1) Gammaglobulins (IgG) will only bind antigens of a specific infection, e.g. measles antibody will only attach measles antigen (virus).

(2) Meu globulins (IgM) will attach (bind) any antigen present in the body, i.e. it is non-specific and is produced early in the immune response.

Note: Immune complexes are produced when IgM or IgG antibodies combine with antigen.

(3) Alpha globulins (IgA) form part of the superficial barrier in all mucous membranes and in body secretions.

(4) IgD occurs in small amounts; it is found on lymphocytes but its exact function is not known.

(5) IgE is the reaginic antibody with an affinity for the mast cells of connective tissue. Atopic persons have an inherited tendency to make IgE antibodies. With increasing exposure to allergens, their bodies build up IgE antibodies.

IgE antibodies become attached to mast cells in the airways and elsewhere in the body. Allergens entering the body will become linked to the IgE on the mast cell. If the sensitised mast cells are located in the airways, contact with allergens will cause an explosive reaction with the liberation of histamine and the symptoms of asthma.

Functions of antibodies

(*a*) Agglutination (aggregation into clumps) and opsonisation (preparation for phagocytosis) of organisations of organisms to facilitate phagocytosis.

(*b*) Lysis of microbes by interaction between antibody and complement.

(*c*) The antibody, antitoxin, combines with toxin to neutralise it.

(*d*) Preventing the adhering of viruses to cells, thus preventing their entry into the cell.

(*e*) Although phagocytic cells can digest and destroy unprepared antigens, they do this much more efficiently if the antigen has been coated by specific antibody and/or complement.

Note: Humoral immunity is especially concerned with extracellular microbes (most species of bacteria and certain susceptible viruses).

The time between initial exposure to the foreign substance and specific antibody production (the primary response) is 2–3 weeks. On subsequent exposure to the antigen, antibodies are produced at a much faster rate and in greater amounts.

Complement activation

The complement complex consists of a group of 9–15 inactive proteolytic enzymes found in normal plasma.

They are activated in sequence either directly by antigen/antibody combinations (immune complexes) or indirectly by endotoxin of Gram-positive bacteria. Activation causes them to activate one another in a serial fashion to cause 'a complement cascade'.

Complement activation aids phagocytosis either directly by causing adherence between micro-organisms and phagocytes to facilitate phagocytosis, or indirectly by attracting neutrophils to the traumatised area and later also lymphocytes if the inflammation becomes chronic. This is called chemotaxis.

IMMUNITY

Immunity means the insusceptibility of the body to infective diseases and conditions. It can be natural or acquired, and specific for a certain disease, or generalised as the 'resistance' of the body. The discussion that follows deals with specific immunity. The immunological process in the body can be described as either humoral or cell-mediated.

Natural immunity

Permanent immunity

Every type of animal is subject only to its own kinds of diseases (species immunity). The human being is insusceptible to the majority of animal diseases, with the exception of anthrax, bovine tuberculosis, rabies, psittacosis and plague. Individuals in a group are relatively resistant to certain infective diseases. This is called group or herd immunity, if a large percentage of the group is immune.

Temporary immunity, for example, in babies

The baby is born with its mother's antibodies and is, therefore, insusceptible to the diseases characterised by humoral immunity to which its mother is immune.

Acquired immunity

This is ensured by the presence of antibodies and lymphocytes in the blood, which are instantly ready to combat pathogenic micro-organisms as they gain entry to the body. Immunity may be acquired as follows:

(1) naturally or artificially;
(2) actively or passively.

Active immunity is achieved when the body manufactures its own immune bodies:

(1) *naturally* — during an attack of an infective disease; or
(2) *artificially* — after inoculation (by injection or scarification) or ingestion of a vaccine. Artificial, active immunity is established only after a few weeks to a few months and lasts from months to many years, even for a lifetime. Artificially acquired immunity is never as reliable as naturally-acquired immunity.

Note: Both humoral and cell-mediated immunity can be acquired actively.

Passive immunity is achieved when the body is given antibodies (gammaglobulins) which have been manufactured by another human being or by an animal, either —

(1) *naturally* — in the breast-fed infant, or
(2) *artificially* — by the injection of human or horse serum, which contains the antibodies. This serum is known as antiserum. It is given immediately after exposure to infection for the purpose of preventing the onset of the infective disease.

Note: Cell-mediated immunity cannot be acquired passively.

Summary of the different kinds of acquired immunity

Active

Natural: by having the disease
Artificial: by inoculation with or ingestion of a vaccine

Passive

Natural: from breast milk
Artificial: by injection of an antiserum

A SUMMARY OF THE DEVELOPMENT OF SPECIFIC IMMUNITY

The specific immune response occurs after the lymphocytes have recognised antigens in the body (i.e. microbes, allergens, donor organ cells). The specific immune response is the interaction of humoral and cellular factors with antigen. An antigen is a foreign protein (dead and live microbes, toxins and more) which have been subjected to the body's immune processes on at least one previous occasion. An antigen stimulates the formation of specific antibodies and/or T-lymphocytes. The response is either predominantly humoral (antibody/complement/phagocyte — the ACP system) or predominantly cellular (the cell-mediated CMI system).

In the CMI system the T-lymphocytes kill antigens to which they have been previously exposed. T-cells also produce a number of soluble mediators on exposure to specific antigens. These so-called lymphokines consist of interleukins, chemotactic factors and interferons which assist the body's immune response. Cell-mediated immunity is limited to a few specific infections, e.g. M. tuberculosis, some viruses, Aspergillus, Candida, Histoplasma, Toxoplasma, Pneumocystis. Tuberculin reactions and contact allergy reactions are also cell-mediated.

In the ACP system, the B-lymphocytes play the dominant role; the B-cells give rise to the plasma cells which are directly responsible for antibody (immunoglobulin) secretion.

A specific antibody is formed against each kind of antigen. Once the body has been stimulated to form a certain antibody, a certain amount remains in the blood. Should the matching antigens gain entry to the body at a later date, the specific antibodies will be mobilised immediately to combat the antigens.

The important protective immunoglobulins are:

(1) Gammaglobulins (IgG) which will only bind antigens of a specific infection, e.g. measles antibody will only attach measles antigen (virus).
(2) Meu globulins (IgM) which will attach (bind) any antigen present in the body, i.e. it is non-specific and is produced early in the immune response.
(3) Alpha globulins (IgA) which form part of the superficial barrier in all mucous membranes and in body secretions.

Functions of antibodies:

(1) Agglutination (aggregation into clumps) and opsonisation (preparation for phagocytosis) of organisms to facilitate phagocytosis.
(2) Lysis of microbes by interaction between antibody and complement.
(3) The antibody, antitoxin, combines with toxin to neutralise it.
(4) Preventing the adhering of viruses to cells, thus preventing their entry into the cell.
(5) Although phagocytic cells can digest and destroy unprepared antigens, they do this much more efficiently if the antigen has been coated with specific antibody and/or complement.

Humoral immunity is especially concerned with extracellular microbes.

The time between initial exposure to the foreign substance and specific antibody production (the primary response) is 2–3 weeks. On subsequent exposure to the antigen, antibodies are produced at a much faster rate and in greater amounts.

REFERENCES

(1) Wood NJ. Fever. *Medicine International* 1984; April: S43–S54.

TEST OF KNOWLEDGE

The student has benefited from studying this chapter if he/she can answer the following questions:

(1) Define the following terms:
    – Incubation period
    – Subclinical infection
    – Fastigium
    – Quarantine
    – Bacteraemia
    – Epidemic and pandemic
    – Enzootic
    – Typhoid state
    – Endemic infective disease
    – Disease carrier
    – Biological vectors of disease
    – Droplet infection
    – Immune contact
(2) Write notes on:
    – Endogenous pyrogens
    – The rash in measles and rubella
    – The prodromal stage of a febrile disease
    – The spread of infection in the body
    – Leucocytosis in infections
    – The resistance of the body to infection
    – The sources of infection
(3) Define immunity and state how it may be acquired.
(4) Distinguish between:
    – Humoral and cell-mediated immunity
    – Active and passive immunity
    – Natural and artificially-acquired active immunity

27

Control of Communicable Diseases

OBJECTIVES

This chapter introduces the student to the public (community) health measures taken to control the communicable diseases, which are South Africa's greatest community health problem amongst blacks. The student must learn about disease surveillance and the role surveillance and immunisation play in the effort to eradicate communicable diseases. The list of legally notifiable diseases must be memorised and the notification process noted.

Regulation 2438 of the Health Act 63 of 1977, relating to communicable diseases, is a very important piece of legislation for local authorities, pupils and teaching institutions, and is aimed at preventing the transmission of communicable disease by animals, insects and parasites and the prevention of malaria.

IN THIS CHAPTER

COMMUNITY HEALTH MEASURES AGAINST THE SPREAD OF INFECTION

Although the Department of Health acts in a subsidising, advisory, supervisory and, if necessary, coercive capacity, the local authorities are essentially the responsible agencies for preventing disease and promoting community health in their areas of jurisdiction. In the absence of a suitable local authority, some other authority may be appointed by the state to take its place, viz. a neighbouring local authority. Local authorities usually appoint medical officers of health (MOH) who may or may not head a health department, depending on the size and complexity of the area. The Health Department of the local authority comprises medical officers, community health nurses (health visitors), health inspectors; its essential functions are maternal and child welfare, family planning and the control of communicable diseases. These functions are included in their overall responsibility for primary health care.

The main function of the community health nurse is the organisation of community health and immunisation clinics and services. The MOH may apply to the Minister of Health to make it compulsory in his area for all births to be reported to the local authority (as well as to the Registrar of Births) so that every mother may be contacted after the birth of her infant and be offered the services of mothercraft experts at the well-baby clinics of the local authority. This contact with

every new mother creates the ideal opportunity for health education, not only with regard to nutrition but also with regard to the prevention of communicable diseases. Every mother is encouraged to subject her infant to a programme of immunisation. (See p. 492.)

According to the Health Act 63 of 1977:

'**20.** (1) Every local authority shall take all lawful, necessary and reasonably practicable measures —

(*a*) to maintain its district at all times in a hygienic and clean condition;

(*b*) to prevent the occurrence within its district of —
  (i) any nuisance;
  (ii) any unhygienic condition;
  (iii) any offensive condition; or
  (iv) any other condition which will or could be harmful or dangerous to the health of any person within its district or the district of any other local authority.
or, where a nuisance or condition referred to in subparagraphs (i) to (iv), inclusive, has so occurred, to abate, or cause to be abated, such nuisance, or remedy, or cause to be remedied, such condition, as the case may be;

(*c*) to prevent the pollution of any water intended for the use of the inhabitants of its district, irrespective of whether such water is obtained from sources within or outside its district, or to purify such water which has become so polluted;

(*d*) to render in its district, subject to the provisions of this Act or any other law, services approved by the Minister for —

  (i) the prevention of communicable diseases;
  (ii) the promotion of the health of persons;
  (iii) the rehabilitation in the community of persons cured of any medical condition,
  (iv) the treatment of diseases and injuries which are normally treated by a general practitioner; and
  (v) the provision of essential medicines, and to co-ordinate such services with due regard to similar services rendered by the Departments of Health or the provincial administration of the province in which its district is situated.'

Note: The prevention of communicable diseases includes all communicable diseases, not only the notifiable ones.

Note: The Health Act 1977 has made provision for provincial health authorities to assume responsibility for all personal health services. This includes the medical care of patients with communicable diseases and the running of ambulance services. The responsibility of the local authority is the prevention of communicable diseases to ensure that the infectious patient does get isolation care, either at home or in a provincial or other type of isolation hospital; the actual medical care of the patient is not the responsibility of the local authority.

The following community health prophylactic measures are, therefore, important tasks of the local authority:

(1) *Education of the public* on the causes and prevention of disease by means of pamphlets, placards, notices in public conveniences and at bilharzia-infested rivers. Health education by community health nurses at clinics and in the community is an important function of the health department of the local authority.

(2) *Extermination of insect and animal (e.g. rat) vectors of diseases.* It is an offence for anyone to harbour these pests on their premises; they can apply to the local authority for advice regarding pest control measures.

(3) *Public water supplies.* The local authority is required by law to prevent the pollution of pure drinking water and to purify water for drinking or domestic purposes, if it has been polluted. (See p. 176.)

(4) *Food.* The sale of unwholesome, diseased or contaminated food (e.g. milk from a tuberculosis-infected herd) is forbidden by law and the local authority must take adequate preventive measures. Dairies, dairy farms, abattoirs and places where food is prepared for public consumption (hospitals, hotels and restaurants) must be controlled. Control includes medical examination of all employees so that carriers of infectious diseases can be traced and prevented from working with food. The inspection of the slaughtering of animals and of meat for public consumption is an important community health control measure. (See p. 168.)

(5) *Sanitation.* The local authority must maintain adequate sanitation services, viz. the disposal of refuse and excreta. Every large local authority disposes of excreta at a sewage farm located on the outskirts of the inhabited areas. (See p. 149.)

(6) *Housing.* The law requires the local authority to ensure the cleanliness of premises and to prevent or get rid of nuisances, by force if necessary. The local authority must also remedy any danger to health arising from unsuitable dwellings, e.g. back to back houses and rooms without cross-ventilation. Overcrowded and bad housing conditions in cities are undesirable and their gradual replacement by economic housing schemes is a health-promotive measure which requires the co-operation of the central government and the local authority. (See Chapter 11.)

NOTIFICATION OF NOTIFIABLE CONDITIONS

The list of notifiable medical conditions is modified from time to time by the Minister of Health. The current list was declared in February 1991 (R328 to the Health Act 63 of 1977). Three diseases were added in April 1994.

- Acute flaccid paralysis.
- Acute rheumatic fever.
- Anthrax.
- Brucellosis.
- Cholera.
- Congenital syphilis.
- Diphtheria.
- Food poisoning (outbreaks of more than four persons).
- Haemophilus influenzae type B(Hib).
- Haemorrhagic fevers of Africa (Congo fever, Dengue fever, Ebola fever, Lassa fever, Marburg fever, Rift Valley fever).
- Lead poisoning.
- Legionellosis.
- Leprosy.
- Malaria.
- Measles.
- Meningococcal infections.
- Paratyphoid fever.
- Plague.
- Poisoning from any agricultural or stock remedy registered in terms of the Fertilizers, Farm Feeds, Agricultural Remedies and Stock Remedies Act 36 of 1947.
- Poliomyelitis.
- Rabies (specify whether human case or human contact).

▪ Rheumatic heart disease (first diagnosis only).
▪ Smallpox and any smallpox-like disease, excluding chicken-pox.
▪ Tetanus.
▪ Tetanus neonatorum.
▪ Trachoma.
▪ Tuberculosis —
  (i) pulmonary and other forms, except cases diagnosed solely on the basis of clinical signs and symptoms;
  (ii) a strongly positive reaction after a tuberculin test in children under 5 years of age (Gr. III or IV Heaf or 14 mm induration or more Mantoux).
▪ Typhoid fever.
▪ Typhus fever (epidemic lice typhus fever, endemic rat-flea typhus fever).
▪ Viral hepatitis A, B, non-A, non-B and undifferentiated.
▪ Yellow fever.
▪ Whooping cough (pertussis).

Any non-notifiable disease can be proclaimed notifiable in the event of a severe epidemic.

Notification of primary tuberculosis on the basis of positive 'skin' tests in children under the age of 5 years and to whom BCG has not been administered was reinstituted in 1982. This measure is a valuable means of tracing contacts.

AIDS, the most dangerous communicable disease in the world today, is not a notifiable disease. It is reportable, however. The essential difference between reporting and notifying is that reporting provides all the epidemiologically relevant information supplied by notification but does not permit identification of the patient concerned.

AIDS, but not HIV seropositivity, has been declared a communicable disease, in terms of Government Notice R2438, 1987 (Act 63 of 1977). The effect of this regulation is that if a patient is suspected of being an AIDS sufferer, the MOH can require him to submit to a medical examination.

Notifications of diseases seldom accurately reflect the true incidence of infectious diseases and can be taken only as approximations of trends. Thus we can be absolutely sure that tuberculosis is our gravest community health problem, notifications reaching approximately 80 000 per year, 80 % of all notifications. It occurs in all regions of South Africa, 40 to 60 times more often than typhoid fever, which is a major problem in areas with a high rainfall.

Western Cape notified 25 636 cases of tuberculosis in 1992, more than a third of all cases of TB in that year, in the whole country. Tuberculosis of other organs is also rising in number. This has been associated with an increase in HIV prevalence.

Malaria, against which there is no vaccine, in 1992 had a notified incidence of more than 2 871. This is greater than that of typhoid (1 316) and viral hepatitis (2 408). It must be remembered, however, that malaria occurs almost exclusively in the Transvaal lowveld, hence its incidence is high in this endemic area, despite the drought in 1992.

Comparatively few cases of trachoma (221 in 1991), endemic in the northern Transvaal, are notified when one considers that approximately 80 % of Africans in the endemic areas get the disease, 25 % in a severe form. Over the age of 50 years, only 5 % of people at risk have no signs of past and present trachoma.

Smallpox has been eradicated from the world (1978). In October 1977 the last case of pox (except for a laboratory accident in the UK) occurred in Somalia. South Africa has been free of smallpox for some years; in 1977 a few hundred cases of smallpox were reported from the horn of Africa. The global eradication of smallpox is a great triumph for the World Health Organisation. The other infectious diseases, unique to man, which will probably receive the attention of the WHO, are measles and poliomyelitis. For the global eradication of an infectious disease to happen, international co-operation is essential.

Typhus, plague and rabies need insect or animal hosts (vectors); in the RSA, these hosts are well controlled; typhus has hardly occurred in South Africa for some years, but rabies is still a danger, over 102 cases (human contacts) being notified in 1981, and only 9 in 1988 and 1991.

Notifications in the RSA in 1991 of polio (2 cases), diphtheria (12 cases) and tetanus (83 cases) indicate that these diseases have been relatively well controlled, but by no means eradicated. Pertussis and measles are still of high incidence in the developing world, including the black people of South Africa. 22 697 cases of measles were notified in 1991 and this number is rising. Meningococcal infection is still endemic in all regions of South Africa; the disease is preventable through the use of vaccines (see p. 554).

Yellow fever is not endemic in South Africa. Yellow fever in Africa is no longer a danger, although sporadic outbreaks still occur.

Until recently cholera was not endemic in the RSA, but in 1980 this formidable disease assumed epidemic proportions in the Transvaal lowveld. Cholera is once more under control, only 6 cases being notified in 1988, and 1 in 1991.

Notification figures for greater South Africa obtained from: *Epidemiological Comments*; **16**(7) and **19**(1).[1]

The purposes of notification:[2]

(1) To set the process of disease control in motion.

(2) To enable local and regional authorities to gain access to special powers, facilities and funds for the control of notified diseases.

(3) To accumulate data over time, thereby determining trends and evaluating intervention strategies.

(4) To serve as a basis for passive disease surveillance.

Surveillance

Surveillance means supervision or monitoring of diseases, or the continuing search for infected persons. It is a community health method used to prevent the outbreak of an acute episode of a disease which is presently under control or to devise an effective control programme for a widespread disease. The purpose of surveillance thus includes the treatment of carriers and sufferers in order to control the spread of infection to other humans, or to animal or insect vectors of human diseases.

The source of infection is traced either from routine notifications (passive surveillance) or by means of surveys which are specially designed for the purpose of the so-called active surveillance, where there is a need for more detailed information or for a quicker response.

Examples of active surveillance:

(1) malaria surveillance of carriers in the malaria endemic areas of the Transvaal lowveld (see p. 656);

(2) population surveillance of sufferers from a zoonosis, e.g. brucellosis, after the disease has been eradicated in the animal hosts;

(3) individual surveillance of infected persons, e.g. typhoid carriers, until they are no longer an infection risk to others;

(4) tuberculosis deaths, incidence and prevalence rates and response to treatment regimens, monitored in order to design an effective TB control programme (see p. 522).

Apart from the collection of data, surveillance also includes the statistical analysis of data and the interpretation of the statistics to provide information. This information is then sent to all who require it for the control of the disease.

Note: Surveillance merely supplies the data on which control measures by the local authority are based.

South Africa was divided in April 1992 into nine development regions. Health services have likewise been regionalised from 7 to 9 regions, with a regional director (RD) in charge of each Regional Health Office (RHO). Two new Regional Health Offices were established at Nelspruit and Klerksdorp.

The present nine health regions and their headquarters (RHO) are:

Western Cape (A) . . . . Bellville
Northern Cape (B) . . . . Kimberley
Free State (C) . . . . Bloemfontein
Eastern Cape (D) . . . . Port Elizabeth
Natal/KwaZulu (E) . . . . Durban
Mpumalanga (F) . . . . Nelspruit
Northern Transvaal (G) . . . . . . Pietersburg
Gauteng (H) . . . . Johannesburg
Northwest (I) . . . . Klerksdorp

Health surveys and disease surveillance cannot be practised in South Africa without access to population data.

The notification process[2]

The occurrence of a notifiable disease must be reported to a Medical Officer of Health (MOH) of the relevant local authority. In the black rural (Section 30) areas under the care of provincial hospital departments, the Director-General: De-

Notification of disease / *Aanmelding van siekte*

(Sections 32, 47(i)(a) and 47(i)(b) of Act 63 of 1977)   *(Artikels 32, 47(i)(a) en 47(i)(b) van Wet 63 van 1977)*

Department of National
Health & Population
Development
——
*Departement van Nasionale
Gesondheid en
Bevolkingsontwikkeling*

Where appropriate, ✔ the correct block / *Waar toepaslik, ✔ die korrekte blok.*

Complete in DUPLICATE. Original to be posted to Local Authority in area where patient stays, copy to remain in book

Voltooi in DUPLIKAAT. Die oorspronklike word gestuur aan die Plaaslike Owerheid van die gebied waar die pasiënt woon, die afskrif bly in die boek.

PATIENT DETAILS / *BESONDERHEDE VAN PASIËNT*

Full name
Volle naam

Age *Ouderdom*	Sex *Geslag*	Male *Manlik*	Female *Vroulik*	Population group *Bevolkingsgroep*	Asian *Asiër*	Black *Swart*	Coloured *Kleuring*	White *Blank*

Residential address*
*Woonadres**

*If resident on a farm, state the farmer's name, name and number of farm. If street address not available, give the name & address of the nearest clinic, school, headman, river.

*Indien woonagtig op 'n plaas, noem die boer se naam, plaasnaam, nommer van plaas. Indien straatadres nie biskikbaar is nie, gee die naam en adres van die naaste kliniek, skool, hoofman, rivier.

District
Distrik

Telephone no.
Telefoon nr.

Occupation
Beroep

DISEASE DETAILS / *BESONDERHEDE VAN SIEKTE*

Disease
Siekte

Date of onset of disease (if known) *Aanvangsdatum van siekte (indien bekend)*	Is the patient symptomatic? *Is die pasiënt simptomaties?*	Yes *Ja*	No *Nee*	Died *Oorlede*

Date of death (if applicable)✦ *Datum van sterfte (indien van toepassing)✦*	✦Was the patient notified when the disease was diagnosed? ✦*Is die pasiënt aangemeld toe die siekte gediagnoseer is?*	Yes *Ja*	No *Nee*	Unknown *Onbekend*

Possible place and district of infection (if known)
Moontlike piek en distrik van infeksie (indien bekend)

LABORATORY INVESTIGATION RESULTS / *RESULTAAT VAN LABORATORIUMTOETSE*

Investigation (excluding TB sputum) *Ondersoek (TB sputum uitgesluit)* ↓	Results *Resultate* ↓	
		Awaiting result *Wag vir resultaat*
		Awaiting result *Wag vir resultaat*
		Awaiting result *Wag vir resultaat*

If TB, give sputum result : *Indien TB, gee sputumresultaat :*	Microscopy positive *Mikroskopie positief*	Microscopy negative *Mikroskopie negatief*	Culture positive *Kultuur positief*	Culture negative *Kultuur negatief*

NOTIFIED BY / *AANGEMELD DEUR*

Medical practitioner *Geneesheer*	Nurse *Verpleegster*	Other *Ander*	Name (please PRINT) *Naam (DRUKSKRIF asb)*

Signature *Handtekening*	Date *Datum*	Telephone no. *Telefoon nr.*

Address
Adres

LOCAL AUTHORITY REPLY / *ANTWOORD DEUR PLAASLIKE OWERHEID*

Local Authority to reply to referring doctor/nurse with brief report of further findings and management.

Plaaslike Owerheid se antwoord aan verwysende dokter/verpleegster oor verdere bevindinge en hantering.

Date / Datum   Signature / Handtekening

Figure 27.1

Notifiable medical conditions
Number of notified cases and deaths January to May 1995 compared to the same period in 1994 (as on 10/07/95)[3]

MEDICAL CONDITION	1994*		1995*†	
	DEATHS	CASES	DEATHS	CASES
Accute flaccid paralysis	0	0	0	6
Anthrax	0	0	0	0
Brucellosis	0	11	0	3
Cholera	0	2	0	0
Congenital syphilis	8	410	2	205
Crimean-Congo haemorrhagic fever	0	4	0	0
Other haemorrhagic fevers of Africa	0	0	0	0
Diphtheria	1	0	0	0
Food poisoning	0	94	0	27
Haemophilus influenzae type B	0	2	0	19
Lead poisoning	0	3	0	0
Legionellosis	0	4	0	0
Leprosy	1	4	0	3
Malaria	7	6 849	0	1 575
Measles	9	1 317	2	1 131
Meningococcal infection	8	103	14	80
Paratyphoid fever	1	4	0	1
Plague	0	0	0	0
Poisoning agric. stock remedies	3	61	0	30
Poliomyelitis	0	0	0	0
Rabies	0	3	0	1
Rheumatic fever	0	20	0	3
Tetanus	6	19	4	11
Tetanus neonatorum	3	8	1	1
Trachoma	0	32	0	25
Tuberculosis primary	7	2 875	10	2 119
Tuberculosis pulmonary	865	31 977	648	18 769
Tuberculosis of other respiratory organs	2	645	4	348
Tuberculosis of meninges	38	133	18	89
Tuberculosis of intestines, peritoneum	0	34	2	28
Tuberculosis of bones and joints	1	43	2	35
Tuberculosis of genito-urinary system	1	41	2	11
Tuberculosis of other organs	5	277	6	152
Tuberculosis miliary	18	90	11	42
Tuberculosis total	937	36 115	703	21 593
Typhoid fever	8	620	12	304
Typhus fever (lice-borne)	0	0	0	0
Typhus fever (ratflea-borne)	0	0	0	1
Viral hepatitis type A	1	443	11	188
Viral hepatitis type B	4	147	10	108
Viral hepatitis non-A non-B	1	35	1	16
Viral hepatitis unspecified	5	110	0	50
Viral hepatitis total	11	735	22	362
Whooping cough	0	19	0	11
Yellow fever	0	0	0	0

*Notifications are coded according to date of onset (if known), else date of notification
†The data for this year are still incomplete

partment of Health, represented by the regional director (RD), serves as the 'local authority' to whom notifications must be made.

Diagnosis, treatment and notification are made by the doctor attending the patient at the clinic, hospital or in private practice, or by any other person legally competent to diagnose and treat (e.g. PHC nurse). A formidable epidemic disease (plague, viral haemorrhagic fever, cholera) must be reported to the RD concerned by telegram or telephone by the MOH. The RD notifies Head Office immediately.

The primary notification form is GW 17/5. This form makes provision for a person who is 'suffering from' and who 'has died from' a notifiable disease. The patient who dies is notified twice, once as a 'case' and once as a 'death'.

The local authority which is legally, administratively and functionally equipped and charged to execute control measures, summarises all notifications once a week on two summary sheets (GW/17/3 and GW 17/4), one for cases and one for deaths. He sends them to the relevant regional office (of one of the nine health regions, see p. 483). The regional office conducts surveillance and keeps copies, while the originals are sent weekly to Head Office in Pretoria for processing and entering into the computer file for statistical analysis. Apart from the mainstream file (the Notifiable Diseases), there are also special disease files for special detailed surveillance systems.

The Head Office conducts surveillance and provides feedback through its publication, *Epidemiological Comments*, which is sent to primary notifiers.

Note: All dangerous infections, including those caused by multiple resistant pneumococcus, are notified to the 'Centre for Disease Control' in Atlanta, USA.

CONTROL OF COMMUNICABLE DISEASES

Quarantine of contacts

Quarantine means the restriction of the free movement of healthy people or domestic animals that have been exposed to a communicable disease, in order to prevent such disease from spreading. (Act 63 of 1977.) The quarantine period is two days longer than the maximum incubation period and is compulsory for adults in cases of the dangerous viral haemorrhagic

diseases, plague and yellow fever. Quarantine is instituted at schools for other dangerous diseases and strongly enforced in nursery schools. Refer to R2438.

Control of carriers

Refer to R2438.

Isolation

Isolation of the patient while he is infectious not only prevents the spread of bacteria but also provides an opportunity for treatment. It is the duty of the local authority to see that isolation is carried out in one of the following ways:

(1) At home if the facilities for isolation are satisfactory and if consent has been granted by the Medical Officer of Health.

(2) In a provincial hospital if the disease is of a serious nature or if home facilities are unsatisfactory. The patient may be isolated in one of the following ways:
   (a) by barrier nursing in a general ward;
   (b) in a large ward with cubicles which makes it possible to isolate more than one type of infectious disease;
   (c) in a large ward in which only one type of infectious disease is nursed, e.g. measles, tuberculosis.

(3) In special isolation hospitals, e.g. SANTA hospitals for tuberculosis patients and provincial hospitals in which 'containment nursing' is practised during the occasional outbreaks of the dangerous viral haemorrhagic fevers of Africa (refer to R2438).

Disinfection and disinfestation

The local authority is empowered to disinfect premises and articles and to disinfest verminous persons, if they are unable to carry out this service for themselves. Delousing of schoolchildren is supervised by school nurses, and is done preferably by the parents. Refer to R2438.

Immunisation

See Chapter 28 and refer to R2438.

EXTRACTS FROM R2438 (OCTOBER 1987) OF HEALTH ACT 63 OF 1977

'The Minister of National Health and Population Development has promulgated the regulations contained in the Schedule hereto in terms of Section 32, 33 and 34 of the Health Act, 1977 (Act 63 of 1977).

2. (1) A local authority may, when it comes to its notice that a communicable disease is present or has occurred in its district:

(*a*) close any teaching institution, place of public entertainment or place used for public receptions, recreation or amusement that is situated within its district;

(*d*) place under quarantine in order to prevent the spread of such disease or in order to control or restrict such disease —

(i) any person or persons actually suffering or suspected to be suffering from such disease, in cases where such person or persons are not removed to a hospital or place of isolation —

(ii) any person who is in contact with or who has, within the period determined by a medical officer of health or a medical practitioner in the employ of the State, been in contact with any person or persons referred to in subparagraph (i).

3. (1) A medical officer of health may, if he is satisfied that the incidence of a communicable disease in his district is of such a nature that the spread of such disease constitutes or will constitute a real danger to health . . . exercise the powers of a local authority as referred to in regulation 2(1).

5. The chief administrative officer of a local authority

(*a*) immediately after an order is issued by the local authority concerned in terms of regulation 2;
inform the Director-General by telegraph, by telex or by telephone of the issuing of and the reasons for the issuing of the order concerned.

6. (1) A medical officer of health or a medical practitioner in the employ of the State may, at his discretion, in order to prevent the spread of a communicable disease referred to in Annexure

1 [see p. 487] or in order to control or restrict such disease —

(*a*) require that he be furnished with the names and addresses —

(i) of pupils or employees at any teaching institution;

(ii) of persons present at any meeting, place of public amusement or place used for public receptions, recreation or amusement;

(iii) of patients, medical practitioners, nurses, employees and visitors at any hospital, nursing home, maternity home or similar institution;

(*b*) question or medically examine or have examined any person;

(*c*) restrict any person or group of persons found on any premises to those premises for a period of not more than 12 hours for the purposes of questioning or medical examination.

Specific measures relating to pupils and teaching institutions

7. (1) A principal —

(*a*) who is aware or has reason to suspect that a pupil at the teaching institution of which he is principal or a person employed at or who happened to visit such institution —

(i) suffers from a communicable disease referred to in Annexure 1; [see p. 487]

(ii) was in contact with any person suffering from such disease; or

(iii) is infested with fleas, lice or similar external parasites, shall without delay—

(*aa*) in cases where such institution falls within the district of a local authority, inform the medical officer of health or, if he is not available, the chief administrative officer of such local authority; or

(*bb*) in cases where such institution is situated outside the district of a local authority, inform the regional director of the district in which such institution is situated,
by telegraph, by telex or by telephone of such condition;

(2) The parent or guardian of a child who attends a teaching institution as a pupil, . . . of whom to

the knowledge of the parent or guardian a condition referred to in subregulation (1)(a)(i), (ii) or (iii) . . . applies, shall inform the principal of the teaching institution concerned immediately of such condition.

Quarantine

8. (1) A person who is placed in quarantine in terms of an order referred to in regulation 2(1) or who is isolated in terms of regulation 13(5)(b) shall be obliged to satisfy the provisions of that order.

(2) Any person who is present on premises or in an area placed under quarantine in terms of regulation 2(1) or who enters such premises or area after such quarantine has been imposed without the authorisation of the Director-General, a medical practitioner in the employ of the State or a medical officer of health —

(a) may not leave such premises or area before the expiry of the prescribed quarantine period without the prior authorisation of the Director-General, a medical practitioner in the employ of the State or a medical officer of health;

(b) shall subject himself during such period to any medical observation, examination or supervision determined by a medical practitioner in the employ of the State or a medical officer of health.

Conveyance of bodies of persons who have died of communicable diseases

9. The body of any person who has died of acquired immuno deficiency syndrome (AIDS), cholera, a haemorrhagic fever of Africa, meningococcemia, plague, poliomyelitis, rabies or typhoid fever may not be conveyed by train or in any other way unless —

(a) such body is screened off according to the directions of a medical practitioner and such medical practitioner has stated in writing that in his opinion the conveyance of the body will not constitute a danger to health; and . . .

Prevention of the transmission of a communicable disease by animals, insects, and parasites and the prevention of malaria

11. In order to prevent the transmission or development of a communicable disease among people a medical officer of health may, by means of a written notice, order the owner or occupier of any premises situated within his district, within the period specified in such notice, to —

(a) furnish such medical officer of health with all the information at the disposal of such owner or occupier or readily obtainable by him with regard to the occurrence, spread, extermination or reduction of any animal, animal carcass, animal product, animal parasite, arthropod, plant or plant material, plant parasite or micro-organism referred to in the notice, on such premises;

12. (1) An owner or occupier of land shall take all reasonable measures to treat any collection of water or any other habitat in which mosquitoes can breed or live on such land in such a way that the breeding of mosquitoes is prevented or kept to the minimum.

(2) An owner or occupier of land shall, if ordered to do so in writing by the local authority in whose district such land is situated, or by the Director-General, within the period determined in the order, in respect of any building or structure on such land that is used as a residence or that is intended to be used as such or in which people gather, whether for work or otherwise —

(a) spray such building or structure or have it sprayed with such insecticide in such a way and with such strength of application and at such application intervals as determined by the local authority concerned or the Director-General;

(b) screen the outer doors, windows and other openings with gauze screens with not less than five openings per centimetre of the surface, and maintain such gauze screens in good condition in order to prevent the entry of mosquitoes.

(3) The owner or occupier of any building or structure that has been treated with a residual insecticide as referred to in subregulation (2) shall ensure that such insecticide is not plastered

over, painted over, removed or rendered harmless during the effective period.

Immunisation and emergency measures

13. (1) If the Director-General is satisfied that there is sufficient reason on medical scientific grounds to suspect that the health of the population of the Republic or any part of the population may be affected by a medical condition against which people can be immunised, he may by means of a notice in the *Gazette*—

(*a*) demarcate an area referred to in the notice for compulsory immunisation of all inhabitants or of a specific group or category of inhabitants, as referred to in the notice, of such demarcated area;

(*b*) designate the government body, person or persons that must carry out such immunisation, and determine the period during which the immunisation is to be done.

(5) (*a*) No person may disregard or fail to comply with an instruction from the government body or person or immunisation officer referred to in subregulation (2).

(*b*) Any person who, when instructed to do so, cannot or will not undergo immunisation for a medical or any other reason may by order of the regional director concerned be placed and detained in a place of isolation for a reasonable period.

Carriers of communicable diseases

14. (1) Any person a medical officer of health suspects on reasonable grounds to be a carrier of a communicable disease and who as such constitutes a danger to the public health shall, if so instructed by such medical officer of health, subject himself to a medical examination at a time and place determined by the medical officer of health in order to establish whether such person is in fact a carrier as suspected.

(2) Every carrier so instructed in writing by a medical officer of health shall —

(*a*) at all times comply with and carry out all reasonable and feasible instructions given to him by the medical officer of health in respect of the disposal of his excrement, the cleansing of himself and of articles used by him, or other precautions to prevent the

spread of an infection or to restrict it to the minimum;

(*b*) Inform such medical officer of health of his intention to change his place of residence or place of work and, after such change, of his new place of residence or place of work, and such medical officer of health shall inform the regional director of the region if which such a carrier finds himself of such new address.

(3) A medical officer of health may, when he is satisfied on medical scientific grounds that the danger exists of a carrier of a communicable disease transmitting such disease to other people, order in writing that such carrier —

(*a*) go or be removed to a hospital, other place of isolation or area referred to in the order so as to remain there under medical supervision for a period determined in such order;

(*b*) report for medical examination and treatment at the times and places determined in the order.

(*c*) (i) not prepare any food intended for other persons;

(ii) not handle any food or water intended for other persons;

(iii) not handle any container for such food or water;

(*d*) comply with such other requirements as are deemed necessary by the medical officer of health in order to safeguard public health.

(4) A parent, guardian or person who has legal custody and control of a child who is a carrier, shall render all reasonable assistance in the implementation of this regulation or of any order issued in terms thereof in respect of such child.

Disinfecting of premises

15. (*a*) If a medical officer of health is of the opinion that any premises or object is in such a condition that it is likely to give rise to the development of a communicable disease, he may disinfect or have disinfected such premises or object after the owner or occupier has been given reasonable notice thereof.

Compulsory evacuation of premises

16. (1) (*a*) If the Director-General or a local authority is satisfied on medical scientific grounds that there is sufficient reason to suspect that the occupation or use of premises or any part thereof is likely to favour the spread or impede the eradication of a communicable disease he may by written order direct the evacuation of such premises.

Compulsory medical examination, hospitalisation or treatment of persons

17. Any person who in the opinion of a medical officer of health is or could be suffering from a communicable disease referred to in Annexure I [see p. 487] shall, if so instructed by the medical officer of health —

(*a*) subject himself at the time and place determined by the medical officer of health to such a medical examination and such treatment as prescribed by the person undertaking the examination;

(*b*) go or be removed to a hospital or other place of isolation determined by the medical officer of health in order to remain there under medical supervision and receive treatment;

(*c*) subject himself to the medical treatment prescribed by the medical officer of health or the person assigned by the medical officer of health,

until he is free of infection or may be discharged without in any way endangering public health.

Compulsory removal, cleansing and disinfecting of persons infested with fleas, lice or similar parasites

18. A medical officer of health who is aware of any person infested with fleas, lice or similar external parasites, may by written order —

(*a*) direct that —

(i) the infested person himself, or

(ii) a person with legal custody or control of the infested person, cleanse or disinfect such person under the supervision of the health officer designated by the medical officer of health or have such infested person cleansed or disinfected by such designated health officer at a time and place determined by the medical officer of health; or

(*b*) direct any person designated by such designated health officer to remove the infested person to a place mentioned in the order so that he may be cleansed or disinfected there by or under the supervision of a health officer.

Notification of notifiable medical conditions

19. (1) When a medical practitioner, a practitioner registered as such in terms of the Associated Health Service Professions Act, 1982 (Act 63 or 1982), or any other person legally competent to diagnose and treat a person with regard to notifiable medical conditions, for gain, diagnoses a notifiable medical condition in a person he shall report his findings —

(*a*) in cases where the condition concerned is also a communicable disease, without delay orally, and this must be confirmed in writing within 24 hours; or

(*b*) in any other case within seven days orally and, if so requested by the body to which the report must be made, in writing to —

(i) the office of the health section or any other appropriate section of the local authority concerned; or

(ii) the appropriate regional director in cases where the Director-General acts as a local authority in terms of Section 30 of the Act.

(2) On making a report referred to in subregulation (1) the following shall be furnished: Name, age, sex, population group, identity number or if the identity number is not available, the date of birth, and the address, place of work or school of the person in respect of whom the report is made, as well as the date of commencement of the notifiable medical condition and any available information concerning the probable place and source of infection.

(3) The local authority concerned shall forward, weekly via the regional director, particulars of all reports referred to in subregulation (1) in respect of the preceding week to the Director-General on a form drawn up and made available by the Department of Health.'

ANNEXURE 1
(See page 486.)

Communicable disease	Patient may return to teaching institution	Contact may return to teaching institution
Acquired immuno-deficiency syndrome (AIDS)	On submission of a medical certificate	Immediately.
Chicken-pox	14 days after appearance of rash or on submission of a medical certificate	Immediately.
Cholera	On submission of a medical certificate	According to quarantine measures.
Diphtheria	On submission of a medical certificate and after two nose and two throat swabs, at appropriate intervals, prove negative	*Non-immune contacts*: Eight days after removal from source of infection. *Immune contacts*: Immediately.
Epidemic typhus	On submission of a medical certificate	Immediately.
German measles (rubella)	Seven days after appearance of rash	Immediately.
Haemorrhagic fever diseases of Africa	On submission of a medical certificate	According to quarantine measures.
Haemorrhagic virus conjunctivitis	Seven days after beginning of symptoms	Immediately.
Hepatitis A	Seven days after appearance of jaundice or on submission of a medical certificate	Immediately.
Leprosy	On submission of a medical certificate	Immediately.
Louse infestation	After complete cleansing and delousing and removal of nits on head, body and clothing	Immediately
Measles	Seven days after appearance of rash	Immediately.
Meningococcaemia	On submission of a medical certificate	Immediately, provided the necessary prophylactic medicine is taken.
Mumps	Nine days after appearance of swelling	Immediately.
Plague	On submission of a medical certificate	According to quarantine measures.
Poliomyelitis	On submission of a medical certificate	Immediately.
Scabies	After proper treatment	Immediately.
Tuberculosis of the lungs	On submission of a medical certificate	Immediately.
Typhoid fever	On submission of a medical certificate. After three negative stool and urine tests have been done at appropriate intervals (at least 48 hours) and not less than 72 hours after cessation of antibiotic therapy	Immediately.
Whooping cough	21 days after beginning of paroxysms or on submission of a medical certificate	Immediately.

REFERENCES

(1) *Epidemiological Comments* 1989; **16**(7), and 1992; **19**(1).

(2) *Epidemiological Comments* 1988; **15**(4).

(3) *Epidemiological Comments* January 1994; **21**(1).

TEST OF KNOWLEDGE

The student has benefited from studying this chapter if he/she can answer the following questions:

(1) Discuss the purposes of notification and surveillance of communicable diseases.

(2) Discuss the responsibilities and tasks of local authorities with regard to infection control in their areas of jurisdiction.

(3) Write notes on:
    – the carrier state and its control;
    – isolation of an infectious patient;
    – quarantine of contacts;
    – disinfestation.

28

Immunisation

IMMUNISATION

Immunisation is an inoculation, orally or parenterally, with vaccines. The inoculation is called
vaccination.

Vaccines

A vaccine is a suspension of antigens in a base.
The antigens are too weak to cause the disease;
they nevertheless stimulate an immune response. The following antigens are used for the
manufacture of vaccines:

(1) attenuated (weakened) live microbes;
(2) an avirulent harmless strain of the live mi-
    crobe;
(3) dead microbes;
(4) toxins rendered non-poisonous.

Kinds of vaccines

(1) Vaccines can be prepared from detoxified
    toxins, for example, those used in diphtheria
    and tetanus. Immunisation is done by intra-
    muscular or subcutaneous injection of
    toxoid, i.e. toxin which is detoxified by the
    addition of formalin. The prophylactic
    toxoids are: APT (Alum Precipitated
    Toxoid), and Diphtet (diphtheria and teta-
    nus), tetanus toxoid (fluid and adsorbed).

(2) Vaccines can be prepared from harmless,
    live microbes, e.g. those used in smallpox
    and poliomyelitis.

    The Sabin polio vaccine is given orally
    in a syrupy base. The harmless strain of live
    polio virus from which it is grown at the
    National Institute of Virology in Johannes-
    burg was originally imported from the USA.
    It is a very efficient vaccine, for not only
    does it immunise the person who ingests the
    vaccine, but immunity is spread to non-im-
    munised persons by virtue of the discharge
    of the harmless polio virus in the stools.
    Vaccination against smallpox is done by
    applying the live vaccinia (cowpox) virus to
    the scarified skin, with subsequent develop-
    ment of a pustule. The virus is obtained from
    a pustule of an inoculated animal. The
    lymph stimulates the formation of antibod-
    ies which also neutralise the smallpox virus,
    in this way affording protection against
    smallpox.

    Note: Smallpox vaccination is no longer practised.

(3) Vaccines can also be prepared from dead
    microbes, for example dead microbes form
    the antigens for whooping cough, enteric
    fever (TAB vaccine), plague, cholera, ra-
    bies, influenza, hepatitis B and polio (Salk)
    vaccine. Immunity lasts only a few years
    and needs to be boosted whenever there is a
    danger of contracting the disease.

(4) Live, attenuated (weakened) microbes form the vaccines for yellow fever, tuberculosis (BCG vaccine), measles and mumps, rubella, Sabin polio, varicella.

Note:
(1) Recently more stable, lyophilised (freeze-dried) vaccines have been produced.
(2) There are no contra-indications to the simultaneous administration of a number of live vaccines.

We are on the brink of a large revolution in vaccine production — the era of biologically engineered vaccines, such as 'cloned' hepatitis B, herpes, influenza, rabies, respiratory syncytial vaccines, vaccinia recombinant vaccines and many more.

Antisera (immunoglobulins) confer passive immunity. Some are invaluable as therapeutic agents. Some immunoglobulins are made from horse serum, others from human serum. The antiserum carries the antibodies (immunoglobulins).

(1) Antitoxic immunoglobulins in refined horse serum, e.g. anti-diphtheritic serum and antitetanus serum. Dangers of horse serum: sensitivity reactions. (See p. 509.)
(2) New high-titred human gammaglobulins are available for measles, rubella, hepatitis B, varicella-zoster, rabies. These preparations provide immediate antibody for patients who need rapid prophylaxis against these diseases.

Care of vaccines

Vaccines are labile biological substances and can lose their potency during storage and transportation if suitable measures for refrigeration are not taken. They must be stored in a refrigerator at 0–8 °C. Excess cold and heat damage vaccines. Every vaccine refrigerator must have a thermometer and its temperature recorded daily. The refrigerator may never be turned off and notices to that effect must be placed at the switches. No food or drinks may be stored in the fridge which should carry bottles of cold water in its lower racks. Vaccines are stored in the upper half of the fridge, never in its door or against the freezing plate. The space between vaccine packs must be greater than 1 cm to allow for circulation.[17]

It is absolutely essential to ensure a continuous cold-chain from producer to the person vaccinated. A break in this chain can adversely affect the potency of the vaccines, especially those containing live organisms, e.g. BCG, Sabin. It is especially important that mobile units conducting mass immunisation campaigns have refrigerator space on their vans, and that country clinics without electricity maintain their paraffin refrigerators in good working order. The vaccine must be transported in insulated containers in which the vaccine is held at the correct low temperature. Deep-frozen cooling packs can be used for the purpose, but they must not be used in the unfrozen state.

Keeping vaccines continuously cold while transporting and storing them is a very difficult task. The so-called 'cold-chain' is easily broken, resulting in loss of potency of the vaccine. A break in the cold-chain is dependent on length of storage and absolute heat exposure. The weakest links in the cold-chain are transportation and maintenance of vaccine viability at the end-point.

The commonly used cold-chain monitor is a thermo-sensitive chemical indicator in a card e.g. WHO Vaccine Cold-Chain Monitor. It turns blue on exposure to a temperature of more than 10 °C. It gives a different reaction when the temperature rises above 34 °C. These cards are activated and dispatched with batches of vaccines from the central stores to the hospital stores and finally to the point of use in the clinic. At each point of arrival and departure at an intermediary stop, the card should be checked and information filled in. Finally, it is sent to a predetermined laboratory for checking of weak spots in the cold-chain.

Feedback is given in order to improve preservation techniques. Although the clinics are requested not to keep their stock of vaccine for longer than a fortnight, it may take months for a batch of vaccine to reach the user after dispatch from the central store. In a study done in Gazankulu, De Swardt *et al.* found that, owing to the cumulative effect of heat exposure, up to 90 % of all vaccine batches were exposed to temperatures high enough and for a sufficient period of time potentially to have affected their potency.[6]

The status of the cold-chain is therefore of the utmost importance in any vaccination programme. A poor cold-chain which affects the potency of the vaccine severely may cause vaccination to have no effect on the immunity of the 'immunised' person.

When reconstituting freeze-dried vaccines, the diluent should be chilled; if at ambient (room) temperature in a warm climate, the diluent may destroy the potency of the vaccine. Care must be taken that vaccines preserved with antiseptics (e.g. DPT, cholera, typhoid) are not allowed to freeze.

A sterile abscess may form at the site after vaccination with DPT vaccine that has been frozen. Freezing causes permanent changes in the phosphate gel with resultant flocculation.

Skin disinfection before injections is usually done but is not essential. If dirty, the skin should be washed. If 70 % alcohol is used, it should either be allowed to dry or should be wiped off before the skin puncture is made. In caring for the immunising equipment, the possibility of carrying hepatitis B virus from one vaccine to another must be borne in mind. This virus resides in tissue fluids.

A Gazankulu experience with the organisation of cold-chain maintenance [5]

One of the important aims of the Gazankulu immunisation policy was the organisation of cold-chain maintenance. Vaccines were treated as follows to maintain their potency:

(1) Centralisation of vaccine ordering and bulk storage in a central (Letaba Hospital) cool room. Supply calculations are done for each vaccination point and for each vaccine individually. Fresh vaccine is transported from the central depot to hospital refrigerator. In the hospital storage refrigerator, storage time is long.

(2) Vaccine distribution from hospitals to clinics by community health nurses, every 14 days. Only good quality cool boxes with lockable lids and an adequate number of ice packs were used for transport. Clinics may not store more vaccines than that needed for a fortnight.

(3) Vaccines were stored in the hospitals and clinics in chest-type refrigerators with locks. These refrigerators were used for vaccine storage only.

(4) Responsible persons should be in charge of vaccine refrigerators and of refrigerator maintenance. Refrigerators must be repaired as soon as they break down or an alternative cooling space found for the vaccines to maintain their potency.

(5) At the point of use, either a fixed primary health care clinic or special mobile immunisation clinic staffed by a driver and 2 nurses, vaccines were dispensed to patients from 'stock rotation trays'. Trays are made of blocks of wood with holes drilled in them to accommodate the correct number of vials. The vials are gradually moved from the back row to the front row where they are used. In this way stockpiling of vaccines is virtually impossible.

IMMUNISATION — THE EPI PROGRAMME

Immunisation is one of the most powerful and cost-effective methods of preventing communicable diseases. Yet in South Africa much remains to be done to reach the target of immunisation cover (i.e. child immunisation) to EPI diseases set by the WHO of 80 % or more by 1990.[1]

EPI is the acronym for Expanded Program on Immunisation, 'expanded' referring to the addition of more antigens (vaccines) to vaccination schedules and the increase of geographical and socio-economic coverage and accessibility of vaccination services.[2]

The WHO target for 1990 is: 3 doses DPT, 3 doses polio, and one each measles and tuberculosis for all children before their 1st birthday. In addition, where neonatal tetanus is rife, every pregnant woman must be adequately immunised against tetanus.

The WHO expanded programme on immunisation, initiated in 1974, aims to reduce morbidity and mortality for 6 vaccine-preventable diseases of childhood: diphtheria, pertussis (whooping-cough), measles, tetanus, poliomyelitis and tuberculosis. EPI is an essential component of Maternal and Child Health Care or Primary Health Care which is of special but not exclusive relevance to Third-World countries.

In South Africa, a new childhood vaccination schedule has been adopted by the Minister of Health, Dr N D Zuma, following the recommendations of the review of the national immunisation programme in September 1994. The new schedule will protect children by 14 weeks of age against poliomyelitis, hepatitis B, diphtheria, tetanus and whooping cough. This is concurrent with international thinking and recommendations by the WHO's Expanded Programme on Immunisations (*S Afr Med J* April 1995; 85(4).

Main strategies used by the EPI to reach its target:[2]

(1) Management training to organise national programmes with central co-ordination and clear lines of responsibility and accountability. Henderson (quoted by Ysselmuiden and Gear[2]) states, *inter alia*, 'it is the lack of human resources, in general, and the lack of management skills in particular, that pose the most severe threat to the achievement of the EPI's goal'.

    It is important that health professionals be thoroughly grounded in the principles and management of immunisation, especially cold-chain management, to ensure the potency of the vaccine at the point of use — the body of the child.

(2) Improving the supply of better vaccines locally and the materials used to maintain the cold-chain in the storage and transport of vaccines.

(3) Increasing the demand for greater immunisation coverage by health education and community-based (locally organised) immunisation programmes, which ensure that vaccination is provided at every point of contact between children and health caregivers.

(4) Improved monitoring of: the incidence of EPI target diseases, cold-chain maintenance and immunisation coverage.

Disease surveillance by notification at local and central level is very important. Thus the effectiveness of an immunisation programme can be evaluated by its national long-term trends. But data must also be made available at local level to allow for the identification and containment of local epidemics and to provide feedback to health workers. These small areas of high risk prevent the formation of herd immunity. Such areas merit special attention: the local authority can set its sight on specific and attainable goals.

In South Africa it has become mandatory to vaccinate all at risk against the 6 EPI target diseases. The solution of the problem of continuing infection by EPI target diseases seems simple: use effective, constantly cooled vaccines from the coolbox on all children at risk, at the correct age and for the requisite number of doses. The primary health care team of the local authority must have an estimate of the size of their target group for a given year. Both the number of children to be vaccinated and the number of vaccinations given must be recorded on a special data-capturing form (the so-called 'yellow pages'). Thus the percentage coverage can be obtained per population group, region, disease and year. The size of the target group is calculated from the number of births notified in the target area for that year. Another method of computing the size of the target group is to get an estimation of the population under the age of 1 year (statistical computation from census figures).

If the percentage coverage is more than 100 %, then children from another local authority have been included. If the percentage obtained is persistently low, i.e. under 70 %, year after year, then a problem exists which must be addressed by high priority primary health care.

A community is well guarded against the EPI target diseases if over 80 % of its children under the age of 5 years have been fully vaccinated. The herd immunity which thus has a chance of developing will prevent the outbreak of epidemics.

Ysselmuiden *et al.*[3] studied municipal vaccination coverage and central notification of 5 of the EPI target diseases, viz. measles, tuberculosis in children, diphtheria, tetanus, poliomyelitis. They used the following data:

(1) Incidence rates up to the middle of 1987 of the 5 target diseases as supplied by the Department of National Health and Population Development.

(2) Number of vaccinations done by 13 of the larger municipalities (covering 26 % of the population in the Health Regions of the

RSA), to assess the vaccination coverage in these areas. Municipalities are responsible for the adequate vaccination of most children in the RSA.

Evaluation of vaccination against EPI target diseases in the RSA

They found that the incidence of the 5 target diseases is linked to vaccination coverage and came to the following conclusions:

'On a nationwide scale, vaccination programmes have probably reduced diphtheria, have possibly influenced poliomyelitis, but have had no discernible effect on measles, tetanus and tuberculosis, despite the proven high efficacy of polio, measles and tetanus vaccines. The main reason seems to be inadequate coverage of the target population . . .'[3]

Measles, neonatal tetanus and tuberculosis are the major notifiable causes of child morbidity and mortality in South Africa and measles and tetanus show no signs of decreasing. For every death from one of the EPI target diseases, at least one other child will be permanently disabled, blinded or mentally retarded by the complications.[2]

Gazankulu is attempting to deal with the prevention of EPI target diseases.[5]

In Gazankulu, legislation delegates responsibility for the provision of all health services to the superintendent of the 6 hospitals of the 6 health wards. The hospitals also act as local authorities for the prevention of communicable diseases. In 1986 a new immunisation policy was planned. A nurse, appointed at Head Office level, is the programme co-ordinator.

The aim of the immunisation policy was to provide an effective immunisation service for Gazankulu in respect of the 6 EPI target diseases and to have 97 % coverage by the year 1990.

The organisation of the cold-chain in order to ensure the potency of the vaccine at the endpoint — introduction into the body of the child — was an important aim of the policy (see p. 491).

Care groups and village committees, encouraged and organised by chiefs, were involved in the mobile clinic service. Care group members have their own children vaccinated and also encourage the vaccination of the children in 10 neighbouring families. Thereby they create the demand for vaccination.

Training courses for all staff are held at the hospitals, the Nursing Colleges and headquarters of the Department of Health.

Recording of vaccination was done on Road-to-Health cards for the patient to retain, thereby placing vaccination in the minds of the public with general child health care. Raw data in the field must be reported for data input and control of satisfactory coverage to the vaccination programme co-ordinator.

Thus, if vigorous efforts are made to ensure vaccine potency, to use the correct vaccination technique and to supply a regular and timely, well-co-ordinated vaccination service, widely spread rural areas can be satisfactorily immunised.[5]

THE MEASLES STRATEGY (MS) OF THE DNHPD — 1990[14]

The DNHPD committed itself to improve primary health care (PHC) services in the RSA. In line with the WHO's target for universal immunisation coverage in 1990, the DNHPD chose the WHO's EPI (see p. 494) as its way of showing its commitment to PHC. This study is called 'The Measles Strategy' (MS). The Measles Strategy covers all the EPI diseases.

The MS was started in January 1990 and became fully operational in 1991. It comprised a pre-campaign evaluation of the vaccination levels of children aged 12–13 months, the mass vaccination campaign, and a post-campaign evaluation. The vaccination coverage surveys were conducted (1988–1990) by the Departments of Community Health of the seven Medical Schools and some RHOSA (see p. 434) members.

The following vaccination coverage levels were found prior to the implementation of the Measles Strategy:

BCG . . . . 85 %
DPT3 . . . . 67 %
Polio3 . . . . 69 %
Measles . . . . 63 %

The objectives of the measles campaign were wider, however, i.e. to raise the immunisation levels of all susceptible children against all the EPI diseases before their first birthday and to maintain these high levels in subsequent groups of children.

Vaccinations were available every day and at every opportunity.

An evaluation in 1991 of its effect

The primary objective of the MS was to determine its effect on the morbidity, mortality and disability associated with measles in the RSA. The estimated increase in vaccination coverage was only 8 %, i.e. from 63 % to 71 %, yet there was a decline in case notification of over 70 % and of notified deaths of more than 90 %. In 1991, 3 847 cases of measles were notified and in 1990, 10 623.

Although somewhat inexplicable, it would seem that the MS was a great success, especially in highlighting the effectiveness at low cost of the PHC services within whose ambit the MS was planned and executed.

The Measles Strategy — what happened?[16]

In August 1992 it was reported that the good effects of the MS were beginning to slide to pre-campaign levels, and even further. From all corners of the country increasing numbers of measles cases were being notified. The RSA experienced an epidemic of measles, especially during the second half of 1992. More whites and Asians than before the MS were being affected. More older children developed measles. Deaths from measles remained at a low level, however. It would seem that the herd immunity of older children was insufficient to prevent the 1992 epidemic (22 745 notified cases).

In November 1992 the DNHPD recommended the administration of 3 doses of measles vaccine, at 6–9 months, at 18 months and at school-entry, in order to raise herd immunity. It would seem that measles amongst the immunised children occurred at 6 years and older and in the unimmunised children at 3 years and younger. During the year 1993, 11 762 cases of measles were notified and 19 deaths from measles occurred. (See 'Childhood immunisation schedule' below.)

COMMUNITY HEALTH IMMUNISATION PROGRAMMES

Infectious diseases are the most important community health problem in the developing world. In order for an immunisation programme to attain success, cognizance must be taken of local conditions, beliefs and customs. In most cases, the immediate objective of the immunisation programme is to reduce morbidity and mortality, but in the case of smallpox, eradication was aimed at and was achieved.

Active immunisation against a number of bacterial and viral infective diseases should be started in infancy. According to regulation No. 1754 published in the *Government Gazette*, September 1973, the law requires every infant to be vaccinated with BCG vaccine before the age of 6 months (subject to the provisions of regulation 12). This regulation has since been repealed (1987).

Immunisation against poliomyelitis is no longer compulsory in childhood. Immigrants up to the age of 40 years should receive 4 doses of polio vaccine (Sabin).

Strong pressure is put on parents by local authorities to have their infants immunised against the following diseases: diphtheria, tetanus, whooping cough (pertussis) and measles. Vaccines against these four diseases can be administered simultaneously without ill effect, the body being able to manufacture antibodies against a number of antigens at the same time. The customary pattern followed is to do the primary vaccination during the first year of life and to give booster doses of the vaccines at times when the child is likely to be exposed to infection, i.e. on going to nursery school and on going to 'big' school.

Vaccines have also been prepared against the following diseases: cholera, plague, typhus, rabies, yellow fever and typhoid. These vaccines are administered only when people are at risk, e.g. yellow fever vaccination is sometimes required of travellers proceeding beyond the borders of South Africa. Typhoid vaccination is used during epidemics of typhoid fever, and is also given to workers at risk.

Rabies vaccine is given after a bite by a rabid animal.

CHILDHOOD IMMUNSATION SCHEDULE

Age of Child	Vaccines		
Birth	TOPVO	BCG	
6 weeks	TOP1	DTP1	HBV1
10 weeks	TOP2	DTP2	HBV2
14 weeks	TOPV3	DTP3	HBV3
9 months	Measles 1		
18 months	TOPV4	DTP4	Measles 2
5 years	TOPV5	DT	
TOPV	Trivalent oral polio vaccine		
DTP	Diphtheria. Tetanus, Pertussis vaccine		
HBV	Hepatitis B vaccine (derived from plasma)		
DT	Diphtheria, Tetanus vaccine		
BCG	Bacille Calmette-Guerin (TB vaccine)		

S Afr Med J, April 1995; **85**(4):298

Every subsequent 10 years and whenever there is special danger of contracting tetanus, the vaccine should be given. Pregnant women should be immunised against tetanus.

No immunisation procedures are allowed to be done without written consent of parent or guardian.

Note: HIV-infected infants have a lower level of protection from the vaccines that non-infected infants.

Non-immunised children with symptomatic AIDS should not receive BCG-, Mumps- and Rubella vaccines. They should, however, receive the other childhood vaccines, namely trivalent oral polio-, DTP/DT- and measles-vaccine, the latter excluded only if the medical practitioner rules against such on grounds of severe immunosuppression.

Inactive vaccines such as Hepatitis B, Influenza, H. Influenza and Pneumococcal vaccines may be administered. The latter vaccines, however, are not supplied by the Department.[13]

Contra-indications to immunisation

Serious side-effects are rare, with different vaccines holding different risks.

DPT must not be given if there is a severe local or general reaction, e.g. anaphylaxis to a previous dose, or if the patient is acutely ill with a high temperature, or if he is sensitive to egg protein, or has a history of convulsions and neonatal brain damage.

Live vaccines (e.g. BCG, polio (Sabin) and measles) should not be given to immuno-compromised persons or pregnant women.

Oral polio vaccine must not be given during an attack of gastro-enteritis.

High-risk vaccinations but not total contra-indications

When giving measles, mumps and rubella vaccines, the child must be monitored; the nurse must be prepared to treat expected reactions, e.g. anaphylaxis. The doubtful conditions are:

- Acute febrile illnesses.
- Allergy to eggs.
- A previous seizure or epilepsy in the close family. Should the child develop a fever, bring the temperature down with paracetamol before giving the vaccine
- Hypersensitivity to neomycin.

No contra-indication to immunisation

- All sensitivities (asthma, eczema, migraine, food allergy) except *anaphylaxis* to egg *protein.*
- Antibiotics, other medicines including topical and low-dose oral steroids.
- Chronic illness.
- PEM and failure to thrive — prematurity.
- Pregnancy and breast-feeding
- Uncertainty about previous measles vaccination.
- Previous history of pertussis.
- Prematurity.

Reference: Kibel MA, Hay I, Donald P. Immunisation. *Nursing RSA Verpleging* 1990; **5**(3).

TUBERCULOSIS VACCINE

Tuberculosis is well controlled in developed countries, but in most parts of South Africa the incidence is still very high because of the difficulty in controlling pre-treatment disease transmission, and because of poor socio-economic conditions. In 1981, 52 013 cases were notified and in 1991, over 80 000. The Tuberculosis Research Institute of the MRC found a prevalence of 120 000 infectious tuberculosis cases in the RSA at any point in time and a reservoir of 10 million infected cases, viz. persons with a dormant infection.[7]

BCG vaccination before the age of 6 months was compulsory in the RSA from 1973. Since October 1987 it is no longer compulsory.[11] All children should be vaccinated, however, since it offers them a great deal of protection. Coverage has reached more than

80 %. It is given to infants, a second dose being given at 3 months if there is no scar from the vaccination done at birth.[7] Booster doses of the vaccine are advocated at the age of 5 to 6 years (i.e. at school-entry) and again at school-leaving, as the protective effect of BCG wanes after approximately 5–10 years. It is also given to tuberculin-negative contacts of infectious patients. Acquired immunity to tuberculosis gives only about 80 % protection even under ideal conditions; therefore, a person may succumb to a virulent infection even after BCG vaccination. BCG may, therefore, not prevent tuberculosis. An immunisation programme started in infancy may prevent the tuberculous meningitis of infancy. It has been found that, although BCG vaccination does not prevent pulmonary tuberculosis on exposure to infection, the disease is usually milder and cavities do not usually form in the lungs; the TB is, therefore, not infectious. BCG, therefore, helps to reduce the reservoir of infection.

Immunity to tuberculosis is not dependent on antibody formation, i.e. the newborn does not get a passive immunity from its mother; BCG causes a cellular immune response which is effective from birth. Resistance to tuberculosis is, however, adversely affected by malnutrition, virus infections (especially AIDS), steroids, stress (emotional and physical) and age (low and high).

BCG vaccine can be given at any age and in conjunction with any other vaccine, the BCG induced protection against tuberculosis being gauged by the skin sensitivity which develops within 6 weeks of vaccination. The aim of vaccination is to convert a negative PPD (tuberculin) reaction to a positive one. In principle, it is given only to non-infected individuals, hence the rationale of vaccinating newborn infants.

The Bacille Calmette-Guèrin (BCG) vaccine is a freeze-dried preparation of live, attenuated (weakened) bovine tubercle bacilli, different varieties of the vaccine being made from different strains of the bacillus. Because the vaccine is made from live organisms, it is easily destroyed by light and heat. The vaccine must, therefore, be protected against light and is supplied in either red or brown ampoules, together with fluid (saline) used for reconstituting the solid vaccine before use. The vaccination must

never be done outside in direct sunlight and, if done in the shade under trees, the multiple dose vial must be kept covered between injections. The vaccine must be kept under ordinary refrigeration and transported under cold conditions, e.g. a freezer bag with ice blocks which are renewed daily. The vaccine is kept cold until the moment of use. Only one vial of the vaccine is reconstituted with diluent at a time and any left-over mixed vaccine is discarded.

Note:
(1) The Japanese percutaneous BCG vaccine, Tokyo Strain 172, has special advantages in that it is heat stable.
(2) BCG vaccine is distributed and supplied free of charge by the Department of Health to local authorities. Private doctors may not give the vaccine.
(3) The freeze-dried vaccine can be stored at 8 °C for 12 months.

Vaccination is done by either an intradermal or a percutaneous, multiple puncture injection, different strengths of the vaccine being used for intradermal and percutaneous injections. For practical reasons, the percutaneous route is preferred.

Method of intradermal vaccination

A plastic tuberculin syringe, checked for tightness of fit, is filled with one dose (0,1 ml) of the correctly reconstituted vaccine. The syringe can be reused 10 times, but a fresh sterile 25-gauge needle must be used for each person. The injection is given into the skin of the front outer aspect of the left forearm. The arm must be clean.

Note: The intradermal BCG vaccine is also used in the treatment of cancer for the purpose of raising the body's immune responsitivity to cancer cells.

Method of percutaneous (multiple puncture) vaccination

Percutaneous vaccination with the special Japanese percutaneous vaccine is used in routine immunisation programmes. The advantage of this method of vaccination is its ease of administration, especially in infants. The 50 dose vial is mixed with 1,5 ml of saline and the 10 dose vial with 0,3 ml. It is important to check that the correct vaccine is used, as severe ulceration may be caused if, for example, the vaccine meant for percutaneous injection is used intradermally. The BCG vaccine must be placed on ice after dilution and protected against sunlight. The vial must be shaken before use.

Immunisation is done either with the Heaf 'gun' apparatus, using the East Mark VI model or the Allen and Hanbury's model with 20 needles, or with the Japanese plastic vaccinating tool (needle-planted cylinder). The essential part of the Heaf 'gun' is a spring which can be triggered to shoot forward for a controlled pre-set distance, short even needles (tines) fixed in a circle to the gun head, through holes in a metal shield, the end plate. For infants the needles are set to penetrate 1 mm, but in children a deeper penetration of 2 mm is required.

The gun is periodically oiled, kept in alcohol and flamed before use. It must, however, be cool before use, as heat destroys the vaccine. When doing vaccination, the right arm is held horizontally and the skin of the upper arm is tensed by gripping the undersurface of the arm between thumb and fingers. After cleaning and drying the skin, one drop (0,5 m) of the vaccine is applied either with a syringe needle or a glass rod to the upper arm, in the region of the insertion of the deltoid muscle.

The end plate of the gun is rotated on the drop in order to spread the vaccine. Holding the gun perpendicularly to the skin, the gun is fired. The needles (tines) are drawn up, the end plate is rotated slightly and the needles are fired a second time to give 40 penetrations through the skin area covered with the vaccine. The needles are drawn up again and the end plate rotated to force the vaccine into the punctures. No dressing is necessary. The vaccinated person should stay out of the sun for 5 minutes.

Note: In infants, one firing, i.e. 20 penetrations, is sufficient. Some authorities claim that it is unnecessary to use more than one firing in children. The needles must be drawn up before rotation of the end plate, otherwise painful tearing of the skin will result.

The Japanese multipuncture BCG vaccinating tool has 9 fine steel needles fixed in an inner disc near one end of the cylinder which is surrounded by a depth-controlling flange. A drop of BCG vaccine is spread out in a film on the cleaned, dry outer part of the upper arm and the cylinder pressed down vertically until the sides of the flange touch the skin; thus 9 punctures are made. This manoeuvre is repeated once for neonates (i.e. 18 punctures) and twice for older children (i.e. 27 punctures) by lifting the cylinder and either rotating it slightly or moving it to slightly overlapping adjacent sites. The skin area to be punctured must be covered with a film of the BCG vaccine, so that no punctures are made through dry skin.

The Japanese BCG vaccinating tool can be used for more than 100 vaccinations. Sterilisation of the cylinder between vaccinations (to eliminate infection with hepatitis B virus) can be done either by autoclaving (115 °C for 20 minutes or 121 °C for 15 minutes) or by placing the needle end of the cylinder in 10 % formalin for 10 minutes and rinsing it afterwards in running water.[8]

Reaction to BCG vaccination occurs approximately 2 weeks later and may persist for 5 to 6 weeks. The mother should be warned about the reaction and told that scratching must be avoided. If the child is not co-operative, a dressing is applied over the area.

BCG vaccination lesions will be found to range from: no reaction, to small and large red pustules often on a red indurated base. Minute hypopigmented scars remain as evidence of vaccination. If ulceration occurs, neomycin ointment is applied and a doctor consulted. A tuberculin (PPD) skin sensitivity Mantoux test (see p. 527) can be done on the left arm, 7 to 14 (average 10) weeks after BCG vaccination, to estimate the success of vaccination.

BCG vaccination is deemed to have been successful if the red induration (hardened area) at the site of the sensitivity test is 10 mm or more in diameter. Tuberculin testing is done to find out if conversion from a negative pre-vaccination to a positive post-vaccination reaction has taken place. If the BCG vaccine has induced hypersensitivity to tuberculin (PPD), the criterion of successful vaccination has been met.

Ysselmuiden *et al.* state:

'In relation to tuberculosis, no influence of BCG vaccination programmes could be shown. This cannot be interpreted as meaning that BCG vaccine is ineffective. It does mean, however, that BCG vaccination plays only a minor role, if any, in the overall control of tuberculosis and that the provision of appropriate primary health care services to all people in South Africa is the main contribution that the health services can, and must, make in order to have an impact on tuberculosis control.'[3]

In spite of the rather negative finding above, Fourie[4] of the Tuberculosis Research Institute of the SAMRC advocates that BCG vaccination should remain compulsory at birth (see p. 497), should be repeated at 3 months in children without evidence of reactivity at the vaccination site, as well as at school-entry and school-leaving.

HEPATITIS B VACCINE

Hepatitis B vaccine became available in the RSA in 1983. At this stage it was intended for health care workers exposed to blood and blood products and for patients involved in dialysis programmes. The vaccine was originally tested in New York on homosexual males — a population at high risk of getting hepatitis.

The development of the vaccine began with the finding that if dilute hepatitis B infective serum is boiled for a short period, it loses its infectivity but not its antigenicity. The vaccine consists of highly purified, formalin-inactivated antigenic particles as derived from the plasma of chronic hepatitis B carriers. The immune response is confirmed by the appearance of antibodies in the serum. The vaccine is given by injection in three doses, the first two at a monthly interval and a booster dose after 6 months. Immunity will probably last for at least 5 years.

Smith Kline Pharmaceuticals have recently developed Engerix-B recombinant DNA vaccine against hepatitis B. It is the first genetically engineered and yeast-derived vaccine. This vaccine, an antigen protein, is not only very effective after the final dose but also very safe. Engerix is given in 3 separate doses of 20 micrograms each at the following intervals: 0, 1 and 6 months. This standard schedule confers immunity for approximately 5 years, after which a booster dose is needed. For those persons at more immediate risk a schedule of 0, 1, 2 months requires a booster dose after 1 year.

Engerix is highly immunogenic when given at birth to infants of carrier women (found positive for hepatitis B surface antigen (HB_sAg) and hepatitis B_e antigen (HB_eAg)). In some areas perinatally acquired infections account for many cases of chronic infection. Engerix blocks virus transmission, both perinatally and in early childhood.

POLIOMYELITIS VACCINES

Since 1987 polio vaccination in the RSA is no longer compulsory. All children should be vaccinated, however.[11] The vaccination coverage of the under-five group was 76 % in 1985.

Susceptible contacts of a polio case should be vaccinated immediately. The OPV (Oral Polio Vaccine) provides immediate protection as it interferes with the 'wild' poliovirus.

There are two types of polio vaccine in use throughout the world.[12]

Salk vaccine

The original vaccine is the Salk inactivated polio vaccine (IPV) given by injection and made from dead polioviruses. IPV stimulates humoral immunity resulting in IgM, IgG and IgA serum antibodies, but no immune activity in the gut. IPV has been used with complete success in some European countries with high socio-economic standards in which faecal/oral spread plays a minor role. It requires wide vaccine coverage to provide herd immunity.

Sabin vaccine

In the RSA the Sabin vaccine is generally used for community health immunisation programmes. It is an oral live attenuated (avirulent) vaccine (OPV) which results in an active infection of the oropharynx and intestinal epithelium by the attenuated vaccine virus. Special local antibodies in addition to the serum antibodies (as with IPV) are produced. The virus is excreted in the faeces and secondary spread occurs to susceptible contacts, thus bringing about herd immunity even if the coverage is only 66 %. One in 3 million doses of the OPV can cause paralytic polio, usually because of immunosuppression of the recipient.

The OPV is less expensive than the IPV and easier to administer. The live attenuated virus is sensitive to destruction by both heat (necessitating storage at below 10 °C) and enteroviruses in the intestine which may prevent the attenuated vaccine virus from multiplying in the gut to elicit a strong antibody reaction. To ensure effective immunity, the number of doses for primary vaccination was recently increased from 3 to 4, the last dose being given at 12 months. This is the 'safety' dose in case one of the first 3 doses failed.

The Sabin vaccine is administered from the age of 3 months by placing 3 drops on syrup or sugar which is dropped directly on to the tongue. No breast milk is to be given for half an hour before or two hours after the OPV as it may kill the virus.

The Salk vaccine is used where there are contra-indications to the use of the Sabin vaccine.

Contra-indications to the use of all live, attenuated virus vaccines, i.e. measles, mumps, rubella and polio:

(1) Immunodeficiency or -suppression for whatever reason.
(2) Leukaemia, lymphoma.
(3) The administration of gammaglobulin or plasma in the preceding 8 weeks.
(4) Pregnancy.

DIPHTHERIA, PERTUSSIS, TETANUS (DPT) VACCINE

A combined diphtheria, pertussis, tetanus (DPT) vaccine given by intramuscular injection is used in community health immunisation programmes, this primary immunisation usually being started at the age of 2–3 months. In tetanus and pertussis, there is no herd immunity, every person requiring individual protection. This is not the case in diphtheria (and poliomyelitis); if 80 % of the population has been immunised against diphtheria, there will be no spread of the infection in a closed community and the disease will disappear.

The coverage in the RSA with DPT vaccine was 74 % in 1985.

The four doses are given respectively at 3, $4\frac{1}{2}$, 6 and 18 months.

Single preparations of these vaccines are also available.

Pertussis (whooping-cough) vaccine

Pertussis vaccine is made from killed whole organisms (Bordetella pertussis) and can be given by deep intramuscular injection to prevent skin reactions.

Early immunisation of infants in developing countries, i.e. at 1 month, is advocated by some authorities, as these infants may develop fatal pertussis before the age of 3 months. As the body's defences are immature at this age, however, the immunisation may not be effective. Young infants should, therefore, not be exposed to older children with pertussis until primary vaccination has been commenced. No child should be given a pertussis vaccine after the age of $2\frac{1}{2}$ years as there is increased danger of encephalopathy with seizures and brain damage. No child who has been affected thus should have any further injections against pertussis. As whooping cough is such a dangerous disease in infancy, a pertussis epidemic is an indication for the rapid immunisation (i.e. three weekly doses) of unvaccinated infants, especially those under the age of 3 months.

Note: Pertussis became a notifiable disease in 1994.

Mild reactions to pertussis vaccine: redness, pain, swelling at the site of the injection, pyrexia and fractiousness (peevishness).

Contra-indications to pertussis immunisation:

(1) neurological signs in the neonatal period; history of convulsions;
(2) family history of diseases of the nervous system;
(3) during a febrile illness.

Diphtheria vaccine

See p. 545.

Active immunisation against diphtheria can also be started soon after birth in the event of a diphtheria epidemic, but as in the case of pertussis, it is not as effective as later in infancy. Infants are not hypersensitive to diphtheria toxoid, but as children over 10 years and adults may be hypersensitive (exhibiting pyrexia, vomiting, headache and local swelling and erythema), they should be Schick-tested before receiving a booster dose. A negative Schick test will contra-indicate the giving of the vaccine. If the Schick test is positive, blood is taken for diphtheria antitoxin assay and medical advice followed regarding immunisation.

Tetanus vaccine

Active immunisation: In family health centres (well-baby clinics), primary immunisation against tetanus is started at the age of 2 to 3 months. The second dose is given at 4 to 5 months and the third at 5 to 6 months. A booster dose is given at 18 months and another at 5 to 6 years. Tetanus vaccine should be repeated (booster dose) at the age of 10 years and every subsequent 10 years in persons at special risk (e.g. sportsmen), or whenever there is special danger of contracting the disease, e.g. after deep wounding or a septic abortion. Active immunisation is done with adsorbed tetanus toxoid. It is an effective antigen which can be used in very small doses.

There is a measurable increase in antibody titre within 4 to 7 days after the first dose of the tetanus toxoid.

Antenatal immunisation of the pregnant woman against tetanus is advocated to protect an infant against neonatal tetanus — a possibility where cultural practices cause infection through the umbilical cord. Immunisation against tetanus is important in children as they are frequently exposed to minor cuts which become unexpectedly infected by *Cl. tetani*.

Note:
(1) Human tetanus immunoglobulin can be used for passive immunisation. It can be used intrathecally early in tetanus to neutralise toxin (tetanospasmin) and lower mortality.
(2) The incidence of tetanus (notifications), of which 60–80 % are in children less than 1 year old (probably due to tetanus neonatorum), has remained largely unchanged in the 1980s. Over 92 % of tetanus notifications occur amongst blacks.
(3) Tetanus neonatorum was made notifiable in 1991.

RUBELLA (GERMAN MEASLES) VACCINE

The rubella vaccine is usually given to pre-puberty girls in their last year in primary school, to prevent the teratogenic effects of rubella during the early weeks of pregnancy, when these girls reach adulthood. Infants born with the defects of the rubella syndrome are a danger to others as they may excrete the virus for months and thus infect pregnant women in their environment.

The first rubella vaccine was licensed in the USA in 1969. Vaccination with the attenuated rubella live-virus vaccine is used in community vaccination campaigns. It is not administered in cases of pregnancy (when it may be teratogenic), febrile illness or defective immunological responses for whatever reason, and vaccination is not done routinely in women of childbearing age (in case the woman is pregnant or about to become pregnant within 8 weeks) except in special groups of women, e.g. health workers, at risk, but only if they are seronegative and not pregnant.

It can also be given to a woman during the puerperium if blood tests done during pregnancy show an absence of immunity to rubella (by rubella-specific IgM determinations).

The freeze-dried vaccine is stored in a refrigerator (4 °C) and immediately before use by subcutaneous injection reconstituted with cold sterile water; it is used within an hour.

MEASLES (MORBILLI) VACCINE

Two types of vaccines against measles recently came into use, one prepared from dead viruses and one prepared from live attenuated organisms. The former vaccine is safer yet less effective than the one made from live viruses; the latter probably gives immunity for life if the child's immunological reactions are normal. This effective vaccine may, however, cause side-effects which resemble a mild attack of the disease. The attenuated, live-virus vaccine should not be administered to women who are pregnant, or likely to become pregnant, to patients suffering from any chronic infectious (e.g. active untreated tuberculosis) or malignant disease or to people whose immunological responses are defective for any reason. It can, however, be given to all severely malnourished children and those with gastro-enteritis and bronchopneumonia when admitted to hospital with these conditions.[9]

Vaccination of infants against measles is especially important in the lower socio-economic communities where infants have little resistance and easily succumb to its complications. These are the high-risk groups.

In May 1991 a new measles vaccine based on a different strain of the virus, the high-titre Edmonston-Zagreb (HTEZ), was introduced. Although four times as expensive as the old (Schwartz) vaccine, it is active from 6 months of age, whereas the Schwartz is active from 9 months of age. The alternative use of these two vaccines will depend upon the availability of HTEZ (high-titre) and on whether the child is at high risk and immunisation at 6 months of age is mandatory.

Man is the only host of the virus and a single dose of effective vaccine will provide long-lasting immunity in 90–95 % of vaccinated persons.

The 1993 Measles Immunisation Policy

It is Departmental policy that all children be immunised against measles at the age of 9 months and 18 months of age. However, children in high-risk areas (low measles immunisation coverage (< 70 %) and reported cases of measles under 9 months of age) should receive *an additional dose* of measles vaccine at 6 months, i.e. 6, 9 and 18 months of age.

The measles immunisation status of every child who attends a health-care delivery point, should be assessed. All children in the age group 2–5 years who do not have a definite history of measles or who have not had at least two doses of measles vaccine, should receive measles vaccine. If in any doubt whether an infant has been immunised, it is far safer to carry out immunisation.

In order to raise herd immunity, a dose of measles vaccine is also recommended at school-entry age (see p. 560).

The live-virus vaccine is a freeze-dried suspension of live, attenuated measles viruses which requires reconstitution with cold, sterile water immediately before use. The dried vaccine is stored in a refrigerator (4 °C). In freeze-dried form it has a half-life of 37 months at 4 °C, 31 days at 25 °C and 16 days at 37 °C. The reconstituted vaccine must be kept in the dark and used within the hour. It is given by intramuscular or subcutaneous injection.

Reactions, simulating a subclinical attack of measles, may occur 5 to 12 days after inoculation. Some authorities feel that a child with an existing temperature and upper respiratory tract infection should not be inoculated against measles. Others again aver that a mild indisposition is not a contra-indication to inoculation with vaccines.[10]

Measles vaccine can be given in combination with other vaccines, but the vaccine affects tuberculin sensitivity test reactions; therefore, the Mantoux and Heaf PPD tests should be done either before or two months after measles inoculation.

MUMPS VACCINE

The live, attenuated mumps virus vaccine is cultivated in chick embryos; it is given subcutaneously and the dangers from toxic side-effects are minimal. The duration of induced immunity is not certain, but immunity has been found to last for at least ten years.

The use of the mumps vaccine in community health immunisation programmes is not essential; if used for this purpose, however, a single dose in combination with measles and rubella vaccines is sufficient. It should not be administered before the age of 12 months as maternal anti-mumps antibodies may prevent the immune reaction from taking place. Its use as a single vaccine in pre-adolescents and adolescents who are in danger of developing orchitis or oophoritis (complications of mumps) is considered advisable. It will, however, not prevent mumps if given after the susceptible patient has been exposed to mumps virus infection.

The use of mumps vaccine is contra-indicated as for rubella vaccine.

INFLUENZA VACCINE

For each expected influenza epidemic, certain vaccines are recommended by the Department of Health, based on information provided by the World Health Organisation as well as information derived from influenza surveillance programmes carried out by the National Institute of Virology and the Department of Medical Microbiology, University of Cape Town.three virus strains with different antigenic structures. The vaccine usually changes yearly to include the most commonly occurring virus strains for a specific year. If there has been no antigenic change in the virus strains, then no new vaccine will be made that year.

Flu vaccines have a prophylactic value only if they are prepared from the current antigenic strains.

The vaccine is made either from killed whole organisms (given by hypodermic injection) or from live, attenuated organisms (given by inhalation).

Note:

(1) 'The vaccines can only protect sufficiently against virus strains they contain. No enduring protection can be expected against other viruses or other respiratory diseases such as colds. Many other respiratory diseases not due to influenza viruses occur and are also commonly termed "flu". It cannot be expected of the influenza vaccines that they should protect patients against the latter diseases.'

(2) No influenza epidemics occurred during 1982 because of the absence of antigenic change during this period.

REFERENCES

(1) Editorial. *S Afr Journal of Epidemiology and Infection* 1989; **4**(1).

(2) Ysselmuiden CB, Gear JSS. Editorial. Expanded Programme on Immunisation for South Africa. *S Afr Med J* 1987; **72**: 305–306.

(3) Ysselmuiden CB, Kustner HGV, Barron PM, Steinberg WJ. Notification of five of the EPI target diseases in South Africa. *S Afr Med J* 1987; **72**: 311–317.

(4) Fourie PB. BCG vaccination and the EPI. *S Afr Med J* 1987; **72**: 323–326.

(5) Crisp NG, Ysselmuiden, CB, De Swardt R, *et al*. Provision of immunisation — The Gazankulu experience. *S Afr Med J* 1987; **72**: 345–348.

(6) De Swardt R, Ysselmuiden CB, Edginton ME. Vaccine cold-chain status in the Elim health ward of Gazankulu. *S Afr Med J* 1987; **72**: 334–336.

(7) Glatthaar E. Editorial. *S Afr Med J* 1981; **59**: 550.

(8) Glatthaar E, Kleeberg HH. *S Afr Med J* 1977; **52**: 633.

(9) Harris MF. *S Afr Med J* 1979; **55**: 38.

(10) Prozesky OW. *Curationis* 1978; **1**: 8.

(11) *Government Gazette* No. 11014, October 1987 Regulation No. 2438 of 31 October, 1987.

(12) SAMJ News. *S Afr Med J* 1989; **76**: xvi.

(13) Childhood immunisation of HIV-infected infants and children. *Epidemiological Comments* 1991;**18**(5).

(14) The measles strategy. *Epidemiological Comments* 1991;**18**(5).

(15) The measles strategy, South Africa, 1991 — An evaluation of its effect. *Epidemiological Comments* 1992;**19**(7).

(16) The measles strategy revisited — What happened? *Epidemiological Comments* 1993;**20**(9).

(17) Benadé JG. Compliance with code of practice for vaccine storage, transportation and handling. *S Afr Journal of Epidemiology & Infection* 1994;**9**(2).

TEST OF KNOWLEDGE

The student has benefited from studying this chapter if he/she can answer the following questions:

(1) Distinguish between:
  – Sabin and Salk polio vaccines;
  – vaccines and gammaglobulins.

(2) Define:
  – immunity
  – status of the cold-chain of a vaccine
  – prophylactic toxoids

(3) Write notes on:
  – The definition of, and contra-indications to, live-virus vaccines
  – The evaluation of BCG vaccination
  – The low incidence of diphtheria in the RSA
  – The influenza vaccine
  – The immunisation programme for primary immunisation used by Child Health clinics in the RSA

(4) Prepare the outline of a lecture for a group of enrolled community health nurses on the subject of the maintenance of the cold-chain in caring for vaccines.

(5) What is meant by the WHO's EPI? What are its aims and what strategies can be used in South Africa to reach the EPI target by 1990?

(6) Describe how immunisation against the following diseases may be done:
  – tuberculosis
  – poliomyelitis
  – pertussis
  – hepatitis B
  – tetanus
  – measles.

29

The Control of Infection by Antimicrobial Agents (AMA)[*]

OBJECTIVES

The nurse must:

(1) learn about the vast field of antimicrobial agents (mainly antibiotics) which control infection inside the body and which are prescribed by the doctor and the PHC nurse and administered by the nurse;

(2) grasp the fact the there are no innocuous antimicrobials and that every patient receiving these medicines must be observed for untoward signs and symptoms. He/she must know the main toxic effects of every group of antimicrobial agents;

(3) be especially aware of the hypersensitivity reactions to penicillin, cephalosporins, amphotericin B and streptomycin, and know what emergency steps to take in the case of an anaphylactic reaction;

(4) understand the concepts 'immunocompromised patient' and 'opportunistic infections';

(5) understand the concept 'antimicrobial agent resistance' (AMAR).

---

* Extracts from Chapter 26 of Vlok ME *Manual of Nursing* vol. I *Basic Nursing* (with kind permission of the publishers).

IN THIS CHAPTER

INTRODUCTION

Chemotherapy or pharmacotherapy means the treatment of disease by means of chemical substances which may be introduced orally or parenterally or may even be used topically and in body cavities.

Antimicrobial means against microbes, i.e. the microscopic bacteria, fungi, viruses and protozoa which cause infective diseases in man.

Antimicrobial chemotherapy, therefore, means the treatment of infective conditions by means of medicines (agents).

Although chemotherapy has been practised since time immemorial, the antimicrobial chemotherapeutic era started with the advent of sulphonamides (M & B 693, Prontosil) shortly before World War II. The discovery of penicillin by Fleming, Florey and co-workers soon after, heralded the start of the antibiotic era. The effects of sulphonamides and antibiotics on infection were dramatic; their promise has been disappointing to some extent, as microbes developed resistance to them and dangerous side-effects became apparent.

Antibiotics (*anti* = against, *bios* = life) are substances secreted by living organisms, especially branched fungi and bacteria. Antibiotics are antagonistic to the growth of other microbes and may even kill them; antibiotics are, therefore, either bacteriostatic or bactericidal. Penicillin, bacitracin and vancomycin, for instance, inhibit bacterial cell wall synthesis, thus causing bacteria to burst and die. Erythromycin, chloramphenicol and the aminoglycosides inhibit bacterial cell protein synthesis and thereby stop cell replication. The polymyxins are cationic detergents that make bacterial cells permeable and cause them to burst.

Historically a distinction was made between synthetic chemotherapeutic antimicrobial agents (e.g. metronidazole, sulphonamides) and biologically produced antimicrobial agents (e.g. antibiotics), but the modern trend is to use the term antimicrobial agent (AMA) to include antibiotics, semisynthetic congeners (agents akin to) of antibiotics and synthetic chemotherapeutic agents.

NATURAL AND ACQUIRED RESISTANCE OF MICRO-ORGANISMS TO ANTIBIOTICS

Antimicrobial agent resistance (AMAR)

Natural resistance by selection

When an antimicrobial agent (AMA) is administered, most of the susceptible microbes are affected (killed or growth inhibited) and thus infection is brought under control. A small percentage of the organisms will not be affected — they possess natural resistance. They survive, multiply and soon predominate over the susceptible class of organisms in their neighbourhood, e.g. in a hospital ward. Thus the antibiotics which were originally used effectively lose their power over the organisms through a process of natural selection. The microbes have developed resistance to the antibiotics.

Acquired resistance

This is a more common and persistent kind of resistance of microbes to a class or classes of antibiotics and is the reason why scientists are constantly doing research to discover new antimicrobial agents.

There are many ways in which micro-organisms can change (adapt) in order to protect themselves against antibiotic threats. Each antibiotic has its unique target site in or on the microbe. For any antibiotic to be effective, there must be an affinity between the antibiotic and its particular site of action. If there is any change in the target site on the microbe, affinity is lost and the antibiotic will lose its effectiveness.

Resistance may depend on the ability of certain microbes to develop enzymes against some antibiotics which render the latter inactive. Penicillins and cephalosporins, the safest and, before inactivation, the most effective of all antibiotics, are especially liable to become inactivated by enzymes collectively known as beta-lactamases. (This enzyme was formerly known as penicillinase, the new term, -lactamase, denoting resistance to the very similar cephalosporins as well.)

Organisms that have become resistant will render a 'good' antibiotic absolutely useless.

The following organisms are especially liable to build up resistance to antibiotics:

Gram-negative bacilli, e.g. Klebsiella, Serratia, Pseudomonas.

Gram-positive cocci, e.g. Staphylococcus aureus, Streptococcus pneumoniae, enterobacteriaceae. Gram-negative cocci, e.g. Neisseria gonorrhoeae and meningitidis.

Preventing or retarding resistance

The doctor prescribing, the nurse administering or supervising the latter, and the patient taking the AMA should co-operate to ensure that AMAs are used:

(a) only when necessary, in this way preventing the natural selection of resistant organisms;

(b) adequately with regard to dose and duration of therapy;

(c) selectively, i.e. reserving key AMAs for dire necessities only, e.g. vancomycin;

(d) only for infections which are susceptible to the AMA;

(e) in combination therapy of various classes to ensure destruction of all the microbes present, where the above specificity cannot be assumed. There are advantages (more effective, less chance of developing resistance) and disadvantages (expensive, superinfection, antagonistic effects, more potential adverse effects).

OPPORTUNISTIC INFECTIONS AND THE IMMUNOCOMPROMISED PATIENT

The occurrence of opportunistic infections is a very important problem in antimicrobial chemotherapy. Opportunists are pathogenic microbes which do not normally cause disease in the healthy human host. They invade the body when the host's immune defence mechanisms become 'compromised' or lowered.

Lowered immunity may be due to:

(a) immunosuppressive drugs given to treat cancer or to prevent donor rejection after transplant surgery;

(b) steroid therapy for the relief of symptoms in auto-immune diseases, e.g. rheumatoid arthritis;

(c) concurrent disturbances such as diabetes mellitus, leukaemia, severe burns, etc.;

(d) the presence of foreign bodies, e.g. urinary catheters, intravenous cannulation, endotracheal tubes;

(e) acquired immunodeficiency syndrome (e.g. AIDS) and other immunodeficiency conditions;

(f) malnutrition.

There are many other less definite reasons why the host's immunity is lowered to such an extent that opportunistic infections, for example, the common cold, take place.

When host immunity is compromised for a period, infection is difficult to overcome with the appropriate antimicrobial agents which are usually effective, due to loss of the body's own defences which normally play a very important role in overcoming infection.

The following are examples of microbes which cause infections in patients with immunological deficiency syndromes:

Defect in humoral immunity: meningococcus, pneumococcus, streptococcus, pseudomonas.

Defect in cell-mediated immunity: varicella/zoster virus, vaccinia virus, herpes simplex virus, cytomegalovirus, fungi, including yeasts, *M. tuberculosis*.

SPECIFICITY OF ANTIBIOTICS

Antibiotics are not absolutely specific in their action and vary from being effective against a few kinds of microbes (narrow-spectrum) to being effective against a large number of microbes (broad-spectrum).

The *narrow-spectrum antibiotics* are predominantly active against one of the following classes of microbes:

- Gram-positive microbes, e.g. penicillin.
- Gram-negative organisms, e.g. polymyxin B.

Common pathogenic bacteria classified according to Gram staining:

Gram-positive	Gram-negative
Streptococcus	*Neisseria gonorrhoeae*
Staphylococcus	*Neisseria meningitidis*
Corynebacterium	*Salmonella* and *Shigella*
Bacillus	*Escherichia (coli)*
Clostridium	*Klebsiella* spp.
	Proteus spp.
	Vibrio
	Pseudomonas (aeruginosa) and *(pyocyanea)*
	The parvobacteria (Brucella, Haemophilus (influenzae), Bordetella, Pasteurella, Yersinia, Bacteroides)

The *broad-spectrum antibiotics* have a much wider range of activity, i.e. they are effective against Gram-negative and Gram-positive organisms, as well as some of the larger viruses, chlamydiae, protozoa, rickettsiae and actinomycetes. They are generally given orally and their main hazard is that they may kill off the Gram-negative intestinal flora, thereby causing superinfection of the bowel with organisms which are resistant to their action, e.g. staphylococci and Candida albicans.

These broad-spectrum antibiotics are never used in preference to penicillin which is still the safest antibiotic despite its proneness to elicit hypersensitivity reactions. They are, therefore, used only if penicillin is ineffective or if the patient has an acquired sensitivity to it.

UNTOWARD SIDE-EFFECTS OF AMA

Many effective antibiotics and other antimicrobials are toxic and have dangerous side-effects, e.g. deafness and damage to renal and blood forming tissues. Others again, like penicillin, do not have dangerous side-effects, but may elicit a hypersensitivity reaction, ranging from urticaria to fatal anaphylactic shock. For these reasons antimicrobial agents are legally controlled, being listed in Schedule 4 and obtainable on prescription only.

EMPIRIC (PRESUMPTIVE OR BLIND) INITIAL THERAPY

During the first day or two of the infective illness the doctor prescribes the antibiotic he thinks will be the best one to fight the infection. His choice depends upon his clinical findings, and his surmise as to the nature of the infecting microbe, if the infection is non-specific, and the antibiotic to which the microbe is likely to be susceptible. Penicillin should be the drug of choice except in patients who are known to be penicillin-sensitive, or those who are immunocompromised. If any infected discharges are present (e.g. sputum, pus from a wound, urine, faeces) or if blood or CSF is likely to harbour the microbe, a specimen is immediately obtained and sent to the laboratory for identification of the microbe and for a microbiological sensitivity test to a large variety of antibiotics, e.g. a cephalosporin, a variety of penicillins, erythromycin, a tetracycline, chloramphenicol, and a few aminoglycoside antibiotics. Initial empiric therapy is then followed by definitive (final) therapy.

DEFINITIVE (FINAL) THERAPY

The test result enables the doctor to choose the best antibiotic according to the following criteria:

(a) the infecting microbe must be highly sensitive to it;

(b) the antibiotic must be as non-toxic as possible; the doctor chooses an effective antibiotic which is likely to have as few side-effects as possible and which is not likely to be retained by the body, in case of poor renal function of a very sick patient;

(c) the antibiotic must be relatively inexpensive;

(d) the patient must not be sensitive (allergic) to the antibiotic, e.g. penicillin.

Where microbiological testing facilities are not readily available, definitive therapy is guided by the success or failure of initial therapy and the need to use antibiotics with low toxicity.

Other points to prevent ineffectual antibiotic therapy include:

(1) The antibiotic chosen by the doctor must have the narrowest spectrum possible without sacrificing efficiency, as the side-effects of the broad-spectrum antibiotics are often more harmful than those of the narrow-spectrum antibiotics.

(2) Antibiotics should never be used to bring down a temperature, if a diagnosis of the cause of the pyrexia has not been made. The latter may be due to a virus which will not respond to the antibiotic.

(3) Once started, a course of antibiotics should be completed, the usual length of a course being 5–6 days. If necessary, the course can be extended. The medicines must be taken at the prescribed times to maintain an optimal blood level for the desired effect. If blood levels of the antibiotic are allowed to fall below the therapeutic level, the microbes can build up resistance to the antibiotic and render it useless.

HYPERSENSITIVITY REACTIONS AND ANAPHYLACTIC SHOCK

The introduction of a foreign protein into the body of a sensitive person may cause the following reactions unexpectedly:

(1) Immediate and dangerous. Death may follow as a result of anaphylactic shock which includes respiratory obstruction due to bronchospasm and angioneurotic oedema. In anaphylactic shock there is sudden peripheral vascular failure due to widespread vasodilation; there may be cardiac and respiratory arrest. The patient may die within a few minutes.

(2) Delayed and dangerous. Symptoms such as urticaria and respiratory obstruction appear 2–5 days after administration of a foreign protein.

(3) Delayed and not dangerous. Serum sickness about 10 days after the administration of horse serum (antiserum).

Causes:

(1) The administration of certain medicines, especially antibiotics such as penicillins, cephalosporins, amphotericin B and strepto-

mycin in those people who have previously had a sensitivity reaction.

(2) The administration of antisera (e.g. antivenin serum (against snake bite), especially if the patient suffers from atopic hay fever or asthma).

(3) (*a*) Insect bites and stings, e.g. bee stings.
(*b*) Snake bite.

(4) Radiographic contrast media injected intravenously.

The treatment of a patient with a hypersensitivity reaction (anaphylactic shock and delayed dangerous reaction):

(*a*) Since the patient often collapses due to cardiac and respiratory arrest, external cardiac massage and mouth-to-mouth respiration is the first requirement.

(*b*) The patient can be intubated and given oxygen if angioneurotic oedema blocks the airway.

(*c*) Adrenaline 1:10 000, 10 ml must be given intravenously at the earliest possible moment if the patient has collapsed. If the patient has not yet collapsed, 5 ml 1:10 000 is given at the rate of 1 ml per minute, or 8 minims 1:1000 at the rate of 1 minim/minute. If possible, intravenous therapy is set up at this stage. Plasma expanders (e.g. plasma PPS) 1 litre is given quickly.

(*d*) The patient is kept flat and the legs are elevated.

(*e*) If the patient is conscious, he is reassured.

(*f*) Solu-Cortef 200 mg may be given intravenously immediately and repeated 4 to 6 hourly for 24 hours, in an attempt to restore the tone of the arterioles.

(*g*) Aminophyllin 250 mg may be given as a bolus dose by slow intravenous injection and 500 mg diluted in 500 ml dextrose water is given by intravenous infusion over the next 8 hours, if bronchospasm is marked.

(*h*) Antihistaminics are given intravenously, e.g. mepyramine (Anthisan) 25 mg followed by 25 mg two to four times a day, if skin manifestations are marked.

(*i*) Acidosis is corrected with sodium bicarbonate given by IV infusion.

Note: Soda bic therapy is fast losing favour.

(*j*) Vital signs must be monitored for at least 24 hours. Observations are made $\frac{1}{4}$-to-$\frac{1}{2}$-

hourly until the patient has responded to the therapy and has recovered from the shock.

(k) Intravenous therapy is maintained for at least 24 hours in case it is suddenly needed and for the correction of the electrolyte balance of the blood.

ORAL DESENSITISATION PROCEDURE FOR SYPHILITIC PATIENTS WITH PROVEN ALLERGY TO PENICILLIN

Pregnant women with syphilis or patients requiring treatment for neurosyphilis, who have a proven allergy to penicillin, should be desensitised to the antibiotic by using the oral method as recommended by the Centers for Disease Control, Atlanta, USA. It is recommended that the procedure be performed in a hospital setting, since serious IgE-mediated allergic reactions can rarely occur. Desensitisation can be completed within four hours, after which the first therapeutic dose of penicillin may be given. The schedule for increasing the dose of penicillin during the desensitising period is shown below.

Dose*	Penicillin V suspension	Amount†		Cumulative dose (units)
		ml	units	
1	1 000	0,1	100	100
2	1 000	0,2	200	300
3	1 000	0,4	400	700
4	1 000	0,8	800	1 500
5	1 000	1,6	1 600	3 100
6	1 000	3,2	3 200	6 300
7	1 000	6,4	6 400	12 700
8	10 000	1,2	12 000	24 700
9	10 000	2,4	24 000	48 700
10	10 000	4,8	48 000	96 700
11	80 000	1,0	80 000	176 700
12	80 000	2,0	160 000	336 700
13	80 000	4,0	320 000	656 700
14	80 000	8,0	640 000	1 296 700

Observation period: 30 minutes before parenteral administration of penicillin.
* Interval between doses: 15 minutes. Elapsed time, 3 hours and 45 minutes. Cumulative dose, 1,3 million units.
†The specific amount of drug is diluted in approximately 30 ml of water and then given orally.
Adapted from *New England Journal of Medicine* 1985; 312:1229–32.

REFERENCES

(1) Parkin D P. Antimicrobial agent resistance (AMAR). *SA Journal of Continuing Medical Education* June 1986;**4**.

(2) Klugman KP. A rational approach to empiric antibiotic use in the hospital setting. *Specialist Medicine* July 1993.

TEST OF KNOWLEDGE

The nurse has grasped the contents of this chapter if he/she:

(1) appreciates that a good antibiotic may be rendered useless by the ability of microbes to build up resistance to them, and appreciates the urgent need not to misuse antibiotics by unnecessary and ineffectual use and not to increase AMAR nosocomial infections by poor hygiene and isolation practices in hospitals;

(2) knows what precautions can be taken to prevent the abuse of antibiotics and the development of AMAR;

(3) knows the causes and emergency treatment of anaphylactic shock;

(4) knows how to prevent congenital syphilis in a pregnant woman with syphilis and a proven allergy to penicillin;

(5) understands that the developed resistance of microbes to antibiotics in current use is causing billions to be spent annually on the search for new antibiotics to which microbes will be sensitive.

30

The Mycobacterial Infections

OBJECTIVES

The main objective of this chapter is to present to the student the two mycobacterial infections which are associated with poor socio-economic conditions — leprosy and tuberculosis. They have caused much misery for mankind through the ages. Leprosy has filled men's hearts with horror since biblical days through its association with maiming and banishment from society. Its intensity has, however, abated to such an extent in South Africa that it has become a minor disease, curable and no longer requiring isolation in institutions. Tuberculosis, on the other hand, although fairly easily curable, is the greatest community health problem in the RSA, especially amongst black and coloured people.

These two diseases have much in common yet differ epidemiologically in their containability by community health preventive measures. While few students are likely to have contact with leprosy patients, tuberculosis is every nurse's problem.

STUDY OBJECTIVES

The student must:
(1) become familiar with both leprosy and tuberculosis control programmes which are supported by the Department of Health;
(2) know the role BCG vaccine plays in the prevention of both leprosy and tuberculosis, as well as the similarities and differences in their curative chemotherapy;
(3) understand that poor socio-economic conditions — poverty, overpopulation, malnutrition, crowded living conditions, ignorance and alcohol abuse — conditions commonly found among developing nations — form the breeding ground for mycobacterial infections;
(4) find out why, apart from adverse socio-economic conditions, tuberculosis in the RSA is such a great community health problem, despite the free availability of effective anti-TB drugs;
(5) become familiar with the advantages and disadvantages of hospital versus ambulatory (clinic) treatment of tuberculosis; and
(6) become familiar with all the efforts made by the national tuberculosis control programme (primary and secondary prevention) to reduce the incidence and prevalence of TB in South Africa;
(7) understand why tuberculosis is a common accompaniment of HIV/AIDS infection.

THE MYCOBACTERIAL INFECTIONS

Both leprosy and tuberculosis are caused by mycobacteria, leprosy by the *M. leprae* and tuberculosis by the *M. tuberculosis*. In both diseases there is a genetic predisposition to acquire the infection. In both diseases immunity is decreased by malnutrition, intercurrent infection (especially AIDS) and overcrowding, i.e. poor socio-economic conditions.

In both diseases cell-mediated immune reactions constitute the body's main defence against the organism.

Both leprosy and tuberculosis are notifiable conditions. Leprosy is a minor disease in South Africa, but tuberculosis is this country's most devastating infectious disease.

BCG vaccine can be used in both conditions, there being some evidence that if used in leprosy contacts it affords some protection. There is no other vaccine for use in leprosy.

In both leprosy and tuberculosis the emergence of drug resistance has necessitated multidrug therapy. Rifampicin is the most potent bactericidal drug in both diseases.

LEPROSY (HANSEN'S DISEASE)

Prevalence: The WHO estimates that there are at least 10–12 million cases of leprosy in the world, 5 million being registered cases, i.e. patients receiving chemotherapy and therefore properly diagnosed.[4] In South Africa there were 962 registered cases in 1988, i.e. this endemic disease is of low prevalence in the RSA. There were 124 new patients at Westfort Hospital in 1983, of whom 2 were white, 1 coloured and the rest black.[3] In 1989, 132 cases of leprosy were notified in the total RSA and 113 in 1991. In South Africa the prevalence is usually taken as 10 times the incidence.[28]

Incubation period: 3–4 years; the range is 6 months to 20 years and longer.

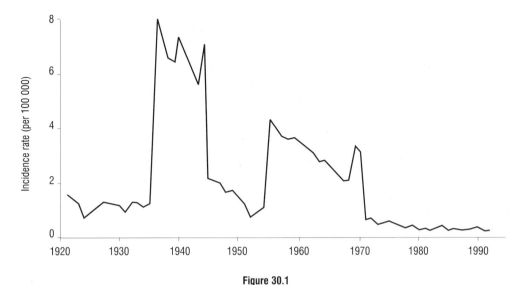

Figure 30.1

Incidence rate of leprosy

Source: *Epidemiological Comments* 1994; **21**(3)

Method of culture: The *M. leprae* has not yet been grown in artificial media; for culture outside the body, it must be grown in mice.

Modes of transmission:

(1) Droplet infection from nasal secretions.

(2) Direct contact through traumatised skin.

(3) Through the placenta.

Most known cases of leprosy in the RSA are found in the eastern regions, extending from there into the metropolitan areas of the Witwatersrand. The majority of patients are in the Gauteng Health Region and KwaZulu/Natal.

Since biblical days leprosy has been viewed with such dread that all lepers were formerly isolated in state-supported institutions. Since 1977 hospitalisation of leprosy patients in South Africa has not been compulsory, and the only remaining leprosy institution is Westfort State Hospital in Pretoria. Here the following care is given:

(1) Confirmation of diagnosis.

(2) Initiation of treatment for approximately 6 weeks, unless treatment for complications is required.

(3) Patients are registered for follow-up and medicines are supplied free for a period of either 6 months or 2 years when the patient

should be cured, depending upon the type of leprosy.

The Westfort treatment plan is assisted in a voluntary capacity by the Leprosy Mission of Southern Africa — a charity organisation caring for leprosy patients in the community. The priorities of the Mission are: case-finding, follow-up care and rehabilitation of the cured patient in his community.

DIAGNOSIS AND TYPES OF LEPROSY

The *M. leprae* may attack any tissues of the body through ingestion of the bacillus by macrophages and their neural equivalent, the Schwann cell,[3] which then become infected. The disease is diagnosed on clinical signs and smears taken from skin lesions and from the nasal mucosa. If the diagnosis is in doubt, skin and nerve biopsies may be specifically requested.

Pathogenesis

If the cell-mediated response to the infection of macrophages is effective, a tuberculoid granuloma forms, the bacilli in the granuloma being killed. This type of leprosy is called tuberculoid leprosy. Skin lesions are macular with raised edges and the surface may be scaling. As cutaneous nerves are involved, sensation of the lesions is decreased.

If cell-mediated immunity is ineffective, the bacilli multiply in the macrophages and the infection spreads to cause infectious nodular or lepromatous leprosy ENL (erythema nodosum leprosum). Nodules (leproma) develop in the skin of the face, hands and feet. The overlying skin ulcerates and extensive tissue necrosis occurs if the infection is severe. The *M. leprae* may invade any and all tissues of the body.

Between these extreme types of leprosy, intermediate or borderline types occur, depending upon the degree of cell-mediated immunity and the severity of the infection.

Nerve involvement in leprosy

Neuritis is always present in human leprosy, although it is usually asymptomatic.[4] Sensory, motor and autonomic nerves can be affected in all types of leprosy. The bacilli are more common in the nerves than in the skin.

In tuberculoid leprosy, peripheral nerve trunks are involved early, the nerve feeling thicker and harder than normal. Nerves may be tender and painful.

Nerve involvement in lepromatous leprosy starts in the cutaneous nerves and develops slowly.

Nerve involvement without skin lesions is rare in the RSA, but does occur elsewhere in the world.

Nerve involvement may cause sensory loss (leading to injury), and motor disturbance with weakness, wasting and paralysis of muscles and contractures. Sympathetic nerve dysfunction may cause dryness of skin with ulceration and infection.

Leprosy may cause blindness as a result of glaucoma or through involvement of the cornea, iris or lens.

LEPROSY CONTROL

As active cases of leprosy are the reason for the continued existence of leprosy, case-finding and treatment are the most important control measures.

Case-finding

Cases are found amongst the contacts of leprosy patients. Because of the long incubation period and slow development of signs and symptoms, this is a difficult task. Unfortunately most cases are only discovered at a late stage, when mutilation has already taken place.

Surveillance of contacts

All known contacts of every new leprosy patient should be listed and regularly interviewed and examined for: new skin lesions, discolouration and/or paraesthesias of the skin. These are the early signs of leprosy.[28]

Treatment

Multidrug therapy (MDT) has been the treatment of choice since the early 1980s and has resulted in many patients being discharged from therapy and taken off registers.[4] Monotherapy, practised especially with dapsone before this era, caused the *M. leprae* to become drug resistant.

MDT consists of rifampicin, dapsone and clofazimine.

Dapsone is a sulphone which is given by mouth in daily doses during the entire course of treatment. Dapsone is the important anti-leprosy drug, the use of rifampicin and clofazimine being to overcome resistance to dapsone. Rifampicin is discussed on p. 530. It renders patients non-infectious within a few weeks. Clofazimine (e.g. Lamprene) has both an antibacterial and anti-inflammatory action in leprosy, its main use being to overcome resistance of the *M. leprae* to dapsone. For the purpose of MDT (according to the WHO) patients are divided into 2 groups: multibacillary (heavily infected) (MB) and paucibacillary (not heavily infected) (PB). They are treated differently: PB for 6 months and MB for 2 years, in order to treat as many patients as possible in underdeveloped countries with a heavy load of leprosy patients. Patients are followed up for relapses, in which case therapy is repeated.

The WHO's suggested adult treatment schedule[4]

PB patients are treated for 6 months with:

- Rifampicin 600 mg once monthly (pulse therapy)
- Dapsone 100 mg daily

MB patients are treated for two years with:

- Rifampicin 600 mg once monthly
- Dapsone 100 mg daily
- Clofazimine 50 mg daily and 300 mg once monthly

Note:

(1) Monthly doses of rifampicin and clofazimine are given under supervision to ensure compliance.

(2) If patients are smear-positive on completion of a course of therapy, the latter is continued.

(3) Duration of treatment varies, some experts treating tuberculoid leprosy with dapsone for 5 years and lepromatous leprosy indefinitely.[3]

(4) Rifampicin and clofazimine are often given in larger doses, e.g. rifampicin 600 mg/d for 6 weeks,[3] clofazimine 300 mg weekly for 3 months.[3]

Follow-up

Follow-up of discharged patients in therapy must be done to ensure continued compliance with out-patient therapy.

Prevention

As leprosy is a disease of developing countries, improvement in environmental hygiene and socio-economic development are the best primary preventive measures.

Research has shown that the BCG vaccine has a protective effect in the non-lepromatous (i.e. tuberculoid) form of leprosy which is capable of mounting an effective antimycobacterial cellular immunity.

Education

Health education of community health nurses, especially those working in high-risk areas, to help them recognise leprosy in the early stages before the development of mutilating complications. Patients also need education about their role in ensuring a cure, i.e. compliance with treatment. The WHO recommends that the leprosy treatment programme be integrated into community health services, not only to save labour resources but also to banish fear of the disease and its association with erstwhile isolation in leper colonies.

Surveillance of cured leprosy patients

It is recommended that MB patients be kept under surveillance for 10 years since the optimal length of treatment needed to eliminate organisms and to prevent relapse is not yet known.[4]

TUBERCULOSIS

Introduction

Tuberculosis is South Africa's greatest community health problem, despite its vastly improved prognosis since the discovery of the tuberculostatic drugs in the 1950s. There are probably 150 000 TB sufferers in South Africa. Yet, tuberculosis is both curable and preventable.

Tuberculosis accounts for 83 % of all cases of communicable diseases notified to the Department of Health.[5]

When correlating the incidence and prevalence of tuberculosis of whites and non-whites in the RSA with their overall living standards, there can be no doubt that tuberculosis is associated with poverty and all the evils that result from it.

Tuberculosis is a disease of poverty and poor living conditions — malnutrition and alcoholism lower resistance and overcrowding favours close contact of susceptible persons, especially children, with infected persons. Protein energy malnutrition (PEM) has a suppressive effect on cell-mediated immunity. Malnourished children who have been immunised with BCG develop a relatively poor immunity, as shown by depressed conversion rates with tuberculin (PPD) testing.[6] For the modern approach to tuberculosis as a socio-economic and environmental problem to be accepted, what is required is the education of the public and especially employers of ambulant cases of tuberculosis who are encouraged to continue in employment.

Because tuberculosis is associated with cell-mediated immunity, it is also closely associated with HIV/AIDS in which there is a severe destruction of lymphocytes (acquired immune-deficiency syndrome). TB is the most important opportunistic disease in AIDS.

A report of a joint IUAT (International Union Against Tuberculosis)/WHO study group on tuberculosis control (September 1981)[7] states that technically advanced countries have controlled tuberculosis to a remarkable degree over the past thirty years due especially to the effective application of chemotherapy and mass BCG vaccination of children. In developing countries, however, there is no improvement in the epidemiological situation, especially in the light of the fact that the population has doubled during this period of thirty years. IUAT/WHO estimate the incidence and mortality of TB in developing countries to be as follows:

Between 4 and 5 million highly infectious cases of smear-positive TB occur each year.

Between 4 and 5 million less infectious cases (positive on culture only and culture negative cases (children)) occur each year.

Three million die from TB each year.

Annual 'risk of infection' is 2–5 % (20–50 times greater than in technically advanced countries).

Dr A Kochi, Manager, WHO TB programme said:[34] 'Tuberculosis is humanity's greatest killer and it is out of control in many parts of the world.' World-wide there are 8 million new cases of TB each year and 3 million deaths. This serious situation can be blamed partly on increasing HIV infection and partly on the emerging Multi-Drug Resistant Tuberculosis (MDR TB).

The malignant onslaught of TB in the RSA is already evident in the Western Cape, with its incidence rate of 610/100 000 (average in the RSA is 364/100 000). At present (1993) up to 15 % of all TB cases are HIV positive.[34]

The study group is adamant that the most powerful weapon in tuberculosis control is the combination of case-finding, case-holding and chemotherapy, case-finding and case-holding being necessary for treatment and cure. The more people cured, the smaller will be the reservoir of infection to which highly susceptible children are exposed. These are the principles on which the modern tuberculosis control programme of the RSA is built.

An editorial of the *South African Medical Journal* (30 August 1986) sums up the essentials of tuberculosis control in South Africa:

'Without doubt the most important factor in the control of tuberculosis is improvement in living standards. Unless there is improvement in nutritional status, reduction in overcrowding, and improvement in the overall level of education no tuberculosis programme can hope to be more than marginally effective. Socio-economic factors aside, the essence of tuberculosis control lies in identifying all patients with the disease and treating them fully. This requires screening of high risk groups, education of the public to ensure early diagnosis, adequate tracing of contacts, and the implementation of an effective antituberculous treatment regimen.'

The cause of tuberculosis is the *Mycobacterium tuberculosis* (Koch's bacillus) — an obligate aerobe. There is also a bovine type *(M. bovis)*, but this type is of minimal importance in the RSA. *M. bovis* is transmitted to man mainly through milk and causes cervical lymphadenopathy. Infection with the avian (bird) strain does not cause tuberculosis in man but may give a slightly positive reaction to tuberculin tests. The tubercle bacillus is covered with a waxy envelope which protects it against desiccation (drying); therefore it can remain viable (alive) for months in dried sputum. The mycobacterium infects practically any tissue in the body, where the tissue oxygen tension is high, but its two most feared targets are the apices of the lungs (pulmonary tuberculosis, consumption or phthisis) and the meninges in children. The *M. tuberculosis* is either inhaled in sputum droplets or dust, or it is ingested in infected milk *(M. bovis)*. Untreated, open tuberculosis, in which case microbes are discharged to the outside, is very infectious but, once effective chemotherapy has been commenced, infectiveness is reduced. When the sputum is negative on repeated smear examinations, the patient can return to work which brings him into contact with people. Infection of contacts usually occurs in the pre-diagnosis, pre-treatment period.

As a result of clinical or subclinical infection, or after successful BCG vaccination, the body develops a hypersensitivity to the

M. tuberculosis due to the presence of immunoreactive lymphocytes. This cell-mediated response is the type of immune response elicited by the tubercle bacillus. The hypersensitivity is manifested as an inflammatory reaction of the skin at the site of testing with tuberculin.

The incubation period of a primary infection is a minimum of 4–6 weeks, during which time the body develops cell-mediated immunity. The incubation period of the secondary infection is potentially lifelong.

Notification of tuberculosis deaths and cases was made compulsory in South Africa in 1920, and BCG vaccination of newborns in 1973. Although BCG vaccination is no longer obligatory, the practice continues.

All forms of tuberculosis are notifiable, except cases diagnosed solely on the basis of clinical signs and symptoms and/or a positive tuberculin test (R.1802 of Act 63/1977).

A strongly positive reaction after a tuberculin test in children under 5 years of age (Gr. III or IV Heaf or 14 mm induration or more — Mantoux) legally requires notification as tuberculosis.

EPIDEMIOLOGY OF TUBERCULOSIS

The mortality rate, the incidence and prevalence of tuberculosis, estimates of annual risk of infection, as well as response to different treatment regimens, should be monitored for the different population groups in the RSA in order to design effective TB control programmes.

According to Retief,[9] the TB death-rate was 30–35 % in the early 1950s. In 1986 it was between 4 % and 5 %.

Incidence

The incidence of TB is obtained from notification data.

Incidence in this chapter refers to the number of new cases notified during one year, from midyear to midyear. It is expressed as the rate (number) per 100 000 of the population.

Except for the Western Cape, the TB incidence of the RSA has declined since 1982. Incidence rates for all forms of tuberculosis declined in children aged 0 to 4 years from 321 in 1971 to 132 in 1984, from 187 to 67 for 5–9-year-olds and from 124 to 49 for 10–14-year-olds.[10]

The incidence of TB is high amongst blacks (194/100 000) and coloureds (660/100 000). In 1992 the rates amongst blacks and coloureds

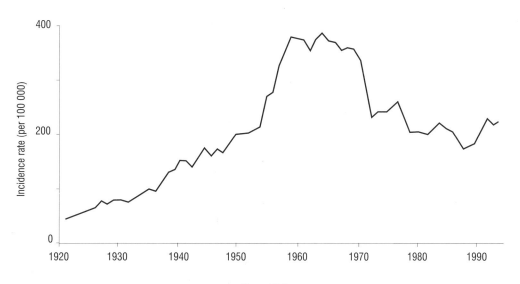

Figure 30.2

Incidence rate of tuberculosis
Source: *Epidemiological Comments* 1994; **21**(3)

were even higher in the Western Cape. The increased incidence rate for blacks is in part due to the migrant labour force entering Cape Town from the rural areas, and infected people not on treatment.

The disruption in routine services due to unrest in many parts of the country may have contributed to this problem.[31]

In 1992 the number of notifications in the entire South Africa increased to 82 103 and in 1993 to 88 319. This represents more than 80 % of all notifications of medical conditions.

In 1987 whites had an incidence rate of 14/100 000, except in the Western Cape where it rose to 25/100 000.[11]

Prevalence

Prevalence of TB (the disease) is the number of registered cases of TB according to specific diagnostic criteria at a specific time in the specific population, per 100 000 of the population.

Note: Prevalence of TB infection (not necessarily the disease), on the other hand, is the number of infected persons in a specific population at a specific time, based on an estimate of the proportion tuberculin sensitivity which can be ascribed to natural infection.[11] It is indicated as the percentage strong tuberculin reactors in a specific age group.

The prevalence rate increased from 590/100 000 in 1990 to 622/100 000 in 1991. As there has not been much change in the incidence rates between 1990 and 1991, this suggests that the duration of disease is increasing, i.e. patients are on treatment for a longer time. (See p. 535 . . . resistance of TB to drugs.)

Prevalence surveys are conducted occasionally by the Tuberculosis Research Institute of the SA Medical Research Council to identify all cases of tuberculosis in defined communities, e.g. Transkei, KwaZulu/Natal. Results of prevalence surveys are compared with notification rates to find out what percentage of open tuberculotics are diagnosed and notified annually. Prevalence surveys are difficult to conduct and expensive; therefore, annual 'risk of infection' indices are commonly used to assess trends in tuberculosis.

Risk of infection

The most useful and reliable indicator of the TB status of a community is its annual risk of infec-

tion. It is a sensitive measure of the progress of a tuberculosis programme.

'Risk of TB infection' indicates the probability that the person will become infected during the following period of a year.

Annual 'risk of infection' is computed by tuberculin-testing a representative sample of schoolgoing children. The significant positive reactors are at risk as they have already acquired a primary infection.

If the risk of infection is high, new cases of TB arise as a result of reinfection (i.e. not reactivation of an old lesion). If the risk of infection decreases due to fewer infectious cases, the incidence of TB will decline.

Method of calculating risk of infection[12]

The TB surveillance research unit developed a mathematical model to calculate 'risk of infection' from data obtained from tuberculin surveys of schoolgoing children.

In the RSA these surveys are done at intervals of a few years for each ethnic group in defined areas, e.g. Pretoria district, in order to detect trends. The sample to be given Mantoux tests is obtained by randomly selecting a number of schools from six strata of differing socioeconomic standards. Within each school, school beginners, and Standards 2, 5 and 8 scholars are used, thus excluding recently vaccinated children.

Some 'risk of infection' statistics:[13]

South Africa (blacks)	2,2 %
Transkei	4–5 %
Botswana, Swaziland	5–7 %
Sowetan blacks	0,3 %
South African whites	0,1 %
Coloureds	0,6 %
Asians	0,4 %

Once the risk of infection has been reduced (by case-finding and chemotherapy), an effort should be made to reduce endogenous reactivation by attention to immunity-reducing environmental factors and by reducing the number of infected (i.e. non-infectious) persons by means of secondary chemoprophylaxis with INH. The aim of the National TB Control Programme is to reduce the risk of infection by 10 % annually. The annual risk of tuberculosis infection, determined by the Tuberculosis Research Institute by survey of tuberculin reactivity, is declining. The annual change in risk in 1985 was — 11,1 % for the Asian group — 2,2 % for the coloured group and — 6,2 % for blacks.[10]

The progress in TB control amongst the white and Indian populations equals that amongst the advanced technical nations of the world. The general rate of infection decreased by 5–8 % per year until 1977 and since then by 11–13 % per year. This is due to mass BCG vaccination, improvement in urban living standards of Asians and the effects of case-finding and chemotherapy.

Note: In the 10 years 1972–1982 30–35 million BCG vaccinations have been done; approximately ½ million patients have been rendered non-infectious by chemotherapy.[14]

Glatthaar[13] states the extent of the TB problem in South Africa to be as follows:

(1) about 1 in every 200 persons in the RSA suffers from tuberculosis;
(2) 6–10 persons die of TB daily;
(3) the pool of infectious cases is 70 000–100 000 (this is probably a conservative estimate);
(4) the pool of infected (dormant/latent infections) cases comprises 5,5–7 million people.

Distribution of tuberculosis in the RSA:

Blacks . . . . 82 %
Coloureds . . . . 15 %
Asians . . . . 1,5 %
Whites . . . . 1,0 %

Age distribution: the disease affects mainly the very young, the 20–30-year-old group and the elderly.

Of every 1 000 children born in South Africa, one will get TB before the age of 1 year. In the Western Cape, 5/1 000 will be affected thus and 9/100 000 children will develop tuberculous meningitis.

During 1988 nearly two thirds of all new cases were diagnosed in the Western Cape (33 %) and Southern Transvaal (27 %). *Epidemiological Comments* **17**(1) reports in January 1990 that the TB problem in the seven health regions of the RSA had not improved between 1987 and 1988. The total case-load had increased and the outcome had worsened. Management varied from region to region, the fol-

lowing extremes being found: the Western Cape, with the greatest number of patients (31 342), admitted 40 % to hospital for treatment, whereas Natal, with 16 626 patients, admitted 47 % to hospital. The relative costs of treating patients in these two regions, therefore, vary tremendously. In both instances the fatalities were 4 %, the cure rate differing by 1 %.

THE PATHOGENESIS OF TUBERCULOSIS

The *Mycobacterium tuberculosis* may infect any tissue of the body, but infects mainly the lungs as the *M. tuberculosis* thrives in an oxygen-rich environment. The proportion of extrapulmonary forms of tuberculosis (TB) has recently increased to 6 % in the RSA, especially in the Western Cape Health Region where tuberculosis is rampant amongst the black and coloured sectors of the population.

Tuberculosis is characterised by the acquisition of a primary infection in childhood (if exposure to infection has occurred) to which the child builds up cell-mediated immunity. The primary lesion usually heals, but the infection may become dormant. The reason why primary TB is usually acquired only in childhood is because cell-mediated immunity is minimally effective at this stage. The infant is not passively immune against tuberculosis at birth, even if its mother is immune, as immunity does not depend upon antibodies which cross the placenta from mother to child.

An adult patient can infect another person whose resistance to infection is low and who has repeated contact with the adult patient, for example children in a family can be infected by their mother or father. Infrequent contact does not transmit the infection. Adult persons often succumb to their own dormant endogenous infection if their resistance is lowered. This is the common method of infection in adults.

The susceptible contact becomes infected via droplets of sputum (liberated by coughing or speaking) from an infectious ('open') tuberculosis patient after repeated exposure. The inhaled mycobacteria multiply to cause a primary infection (small area of bronchopneumonia) in the lung. The microbes disseminate to infect the regional lymph nodes (lymphadenitis) and from there to the bloodstream (bacteraemia) and to many organs throughout the body (causing a secondary infection). The small primary pulmonary inflammatory area with its regional lymphadenitis constitute the primary complex which commonly heals with minimal scarring and calcification. During the above process the patient, although asymptomatic, is developing a cell-mediated immune reaction which can be detected as a positive (hypersensitivity) tuberculin skin reaction within 4–6 weeks of the infection. The immune reaction kills off most of the mycobacteria in the primary complex and in secondary sites in the body (meninges, lung apices, spine, glands, kidneys, bones), some remaining alive but dormant (inactive) in foci of high O_2 tension.

To repeat, in 85–95 % of cases complete healing (sterilisation of secondary lesions) takes place, leaving the patient with a naturally acquired immunity. In 5–15 % of cases the dormant mycobacteria remain viable, however, walled off in a capsule of fibrous tissue, the infection being 'closed', i.e. non-infectious to other people. The infected, clinically healthy person will have a relative immunity to subsequent reinfection by inhaled mycobacteria and his skin tuberculin test will be positive. Reactivation of this dormant infection may occur, the risk being greatest in the first few years after the primary infection. Endogenous reactivation accounts for most cases of tuberculosis in adults. The infected person carries the risk of developing tuberculosis for a lifetime. Most tuberculosis infections will lie dormant while there is a balance between the pathogenicity of the *M. tuberculosis* and the host's defence mechanisms (cell-mediated immunity).

The cause of endogenous reactivation is the lowering of cell-mediated immunity by various factors. Consequently the barrier breaks down and the microbes are liberated in the tissues. The disease is then reactivated and a chronic, infectious tuberculosis develops.

The causes of the lowered cell-mediated immunity which reactivates an earlier, dormant TB infection are:

(1) stress (both physical, e.g. socio-economic, and emotional);
(2) immunosuppression by malignant disease, cancer chemotherapy, long-term steroid therapy and AIDS/HIV infection;

(3) malnutrition and alcoholism which lower cell-mediated immunity;
(4) the extremes of age;
(5) viral infections; silicosis; diabetes mellitus;
(6) continuous exposure to tuberculosis mycobacteria.

To sum up, there are two sources of infection:

(1) The exogenous source — the infectious pool — consisting of untreated patients with open TB: this source gives rise to the primary infection of childhood and to later reinfection.
(2) The endogenous source — the infected pool — consisting of tuberculin positive persons who are at risk of endogenous reactivation of a latent (dormant) childhood infection. This risk is 10–15 % in South African blacks. The bigger the pool of infected persons, the longer it will take to eradicate tuberculosis. In the RSA there may be 5,5–7 million black dormant carriers of TB — the infected pool.[13]

Amongst whites, only 1–2/1 000 per year become infected and of these only 2 % break down, i.e. become reactivated. Amongst the Asians, 3–4/1 000 children per year become infected.

HIV and tuberculosis

It has been estimated[29] that between 3 and $4\frac{1}{2}$ million persons in sub-Saharan Africa are co-infected with HIV and TB. As HIV infection causes a decline in cell-mediated immunity, a large number of persons will undergo endogenous reactivation of the dormant tuberculosis. This danger is especially great in cases of extrapulmonary TB which is associated with an increase in HIV prevalence. HIV should, therefore, be monitored in TB patients.

EXTRA-PULMONARY TUBERCULOSIS

Extra-pulmonary TB refers to all TB infections outside the lung parenchyma. Infection may reach non-respiratory sites by lymphatic and haematogenous spread from a primary site or by contiguous spread, e.g. from mediastimal glands to pericardium.

The following nine syndromes caused by *M. tuberculosis* are recognised by the ICD (9th revision, 1975). All are notifiable in the RSA.

1. Primary tuberculous infection with enlarged hilar nodes

Primary TB may co-exist with TB lymphadenitis.

A child under 5 years of age with a strong tuberculin reaction plus symptoms of tuberculosis is also considered to be a TB 'case'.[11]

Note: For notification purposes, a clinical diagnosis of TB adenopathy is not acceptable. Confirmation of diagnosis must be obtained by biopsy.[16]

2. Pulmonary TB

3. Other respiratory TB

For example, pleural effusion, mediastinal glands. In a pleural effusion with doubtful diagnosis (i.e. pleural biopsy and tuberculin test negative) a course of anti-TB therapy should be given. If there is radiological evidence of improvement after a month, the diagnosis of tuberculous pleural effusion is certain.

4. TB of the meninges and CNS

(1) TB meningitis (TBM) usually develops within six months of acquiring primary TB and is commonest in infancy and early childhood. The symptoms usually manifest slowly with headaches and personality changes. Later there are classical signs of meningitis with cranial nerve damage, raised intracranial pressure and neurological defects (e.g. cerebral palsy and intellectual impairment). Diagnosis may be difficult as the CSF may reveal no bacteria. Chest X-rays may be positive for TB.
(2) TB tuberculoma may form in the brain, giving rise to headaches, convulsions and paralysis.

Case-fatality rate for TB of meninges and CNS was 27,7 % (1987).[11]

5. TB of intestines, peritoneum and mesenteric glands

Any part of the gastro-intestinal canal, from the stomach to the anus, may become infected, the common sites being the distal ileum and caecum.

Abdominal distension occurs generally and in approximately half the cases there are signs of pulmonary TB and abdominal masses.

6. TB of bones and joints

Bone TB may lead to severe skeletal deformities, e.g. Pott's disease of the spine (tuberculous spondylitis) in which multiple vertebrae and discs in any part of the spine may be affected. The vertebral bodies and discs are destroyed and collapse forward to cause spinal curvature (kyphosis). The spinal cord is compressed or angulated and thus paraplegia and complete sensory loss may occur. Paravertebral abscesses may also form, e.g. a psoas abscess where pus tracks down the psoas muscle to point as a cold abscess in the groin. A lumbar paravertebral abscess may present as an abdominal mass.

TB may also affect joints, especially the knee, hip and ankle, causing their destruction unless timely chemotherapy is instituted. Bone and joint TB is also treated by immobilisation and surgery, e.g. evacuation of abscesses and spinal canal decompression, followed by spinal fusion.

7. TB of the genito-urinary system

TB may start in the kidney and spread to cause chronic urinary tract infection. An obstructive ureteric lesion may need surgical intervention after the infection has yielded to chemotherapy. Men may develop chronic epididymitis and in women the ovaries, Fallopian tubes and endometrium may be involved with resultant infertility.

8. TB of other organs

For example, larynx, middle ear, conjunctiva and liver. TB pericarditis is the commonest cause of pericardial effusion in the black population of South Africa, particularly in Transkei.[28]

9. Miliary TB

This is the acute disseminated form of tuberculosis. It is relatively rare as the cell-mediated immunity elicited by the primary infection usually causes the infection to become chronic.

Childhood malnutrition, measles and repeated heavy re-exposures to infection, however, cause low tuberculin sensitivity and poor response to BCG immunisation. These are signs of failure of the cell-mediated immune response. Thus, the mortality from acute disseminated tuberculosis amongst these children is high. In disseminated tuberculosis, the circulation becomes flooded with mycobacteria (e.g. from a mediastinal TB gland abscess rupturing into the thoracic duct) causing miliary tuberculosis. This is an acute tuberculosis with widely disseminated, countless, minute, discrete tubercles in the tissues and with profound toxaemia. Case-fatality rate was 19,3 % in 1987.[11]

Note: Disseminated tuberculosis can also occur in adults, being characterised by wasting, pyrexia, with chest signs and symptoms. The chest X-ray may present a typical miliary-like appearance. Tuberculin skin tests are often negative.

TB lymphadenitis of the superficial lymph nodes may accompany primary tuberculous infection. At first single or multiple lymph nodes start swelling slowly. They feel rubbery and are painless unless secondarily infected. Their usual locus is the neck (cervical) but they also appear in the axilla. The contents of the affected gland may break down to a fluctuant, caseous (cold) abscess which discharges to the skin through a chronic sinus.

PULMONARY TUBERCULOSIS (PTB)

The pathogenesis of PTB

Chronic, adult type tuberculosis usually affects the lungs to cause PTB. In the RSA 89 % of all reported tuberculosis in 1992 was pulmonary.[17] The pathological process, which may continue for years, is the following:

(1) Tubercles (granulomata) form and coalesce. Central necrosis takes place with the formation of a cheese-like pus. This process is called caseation. Tissue destruction may be widespread and in some patients cavities develop in the lung (cavitation) when the lesion erupts into a bronchus. The rupture causes heavily infected nummular sputum to be coughed up. There may be haemoptysis from the erosion of small blood vessels. Bronchogenic spread of mycobacteria to other parts of the lung takes place.

(2) Healing takes place by fibrous tissue encapsulation, the capsule forming a defensive barrier which prevents progression of the disease. Caseation, cavitation and encapsulation continue side by side for many years, the extent of necrosis depending upon the rate of development of the enveloping capsule. The spaces become filled with reticular and lymphoid tissue which harbour dormant mycobacteria. The viable mycobacteria in these TB scars may even, in this advanced stage of healing, be released into the bronchi and from there to other parts of the lung under conditions of stress or because of premature cessation of therapy. This accounts for the relapses that are common in chronic tuberculosis.

Radiological findings in PTB

Radiography of the lungs is frequently done for screening purposes by mass miniature X-rays. This is not found to be cost-effective. Radiological diagnosis of PTB on the large screen is useful if progressive changes occur on repeated radiography every 1–3 months. The radiographs have a 'cotton wool' appearance and there may be thick-walled cavities. Healing and healed lesions are seen as fibrotic and calcified patches.

In primary PTB the radiographs are usually normal, but there may be hilar and paratracheal lymph node enlargement.

Bacteriological findings in PTB

In order to confirm a diagnosis of pulmonary tuberculosis, the *M. tuberculosis* must be found in the sputum, by direct smear or by culture. Direct microscopy is quick but it detects only one-third of cases with a positive culture and must, therefore, be repeated, if the test result is negative.

THE CONTROL OF TUBERCULOSIS IN SOUTH AFRICA

Tuberculosis is controlled by the national tuberculosis control programme — the TBCP of the Department of Health. The determination of the

TB control policy is guided by the following bodies in the RSA:

(1) The Research Evaluation Committee for Institutes of the Tuberculosis Research Institute (TBRI) of the SA Medical Research Council.

(2) The TBRI.

(3) Numerous experts in the field of tuberculosis management, both abroad and local (e.g. epidemiologists of the Department, regional directors).

(4) Various academic departments of faculties of medicine of medical schools.

(5) The Medical Officers of Health of the larger local authorities.

(6) Other recognised and concerned experts and organisations, e.g. the SAIMR, SANTA.

A national register for standardising the recording of information on diagnosis and treatment of TB will be implemented by the DOH at all clinics in South Africa in 1995. This will enable the DOH to accurately interpret TB statistics, thus promoting control. (Statement by DOH and Medical Research Council in *Nursing News*, March 1995.)

Local authorities are expected to control tuberculosis in their areas in conformity with the policy of the Department of Health. The Department carries the financial burden of the tuberculosis control service from funds allocated by the treasury.

The control of tuberculosis has become largely a management problem to find infected cases in the community and to hold these cases in therapy long enough (6 months) to bring about a cure. If the management of TB patients can be improved, the infectious pool of cases, which causes an alarming annual incidence of TB cases in the RSA, will be reduced. Despite the large amount of money spent annually on effective anti-tuberculosis drugs, the prevalence of TB is slowly rising (see p. 520). Apart from adverse socio-economic conditions, this can be ascribed to therapy defaulting (to the tune of 10 000 in 1987); cases being retreated because of treatment and case defaulting have 4,6 times more positive smears and 6,1 times more positive cultures than new cases, because of acquired resistance to anti-tuberculosis drugs, especially INH. There appears to be a pool of

chronic TB cases which is likely to infect healthy persons with drug-resistant bacteria.[11]

Goals

The goals of the TB control programme (TBCP) are:[18]

(1) to reduce the incidence of infection;
(2) to reduce the prevalence of tuberculosis;
(3) to reduce mortality from tuberculosis.

To accomplish these goals the following operational objectives have been set:

(1) Primary prevention
  – Health education
  – BCG immunisation
(2) Secondary prevention
  – Diagnosing tuberculosis.
  – Case-finding by screening (bacteriological, X-ray, tuberculin testing) and contact tracing.
  – Notification.
  – Chemoprophylaxis of infected persons.
  – Curative chemotherapy of persons with tuberculous disease, for the appropriate period, usually 6 months.
  – Case-holding during anti-tuberculosis drug therapy — prevention of defaulting.
  – Sensitivity tests to find those resistant to standard treatment regimens. They are given special treatment. (See p. 533.)

To evaluate the success of the TBCP, the following assessments are done by means of epidemiological research:

(1) The cure rate
(2) The absconding rate
(3) The case-fatality rate[30]

These rates are established by epidemiological research on a sample of TB cases. The denominator of the rates is the number of cases diagnosed, i.e. the total annual case-load.

PRIMARY PREVENTION OF TUBERCULOSIS

Although a majority of adults have been infected in childhood, the tubercle bacillus is destroyed by the body's defences in 85 % (95 % in whites) of infected cases and the body builds up resistance which prevents the development of the disease. Tuberculosis in the 5–15 % of persons with a dormant infection becomes destructively active when resistance is lowered, primarily by poor socio-economic living conditions and malnutrition. The people especially at risk are infants and young children, young people, expectant mothers and adults under stress for a variety of reasons. TB control is directed at the protection of the people at risk, especially children. Control measures are applied not only by professional, technical staff but also by members of the community who work on a voluntary basis (SANTA) directly with the people whose resistance and socio-economic circumstances need to be raised.

Primary prevention of tuberculosis depends mainly on anti-tuberculosis health education (including positive steps towards socio-economic upliftment, better nutrition) and BCG vaccination.

Health education

Officially, health education is regarded as the single most important measure in the control of TB.[19] The aim of TB health education is to motivate the community to assist with therapy, case-finding and improvement of socio-economic factors. The department has launched a TB education and motivation programme in co-operation with the SA National Tuberculosis Association (SANTA) and the SA Christmas Stamp Fund. Lay educators are trained to recognise symptoms of TB and to teach this to their communities.

In South Africa (1982) fifty tuberculosis lay educators were trained by SANTA. This is the beginning of what, hopefully, will become a large task force to educate the black population in scientific concepts regarding tuberculosis.

The anti-tuberculosis education programme can be augmented with assisted self-help feeding schemes in areas where the nutritional standard of the people is low. Optimal nutrition strengthens the body's immunological systems and prevents the occurrence of active tuberculosis.

Education should be started at school and should be a continuous process. The establishment of SANTA Voluntary Worker Committees serves to educate the adult population. People from all walks of life are invited to meetings at which films on tuberculosis are shown, and at which talks are given by health educators on various health topics.

People are made aware of the existence of preventive health clinics.

Health educators, including community health nurses, can go into schools to show films on tuberculosis and give formal education to school principals, teachers and students. This is done to get the teachers involved and to motivate them and the affected children on the need for uninterrupted INH prophylactic therapy.

Formal education in tuberculosis consists of:

(1) The teaching of natural causes based on anatomical knowledge of the lungs and the microscopy of infected sputum. For this, the following teaching aids are needed: torso with removable lungs, line drawings, films, pamphlets, posters.

(2) Demonstration of the instruments used for tuberculin testing and BCG vaccination.

(3) Explanation of these procedures and why they are done.

Patients with infected sputum must be educated in safe sputum disposal. There is a law against expectoration in public places, as the mycobacterium can live for a long time in dried sputum and dust.

The patient with pulmonary TB is taught to cover his mouth when he coughs.

Use can be made of the public media (radio, newspapers, television) to cover tuberculosis and explain treatment. An appeal can thus be made to employers to release their staff for diagnostic procedures (mass chest X-rays) and to re-employ affected workers once they are under effective chemotherapeutic cover.

It would appear, however, that exposure to TB health education programmes has not led to significant differences in TB knowledge among the general black population.[18]

A study on traditional attitudes towards TB was done by Moloantoa[20] in 1982 on 50 TB patients at Ga-Rankuwa Hospital and 50 TB out-patients attending at Boekenhout Clinic. She found that the people interviewed had not yet received the 'scientific message' on TB. Traditional beliefs and attitudes persist.

Moloantoa suggests an improvement in the nurse-patient relationship to promote effective communication.

It has been suggested that TB health education programmes can be useful for improving knowledge, as long as they have a built-in evaluatory component.[18]

Ignorance about tuberculosis contributes greatly to its high prevalence. It causes patients to delay seeking help and to grasp the importance of completing treatment. Ignorance on the part of employers leads to sufferers losing their jobs. Apart from causing poverty, a valuable opportunity to help the sufferer obtain therapy is lost.

BCG vaccination

BCG vaccination of the uninfected (i.e. tuberculin negative) section of the population which is at risk, especially children and people whose nutritional standards are poor, is done. It is no longer compulsory by law to vaccinate against tuberculosis before a child is 6 months old, but the practice continues. Although BCG immunisation of the newborn does not confer absolute immunity, it is of great value. Cartwright[21] found that, although BCG vaccination gives only 60 %–80 % protection to the newborn for about 5 years, tuberculous meningitis and miliary (acute, generalised) tuberculosis do not occur frequently. BCG vaccination also decreases the incidence of cavitating infective cases. The immunisation programme is continued in the schools (see p. 496 for BCG immunisation).

Successful vaccination is judged by the conversion of a negative tuberculin reaction to a positive one. The immunised person becomes hypersensitive to PPD (antigen/lymphocyte reaction) — a sign that he is developing a cell-mediated immune response against the *M. tuberculosis*.

SECONDARY PREVENTION OF TUBERCULOSIS

Diagnosing tuberculous disease

Tuberculosis is an insidious (secretly progressing) disease which can infect any organ of the body. In the early stages it may be asymptomatic. As 89 % of tuberculous disease in South Africa is pulmonary, the diagnosis of PTB will be discussed.

Clinical features of pulmonary tuberculosis (PTB):

(1) Tuberculous toxaemia is characterised by drenching night sweats, anorexia and mass loss, weakness and malaise, intermittent pyrexia (sometimes) and tachycardia.

(2) Tuberculous lesions of the lung are characterised by a chronic productive cough with purulent sputum (greenish-grey, sometimes bloodstained) becoming nummular (discrete discoid masses like coins) in the advanced stage, dyspnoea and haemoptysis; pneumothorax.

(3) In far advanced cases there may be clubbing of the fingers, erythema nodosum, phlyctenular conjunctivitis, bronchiectasis, cor pulmonale.

(4) In children the following signs and symptoms should arouse the suspicion of tuberculous disease:

   (*a*) failure to gain mass or mass loss (as reflected on the Road-to-Health cards);

   (*b*) wheezing resulting from enlarged hilar or paratracheal lymph nodes.

The tuberculin diagnostic tests will be strongly positive in a patient with active tuberculosis, but a positive reaction does not necessarily indicate that a patient is suffering from the disease; healthy infected persons who have been exposed to infection exhibit a similar kind of reaction. Persons with positive tuberculin reactions not induced by BCG vaccine are at risk and the danger of developing tuberculosis is greatest in the period immediately following exposure to infection.

With the above signs and symptoms, the diagnosis of pulmonary tuberculosis is more suspect if: the patient comes from a high-TB-prevalence or a low socio-economic group, has had tuberculosis before, has had contact with tuberculosis or suffers from any predisposing illness, e.g. AIDS, silicosis, diabetes mellitus, or abuses alcohol.

The diagnostic criteria used here[31] are those of the WHO, amended by, *inter alia*, the Center for Disease Control, Atlanta, Georgia.

All cases of tuberculosis, i.e. those with sufficient clinical signs and symptoms to warrant investigation, can be categorised as 'confirmed', 'suspect' or 'probable'.

A confirmed case

All cases with positive direct microscopy, culture or histology reported on any clinical specimen.

A suspect case

(a) All ages
- Evaluation of pleural, ascitic or pericardial fluid that is suspicious of TB.
- A 'suspicious' chest radiograph.
- All cases with clinical signs suggesting PTB or TB of the meninges and the CNS.
(b) Children (under 14 years)
- Contact with TB and weight loss or failure to gain.

A probable case

(a) All ages
- 'Diagnostic' chest radiograph findings.
- 'Probable' pleural, ascitic or pericardial findings.
- Cerebrospinal fluid findings typical of TB meningitis.
- All other cases of extra-pulmonary TB.
(b) Children (under 14 years)
- Significantly positive tuberculin reaction (and clinical signs of TB), or
- Positive response to a therapeutic trial, or
- Any child with a 'suspicious' chest radiograph and any of the following: strongly positive tuberculin reaction, history of contact with TB and weight loss or failure to gain sufficiently, or
- Diagnosis of TB of the meninges and the CNS and preceding loss of weight or failure to gain.
(c) Children under 5 years
- A significantly positive tuberculin reaction.

Case-finding

Active and passive case-finding is essential for reducing the infectious reservoir. To promote the secondary prevention of tuberculosis, it is necessary for the community to be educated and motivated to co-operate with the helping authorities.

Patients with tuberculosis are often diagnosed when they attend clinics or hospitals for their indisposition (passive case-finding). The latter can also be done by referral of persons by enlightened members of the public. Many, however, and especially the pre-school child from 0 to 5 years, are not diagnosed and treated; these patients need to be discovered by an active case-finding survey in at-risk communities, not only to bring them to therapy but also to reduce the source of infection in the community, i.e. the infectious pool (reservoir).

The community must assist in case-finding. Primary health care workers must be able to recognise the clinical picture of active TB, after education by trained educators.

Before conducting a case-finding campaign, the leaders of the community must be educated by health educators and TB information officers (SANTA educators) and their co-operation gained in order that they may help the teams of tuberculosis workers of the health departments (local authority or state) or SANTA by persuading the people to come forward with information and to co-operate with the workers. The important leaders who are indispensable for such a campaign are the church ministers, school principals, social workers, businessmen and members of local government. These leaders are enlightened as to the nature of the campaign and their help is enlisted to motivate the people to come for examination.

The case-finding programme can be implemented as follows.

Investigation of suspect cases

Suspected cases who are referred either passively (i.e. by the community doctors and hospitals) or actively via search campaigns, e.g. interviewing community leaders to identify suspects, must be investigated. A case is suspected of having TB if he has a cough for more than three weeks, has an haemoptysis and has lost weight and appetite.

All patients attending hospitals and health centres in black areas should be examined for tuberculosis if they present with respiratory symptoms.

The screening investigations carried out on suspect cases are:

Sputum

Sputum specimens are taken for culture and microscopy (smear) for rapid diagnosis. Culture is more accurate than microscopy but takes much longer (3–6 weeks). State laboratories are available to cope with mass bacteriological case-finding. Satisfactory sputum specimens can be obtained either by irritating the throat or by getting subjects to inhale a nebulised saline aerosol. In children a gastric aspirate, neutralised with sodabic, is submitted.

X-ray

The chest is X-rayed to confirm evidence of TB. In children, mediastinal adenopathy may be discovered in this way.

X-ray screening by mass miniature radiography is done to detect tuberculosis in adults and children over the age of 10 years. Arabin *et al.*[22] found mass radiography in active case-finding campaigns to be impracticable and too costly and advised that they be used only in prevalence surveys and for high-risk groups in cities (e.g. workers, work seekers, adult contacts of scholars with significant tuberculin reactions).

Tuberculin skin testing

All pre-school children without BCG scars under the age of 5 years and those older children not at school are tuberculin tested. This is done by house-to-house visiting by the anti-tuberculosis team (professional and voluntary). Significant reactors of 5 years and under are sputum-tested and X-rayed (large plate) at a hospital to diagnose tuberculosis. If negative, they are treated with INH and ethambutol (or ethionamide) for one year. If positive they are given full anti-tuberculosis treatment.

Note: There is no indication for the routine tuberculin testing of adults. The test is used only for diagnostic problems.

Tuberculin skin testing is done on all children between the ages of 5 and 16 years at school to find significant tuberculin reactors; these significant reactors are sputum-tested and then X-rayed to detect active tuberculosis. Only then are they notified. The insignificant reactors must be BCG vaccinated. The significant reactors (infected healthy subjects) receive long-term (6 months) INH chemoprophylaxis (see

p. 530). The significant reactors with positive sputum tests and chest X-rays are given full anti-tuberculosis treatment.

Tuberculin PPD testing

The tuberculin used for sensitivity tests (PPD — purified protein derivative) is an antigen derived from the tubercle bacillus, either the human or the avian strain.

Note: Tuberculin must not be confused with BCG vaccine which is made of attenuated (weakened but live) bovine (cattle) tubercle bacilli.

The most important tuberculin tests are the Mantoux intradermal test and the Heaf multiple puncture (or tine) percutaneous test.

Mantoux test. A small amount of tuberculin PPD (2 units of human PPD in 0,1 ml) is drawn up in a tuberculin syringe and injected intradermally in the proximal anterior surface of the forearm which has been cleaned with 70 % alcohol and dried with a sterile swab. The test is read after 2–3 days, the measurement being made with calipers. A positive Mantoux reaction is a red, raised and hard (indurated) area with a diameter of at least 10 mm. This is the finding in a healthy infected person who has not had BCG vaccine. A child who has had BCG would be expected to have a Mantoux reaction of up to 5 mm. If the induration is 15 mm, the child has a TB infection. If the child has not had BCG, an induration of 10 mm is accepted as a positive response needing therapy, in the 0–5 age group.

The patient who is actually suffering from tuberculosis should have a much larger indurated area. If the Mantoux test is done 7 to 14 weeks after BCG vaccination, a positive Mantoux reaction will indicate that conversion from a negative pre- to a positive post-vaccination reaction has taken place, i.e. that BCG vaccination has been successful.

Heaf multiple puncture (tine) percutaneous test is done with a Heaf 6-needle gun and 2 to 5 TU undiluted tuberculin PPD. The proximal anterior surface of the left forearm is cleaned as above, a small drop of PPD is placed with a syringe on the chosen site and the gun is flamed after dipping it in a special flammable solution. Holding the gun shield flush with the skin on the drop of PPD, the end plate is rotated slightly to spread the PPD and then slight pressure is exerted to release the head with the needles (tines). In this way the skin is punctured percutaneously to introduce the tuberculin.

After 3 days, i.e. on the 4th day, the test results are read.

Tuberculin tests can be performed and interpreted (read) by nurses with special training. Multiple puncture reactions can be interpreted according to 4 Heaf grades.

Grade 0. No palpable reaction to minute papules at each puncture site — there is no tuberculous infection.

Grade I. Discrete papules (induration) at the site of each puncture; papules may tend to coalesce, but do not form a uniform inflammatory ring. This indicates an insignificant non-specific infection — there is no tuberculous infection.

The grades above are the non-reactors who need BCG vaccination.

Grade II. A continuous confluent inflammatory ring, i.e. coalescence of indurations to form a ring. This may or may not be a positive reaction, confirmation being obtained by doing a Mantoux test. A false positive reaction may be due to the presence of non-tubercular mycobacteria.

Grade III. A confluent inflammatory ring involving the central area which swells more and more, forming a smooth dome-shaped swelling (disc formation).

Grade IV. In this reaction the swelling starts ulcerating from the periphery; the severest reaction is extensive ulceration or vesiculation of the entire swelling.

If the Heaf test is used in a TB control programme, the positive tuberculin reactors in grades III and IV require chemoprophylaxis.

Note:
(1) The multiple-puncture method is easier but less accurate than the Mantoux test. It is considered suitable for field screening of tuberculin reactors, provided that the doubtful grade II positives are retested with the Mantoux test in order to decide whether to institute a course of chemoprophylaxis or BCG vaccination.
(2) In positive PPD reactors, i.e. those with a TB infection and those who have been successfully vaccinated with BCG, a negative PPD reaction may occur once the TB is completely cured with all TB lesions sterilised, or after waning of the effects of BCG. These persons have lost their relative immunity and, if exposed to TB infection, should be vaccinated with BCG vaccine.
(3) Glatthaar and Donald[16] are of the opinion that the multipuncture Heaf apparatus should be discontinued, as it poses a risk in the spread of AIDS and Hepatitis B infections.
    The percutaneous test can be done with a small disposable plastic instrument. This small apparatus has several tines (prongs) which are covered with dry tuberculin and are pushed into the skin to give one multiple puncture percutaneous injection.

TB contact tracing

A TB contact is a person who has had intimate contact with someone who, at the time of contact, had open TB and was not yet receiving treatment, by:

(1) living in the same room or house as an active TB patient; especially if there is overcrowding;
(2) sleeping within 5 metres of an active TB patient, in a compound or hostel;
(3) working daily in the same room as an active TB patient;
(4) having an intimate relationship which is repeated or continuous, e.g. lovers, a child and his nursemaid, teacher and pupils in a classroom.
(5) being born to a mother who has tuberculosis.

Chemoprophylaxis

Child contacts are given chemoprophylaxis for three months. If they are tuberculin negative after this course, they are vaccinated with BCG.

If they are tuberculin positive, INH prophylaxis is continued for a further three months. Adult contacts are treated as suspect cases, i.e. a chest radiograph is taken and/or a bacteriological investigation is done. Re-evaluation is done after three months.

The notification of tuberculosis

(See also p. 477.)

Tuberculosis is a notifiable disease and all notified patients (cases) should submit to treatment. Their contacts at home and at work must be traced and investigated and either curative or prophylactic treatment applied. In PTB diagnostic criteria are confirmed by a positive sputum and chest X-ray (see p. 534 for chemotherapy surveillance).

In 1979 the Department of National Health and Population Development abolished the notification of positive tuberculin reactors under 5 years of age, in line with international practice and on the advice of its policy guiding bodies. It has since been reinstituted.

In the revised list of notifiable medical conditions (December 1989) notifiable tuberculosis is defined as follows:

'Tuberculosis —

(1) pulmonary and other forms, except cases diagnosed solely on the basis of clinical signs and symptoms;
(2) a strongly positive reaction after a tuberculin test in children under 5 years of age (Gr. III or IV Heaf or 14 mm induration or more Mantoux).'

Note: As the Department provides treatment, examination and follow-up of contacts of every person with suspected TB referred to a clinic or hospital, at-risk children under the age of 5 years will receive care.[23]

Notification is essential for the planning of the tuberculosis control programme (TBCP).

Special notification of TB in areas covered by the nine health regions of the RSA

Apart from, and independent of, normal TB notification procedure, the Department of National Health and Population Development issued a new data-capturing form (Tuberculosis Statistics GW 20/10) in 1991, to be filled in by every TB clinic, hospital or treatment point (LA clinics, mobile clinics or employers administering therapy). The information thus gathered is intended to provide detailed information on the functioning of the national TB control programme, thus enabling the Department to compute total case-load, incidence rates, the number of suspects and contacts investigated for TB, the number of people receiving different treatment regimens, the place of treatment and the cure, default and death-rates.[10]

Departmental policy in 1991[36]

All proven relapsed patients should be renotified.

Definition of relapsed PTB patients:

'The reappearance of TB bacilli in the sputum of a patient after completion of a full period of successful treatment. Bacteriological proof by microscopy and/or culture is essential — radiological diagnosis only is not accepted.'

PTB cases lost to the TBCP, for whatever reason, before completing a full course of treatment successfully and subsequently found, are not to be renotified. Similarly, any PTB patient whose sputum has converted to negative while on treatment, then again becomes positive while still on

the same course of treatment, should not be renotified.

During the completion of the monthly GW 20/10 statistical form, the number of proven relapse cases should be recorded under Section A in Column 'Patients gained — relapse/re-infection'.[36]

Chemoprophylaxis of infected persons

Chemoprophylaxis by isoniazid-INH (6 months) or Isoprodian (4 months) therapy for infected healthy subjects, i.e. those with a significant positive tuberculin reaction and no clinical bacteriological or radiological signs of tuberculosis. It aims at eradicating dormant organisms in recently infected contacts, thus preventing reactivation 1–3 years later.

Collins,[24] quoting USA experience, recommends that a multidrug regimen of rifampicin and pyrazinamide (with or without INH) might permit preventive treatment to be as short as two months in schoolgoing children with Grade IV (blistering) Heaf test reactions.

INH chemoprophylaxis is indicated for intimate contacts of infectious tuberculosis patients, e.g. family members and traders in stores, where many TB patients congregate. Most con-

Notified cases and deaths due to TB in the RSA
(TBV countries excluded but other homelands included) for 1987.[11]

TB Category	Number of cases	Number of deaths	Incidence per 100 000	Case-fatality (percentage)
Primary infection	2 079	3	7,2	0,1
Pulmonary	50 243	2 168	173,6	4,3
Other respiratory	71	6	0,2	8,5
Meninges and CNS	242	67	0,8	27,7
Intestines, peritoneum and mesenteric glands	403	13	1,4	3,2
Bones and joints	177	8	0,6	4,5
Genito-urinary	58	0	0,2	0,0
Other organs	204	6	0,7	2,9
Miliary	150	29	0,5	19,3
TOTAL	53 627	2 300	185,0	4,3

Estimated population of the RSA in 1987: 28 934 000
Source: Directorate Epidemiology. Department of National Health and Population Development.

tacts receiving INH are children. INH prophylaxis for contacts is usually given for three months.

As soon as an adult case has been notified and put on treatment, all small children in the house should be put on prophylactic INH until danger of infection has ceased.

Curative chemotherapy for tuberculous disease

Tuberculosis is treated with drugs, modern tuberculosis chemotherapy being given either at home or at community health or special tuberculosis clinics, or by the occupational health nurse at work. The erstwhile long periods of rest in sanatoriums are no longer deemed essential, neither is it necessary to isolate the sufferer from his family and the community, provided he submits to regular therapy. Even new cases can be treated on an intensive out-patient regime, as they are not likely to be infectious after a month of regular treatment on a daily or thrice weekly basis (see p. 532). Furthermore, the family members exposed to the infection can be protected by INH prophylaxis.

During 1985 approximately 88 000 TB cases were cared for by the national TB control programme (seven health regions of the RSA). This increased by 5 % in 1986. Western Cape had an increase of 23 % to 25 000 cases. The region with the highest incidence and prevalence rates in 1991 was the Western Cape, followed closely by the Orange Free State.

All therapy must be administered under supervision; the community must assist with supervision at home and at work. They are taught to do this by trained educators. The clinic sister must choose a suitable, short-course regimen and home therapy can be supervised by lay workers (care groups). TB therapy can also be dispensed at clinics, or from mobile clinics at bus-stops or casualty departments.

Supervised ambulatory treatment is thus encouraged. Patients are hospitalised only in exceptional circumstances, e.g. if they are too ill to attend a clinic, if they have an associated illness, e.g. diabetes mellitus, cardio-vascular disease, malnutrition; or if treatment cannot be supervised either at work or at home and the patient lives far from a clinic and is not responsible enough to take his medication regularly.

Where hospitalisation is imperative, use is made of general hospital facilities in the patient's own area, or in a SANTA or Life Care Group hospital.

Overall about 75 % of all cases receive treatment in clinics and 25 % in hospitals.[10]

In Natal, however, 53 % of TB patients were treated in hospitals in 1986.

The cost per patient/treatment/month is 11 times greater in a hospital than when a patient is treated by a clinic on an out-patient basis. To cure a patient costs almost 5 times more in a hospital than via clinic services.

The principal standard, primary tuberculostatic drugs are **isoniazid, rifampicin** and **pyrazinamide**. Streptomycin used to be included here. **Streptomycin** is given by injection and is not used for longer than 3 months and not at all for people over the age of 50 years because of the danger of renal and VIIIth cranial nerve damage. It is potentially teratogenic and must not be used in pregnancy. Streptomycin acts on extra-cellular and rapid-growing bacilli and affects mainly the bacilli in TB cavities. The use of streptomycin is no longer recommended (1989) for the routine use of new cases, especially not for children.[16]

Isoniazid (INH) is a specific tuberculostatic drug which is more effective than streptomycin because it penetrates through the pathogenic tissue to reach the tubercle bacilli. Although it is a cheap and safe drug, INH may have many toxic side-effects if given in high dosage; massive overdosage may be lethal. It is not teratogenic and can thus be used in pregnancy.

Special INH preparations:

- Rifater — the ideal combination drug for ambulant therapy, which consists of INH, rifampicin and pyrazinamide.
- Rifinah — a combination of INH and rifampicin.
- Tebesium — delayed-release INH tablet used for intermittent therapy.
- Isoprodian — a combination of INH, diaphenylsulphone and protionamide.

Rifampicin is a rifamycin with truly bactericidal properties even on dormant bacilli. It is an essential component of multidrug TB chemotherapy, cutting down the duration of erstwhile lengthy therapy periods. Its action commences two hours after ingestion.

Rifampicin is a component of Rifater and Rifinah.

Rifampicin has many toxic side-effects, of which hepatotoxicity can be serious.

Pyrazinamide (PZA) is one of the principal, standard tuberculostatic drugs as it shortens therapy to 6 months. It is as hepatotoxic as rifampicin. Pyrazinamide is a component of Rifater.

The three standard drugs, rifampicin, INH and pyrazinamide are combined in a single tablet called *Rifater*. For modern ambulant therapy one tablet Rifater/10 kg body mass can be given instead of a variety of different preparations which can be very confusing and lead to mistakes, i.e. treatment defaulting. Administration of Rifater is simple and safe, for example, 5 tablets once a day for a patient weighing 50 kg and more. Rifater, therefore, aims to improve patient acceptance and compliance with therapy.

Ethambutol is an expensive drug which is readily accepted by patients because it does not cause gastro-intestinal upsets. It is mainly a bacteriostatic drug and minimises the emergence of drug resistance when used in combination with the standard tuberculostatic drugs. Its greatest drawback is that it may cause retrobulbar neuritis and green/red colour blindness. It appears to be safe in pregnancy. In combination with INH, ethambutol is known as Mynah.

Thiacetazone is frequently used as a companion drug to INH, but not in children and pregnant women. If given in high dosage it has frequent toxic effects, therefore a low dosage of 150 mg per day (on a daily regimen) is used. It is bacteriostatic.

Ethionamide can be used where standard drugs are excluded because of toxic symptoms. It is not well tolerated and may cause nausea and vomiting. It is bacteriostatic and is possibly teratogenic.

The Department of National Health and Population Development designed four short-course drug regimens in 1979. These courses last from 6–9 months. One of the aims of these regimens is to make it possible to obtain a high compliance rate for primary treatment, e.g. short continuous courses, or longer intermittent courses, depending upon socio-cultural factors. If a patient defaults despite being given the most accommodating treatment regime, then he should be admitted to hospital for in-patient therapy.

These regimens have recently been simplified by the exclusion of streptomycin which, however, can still be used at the discretion of the physician. Streptomycin in combination with ethambutol and ethionamide are also used as substitute therapeutic agents if the standard drugs cause hepatotoxicity.

In pregnancy, the safest anti-tuberculosis drugs are isoniazid, rifampicin and ethambutol used in combination.

The anti-tuberculosis drugs (except streptomycin) are given daily (e.g. 5 times per week — Mondays to Fridays) by mouth. In the intermittent schedule (regimen 3) the drugs are given 2 or 3 times per week. Courses containing pyrazinamide last 6 months. A course has been completed if 80 % of the scheduled doses have been taken.

Infectiousness of patients on therapy

Although the patient on regular therapy may excrete viable bacilli for a month after starting therapy, he is relatively non-infectious within 24 hours after onset of treatment, as the bacilli are too weak to induce active disease. This does not apply to young children, especially if malnourished, who are as yet unable to build up cell-mediated immunity. It is thus advisable to keep patients with open tuberculosis away from children for at least the first month of therapy.[16]

TB meningitis and uncomplicated primary TB are never infectious.

For adults and children 7 years of age and older (new cases) one of regimens 1, 2 and 3 is used, and regimen 4 for children 6 years of age and younger. If isoniazid resistance is expected, ethambutol may be added to regimen 1.

Treatment regimen/s are to be selected carefully to suit the patient and local needs and taking into account factors such as distance from clinic, place of employment, available funds and infrastructure.

Treatment of pulmonary tuberculosis: new cases[16]

DRUG	DOSAGE	ADMINISTRATION	DURATION
A. TREATMENT OF ADULTS AND CHILDREN 7 YEARS OF AGE AND OLDER			
Regimen 1 (Recommended treatment of choice)			
Rifater (Rifampicin 120 mg; Isoniazid 80 mg; Pyrazinamide 250 mg)	1 tablet per 10 kg body mass Average adult dose: 4 tablets (body mass under 50 kg) or 5 tablets (body mass greater than 50 kg)	Once daily (Mon.–Fri.)	6 months
Regimen 2 (Optional alternative treatment)			
Rifampicin	450 mg (body mass under 50 kg) or 600 mg (body mass greater than 50 kg)	Once daily (Mon.–Fri.)	6 months
Pyrazinamide	1,5 mg	Once daily (Mon.–Fri.)	6 months
Isoniazid	300 mg	Once daily (Mon.–Fri.)	6 months
Ethambutol	20 mg/kg body mass	Once daily (Mon.–Fri.)	6 months
Regimen 3 (Recommended if intermittent treatment indicated or preferred)			
Rifampicin	600 mg	2 or 3 x /week	6 months
Isoniazid — delayed release*	20–25 mg/kg body mass	2 or 3 x /week	6 months
Pyrazinamide	3 g	2 or 3 x /week	6 months
Ethambutol	30–40 mg/kg body mass	2 or 3 x /week	6 months
B. TREATMENT OF CHILDREN 6 YEARS OF AGE AND YOUNGER			
Regimen 4			
Rifampicin	10 mg/kg body mass	Once daily (Mon.–Fri.)	6 months
Isoniazid	8–10 mg/kg body mass	Once daily (Mon.–Fri.)	6 months
Pyrazinamide	20–25 mg/kg body mass	Once daily (Mon.–Fri.)	6 months

*Delayed release isoniazid preparation available as Tebesium 0,5 g (= 500 mg isoniazid) or Tebesium 0,3 g (= 300 mg isoniazid)
Note: For children 7 years of age and older the following dosages apply:
Regimen 1: Rifater 1 tablet for every 10 kg of body mass
Regimen 2: Isoniazid 8–10 mg/kg, rifampicin 10 mg/kg, pyrazinamide 20–25 mg/kg, ethambutol 20 mg/kg
Regimen 3: Rifampicin 10–15 mg/kg, pyrazinamide 30 mg/kg, Tebesium 20 mg/kg, ethambutol 30 mg/kg.

The consensus appears to be that hospitalisation does not lead to a better outcome than strictly supervised ambulatory chemotherapy.

Unsupervised treatment, with certain exceptions, should be expressly forbidden, as this leads to non-compliance and the problem of drug resistance.[32]

Drug-resistant TB is likely to spread rapidly among HIV-infected persons.

Patients with cavitary or smear-positive disease should be given a 6-month period of treatment and discharged promptly unless their sputum smears are still positive.

Regimen 3 (intermittent therapy) should be considered for supervised, ambulatory treatment as it is as effective and cheaper than continuous therapy and more likely to increase full compliance.[33]

The mother who is breast-feeding her infant while on therapy, may continue to do so. The doctor will probably increase her dose of isoniazid. If the infant is receiving full anti-TB therapy, breast-feeding should be discontinued as the additional medication from the breast milk may have toxic effects.

Treatment of previously treated cases of pulmonary TB

If reactivation or reinfection occurs within 6 months of previous treatment, one of regimens 1, 2 or 3 is used, plus a 4th or a 4th and a 5th drug. If reactivation or reinfection occurs after 6 months, the patient is treated as a new case.

Treatment of extrapulmonary tuberculosis

In general, drug regimens which are suitable for pulmonary tuberculosis are also suitable for extrapulmonary tuberculosis.

Toxic side-effects of anti-tuberculosis drugs

These are legion and are described in package inserts of the drugs. The majority of tuberculostatics are listed in Schedule 3, but all rifampicin products, being antibiotics, are listed in Schedule 4.

Drug resistance

This is one of the major problems encountered in the treatment of tuberculosis.

Primary resistance (i.e. on first contact with the drug) is caused by mutation of a strain of the tubercle bacillus.

Secondary or acquired resistance results from prior therapy which did not effect a cure. The longer therapy lasts, the more likely the patient is to acquire resistance to one or more drugs. Infection with resistant organisms originates from patients with acquired resistance.

The two major factors influencing resistance rates are:

(i) previous unsuccessful anti-TB therapy due to poor compliance and subsequently a protracted period of therapy;

(ii) the presence of cavitary PTB.

In his study of drug resistance on 322 TB patients in the Southern Transvaal 1982–1984, Collins [32] found the following categories of resistance:

Rifampicin only	15	(4,5 %)
Rifampicin + INH	49	(14,8 %)
Rifampicin + streptomycin	6	(1,8 %)
Rifampicin + INH + streptomycin	262	(78,9 %)
Total	332	(100 %)

The situation of the patient with resistance to both rifampicin and INH is serious. Streptomycin is hardly used for TB today. Resistance to rifampicin may develop rapidly when therapy is irregular or inadequate.

Rifampicin is potentially hepatotoxic and may cause gastric discomfort, jaundice and leucopenia. It counteracts the effects of steroidal contraceptives. Besides rifampicin, INH and pyrazinamide are also eliminated by the liver and are potentially hepatotoxic. Therefore, standard anti-tuberculosis therapy should be stopped if it induces hepatitis with jaundice. After recovery of the liver, therapy is resumed with alternative drugs, e.g. thiacetazone, ethambutol and ethionamide.

Straughan[25] writes as follows about dosage schedules for tuberculosis patients:

'We do not endorse the concept of a fixed dosage regimen for anti-tuberculosis drugs. Streptomycin dosage, for example, should be related to age, body mass and renal function. Age is an important determinant of dosage for most drugs. Dosages should also be calculated on the basis of body mass, but for drugs with a narrow therapeutic margin, it is even better to calculate dosage in terms of surface area of the body.

For anti-tuberculosis drugs, about which we are often consulted because of toxicity problems, we regularly advocate more careful calculation of dosage on the basis of body mass.

The package inserts — the official guidelines for the usage of drugs for the products containing PZA available in the RSA — recommend that the daily dose be given in divided amounts. The same recommendation is made for ethionamide. However, for rifampicin, isoniazid and ethambutol, the recommendations are that these agents be given in single daily doses.'

Bacteriological and radiological surveillance of TB patients during chemotherapy

New cases

Initially, three sputum smears are sent to the laboratory on 3 consecutive days for direct microscopy. If this test is negative, one sputum specimen is sent for culture. A chest X-ray is done to confirm the diagnosis.

After 3 months of chemotherapy, three sputum smears are sent on 3 consecutive days for direct microscopy. If this test is positive, sputum is sent once for culture and sensitivity (to anti-TB drugs). After this, 3 sputum smears are sent for direct microscopy at monthly intervals until the test is negative.

Note: The chest is X-rayed after 3 months of chemotherapy and thereafter at 3-monthly intervals. If any of 3 sputum smears taken at the time of X-ray is positive, the same procedure is followed as above.

Old cases (relapses and reinfections)

Initially, three sputum smears for direct microscopy and one sputum specimen for culture and sensitivity are sent to the laboratory.

After 3 months of chemotherapy, three sputum smears are sent for direct microscopy. The chest is X-rayed at this time and thereafter at 3-monthly intervals. If any of the 3 sputum smears taken at the time of X-ray is positive, treatment is reviewed.

(Procedure followed by Department of Community Health, MEDUNSA[26])

Case-holding — prevention of defaulting

Case-holding is an organised attempt to treat and cure all known cases with the correct drug dosage, regular drug intake and an adequate treatment duration.[18]

Although hospitalisation ensures case-holding, it is not recommended as it is very expensive and disrupts the normal life of patients and their families. The best form of therapy is supervised ambulatory care at a clinic and is the method of choice of the TBCP in the nine health regions of the RSA where the following percentage of TB cases were treated as out-patients:

1985: 70 %
1986: 75 %
1987: 79 %

The case-holding success of the TB control programme in the nine RSA health regions can be gauged from the following percentages of cured and discharged cases:

1985: 78 %
1986: 77 %
1987: 75 %

Relapses or reinfections accounted for the following percentages of the total case-load:

1985: 10 %
1986: 11 %
1987: 11 %

In South Africa failure to reach a 100 % cure rate is largely due to breaches in case-holding caused by non-compliance (defaulting) with curative TB chemotherapy.

Definitions

A case that is cured and discharged is one who has completed (up to 75 %–80 % of doses during the 6-month therapy period) a recommended regimen under full supervision. No follow-up is required. A relapse or reinfection may be so classified only if the disease is proven bacteriologically. A defaulter is a case who has not attended for therapy for two consecutive months, or has had less than 75 % of doses during the 6-month therapy period.

Defaulting or non-compliance can be attributed to the following factors:

(1) Lack of hospital beds for those unable to take the responsibility for their own therapy and without social assistance.
(2) Ignorance on the part of the patient of the importance of completing a therapy course.
(3) Unemployment with consequent poverty and inability to pay for transport.
(4) Lack of legislation to enforce treatment.
(5) Lack of co-operation by employers.
(6) Alcohol abuse.
(7) Failure to attend for treatment after having been notified as having tuberculosis.

Defaulters constitute the 'hard core' in the development of resistant strains of mycobacteria (MDR TB). They are also an important source of infection in the community. In 1987 there were 10 000 defaulters. Special efforts are therefore made to reduce the non-compliance rate by health education and by involving the community in actively caring for TB out-patients.

Prevention of defaulting

(1) At the time when tuberculosis is diagnosed, adequate explanation must be given to the patient and his family about chemotherapy: how it works, the duration of treatment and the importance of the regular taking of pills. A family member or voluntary SANTA worker is usually appointed to supervise the taking of medication. If this is not possible and the patient appears somewhat unreliable, the patient is enrolled either for a domiciliary or clinic course of treatment; if the patient's therapy cannot be controlled by these measures, he is hospitalised.
(2) A treatment regimen decided upon should take cognizance of socio-cultural factors which are likely to determine compliance. Example: vast distances in a rural area make it difficult for patients to attend clinics daily. In this case a supervised, intermittent ambulant therapy (SIAT) regimen is more likely to promote compliance.
(3) Clinics must be run efficiently, using an appointment system, so that patients are not kept waiting and also so that the clinic sister is immediately aware of missed appointments. A **register of active tuberculosis patients** must be kept in a given area in order to keep proper control of the disease.
(4) The community must be involved in the anti-tuberculosis programme, and in the formation of voluntary SANTA branches in their community.
(5) As the treatment of tuberculosis is mandatory, all anti-tuberculosis treatment is given free.

Detection of non-compliance in unsupervised chemotherapy

Treatment defaulting can be diagnosed by urine tests, viz. rifampicin, isoniazid, pyrazinamide and ethambutol can be detected in urine as a means of monitoring drug intake.

Handling of defaulting by absenteeism

A patient is declared a defaulter when he has been completely absent from the source of his supervised medication for 2 consecutive months. Absenteeism of more than 2 weeks is handled by sending a TB worker to trace the patient and to ascertain the reason for the absence.

If the patient cannot be found, further attempts at tracing are made 2 weeks and 2 months later before abandoning the search and discharging the patient as a defaulter.

If the defaulter is found after 2 or 4 weeks of absence and can be persuaded to come for therapy, chemotherapy is restarted from the beginning and sputum monitored as with new cases. If the defaulter is traced only after an absence of 2 months and is willing to return for chemotherapy, he is first re-evaluated. His chest is X-rayed and sputum is sent for direct microscopy and for culture and drug sensitivity. Treatment is recommended if these tests are positive and the sputum is monitored as with new cases. (Procedure followed by Department of Community Health, MEDUNSA.)[26]

Post-cure surveillance and relapses

Follow-up surveillance of the TB patient should ideally be carried out, but some authorities are of the opinion that the effective modern treatment of tuberculosis makes it unnecessary to do the time-consuming, long-term follow-up visits to ex-patients who have been discharged from the treatment programme. If patients have a relapse, they will seek help and be given another course of anti-tuberculosis treatment.

A high relapse rate is one of the factors responsible for the high prevalence of TB in the RSA.

A relapse rate of 1–5 % in cured patients can be expected.

THE ROLE OF THE TUBERCULOSIS CLINIC SISTER

The Department of Health runs an intensive training course for nurses, lasting 3 months, in tuberculosis and leprosy control. The TB nurses work under the direction of a Regional Tuberculosis Medical Officer who provides a consultant service for a large region.

In the absence of continuous medical cover at some clinics, especially those in the rural areas of the former black national states, the clinic sister must of necessity **take great responsibilities**, viz.:

(1) Inform the patient of his diagnosis and about the nature, symptoms, complications and treatment of tuberculosis. She must reassure and encourage the patient in order to allay fear and get his co-operation in therapy. The patient is more likely to co-operate if he understands what is happening to him and what is expected from him in therapy.

(2) Inform the family and the patient's employer to get their co-operation. The employer is enlightened as to the nature of TB; management is persuaded to keep the patient in employment and to play an active part in getting the patient to comply with therapy.

(3) Assess the patient and his environment and in consultation with the patient choose a suitable therapy regimen with which the patient is likely to comply. Patient compliance is more likely to be obtained if there is consultation about the following:

(a) home conditions and special problems, e.g. the problem of dependants when contemplating sending a mother or a breadwinner to hospital;

(b) the wishes of the patient;

(c) the patient's ability to work (as influenced by his physical state) and his keenness to continue in employment;

(d) facilities for supervised ambulatory treatment:
(i) at work or at a clinic;
(ii) clinic difficult to reach due to distances.

(4) Request tests of sensitivity of tubercle bacillus to anti-TB drugs when submitting sputum for bacteriological investigation.

The TB clinic sister plays a very important role in *primary TB prevention* (see p. 524 Education and BCG vaccination) and in *secondary TB prevention* (see p. 525). She is also involved in the bacteriological and radiological surveillance of TB patients during therapy, and is responsible for maintaining the cold-chain of BCG vaccine and tuberculin.

The clinic sister must **keep records**; at the end of every year she should be able to state how many patients:

(1) received primary treatment;
(2) were cured;
(3) died;
(4) relapsed and became chronic TB sufferers;
(5) defaulted through either:
(a) non-compliance with therapy (unsupervised) (treatment defaulting); or
(b) absenteeism (case defaulting).

At the end of each month the clinic must fill in a Tuberculosis Statistics form. This form must reach the appropriate DOH regional health office (see p. 479) by the 10th day of the next month. The information required is: TB patients under supervision of the clinic/TB hospital, number gained during the month, number lost, information about bacteriological investigations (including number of patients found to be resistant to INH and/or Rifampicin) and the number of patients on various treatment schedules.

SUMMARY OF CURRENT TUBERCULOSIS FINDINGS IN THE RSA[27]

Tuberculous infection is defined as tuberculin positivity due to contact with tuberculosis. A 'case', 'tuberculosis' or 'tuberculous disease' are all equivalent and indicate clinically evident tuberculosis.

Following the primary infection, 85 % of infections resolve by healing completely. The remaining 15 % resolve with latent foci of living bacilli and of these, 10–15 % will undergo endogenous reactivation in later life and cause the development of overt tuberculosis.

One sputum positive person infects 10 persons per year and can remain infectious for 2 years or longer. One third to two thirds of close contacts of open cases are infected when the latter are diagnosed, but only 8 % of contacts actually suffer from tuberculosis.

Secondary tuberculosis may be due to either endogenous reactivation of infection or exogenous reinfection, the relative importance of their roles in tuberculosis being a controversial point. There is less risk of a tuberculin positive person getting an exogenous infection, yet the incidence of TB in tuberculin positives is 4 times higher than in tuberculin negatives.

The fatality rate of those with untreated disease is 4–10 %. This rate is effectively reduced by case-finding and treatment.

The best and most cost-effective cure rate is obtained by a short (6 months) treatment course of effective anti-tuberculosis drugs given by means of a supervised ambulatory case system.

Every effort should be made to keep the patient employed and productive.

TERTIARY PREVENTION OF TB — REHABILITATION

Tuberculotics who cannot work can obtain a disability grant. These patients are treated daily at clinics. Disability grants are usually cancelled on completion of treatment when the patient should be fit for work. Sick tuberculotics who are entitled to it can draw unemployment insurance and sick pay. The Anti-Tuberculosis Association, assisted by SANTA, helps tuberculotics with legal advice, food and housing.

It is important for community health authorities to enlist the co-operation of employers with regard to re-employment and attendance at out-patient clinics. A TB patient who stays away from work and has no income is not likely to be able to afford the food which is essential for building up his resistance.

THE WORK OF THE SA NATIONAL TUBERCULOSIS ASSOCIATION (SANTA)

SANTA is an association of people who help state and local authority medical services to fight tuberculosis on a voluntary basis. Many voluntary members are doctors and nurses. It was formed in 1947 and its Patron-in-Chief is the State President, its Patron, the Minister of Health. SANTA raises money from the public to carry out its programmes and also receives state subsidies. One of its main fund-raising efforts is the Xmas Stamp Fund. Every ten years or so, it launches National Appeals for funds. SANTA forms a link between the public and the medical authorities and supplies the community with information about tuberculosis, its prevention and cure. SANTA's headquarters are in Johannesburg; the National body controls 425 SANTA branches (SANTA voluntary committees who work actively in the community). In each province or large region, branches are controlled by branch liaison officers. Branch committees ('work or care groups') can liaise with local authorities to launch control schemes in their area, if such an area has not yet been covered by state anti-tuberculosis campaigns.

As tuberculosis is predominantly a problem of the non-white peoples of South Africa, the white committees are more concerned with fund-raising activities while the black voluntary workers are more concerned with visiting black TB patients in their homes and in clinics in black schools.

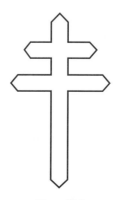

Figure 30.3
International emblem for anti-TB work

SANTA's programme includes the following:

(1) **Prevention:** the protection of children from infection and the promotion of public participation in preventive measures. In urban, rural and former national black state areas, SANTA has established 'Town and Village TB Control Schemes' with the approval of the DOH. Instead of local authority teams, SANTA teams are doing systematic surveys, going from house to house to do Heaf diagnostic tests on pre- and non-schoolgoing children, as well as on elderly adults. The negative reactors are given BCG vaccine and the positive reactors are X-rayed and treated where necessary. These teams are also used for case-finding and tracing foci of infection. Persuading employers to retain their staff with tuberculosis is also a preventive measure done by SANTA members, as continued employment prevents poverty through unemployment — a factor which exacerbates the disease and helps to lower the resistance of contact family members.

(2) **Treatment:** SANTA is operating 30 treatment centres (hospitals) for non-whites only, e.g. the Charles Hurwitz SANTA centre near Baragwanath Hospital. These hospitals have a total of more than 6 000 beds and operating costs are subsidised in full by the state. As emphasis in TB work is on domiciliary treatment, patients admitted to these hospitals are very sick or totally unable to cope with domiciliary treatment because of poor socio-economic circumstances. Patients on oral chemotherapy who live at home can, on the other hand, be supervised with the taking of their medication by volunteer workers, who also persuade employers and teachers to help with supervision where possible.

(3) **Research:** developing effective control procedures and compiling reliable data. TB surveys have been undertaken in various areas to establish the prevalence of the disease.

(4) **Control measures:** pilot TB control schemes have been introduced in several areas, necessitating the use of mobile treatment units for case-finding and their personnel, including registered nurses. The mobile X-ray units of SANTA go where requested and are controlled by the Johannesburg branch of SANTA.

(5) **Health Education:** SANTA trains black health educators at Modderbee (Transvaal) and appoints teams of health educators and TB information officers to work amongst the black people in order to break down the barriers of superstition and ignorance which hamper scientific control measures. One health educator is attached to the Eastern Cape liaison officer. SANTA keeps stocks of educational aids for the health educators.

(6) **Publicity and information services:** these are provided to keep the community informed in regard to tuberculosis. Public support is essential to tuberculosis control.

(7) **Social assistance** by SANTA branches, e.g. 'Friends of the Sick Associations in Durban and Cape Town', are Indian branches which care for the sick tuberculotics. The branches do welfare work for TB families, pay rent or arrange for rent remission of patients undergoing treatment if asked by needy people and apply for disability and maintenance grants where the breadwinner cannot work. They also run soup kitchens at schools where child nutrition is suboptimal as well as crèches. Social assistance is of vital importance as a means of building up the resistance of family contacts to infection, through improved diet and living conditions. Branch members also help to place non-infectious tuberculotics in employment, and persuade reluctant employers to keep non-infectious tuberculotics in employment by acting as educators of the public.

SANTA encourages public-spirited people to form a SANTA branch in their community, the aim being to establish SANTA branches in every city, town and village in South Africa. SANTA branches not only help local TB sufferers and their dependants and liaise with local health authorities in their anti-TB projects but can also apply to the national organisation for the establishment of TB treatment centres and clinics. If the establishment of such a centre or clinic is warranted, the responsibility for its administration falls upon the branch. If a few public-spirited community leaders in a community feel the need for establishing a branch, they must apply to the national office of SANTA in Johannesburg, who will assist with the mechanics of forming such a branch. The branch becomes affiliated to the national organisation and has access to advice, assistance, information, and publicity and propaganda material at all times.

(This section was compiled from information supplied by SANTA national office.)

REFERENCES

(1) Department of National Health and Population Development. *Epidemiological Comments* 1983; **10**: 12.

(2) Department of National Health and Population Development. *Epidemiological Comments* 1984; **11**: 1.

(3) Schultz EJ. Leprosy and cutaneous tuberculosis. South African perspectives. *S Afr J Cont Med Educ* 1984; **2**: 39–51.

(4) Schultz EJ. 13th International Leprosy Congress, The Netherlands. 1988. *S Afr Med J* 1989; **76**: 233–234.

(5) Glatthaar E, Donald PR. Diagnosis and treatment of tuberculosis with special reference to paediatric application. *S Afr J Cont Med Educ* 1989; **7**: 267–281.

(6) Hutt MSR. *J Trop Paediat* 1969; **15**: 153.

(7) WHO *Technical Report Series*, 671.

(8) Fourie PB. Editorial. Tuberculosis, mycobacteriosis and AIDS. *J Epidemiology and Infection* 1988; **3**: 163.

(9) Retief FP. Tuberculosis control and treatment. *S Afr Med J* 1986; **70**: 773.

(10) Department of National Health and Population Development. TB Control Programme. *Epidemiological Comments* August 1987; **14**(8).

(11) Weyer K, Fourie PB. Die epidemiologie van tuberkulose in Suider-Afrika. *S Afr J Cont Med Educ* 1989; **7**(3).

(12) Glatthaar E, Arabin G, Kleeberg HH. The significance of the tuberculosis infection risk and its application in Pretoria. *S Afr Med J* 1978; **53**: 615.

(13) Glatthaar E. Tuberculosis control in South Africa. *S Afr Med J* November 1982; Special Issue.

(14) Kleeberg HH. The dynamics of tuberculosis in South Africa and the impact of the control programme. *S Afr Med J* November 1982; Special Issue.

(15) Department of National Health and Population Development. *Epidemiological Comments* November 1988; **15**(11).

(16) Glatthaar E, Donald PR. Diagnosis and treatment of tuberculosis with special reference to paediatric application. *S Afr J Cont Med Educ* 1989; **7**(3).

(17) Department of National Health and Population Development. *Epidemiological Comments* September 1987; **14**(9).

(18) Westaway MS, Fourie PB. Tuberculosis control. *S Afr J Cont Med Educ* March 1989; **7**(3).

(19) Thomson EM, Myrdal S. Regional variations in tuberculosis policy in the Cape and Ciskei. *S Afr Med J* 1986; **70**: 253–257.

(20) Moloantoa KEM. Traditional attitudes towards tuberculosis. *S Afr Med J* November 1982. Special Issue.

(21) Cartwright JD. *S Afr Med J* 1978; **54**: 65.

(22) Arabin G, Gärtig D, Kleeberg HH. First tuberculosis prevalence survey in KwaZulu. *S Afr Med J* 1979; **56**: 434.

(23) Glatthaar E. Letter to the Editor. Notification of tuberculosis. *S Afr Med J* 1986; **70**: 177.

(24) Collins FFB. Smouldering tuberculous disease not detectable by clinical means. *S Afr Med J* 1987; **72**: 85–86.

(25) Straughan J. Letter to the Editor. *S Afr Med J* 1987; **72**: 440.

(26) Adapted from: Hattingh ME. Tuberculosis management — some aspects of the role of the nurse manager. *Curationis* 1981; **4**: 26.

(27) Department of National Health and Population Development. *Epidemiological Comments* September 1985; **12**(9).

(28) Department of National Health and Population Development. *Epidemiological Comments* April 1993; **20**(4).

(29) Martin DJ. HIV and tuberculosis. *Specialist Medicine* July 1993.

(30) DNHPD. Tuberculosis Control Programme — 1991. *Epidemiological Comments* January 1993; **20**(1).

(31) DNHPD. The degree of diagnostic certainty of notified tuberculosis cases . . . in 1990. *Epidemiological Comments* June 1991; **18**(6).

(32) Collins TF. Study of drug resistance in tuberculosis. *Epidemiological Comments* January 1991; **18**(1).

(33) DNHPD. *Epidemiological Comments* June 1993; **20**(6).

(34) Editor's Comments. *CHASA* April/May 1993; **4**(2).

(35) Shennan DH, Weyer K, Maarsingh H. Evaluation of the standard tuberculosis drug regimens in Transkei . . . *The South Africa J of Epidemiology and Inf* 1991; **6**(1): 5–7.

(36) DNHPD policy about the re-notification of proven relapsed PTB patients. *Epidemiological Comments* May 1991; **18**(5).

TEST OF KNOWLEDGE

The student has benefited from studying this chapter if he/she can answer the following questions:

(1) Discuss the following with special reference to their importance in tuberculosis control:
  – Annual risk of infection
  – Dormant tubercle bacilli in the body
  – Pott's disease of the spine
  – The care and use of BCG vaccine at present (1994)
  – Tuberculin testing of children

(2) Discuss the extent of the TB problem in the RSA.

(3) Distinguish between the following pairs:
  – Incidence and prevalence
  – Prevalence of TB and prevalence of TB infection
  – The infected and the infectious pool
  – Exogenous and endogenous sources of TB infection
  – Primary and secondary prevention of TB
  – The use of anti-tuberculosis drugs for TB-infected persons and for persons with tuberculous disease

(4) Discuss the control of TB in the RSA with special reference to case defaulting as a management problem.

(5) Describe the pathogenesis of TB, with special reference to pulmonary TB and to the causes of endogenous reactivation of disease.

(6) Name the types of extra-pulmonary TB. What is their relative importance in tuberculous disease in general?

(7) Discuss the diagnosis of pulmonary tuberculosis.

(8) Define the following:
  – A case of tuberculosis
  – A suspect case of tuberculosis
  – A case that is cured
  – A relapse or reinfection
  – A case defaulter

(9) Discuss the use of the three standard, primary tuberculostatic drugs used in the state TB clinics, as well as the infectiousness of patients while in therapy.

(10) Discuss the causes, consequences and prevention of TB case defaulting.

31

Bacterial Infections

OBJECTIVES

The objectives of this chapter are to introduce the student to important communicable diseases which are caused by bacteria. In this chapter six bacterial medical conditions are discussed. The sequelae of haemolytic streptococcal infections, acute rheumatic fever (ARF) and rheumatic heart disease (RHD) are important preventive health topics for study. These diseases were made notifiable medical conditions in 1989. The community nurse can help to avert the crippling effects of RHD by timeous attention to the 'sore throat' in children under his/her care, either in health clinics or in schools, and by ensuring that children under his/her care for ARF prevention receive their monthly penicillin injections.

The notified incidence of diphtheria diminished to 7 in 1989 and 5 in 1993. This splendid achievement is attributable to effective childhood immunisation which has brought about relatively good herd immunity. Diphtheria has, however, not yet been eradicated as in the case of smallpox, hence the continued necessity for surveillance, which includes alertness to the possibility of cutaneous diphtheria which may produce contagious virulent throat infections.

The student must be aware that herd immunity to tetanus cannot be built up and that tetanus immunity is short-lived and needs to be boosted at intervals in at-risk persons. Amongst the developing populations antenatal immunisation is especially important in the prevention of tetanus neonatorum, the commonest form of tetanus. Other preventive measures are also outlined.

Whooping cough is a dangerous infection in early childhood; it is now notifiable and the diagnosis may be difficult. Immunisation is not a very effective primary preventive measure, thus babies must be kept away from crowded places and from contact with other children with a cough. These measures apply to the prevention of all respiratory infections which exact a high death toll. Legionnaire's disease is a relatively rare and new disease which was made notifiable in 1989.

Meningitis is the commonest infection of the CNS and can be caused by a wide variety of organisms. Only tuberculous and cerebrospinal (meningococcal) meningitis are notifiable medical conditions. Meningococcal disease may present in sporadic or epidemic form; it is important for the community nurse to recognise this infection in the early, curable stage.

IN THIS CHAPTER

STREPTOCOCCAL INFECTIONS AND THEIR SEQUELAE

A sequela is a disease condition following as a consequence of a disease.

The Lancefield Group A beta-haemolytic streptococcus *(Strep. pyogenes)* can infect any part of the body, but the important infections in children are those of the throat (nasopharynx). In temperate climate countries, streptococcal infections have been undergoing a spontaneous decline in their severity; they respond well to penicillin and the streptococcus has never been known to build up a resistance to this antibiotic. The sequelae to streptococcal infections, viz. **glomerulonephritis and rheumatic fever** (RF) are probably due to an immunological reaction of the body to streptococcal antigens. Whereas any serotype of the *Strep. pyogenes* can cause rheumatic fever, only the nephritogenic haemolytic streptococcus type 12 causes acute glomerulonephritis — a much rarer disease than rheumatic fever and rheumatic heart disease. Acute nephritis is preceded by an acute streptococcal infection such as acute tonsillitis, scarlet fever or upper respiratory infection.

Scarlet fever used to be a great killer in temperate climate countries, but is no longer a community health problem of any magnitude and death-rates are zero. It is no longer a notifiable disease in South Africa. (In 1977, 220 cases were notified.) It is a mild disease and effective chemotherapy with penicillin can prevent the complications: suppurative otitis media and sinusitis. Rheumatic disease and acute glomerulonephritis are rare sequelae which may follow 1 to 3 weeks after the onset of scarlet fever.

In warm climate countries in the tropics and subtropics, however, the sequelae of scarlet fever and streptococcal pharyngitis are prevalent and the cause of much morbidity in children and adolescents. Half the children with RF get carditis and two-thirds of these develop rheumatic heart disease with heart valve lesions. This probably has nothing to do with climatic conditions, but with the fact that the poor developing nations populate these areas. In most developed countries, the reported incidence of rheumatic fever and rheumatic heart disease declined dramatically even before the advent of antibiotics to combat streptococcal infections. This is ascribed in great measure to general improvement in the socio-economic status of the developed countries, especially housing.

McLaren *et al.*[1] state that even in the temperate climate of the Transvaal highveld rheumatic heart disease remains prevalent in all population groups; each year at least 100 whites with rheumatic heart disease report for the first time to the cardiac clinic of the Johannesburg Hospital. Rheumatic heart disease is, however, a special community health problem among the urban black children of Soweto, Johannesburg. This has been attributed to poverty and overcrowding, the latter encouraging the transmission of the streptococcus, mainly by droplet spread. Amongst poor people, sore throats are likely to be neglected and give rise to the high prevalence of rheumatic heart disease. In developing countries RHD is the most important cause of cardiac deaths up to the age of 50.[4]

ACUTE RHEUMATIC FEVER (ARF) AND RHEUMATIC HEART DISEASE (RHD)

RHD is a crippling and killing disease of childhood and adolescence, which is a sequel to some primary infection with any serotype of the *Strep. pyogenes*. The infection is usually in the throat (nasopharynx). Frequently external signs of the antecedent infection are gone by the time the patient complains of the symptoms of rheumatic fever. On the other hand, an attack of rheumatic fever may be so mild that it passes unnoticed; thus half the children with RHD give no history of rheumatic fever.

A positive result of one of the 3 antistreptococcal antibody tests, e.g. the anti-streptolysin O (ASO) level in the blood, will confirm the antecedent streptococcal infection and the probability of an attack of acute rheumatic fever (ARF). Recurrence of an attack of rheumatic fever occurs within 5 years, unless special prophylactic measures are taken. Rheumatic fever is rare below the age of 5 years, the peak incidence being between 6 and 15 years of age. The attack rate is greatest in those who have had a previous attack of rheumatic fever and may also be influenced by familial susceptibility. The chance of recurrence continues until the age of 25 years.

With each attack, damage to the myocardium and heart valves is exacerbated and the child may either die in chronic heart failure or require valvular surgery.

In rheumatic disease, the fibrous tissues of the body, especially those in the joints, muscles and heart valves, are involved in an immunological reaction by antibodies (antistreptolysin O, ASO) against streptococcal toxins (streptolysin). It is the ASO which attacks body tissues in the immunological reaction and causes rheumatic fever and carditis. This immunological reaction is characterised by hyperaemia, oedema of collagen tissues and infiltration with leucocytes.

Prevalence rate in developed countries: 0,5–1/1 000 population.

In 1972 a survey was done in Soweto, Johannesburg, to determine the prevalence of RHD in a sample of 12 050 black children between the ages of 2 and 18 years.[1] The findings were as follows: overall prevalence rate of RHD was 6,9 per 1 000, the highest rate yet found in the world from recent surveys (it is equal in frequency to coronary heart disease in adults); peak prevalence rate of 19,2 per 1 000 children of the seventh school grade; female preponderance of 1,6:1; a rise in the prevalence with increasing family size. The commonest valve lesion was mitral regurgitation.

Lancefield's Group A beta-haemolytic streptococcus was isolated from the throats of 52 per 1 000 Soweto children taking part in the survey, which was done on a stratified random sample.

Incidence of ARF[2] after streptococcal pharyngitis:

- epidemic infections — 3 % of patients;
- endemic infections — 0,3 % of patients.

The true incidence of ARF is unknown, as it is often mild or subclinical.

Projecting the findings of McLaren *et al.* to the total South African population, Bundred and Kitchiner[2] computed that approximately 93 000 people in the RSA will have RHD in the future.

Overcrowding has been shown to be the most important factor contributing to the high incidence of RHD. Poor nutrition, *per se*, does not increase the susceptibility to RF. In Soweto there is much overcrowding in schools and homes due to shortage of accommodation and large family size. No comparable data is available for other ethnic groups or in rural areas.

In a study done from 1981–1984[3] on 46 children admitted to the Coronation Hospital, Johannesburg, with acute rheumatic fever (ARF), 26 were found to have carditis and 35 (76 %) developed RHD (mitral regurgitation) by the end of 1985. ARF recurred in 12 children, half of whom received ARF prophylaxis. The authors came to the conclusion that if this disease is to be eliminated in the area from which the children came, there will have to be considerable improvement in their socio-economic status.

Acute rheumatic fever (ARF) and rheumatic heart disease (RHD) (first diagnosis only) were made notifiable medical conditions in the RSA in December 1989. Notification will give a more accurate reflection of the incidence of ARF and RHD.

Primary prevention

(1) The main prophylactic measure is to **raise the socio-economic status** of underprivileged people; it is important to increase school and housing accommodation and to limit the size of families by attention to family planning programmes.

(2) Outbreaks of **pharyngitis should be controlled** by chemoprophylaxis. A throat swab should be taken to diagnose streptococcal infection. Treatment must be prompt. Generally one intramuscular injection of benzathine penicillin G is sufficient to clear up the infection. The penicillin is very slowly absorbed from the intramuscular depot and produces prolonged antibiotic activity. It is preferred to the oral penicillins (phenoxymethyl penicillin V) which are given for 10 days. It will prevent an attack of rheumatic fever.

Note: Erythromycin, if the child is allergic to penicillin, is the only alternative antibiotic of any use for a sore throat.

The doctor or primary health care nurse should look for and treat reservoirs of streptococcal infection in children: nasal and ear discharges, and acute and chronic pharyngitis. In this way it is hoped to prevent the primary attack of rheumatic fever. Schoolteachers and community nurses can play a part in spotting streptococcal infections and arranging for therapy.

(3) **Education** of the population concerned to seek medical aid for sore throats.

Secondary prevention

(1) For the control of acute rheumatic fever, **early diagnosis** is the first requirement. At least two of the major manifestations must be present for diagnosis to be verified: carditis with tachycardia, cardiomegaly and abnormal ECG; migratory polyarthritis; chorea; subcutaneous nodules on elbows, scalp and over the spine; erythema marginatum (irregular red circles with raised skin edges). There are no laboratory tests diagnostic of acute rheumatic fever; the ESR is raised. Serial determination at weekly intervals of

ASO titre gives an index of recent streptococcal infection; this may help to confirm the diagnosis of rheumatic fever. The C-reactive protein test is positive and there is a leucocytosis and raised temperature. B-haemolytic streptococci may be found on throat swabs, but this is not common.

(2) **Treatment of patients with rheumatic fever** to prevent further damage to the heart. The patient is confined to bed-rest while his temperature and ESR are raised and there is danger of cardiac failure usually for the first 3 weeks of the RF. Penicillin is used to eliminate persisting streptococci and salicylates are given to control the temperature and joint pains. Steroids are used for 3–4 weeks as an anti-inflammatory agent in acute carditis.

Chorea is a neurological reaction to the streptococcus which may occur in the absence of polyarthritis. The patient is weak and 'emotional' and involuntary movements occur. They abate during sleep. Penicillin is given, even where there is no arthritis, to get rid of streptococci and the choreiform movements are calmed with oral haloperidol.

(3) The most important factor in secondary prevention is the **prevention of further attacks** of rheumatic fever by the 4-weekly injection of benzathine penicillin G (1,2 mu) in all children who have had an attack of rheumatic fever. Instead of the IMI, daily oral penicillin or sulphadiazine can be given. This is continued ideally until the age of 25 years. The incidence of RHD rises with each attack of rheumatic fever; therefore, if further attacks are prevented, the child is not likely to suffer from the chronic permanent manifestations of RHD, viz. valvular heart disease, one attack being unlikely to cause RHD.

(4) A **surveillance programme** should be instituted to make sure that every child who has had rheumatic fever comes for his 4-weekly intramuscular penicillin injection. In communities where rheumatic disease is a community health problem, rheumatic clinics should be established to which patients can be referred.

Examples of public health measures[3]

In 1984, the Johannesburg Municipality instituted a free monthly home visit by the community nurse to administer the penicillin injection to all patients who have had ARF. The Transvaal Department of Hospital Services gives free hospital services to all patients who have had ARF.

(5) A **card system** can be used to obtain parental co-operation and regular attendance for the 4-weekly CHD prophylactic injection. Defaulters should be followed up by the community health nurses.

(6) **Case-finding** by screening for heart murmurs. School children can be screened by auscultation of the heart to detect murmurs. In black, Indian and coloured children school nurses use stethoscopes for this purpose. A child with a murmur is referred to a physician or cardiac clinic for the possible diagnosis of rheumatic endocarditis. Treatment will be as in (3).

Tertiary prevention

(1) Patients with valvular lesions are prone to get subacute bacterial endocarditis when exposed to infection with *Strep. viridans*, e.g. after dental extraction and other surgical treatment. In these cases prophylactic penicillin is given before the operation and for two days post-operatively.

(2) If valvular lesions are severe enough to cause cardiac failure, cardiac surgery is done to free the compromised heart from its extra load of work.

(3) Patients with ARF should be treated free at public hospitals and follow-up clinics. This will be cost-effective in the long run. During the period 1982–1987, approximately 8 226 heart valves damaged by rheumatic fever were replaced in the RSA at a cost of R205 million.[4]

DIPHTHERIA

(See also p. 500.)

Diphtheria is an acute infectious disease caused by *Corynebacterium diphtheriae* infection of the pharynx, nose or/and larynx, and skin. It is a notifiable disease, three cases being notified in South Africa in 1992 and five in 1993. Diphtheria is a preventable disease through immunisation which should be started at the age of 2 months. Clinical diphtheria is no longer the feared disease it was in former times. In temperate and cold climates its incidence and mortality have declined to almost zero because of the widespread and effective use of active

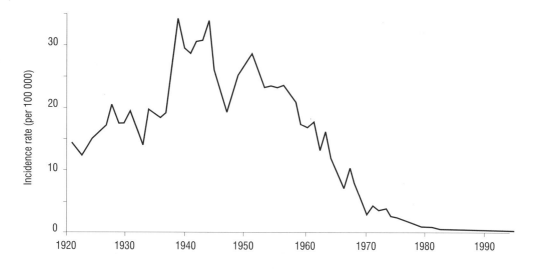

Figure 31.1

Incidence rate of diphtheria

immunisation. A person who has been immunised, as well as a person who has suffered from the disease, may become a carrier, but will not contract the disease.

Incubation period: 2–5 days.

Pharyngeal (or faucial) diphtheria has always been the most virulent form of diphtheria. Virulence or the ability to produce a powerful exotoxin is caused by a viral (bacteriophage) infection of the corynebacterium. The toxigenicity of the corynebacterium causes clinical diphtheria; the toxin causes acute inflammation locally and the formation of a membrane composed of fibrinous exudate which is opaque, adherent and bleeds when forcibly separated from its base. When absorbed by the bloodstream, the exotoxin causes paralysing peripheral neuritis and myocarditis with cardiac failure; it also attacks the adrenal glands and kidneys.

The localised oedema and membrane in **laryngeal diphtheria** may cause asphyxia, necessitating tracheostomy. Severe toxaemia which is not neutralised by prompt treatment usually ends fatally.

Cutaneous (skin) diphtheria is more prevalent in tropical and subtropical regions. The *C. diphtheriae* may cause primary cutaneous diphtheria or may secondarily invade wounds and skin lesions caused by scabies, insect bites, eczema and impetigo. Virulent toxigenic strains of the corynebacterium are found more commonly in the latter.[5]

Cutaneous diphtheria seldom presents as a severe systemic illness with late complications (e.g. myocarditis with cardiac failure) as in pharyngeal diphtheria, but peripheral neuropathies may cause paraesthesias and polyneuritis resembling the Guillain-Barré syndrome.[5]

Cutaneous diphtheria may cause partial or complete immunity to pharyngeal diphtheria.

Infectiveness of diphtheria

Cutaneous diphtheria is more contagious than pharyngeal diphtheria. Skin lesions are the commonest source of diphtheria infections in tropical countries and in overcrowded, impoverished communities in temperate areas.

In cutaneous diphtheria the immediate environment is contaminated (in contrast to pharyngeal diphtheria). The infected environment can be a source of both cutaneous and pharyngeal cross-infection. Infection may be acquired by droplets (from pharyngeal infection) or by direct or indirect contact with infected skin lesions. Milk contaminated with droplets can also be a source of infection. In 20–40 % of patients with cutaneous diphtheria, the corynebacterium is carried in the pharynx (avirulent strain).[5] The period of infectiveness varies. The patient with diphtheria must be isolated and barrier nursed until he has received 48 hours of appropriate antibiotic therapy. The patient is returned to the community after three negative throat, nose or skin smears, taken at one- or two-day intervals consecutively, have been obtained, provided the patient is physically fit for discharge.

Diagnosis

The diagnosis of diphtheria is made by finding the *C. diphtheriae* (and isolating it by culture) in smears taken from the throat or skin lesion. The bacteria are tested for virulence.

Primary prevention

(1) Active immunisation of all children (see p. 497 for the immunisation schedule) and early treatment of carriers.
(2) Prevention of the carrier state by not allowing a diphtheria patient out of isolation until he no longer harbours the infection.

Secondary prevention

(1) *Early detection* (by diagnosis) and notification of diphtheria, and isolation of the patient in an isolation ward. All discharges from the patient are disinfected. Duration of isolation: until cultures from both throat and nose taken not less than 24 hours apart, and not less than 24 hours after cessation of antimicrobial therapy, prove negative. Where culture is impractical, isolation may be ended 14 days after appropriate antibiotic treatment.
(2) *Tracing of contacts.* Throat and nose cultures are taken from them.
   (*a*) Contacts under the age of 10 years:
      if fully immunised: administer a booster;

if not previously immunised: commence prophylactic treatment with erythromycin and continue for a period of 5 days. At the same time a primary diphtheria immunisation course is commenced. Isolation: 8 days after removal from source of infection.

(b) Contacts aged 10 years and older:
if fully immunised: observe for signs of diphtheria for 6 days;
if not immunised: do a Schick test and commence prophylactic treatment as above. Primary diphtheria immunisation (small dose of toxoid) is done only if the Schick test is positive. Three or four doses of toxoid may be necessary, according to a repeated Schick test. Adult contacts may not handle food or associate with children until carrier status has been excluded by bacteriological examination.

(3) *Surveillance of the population at risk*, e.g. a school, and contact tracing to screen for susceptibility and the carrier state.
Susceptibility to infection can be diagnosed by two tests:

(a) antitoxin titres obtained from a sample of blood;

(b) the Schick test: a small amount of exotoxin is injected intradermally. A positive result is characterised by a red patch, 10 mm in diameter, within 24 to 48 hours. It remains red for 4 to 7 days and leaves a brown mark after desquamation.

Susceptibility and diagnostic test results signify the following:

(a) both negative: immune to diphtheria;

(b) susceptibility test negative and smear positive: a carrier of diphtheria;

(c) susceptibility test positive and smear positive: the person is about to go down with diphtheria;

(d) susceptibility test positive and smear negative: the person is susceptible to infection.

Susceptible contacts should be immunised. These children are kept out of school for 8 days in case they contract the disease.

(4) *Treatment of sufferers and carriers.*
Specific treatment of diphtheria:

(a) Intramuscular injection of anti-diphtheritic serum (ADS) (20 000 to 100 000 units) as soon as the patient is admitted, even before diagnosis has been confirmed by the finding of a positive smear. It neutralises the harmful effects of the exotoxins already liberated and helps to prevent complications. Hypersensitivity to serum must first be ruled out.

Note: ADS can also be given to a susceptible contact.

(b) Penicillin or erythromycin is used for 7 days (in combination with diphtheria antitoxin in cases of systemic toxicity).

Healthy carriers are treated with a course of penicillin while they are kept in isolation. If the carrier condition persists, despite the sensitivity of the organisms to antibiotics, a tonsillectomy is advised.

TETANUS

Tetanus is a preventable, non-contagious, endemic, infective disease with world-wide distribution, which never erupts in epidemic form. It is of minor importance in the developed world but is one of the major causes of death in many tropical and subtropical, developing countries. The global trend has been for morbidity and mortality rates to come down as educational and socio-economic standards have gone up. In South Africa, 331 cases were notified in 1981, 204 in 1985 and 300 in 1986.

There are no seasonal variations in the incidence of the disease and 60 % of all notified cases of tetanus occur in children under the age of 1 year, most of these being assumed to be cases of tetanus neonatorum. Ninety per cent of tetanus occurs in the black population, the most severely affected areas being the northern Transvaal and Natal.

Tetanus is caused by the *Clostridium tetani*, a spore-bearing, anaerobic bacterium. The spores of the *Cl. tetani* are present, universally, in any kind of soil and dust and the vegetative form of the toxigenic strain of the organism may be carried in the gut of many domesticated animals (horses, cattle, sheep, goats, dogs) and,

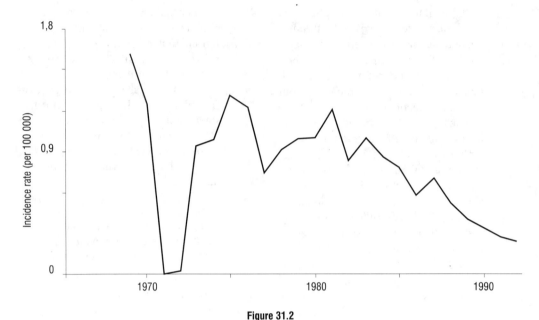

Figure 31.2

Incidence rate of tetanus
Source: *Epidemiological Comments* 1994; **21** (3)

in some countries, of man. The spores enter the
body through a break in the skin or mucous
membrane and if they encounter favourable
conditions (e.g. anaerobic, deep, penetrating
wounds with necrotic tissue, sepsis) the spores
germinate and local infection takes place. A
virulent, potent, exotoxin (tetanospasmin) liberated locally is carried by the peripheral nerves
and bloodstream to the anterior horn cells of the
spinal cord. After a variable incubation period,
tetanospasmin causes muscle spasms, starting
with facial muscles to give the patient trismus
(lockjaw) and risus sardonicus (sardonic smile).
The shorter the incubation period, the more
severe the disease. Facial spasms are followed
by painful, paroxysmal muscle contractions
which may involve the whole body (opisthotonus) in response to any sensory stimulation.
Spasms may last from seconds to minutes; they
prevent breathing and cause the untreated patient to die from exhaustion and respiratory
infection.

Tetanus is a lethal infection, but if recovery
takes place after intensive medical and nursing
care in an intensive care unit of a hospital, there
are no sequelae. The patient is, however, not
naturally immune to further infections by the
clostridium.

Although any susceptible (i.e. non-immunised) person can acquire the disease, the following types of tetanus are well-known entities:

(1) **Neonatal (tetanus neonatorum).** This is
the commonest form of tetanus; it is very
often fatal. In some developing countries, 10
to 30 % of all tetanus occurs in this period
because of the unhygienic treatment of the
umbilical cord stump. The tribal custom of
treating the stump with cow dung reputedly
accounts for many cases of neonatal tetanus.
Fourie[6] reporting on 34 cases of tetanus
neonatorum seen over a period of 2 years at
Ga-Rankuwa Hospital, found no instances
of the use of manure or polish on the cord.
The cords had been cut with scissors, safety
razor blades, surgical instruments and
knives, and the stumps had been treated or
dressed with string, cotton wool, dress material, petroleum jelly, baby powder, newspaper and lard. In February 1991, tetanus
neonatorum (TN) was declared a notifiable
disease. Notification of tetanus was as follows:

1992: Tetanus 68 (deaths 20) TN: 13 (deaths 3)

1993: Tetanus 32 (deaths 10) TN: 16 (deaths 1)

Note: Tetanus neonatorum is a preventable disease due for global eradication (WHO) by 1995.

(2) **Juvenile tetanus** in the age group 1 to 15 years. Children are prone to wounding and to thorn pricks if they walk barefoot in the veld.

(3) **Puerperal (post-partum) and post-abortal tetanus.** The genital tract can be the portal of entry of the *Clostridium tetani*. Criminal abortion, especially if dirty instruments have been used, is the main cause of tetanus in the woman of childbearing age. The retention of necrotic tissue after incomplete abortion may predispose to tetanus. Attempted criminal abortions and septic incomplete abortions are common causes of tetanus in non-immunised women. In the majority of cases of puerperal (post-partum) tetanus, the delivery was done at home under unhygienic conditions.

Primary prevention

(1) Tetanus neonatorum can be prevented by active immunisation of the pregnant woman, especially the black woman, starting early in pregnancy and giving a second injection after 1 month, at least 2 weeks before delivery. Tetanus immunisation should form part of routine antenatal care. The infant will be born with sufficient antibodies (passive immunity) to prevent the disease during the critical neonatal period (first 3–6 days of life).

The mother's third primary tetanus toxoid injection can be given when the infant begins his immunisation. As the mother's immunity will last 40 months, infants born within that period will also be passively immunised.

(2) Active immunisation against tetanus (see p. 503).

(3) Prophylaxis after wounding is further enhanced by the *débridement* of the wound when liberal use is made of hydrogen peroxide to kill the anaerobic clostridium. Likewise, it is important to evacuate the uterus completely by curettage, after a septic incomplete abortion. The modern practice is to use the vaccine even if the patient has not had a course of active immunisation, three injections of the vaccine being given at intervals of 14 days. The vaccine may be given in conjunction with penicillin for 5 days.

Note: Active-passive immunisation with human tetanus immunoglobulin (TIG) in addition to tetanus toxoid is sometimes done in patients with septic incomplete abortions or after deep wounding if previous active immunisation is inadequate or unknown.

(4) Health education of pregnant women regarding the cutting of the umbilical cord and the hygienic care of the stump is important for those women who are likely to deliver at home.

The public must be made aware of the disease.

(5) It is important that all diagnosed cases of, and deaths from, tetanus be notified. Where endemicity of tetanus is thus found to be high, epidemiological surveys can be conducted by the Department of Health and the necessary remedial measures taken to protect the susceptible population. Tetanus being a non-communicable disease, no group immunity is built up; every individual must develop his own immunity. Complete coverage of the susceptible population is, therefore, a tremendous community health task.

Note: As tetanus is a non-contagious, non-epidemic disease, secondary preventive measures are not applicable. The intramuscular injection of human TIG within 24 hours of the start of spasms decreases mortality.

WHOOPING COUGH (PERTUSSIS)

(See also p. 502.)

Whooping-cough is an acute, infectious, respiratory disease characterised by paroxysmal coughing accompanied by 'whooping' and caused by the *Bordetella pertussis*. Its distribution is world-wide and epidemics occur; there is no seasonal variation.

Pertussis starts with coryza, upper respiratory catarrh and a slight cough, which gradually increases in intensity after the end of the second week, to coughing paroxysms with stringy, sticky sputum, cyanosis and vomiting. Between bouts of coughing, which vary in frequency between 5 and 20 per day, the child appears to be normal. Infectiveness is high, the infectious period lasting for 4 weeks (from the first prodromal symptoms) and the disease for 4 to 6 weeks. Vaccinated children may have abortive attacks, but one attack gives lasting immunity.

The incubation period is 5 to 14 days; the infection is spread by inhalation of infected droplets of cases. Quarantine of school contacts is unnecessary.

Half the cases of pertussis occur before the age of 4 years, the earlier the incidence the more dangerous the disease, the mortality rate in babies under 6 months being fairly high. In developed countries with good facilities for early immunisation (i.e. first dose at 2–3 months of age) and early treatment of affected children with antibiotics, whooping-cough is no longer a serious disease. In the poorer countries, however, early occurrence in infancy may lead to sudden, unexpected death, or death may occur from secondary infection: bronchopneumonia, chronic bronchitis, bronchiectasis, encephalopathy and CCF.

The diagnosis of pertussis is difficult. Laboratory diagnosis by antibody assays are unreliable and culture of the B. pertussis in specimens of mucus taken through the nose after a paroxysm of coughing is difficult. Diagnosis depends largely on clinical features, especially the spasmodic cough as the 'whoop' may be absent and, if present, may be due to other infections. Pertussis is characterised by leucocytosis with absolute lymphocytosis. History of contact with a case indicates the possibility of pertussis. During an epidemic, pertussis is diagnosed on prodromal symptoms.

Primary prevention

(1) Primary immunisation of infants during the first year of life, three doses of the vaccine being given in conjunction with diphtheria and tetanus vaccine (see p. 497). Because there have been instances of severe neurological damage after pertussis vaccination and because immunisation does not give perfect protection, the vaccine is not completely acceptable and should not be given in cases of parental objection. It should not be given after the age of 2 years as the danger of encephalopathy increases after this age. It should not be used for infants with a history of convulsions. Booster injections are not given after completion of the primary course.

(2) A young baby should be isolated from contact with a case of whooping-cough.

(3) If isolation of a young baby is impossible, prophylactic erythromycin is sometimes given.

Secondary prevention

Secondary prevention is by the treatment of the pertussis patient from the prodromal stage for 14 days with suitable antibiotics, e.g. erythromycin together with salbutamol. Cough mixtures are ineffective. Patients at school or preschool should be kept at home for a period of 7 days after starting treatment with erythromycin, or 3 weeks if antimicrobial therapy is not given.[15]

As pertussis was not a notifiable disease, the efficacy of current vaccination programmes cannot be assessed. It is known, however, that the pool of infants and young children susceptible to pertussis in the RSA is large because of poor vaccination coverage and relatively low vaccine efficacy.[7] Pertussis was made a notifiable disease in 1994.

Note: Pertussis occurs frequently before the immunisation programme commences, i.e. before 3 months of age.

LEGIONNAIRES' DISEASE (LEGIONELLOSIS)

Legionnaires' disease is caused by the *Legionella pneumophila*, a short flagellated Gram-negative bacillus. In the laboratory it grows best under aerobic conditions and for culture needs special laboratory tests. In nature it grows best in warm, stagnant water and is found in a wide variety of water sources. *Legionellae* have been isolated from, *inter alia*, plumbing fixtures, air-conditioning systems and nebulisers in buildings such as hotels and hospitals. There are many serotypes and species, most being harmless. Both sporadic and epidemic forms of the illness occur. Its major mode of spread is through the air, the bacillus being inhaled and attacking the lungs.

Legionellosis, known only since 1947, is an acute bacterial pneumonia. The first major outbreak of the disease occurred in the USA in 1965, but the impact of this dramatic infection was only felt in 1976.[8] South Africa has had two minor outbreaks in 1982 and 1985/1986, the last one in a Johannesburg hospital. It was made a notifiable medical condition only in December 1989, and therefore its incidence in the RSA was not yet known in 1990. In 1992 two cases were notified and in 1993 two cases, of whom one died.

Incubation period: 2–14 days, mean of 8 days.

People at increased risk of infection: smokers, alcoholics, diabetics, those with chronic obstructive pulmonary disease. Immunosuppressed and renal transplant patients are at particular risk.

Legionellosis may occur at any age, but it is more common in the elderly.

Case definition: a case is defined as a patient with clinical and/or radiological evidence of pneumonia, together with laboratory evidence of legionella infection, viz.

(1) positive staining of sputum or lung tissue or Direct Fluorescent Antibody (DFA) testing for *L. pneumophila*, and/or

(2) a fourfold change in titres to *L. pneumophila* on Indirect Fluorescent Antibody (IFA) testing to a titre of at least 1:128, and/or

(3) a single IFA titre to *L. pneumophila* of greater than 1:256.[9]

Note: The SAIMR has had a Legionella Laboratory in Johannesburg since 1979.

Once the *L. pneumophila* enters the lungs, it multiplies in the alveolar macrophages and causes a patchy bronchopneumonia which may coalesce to form a lobar consolidation. Local and systemic disease manifestations are caused by an endotoxin. Some serotypes of legionella may be more neurotoxic or nephrotoxic because of their particular endotoxin.[8]

Clinical features

Legionellosis may vary from a mild lower respiratory tract infection to a fatal pneumonia. It presents as any other acute pneumonia. The first symptoms are malaise, anorexia, lethargy, headache and myalgia plus coryza-like symptoms. After two days the patient suffers from a pyrexial illness with rigors and bradycardia. The early cough may be moderate and non-productive or productive with scanty bloodstained, mucoid sputum. The patient may appear acutely ill and develop the following complications:

(1) Painless, watery diarrhoea, nausea and vomiting.

(2) Alteration in mental state from mild confusion to disorientation, stupor and coma.

(3) The kidneys are affected and acute renal failure may occur.

(4) The heart may be affected.

These complications clear up once the legionellosis is cured. The disease becomes progressively worse during the first 4–6 days. The patient may require ventilatory support.

The diagnosis can only be made with certainty in the laboratory. The patient may die or the disease may gradually resolve, clinical improvement far outstripping radiographic improvement.

With effective chemotherapy, the fatality rate is much reduced.

Treatment

Treatment is supportive and specific.

Supportive treatment is symptomatic treatment for respiratory failure, shock and renal failure, some patients needing dialysis.

Specific: Erythromycin is the drug of first choice.[8] It is given intravenously for the first week of therapy and then orally for 2 weeks. Curtailment of therapy may cause a relapse. Rifampicin is also active against legionella. It should never be used alone, however, as the organism may rapidly develop resistance to the drug. It is used in patients who are deteriorating on erythromycin.[8]

MENINGITIS

Meningitis — inflammation of the meninges — can be caused by a number of organisms, viz. bacteria (including *M. tuberculosis*) and viruses. For TB meningitis, see p. 521.

Bacterial meningitis with pus-forming organisms is a much more serious disease than viral meningitis which, if correctly diagnosed, can be nursed at home.

Although any organism may cause meningitis in a susceptible host, the most common organisms are the following: *Haemophilus influenzae, Strept. pneumoniae* (pneumococcus), the *Neisseria meningitidis* (meningococcus) and the *Staph. aureus*.

These organisms can live in the nasopharynx of man as commensals and cause the carrier condition — capable of spread. When they colonise a susceptible host, they become invasive, i.e. enter the bloodstream and thus reach the meninges — for which they have an, as yet, unexplained predilection — to cause infection. The blood/brain barrier is breached and the piamater may be destroyed so that an inflammatory exudate forms on the surface of the brain.

Neurological sequelae of severe bacterial meningitis[10]

(1) In severe cases the superficial layers of the cortex may be destroyed *(subpial encephalopathy)*; this gives rise to convulsions and, later, generalised brain atrophy.[10] Breakdown products (pus) from the generalised inflammation enter the CSF pathways which may become blocked.

(2) Subarachnoid venous and arterial thrombosis which may even extend to the sagittal sinus, causes mainly infarction of the cerebral cortex. The serious sequelae are: hemiplegia, decorticate or decerebrate rigidity, cortical blindness, stupor or coma.

(3) Raised intracranial pressure (ICP) due to many causes, e.g. blocked CSF circulation with hydrocephalus, cerebral oedema and space-occupying lesions such as subdural effusions and empyema.

(4) Raised ICP may lead to 'coning', heralded by dilatation of one or both pupils. There will be loss of consciousness, signs of brainstem compression and death (unless decompression is done timeously).

Note: Coning means the impaction of the medulla oblongata in the foramen magnum.

Although acute bacterial meningitis is a curable condition, diagnosis and treatment must be started at an early stage. Once the patient is in a coma, the prognosis is extremely poor, the patient either dying or being crippled by neuro-logical sequelae such as blindness, hydrocephalus or mental retardation.

The meningococcal form of bacterial meningitis is of importance in community health as it can occur in epidemics which are to a certain extent preventable. It is for this reason that meningococcal infections have been made a notifiable medical condition.

In a study done by Donald *et al.*[13] it was found that 'N. meningitidis remains the commonest cause of bacterial meningitis in children (under the age of 13 years) in the Western Cape, and that 21 % of the organisms are now resistant to sulphonamides. It continues to affect mainly young coloured children . . . Among white children *H. influenzae* is the commonest cause of bacterial meningitis.'[13]

MENINGOCOCCAL INFECTION (*N. meningitidis*)

Meningococcal infection is a severe, acute infectious disease which initially causes a bacteraemia or a septicaemia which may be followed by cerebrospinal meningitis (CSM). Instead of developing into meningitis, the disease may end fatally in a fulminating meningococcal septicaemia, known as the Waterhouse–Friderichsen syndrome, especially in children under the age of two. The most susceptible age for CSM is the first 5 years of life.

Meningococcal infection is spread directly from man to man by droplet infection from the nasopharynx (usually from an immune carrier) to a susceptible host whose upper respiratory tract immunity has been compromised by a virus infection. Carrier and infected cases must have been in close contact for infection to take place, the ideal conditions being overcrowding in houses and institutions. Both the carrier and the susceptible states are transient in nature. Many people carry the meningococcus in their nasopharynx and during epidemics the carrier state may go up to 80 % of the population until all the susceptible people have become immune. Then the epidemic ends; it may return in a year or two, however, as natural immunity is transient, and host susceptibility returns. Meningococcal infection epidemics come in cycles.

Mortality rate: the untreated disease has a mortality of 65 % but with effective chemotherapy the mortality may be 1–5 %. Incubation

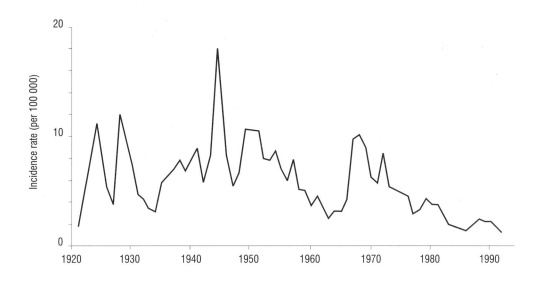

Figure 31.3

Incidence rate of meningococcal infection
Source: *Epidemiological Comments* 1994; **21** (3)

period varies from 2–10 days but is usually 3–4 days. The disease is spread mainly by carriers with nasopharyngeal discharges.

Epidemics may occur in winter (because of people huddling together), seldom in a temperate climate but frequently in warm climate countries, especially in the cerebrospinal meningitis belt of the Sahel in Africa, a belt which lies north of the equator and south of the Sahara. In this region people live in airless mud huts and crowd together in the cold, dry winter nights. The climate in Sahel, a semi-arid zone, plays an important role in the epidemiology of cerebrospinal meningitis (CSM). The degree of air pollution by infected droplets in the small, overcrowded houses, closed against the cold at night, was observed to parallel the incidence of CSM. Although most of the infected persons will become carriers, a few will develop CSM.

In South Africa 533 cases of meningococcal infection were notified in 1992, and 470 in 1993. Of the latter, 60 died. These were mostly sporadic cases or cases occurring in small epidemics.

Over the past 20 years a change has occurred in the epidemiological pattern of CSM. Whereas young adult black males (often mine

workers) used to be the high-risk group, their high-risk status has been taken over by coloured and black children.[12]

Primary prevention

(1) *Environmental sanitation.* In CSM endemic areas where epidemic waves of CSM occur regularly, good ventilation of homes and the prevention of overcrowding should get priority in order to prevent devastating epidemics from occurring. Improvement of housing and socio-economic circumstances are, therefore, essential for eliminating epidemics.

(2) *Immunisation of people at risk.* The meningococcus has a polysaccharide capsule which is antigenic; this determines if the organism is Serotype A, B or C. Vaccines have been devised against Serotype A and C infections, but not against Serotype B infection. Immunity is antibody-mediated. Children at the age of 3 months react feebly to type C antigen and not to type A. From the age of 2 to 6 years, however, they are able to develop good active immunity to both Serotype A and Serotype C vaccine. The

vaccines cause no serious side-effects. It seems to be justified to use this rather expensive vaccine in epidemic areas, but not for routine vaccination of children in non-epidemic areas. The vaccine should be used primarily for the protection of high-risk groups, e.g. children in epidemic areas. Either monovalent (either A or C) or bivalent (A and C) vaccines are given. Group A vaccine is given to children under 18 months (if appropriate); at this age, Group C vaccine is not effective. Generally vaccines are not considered efficacious in the prevention of CSM,[12] especially as the Serotype B meningococcus is dominant in young coloured children, the main at-risk group in the Western Cape.[13]

(3) *Chemoprophylaxis* plays an important role in preventing CSM. Household members are at an increased risk and may be given rifampicin prophylaxis for two days. Daycare centre contacts and close contacts in military barracks, prisons and overcrowded hostels are treated in the same manner. Normal school and work contacts should not be treated. Hospital contacts should only be treated if intensive and intimate exposure has occurred, e.g. giving mouth-to-mouth resuscitation.

Dosage:
Adults: Rifampicin 600 mg twice a day for 2 days.
Children (1 month to 12 years of age): Rifampicin 10 mg/kg body mass twice a day for 2 days.
Infants: (under 1 month of age): Rifampicin 5 mg/kg body mass twice a day for two days.[15]

(4) Spread can best be interrupted by avoiding large gatherings while an epidemic is raging.

(5) The patient is nursed in isolation, but quarantine of contacts is unnecessary.

(6) During an epidemic in an institution, the adequacy of ventilation must be ensured.

Secondary prevention

(1) High-risk contacts of a patient with meningococcal meningitis or septicaemia should show clinically apparent signs and symptoms within 5 days in 50 % of cases.
Early diagnosis of CSM by clinical signs (sudden pyrexia, petechial skin lesions with pink macules, signs of meningeal irritation, convulsions) and positive laboratory findings in the cerebrospinal fluid and blood of *N. meningitidis*. Meningococcal infection must be notified immediately to limit the spread of the infection.

(2) Patients are **treated chemotherapeutically**, penicillin being the drug of choice. Penicillin in large doses for one week, given parenterally, is the most effective drug in use at present. Large parenteral dosage has made intrathecal administration of penicillin unnecessary.

(3) Health education of the general public to get medical help for suspect patients as early in the disease process as possible. This will reduce the rising case-fatality rate.[12]

REFERENCES

(1) McLaren MJ, Hawkins DM, Koornhof HJ, *et al*. Epidemiology of rheumatic heart disease in black children of Soweto, Johannesburg. *Br Med J* 1975; **3**: 474–478.

(2) Bundred P, Kitchiner D. Rheumatic heart disease in South Africa. *S Afr J Cont Med Educ* 1983; **1**: February.

(3) Ransome OJ, Roode H. Rheumatic fever in an urban community. *S Afr Med J* 1988; **73**: 154–156.

(4) Van der Merwe PL. Rumatiekkoors — waarheen? Editorial *S Afr J Cont Med Educ* 1989; **7**: 497–498.

(5) Miller SD. Cutaneous diphtheria at Hillbrow Hospital: A report of 3 cases and review of the subject. *S Afr J Epidemiology and Infection* 1986; **1**: 16–18.

(6) Fourie DT. Some aspects of tetanus neonatorum in the Pretoria area. *S Afr Med J* 1982; **61**: 183.

(7) Ram Kissoon A, Coovadia HM, Loening WEK. Whooping cough — a neglected disease in Southern Africa. 1989; **75**: 560–561.

(8) Marik PE. Legionnaires' disease. *S Afr Med J* 1989; **76**: 265–267.

(9) Department of National Health and Population Development. An outbreak of Legion-

naires' Disease. *Epidemiological Comments* 1986; **13**: 8.

(10) Moodley M, Bullock MR. Severe neurological sequelae of childhood bacterial meningitis. *S Afr Med J* 1985; **68**: 566–570.

(11) Liebowitz LD, Koornhof HJ, *et al.* Bacterial meningitis in Johannesburg 1980–1982. *S Afr Med J* 1984; **66**: 677–679.

(12) Department of National Health and Population Development. Meningococcal infection. *Epidemiological Comments* 1988; **15**: 10.

(13) Donald PR, Burger PJ, Becker WB. Paediatric meningitis in the Western Cape. *S Afr Med J* 1986; **70**: 391–395.

(14) Department of National Health and Population Development. Meningococcal infection — update. *Epidemiological Comments* 1989; **16**: 5.

(15) Departmental policy: Meningococcal meningitis and septicemia: Outbreak control. *Epidemiological Comments* 1991; **18**: 12.

TEST OF KNOWLEDGE

The student has benefited from studying this chapter if he/she can answer the following questions:

(1) (*a*) Define the word sequela(e).

    (*b*) List and describe briefly the sequelae of the following disease conditions:
– Haemolytic streptococcal infections
– Bacterial meningitis

(2) Write notes on:
- Immunisation against meningococcal infection
- Tetanus neonatorum and its prevention
- The diagnosis of cerebrospinal meningitis
- The antistreptolysin O (ASO) level of the blood
- Primary and tertiary prevention of rheumatic heart disease

(3) Describe legionellosis under the following headings:
- Aetiology
- Epidemiology
- Case definition
- Pathology
- Clinical features, including complications
- Treatment

(4) Define:
- Waterhouse–Friderichson syndrome
- Schick test
- Tetanospasmin
- Trismus and risus sardonicus

32

Viral Infections

INTRODUCTION

In this chapter the common viral diseases which occur mostly in children are discussed. Measles, viral hepatitis and poliomyelitis are notifiable.

Encephalitis and encephalomyelitis are no longer notifiable medical conditions. Their aetiology is varied, some viruses causing a benign disease of low infectivity, while others cause severe and permanent brain damage. Encephalitis may be a primary disease, but often it is a complication of systemic viral diseases such as mumps, measles and varicella zoster. Herpes simplex, which is commonly associated with the benign fever blister, can cause severe primary disease conditions and vicious complications in the immunocompromised patient. It causes the most neurologically damaging kind of encephalitis. Some of the viral diseases are teratogenic, e.g. mumps, varicella and rubella. Rubella infection during the first trimester of pregnancy is an indication for therapeutic abortion to prevent the birth of a child with the congenital rubella syndrome.

Only 6 of the 12 primary viral diseases discussed in this chapter are preventable by immunisation: measles, polio, rubella, mumps, influenza and B virus hepatitis. In the last-mentioned 4 diseases, vaccines are given only to at-risk groups.

IN THIS CHAPTER

MEASLES (MORBILLI)

See pp. 496, 504.

Measles, an extremely infectious, mildly acute virus disease of childhood in developed (white) nations, is a very serious, often fatal, disease with multiple complications in developing nations, being especially virulent in the malnourished child with a sluggish immune response to the virus caused by depression of the cell-mediated immune mechanism. In South Africa the coloured and black children are those at highest risk.

Measles also strikes at a much earlier age in the developing countries. Unfortunately about 40 % of urban and peri-urban cases occur before 9 months of age, particularly noticeable in overcrowded areas.[9] For this reason, it is recom-

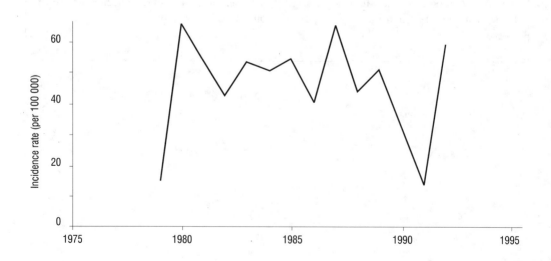

Figure 32.1

Incidence rate of measles

mended that in special conditions of high risk, e.g. refugee camps, squatter camps, the first dose of measles vaccine be given at the age of 6 months and the second dose at 9 months.[9] (See p. 504 Primary Prevention.)

In the developed countries, the greatest incidence of the disease (in unvaccinated children) is between 1–7 years. One attack confers immunity.

In a healthy community infants whose mothers have had measles are protected for the first 6 months of life. Measles can be dangerous, however, between the ages of 5 and 9 months, 'the window period' while the child is building up active immunity.

Epidemiology

Measles became a notifiable disease in 1979. The number of cases notified in the RSA (TBVC countries excluded) varied between 10 799 in 1982, 11 762 in 1993 and 22 745 in 1992. Notified deaths varied with a case-fatality rate between 1 and 6 %.

Reynolds et al.[6] estimate that less than 20 % of cases in the Western Cape are notified, i.e. those who reach the clinics and hospitals because of complications. They ascribe the persistence of measles as a community health problem to rapid urbanisation and overcrowding; poverty and ignorance result in many children not being brought for immunisation. Kettles[8] gives these comparative incidence rates in the Western Cape (1983): 28,1/100 000 (compared with the national 'average' of 60/100 000). When analysed by race, however, the rate for whites is 6,5, for coloureds 20 and for blacks a high 131/100 000.[8]

Measles is the second most prevalent notifiable condition in the RSA after tuberculosis.

After its great success in eradicating smallpox from the globe, the WHO has set its sights on doing the same for measles. According to Fenner,[5] 'The possibility of measles eradication is suggested by the fact that man is the only host of the virus and that a single dose of an inexpensive vaccine provides long-lasting immunity in 90–95 % of vaccinated persons.'

Measles usually occurs in epidemics and is endemic amongst unvaccinated children. Adults are usually immune but when newly introduced into a community, all age groups are susceptible.

In South Africa measles occurs throughout the year with the highest incidence from August to November.

The incubation period of measles is ten days to the prodromal, catarrhal stage which presents with pyrexia, conjunctivitis, coryza and cough and the presence of Koplik's spots on the mucous membrane of the mouth. Koplik's spots are tiny white specks, resembling grains of salt, caused by minute areas of necrosis of the buccal mucosa. They are best seen on the inside of the cheek, near the 2nd upper molar, but may also be on the gums. This stage, which lasts 4 days, is the most infectious stage of the disease, as infection is spread by droplets from the respiratory tract of sufferers, there being no carrier condition in measles. Infectivity ceases about 5 days after the eruption of the rash. The prodromal stage ends with the appearance of the exanthem — a generalised confluent maculo-papular skin rash (see p. 466). The enanthem affects the mucous membrane of the respiratory and gastro-intestinal tracts and the conjunctiva (see complications).

There is a high incidence of respiratory complications during the first few months after recovery from measles. Many children thus affected are malnourished. In poor countries, measles may precipitate children into kwashiorkor and marasmus.

Primary prevention

(1) Improvement in the nutritional and socio-economic status of underprivileged people will reduce the virulence of the disease which is not due to a special virulent strain of the organism in developing countries, but to the poor immunological resistance of underfed people.

(2) Active immunisation against measles. (For a discussion of the vaccine and maintenance of the cold-chain, see Chapter 28.)

Measles vaccination is one of the most cost-effective public health measures available to children in developing countries.[1]

The vaccine is supplied free of charge by the Department of Health to all local authorities, district surgeons, district nursing services, state and provincial hospitals. Mass immunisation campaigns are being carried out in selected areas such as Durban and Soweto, but immunisation is not compulsory.

The vaccine must be freshly mixed and kept in the dark to ensure full potency. In order not to waste any vaccine, arrangements must be made beforehand to ensure that multiples of 10 children attend the clinic to be vaccinated within one hour of reconstituting the vaccine.

(3) It is not necessary to quarantine contacts, but children with the disease must be kept isolated and out of school for 14 days. All susceptible contacts should be vaccinated within 48 hours. After this, and in cases where the vaccine is contra-indicated, measles hyperimmune globulin can be given.

(4) Health education to motivate the community to have their children immunised against measles.

In spite of the fact that a heat-stabilised, effective anti-measles vaccine in the freeze-dried form before reconstitution has been available for the past fifteen years (since 1979), the incidence of measles has not been reduced as significantly as that of diphtheria (5 cases notified in 1993) or poliomyelitis (no cases in 1993). In these two diseases immunisation has conferred 'herd' immunity. High immunisation coverage (95 %) is required for herd immunity in measles. The reasons for the poorer response to primary preventive measures, apart from poverty, overcrowding, and ignorance, are that measles is more easily transmitted and that all children over the age of 1 year, not vaccinated, are susceptible. Cultural factors are often counterproductive to health education. In rural Third-World areas health education may be rendered ineffective by the conservative influence of grandmothers whose beliefs and 'medical' practices are contrary to scientific medical practice.

An example is given by Ysselmuiden.[2] Measles has an incidence of 100/100 000 in Gazankulu (in 1983). In Elim Hospital (Gazankulu) measles accounts for 9,6 % of the admissions to the children's wards; the case-fatality rate is 8,1 % and the mean age of admission 31 months. These statistics point to an unsuccessful vaccination programme, despite vaccine availability since 1977. Mass vaccination campaigns preceded by health education periods have been conducted in Gazankulu since 1980, yet at the clinics (1983) measles vaccinations are given at an annual rate of 15/1 000 inhabitants (birth-rate 40/1 000). This is not enough to influence the heavy toll measles exacts in this developing country.

In an enquiry, the following beliefs and practices emerged:

(1) measles is a 'God-given' disease — essential for the normal development of the child and thus not to be prevented;

(2) some remedies used are a threat to the health of the child;

(3) 73 % of mothers had a positive attitude to vaccination, most mothers preferring the injection when the child is sick 'to hasten the development of the rash' and thus prevent the rash 'falling into the chest' (i.e. the complication of pneumonia).

The reason for vaccination is thus not grasped and the positive attitude is for the wrong reason. Cultural factors appear to play a very important role in the failure of the vaccination programme.

Motivation to accept vaccination is encouraged by —

(1) giving the people reasons for acceptance which, though not scientific, fit in with their beliefs;

(2) not discouraging cultural practices which are harmless.

Secondary prevention

Measles is a notifiable disease and is easily detectable as it usually occurs in epidemics. Children must be nursed at home in bed. If any complications supervene during an attack of measles, the child should be admitted to an isolation hospital with facilities for assisted mechanical ventilation and tracheostomy care.

Complications

(1) Pneumonia is the commonest lethal complication. In 97 % of cases[7] pneumonia is caused by a supervening infection, i.e. not

the measles virus. The infection may be due to a large number of different viruses, bacteria and fungi. Some of the children with pneumonia die after up to 30 days of mechanical ventilation in a special respiratory care unit.

(2) Gastro-enteritis.
(3) Otitis media.
(4) Cardiac and renal failure.
(5) Gingivostomatitis which may give rise to cancrum oris, a gangrenous, ulcerative lesion of the mouth.
(6) Laryngotracheobronchitis which may require tracheostomy.
(7) Acute necrotising bronchiolitis.
(8) Conjunctivitis (enanthem), corneal ulceration and blinding (prevention requires oral vit. A therapy).
(9) Disseminated herpes simplex.

Sequelae may be chronic bronchiectasis and subacute sclerosing panencephalitis (see below).

Peripheral lymphocytopenia and malnutrition are common in fatal cases of measles, suggesting the possible role of depressed T-cell immunity to account for the variety of organisms and frequency of supervening infections. These supervening infections generally occur within 6 to 8 weeks of the onset of the measles rash. Depressed cell-mediated immunity leads to prolonged measles infection; this, in turn, exacerbates the damaged immunity.[7]

Subacute sclerosing panencephalitis (SSPE)

SSPE is a late sequela of measles resulting from measles involvement of the CNS; it has a fatal outcome. The National Institute for Virology keeps a registry of SSPE cases. Over the past 24 years, (prior to 1980) 116 cases have been reported, 73 % appearing in the last 9 years.

The mean incubation period, i.e. time from primary measles infection until onset of symptoms, is 6,4 years.[3]

Association between measles and SSPE is established by finding high levels of measles complement-fixing antibodies in the CSF and serum. Clinical picture: the disease starts with mental and behavioural changes. This is followed by convulsions and progressive cerebral degeneration. The patient dies after 1–3 years, deaf, blind, mute, paralysed and demented. For 'The Measles Strategy', see p. 496.

MUMPS (EPIDEMIC PAROTITIS)

Mumps is an acute communicable disease caused by the paramyxovirus. It is a disease mainly of schoolchildren and young adults, spread by oral contact and droplets of saliva from recognisable and subclinical (25 %) cases. It is endemic throughout the world and localised epidemics occur infrequently. It is not notifiable in the RSA.

The target organs of the virus are the salivary glands, principally the parotid glands.

The incubation period of mumps is 14 to 21 days. There is a short prodromal period with headache, sore throat and pyrexia. Then the salivary glands start swelling in staggered succession. Acid substances in the mouth cause acute pain as the salivary glands respond to the stimulus.

The period of infectivity lasts from 6 days prior to, until up to 9 days after, the onset of parotitis. By this time all gland swellings should have subsided and the temperature returned to normal.

Complications

(1) Meningo-encephalitis may occur even in the absence of parotitis (subclinical mumps) and is a benign disease. During a mumps epidemic the mumps virus can account for up to 25 % of all encephalitis cases in a community.[10] The signs and symptoms of encephalitis occur 3–10 days after the onset of parotitis.
(2) Pancreatitis may give rise to diabetes mellitus. This is a rare complication.
(3) After puberty: orchitis/oophoritis occurs fairly frequently. One or both testes (in orchitis) may become tender, red and swollen. The patient develops a temperature and there is severe testicular pain. Although there may be residual atrophy with shrinkage of one or both testes, sterility seldom results.

Clinical and subclinical cases give long-lasting immunity. The infant whose mother has had mumps is passively protected for the first 6–9 months of life.

Primary prevention

(1) Isolation of cases does not prevent the spread of mumps and quarantine of contacts is not practised.
(2) Immunisation (see p. 504) is done in selected cases, but mumps vaccination is not included in the routine primary vaccination of infants.

Secondary prevention

There is no specific therapy for mumps.

Good mouth hygiene and nursing care of the febrile patient is required.

Local support and warmth are helpful in cases of orchitis.

Mumps meningo-encephalitis requires bed-rest until the pyrexia and headaches have subsided.

ENCEPHALITIS AND ENCEPHALOMYELITIS

Encephalitis means inflammation of the brain and myelitis, inflammation of the spinal cord. They can appear singly or as a combined condition, encephalomyelitis. The encephalitis of public health importance is caused by viral infections, there being many different kinds of infective viral encephalitis.

Viral encephalitis may be either a primary or secondary condition. *Primary encephalitis* is usually a benign disease caused by one of the following viruses: Coxsackie, echovirus, arbovirus, poliovirus. The disease presents with fever, headache, malaise, nausea and vomiting. The level of consciousness is altered with memory defects, seizures, abnormal behaviour and pathological reflexes, but consciousness is not lost.

Infection by these viruses occurs sporadically throughout the year, but may reach epidemic proportions in the late summer.[10]

Secondary encephalitis is a complication of a systemic viral disease such as measles, mumps, herpes simplex type 1 and varicella zoster.

Mumps encephalitis is a benign disease with complete recovery within 2–3 weeks. Very rarely the patient is left with permanent neuro-

logical sequelae. Herpes simplex virus type 1 encephalitis is a very dangerous condition which leaves the patient with serious neurological deficits and may cause death.

Measles can cause an acute viral encephalitis as well as the subacute sclerosing panencephalitis (see p. 563).

Post-infectious encephalitis occurs after childhood viral diseases have healed, and is associated with damage to neurons or their myelin sheath. It is an immunogenic disease with a poor prognosis.

VIRAL HEPATITIS

Hepatitis (inflammation of the liver) can be caused by many agents, but only viral hepatitis poses a community health problem. Viral hepatitis is caused by four main kinds of viruses, hepatitis A virus (HAV) (infective hepatitis), hepatitis B virus (HBV) (serum hepatitis) and the antigenically different non-A non-B viruses (NANBH), which also cause serum hepatitis with its sequelae but are less virulent than the B virus. A fourth hepatitis virus is called unspecified or undifferentiated.

The various hepatitis viruses and their antibodies can be identified in the laboratory.

Epidemiology

Incidence: Viral hepatitis became a notifiable disease in 1979. The incidence of NANBH is low — 86 cases in 1993, when 447 cases of HBV and 1 048 cases of HAV were notified. There were, however, 225 viral hepatitis cases of unspecified or undifferentiated type. Coloured people in the Western Cape are particularly susceptible to HBV infection.

Common features of viral hepatitis

Clinically and pathologically all forms of viral hepatitis are similar. The disease may be mild or severe, acute or chronic and, in some cases, terminates fatally. Serum hepatitis is of slower onset and has a longer incubation period, i.e. 30–180 days as against 15–45 days in the case of infective hepatitis.

Acute viral hepatitis may be mild and without jaundice, but the typical overt attack presents as follows: the hepatitis viruses cause necrosis of scattered liver cells and there is peri-portal infiltration by lymphocytes. The prodro-mal period (2–14 days) is characterised by head-ache, malaise, nausea, anorexia, pyrexia, vomiting, palpable liver and pain in the right hypochondrium.

After 2–14 days, the jaundice (of variable severity) appears with dark urine and pale stools. The prodromal symptoms subside with the appearance of the jaundice and after a few weeks the colour of the skin, urine and stools returns to normal. In most cases the patient recovers completely, but there may be relapses, and, in the case of hepatitis type B, there may be serious sequelae. It is impossible to distin-guish clinically between individual cases of se-rum and infective hepatitis, but serological tests can make the distinction. Epidemiologically there is a big difference between the two main kinds of viral hepatitis.

Hepatitis B virus (HBV) infection

Special features of Hepatitis B virus (HBV) infection (Serum Hepatitis SH)

It used to be called SH because the virus is found in the body fluids, blood, saliva, tears, seminal fluid, of sufferers and carriers. Carriers form a large reservoir for hepatitis B virus. Even sub-clinical forms of the disease may give rise to the carrier state.

Epidemiology of HBV hepatitis

It is estimated that there are over 200 million carriers of HBV globally.

In South African whites the carrier rate is low, but 18 % of blacks are carriers, which is extremely high by world standards.

The clinical picture of HBV infection varies from an asymptomatic illness without jaundice to a fulminant disease with massive hepatic necrosis and a fatal ending. Between these ex-tremes is the acute viral hepatitis with variable outcome; 2 % of blacks and 98 % of whites heal completely. Those who are not healed either become carriers or develop the disease in a chronic form. Years later they may die from the sequelae of the disease: chronic liver failure, cirrhosis of the liver or primary liver cancer (hepatocellular carcinoma — HCC). Rural black HBV carriers, mostly males, die of HCC between the age of 20–30 years, in greater num-bers and at an earlier age than urban blacks,

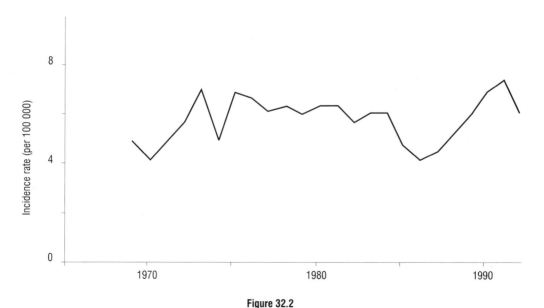

Figure 32.2
Incidence rate of viral hepatitis
Source: *Epidemiological Comments* 1994; **21** (3)

probably because of greater exposure to the cocarcinogen, aflatoxin, found in mouldy grains, groundnuts and beans stored in damp, underground cellars. Lifelong HBV carriers are at high risk of developing primary liver cancer which runs a much more acute course in blacks than in whites and also presents at a much earlier age.

Mode of spread of HBV:

(1) By injection given with syringes and/or needles contaminated by body fluids of sufferers or carriers. This is a special danger in mass immunisations by the parenteral route and in haemodialysis units. Intravenous injections by drug addicts who use communal syringes are a common mode of spread in this group.

(2) By sexual intercourse; serum hepatitis can thus be classed as a sexually transmitted disease. As the virus can be present in saliva, kissing may also cause spread. It is quite common amongst homosexuals.

(3) Through skin lesions and the conjunctiva of persons working with infected body fluids, e.g. nurses while cleaning sharp instruments. Viral hepatitis is an occupational hazard in nurses, doctors and laboratory technicians. It can also be spread by the shared razor and toothbrush and by tattooing and scarification equipment.

(4) Inoculation with the virus during dental and surgical procedures.

(5) Blood transfusions used to be a common cause of post-transfusion hepatitis. With the modern testing of blood donors for the presence of hepatitis B virus (HBsAg) in their blood, this danger from hepatitis B virus has been eliminated.

(6) Carrier mothers can transmit the B virus to their infants during the birth process.

(7) HBV infection is endemic in some areas of Southern Africa with low standard of living and high herd immunity. Here infection is contracted at an early age, mainly through horizontal spread (child to child). The exact mechanisms of horizontal spread are still unknown.

Hepatitis B virus is fairly resistant to the common disinfectants and boiling; therefore, fomites must either be destroyed by incineration or sterilised by means of steam under pressure or formalin and glutaraldehyde disinfectants.

As there are no specific drugs against these viral infections, *primary prevention* of viral hepatitis is the ideal to be aimed at.

Primary prevention

(1) The control of hepatitis B by active immunisation became possible in the RSA in 1983 (see p. 501). A new vaccine, Engerix, is cheaper and therefore more likely to be used on a large scale.

The following at-risk groups should have priority:

(a) Infants in endemic areas, and of carrier mothers. Universal immunisation of infants with 3 doses of vaccine is the ideal.

(b) Hospital staff (medical, nursing and domestic).

(c) Sexually promiscuous persons, mainline drug addicts, homosexuals and commercial sex workers (prostitutes).

(d) Staff, blood donors and recipients and patients exposed to blood and blood products in laboratories, hospitals, blood transfusion services.

(e) Patients and staff in institutions for the mentally retarded.

(f) Immunocompromised patients.

(g) Family and close contacts of HBV sufferers.

(h) Prisoners, prison staff, ambulance and rescue service staff.

Note: Pre-vaccination serological testing for susceptibility to the HBV in high-prevalence groups, especially health care workers, would be cost-effective if immune persons could thus be excluded from vaccination.

HBV vaccine is very expensive. This is probably the reason why mass vaccination has not been initiated in the RSA for, for instance, all infants and all susceptible persons living in poor socio-economic conditions where HBV prevalence may be high.

(2) Disposable syringes and needles which are used as such, are important to halt the spread of the B virus. Health workers and laboratory technicians must take precautions, e.g. by the wearing of rubber gloves, when working with blood and blood products:

(a) to prevent inoculating themselves with the virus by accidental pricks and cuts;

(b) by not exposing existing lesions to these products.

(3) All blood for transfusion must be free of the virus by carefully testing the donors and excluding virus B carriers.

(4) Scarification by sangomas and tattooing must be discouraged.

(5) Post-exposure prophylaxis with hyperimmune hepatitis B-immunoglobin preparations. The major protective indications are: needle-stick injury, risky exposure to infected blood, sexual contact with infected persons and neonates born to mothers with acute or chronic hepatitis B infection. This hyperimmune immunoglobin must be given within 48 hours of probable infection. Safety is enhanced if active immunisation is also commenced.

Note: Even if a person testing positive for hepatitis B is asymptomatic, he should still be notified.[22]

Hepatitis A virus (HAV) infection

Mode of spread: faecal-oral route and by faecally contaminated drinking water. Faeces are infectious during the prodromal period, but infectiveness stops when the serum bilirubin (i.e. the degree of jaundice) is at its peak. In sporadic cases, the danger of spread is greatest before the diagnosis is made. The disease may occur in small epidemics, e.g. in an army camp when people are in close contact. Homosexual spread is also known. In this case diagnosis can be made on prodromal symptoms and serological tests; thus suitable isolation precautions can be taken to prevent spread.

The HAV is endemic among the black population in the RSA; nearly all infants are infected but are largely asymptomatic. By schoolgoing age most black children are immune and remain so for life. Clinical hepatitis A rarely occurs in adult blacks. Because of higher standards of food hygiene, whites acquire immunity much later, therefore clinical hepatitis A is fairly prevalent.[11] The large majority of white viral hepatitis cases are asymptomatic and subclinical. There is no major reservoir of infection, either in human beings or in animals (i.e. no carrier condition), sufferers transmitting the disease through their infected faeces to new cases. Water-borne or food-borne epidemics may occur, especially in developing countries; shellfish may also harbour the virus. Its incidence is decreasing in Western countries.

HAV infection does not give rise to chronic liver disease or liver cancer.

Primary prevention

(1) Improvement of faecal/oral personal hygiene.

(2) Community hygiene with regard to water and food supplies.

(3) Pooled human immunoglobulin, with standard titres of anti-HAV, can be given to control local outbreaks of hepatitis A in young children and pregnant or debilitated adults.

Secondary prevention

Secondary prevention can be practised only during an epidemic when the disease is diagnosed during the infectious prodromal period. The virus is excreted in the stools during the last 2 weeks of the incubation period until 7–10 days after the appearance of jaundice. Immunity after an attack is probably lifelong. Isolation care with special attention to the disinfection of stools should halt the progression of the epidemic.

POLIOMYELITIS

See p. 501.

Poliomyelitis is an acute infectious RNA-virus disease of the central nervous system which has been notifiable in the RSA since 1919. The poliovirus is an enterovirus which can survive for long periods in water, milk and food and can possibly be transmitted by flies and cockroaches; it is well adapted to the faecal/oral mode of transmission by faecally contaminated fingers and eating utensils and is prevalent in overcrowded, insanitary conditions with poor water supplies. Droplet/inhalation transmission is possible in developed communities with a high standard of hygiene.

The poliovirus survives and replicates in the gastro-intestinal tract. There are 3 serotypes of the poliovirus, type 1, 2 and 3.

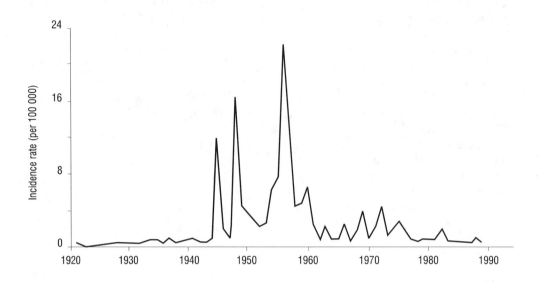

Figure 32.3
Incidence rate of poliomyelitis
Source: *Epidemiological Comments* 1994; **21** (3)

The natural pathogenic poliovirus is called the 'wild' virus; this virus is contrasted with the weakened, usually non-pathogenic, vaccine-derived virus which elicits the antibody reaction after immunisation with the Sabin polio vaccine.

In 1985 the World Health Assembly passed a resolution committing the WHO to the global eradication of poliomyelitis by the year 2000.

Epidemiology of poliomyelitis

Poliomyelitis occurs in all parts of the world, even in the Arctic regions. There are no true seasonal variations, except that extreme cold confines people to their homes, thus preventing interpersonal contact, especially among young children. In temperate and cold climates the spread of the virus is, therefore, limited to the summer and early autumn months when people congregate.

South Africa had a number of large epidemics during the period between 1950 and 1960 before the advent of large-scale polio vaccination with the Sabin vaccine. In 1989 only 11 cases of poliomyelitis were notified in the RSA,

while in 1956 there were 3 000 notifications. In 1992 and 1993 there were no notifications.

The epidemiology of polio has been somewhat modified by immunisation and three patterns can be delineated.

Little or no immunisation

Third-World countries with poor socio-economic and little or no immunisation, with endemic (wild) polio. In these countries the wild virus immunises 80–90 % of the population at an early age, sporadic cases of paralytic polio occurring in young children.

Partial immunisation

Third-World countries with partial immunisation and endemic (wild) polio. The wild virus has to some extent been replaced by vaccine-derived viruses in the environment. Some susceptible persons have not been exposed to either kind of virus and are at great risk of paralytic infection due to opportunities for direct spread (poor sanitation and water supplies). Epidemics can be expected. This pattern operates in the RSA.

In 1982 there was a major outbreak of polio in the eastern and northern Transvaal, with 260 cases of paralytic polio recorded over a 4-month period. Attack (incidence) rate: 32,8/100 000, most under 6 years of age. Case-fatality rate: 13,8 %. Poliovirus type 1 was the causative agent.

In 1987–1988, after 3 years of low incidence and high herd immunity, a polio epidemic (275 persons) broke out in KwaZulu/Natal among blacks. Incidence rate: 4,5/100 000 overall, peaking at 24,2/100 000 in the under-five group who formed 76 % of the polio sufferers.[14] Case fatality rate: 10,2 %. Poliovirus type 1 predominated. Some of the children had been fully vaccinated and some partially.

The epidemic was ended by a vaccination campaign (in addition to the routine vaccination programme) with over 200 000 monovalent vaccine doses (against type 1 virus). The epidemiologists found an association between the September 1987 floods (dissemination of faecal matter) and the epidemic and recommended the following:

- Close monitoring (surveillance) of vaccination coverage.
- Testing of the vaccines in use to ensure their potency and checking the efficiency of the refrigerators which maintain the cold-chain.

Total immunisation

Developed countries with almost total immunisation coverage. In these communities polio is virtually eliminated. Sporadic cases of paralytic polio do occur due to some remaining wild polioviruses and to live attenuated vaccine-derived viruses, i.e. in recipients of vaccines or their close contacts, especially immunosuppressed persons.

Note: These immunosuppressed persons and any close contacts should receive the Salk inactivated polio vaccine (IPV).

Clinical features of poliomyelitis

Poliovirus infection of a susceptible person may manifest in three ways:

(1) Unapparent infection in 90–95 % of persons during the incubation period of 7–14, up to 21 days. The virus enters the mouth and replicates in the oropharynx, tonsils, intesti-

nal mucosa and Peyer's patches. The infection goes no further. In this stage the immune system is stimulated to produce specific, lifelong immunity.

(2) Abortive illness in 4–8 % of cases whose illness progresses beyond the incubation period. The virus spreads to the draining lymph nodes, multiplies and enters the bloodstream to cause a transient viraemia and a mild, self-limited flu-like disease.

(3) Classical paralytic poliomyelitis in 1–2 % of cases. This consists of a minor flu-like illness (prodromal stage) culminating in a major paralytic illness.

If the virus replication is not stopped by the body's defences, the virus spreads to the reticulo-endothelial cells of a number of organs and multiplies extensively to cause a persistent severe viraemia with symptoms of fever, headache, neck stiffness indicative of aseptic meningitis, and photophobia. The patient is restless. After a few days the paralytic stage sets in.

The virus enters the central nervous system either by haematogenous spread or by neurological spread (via the autonomic nervous system) and attacks the anterior horn cells of the spinal cord. The involved muscles become painful and stiff. This is followed within a few days of onset by flaccid paralysis which may be either permanent (if the nerve cell is destroyed) or temporary (if the nerve cell is put out of action by toxins or swelling). Depending on the extent of nerve cell involvement, paralysis may be slight or massive, i.e. parts of muscles or groups of muscles on one or both sides of the body and even paraplegia. The infection may spread upwards to involve the brain stem (bulbar polio) and affect the vital centres of respiration, coughing and swallowing, and even to the motor cortex to cause polio-encephalitis.

There is no loss of muscle sensation; the spastic non-paralysed muscles are painful. As the paralysed muscles are flaccid, the non-paralysed muscles go into spasm thereby causing deformities which, if not corrected after muscle pain has ceased, cause orthopaedic problems. The paralysed muscles waste. There may be improvement in muscle activity for up to a year as unaffected muscles are strengthened by physiotherapy and temporarily paralysed muscles recover their power.

Paralysis is a rare complication of polio, the following factors affecting its severity:

(1) Age: paralysis is more common and extensive in adults than in infants.
(2) Injuries to muscles and hypodermic injections tend to localise paralysis to relevant areas.
(3) Tonsillectomies and tooth extractions increase the likelihood of bulbar polio which is frequently fatal or requires permanent respiratory support.
(4) Pregnancy and immunosuppression affect the incidence and severity of paralysis.

Period of infectiveness and isolation: from the prodromal period until three weeks after the onset of paralysis.

Diagnosis

During an epidemic, paralytic polio is easily recognised clinically. For notification purposes, EPI suggests the following case definition:[21]
'A case of poliomyelitis is defined as any patient with acute flaccid paralysis (including any child less than 15 years of age diagnosed to have Guillain-Barré syndrome) for whom no other cause can be identified.'

In 1994, however, acute flaccid paralysis (AFP) was made a separate notifiable medical condition. The reason for this is tied up with the WHO campaign for the eradication of poliomyelitis by the year 2000. Notification of AFP implies the necessity for the investigation of all cases of lameness (paralysis) when accompanied early in the onset of the illness (acute), by reduced muscle tone and reduced reflexes, (flaccid) and without sensory loss. Besides poliomyelitis, AFP may also be caused by the Guillain-Barré syndrome, transverse myelitis, and may be a complication of oral polio vaccine. A full investigation of AFP may thus exclude polio as a cause of the paralysis. The campaign for the eradication of polio will thus not be hampered by a false diagnosis of polio.[23]
Sporadic paralytic polio is diagnosed by:

(1) Isolation of the virus in stools and rectal swabs with faeces up to 5 weeks after the onset of paralysis, as well as naso-pharyngeal swabs during the first 5 days. The specimen must be fresh and kept cold or frozen. Two kinds of poliovirus may be identified: the wild natural virus or the attenuated Sabin vaccine-derived virus. The latter as a cause of paralysis is possible in immunosuppressed patients.
(2) After isolation the virus must be serotyped. Type 1 is the most paralytogenic kind of virus and is often associated with epidemics.
(3) Serological diagnosis to:
    (a) identify the virus as a wild-type or vaccine-derived;
    (b) identify specific antibodies. Outbreaks of polio in Third-World countries usually show a moderate to high titre of antibodies to type 1 poliovirus, an indication of the presence of type 1 polio in children who have not been previously immunised. Type 2 antibodies is the sensitive indicator of immunisation.

Note: the detection of antibodies to the 3 polio types is important in assessing individual and community immunity.[13]

Immunity to poliomyelitis is obtained as follows:
Active:

(1) Subclinical, abortive or clinical attack of the disease.
(2) Immunisation (see p. 501).

Passive:

(1) The injection of contacts with human immunoglobulin.
(2) It may be present at birth because maternal antibodies pass the placental barrier; neonates have an immunity which is as strong as that of their mothers. This immunity lasts six months.
(3) As breast milk contains the polio antibodies of the mother, breast-fed infants are doubly protected if their mothers are immune to polio.

Immunity after infection is lifelong, but only against the type that caused the infection. The vaccine highly recommended for community immunisation in the RSA is the Sabin oral trivalent vaccine which immunises against all three serotypes.

Vaccination against polio forms part of the EPI (expanded programme of immunisation) followed in South Africa. It was made compulsory in 1963 but this requirement was rescinded in 1987. Many children are protected against the disease by 'herd' immunity (which operates after 66 % of the population have been vaccinated) or by having had a subclinical attack of polio during early childhood.

Prevention

Primary prevention

This is obtained by:

(1) Raising the standards of personal and environmental hygiene of developing countries.
(2) Immunising against polio with the live, trivalent Sabin vaccine. This is a very effective vaccine and, if used correctly, should give complete protection to a community. The oral vaccine is cheap and easy to administer; when first introduced into a community, all age groups should be vaccinated.

Mass immunisation campaigns have been very successful in some Third-World countries, e.g. Cuba and Brazil, where, amidst great publicity, all children under 3–5 years are immunised with the oral Sabin vaccine annually on two days of the year separated by two months. This causes the environment to be flooded with live vaccine-derived viruses; repeated exposure of the people ensures high levels of immunity.[13]
(3) Surveillance is essential in Third-World (developing) countries experiencing outbreaks of paralytic polio, in order to prevent a build-up of susceptible individuals.[13] This is done in two ways:
   (*a*) serological monitoring of population immunity by collecting statistically planned (random) blood samples of the population to test for the presence of protective poliovirus antibodies (vaccination coverage);
   (*b*) strictly-controlled vaccine recall from peripheral parts of the cold-chain (see p. 493) to the laboratory to test the potency of vaccines in use in community immunisation programmes.
(4) Prohibiting large gatherings of people and advising people against strenuous exercise and tonsillectomies when an epidemic is raging.
(5) Zero reporting must be done monthly when there are no cases.

Secondary prevention

This is obtained in the following ways:

(1) Early detection and notification of infected persons. Diagnosis rests on the presence of the virus in stools, rectal and nasal swabs, pyrexia, meningeal irritation and flaccid paralysis of muscles (see p. 568).
(2) Contacts are sometimes quarantined for three weeks (highest limit of the incubation period). During this time, contacts must not be subjected to surgery or injections. All contacts are immediately immunised with Sabin vaccine.
(3) Cases of poliomyelitis are isolated for at least three weeks. Isolation care is given in a hospital with facilities for aiding failing vital functions. There is no specific drug treatment for polio. Muscles and vital functions are supported where necessary and pain is usually alleviated with heat treatments. Physiotherapy is commenced when the temperature returns to normal and muscle pain subsides.
(4) The need for psychological support is paramount.

Tertiary prevention

Severely paralysed patients remain invalids for life and need rehabilitative care. Sheltered employment may be necessary. Physiotherapy becomes a way of life to strengthen healthy muscles and help them to take over some of the functions of the paralysed ones. Where respiratory muscles have been affected, regular physiotherapy is necessary to prevent respiratory infection. Orthopaedic aids and surgery may be necessary to help the patient become ambulatory.

GERMAN MEASLES (RUBELLA)

For rubella vaccination, see p. 503.

Rubella is a mild infectious disease caused by the rubellavirus, which occurs throughout the world either sporadically or in localised epidemics. The incubation period is 14 to 21 days and, after a short prodromal period of upper respiratory indisposition, it is characterised by enlargement of posterior cervical lymph glands, polyarthritis sometimes and a rash (see p. 466), although sometimes the rash is not apparent. Antibodies appear in the blood 1–3 days after the rash has appeared. Rubella is most infectious in the week before the rash appears, direct spread being from case to case by droplets from the upper respiratory tract. The virus is also present in urine and blood and crosses the placental barrier. Past infection is detected by serological (antibody) evidence and diagnosis depends on finding a rising antibody titre against the rubella virus in the blood, and culture for the presence of the virus in pharyngeal secretions and urine.

The **community health problem** posed by rubella is its teratogenic effects when a woman gets rubella in the first three months of pregnancy or if she becomes pregnant within three months of having an attack of rubella. The earlier the infection occurs in the pregnancy, the greater is the likelihood of damage to the foetus; this is called the **congenital rubella syndrome** (CRS). The most common congenital foetal defects, which may be multiple, are: (*a*) cataracts; (*b*) perceptual deafness; (*c*) cardiac abnormalities.

Some sequelae are of late onset; these include mental retardation. Deafness and other defects may be noticed for the first time years after the infant's birth, in the case of a susceptible pregnant woman who had clinically unrecognised rubella. Infants born with the rubella syndrome may excrete the virus for months in their urine or harbour it in their throats, thus becoming an infection hazard to pregnant women in their environment. Rubella infection early in pregnancy, when confirmed serologically, is an indication for therapeutic abortion.

In a Cape Town study done by Kipps *et al.*[15] during the years 1975 to 1977, it was found that 92 % of women of three races in the age group 18 to 25 years had rubella antibodies in their blood, i.e. they had been exposed to rubella infection (or had been immunised against rubella) and were therefore immune. The high prevalence of the disease in the Cape Town women may apply to other parts of the country

as well and may possibly be due to the 1975 rubella epidemic. The implications of these findings were that children born in Cape Town at that time were at small risk of having the congenital rubella syndrome.

It is doubtful if lifelong immunity to rubella is obtained. Second, 'break-through' infections occur, either after a primary infection or after successful vaccination. No case of CRS has, however, been documented as a result of break-through infection which is, moreover, not an indication for termination of pregnancy.[17]

Rubella is not notifiable.

Prevention

Primary prevention of the congenital rubella syndrome

This is possible by ensuring that all women of childbearing age are immune to rubella.

This can be brought about by immunising all non-immune pre-adolescent schoolgirls between the ages of 11 and 14 years. To find these non-immune girls requires continued serological surveillance of all schoolgirls as they reach the stated age group. Serological surveillance requires extensive laboratory services, as well as extensive health teams to take blood specimens and, after screening, to vaccinate the non-immune girls. As the service would be based on voluntary co-operation of the schoolgirls and their parents, a health education programme for the public must first be launched.

Selective immunisation of seronegative schoolgirls is at present not yet practised, many local authorities having introduced rubella vaccination programmes for all volunteer pre-pubertal girls in the schools which come under their jurisdiction.

Nurses and female paramedical staff working in hospitals are at risk of contracting rubella and of infecting susceptible pregnant patients. They should, therefore, be immunised when they enter hospital service.

Secondary prevention of the congenital rubella syndrome (CRS)

Secondary prevention is by the recommendation for therapeutic abortion of all those pregnant women in whom rubella has been diagnosed by serological testing during the first trimester, or during the three months before conception.

Keen *et al.*[16] of the National Institute for Virology recommend the following testing procedures for detection of rubella antibodies for specific purposes:

(1) Contact with rubella by a pregnant woman: a specimen of clotted blood (or serum) must be sent as soon as possible after contact to detect the presence of previously present antibodies. If found, the woman is immune and there is no danger of CRS and no further blood samples are required. If no antibodies are found at this stage, the woman is susceptible to infection and a second blood sample is required 3 weeks after the contact.

(2) Confirmation of a rubella-like illness with rash: two blood samples are required: one as soon as rubella is suspected and one 7 or more days after the appearance of the rash.

(3) Determination of immune status of any woman at any time to determine if rubella vaccination is necessary: a single blood sample is sufficient.

Note: In all cases where an attack of rubella is suspected, full details regarding dates of contact, rash and blood sample collection are required. It is very difficult (but not impossible) to make a retrospective diagnosis some time after the illness. Retrospective diagnosis should never be resorted to as a routine measure.

INFLUENZA

For vaccine, see p. 504.

Influenza is a highly infectious, epidemic disease caused by a myxovirus, Influenza virus type A, type B and type C. The B type is endemic to an area and causes small local epidemics of mild flu, or the sporadic case. The A type causes epidemics which may assume pandemic proportions with high mortality, e.g. the flu pandemic of 1918 which caused more than 20 million deaths from complications, throughout the world. Type C is a very common, but mild, pathogen.

The epidemics of 'Asian', 'Hong-Kong', New Jersey', 'Victoria' flu which occurred during the past two decades, causing ripples of fear in South Africa, were caused by variant strains of Influenza A.

The influenza virus may change its antigenic structure, i.e. may form new variants; thus one person can have many attacks of flu in a lifetime, but immunity to each type and variant is long-lasting, i.e. for up to sixty years.

The variation affects the duration of immunity acquired either naturally or artificially by immunisation.

Incubation period: 1 to 3 days. It is not notifiable.

The incidence of flu is higher in the winter than in the summer; it is spread by droplet infection and infected fomites. Subclinical infections occur and infectivenss is high, extending from before onset of symptoms (abrupt pyrexia, pains in body, head and throat, cough) until after the temperature returns to normal, approximately 3 days in the absence of complications.

The important **complication** is a bacterial infection (with either *Strep. pneumoniae* or *H. influenzae*) of the respiratory tract, 1 to 2 days after onset of symptoms. The infection varies from a mild bronchitis to a fatal pneumonia. The fatal complications of influenza strike mainly elderly people with respiratory and cardiac diseases.

Primary prevention of influenza epidemics

An epidemic of type A flu may spread to South Africa from overseas, after an influenza season (end of winter) in the northern hemisphere. Thus the Department of Health is alerted in good time to make available on a preset date sufficient prophylactic vaccine against the specific type or variant of virus to avert a major epidemic in the RSA. It advises on the advisability of launching a mass public immunisation campaign or whether to use available stocks of the vaccine only for at-risk patients.

The following patients are 'at risk':

(1) those with chronic pulmonary disease;
(2) those with cardiac diseases;
(3) those with chronic renal diseases;
(4) frail, elderly people;
(5) those with diabetes mellitus;
(6) immunocompromised patients.

Note: Haemophilus influenzae type B (Hib) was made a notifiable medical condition in 1994. The Haemophilus influenzae (Koch–Weeks) bacillus, is a species of the haemophilus found in the respiratory tract. It causes acute respiratory infections, acute conjunctivitis and purulent meningitis in children.

Haemophilis influenzae type B is notifiable if it is isolated from a normally sterile site.[23]

Haemophilus influenzae type B is not the usual cause of influenza which is caused by a virus (see above).

THE ACUTE HAEMORRHAGIC CONJUNCTIVITIS SYNDROME

Acute haemorrhagic conjunctivitis (pink eye) occurred in 1982 as a second pandemic affecting Africa, Asia and the Americas. The first pandemic originated in Ghana in 1969. It is caused by enterovirus 70 (EV 70), a new member of the picornavirus family, and the Coxsackie virus A24 variant; it is easily spread by direct contact via hands, or indirectly, via fomites.

Incubation period: 12–72 hours.

Immunity: short-lived (a few weeks).

Extent of problem in RSA

The first pandemic reached Johannesburg in 1973, and the second in 1982, affecting large areas of the RSA. The estimated incidence was tens of thousands of cases,[18] an estimated 5 % of the population.

Small foci of infection remain between epidemics, mainly in black townships, and sporadic cases appear.

In 1984–1985, a large outbreak occurred over large areas of the RSA, and in 1988–1989, a small outbreak in Mamelodi, near Pretoria.[19] The incidence is highest in overcrowded, low socio-economic areas.

Signs and symptoms

Itching of eyes, pain and swelling of eyelids, gravelly sensation; photophobia, profuse watery discharge, congestion of conjunctiva with subconjunctival haemorrhages. The condition is self-limiting, lasting 3–4 days. Punctate keratitis and reactivation of a latent herpes simplex virus infection may complicate the condition. Neurological complications have not occurred in the RSA.

Treatment

Treatment is symptomatic: frequent bathing with saline and instillation of anti-histamine drops and artificial tears. Local anaesthetics should not be used for pain as this may lead to epithelial ulceration. Antibiotics are useful only if secondary infection causes a purulent discharge. Vasoconstrictor drops may be used to reduce swelling.

The patient should refrain from touching and rubbing his eyes and contact lenses should not be worn. Steroid drops must not be used.

Infectiveness: Although very infectious, the period of infectiveness is not known. Spread is prevented by isolation, i.e. staying off work or away from school for 4–6 days. Good personal hygiene must be observed with isolation of towels and face-cloths and appropriate hand-washing.

THE HERPES VIRUS INFECTIONS

The herpes viruses (types I, II, III, IV and V, see p. 461) are important causes of infection in man, their only host. The STD herpes virus (type II herpes virus genitalis) is discussed in Chapter 33.

Herpes viruses share the following pathogenic properties: primary infection, latency period in sensory ganglia and reactivation (see p. 595) when cell-mediated immunity is lowered by sunlight and fever (fever blisters), emotional stress, local trauma and other unknown factors.

Herpes simplex virus (HSV-1) infections[20]

The main sites of herpes simplex virus (HSV-1 or herpes labialis) attack is the mouth, lips and surrounding skin. Primary HSV-1 infection usually occurs in childhood and more readily in the lower socio-economic groups.

The following primary HSV-1 infections may occur:

(1) Gingivostomatitis. Prodromal pyrexia and sore throat are followed by the eruption of small vesicles on the mucosa of the mouth, pharynx, gums, tongue, lips and cheeks, usually accompanied by cervical lymphadenopathy. This painful condition clears up completely after 10–14 days and may later be reactivated to appear as the much milder labial herpes (fever blisters) on or around the lips.

(2) Eye infections — unilateral conjunctivitis with oedema, photophobia and lacrimation,

as well as corneal involvement (e.g. den-
dritic ulcers), which usually clear up after
2–3 weeks. This infection may recur as a
superficial keratitis with corneal ulcers.
More serious infections involve the uvea
and produce permanent visual damage.
(3) Herpetic whitlow, which may attack health
care workers.
(4) Genital herpes.

Complications of primary or recurrent HSV infections:

(1) Encephalitis in adults. The temporal lobes
are involved in a haemorrhagic inflammation. The patient may die or be left with a
serious neurological deficit.
(2) Eczema herpeticum — herpes infection superimposed on an eczema rash.
(3) Immunocompromised patients may develop
severe and prolonged recurrences of the
HSV infection which may spread to the
respiratory or gastro-intestinal tracts.

Treatment

Some antiviral drugs are used in severe HSV
infections, e.g. idoxuridine, vidarabine, acyclovir.

Chicken-pox (varicella) (HZV)

Varicella zoster virus (HZV — herpesvirus
varicella or type III) infections.[20]

Primary infection with HZV causes
chicken-pox (varicella).

This disease commonly occurs in children
under the age of 10, but can be a serious disease
in immunosuppressed adults.

Spread is by air-borne droplets either from
the respiratory tract (in the prodromal stage) or
from vesicle fluid which contains infectious
viruses.

After the primary infection the virus remains dormant in dorsal (sensory) root ganglia.

Signs and symptoms

Fever and an itchy rash (see p. 466). Lesions are
seen at different stages in the same area and may
also appear on mucous membranes. The illness
usually lasts a week when the last vesicles dry
up and the crusts separate.

Complications

(1) Cellulitis or impetigo due to secondary
streptococcal or staphylococcal infection.
(2) Pneumonitis with widespread nodules in the
lungs which last several weeks.
(3) Acute meningitis or encephalitis; cerebellar
ataxia may appear 1–2 weeks after the rash.

Varicella in the early stages of pregnancy has
been associated with congenital abnormalities.

To prevent an attack of varicella in these
high-risk persons, specific zoster immune
globulin can be given within 3 days of exposure to infection to modify or prevent the
disease.

Herpes zoster (shingles)

Secondary infection by reactivation of the HZV
causes herpes zoster (shingles). This is a sporadic disease occurring more frequently in old
age. Herpes zoster is not contracted after exposure to chicken-pox or shingles, i.e. it is not a
contagious disease and the reason for reactivation is usually unknown.

Clinical features

Shingles is characterised by a unilateral painful rash, usually in a lumbar, thoracic or facial
(trigeminal) dermatomal distribution. The
rash is preceded by several days of superficial
pain and hyperaesthesia of the overlying skin.
The rash begins as intense erythema on which
groups of large vesicles continue to appear for
several days. Crusts form which separate after
8–10 days. Trigeminal shingles of the face
may be accompanied by oral, palatal and pharyngeal lesions, or keratitis and uveitis, depending upon which branch of the nerve is
affected.

Shingles is frequently accompanied by viraemia and a thinly scattered chicken-pox rash.
In the immunocompromised patient this may
disseminate to skin and viscera. Cranial nerves
may be affected.

The prognosis for recovery is good.

Complications

(1) Post-herpetic neuralgia with prolonged and sometimes intolerable burning or stabbing pain.

(2) Meningitis, encephalitis and myelitis.

Treatment

Antiviral drugs are useful, especially in immunocompromised patients. They do not mitigate the frequency or severity of post-herpetic neuralgia, however.

Infectious mononucleosis (glandular fever)

This disease is caused by the Epstein-Barr virus (EB virus) which is the herpesvirus type IV.

Spread occurs from man to man through saliva (often through kissing) or respiratory droplets.

Epidemiology

Subclinical attacks in childhood are common among South African blacks. The majority of blacks are, therefore, immune (seropositive for the specific cell-mediated immune response against virus-infected B cells) by the time adolescence is reached.

Note: There is a strong association between the EB virus and Burkitt's lymphoma in tropical Africa.[17]

Diagnosis

Atypical lymphocytosis (hence the name, mononucleosis). A specific serological test, the immunofluorescence test, is done for antibodies to the viral capsid (shell) antigen (VCA) of the EB virus. VCA IgM antibodies indicate recent infection and VCA IgG antibodies, past infection.[17]

Clinical features

There is gradual onset with malaise, anorexia, pyrexia, sore throat, lymphadenopathy and, frequently, splenomegaly. The cervical, axillary and inguinal glands become noticeably enlarged and painful by the third week of the illness. Occasionally the patient develops a maculopapular rash.

Treatment of the sore throat

In the absence of a definitive diagnosis, antibiotics for sore throat should not be prescribed until streptococcal infection has been bacteriologically confirmed. If the sore throat is due to mononucleosis, ampicillin and penicillin will cause a rash.[17] The lengthy course of the illness is characterised by relapses and intermittent fever, but recovery eventually takes place and one attack confers immunity.

The patient can be nursed at home. Due precautions must be taken to prevent spread by droplets and saliva.

There is no prophylactic vaccine and no specific chemotherapeutic medicine.

The herpes virus infections are not notifiable.

REFERENCES

(1) Morley D. *Paediatric Priorities in the Developing World.* London: Butterworths, 1979.

(2) Ysselmuiden CB. Beliefs and practices concerning measles in Gazankulu. *S Afr Med J* 1983; **63**: 360–3.

(3) Moodie JW, Mackenzie DJM, Kipps A. Subacute sclerosing panencephalitis (SSPE) in Southern Africa. *S Afr Med J* 1980; **58**: 964.

(4) Department of National Health and Population Development. Eight years of measles notifications. *Epidemiological Comments* 1988; **15** (6).

(5) Fenner F, Henderson DA, Arita I, *et al. Smallpox and its Eradication.* Geneva: World Health Organisation, 1988.

(6) Reynolds LG, Hussey G, Kettles AN. The continuing scourge of measles. *S Afr Med J* 1987; **71**: 611.

(7) Beckford AP, Kaschula ROC, Stephen C. Factors associated with fatal cases of measles. *S Afr Med J* 1985; **68**: 858–863.

(8) Kettles AN. *The incidence of measles in the Western Cape Region. Interim Report.* Department of Community Medicine. University of Cape Town, 1985.

(9) Coovadia HM, Loening WEK, Yach D. National Workshop on measles immunization. *S Afr Med J* 1989; **76**: 82–83.

(10) Department of National Health and Population Development. Encephalitis in the South Rand area. *Epidemiological Comments* 1986; **13** (4).

(11) Prozesky OW. *Viral hepatitis in Southern Africa*. Supplement to *S Afr Med J* 11 October 1986.

(12) Maynard JE. World-wide control of Hepatitis B. *International Journal of Epidemiology* 1984; **13**: 406–407.

(13) Schoub BD. Poliomyelitis. *Medicine International* 1984; June Core 91–96.

(14) Department of National Health and Population Development. *Epidemiological Comments* 1988; **15** (3).

(15) Kipps A, *et al. S Afr Med J* 1977; **52**: 956.

(16) Keen GA, Naude W du T, Kipps A. *S Afr Med J* 1978; **54**.

(17) Scoub BD. Adviser's comments on rubella. *Medicine International* April 1984.

(18) Hoffman. Acute haemorrhagic conjunctivitis. *S Afr Med J* 1982; **62**: 311–12.

(19) Department of National Health and Population Development. Acute Haemorrhagic Conjunctivitis (AHC) 'Pink Eye'. *Epidemiological Comments* 1989; **16** (8).

(20) Wood MJ. Herpes simplex and varicella zoster infections. *Medicine International* June 1984.

(21) The Eradication of Poliomyelitis from South Africa. *Epidemiological Comments* 1990; **17** (8).

(22) Robson SC, Kirsch RE. National strategy for viral hepatitis. *S Afr Med J* 1991; **80**: 347–356.

(23) New notifiable medical conditions. *Epidemiological Comments* 1994; **21** (5).

TEST OF KNOWLEDGE

The student has benefited from studying this chapter if he/she can answer the following questions:

(1) Discuss the epidemiology in the RSA of the following diseases:
  – Measles (morbilli)
  – B virus hepatitis
  – Poliomyelitis

(2) Discuss immunisation in the following diseases (refer also to Chapter 28):
  – Rubella
  – Poliomyelitis
  – Influenza
  – B virus hepatitis
  – Mumps

(3) Describe the following complications of virus diseases:
  – Subacute sclerosing panencephalitis
  – Classical paralytic poliomyelitis
  – Congenital rubella syndrome

(4) What are the main complications of:
  – Measles
  – Rubella
  – Mumps
  – Varicella
  – Herpes simplex infection?

(5) Define the following terms:
  – Infectious mononucleosis
  – Gingivostomatitis in HSV infections
  – Koplik's spots
  – Reactivation of herpesvirus infections
  – The immunocompromised patient
  – Uveitis and keratitis
  – Haemorrhagic conjunctivitis
  – Encephalomyelitis
  – Herpes zoster

33

Trachoma and Sexually Transmitted (Venereal) Diseases

OBJECTIVES

Sexually transmitted diseases (STDs), including AIDS (see Chapter 34), rank with diseases of poverty, such as tuberculosis and malnutrition, as the most important community health problems in South Africa.

The extent of the STD problem has broadened to include young people in their teens on whom the STDs may impose a life sentence of human misery.

The modern age of sexual liberation launched by the free availability of contraceptives has exacted a heavy toll in youthful infertility, early cancer and chronic venereal lesions which spoil the enjoyment of mature heterosexual relationships. The problem of AIDS is not yet very obtrusive in South Africa, but statistics of its rapidly multiplying incidence point to the threat of a decimation of the peoples of Africa, including South Africa. See p. 522 for its role in the prevalence of tuberculosis.

The medical profession is acutely aware of the rampant incidence of STDs for which there are no preventive vaccines and against which medication is becoming more and more powerless as microbes build up resistance to formerly powerful antibiotics. The objectives of this chapter are to give the student an understanding of the medical and social problems encountered in the fight against STDs. The nurse's role is mainly that of educator. To be successful as a health edu-cator the nurse needs to understand the immense social and personal problems which underlie venereal diseases: sexual promiscuity; immature sexual relationships which confuse sexual licence with sexual freedom and momentary passion and pleasure with happiness; and inability to take responsibility for ill-considered, impulsive actions. The modern increase in promiscuity is a cultural phenomenon and is closely related to the breakup of monogamous family ties. It cannot be expected from the nurse to reverse these strong cultural tides which are sweeping First-World and Third-World countries. The nurse can, however, help to educate her at-risk clients in the use of safe coital practices, e.g. the use of a condom, and she can see to it that women at risk attending antenatal clinics are tested for syphilis at appropriate intervals to ensure that timeous treatment will prevent congenital syphilis. It is also very important for a well-informed nurse to counsel groups of adolescents about the dangers of early and promiscuous sexual practices, where he/she gets the opportunity to educate this vulnerable group. Health education in safe sexual practices and the inculcation of feelings of concern for the welfare of sexual partners are some of the ways in which a community nurse may contribute to the alleviation of the grave community health problem posed by the sexually transmitted diseases.

IN THIS CHAPTER

TRACHOMA

Trachoma is a mildly contagious, chronic infection of the eyes (conjunctiva, especially that of the upper lid) with the *Chlamydia trachomatis* which also causes a sexually transmitted disease. Its distribution is almost world-wide, but whereas sporadic cases generally occur, it is endemic in some warm, dry areas, e.g. amongst the indigenous peoples of the northern Transvaal and north-western Transvaal. Although trachoma is endemic in the whole of this area and most people are affected by the disease, only 25 % of the inhabitants of the Bungeni area of north-western Gazankulu, where a survey was done, have intense upper tarsal disease.[1] It is found that in the endemic areas only 5 % of people over the age of 50 years have no signs of past or present trachoma.

Trachoma is today the most important single cause of preventable blindness in the world and is an important stumbling-block to economic progress in those areas which are extensively affected.[2]

Trachoma is a strictly human disease spread either directly (by intra-familial contact) or indirectly by flies and fomites, especially the communal family face-cloth, or by the fingers from infected genitalia or eyes, to healthy eyes. Bacterial infection is often superimposed on trachoma infection and causes increased discharges which are attractive to flies.

Trachoma is a community health problem which is intimately linked to poor socio-economic and hygiene standards. Its prevalence and severity are related to poor personal and environmental hygiene which enhances the fly menace. Lack of clean piped water in homes and lack of toilet facilities are the factors responsible for high morbidity rates, as well as the dissemination and persistence of the infection.

The outcome of a trachomatous process will depend upon the frequency and severity of re-infections. There are thus two separate patterns of trachoma:

(1) blinding trachoma in hyperendemic areas where there is a scarcity of water and personal hygiene is poor; reinfections are common and severe;

(2) non-blinding trachoma in endemic areas with better personal hygiene and a better supply of uncontaminated water. Reinfections are less common.

Children of pre-school age are very susceptible to trachoma infection; they form the main reservoir of repeated infections of their elders — to cause chronic adult trachoma with blinding sequelae — but infection in childhood generally clears up, even without treatment. The disease usually spreads within the family unit.

There is, however, no lifelong immunity to the disease. Trachoma is liable to relapses and reinfections and to become chronic; this leads to the following sequelae in adulthood: entropion, trichiasis and blinding. Eventually the eye is destroyed altogether, becoming a mass of scar tissue which is beyond the help of surgery. Old ladies appear to get the disease in its chronic form more often than old men, probably because of their greater contact with pre-school children, the main reservoir of infection.

Trachoma is a notifiable disease in South Africa. In 1981, 1 089 cases of trachoma were notified, and in 1989, 572 cases. Ballard[3] et al. state that since trachoma became notifiable in 1925, few cases have actually been notified to the Department of National Health and Population Development. As a result, the disease receives little attention when health priorities for the region are determined. The authors estimate that in northern Lebowa alone 20 000 people are suffering (in 1981) from visual disability due to trachoma and that 150 000 people in the area have active inflammatory trachoma.

Primary prevention

Health promotion by improved environmental and personal hygiene. See p. 708 for community measures taken in the northern Transvaal. Here, trachoma care is part of a comprehensive, community health care programme.

Secondary prevention

(1) Early diagnosis and notification.
(2) Surveillance and case-finding by house-to-house search. This is done in the northern

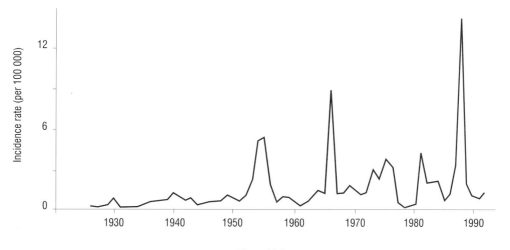

Figure 33.1

Incidence rate of trachoma
Source: *Epidemiological Comments* 1994; **21** (3)

Transvaal by voluntary community health workers (care groups) chosen from the community affected by trachoma. These workers are trained to recognise trachoma in its early stages by a professional health team based at Elim Hospital. Their work, which includes primary care of trachoma in the individual household, is supervised by the professional health team. For financial and other reasons this kind of community care, which reaches each affected household, would be impossible if professional health personnel were used for the purpose.

(3) Treatment of trachoma. Treatment with 1 % tetracycline ophthalmic ointment may be done successfully on an intermittent schedule. The ointment is inserted into both eyes, twice daily, on five consecutive days in one month, for a period of six months. A course may need to be repeated. Hospitals and clinics refer patients to the care groups and they, in turn, send cases that do not respond to treatment to the clinics or hospitals.

The voluntary involvement of the community in the control of trachoma has proved to be very successful, not only in Gazankulu but also in other parts of the world. But mass antibiotic treatment schemes in badly affected endemic areas are successful only where economic development and improvements in the standard of hygiene have risen concomitantly.[1] The erstwhile treatment at school level alone is inadequate, as it reaches only a small proportion of the reservoir of infection.[3]

Tertiary prevention

Rehabilitation and social assistance

(1) Eye operations are done to prevent the blinding sequelae of entropion and trichiasis. These operations can be done only if the visual structures have not yet been destroyed by scarring.

(2) Training of blind people to enable them to earn a living or to run a home is done under the aegis of the SA National Council for the Blind.

(3) Social assistance from the state is available for those who are unable to earn a living because of the blindness, in the form of a government disability grant (Blind Pension).

SEXUALLY TRANSMITTED (VENEREAL) DISEASES (STDs)

The group of sexually transmitted diseases (STDs), formerly called venereal diseases (VD) includes not only the specific venereal diseases, gonorrhoea and syphilis, but also a large number of newer sexually transmitted diseases.

The incidence of sexually transmitted diseases has increased during the past twenty years. Syphilis and gonorrhoea are no longer the only bogymen of promiscuous sexual intercourse; a long list of other diseases, some of them uncontrollable, are sexually transmissible. The sexually transmitted diseases have become a major public health problem.

The extent of the problem

No accurate statistics are available but flashpoints warn of a high prevalence. One such pointer is the fact that the City Health Department clinics of Johannesburg treated 112 000 cases in a year,[4] i.e. 5 % of the white population.

Many patients are treated privately. The WHO estimates that there are 50 million new cases of syphilis and 250 million new cases of gonorrhoea in the world annually.

The epidemiology of the sexually transmitted diseases is largely that of sexual behaviour. In both Western and Third-World countries, the incidence of STDs is increasing, even in countries with adequate treatment facilities. Venereal diseases differ from other communicable diseases in that they are spread by direct contact between two human beings while they are engaged in an intimate social relationship. High incidence is not dependent upon environmental factors which yield to public health measures, but on promiscuous sexual intercourse — a social practice which has its roots in the social structure and the value system of the society. With the imminent population explosion facing the younger generation, the past attitude to sex as essentially a procreative function is changing to the concept of sex as mainly a recreational activity.

The rapid decline in the incidence of the venereal diseases which followed the introduction of curative antibiotics in the early 1950s has been offset by an equally rapid rise in incidence in the 1960s due to the modern trends towards sexual permissiveness and promiscuity in adolescents and young adults. The restraints of close family ties and of religion on extramarital sexual intercourse are gradually disappearing; in addition, the efficacy of modern contraceptives has removed the fear of pregnancy which used to have a restraining influence on premarital sex. Extramarital sex in itself does not cause sexually transmitted disease, but the risk of getting the disease is greater if there is exposure to many sexual partners whose sexual habits and state of health are unknown.

Prostitutes have always played a role in the spread of sexually transmitted disease; they form the main reservoirs of infection. Social factors which encourage prostitution will raise the incidence of sexually transmitted disease, the main prostitute-encouraging factors being abnormal movements of people, which cause a break-up of normal family living. In wars, large numbers of men are separated from their wives and girl friends, therefore, promiscuity and sexually transmitted diseases increase during these times of crisis. Any system of migrant labour which separates spouses will also cause an increase in the incidence of sexually transmitted diseases.

At coastal towns prostitution is always rife because of the periodic influx of sailors. In industrial cities migratory labour causes a tremendous demand for prostitutes. On his return home, a promiscuous husband may infect his wife; all persons with venereal disease are, therefore, not necessarily promiscuous.

Promiscuity may be due to other causes, viz. the consumption of alcohol and addictive drugs may lead to casual sexual relationships. Personality disorders (e.g. the Don Juans and the nymphomaniacs) may give rise to compulsive promiscuity. Male homosexuals are coming to the fore as sexual spreaders of disease, viz. AIDS and shigellosis, hepatitis B and protozoal infections of the large intestine.

Fehler et al.[5] investigated the sexually transmitted diseases amongst two groups of black urban women, one group attending an STD clinic and the other group a family planning clinic in Johannesburg. With the exception of gonorrhoea, which was higher in the STD group, there were no significant differences in the prevalence of other sexually related infections, the prevalence being high. The STDs common to both groups included the human papillomavirus (HPV) (see p. 804). The women in the family planning group were asymptomatic at the time, therefore they were not seeking treatment for STDs. Markowitz et al.[6] ascribe the enormous burden of sexually transmitted pathogens within this community 'to the specific socio-economic and behavioural factors resulting from disruption of normal family units, migratory labour, and lack of recreational facilities'.

In sum, the important factors responsible for the increase in sexually transmitted diseases, despite modern antimicrobial treatment, are:

(1) The emergence of strains of gonococci which are resistant to antibiotics.

(2) Mobility of people in transitional societies leading to social disorganisation and the break-up of stable family life. The loneliness that results from this leads to prostitution.

(3) In South Africa the venereal health of prostitutes is not controlled.

(4) The modern permissive trend towards extra- and premarital sexual relationships and promiscuity, and the increasing use of sex as a recreational activity.

(5) The efficiency of modern contraceptive techniques to prevent unwanted pregnancies which has encouraged the permissive attitude of the youth to premarital intercourse.

(6) The lesser known STDs are often undiagnosed and therefore inadequately treated.

Persons who are at risk of contracting and spreading STDs are:

(1) prostitutes and their clients;

(2) sexually promiscuous persons, i.e. those who have had multiple sexual partners during the recent past and who are not selective about their partners;

AETIOLOGICAL CLASSIFICATION
OF THE SEXUALLY TRANSMITTED DISEASES

ORGANISMS	*DISEASES*
The older sexually transmitted diseases	
BACTERIA	
Treponema pallidum	Syphilis
Neisseria gonorrhoeae	Gonorrhoea
Haemophilus ducreyi	Chancroid
Chlamydia trachomatis (LGV strains)	Lymphogranuloma venereum (LGV)
Calymmatobacterium granulomatis	Granuloma inguinale (donovanosis)
PROTOZOA	
Trichomonas vaginalis	Trichomoniasis
ECTOPARASITES	
Phthirus pubis	Pediculosis
Sarcoptes scabiei	Scabies
The newer sexually transmitted diseases	
BACTERIA	
Gardnerella vaginalis	Bacterial vaginosis
Chlamydia trachomatis (genital strains)	Non-gonococcal urethritis
	Epididymitis
	Cervicitis
	Salpingitis
	Neonatal disease
	Chlamydial Ophthalmia
VIRUSES	
Herpes simplex virus	Genital herpes
Human papillomavirus	Genital warts
Cytomegalovirus	Neonatal disease
Hepatitis A + B virus	Hepatitis
Human immunodeficiency syndrome	AIDS
FUNGI	
Candida albicans	Candida infections (thrush)
MYCOPLASMAS	
Ureaplasma urealyticum	Non-gonococcal urethritis

(3) persons with a previous history of an STD;

(4) drug addicts who use sex for acquiring drugs;

(5) inmates of prisons (homosexual spread).

The general principles of management of STDs:

(1) Accurate diagnosis by:
   (a) taking a full sexual history, including preferred site of sexual contact with male or female;
   (b) making a full physical examination, with special attention to genital organs;
   (c) doing the necessary microbiological and serological investigations.

(2) The diagnosis of an STD reflects unprotected and unselective sexual activity and the possibility of being infected with other STDs, e.g. HIV. Screening for other STDs is, therefore, justified.

(3) Prescribing effective antimicrobial treatment.

(4) The tracing and following up of sexual contacts. Sexual partners must be treated.

(5) Health education of persons at risk, on modes of transmission and their reduction to prevent reinfection. The use of the condom plays the most important role in preventing the spread of STDs, either in the case of the man using the condom or in the case of his partner (male or female).

STDs pose a socio-medical problem which requires for its continued existence sexual contact between two people, one of whom is infected. The sexual contact involves genital organs, including the ano-rectal and oropharyngeal openings into the body. Non-sexual spread, e.g. by toilet seats, is so uncommon that it can be disregarded in the aetiology of most venereal disease. Notable exceptions are syphilis and AIDS, systemic infections which can be introduced into the body by the prick of an infected needle and by blood-transfusions, as well as congenitally.

The aetiological classification of the sexually transmitted diseases is shown on page 582.

Promiscuity and prostitution give rise to a multiplicity of venereal diseases in one person.

STDs commonly present with the following signs and symptoms:

- urethral discharge, especially in men;
- genital ulceration;
- vaginal discharge with or without vulval irritation.

STDs also affect other systems of the body and may present either as an acute or chronic infection.

The main and specifically sexually transmitted diseases are gonorrhoea and syphilis. Both are contact communicable diseases.

The interaction of HIV infection with conventional sexually transmitted diseases

The rates of HIV infection are highest amongst the clientele of STD clinics who generally indulge in indiscriminate, unprotected sexual activity. The STDs actually increase the rate of heterosexual transmission of HIV, especially where there is genital ulceration, e.g. chancroid, or chlamydial inflammation of the genital tract.

HIV infection may lead to treatment failure among patients with early syphilis who are treated with single-dose, long-acting benzathine penicillin.

PRIMARY PREVENTION OF GONORRHOEA AND SYPHILIS

Although essentially curable, the sexually transmitted diseases are very difficult to prevent. There is no vaccine to guard those at risk, there is no immunity against gonorrhoea and the cured patient may reacquire the disease immediately after he has been cured. In syphilis, the cured person is immune for a little while only.

As it is not an easy task to change the social structure of a society in order to get rid of a specific problem, the most practical way to reduce the incidence of venereal disease is by health education. In order to do effective health education, the educator must make a diagnosis of the sexual attitudes of the community in which he works, as well as of the social pathology which encourages sexual promiscuity.

The objectives of health education with regard to the prevention of sexually transmitted diseases may be one or more of the following:

(1) To persuade young people to practise abstinence from, or reduction of, premarital sexual intercourse.

(2) To persuade males to use condoms in order to prevent direct contact with infectious discharges during sexual intercourse, if there is any doubt about their own or their partner's freedom from venereal infection.

Condoms can be used for the prevention of pregnancy and for the prevention of the transmission of STDs. They reduce the risk of infection. This statement applies to condoms only and this fact must be stressed by the educator, as there is widespread belief that the 'pill' and the 'injection' prevent the spread of STDs (with tragic consequences in the case of AIDS).

Any STD service should provide undamaged, reliable, latex (rubber) condoms and instruct their clients in their proper care and use, as little can be done to promote their preventive functions if they break *in situ* after ejaculation has occurred.

Therefore:

(*a*) No potentially damaged or weakened (old, previously used, pricked, or torn, or deteriorated (from exposure to mineral-based lubricants, heat or sunlight)) condom should be used.

(*b*) The putting on and removal of condoms should be done on an erect penis.

The condom is put on before any genital contact occurs between the penis and the participating partner, to prevent exposure to infectious fluids. The tip of the condom is held while the latter is rolled on to the shaft of the penis, leaving enough space to collect the semen in the tip. A water-based lubricant, which preserves the latex, is used.

After ejaculation, the penis is withdrawn while holding on to the base of the condom to prevent it slipping off and spilling its contents.

(3) Counselling and education with regard to the aetiology and effects of sexually transmitted diseases. Education includes information about methods of spread, characteristics and dangers of sexually transmitted diseases, the dangers of sexual promiscuity, and the importance of reporting for early treatment, not only for a quick cure but also to avoid infecting others. The only effective way to encourage those infected to present themselves for early treatment and to divulge the names of their contacts, is to remove the stigma attached to sexually transmitted disease. This requires a broadminded attitude to sex from the educators. Antiquated ideas that a sexually transmitted disease is a punishment for sexual sin have no place in health education, which seeks to get the co-operation of people to participate in the prevention of the spread of the disease. Counselling is successful if it helps people to change their sexual style by adopting safer sex practices.

The purpose of primary prevention is to motivate the risk-taker or potential risk-taker to take reasonable precautions to avoid contracting sexually transmitted diseases or to infect others. This education should be started early in adolescence, i.e. in the schools; it should be part of organised sex education which includes not only basic sex education but also family planning and the importance of emotional involvement of the sexual partners in their relationship.

For the primary prevention of congenital syphilis adequate treatment and monitoring of the infected pregnant woman are necessary.

SECONDARY PREVENTION OF GONORRHOEA AND SYPHILIS

(1) In the absence of vaccines, early diagnosis and appropriate treatment are the most important preventive measures.

A person may have both syphilis and gonorrhoea at the same time; both are cured by penicillin, but the curative dose for gonorrhoea is too small to cure syphilis. These smaller doses of penicillin render the syphilitic patient non-infectious; one injection of high-dosage benzathine penicillin is required to cure syphilis of less than two years duration.

In treating gonorrhoea, it is very important to test for resistance of the *N. gonorrhoea* to penicillin. Penicillin therapy is totally inadequate for PPNG strains of the gonococcus which may, however, respond to tetracycline, spectinomycin, rosoxacin, ceftriaxone according to sensitivity tests. (see p. 508).

(2) Sexually transmitted disease is perpetuated by infected persons who do not receive treatment. It is important for health personnel to get the names of contacts from persons who present themselves for treatment, so that these contacts may be traced and persuaded to come for treatment.

It is especially important to trace the sexual partners of infected pregnant women in order to prevent reinfection. Contacts should be diagnosed. Undiagnosed contacts exposed to infectious syphilis within the preceding three months should be treated as for early syphilis.

An attitude of concern about individual responsibility for the dissemination of sexually transmitted diseases is encouraged in patients.

(3) Women can be screened for gonorrhoea and syphilis at antenatal clinics, family planning clinics and gynaecological clinics, by taking swabs from the urethra, endocervix and rectum (for the diagnosis of gonorrhoea) and by taking blood for the diagnosis of syphilis.

(4) It is very important for every community to recognise and acknowledge the existence of prostitutes and to require them to be examined and treated for sexually transmitted disease. Repressive legislation drives prostitutes underground and beyond the control of health authorities.

(5) Specific machinery for combating sexually transmitted disease in South Africa was set up by the Public Health Act of 1919. This Act provided for the establishment of special clinics and free treatment centres; for the supply of specific drugs by the government to all free patients; for the establishment of free diagnostic facilities for all, and for the subsidising of publicity and social hygiene societies. The Act specified that the conveyance of infection is an offence. Although syphilis and gonorrhoea are not notifiable diseases, the provision of the Act made it compulsory for every person suffering from a sexually transmitted disease to undergo treatment, if the disease is in a communicable form, at least until he/she is rendered non-infectious.

GONORRHOEA

Gonorrhoea is one of the most common infectious diseases in the world, probably because its incidence is not stemmed by immunity and it cannot be prevented by a prophylactic vaccine. It is symptomless in 10 % of men and 60 % of women. These cases are diagnosed by contact tracing from patients.

It is caused by the *Neisseria gonorrhoeae*, a Gram-negative diplococcus which infects mucosal surfaces lined by columnar epithelium. Smears from the urethra, cervix, rectum and eyes are sent for culture to identify the organism.

Gonorrhoea usually causes localised inflammatory reactions, but infections may become disseminated.

The following diseases are caused by the *N. gonorrhoeae*:

Women

- Bartholin's abscess
- Urethritis
- Cervicitis
- Proctitis
- Salpingitis (pelvic inflammatory disease)

Men

- Urethritis
- Proctitis
- Epididymo-orchitis

Both sexes

- Conjunctivitis (ophthalmia)
- Pharyngitis
- Disseminated gonococcaemia with pyrexia and acute arthritis

Infants and young children

- Conjunctivitis
- Pharyngitis
- Proctitis
- Vulvovaginitis

Gonorrhoeal infection is characterised by a purulent discharge approximately three days after exposure to infection. In the woman infection can become chronic and cause ophthalmia neonatorum, an infection of the eyes of the newborn (acquired during the birth process) which may lead to blindness. The inflammatory sequelae of gonorrhoea are an important cause of infertility in both sexes.

During the past thirty years gonorrhoea has been on the increase everywhere in the world, except in those countries where no profound changes in social behaviour have occurred. The risk chances of a man becoming infected if his partner has gonorrhoea is 20 %.

Women are much more readily infected (75 % to 90 %). Both men and women are often not aware that they are infected and therefore do not go for treatment. These asymptomatic carriers with infective gonorrhoea are a great infection hazard to others and act as a reservoir of the gonococcus. They do develop some of the complications of the disease in due time, however, such as arthritis and salpingitis. The pattern of gonorrhoea'has changed recently with increasing involvement of the younger age groups, i.e. from 15 to 19 years, in line with the changed sexual behaviour patterns of this age group.

Disseminated gonorrhoea (gonococcaemia)

The *N. gonorrhoeae* may circulate in the blood (gonococcaemia) and affect joints (arthritis). It is a benign condition. In rare cases gonococcaemia causes the dangerous complications, endocarditis and meningitis. Gonococcal arthritis can be difficult to diagnose as there are usually no venereal signs. The patient gives a history of recent exposure to infection and *N. gonorrhoeae* can be cultured from a mucosal lesion. Temperature, white cell count and ESR are elevated. The arthritis is acute, asymmetrical and may be migratory and purulent. It responds promptly to antibiotic treatment for 10–14 days.

Neonatal conjunctivitis

Gonococcal ophthalmia neonatorum appears within 48 hours of birth with swelling of the eyelids and a profuse purulent discharge. It can be prevented by the instillation of silver nitrate eye drops or 0,5 % erythromycin or 1 % tetracycline eye ointment immediately after birth. If left untreated, corneal ulceration or panophthalmitis may cause serious loss of vision.

Neonatal conjunctivitis caused by the *Chlam. trachomatis* is characterised after 5 to 24 days by papillary hypertrophy of the tarsal conjunctiva and a slight watery discharge. Later the discharge becomes purulent and the eyelids swollen. Normally the ophthalmia is self-limiting. It cannot be prevented by the instillation of silver nitrate drops.

Acute urethritis (GU and NGU)

Acute urethritis is the commonest manifestation of sexually transmitted diseases in men.[12] It is uncommon in females. In males there are two forms of urethritis: gonococcal and non-gonococcal (NGU). Gonococcal urethritis (GU) is common amongst male homosexuals and is more prevalent amongst the lower socio-economic groups. Acute GU presents with a purulent urethral discharge with painful and frequent micturition within a few days after exposure to infection.

NGU is caused mainly by *Chlamydia trachomatis* and *U. urealyticum*. The incubation period of NGU is usually 1–3 weeks. The signs and symptoms are milder than in GU, the discharge being mucoid or mucopurulent. The 'first-catch' urine usually shows threads of pus.

Although pure GU and pure NGU infections can be distinguished, urethritis is often caused by mixed infections. In this case chemotherapy aimed solely at eliminating the gonococcus does not kill *Chlam. trachomatis* and *U. urealyticum* but leaves the patient with a post-gonococcal urethritis (PGU).

Urethritis will not clear up if the man's sexual partner is not treated simultaneously. Most women infected with *Gonococcus* or *Chlamydia* have no symptoms. Infected men and their partners should abstain from sexual intercourse during therapy, or use a condom.

Both gonococcal and *C. trachomatis* urethritis may affect other organs causing acute epididymitis and prostatitis in males, salpingitis associated with acute pelvic inflammatory disease (PID) in females and conjunctivitis in male and female adults and neonates.

Epididymitis (epididymo-orchitis)

Infection of the epididymis (and testis) may occur as a complication of urethral infection with *N. gonorrhoeae* and/or *Chlamydia trachomatis*. (It may also be caused by other organisms, including *M. tuberculosis*.)

The patient needs symptomatic treatment of pain, as well as scrotal elevation to provide maximal lymphatic and venous drainage.[14] Sexual partners must also be treated.

Gonococcal proctitis

Is usually asymptomatic in both sexes exposed to anal intercourse. There may, however, be rectal discharge and burning pain in the rectum and peri-anal irritation.

Gonococcal pharyngitis

Caused by oral intercourse, is usually asymptomatic in both sexes but the patient may complain of sore throat and a slight muco-purulent exudation.

Acute pelvic inflammatory disease (Acute PID)

This is an inflammation of the female genital organs above the level of the internal os.[17] PID is used synonymously with salpingitis. In South Africa it is probably the commonest gynaecological condition in black women.

Primary acute PID is usually a venereal condition (infection from cervix to tubes), but infection may also be introduced by abortion, delivery or surgery. Only 20 % of women with gonorrhoea develop acute PID, the risk being increased by IUCDs. PID coincides with menstruation.

Infective agents in acute PID:

(1) Non-gonococcal
Chlam. trachomatis, H. influenzae, and others.
(2) Gonococcal.

Diagnosis is made on:

(1) Organisms cultured from swabs taken from endocervix and urethra. Intra-abdominal swabs are obtained by laparoscopy.

(2) Main clinical features: bilateral lower abdominal pain; profuse vaginal discharge; dysuria; pyrexia; pelvic peritonitis and pelvic masses. Most infected women are asymptomatic, however, and do not need hospitalisation.

Sequelae: tubal occlusion and infertility.

Treatment is on an in- or out-patient basis, depending on the severity of the condition. IUCDs are removed. Sexual partners should also be treated. As out-patient chemotherapy is usually continued for 10 days, compliance is a major problem.

As the causative organism is not always known, antimicrobial treatment should cover all aetiological agents.

TREATMENT OF GONOCOCCAL AND CHLAMYDIAL INFECTIONS

The current treatment guidelines provide for combination therapy for concomitant chlamydial infection which may be masked by the gonococcal infection. Likewise, treatment of acute epididymo-orchitis and pelvic-inflammatory disease also allows for possible multiple aetiological agents. Below follows a shortened version of Prof. RC Ballard's treatment schedule for gonorrhoea.[25]

Uncomplicated, urethral, endocervical and rectal infections in adults

Patients with gonococcal infections should be treated with antibiotic regimens effective against both *N. gonorrhoeae* and *C. trachomatis.* Such treatment may also lessen the possibility of emergence of antibiotic-resistant strains of *N. gonorrhoeae.*

- Ceftriaxone, 250 mg, intramuscularly as a single dose, or
- Ciprofloxacin, 500 mg. as a single oral dose.

Treatment of gonococcal infections in pregnancy

- Ceftriaxone, 250 mg, intramuscularly as a single dose, or
- Spectinomycin, 2 g, intramuscularly as a single dose, plus
  Erythromycin base or stearate, 500 mg, four times daily for ten days by mouth.

Treatment of disseminated gonococcal infection (DGI)

All patients with DGI should, ideally, be hospitalised and examined for clinical evidence of endocarditis or meningitis.

Treatments for DGI are (for one week):

- Ceftriaxone, 1 g, intramuscularly or intravenously, once daily, or
- Spectinomycin, 2 g, intramuscularly twice daily.

Patients with uncomplicated DGI can be discharged from hospital 24–48 hours following resolution of symptoms. As an alternative, oral therapy with either Amoxycillin 500 mg with clavulanic acid (Augmentin) three times daily or, if not pregnant, Ciprofloxacin 500 mg, twice daily may be given.

Patients with gonococcal meningitis or endocarditis require prolonged intravenous therapy. Ceftriaxone 1–2 g intravenously twice daily for 10–14 days has been recommended for the treatment of gonococcal meningitis. In cases of endocarditis, treatment should be continued for at least four weeks.

Patients with recurrent DGI should be evaluated for complement deficiencies.

Treatment of gonococcal ophthalmia

Adults with uncomplicated gonococcal ophthalmia should be treated with: Ceftriaxone, 250 mg, intramuscularly as a single dose, and neonates likewise with 50 mg/kg.

The eyes should be irrigated frequently with sterile saline to prevent build-up of purulent discharge. Topical antibiotics alone are not considered sufficient therapy and should be avoided. Patients failing to respond fully may have concomitant infection with *C. trachomatis*. Both parents of neonates with ophthalmia must be treated appropriately.

Treatment of acute epididymo-orchitis

- Ceftriaxone, 250 mg intramuscularly as a single dose, plus any 10-day course of tetracycline

Treatment of acute pelvic inflammatory disease (PID)

The treatment regimens suggested have been designed to provide cover for the entire spectrum of possible aetiological agents. This is necessary because it is rarely possible to obtain tubal specimens for culture and anti-microbial susceptibility testing.

Out-patient therapy for PID

- Ceftriaxone, 250 mg, intramuscularly as a single dose, plus Doxycycline or minocycline, twice daily for 10 days by mouth, plus Metronidazole, 400 mg, twice daily for 10 days by mouth.

Hospitalised patients with PID

Two regimens are recommended by the Centers for Disease Control, Atlanta, Georgia. These regimens have been designed to provide empirical therapy, recognising the multi-aetiological nature of the disease.

Regimen A:

- Cefoxitin, 2 g intravenously four times daily, plus
- Doxycycline, 100 mg intravenously twice daily

The above regimen is given for at least 48 hours after the patient clinically improves. After discharge from hospital, the patient continues oral therapy with:

- Doxycycline or minocycline, 100 mg twice daily for 10 days, plus
- Metronidazole, 400 mg twice daily for 10 days.

Regimen B:

- Clindamycin, 900 mg intravenously three times daily, plus
- Gentamicin, loading dose of 2 mg/kg followed by 1,5 mg/kg intravenously, three times daily.

The above regimen is given for at least 48 hours after the patient clinically improves. After discharge from hospital, the patient continues oral therapy with:

- Doxycucline or minocycline, 100 mg twice daily for 10 days, plus
- Metronidazole, 400 mg twice daily for 10 days.

The most common reason for apparent relapse is reinfection, therefore it is important to treat all sexual contacts to cover reinfection with *N. gonorrhoeae*, *C. trachomatis* and *M. hominis*.

SYPHILIS

Syphilis, a chronic sexually transmitted infection which is caused by a spirochaete Treponema pallidum, is a more generalised systemic disease than gonorrhoea; it may be contracted by extra-genital contact, e.g. infected needles or kissing, although the common method of spread is by sexual congress, the spirochaete entering the body through a scratch or abrasion in the skin or mucous membrane. The spirochaetal antigen elicits two kinds of antibodies, non-specific (reagin) and specific IgG and IgM.

The disease may be acquired any time after birth, or it may be congenital, the spirochaetes of a syphilitic mother penetrating the placental barrier to infect the foetus.

Incubation period: from 10 days to 10 weeks, with a mean of 3 weeks.

The course of the disease can be divided into three stages, in both the congenital and acquired forms of the disease: primary, secondary and tertiary. The lesion of the *primary stage* is the chancre — a small, painless, highly infectious swelling — which develops at the site of infection, viz. genital or non-genital skin or mucous membrane, after a variable incubation period and, if left untreated, will resolve spontaneously in 3–8 weeks, usually without leaving a scar. The chancre is associated with enlarged, bilateral lymph nodes.

If it occurs on the cervix, the woman may be unaware of the infection. Anal and rectal lesions occur in male homosexuals.

In the *secondary stage*, 6–8 weeks later, there is a generalised infection of the body with signs of low-grade toxaemia, patchy alopecia, rashes, enlarged glands (generalised lymphadenopathy) and infectious snail-track buccal ulcers and *condylomata lata* (warty growths) on the perineum.

The spirochaete is also present in the blood, and the serological tests are positive. This stage gradually disappears and the disease then becomes hidden (latent) for a variable number of years, during which time the victim is unaware that there is anything wrong with him.

The *tertiary stage* is characterised by the formation of painless, destructive swellings — gumma(ta) — in any part of the body. The most common site is the central nervous system, neurosyphilis being manifested in several forms of which GPI (general paralysis of the insane or *dementia paralytica*) and *tabes dorsalis* are well known. The outstanding features of neurosyphilis are mental deterioration, Argyll Robertson pupils and abnormalities of the cerebrospinal fluid. The serological tests may be positive in the blood or CSF or both, but this is not always the case. The patient may also develop cardio-vascular complications.

The manifestations of the *tertiary stage* are seldom seen today due to the curability of the disease and therefore syphilis no longer inspires the terror it did formerly.

Diagnosis[8, 9]

The diagnosis of syphilis depends on contact tracing, clinical diagnosis of typical lesions and serological testing.

1. Serological tests

Serological (serodiagnostic) tests for syphilis (STS) are of two main kinds:

(1) Tests to detect non-specific antibodies (reagin) to non-treponemal lipoidal antigens.
The erstwhile complement fixation tests (e.g. Wassermann) and the *Treponema pallidum* immobilisation (TPI) test are no longer used. The modern flocculation (agglutination) tests (e.g. the VDRL) and RPR (rapid plasma reagin) agglutination (flocculation) tests are much simpler, quicker and cheaper. The VDRL (Venereal Disease Research Laboratory) is generally preferred. These tests reflect disease activity and are the most widely used screening tests for syphilis. They may be negative in latent and tertiary syphilis. Adequate treatment will also reduce or eliminate their reactivity. The screening of pregnant women, blood donors and 'at-risk' groups helps to control syphilis in a community.

Results can be quantitatively expressed in dilutions (titres), the higher the dilution, the greater the antibody activity. A rising titre of at least fourfold or greater (VDRL and RPR serial tests) suggests active syphilis.

Note:

(i) A biologically false positive reaction (BFP) is indicated by a VDRL titre from 1:8 to 1:16 (positive reaction) and a negative FTA–ABS test (see below).

(ii) No patient should be diagnosed as having syphilis on the basis of a single test. A VDRL test with 1:8 titre should be repeated 10 days later and confirmed with a FTA–ABS test.

Used serially these tests can also be used to measure response to treatment, especially in the primary and secondary stages. The non-treponemal tests may be negative in the early stages of primary syphilis when the FTA–ABS test is positive.

(2) Tests to detect antitreponemal antibodies (IgG and IgM), i.e. specific antibodies against *T. pallidum* antigens. Two tests are used: TPHA (*T. pallidum* haemagglutination assay) and FTA–ABS (fluorescent treponemal antibody absorption).

The TPHA test is commonly used for screening; it is particularly sensitive to detect late treponemal disease. The FTA–ABS (IgM) test is used for the diagnosis of sera which give a discrepant result with the VDRL and TPHA tests. The diagnosis of syphilis is made if the FTA–ABS test is positive.

2. Tests for neurosyphilis

(1) CSF examination: the cell count and total proteins indicate non-specific inflammation in the CNS.

(2) If there is a positive serological IgM-specific-FTA–ABS test, the CSF FTA–ABS will be positive in the presence of neurosyphilis.[9] Likewise, the VDRL test will be positive.

3. Darkfield microscopy of the treponema[7]

In the infectious stages of syphilis, serous exudates are expressed from suspected primary and secondary lesions and the wet preparation is examined microscopically under darkfield illumination.

Screening for syphilis in pregnancy and in the neonate

Naicker *et al.*[9] recommend:

(1) Screening test with TPHA on admission; to be followed by a FTA–ABS confirmatory test.

(2) Repeat TPHA after the 36th week of pregnancy, to detect late infections.

(3) Serological FTA–ABS testing of neonates of syphilitic mothers; if this test is positive (a reliable indicator of congenital syphilis), the CSF should be examined to confirm or exclude neurosyphilis.

(4) All unbooked mothers and their infants should be subjected to (2) and (3).

(5) The FTA–ABS should be used to detect syphilis in patients with unexplained still-births, neonatal deaths and abortion.

Congenital syphilis

Congenital syphilis was only recently added to the list of notifiable diseases. It includes cases (confirmed and presumptive) of congenitally acquired syphilis in infants and children, as well as syphilitic still-births.

A **syphilitic still-birth** is defined as a foetal death in which the mother had untreated or inadequately treated syphilis at delivery, the latter including penicillin given less than 30 days prior to delivery.

A **confirmed** case of congenital syphilis is an infant in whom *Treponema pallidum* is identified by darkfield microscopy or fluorescent antibody, in specimens from lesions, umbilical cord or autopsy material.

A **presumptive** case of congenital syphilis is either of the following:

(a) any infant whose mother had untreated or inadequately treated syphilis at delivery; or

(b) any infant or child who had a reactive treponemal test for syphilis and any **one** of the following:

(i) X-ray evidence on long bones in infants.

(ii) Any physical evidence of congenital syphilis.

Signs in the infant: hepatosplenomegaly, characteristic skin rash (vesicobullous), condylomata lata, snuffles (rhinitis), jaundice or oedema (nephrotic syndrome).

Stigmata in older children: interstitial keratitis with blindness, nerve deafness, saddle-nose, notched upper front permanent teeth, sabre-shaped tibiae and other osseous manifestations, e.g. enlarged epiphyses of bones, thickening of frontal cranial bones, bald patches in hair, mental retardation and neuro-syphilis.

(iii) Abnormal blood and/or CSF tests.

In a study carried out in 1978 by Ross *et al.* [10] at King Edward VIII Hospital in Durban, the perinatal mortality due to syphilis was 3,2/1 000 births, of which 72 % were stillborn and 28 % died soon after birth. Those born alive were apparently healthy and only started developing the stigmata after 2–8 weeks (osseous lesions).

Naicker *et al.*[9] in their King Edward VIII Hospital study of 500 antenatal patients found that the prevalence of active syphilis was 7,4 %, i.e. 1:13 of the women presenting at their ante-natal clinic.

The serodiagnosis of congenital syphilis is based on a rising titre of reagin antibody (VDRL) and the presence of antitreponemal IgM antibodies (FTA–ABS).[8]

Note: In 1993, 989 infants with congenital syphilis were notified, 19 died.

Naicker treatment regimes of pregnant women and neonates[9]

Treatment of pregnant women: 2 doses of ben-zathine penicillin 2 400 000 IU given 7 days apart. After treatment, VDRL tests should be done at monthly intervals until delivery to moni-tor reinfection or relapse. If mothers are ade-quately treated and do not have a reinfection, the infant should not have syphilis.

Treatment of neonates with proven infection of blood and CSF: penicillin G (which crosses the blood-brain barrier) 100 000 U/kg/d for 10 days. If only the serological FTA–ABS test is positive, or if the FTA–ABS test is not available to the infant of a syphilitic mother, then a single dose of benzathine penicillin 50 000 U/kg is given. All infants of sero-positive mothers who were adequately treated, should be serologically examined at birth and at monthly intervals for 3 months.

Note: Penicillin reactions should be prevented. If this is not possible, materials for treating anaphylactic shock should be readily available. See p. 512 for penicillin desensitisation technique.

TABLE 1
WHO treatment schedules[7]
Penicillin-based treatment schedules for venereal syphilis

	Benzathine penicillin G		Aqueous procaine penicillin G	
	Total dose million units	Total number of injections (one a week)	Total dose (million units)	Total number of injections (one a week)
Early syphilis (primary, secondary, early latent, i.e. of *not more than* 2 years' duration)	2,4	1	6,0	10
Late latent syphilis and late benign syphilis	7,2	3	9,0	15
Cardio-vascular syphilis and neurosyphilis	—	—	12,0	20

TABLE 2
Treatment schedules for patients with venereal syphilis who are allergic to penicillin
(See also Penicillin oral desensitisation procedure for pregnant women, p. 510)

	Tetracycline hydrochloride (500 mg by mouth, 4 × daily)		Erythromycin* (500 mg by mouth, 4 × daily)	
	Total dose	Days	Total dose	Days
Syphilis of not more than 2 years' duration	30 g	15	30 g	15
Syphilis of more than 2 years' duration	60 g	30	60 g	30
*Not the estolate.				

The WHO 1982 dosage should be doubled according to Philcox *et al.*, i.e. the total aqueous procaine penicillin G dosage for neurosyphilis should be 24,0 million units[11] (20 doses), i.e. one daily intramuscular injection of 1,2 million units.

Pregnant women are treated as in table 1 or 2, except that they are not given tetracycline or the erythromycin estolate because of potential toxic effects on mother and/or child.

Follow-up of patients treated for syphilis:[7]

(1) Patients with early syphilis are followed up after therapy, at 3 (and then 6–12) months for clinical and serological evaluation (if treated with penicillin), and more frequently if tetracycline and erythromycin were used.

(2) Patients with cardio-vascular and neuro-syphilis should be followed up for many years, if this is possible, as patients are easily lost to follow-up.

(3) Retreatment is necessary if:
   (*a*) active syphilis persists or recurs;
   (*b*) there is a 4-fold rise in the VDRL titre;
   (*c*) an initial high-titre VDRL persists for a year.

(4) Unless reinfection has occurred, CSF should be examined before retreatment.

(5) Retreatment schedules are the same as those recommended for syphilis of more than 2 years' duration; only one retreatment course is indicated.

CHLAMYDIAL INFECTIONS-LYMPHOGRANULOMA VENEREUM (LGV) ('CATSCRATCH' DISEASE)

Chlamydia trachomatis (oculogenital strain) is a common cause of non-gonococcal urethritis in the male. In the female consort of the infected male, it is an important cause of cervicitis, salpingitis and pelvic inflammatory disease (PID), leading to infertility. Chlamydia can also cause trachoma, upper respiratory infection (secretary otitis media, pharyngitis), neonatal inclusion conjunctivitis and pneumonia. In the male it may cause sterility (due to prostatitis or epididymitis) and, in male homosexuals, proctitis. Genital chlamydial infections (e.g. NGU and LGV) are a large and increasingly important problem in developed countries, as well as in developing countries.

Lymphogranuloma venereum, uncommon in the RSA, is caused by special serotypes of the chlamydia which are more invasive. It is painful lymphadenopathy of regional lymph nodes draining the genitalia and affects mostly males, females being asymptomatic carriers.

The onset of lymphadenitis may be accompanied by pyrexia, malaise and headache.

The primary lesion is a small non-painful transient ulcer on the penis in men and on the vulva or lower vagina in women. The ulcer may go unnoticed. In untreated cases the lymph nodes (inguinal and femoral) become matted and adherent to the surrounding tissues; they eventually suppurate. The rectal wall may become involved (ulcerative proctitis) with many localised sequelae.

Incubation period: 1–6 weeks, usually 3 weeks.

LGV presents a diagnostic problem; a positive chlamydia complement fixation test confirms clinical suspicions, i.e. painful inguinal adenopathy in the near absence of genital ulceration. Syphilis must always be excluded by appropriate laboratory tests (e.g. VDRL and FTA–ABS).[15]

Treatment: see p. 587— the treatment of gonorrhoea. The dose of tetracycline or erythromycin is doubled for LGV.[19] Suppurating lymph nodes may need drainage.

CHANCROID (SIGNIFICANT GENITAL ULCERATION)

The infecting organism is the Haemophilus ducreyi. It causes genital ulceration. It is a disease of developing countries with low hygiene standards, but it may occur sporadically and in epidemic form in westernised countries, predominantly among young uncircumcised, sexually active males. Prostitutes are thought to be the carriers.

Clinical presentation

After an incubation period of 3–5 days, a painful ulcer (2 mm–2 cm in diameter), develops:
- *In males:* on internal surface of prepuce, frenulum.
- *In females:* on labia, fourchette, perianal area.

The ratio of occurrence in males 20 : females 1.

Ulcers may become multiple and are painful; inguinal adenopathy may develop. This may lead to a suppurative bubo which may ulcerate.

Prevention

Prompt treatment of cases and their contacts and improved genital hygiene.

Early treatment

Erythromycin 500 mg given three times daily for 5 days is the treatment regimen in use since 1986.[16]

GRANULOMA INGUINALE[18] (DONOVANOSIS)

The causative organism of donovanosis is the Calymmatobacterium granulomatis. It causes a chronic infection of the genitalia of males and females, characterised by genital and inguinal ulcers which become destructive and mutilating if the disease is not treated. It is distributed over parts of southern USA, India, tropical and subtropical Africa. Only sporadic cases have presented in the RSA. It is associated with the lower socio-economic strata and poor personal hygiene. The exact method of transmission is still in doubt.

▨ *Incubation period:* 8–80 days.
▨ *Diagnosis:* microscopic examination of smears of deep scrapings of the floor of the ulcer. Biopsy of ulcer and histological examination.
▨ *Treatment:* antibiotics other than penicillin, e.g. tetracycline, chloramphenicol, until the lesions have healed.

THE ROLE OF VIRUSES IN STDs

A. Hepatitis A and B viruses

Both these viruses are sexually transmissible. Amongst male homosexuals in Western countries, hepatitis B is a leading sexually transmitted disease, but sexual transmission of hepatitis A is also possible.

Hepatitis B is also spread by heterosexual contact, spread occurring more frequently from male to female, but also occurring from female to male. There is a high incidence of Hepatitis B amongst the sexually promiscuous patients with other sexually transmitted diseases and male homosexuals. As the virus may be found in saliva, semen and all body fluids, spread can occur with any type of sexual contact where there is a break in the mucous membrane.

For a discussion of viral hepatitis, and its prevention, see p. 562.

B. Herpes viral diseases

There are four main kinds of herpes viruses:

(1) Herpes zoster virus causing chicken-pox and shingles.
(2) Cytomegalovirus, which is potentially pathogenic to infants, causing neurological disease and mental retardation. Route of infection may be both sexual and non-sexual.
(3) The Epstein-Barr (EB) virus — the commonest cause of glandular fever. It can be transmitted by kissing.
(4) The herpes simplex virus or hominis type I (labial) and type II (genital). They are 2 strains of the herpes simplex virus (HSV). Both may cause true genital herpes. Venereal herpes is contracted through genital, oro-genital or genito-anal contact.

Genital herpes

The HSV enters the body via abrasions or defects in the integrity of the contact mucous membranes, the cervix, in the urethra, in the anus (homosexual men), on the prepuce, the labia minora and majora, other parts of vulva, and even the skin of the surrounding areas (penile shaft, buttocks and thighs). At the site of entry a local reaction develops with a characteristic cluster of herpetic lesions (the primary disease). In a true primary infection there are systemic symptoms of varying severity with headache, neck rigidity, photophobia and a self-limiting aseptic meningitis.

Infection elicits a cell-mediated immune response which heals the lesions in about 12 days. The virus is not eliminated, however. It travels up the axons of the nerves supplying the area to the posterior root ganglia in the sacral plexus. Here the virus becomes inaccessible to the body's immune mechanisms; the disease thus becomes latent for variable periods of time. The disease may be reactivated by trigger stimuli to cause secondary herpes (reactivation disease). These triggers are: menstruation, stress, sexual intercourse, raised temperature. As the virus travels down the axon to produce reactivation herpes, the patient experiences the following prodromal symptoms: an itching or burning sensation and localised erythema. The onset of herpes is recognised by a cluster of papules which change into painful herpetic vesicles. The vesicles rupture and coalesce into superficial painful ulcers. Patients frequently complain of perineal pain, dyspareunia, pruritus, vaginal discharge or bleeding and dysuria. Reactivation infection is milder and of shorter duration than the primary infection. The attack lasts about 12 days, re-epithelialisation taking another 6 days. Moist ulcers heal without scarring; so do dry ulcers which heal by encrustation.

Over 80 % of men and women with primary herpes develop recurrences. The frequency and severity of attacks decline with time, but the absolute number of attacks cannot be predicted.[19]

Incubation period: 2–20 days, average 7 days.

Complications

(1) From infection during pregnancy and birth: although transplacental infection with serious consequences may occur in rare instances, infection of the neonate during the birth process or after rupture of the membranes occurs in 50 % of mothers with genital herpes. Half of these infants will either die or be neurologically damaged.[19] This can be prevented by timely diagnosis of the disease and Caesarean section to avoid the source of infection. 'High-risk' women should be checked twice during the last six months of pregnancy by clinical inspection and virological confirmation of the herpes infection, if necessary.

(2) There is an association of HSV type II and carcinoma of the cervix, but the causal connection has not yet been proved. Epidemiological factors which expose a woman to the risk of contracting STDs, viz. early age of first intercourse, multiple sex partners and poor personal hygiene, are also important in the aetiology of ca cervix later in life.

Herpes is found globally and in all socio-economic strata. Patients with genital herpes form 8 % of patients attending STD clinics in the USA and Scandinavia.[21]

Diagnosis of genital herpes

(1) Characteristic clinical picture and history of recurrent attacks.
(2) The virus can be cultured from smears obtained from lesions. The virus can be grown in a variety of cell cultures.
(3) Direct electron microscopy of vesical fluid or PAP smear.
(4) Complement fixation tests are of little value.

Treatment[19]

▪ There is no known cure for genital herpes. Patients are advised to abstain from sexual contact while lesions are present, and to keep the lesions dry and clean.
▪ Topical therapy with the antiviral agent, idoxuridine with dimethylsulphoxide. Application must be started before the vesicles appear, before the infection has reached its peak. Recurrent episodes of herpes may be treated with prophylactic oral acyclovir, a tablet (200 mg) being taken 4 times per day. It can prevent or reduce the recurrence rate. This beneficial effect stops on cessation of therapy.
▪ Women with proven genital herpes are advised to have PAP smears taken at 6-monthly intervals.
▪ Pregnant women with a history of genital herpes should be monitored as discussed above.

C. Human papillomavirus (HPV) infection

The DNA-containing HPV has been recognised as a common cause of both papillomas and carcinomas.[24] HPV is the promoter/initiator of the cancer. HPV infects keratinised epithelia and induces abnormal cell growth to form localised or spreading tumours which are usually benign but may become malignant.

There are at least 18 types of HPV.[24] They give rise to, *inter alia*, the following:

(1) Benign warts of the skin. They may regress on their own.

(2) Infections of the lower genital tract, e.g. the penis in the male, and the vulva and cervix in the female. In this case the HPV causes warty sexually transmitted diseases: condylomata acuminata and condylomatous squamous cell lesions.

Condylomata acuminata — genital warts are caused by type 6 HPV. These benign growths flourish in moist areas on the vulva and perianal areas, especially in association with Trichomonas vaginalis infection. These cauliflower-like growths can become large and recur after removal. They are highly contagious and difficult to eradicate.

Treatment

(1) Surgical removal by cryosurgery, electrocautery or laser treatment. These treatments are painful and may leave scarring.
(2) The injection of interferon into the base of each wart. This is done twice a week for 8 weeks or until the treated warts disappear.[22]

Condylomatous squamous cell lesions (flat warts) of the penile shaft and the uterine cervix are caused by types 11, 16 and 18 HPV. They are frequently accompanied by CIN 111 and even invasive cancer of the cervix. It has been established that there is a relationship between these premalignant cervical intra-epithelial neoplasias (CIN) and HPV infection, the infected epithelium being 'primed' to become malignant. CIN is the precursor of CIN 111 (carcinoma *in situ*). HPV is, therefore, an important aetiological factor in cancer of the uterine cervix, which is especially prevalent in young promiscuous women.

Markowitz *et al.*[6] found a 100 % association between HPV infection and CIN 111 in a population with an HPV infection prevalence of 66 %, the highest yet reported in the world.

Treatment: Excision of affected area by cone biopsy, or surgical removal of affected area by cryosurgery, electrocautery or laser treatment.

The role of the male sexual partner in cervical carcinogenesis has only recently been investigated. Hudson *et al.*[23] quote studies which suggest that men may be vectors for the aetiological agent (HPV) of cervical neoplasia. In nearly all the men found positive for HPV in the study by Hudson *et al.*, the infection was subclinical, i.e. warts were not seen and special staining techniques had to be used to identify the HPV lesions.

TRICHOMONIASIS

Trichomoniasis is the commonest sexually transmitted urogenital infection in human beings. It is caused by a flagellated protozoan, *Trichomonas vaginalis* — a pathogen recoverable from the vaginal exudate of infected women whose sexual partners are also infected.

Symptoms in infected women: Frothy or watery, purulent, occasionally offensive, green, white or cream vaginal discharge with pruritus and frequency of micturition. Sometimes there is erythema of the vagina with punctate haemorrhages, the so-called 'strawberry' vagina. This acute inflammatory condition may cause dyspareunia. Symptoms increase during menstruation and pregnancy.

Symptoms in infected men: Usually there are none, but the trichomonas may be found in the urethra, epididymus and prostate gland, only sometimes causing inflammation and a slight urethral discharge.

In males the infection clears up spontaneously. There are thus many more symptomatic females than symptomatic males. *T. vaginalis* infection in women is often associated with gonococcal and monilial infections. The trichomonas can also remain dormant in the vagina for months and years, causing a symptomless carrier state. In such women it may become activated during pregnancy and the use of broad-spectrum antibiotics which change the vaginal flora. Although the trichomonas is usually sexually transmitted, it can remain alive in urine for up to 45 minutes and in a wet cloth used for wiping the vulva for up to 23 hours.[21] Transmission in the female can thus be by non-sexual means, e.g. the use of public toilets and communal washcloths.

Diagnosis

(1) By clinical appearance:
In women: the presence of a 'strawberry' vagina, frothy greenish vaginal discharge.
In men: a mild urethritis or prostatitis in the

male sexual partner of an infected woman is suggestive of trichomoniasis.

(2) By laboratory methods: A fresh vaginal smear suspended in saline is subjected to immediate direct microscopy. Culture or microscopic examination of stained slides can also be done. In males, urine and prostatic fluid are examined.

Treatment

Single dose (2 g) oral metronidazole is given concurrently to both sexual partners. If the male refuses medication, the female is treated, with the proviso that the couple refrain from sexual intercourse for 7 days, or use a condom.

REFERENCES

(1) Quoted by Sutter EE, *et al. S Afr Med J* 1978; **53**: 622.

(2) Chairman's report. The South African National Council for the Blind, 1976.

(3) Ballard RC, *et al.* The epidemiology and geographical distribution of trachoma in Lebowa. *S Afr Med J* 1981; **60**: 531.

(4) Editorial. Sexually transmitted disease in South Africa. *S Afr Med J* 1981; **59**: 923.

(5) Fehler HG, Duncan MD, Bilgeri, YR and Ballard RC. Sexually transmitted diseases among urban black women. *S Afr J Sexually Transmitted Diseases* Sept/Nov. 1984; **4** (3).

(6) Markowitz S, Leiman G, Margolius KA. Human papilloma virus and cervical intra-epithelial neoplasia in an African population. *The S Afr J Epidemiology and Infection* 1986; **1**: 65–69.

(7) WHO Technical Report Series 674 *Treponemal Infections* (1982).

(8) Sher S. Sero-diagnosis of syphilis. *The SA Journal of STDs* 1982; **2**: 7.

(9) Naicker SN, *et al.* Serological diagnosis of syphilis in pregnancy. *S Afr Med J* 1983; **63**: 536–7.

(10) Ross SM, *et al.* Unsuccessful pregnancies — report on 200 perinatal post mortems. *S Afr Med J* 1978; **53**: 828–9.

(11) Philcox DV, Callanan JJ, Forder AA. Treatment of neurosyphilis. *S Afr Med J* 1978; **72**: 110–113.

(12) Ballard RC. Acute urethritis and associated infections. *S Afr J Cont Med Educ* 1984; **2**: 53–60.

(13) Editorial. Single dose therapy of gonorrhoea: The role of the cephalosporins. *S Afr J Epidemiology and Infection* 1987; **2** (1).

(14) Editorial. Epididymitis. *S Afr J Epidemiology and Infection* 1989; **4**: (2).

(15) Mauf AC, *et al.* Problems in the diagnosis of lymphogranuloma venereum. *S Afr Med J* 1983; **63**: 55.

(16) MRC's Emergent Pathogen Research Unit (SAIMR). *S Afr J Epidemiology and Infection* 1986; **1** (2).

(17) White RG. Acute pelvic inflammatory disease — a review. *S Afr J of Sexually Transmitted Diseases* 1982; **2** (2).

(18) Freinkel AL, Counihan RJ. Granuloma inguinale (donovanosis) in South Africa. *S Afr Med J* 1983; **63**: 599–601.

(19) Ballard RC. Sexually Transmitted Diseases. Part 2. *S Afr J Cont Med Educ* 1984; **2**: 63–73.

(20) Technical report series 660: World Health Organisation, Geneva, 1981.

(21) Ross SM. Trichomonas vaginalis–A review. *The SA Journal of STDs* 1982; **2** (2).

(22) Friedman-Kien AE, *et al.* Condylomata acuminata — a new treatment. *JAMA* 1988; **259**: 533–539.

(23) Hudson S, Dehaeck K, Soeters RP, Bloch B. Penile human papillomavirus infection in consorts of women with genital human papillomavirus infection. *S Afr Med J* 1988; **74**: 511–512.

(24) Editorial comment. Human papillomavirus — a burgeoning clinical problem. *S Afr J Epidemiol Infect* 1986; **1**: 64.

(25) Ballard RC. Treatment of gonococcal infections in Southern Africa. *S Afr J Epidemiol Infect* 1992; **7** (2).

(26) Ballard RC. Interaction of HIV infection with conventional sexually transmitted diseases. *Specialist Medicine* July 1993.

TEST OF KNOWLEDGE

The student has benefited from studying this chapter if he/she can answer the following questions:

(1) Discuss the effects of Chlamydia trachomatis infections on the eye, the male urethra and the female pelvic organs, as well as their primary and secondary prevention.

(2) (*a*) Prepare the main points of an informal talk to a class of Std VIII girls on the dangers and disadvantages of:
Early sexual relationships during adolescence; Promiscuity in sexual relationships; Prostitution.

(*b*) Name the primary and secondary preventive measures against gonorrhoea and syphilis.

(3) Discuss the social and pharmacological problems which are responsible for the great increase in STDs over the past 30 years.

(4) Write notes on:
– Post-gonococcal urethritis in males;
– PPNG (penicillinase-producing *N. gonorrhoeae*). Name 4 antibiotics to which PPNG may be sensitive.

(5) Discuss the general principles of the management of an STD clinic. What medication would be prescribed for:
– gonococcal ophthalmia neonatorum;
– venereal epididymo-orchitis?
Give reasons for your choices.

(6) (*a*) How may syphilis be diagnosed in Stages 1 and 2?

(*b*) What is neurosyphilis and how can it be treated?

(*c*) How is congenital syphilis recognised and treated during the neonatal period?

(7) Discuss cancer of the uterine cervix as a sexually transmitted disease.

34

Acquired Immunodeficiency Syndrome (AIDS)

OBJECTIVES

To educate the student about this modern scourge caused by the HIV — human immunodeficiency virus — which has swept across the globe unchecked by specific chemotherapy and without the boundaries imposed by immunisation in other communicable diseases. Thus HIV/AIDS is essentially a behavioural and social problem which requires community education for its primary prevention.

STUDY OBJECTIVES

The student must learn:

(1) What HIV/AIDS is, its definitions, aetiology, pathology, clinical stages and the treatment of opportunistic conditions (complications).

(2) The two patterns of AIDS in Western and African countries and how it is spread by homosexual and heterosexual transmission. The student must learn to discriminate infection routes that apply to AIDS and those which do not, so that she may nurse her AIDS patient with confidence.

(3) The epidemiology of AIDS and how HIV infection data are obtained in the RSA. She must take note of the projections for further growth of the AIDS epidemic/pandemic in South Africa.

(4) The measures (strategic plan) taken by government and medical groups in the RSA to contain the AIDS epidemic. These include disease surveillance, HIV testing, control of blood products for donation purposes, identification of high-risk groups, health education and the dissemination of information on AIDS, as well as the provision of health services for the HIV-infected person with AIDS.

(5) The various methods by which AIDS is diagnosed, not only the clinical features of the various stages but also the results of laboratory tests.

(6) The counselling of the HIV-positive patient (considered ethically mandatory for all persons who undergo HIV testing), and the ideal AIDS clinic where HIV-positive patients can be helped.

(7) How to care for AIDS patients without danger to the health care worker, thereby eliminating fear of AIDS patients, which may lead to neglect of very sick people.

(8) Health education in the most important ways of preventing AIDS and stopping the AIDS epidemic, for which there is no vaccine. The student must learn about safe and dangerous sex practices, as well as safe therapeutic and nursing practices.

(9) The way in which blood and blood products — formerly transmitters of HIV — have been made safe in the RSA.

(10) The medico-legal aspects of AIDS, and an ethical strategy for nursing (SANA).

Note: For those primary health care students who want a full description of primary aids care, Dr Clive Evian's *Primary Aids Care* (published in 1993 by Jacana, Private Bag 2004, Houghton 2041) is strongly recommended. It is a practical guide for primary health care personnel in the clinical and supportive care of people with HIV/AIDS.

INTRODUCTION AND DEFINITIONS

More has been written about AIDS since 1981 (when it was recognised as a clinical entity by the Centers for Disease Control, Atlanta, USA) than about any other disease in such a short space of time. The immunodeficiency is caused by viral destruction of lymphocytes (helper T-cells CD4+). AIDS is called a syndrome as the immunodeficiency eventually manifests itself as one or more of a large number of different diseases. The new sexually transmissible virus has swept across the world.

AIDS has been defined as follows: AIDS is a syndrome of opportunistic diseases, infections and certain cancers occurring in people with acquired immunodeficiency following infection with HIV.[4] For purposes of surveillance the Centers for Disease Control, Atlanta, USA, in 1987 defined AIDS as: an illness characterised by the presence of one or more specified opportunistic infections or malignancies, or encephalopathy, in a patient with immunodeficiency that is not due to other known causes. If there is laboratory evidence of HIV infection, a more extensive list of diseases constitutes the diagnosis of AIDS. The diagnosis of AIDS in children is more difficult, since maternal antibodies may be present up to 15 months postpartum, and children with AIDS may have indicator diseases other than those seen in adults.[8]

Adult AIDS in Africa has been given a separate clinical case definition: at least two major signs, e.g. weight loss greater than 10 % and chronic diarrhoea, and at least one minor sign (e.g. oropharyngeal candidiasis), provided other known causes of immunosuppression are absent.[8] (See discussion on AIDS in Africa pp. 604, 606.)

The term **HIV positive** describes a person who is infected with the HIV(virus) and whose blood tests show the presence of antibodies to the HIV. He has, however, not contracted any of the opportunistic infections or cancers associated with immunodeficiency.

The term **AIDS** describes a person who is HIV positive and who has also contracted an opportunistic infection or cancer as a complication of the immunodeficiency.

AIDS is always a fatal disease due to the complications.

The AIDS UNIT of the DOH is the recording body on AIDS in South Africa. Data are made available regularly by this body to the medical profession, the media and the World Health Organisation.[21]

Data are supplied (reported) to the AIDS unit by centres where AIDS patients are treated, and by Blood Transfusion Services, Chamber of Mines, Prisons' Department, by whom continuous surveillance of HIV antibodies is done. Although AIDS is reportable as a communicable disease and strict AIDS records are kept, it is not a notifiable condition in terms of Section 45 (Act 63 of 1977), notification requiring the disclosure of the patient's name (see p. 488). The consensus is that because of the severe social stigma attached to AIDS, notifiability with subsequent loss of confidentiality would drive the disease underground in that sick people would hide their condition from the medical profession. This would make the patient unavailable for health education which helps to combat the spread of the disease.

To repeat, although AIDS is not a notifiable disease, every clinically recognised case is fed by a medical practitioner or a dentist to a confidential AIDS centre — the AIDS UNIT of the DOH in Pretoria, via the regional offices of the Department.[32] Doctors are urgently requested to report all newly diagnosed AIDS patients and all deaths from AIDS to the relevant regional director by using the ANONYMOUS AIDS REPORT form available from the regional offices (see p. 481).

The Minister of Health has stated that the HIV infection in South Africa has been virtually doubling every year since 1991.

AETIOLOGY AND PATHOLOGY OF AIDS

AIDS is caused by a retrovirus — HIV (human immunodeficiency virus) of the species *lentiviruses* (slow viruses) which are associated with slowly progressive disease conditions. There are two main kinds, HIV–1 and HIV–2. West African countries, e.g. Ivory Coast, have the highest prevalence of HIV–2 infections. The degree of AIDS caused by this virus is not known. It has not been studied as well as HIV–1, as it appears to be of lesser importance.

Retroviruses are RNA viruses which contain an enzyme, reverse transcriptase (see p. 111), which transcribes viral RNA into the DNA of the infected host cell so that it forms part of the DNA of the host cell.

Infection occurs into and in the body if the HIV meets CD4 receptor sites: on CD4+ (T-lymphocyte) cells, macrophages, monocytes, tissue cells in the genital tract and anorectal region and glial cells in the brain, the target cell being the helper T-lymphocyte (CD4+).

Besides spread by sexual intercourse, infection is introduced directly or via the placenta into the blood, or into the body via an ulcer or inflamed mucous membrane in STDs. The HIV is found in bone marrow and lymph nodes and in most body fluids, in large amounts in semen, cervical secretions and blood and in lesser amounts in body fluids such as cerebro-spinal fluid, tears, alveolar fluid, saliva and breast milk — apparently not enough to cause infection.

The virus replicates by budding from the infected cell membrane of the host cell and elicits the formation of antibodies (gamma–globulins) by the natural defence system (B–lymphocytes). The HIV has a direct lethal effect on its target cell, the T–helper lymphocyte (CD4+), but its lethal effect may be kept at bay for many years (latent or incubation period) by the antibodies and the cytotoxic T–lymphocytes (CD8+).

Sensitivity

The HIV is an intracellular organism and does not live outside the body. It is easily killed by disinfectants, including household detergents and bleaches, as well as temperatures above 56 °C.

Infectiveness

HIV disease is always infectious, but its most infectious stages are:

(*a*) soon after the person becomes infected in the pre-antibody stage;

(*b*) much later when antibody production falters and CD8+ are no longer made in the bone marrow and the lymph nodes.

When opportunistic infections start to occur, the body has lost its ability to fight the HIV infection and the virus replicates unhindered.

After a variable period after infection, seroconversion from negative to positive takes place. The serum tests become positive for HIV antibodies. Immunity may be so depleted during the seroconversion phase (due to loss of immune regulation) that 50 % of patients develop a flu-like kind of sickness with fever and myalgia, oral and oesophageal ulceration, sore throat, malaise and some swelling of lymph nodes. The patient may be unwell for 2–4 weeks, but recovers completely.

He/she now enters the **asymptomatic** stage with no symptoms of disease. His/her blood is positive for HIV antibodies and the number of CD4+ cells are within the normal range, i.e. 500–800 CD4+ cells/mm^3. (Only 1–100 circulating CD4+ cells is HIV infected; the viraemia is thus mild.)

There is some hyperplasia of B–lymphocytes in the lymph nodes and the CD8+ cells are still increasing in an attempt to fight the infection. The disease may remain asymptomatic for many years, the HIV infection being balanced by the body's relatively competent immune system. The HIV antibody test may be the only sign of HIV infection. Eventually this balance is disturbed as the HIV disease progresses inexorably towards its lethal end.

CLINICAL AIDS CASE DEFINITION[37]

At a meeting of the DNHPD AIDS unit, the S A I M R, and a number of clinicians, epidemiologists and medical researchers, it was proposed that the CDC (Centers for Disease Control, Atlanta, Georgia, USA) surveillance case definition for AIDS should be used, but extended to include modifications suited for Africa and formulated in Abidjan. Thus, a person is considered to have AIDS if:

(1) the CDC surveillance case definition for AIDS is fulfilled;

(2) in adults (older than 12 years):
   (*a*) a test for HIV is positive (see p. 608), and
   (*b*) (i) pulmonary tuberculosis in conjunction with oral thrush (candidiasis) with the features in (ii); or tuberculosis that is disseminated (involving at least two different organs) or miliary; or extra-pulmonary tuberculosis (which may be presumptively diagnosed);
       (ii) more than 10 % body mass loss or cachexia, with diarrhoea and/or fever, intermittent or constant, for at least one month, not known to be due to a condition unrelated to HIV infection.

As the CDC case definition is very cumbersome, it was decided to use the WHO staging system for HIV infection and disease in this manual and to show the correlation of these stages with immunodeficiency as measured by CD4+ counts.

Staging of AIDS (WHO staging system for HIV infection and disease)

Clinical stage I

▪ Asymptomatic — 3–7 years CD4+ count 500–800 cells/mm^3
▪ Persistent, generalised lymphadenopathy

(Performance scale 1: asymptomatic; normal activity)

Clinical stage 2 — CD4+ count 350–500 cells/mm^3

Minor symptoms

▪ Unintentional loss of mass (less than 10 % body mass)
▪ Minor mucocutaneous manifestation — skin rashes, recurrent oral ulcerations
▪ Herpes zoster (recurrent)
▪ Recurrent upper respiratory tract infections and cough for more than one month.

(Performance scale 2: symptomatic; normal activity)

Clinical stage 3 — CD4+ count 200–300 cells/mm^3–AIDS-RELATED COMPLEX (ARC)

▪ Unintentional loss of mass (more than 10 % body mass). This loss may be associated with fever or with diarrhoea
▪ Chronic diarrhoea for more than a month
▪ Oral or vaginal candida infections (thrush)
▪ Pulmonary TB (reactivated) within the last year, with or without loss of mass
▪ Severe bacterial infections (opportunistic)
▪ Skin rashes (pruritic)
▪ Recurrent disseminated herpes simplex infection
▪ Persistent PUO and night sweats, for more than a month

Minor HIV-related symptoms

(Performance scale 3: bedridden less than 50 % of the day during the last month)

Clinical stage 4 — CD4+ count less than 200 cells/mm³ — AIDS PROPER

- HIV wasting syndrome: ongoing diarrhoea with weakness and fatigue
- Oesophageal candidiasis (thrush)
- Extra-pulmonary TB
- Toxoplasmosis of brain
- Kaposi's sarcoma and lymphomas
- HIV encephalopathy with neurological impairment (dementia and confusion)
- Respiratory infection (especially Pneumocystis carinii pneumonia), with fever, cough and chest pain
- Cytomegalovirus infection of lungs, retina, GIT and liver

(Performance scale 4: bedridden more than 50 % of the day during ten last months)

Of these illnesses (among black patients) tuberculosis, both pulmonary and extra-pulmonary, is by far the most common. One of the important co-factors of AIDS is the presence of other sexually transmitted diseases, especially genital ulcer, syphilis and gonorrhoea. (See p. 583.)

Paediatric AIDS

The clinical manifestations of AIDS in children differ from those in adults and may resemble common childhood illnesses, viz. recurrent bacterial, viral and candidal infections, encephalitis and failure to thrive or mass loss, chronic diarrhoea, persistent cough or prolonged fever, all for more than a month, generalised lymphadenopathy. Where infection is not acquired through blood or blood products, the child's mother will either have AIDS, or be positive for AIDS antibodies, or belong to a high-risk group (e.g. prostitute, mainline drug addict).

Most paediatric cases of AIDS in Africa occur under the age of 2 years.

Route of transmission

Children can be infected by contaminated needles and blood transfusions, but the most com-

mon route is maternofoetal transmission which takes place as follows:

(1) By infection of the foetus *in utero*. The virus crosses the placental barrier. This is called vertical HIV transmission.

(2) Perinatally, while the foetus is exposed to infected maternal fluids.

(3) Through breast-feeding. There is scanty evidence for this.[30] The mother should be encouraged to continue breast-feeding her infant, where stopping means the infant will suffer malnutrition.

Note:

(i) A neonate may be born with its mother's HIV antibodies without having contracted the infection. In this case it will become HIV negative by the age of 15–18 months.

(ii) Children do not, under normal circumstances, pass HIV infection to other children.

(iii) HIV-infected children die much sooner than adults from AIDS.

(iv) Fourteen per cent of the reported AIDS cases in South Africa in 1992 were African children, according to a report by the UN Children's Fund. A hundred infected babies are born each week (information to UNICEF by AIDS unit of DNHPD). (*The Star*, June 1994.)

TREATMENT OF AIDS INFECTION

Several anti-retroviral drugs have been used with limited success to inhibit viral replication and thereby restore immune function with regression of opportunistic conditions. The most successful drugs are zidovudine (Retrovir, AZT) and didanosine (DDI, Videx). They are given by mouth and cross the blood-brain barrier. They are, however, very expensive and are toxic to the bone marrow. Their use is, therefore, limited. AZT does not cure AIDS; it postpones the fatal outcome and enhances the quality of life by alleviating opportunistic conditions, i.e. complications of AIDS. These medicines should be started when there is moderate immune-deficiency, i.e. when the CD4+ count drops below 500 cells/mm³ — clinical stage 2.

Treatment of complications of AIDS

Patients with AIDS can be medically treated for their opportunistic infection, although the immunodeficiency does not clear up and another opportunistic disease may eventually prove fatal. Some medicines used for opportunistic infections are:

- *Pneumocystis pneumoniae (carinii)*: Co-trimoxazole, pentamidine isethionate.
- *Toxoplasmosis:* Sulphadiazine, pyrimethamine and clindamycin.
- *Candidiasis:* Ketoconazole, amphotericin, flucytosine, and nystatin.
- *Bacterial infections:* Antibiotics.
- Herpes simplex and varicella zoster: Acyclovir.
- *Cytomegalovirus:* Ganciclovir (Compound BWB759U).

THE SPREAD OF AIDS/HIV

At first AIDS was considered a disease of homosexual males but it has now become clear that it is a sexually transmissible disease which also affects heterosexual men and women. Venereal spread is mainly through semen but cervical secretions can also be infectious. AIDS can also be spread non-venereally through blood contact between infected and non-infected persons, either through blood transfusions, infected needles (especially in mainline drug addicts), blood products used in haemophilia and from an infected mother to her child. The only modes of transmission are, therefore, sexual, parenteral, transplacental and perinatal.

Anyone who harbours the virus can pass it on even if he/she looks and feels completely well. The only way to catch AIDS is for infected blood, semen, cervical secretions and probably breast milk to get into the body of a non-infected person.

Blood transfusions and blood products are no longer the dangers they were earlier as these products have been rendered safe in Western countries. In Africa, however, there is still a danger. The bisexual male has come to the fore as an important link in the transmission of HIV from the infected male homosexual population to females who, if promiscuous, provide a reservoir of infection for the heterosexual male.

Female prostitutes are an important source of infection in the heterosexual spread of the disease. Heterosexual spread may not occur as readily as homosexual spread, but the HIV can pass from men to women and from women to men during vaginal intercourse.

The main risk factors include prostitution, multiple sex partners and genital ulcer diseases such as syphilis, herpes and chancroid (see p. 583). Social factors, such as urbanisation and disruption of the traditional way of life, are important in the spread of AIDS in Africa.

Note: Although the spread of AIDS is commonly described as being Pattern I (mainly homosexual) and Pattern II (mainly heterosexual and paediatric), there is only one HIV/AIDS disease which may be spread as a sexually transmissible disease (either homosexually or heterosexually) or through the blood of an infected person to a non-infected person by needles, blood transfusions, the placenta or perinatally.

Infection is NOT spread by the following:

- Normal social contacts such as shaking hands, hugging and dry kissing.
- Swimming pools, restaurants and other public places.
- Coughing, sneezing and spitting.
- Clothing, toilet seats, door knobs, nursing procedures in which no contact is made with the infected person's blood.

The venereal spread of AIDS has caused its pandemic proportions and created immense social problems which cannot be conquered medically as there is no cure for AIDS and no vaccine to prevent the infection. Health education to bring about a change in personal behaviour seems to be the only weapon available to prevent the spread of the human immunodeficiency virus. AIDS strikes terror into the heart of man. It is a life-threatening, comparatively new disease which is still imperfectly understood. It is incurable and its presence is a death sentence. Its main mode of transmission is related to the sex drive which has found such free expression in modern permissive societies. Its incidence rate is increasing rapidly.

HIV is an infection of low heterosexual transmissibility — probably less than 1 % per episode of intercourse versus 80 % for gonorrhoea, 50 % for chlamydial infection and more than 5 % for rectal transmission of HIV among homosexual men.[40]

The epidemiology of AIDS is, however, a very inexact science and prognostic figures are guesstimates.

THE EPIDEMIOLOGY OF AIDS

In 1986 the United States Surgeon General stated that nearly 100 million people world-wide could die from AIDS by the end of the century if a cure or a vaccine is not found (quoted by *The Star*, 21.01.1987). At present this problem is being addressed on a co-operative international scale by the world's scientists.

World guesstimate

WHO figures released 12 December 1993 show that the number of HIV infections since the start of the HIV/AIDS pandemic has topped 15 million world-wide. The largest number of new infections has been in Africa where the cumulative total is now close to 10 million.

AIDS first appeared in 1979 among homosexual males in Canada and the United States of America. Within seven years it had spread across the globe with 140 countries reporting its presence in 1988. It surfaced in South Africa in 1982 when two whites, who had had homosexual contacts in New York, died from opportunistic pneumonia in Pretoria. The overwhelming infections were ascribed to AIDS.

About five years later the first woman with AIDS was reported and thereafter cases of paediatric AIDS followed.

AIDS statistics in South Africa[35]

Group	Cases	
Men	556	
Women	506	Total: 3 061
Children	104	from 1982–1993
TOTAL in 1993	1 188	

Mode of transmission	Cases	
Homosexual	449	
Heterosexual	1 986	Total: 3 061
Haemophiliac	22	(some unknown)
Blood transfusion	26	Some from other
IV drug use	2	countries
Mother to child	461	
AIDS deaths:	250 in 1993;	
	793 from 1982 - 1993	

Comments on the above statistics

Over a period of twelve years, only 3 061 cases of AIDS have been reported in South Africa;

793 cases have died from AIDS. These cases are incurable and cannot be prevented by vaccines. It would seem that the AIDS epidemic is very small when we compare the numbers with the annual incidence for tuberculosis (78 654), measles (11 762), malaria (10 862) and typhoid (1 414), all of which, however, are curable and preventable by immunisation or other prophylactic measures, and all of which exact a heavy toll in human morbidity and mortality.

Sexually transmitted diseases are not notifiable (except congenital syphilis, with 893 cases and 17 deaths in 1993) and are statistically not numerated, but we know from clinic attendance that they far outstrip AIDS in number of cases. Again they are curable and their fatality rate is low.

AIDS is the greatest global medical disaster of the present age. Millions of persons are infected with the HIV. Because there is no cure and no chemical means of prevention, these millions of infected persons, and many more likely to become infected, may die in the next decade as their immune system becomes destroyed by the virus.

As a result of their immunodeficiency, patients may finally succumb to any disease (opportunistic infection or cancer) which is endemic (either common or unusual) in their environment, for example Pneumocystis carinii pneumonia in the USA (63 %) and diarrhoea (slim disease) and tuberculosis in South Africa. People do not die from AIDS but from the complications (opportunistic infections, cancer) caused by the depletion of their immune system. The AIDS pandemic is thus still in its infancy — the disaster is yet to come.

Duh[38] is of the opinion that the HIV has probably always existed, somewhere in the West, but had not assumed epidemic proportions because the right conditions had not existed. As with the other STDs, the transmission and propagation of the HIV were favoured by the sexual revolution and 'the sharing of needles and bodies' characteristic of the Western drug culture since the 1960s.

The HIV was probably introduced into Africa via the Ivory Coast and a few central African countries where the virus flourished in the fertile soil of populations in poor socio-economic circumstances which led to cross-boundary movement of migrant workers, trucking, break-up of family life, prostitution of women, promiscuity and heavy infections with the sexually transmitted diseases, especially genital ulcers, syphilis and gonorrhoea, for which the infected persons lacked access to adequate medical care.

The medical 'needle', whether for blood transfusions or other injections (medicines, vaccinations), is another source of cross-infection as poverty causes a reluctance to dispose of medical hardware after single use. Blood for transfusions may not have been screened for HIV. Many Africans insist on parenteral medication with the infection hazard of unsterilised needles. Prostitution is greatly supported by tourism. The bisexual male is a means of forming a bridge between the original homosexual spread of HIV/AIDS in the West (with its ratio of male 13 : female 1) and the heterosexual spread in Africa (with its ratio of male 1 : female 1). Paediatric HIV/AIDS follows the infection of women.

HIV/AIDS spread rapidly south from the central African states as a heterosexual disease.

Its mode of transmission is similar to that of syphilis: homosexual, heterosexual, congenital, the prick of an infected needle, infected blood transfusions.

Drug abusers have not yet become a risk group in the RSA. Transfusion and haemophiliac spread has almost ceased.

It must be remembered that epidemiological data on AIDS cases have been assembled by voluntary reported AIDS figures. Only cases are reported — not the large numbers of asymptomatic infected carriers who are likely to develop the disease within years. The inevitability that the infection will culminate in AIDS is a controversial subject. The extent of HIV infection provides far more important information about the AIDS epidemic than AIDS data, but this type of data is even more unreliable.

HIV/AIDS serosurveillance in South Africa at sentinel sites

In South Africa the AIDS epidemic is spreading rapidly. As AIDS is not a notifiable disease (1994), passive surveillance by notification is not possible. In order to gather prevalence, mor-

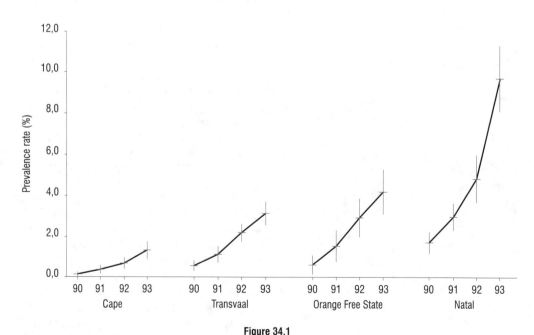

Figure 34.1

National HIV surveys, 1990–1993[34]

Estimated prevalence of HIV infection in women attending antenatal clinics by province
(estimates shown with 95 % confidence intervals)

tality, social, economic and health care data, the need for a serosurveillance system of sentinel (selected group) sites in South Africa is obvious. At these sites blood specimens are taken by health care workers in large numbers for other purposes, i.e. antenatal clinics, STD clinics, TB clinics, blood transfusion services, National Institute for Virology, City Health Departments. This blood is then also tested for HIV positivity (seroprevalence of HIV infection) without divulging the name of the donor, i.e. the blood tested for HIV is anonymous. These sites must represent the spectrum of South African society — urban, peri-urban and rural — and their population must have been enumerated at the recent census. As all people with positive HIV blood do not attend at these AIDS sentinel serosurveillance sites, the statistical results issued by the DNHPD are merely approximations of the severity and direction of the AIDS epidemic.

Seroprevalence data were gathered by means of the first four national HIV surveys of antenatal clinics of 1990, 1991, 1992 and 1993, conducted by the DNHPD. Blood was taken for serum HIV tests of an anonymous representative sample of women attending antenatal clinics throughout South Africa. Although the findings cannot be extrapolated to the entire SA population or even male sexually active population, the surveys do monitor the progress of the HIV/AIDS epidemic for each population group and for each age group. The results (see fig. 34.1) tell us that the HIV/AIDS prevalence rates are the highest in KwaZulu/Natal and that the epidemic is spreading rapidly in the heterosexual group. We can also expect an increase in the number of children born with HIV infection.

HIV surveys of antenatal clinics were done annually by the DNHPD. The latest statistics show that the HIV/AIDS epidemic has definitely spread to the white heterosexual community. Whereas the main victims of HIV infection in the white group were formerly male homosexuals and drug abusers, at present (1994)1:200 sexually active white women could be HIV positive. (See table.)

The HIV prevalence estimates among white women are up from 0,09 % in 1992 to 0,52 % (1:200) in 1993. HIV/AIDS has thus assumed epidemic proportions in the sexually active

white population. The current prevalence rate for black women is more than 5 %(1:20), with a natural doubling time of 13 months. The black heterosexual prevalence rate is probably exacerbated by the very high STD rate, up to 20 % (1:5) among some black groups. The presence of STDs increases the probability of contracting HIV infection up to 10 times.

National HIV surveys 1990–1993[34]
Estimated prevalence of HIV infection in women attending antenatal clinics (by population group).

	Prevalence rate %			
	1993	1992	1991	1990
Asian	0,10	0,33	0,11	1,53
Black RSA[*]	5,55	3,22	1,84	0,89
Black SA[†]	4,90	2,80	1,60	—
Coloured	0,74	0,33	0,14	0,16
White	0,52	0,09	0	0,06

[*]RSA excluding TBVC
[†]SA excluding Bophuthatswana

THE AIDS PROGRAMME

Early in 1985, the DNHPD established an Advisory Group on AIDS to plan and implement effective control measures. In 1993 the AIDS programme was established at the DNHPD in order to broaden the structures responsible for the control of AIDS in the RSA. The former 'AIDS unit' of the DNHPD now includes the 9 regional offices of the DOH as well as the 17 AIDS training and information centres (ATICCs). (See p. 614.)

The AIDS programme is an integral part of health promotion of the Chief Directorate: Primary Health Care. It is supported by, *inter alia,* the Family Planning Programme, local authorities and STD clinics.

The strategic plan for controlling AIDS includes the following measures:[7]

(1) Infection and disease surveillance, including HIV testing.
(2) Monitoring of blood donations, blood products and tissue donations.
(3) Identification of at-risk groups. Groups of highest risk of acquiring AIDS are:
    – homosexual and bisexual men;
    – haemophiliacs and recipients of untested blood transfusions;

- heterosexual (male and female) contacts of AIDS cases;
- children of infected mothers; and
- intravenous drug abusers.

Potential high-risk groups include:

- visitors to and from central Africa who may have been exposed to AIDS through heterosexual contact;
- prostitutes.

The tracing of new cases of HIV infection is done by testing members of high-risk groups free of charge. Successful tracing depends upon the co-operation of the people concerned.

(4) Health education and dissemination of information on AIDS to the public, schools and health professions. The Advisory Group communicates with the media and with the lay public through the production, printing and distribution of educational material.

(5) Provision of health services for HIV-infected persons. Treatment of AIDS cases takes place ideally in academic hospitals, but also in private and church hospices and in the many Hospice Association homes.

(6) Evaluation of antibody testing methods. Research in the RSA is being carried out at the National and other Virology Institutes.

The Department of Health co-ordinates the measures taken to fight AIDS and co-operates in this respect with other countries. An extensive survey of migrant labourers has recently been completed and high-risk countries identified. This has made it possible to restrict the entry of mineworkers from such areas.

The Advisory Group on AIDS instituted the means of recording cases of AIDS and also the numbers of HIV-infected persons[7] to estimate the carrier rate among high-risk groups. This information is contained in a National Register of AIDS. The National Register of AIDS Cases of the Department is confidential and anonymous. A country-wide telephone service has been instituted by the Department of Health as part of the public education plan on AIDS. The so-called AIDSLINE to regional and central offices of the Department is manned by experts who will advise and counsel people telephonically.

LABORATORY TESTS FOR HIV INFECTION

1. Laboratory evidence of immune deficiency

(1) Full blood count for lymphopenia (depletion of T4+ cells) and thrombocytopenia. The quantitative and qualitative defects of T4+ cells are the most important indications of an immune defect.

(2) Skin test for delayed hypersensitivity. Impairment indicates an immune deficiency.

(3) Estimation of the absolute number of T4+ (helper) and T8+ (cytotoxic) T-lymphocytes to get the T4:T8 ratio. Normally this is 5:3; in AIDS the ratio is reversed.

(4) Blood tests for T- and B-cell estimations are done when there is a low total lymphocyte count.

(5) Measurement of serum immunoglobulins for raised values, especially raised IgG.

Immunological abnormalities become severer with clinical progression from an asymptomatic state to the symptomatic AIDS.

2. Laboratory evidence of HIV infection — Antibody detection

This must always be accompanied by pre- and posttest counselling, if testing takes place on a voluntary named basis.

Tests for antibodies against the HIV have been used since 1985. Antibodies take 6–12 weeks (also thought to be 1–6 months) to form, therefore false negative results may be obtained if antibody tests are done too early. During this incubation period after HIV infection the patient is, nevertheless, infective (see the 'window period' pp. 609, 615).

There is also a high incidence of false positive antibody test results. A positive antibody test simply indicates exposure to the virus, i.e. not that the person concerned has or will develop the disease.

Testing for HIV antibodies

(1) Definitely indicated:
   (a) All donors of sperm, tissues and organs.
   (b) Patients with clinical features of HIV infection.
   (c) Blood and bone marrow donations.

(*d*) Persons about to undergo immunosuppressive treatment, e.g. recipients of renal transplants.

(*e*) Patients attending sexually transmitted disease clinics.

(2) High-risk groups (for diagnosis of HIV infection):

(*a*) On request by homosexual and bisexual males, haemophiliacs treated with blood products, intravenous drug abusers, prostitutes (female) and the sexual partners of high-risk persons, who have been counselled and promised confidentiality.

(*b*) If pregnancy is desired by a high-risk person who seeks advice.

(3) Testing in special circumstances:

(*a*) Victims of sexual abuse, e.g. rape.

(*b*) Violent mentally handicapped patients who could injure staff.

(*c*) Mothers from high-risk groups offering their child for adoption or fostering, or the child himself if AIDS is suspected and the mother is not available.

(4) Research, especially HIV surveys for prevalence rates. Voluntary testing for epidemiological, clinical and virological studies.

Testing NOT recommended

(1) Health care workers. There is no evidence that staff who are HIV positive pose a threat to their patients.

(2) Hospital patients for infection control purposes.

(3) As a condition of employment. Employers should be educated and reassured that testing is unnecessary. If they insist, testing will be carried out.

(4) Patients on dialysis.

(5) Persons seeking life or health insurance.

The AIDS Advisory Group of the DOH, from data supplied by the WHO, has recommended testing strategies for serological (antibody) diagnosis of HIV infection according to the prevalence of infection in the population.[33]

The tests must be sufficiently accurate for their objectives, the cost must be low and the technique simple enough to perform with commercially available test kits on a primary health care level. Accuracy of a test depends upon its sensitivity (few false-negative results) and specificity (few false-positive results).

The most commonly used tests are the ELISA tests (enzyme-linked immunosorbent assay) graded as first-, second- and third-generation according to increased sensitivity and specificity. There are many different ELISA tests. The higher the prevalence of HIV infection in a community, the greater the probability that a person who tests positive is truly infected, and vice versa. Some test results are difficult to interpret and sera from such a subject need to be referred to regional and even reference laboratories where testing facilities are much more sophisticated and specialised. The WHO recommends three testing strategies for the various testing objectives (safety of blood transfusion/organ donations, surveillance, diagnosis) to get the most accurate results while keeping the costs low.

Strategy I
(for safety of blood)

All sera are tested with one ELISA. Reactive sera are HIV antibody-positive and non-reactive sera are HIV antibody-negative. The ELISA must be highly sensitive to both HIV-1 and HIV-2.

Strategy II
(for surveillance and diagnosis of HIV infection)

All sera are tested first with one ELISA. Non-reactive sera are antibody-negative. The subjects are requested to return after a period in case antibody build-up is not yet sufficient (**window period**). Reactive (positive) serum is retested with a second ELISA, based on a different preparation, e.g. ELISA competitive binding assay. Serum that is reactive on both tests is considered HIV antibody-positive. If the reactive serum (first test) is non-reactive on the second ELISA test, it is considered antibody-negative. Further tests may, however, be required.

Strategy III
(for diagnosis of asymptomatic persons)

As in Strategy II, all sera are tested first with one ELISA and any reactive samples are retested with a different ELISA. If this serum is reactive, a third test with a different ELISA is required. Serum which is reactive on all three tests is considered HIV antibody-positive. Serum which is reactive on the first two tests, but non-reactive on the third, is considered discrepant and should be referred to a reference laboratory.

3. Laboratory evidence for virus

Antigen detection test

This test was devised in 1986; it is a cumbersome test which can be used to detect infection in the early stages before the antibody screening tests are positive, i.e. during the first 3–6 weeks after infection, before there is a measurable antibody response. It can also be used late in the disease when antibodies are no longer produced.

Virus isolation test

Infection can be detected by the culture of the virus from circulating monocytes. It is a very laborious test. Large samples of uncoagulated blood are taken for the harvesting of monocytes for culture in a special laboratory. Lymphocyte culture tests are even more difficult. These tests take many weeks to complete and are used for research purposes.

Obtaining and handling blood specimens for HIV antibody

The blood must be handled with extreme care as it is potentially infectious. Gloves must be worn and the blood tube marked 'Blood Precautions' to guide the laboratory workers. A specimen of 5 ml coagulated blood in a plain tube is taken and the needle safely disposed of in a closed 'sharps' container.

In order to ensure confidentiality, a coded name may be used for patient identification. In transporting the blood specimen to the laboratory, the outer wrap is marked with a warning label with the biohazard symbol and the words, 'H/A precautions'. Specimens must be placed in a waterproof bag or container before transport. For transport between institutions, even more stringent covering measures are observed.

Note: Informed consent must be obtained for voluntary named HIV testing. This is part of the pretest counselling procedure.

Patients found to be HIV positive are never notified by telephone or letter. Informing the patient forms part of the person-to-person post-test counselling procedure. The infected person is also referred to a support group, e.g. the Gay Association in the case of a homosexual male.

GASA–6010, the Counselling Service of the Gay Association of SA , is not restricted to homosexuals. Heterosexual men and women of all races from several southern African countries make use of the counselling services.

COUNSELLING OF HIV-POSITIVE PATIENTS

The success of voluntary screening for HIV infection as a primary preventive measure will depend on the establishment of testing sites that ensure adequate individual counselling and strict confidentiality. Primary prevention includes the tracing of sexual contacts of HIV-infected persons from any risk group. Success in tracing contacts for screening and health education purposes will depend entirely on the infected person's co-operation, as names are not divulged to the authorities as is the case with notification of notifiable diseases.

Medical counselling and management should be the responsibility of the consulting primary care physician who is ethically bound to preserve confidentiality. If the private doctor feels unable to do justice to the demands of this service, he should refer the patient to the local authority or hospital AIDS clinic. Testing and counselling of the patient's sexual contacts should also be managed by the doctor (private or clinic) with the consent and co-operation of the infected person.

Counselling aims at the establishment of a relationship of trust between the counsellor and the counselled. Counselling is done to help seronegative persons avoid further risky behaviour and seropositive patients to behave responsibly regarding infection of others. Seropositive patients may need repeat counselling sessions. The counsellor should be well informed about homosexual practices and should feel comfortable discussing these with the client in order to persuade him to adopt 'safe sex' practices. In

1991 the counselling service was offered to two main groups:

(1) seropositive haemophiliacs;
(2) homosexual clients.

Both groups suffer traumatic stress and may use the mechanism of denial which renders them inaccessible to counselling. The counsellor advocates a change of behaviour and in the management of their lives socially. Guilt and depression, or anger in the case of haemophiliacs, are negative emotions which prevent the patient from accepting his affliction and adapting to the implications of his illness. Patients who respond positively to counselling will not only avoid infecting others but will also make the best of their curtailed life span by attending to health principles with regard to avoidance of smoking and alcohol abuse, a prudent diet, rest and relaxation alternated with periods of activity and exercise. The patient must be supported to prepare for death in the terminal stages of AIDS.

The advantages of the patient having contact with medical services are that he/she is educated to protect his/her sexual contacts and can help to prevent the further spread of AIDS. The disadvantages of a possible breach in confidentiality through contact with the Health Services are:

(1) Suboptimal medical and dental care. Some doctors and dentists are reluctant to treat HIV-positive patients. Nurses have been known to avoid nursing patients with AIDS. Thus, AIDS patients may be neglected when they need optimal medical and nursing care.

(2) The patient may be subjected to social ostracism and unemployment.

(3) The patient may have difficulty in obtaining medical insurance. When completing medical insurance certificates, the doctor should not divulge HIV status (negative or positive) on request, unless the patient gives consent.

The nurse, as a member of the health team which has contact with the HIV-positive patients, must do everything in her power to preserve confidentiality. By her sensitive handling and support of a patient who has been given a 'death sentence', she must attempt to gain the patient's co-operation in striving for the good of society by preventing the spread of AIDS.

The SAMDC has decided that the Blood Transfusion Services (BTS) may not reveal the results of blood tests for AIDS to insurance companies. In terms of the Human Tissue Act (1983), all BTS records are confidential. Should the results of a particular donor be AIDS-positive, they are communicated to his private doctor who is then responsible for counselling the patient.

THE PROTOTYPE OF AN AIDS CLINIC

In 1987 the first special AIDS clinic[19] was opened under the auspices of the SAIMR's National Institute for Virology. The clinic is sited in the Rietfontein Hospital in Johannesburg and is staffed by two clinicians, one clinical psychologist and one nursing sister. People who attend the clinic are the 'worried well', those referred by their private doctors and those who respond to media advertisements.

The functions of the clinic are:

(1) HIV antibody testing on request.
(2) Counselling before and after testing.
(3) HIV-seropositive patients undergo further clinical and psychological testing.
(4) Follow-up consultations and counselling of the psychosocially assessed patient. The HIV-positive patient is supported in coming to terms with the implications of the results.
(5) The nursing sister does home visiting to assess the patient's social conditions.
(6) If the need arises, the patient is admitted to Rietfontein Hospital — a community hospital.

The authors[19] stress the importance of confidentiality and anonymity. Records are identified by the patient's first name and date of birth.

HEALTH CARE WORKERS (HCWs) AND AIDS

In South Africa the first two cases of AIDS or of seroconversion from negative to positive antibody status in HCWs were reported on 17 November 1990 — they had been pricked by infected needles in a Natal hospital.

Globally there is extensive evidence of a low but measurable and significant risk of nosocomial transmission of HIV to health care workers (HCWs). Infection is related to percutaneous exposure to the HIV and not to casual contact.

Precautions are, therefore, necessary and it is recommended[22] that infection control practices be used routinely when handling all potentially infected patients. The HIV is very sensitive to heat and disinfectants and does not penetrate surgical gloves. Sharps and needles contaminated with the infected patient's blood can be hazardous if they penetrate the HCW's skin. Safe therapeutic practices include routine hygiene, the wearing of gloves during dental and invasive treatments, the careful handling of sharps and syringes, and the sterilisation of instruments after use. Dentists should wear masks and protective eye gear when working with an infected person. The same applies in ophthalmology, where tears may be infected.

The HCW-group of surgical specialists is at risk of becoming infected during obstetric and other types of surgery, and especially during emergency trauma operations where there may be temporary uncontrolled bleeding, e.g. a spurting artery. Surgeons are, therefore, advised to wear adequate protective clothing, e.g. masks incorporating goggles to protect the eyes and mouth, full-length waterproof aprons under their gowns and gloves extending to above the elbows. The passing of sharp instruments during operations is reduced to the minimum by using electric cutters internally. In the case of an accidental needle prick injury while working with an AIDS patient, the HCW should be tested for HIV antibody status immediately to find out what the present status is. Tests should be repeated at regular intervals for six months to monitor the development of antibodies to HIV.

Health care workers infected with HIV must be adequately compensated and their HIV status must remain confidential.[22] There is no reason for their service contracts to be terminated as safe therapeutic practices will not afford any routes of transmission. They must be reassured that HIV infection does not necessarily lead to AIDS.

Fear of HIV infection among HCWs is common and is largely due to ignorance about the mode of spread of the disease and uncertainty about risk factors. The fear of contracting AIDS is the main factor contributing to the prejudice sometimes found amongst HCWs. Nurses could do much to counter any hysteria over AIDS as an occupational hazard among health care workers.

HEALTH EDUCATION IN THE PRIMARY PREVENTION OF AIDS

It is generally believed that education, as opposed to legislation, is the only way to prevent AIDS and to put a stop to the AIDS epidemic. The most effective educational programme to date has been the one initiated by the male homosexual group for its members. 'Safe sex' has virtually stopped the spread of HIV in homosexual men in San Francisco. The seroconversion rate from HIV-negative to HIV-positive antibody results, among the uninfected homosexual males of San Francisco was 21 % in 1982. In 1983 the figure dropped to 2 % and in 1986 it was a mere 0,8 %. The number of new cases of AIDS diagnosed in the city tells a similar story. After increasing steadily since 1981, it reached a peak of about 126 per month in 1986 and is now static.[17]

Education should be aimed at the general public, high-risk groups, health care workers and particularly the youth, who must be taught to protect themselves.[20]

A workshop on AIDS and children's education was held by the AIDS unit of the DNHPD and representatives of all fourteen education authorities. They decided that Health and Education Departments should work together in AIDS prevention and that all children should be AIDS-literate by standard five.[37]

It is important to direct education towards meeting the needs of the high-risk group by bodies within the group. Culture-specific intervention is the major approach to primary prevention.[20] Educators must be aware of the deep-rootedness of the sex drive and not impose on those to be educated their own moralistic and judgemental views on sexual behaviour which is outside the norm.

Ysselmuiden et al. state 'the only way in which HIV transmission in the population at large can be contained is by reducing or eliminating sexual contacts which carry the risk of HIV transmission (e.g. casual) and by reducing the transmissibility of HIV during such contacts. Education must reach all persons engaged in, or likely to become engaged in promiscuous sexual relationships.'[13]

The main principles of preventive therapy are:

(1) The use of the condom during anal or vaginal intercourse in high-risk groups.

> *Note:* For those who cannot afford to buy condoms, they can be obtained free from certain clinics and from ATICCs (AIDS training and information centres) of which there are many in South Africa.

(2) The avoidance of promiscuity and dangerous sexual practices. Promiscuity plays the most important role in the AIDS epidemic, especially in the promiscuous heterosexual population. The return to monogamous sex, i.e. sexual morality, is very important in the control of AIDS and the survival of a community. Casual sex is always risky.

Great care must be taken in the choice of a sexual partner, always remembering that promiscuous partners, those who have other sexually transmitted diseases and prostitutes are at high risk of being HIV infectious. These recommendations apply to males and females.

Dangerous sexual practices such as 'wet kissing', oral sex, receptive anal intercourse (sodomy) and mutual masturbation in males, must be avoided.

Sexual acts with infected persons which damage the anus, penis, mouth or vagina are extremely risky. Anal sex involves the greatest risk for the person receiving infected semen.

The practice of dangerous sex may be as difficult to give up as giving up smoking is to the tobacco addict.

Education alone will not eliminate disease caused by behaviour.[27] Changes in behavioural patterns are often the result of a combination of peer pressure and perceived personal risk. Change may be possible in a supportive environment, as has been found in the gay community.

In order for education to be effective, it is important for information to be complete and accurate, i.e. it must be 'open'. The educator who cannot discuss homosexual practices because they are too revolting in his opinion, is not likely to meet the educational needs of the homosexual community. Likewise, the educator who is judgemental in his/her attitudes towards prostitutes, will have no success in persuading the prostitute to use condoms or to persuade her clients to use them, i.e. to practice 'safe sex'.

Safe sex

The term 'safe sex' was coined to describe the means by which the risk of HIV transmission during sexual contact can be reduced. Safe sex includes the use of condoms and water-based spermicides which are also virucides.

AIDS education for children

The question is often asked: should children (teenagers) be educated about AIDS? Knobel[16] writes as follows: 'To withhold from teenagers all-important information on the grounds of moral and conscientious objection is in my opinion itself immoral because pregnancy and disease, including HIV infection, may occur with the first uninformed and unsafe sexual contact.'

At a conference on AIDS held in Johannesburg in 1988,[25] the opinion was expressed that 'the battleground of AIDS is in the classrooms'. Children should be exposed to 'preventive lifestyle education' to help them deal with sexual urges and promiscuity which is rife amongst adolescents in our modern permissive society. Children should be made aware of the dangers of unguarded sex, not only unwanted pregnancies but also venereal diseases which may blight young lives.

It is, therefore, necessary to obtain the co-operation of the Department of Education to introduce education programmes about sexually transmitted diseases (STDs), including AIDS, into schools. This has been a thorny issue, with some principals and parents' groups refusing access to health educators from outside their schools.

Health education in HIV-infected persons

The education of persons with a HIV infection with accurate and up-to-date medical information is important. Education includes measures which can be taken to prevent further spread of the disease.

Counselling for the infected should be readily available through hospital-based clinics and private doctors.

Condoms play an important role in preventing the transmission of HIV infection, as the virus cannot pass through the condom membrane, providing it is made of latex, is used once only and has not perished from age or exposure to the sun.

Condoms are essentially contraceptive devices (see p. 351) which prevent semen from making contact with the vagina and cervix. They are made of thin stretchable material such as latex, which is strong enough to prevent tearing during intercourse, yet thin enough not to dull sensation. Their use in the prevention of AIDS is to prevent the transmission of the HIV virus so they must be used although the woman may be using another kind of contraception.

The male condom, in the form of a penile sheath, is the commonly used type of condom, but female condoms are also available. A British company recently introduced Femshield, a polyurethane shield which is used like a sanitary tampon. It consists of a loose-fitting sheath and a flexible outer ring which facilitates insertion and holds the sheath in position in the vagina and over the cervix. Sexual intercourse takes place inside the self-lubricating sheath. Femshield purports to protect the wearer against HIV infection, as well as other STDs.

The use of male condoms does not afford 100 % protection against HIV infection as condoms may split if not made of good quality material. The simultaneous use of the spermicide and virucide, nonoxynol-9, is recommended for absolute safety.

It is generally agreed by AIDS educators that condoms should be freely available, even in prisons where anal sex may be practised. At present attention is being given to condom-dispensing machines in public places. The so-called sexual moralists strongly disapprove of such practices, averring that freely available condoms may lead to licentiousness and lowering of moral standards amongst the youth.

Note: The transmission pattern (sexual activity and blood) of HIV is similar to that of the hepatitis B virus, the latter being much more infectious.[18]

The Gay Association of South Africa (GASA), which has played a very important educational role for its members, has even prevailed upon its members to enter into a morally binding 'marriage' with their partners in order to avoid the dangers of promiscuity.

ATICC

(See p. 607.)

In January 1988 the private sector (Chamber of Mines) became involved by sponsoring the establishment of an AIDS Training, Information and Counselling Centre (ATICC). This is sited in the SAIMR, Johannesburg, and was run by full-time employees of the Advisory Group on AIDS. The Department of National Health and Population Development established seventeen similar centres in Cape Town, Port Elizabeth, Durban and Bloemfontein. These centres serve as information bureaux and training centres for training health educators. Prospective educators who are in a position to influence others are health workers, ministers of religion, teachers, cultural organisations and a well-informed public.

Even though the local authority is responsible for the control of, *inter alia,* AIDS and for health education and promotion, the government is subsidising these centres.

ATICC has pioneered AIDS training for the dissemination of informed and accurate up-to-date information and condoms to all sectors of the population.

The functions of ATICC:[14]

(1) To train trainers and educators (lay and professional) in the education and counselling of affected patients and their families and to provide free psychological counselling.

(2) To train educators to give talks on AIDS to schools, industry, hospitals, etc.

(3) To provide advice and guidance in industry, hospitals, insurance companies, etc.

(4) To take AIDS education to black homelands and townships, and to supply free condoms.

(5) To act as a resource centre (for pamphlets, videos, tapes, etc.) and as a referral centre for patients requiring specialised care. Centres referred to, e.g. academic hospitals, should supply full diagnostic and therapeutic back-up, including intensive care facilities, dentistry, bronchoscopy, endoscopy and consultation services in dermatology,

neurology and psychology. The basic education course lasts 1 day and the course for lecturers 2–3 days.

The following is a list of addresses of the Aids Traning, Information And Counselling Centres in the major regions of South Africa. The list is included for persons wishing to be provided with information relating to AIDS and is an extract from the *Resource Directory for HIV and AIDS* provided by ATICC.

Bloemfontein

PO Box 3704
Bloemfontein
9300

Tel: (051) 405-8544/8528
Fax: (051) 30-4573

Brakpan

PO Box 15
Brakpan
1540

C/o Park St & Kingsway Avenue
Brakpan

Tel: (011) 741-2261
Fax: (011) 741-2262

Cape Town

PO Box 2815
Cape Town
8000

12 Hertzog Blvd
Foreshore
Cape Town

Tel: (021) 400-2682/400-3400
Fax: (021) 25-1497

Durban

PO Box 2443
Durban
4000

9 Old Fort Place
Durban
4000

Tel: (031) 300-3104/300-3020
Fax: (031) 300-3030

East London

PO Box 134
East London
5200

39 Cambridge St
East London

Tel: (0431) 34-2382/9743
Fax: (0431) 34-2383

Empangeni

PO Box 115
Empangeni
3880

Tel: (0351) 21131
Fax: (0351) 27465

BLOOD TRANSFUSIONS AND AIDS

Blood is a source of infection if carriers, either in the seropositive or early seronegative stage, donate their blood for transfusion. The recipients of HIV-infected blood have an almost 90 % chance of becoming infected.

From the second half of 1985, routine testing of blood donations for HIV antibodies was started in South Africa by the Blood Transfusion Services. While the screening of donated blood will help to limit the spread of infection, the possibility that donated blood may be in the incubation period of AIDS before seroconversion has taken place (and thus infective) is a blind spot in diagnosis.[23] This is called the 'window period'.

Note: The Antigen Detection Test can be used in the high-risk group to detect HIV infection in the early stages before seroconversion has taken place. This is not routinely done, however. (See p. 610.)

Since the start of the AIDS epidemic in South Africa, 20 patients have been diagnosed with full-blown AIDS as a result of blood transfusion-related HIV infection.

According to reports received, all were infected prior to the time when the seven Blood Transfusion Services operating in South Africa started to screen blood donations.[36] Sixteen persons became infected with HIV as a result of receiving mainly imported blood products.[37]

Blood transfusion-related AIDS cases by year of diagnosis, population group and sex[36]

Year of diagnosis	Black		Coloured		White		Total
	M	F	M	F	M	F	
1985	—	—	—	—	—	—	1
1986	—	—	1	—	1	—	2
1987	—	—	—	—	—	1	2
1988	1	—	—	—	3	—	4
1989	3	—	—	1	3	2	9
1990	—	—	—	—	1	1	2
1991	—	—	—	—	1	—	1
Total	4	—	1	1	10	4	20

The following measures can be taken to reduce the risk of HIV transmission by blood transfusions:

(1) The use of blood for therapeutic purposes must be reduced to the minimum compatible with good medical practice.

(2) The donor population is made safer by:

   (a) Discouraging people from the high-risk group from giving blood. This is not a great problem in the RSA as donors are not paid for their blood. High-risk group donors may, however, erroneously consider themselves no longer a potential danger if they have changed their life-style and an earlier blood test was negative, i.e. seroconversion had not yet taken place.

   (b) Testing all blood donations for HIV antibodies. If antibodies are found, the blood is discarded.

(3) Blood and blood products used in the RSA are comparatively safe:[24]

   – Whole blood and red cell concentrates: very low infectiveness rate.

   – Albumin: completely safe as it is pasteurised after bottling.

   – Plasma containing Factors VIII and IX, in heavy demand for haemophiliacs, is made from large pools of donations. This is imported from the USA because the product made from small pools of donations in the RSA cannot be properly standardised.

Note: Autotransfusion — the use of own stored blood — is demanded by some patients who undergo elective surgery. The amount that can be taken and the difficulties in storing the blood outweigh the advantages of absolute safety.

THE MEDICO-LEGAL ASPECTS OF AIDS

The ethical issues in AIDS have been defined as 'the rights of the individual and the protection of the public'.[20] Sometimes measures which are legally right in that they are taken to protect the public may be wrong according to medical ethics in that they breach patient/doctor confidentiality. This conflict of interests is nowhere more apparent than in the management of patients with AIDS where the patient may refuse to alter his life-style to avoid the spread of HIV infection and the doctor feels he should reveal the patient's HIV status to those who are in danger of being infected, especially his spouse or other sex partner.

Both private and public interests are best served by the same approach, namely, voluntary co-operation through education. The public, including the medical and nursing professions, should be taught that AIDS is a disease and not a judgement. It is a medical and public health problem and not a moral issue. Scapegoating, stigmatisation and rejection of persons with an HIV infection merely exacerbate the problem in that they drive the HIV carrier underground, thereby causing the unchecked spread of the infection. At present the global epidemic of prejudice is spreading as fast as the virus itself.[20] Knobel states: 'AIDS may kill all people, but attitudes and ignorance about AIDS kill the integrity, compassion and care of uninformed health care workers.'[26]

The approach to the high-risk person should involve confidential testing for HIV status with the informed consent of the patient, preceded and followed by counselling, not only to help the seropositive patient cope with his virtual death sentence but also to persuade him to change his life-style to avoid the spread of AIDS. Persons engaged in high-risk sexual practices have an obligation to know their antibody status, to inform their sexual partners and to modify their behaviour if they are found to be HIV seropositive.[8]

Confidential testing by informed consent and reporting (i.e. not notifying) positive results to maintain the patient's anonymity and the confidentiality of positive results, have been adopted globally by those countries with adequate medical and laboratory services, in order to prevent the clandestine spread of the infection. The essential difference between reporting and notifying is that reporting provides all the epidemiologically relevant information supplied by notification but does not permit the identification of the patient concerned. Thus high-risk persons are encouraged to participate in strategies purported to stop the spread of AIDS. AIDS (but not HIV seropositivity) has, however, been declared a communicable disease in South Africa, in terms of government notice R2438, 1987 (Act 63/1977). The effect of this regulation is that if a patient is suspected of being an AIDS or ARC sufferer, the MOH can require him to submit to a medical examination. Thus the element of voluntary co-operation is replaced by compulsory co-operation, to serve the best interests of the public.

At present neither informed consent nor counselling is legally required in cases of compulsory screening in terms of R2438.[8]

At the same time as the above regulation, R3439 was promulgated by the Minister of Home Affairs. This regulation declares AIDS and HIV seropositivity as one of the five diseases which will render a person who is infected and not a South African citizen a 'prohibited' person for the purpose of being allowed entry into the RSA. Act 59/72 (Admission of Persons to the Republic) empowers immigration officers to require aliens who are suspected of being infected to undergo a compulsory medical examination.

This regulation has empowered the Chamber of Mines to test foreign mineworkers (from high-risk African countries) for HIV status. Those found to be HIV seropositive will not have their contracts renewed after they expire, i.e. they will become 'prohibited' persons. This measure has been taken to serve the best interests of the South African population.

Medico-legal issues in caring for people with HIV infection[26]

Refusal to treat a patient with HIV infection on moral grounds is medically unethical and totally unacceptable. This also applies to refusal on the grounds of risk of infection; international experience clearly shows the virtual absence of risk in treating HIV-infected patients using sound nursing and medical practices, even after needle-prick injuries to health care workers treating AIDS patients. By the same rule hospitals are not legally allowed to refuse to admit AIDS patients, unless there are valid and reasonable grounds.

Breach of the patient's confidentiality is not only unethical but also illegal as it is a violation of the patient's right to privacy. Disclosure of positive HIV status to the patient's family or employer without the patient's consent is, however, permitted to parents or guardians in the case of a minor who is treated at their request, or where industrial legislation requires an employee to undergo medical examination (see R3439 above). It is also mandatory for members of the health care team involved with the care of an AIDS patient to be given this information by the doctor. Members of the health care team are, in turn, legally and ethically bound not to disclose this knowledge without the permission of the patient.

Two important publications on AIDS (HIV infection) are available from the Publication Department of the South African Nursing Association:

- SANA's position paper on AIDS: A strategy for nursing.
- SA Strauss: *The Nurse and AIDS: Legal Issues.*

The South African Nursing Association's position paper on its AIDS policy is summarised below:

(1) All nurses should inform the public about preventive measures.

(2) It is incumbent upon nurses in clinical practice to be scientifically informed about AIDS, to educate their patients to understand their responsibility regarding the disease, to observe the patient's right to strict confidentiality, to treat the infected patient according to the highest professional nursing standards and to practise strict infection control measures to prevent parenteral spread of the disease.

(3) No nurse will refuse to nurse a patient with AIDS on ethical grounds.

(4) Nurse managers have the responsibility of ensuring that educational material on all aspects of AIDS and its nursing care is read-

ily available and included in informal training programmes, and that nurses caring for AIDS patients are informed as early as possible regarding the diagnosis.

(5) Nurse educators have the responsibility to ensure that educational material on all aspects of AIDS and its nursing to prevent self-contamination and cross-infection is included in the Nursing Science and Education curricula.

Strauss discusses the following questions about AIDS put to him by the South African Nursing Association in his booklet *The Nurse and AIDS: Legal Issues.*

(1) Professional secrecy, i.e. the extent to which the nurse is bound by her obligation to maintain professional secrecy if she is aware of the fact that a patient who has AIDS nevertheless continues to indulge in a wide sexual practice (unsafe sex).

(2) The position of the health care worker suffering from AIDS with regard to continuing nursing practice, informing patients/employers of the HIV status of the infected caregiver/employee and, generally, his/her employability.

(3) Should AIDS be a notifiable condition?

(4) The potential liability of employers if they compel a nurse to nurse patients with AIDS and the nurse becomes infected.

(5) May a nurse refuse to nurse a patient with AIDS?

(6) May a nurse required to nurse a patient with AIDS insist upon special remuneration?

(7) May the attending doctor keep the nursing staff in the dark as to the diagnosis of AIDS?

AIDS ISSUES IN THE BUSINESS COMMUNITY

The impact of AIDS on the business community and the serious practical, legal and ethical issues which confront employers are discussed in a NIPR report: Duckitt, J H (1988). AIDS in South Africa: Issues for business and employers. NIPR report PERS428.

Issues of importance are: recruitment policy regarding AIDS sufferers or infected persons, how to respond to employees who are afraid of working with AIDS sufferers, and many more topics including the legal status of the AIDS

sufferer or HIV-infected person as an employee, legal implications of issues such as dismissals, change in employment conditions, employment contracts and AIDS testing of present and prospective employees. The position with regard to medical aid, insurance and pension schemes is discussed. The NIPR report helps employers to formulate clear policy guidelines with regard to AIDS-related issues (and to life-threatening illness in general).

REFERENCES

(1) SAMJ News. *S Afr Med J 1989;* **75**: X.

(2) The Advisory Group on AIDS. Update on AIDS: HIV antibody testing. 1986; **7**: 13 September.

(3) Moodie JW. Serology of AIDS. *S Afr J Cont Med Educ* 1988; **6**: 58–63.

(4) Sher R. AIDS — clinical diagnosis and treatment. *S Afr J Cont Med Educ* 1988; **6**: 31–35.

(5) More about AIDS — AIDS in the world and South Africa. *S Afr J Cont Med Educ* 1988; **6**: 64.

(6) Stulting AA, Hendricks MC, Marais AF. Ophthalmological finding in AIDS. *S Afr Med J* 1987; **72**: 715–716.

(7) The Advisory Group on AIDS. Strategic plan for the containment of AIDS in South Africa. *S Afr Med J* 1988; **73**: 495–497.

(8) Ysselmuiden CB, Steinberg MH, Padayachee GN, *et al.* Part I. AIDS and South Africa — towards a comprehensive strategy. *S Afr Med J* 1988; **73**: 455–460.

(9) Goddard J. AIDS. *Nursing RSA Verpleging* 1989; **2**: 17–20.

(10) Schoub, BD, *et al.* Epidemiological considerations of the present status and future growth of the acquired immunodeficiency syndrome epidemic in South Africa. *S Afr Med J* 1988; **74**: 153–157.

(11) Update: AIDS in South Africa. *South Afr J Epidemiol Infect* April–June 1989; **4**: 24.

(12) World Health Organisation: *Update: Aids Cases Reported To Surveillance, Forecasting and Impact Assessment Unit (SFI).* Global Programme on AIDS, 30 July 1988, 1211 Geneva 27 Switzerland.

(13) Ysselmuiden CB, *et al.* AIDS and South Africa — towards a comprehensive strategy. Part III. *S Afr Med J* 1988; **73**: 465–467.

(14) SAMJ News. AIDS education in the RSA. *S Afr Med J* 1988; **74**: IX.

(15) Knobel GJ. An urgent warning — Contraction of HIV infection during mutual masturbation. *S Afr Med J* 1988; **73**: 617.

(16) Knobel GJ. Letter to the Editor. *S Afr Med J* 1988; **74**: 470.

(17) More about sex. Safe sex may stop the spread of HIV in homosexual men. *S Afr J Cont Med Educ* 1988; **6**: 64.

(18) Update on AIDS from the Advisory Group on AIDS. *S Afr Med J* 1986; **70**: 304.

(19) Martin DJ, Tilley JFG, Smith AN, Schoub BD. AIDS clinic — a year on. *S Afr Med J* 1989; **75**: 381–383.

(20) Congress Reports. Third International AIDS Conference. *S Afr Med J* 1987; **72**: 445.

(21) The Advisory Group on AIDS: Activities during 1987. *S Afr Med J* 1988; **73**: 319.

(22) Ysselmuiden CB, Steinberg MH, Padayachee GN, *et al.* AIDS and South Africa — towards a comprehensive strategy. Part II. *S Afr Med J* 1988; **73**: 461–464.

(23) Becker WB. HTLV-III infection in the RSA. Supplement to the *S Afr Med J* 11 October 1986.

(24) Brain P. Blood transfusion and AIDS. *S Afr J Cont Med Educ* 1988; **6**: 47–49.

(25) Conference on AIDS, 1988. *Nursing RSA Verpleging* 1988; **3**: 8.

(26) Knobel GJ. Medicolegal issues in caring for people with HIV infection. *S Afr Med J* 1988; **74**: 150.

(27) Metz J, Malan JM. The impact of AIDS on society. *S Afr J Cont Med Educ* 1988; **6**: 23.

(28) Strauss SA. *The Nurse and AIDS: Legal issues.* SANA. 1989.

(29) Shapiro M, Crookes RL, O'Sullivan E. Screening antenatal blood samples for human immunodeficiency virus antibodies by a large-pool enzyme-linked immunosorbent assay system. *S Afr Med J* 1989; **76**: 245–247.

(30) Van Ammers PM. Human immunodeficiency virus in obstetrics. *S Afr J Cont Med Educ* 1990; **8**: 303–310.

(31) Department of NHPD. The truth about AIDS. *Epidemiological Comments* 1990; **17**: 3–14.

(32) AIDS in South Africa. *Epidemiological Comments* 1993; **20**:12

(33) Fleming AF, Martin DJ. National Strategy for serological diagnosis in HIV infection. *S Afr Med J* 1993; **83**: 685–688.

(34) AIDS in South Africa. *Epidemiological Comments* 1994; **21**: 4

(35) AIDS in South Africa. *Epidemiological Comments* 1994; **21**: 2

(36) HIV screening results of blood transfusion services. *Epidemiological Comments* 1991; **18**: 4

(37) Carswell JW. The response of the AIDS UNIT to the HIV pandemic. *Epidemiological Comments* 1991; **18**: 11

(38) Duh S. *Blacks and AIDS.* Sage Series on Race and Ethnic Relations. 1991, vol 3.

(39) Head of AIDS unit in the DNHPD. *Race Relations Review.* South African Institute of Race Relations. 1993/1994, p. 105.

(40) Ballard RC. Interaction of HIV infection with conventional sexually transmitted diseases. *Specialist Medicine* July 1993.

TEST OF KNOWLEDGE

The student has benefited from studying this chapter if he/she can answer the following questions:

(1) Give a comprehensive definition of AIDS which is useful for purposes of surveillance.

(2) Discuss AIDS under the following headings:
   (*a*) aetiology
   (*b*) spread
   (*c*) the growth of the AIDS epidemic in the RSA
   (*d*) the obtaining of epidemiological data on AIDS and HIV infection
   (*e*) treatment

(3) Describe the stages of HIV infection with special emphasis on AIDS-proper in adults and in children.

(4) Distinguish between notification and reporting of communicable diseases. Why has AIDS not been made a notifiable condition?

(5) Which groups of people are at high risk and at potential high risk of acquiring HIV infection?

(6) Discuss the primary prevention of AIDS by health education and the counselling of HIV-positive patients.

(7) Discuss the functions of the Advisory Group on AIDS.

(8) Discuss the diagnosis of AIDS under the following headings:
   (a) The signs and symptoms of ARC and AIDS complications.
   (b) Laboratory evidence of immune deficiency.
   (c) Laboratory evidence of HIV infection.

(9) (a) What are the indications for HIV antibody testing?
   (b) When is HIV antibody testing not recommended?

(10) Describe the precautionary measures health care workers (including nurses and doctors) must take to prevent self-contamination and the parenteral spread of AIDS.

(11) Enumerate the measures taken by the Department of Health to combat the spread of AIDS in the RSA.

(12) What measures have been taken in the RSA to make blood and blood products relatively safe from HIV infection?

(13) Discuss the main medico-legal issues in AIDS.

35

Schistosomiasis and Intestinal Helminthiasis

OBJECTIVES

The terms metazoa (multicellular animal organisms), visible parasites, helminths (hence helminthiasis) variously describe the worms which may cause pathological conditions in man. Schistosomiasis (bilharzia) is a metazoonosis in that its causative blood fluke (trematode) requires both a vertebrate host (man or animal) and an invertebrate host (snail) to complete its life cycle.

Tapeworm infestations are zoonoses caused by cestodes which require both man and animal for the completion of their life cycles. The nematodes or roundworms are human intestinal parasites which are soil-transmitted. The filarial roundworms (Wucheraria), which live in human blood, lymphatic tissue and viscera and are mosquito-borne, cause a metazoonosis (filariasis) and will not be discussed.

The invasion of the outside of the body by metazoal parasites is called an infestation. The presence of cestodes and nematodes in the bowel is frequently referred to as 'infestation with worms' as the bowel is, strictly speaking, 'outside' the body. The word 'vermes' is an old term for worms, hence the derived terms vermicide and vermifuge for medicines that kill intestinal worms and drive them out. The equivalent term, anthelmintic, means 'against helminths or intestinal worms'. The medicines used against bilharzia are called antischistosomal medicines or bilharzia medicines.

Metazoal parasitic diseases are associated with poor sanitary living conditions and overcrowding in hot, humid climates. In endemic areas the prevalence of trematode and nematode infections may be extremely high, yet only about 10 % of the population are heavily infected.[1] These 'worm-rich' individuals contaminate the environment with their excreta and so keep the infection alive.

IN THIS CHAPTER

COMMON METAZOAL PARASITES OF MAN

The metazoa of medical importance can be classified as follows:

(1) The **platyhelminths or flat worms**, e.g.:
   (a) The trematodes (flukes), e.g. the blood fluke, *Schistosoma*, which causes schistosomiasis (bilharzia) in man. The main blood flukes are:
   S. haematobium which causes urinary bilharzia;
   S. mansoni which causes urinary and rectal bilarzia.
   (b) The cestodes or tapeworms, e.g.:
   Taenia solium — tapeworm of pigs;
   Taenia saginata — tapeworm of cattle;
   Echinococcus granulosus — tapeworm of dogs.

(2) The **nematodes or roundworms** (which are soil-transmitted), e.g.:
   Ascaris lumbricoides;
   Ancylostoma duodenale (hookworm);
   Enterobius (pinworm);
   Trichuris trichiura (whipworm).

(3) The **arthropods**
   Although the majority of arthropods (see p. 653) of medical importance act either as disease vectors or as intermediate hosts to unicellular micro-organisms, some are ectoparasites, i.e. they live in the skin of man, e.g. the mite, *Sarcoptes scabiei* which causes scabies.

SCHISTOSOMIASIS (BILHARZIA)

Schistosomiasis is a parasitic disease caused by the blood fluke (trematode), *Schistosoma*. A high prevalence of bilharzia in a community can be considered an index of poor socio-economic standards. The prevalence rate is 100 % in some South African endemic localities.

Schistosomiasis is essentially a disease of rural and peri-urban communities with poor sanitary facilities and poor hygiene habits, who make use of unpurified, natural supplies of water either for domestic or recreational (swimming, fishing, boating) purposes. Infected people who urinate in the water while they swim, or defaecate on the banks of rivers and dams in the rainy season, are responsible for the continued existence of the disease.

Schistosomiasis is a community health problem in that it causes loss of productive capacity by sapping vitality and causing ill-health. Walker[2] investigated the health handicap of schistosomiasis to black and white children in South Africa. 'Although schistosomiasis can be a fatal disease or have many crippling sequelae, knowledge about the overall ill-effects and the public health burden of schistosomiasis is still inadequate.' Walker is of the opinion that although the combating of bilharzia does not have high public health priority, control measures are required in areas of high endemicity in order to decrease the frequency and intensity of infection, eradication not being the aim of these measures.

At present there is no national control programme by the Department of Health. Treatment is often considered to be of little value due to the high risk of reinfection. Much research is done in the RSA on bilharzia and its snails by the SAMRC and the SAIMR.

Schistosomiasis is a very real risk factor for water sportsmen and water-loving visitors to endemic areas, who make use of inland bodies of fresh water in rural endemic areas. Dams fed by bilharzia-free streams are not exempt from causing heavy bilharzia infection. Gear *et al.*[3] are of the opinion that bilharzia must be suspected in patients who, about 2–4 weeks after a visit to the dams or rivers of an endemic area, feel unwell and develop pyrexia, signs of lung irritation (irritating non-productive cough), followed by signs and symptoms of hepatitis.

Epidemiology of schistosomiasis

Bilharzia is endemic in the densely populated rural areas of the eastern and north-eastern parts of South Africa, including the former national states and Swaziland. Endemic areas adjoin the rivers which run into the Indian Ocean, excluding those from Plettenberg Bay to Cape Agulhas. The non-bilharzial areas are: the Cape (except between the Transkei and Humansdorp), Lesotho, Free State and the greatest part of southern Transvaal.

The *S. haematobium* is much more widely spread than the *S. mansoni,* the latter being found in only 20 % of bilharzia endemic areas, i.e. east of the Drakensberg, north of the Soutpansberg, Swaziland lowveld and a few localities in Natal.[1]

Bilharzia is also endemic in large areas of Africa, especially Egypt. It is estimated that 75 million people in Africa are infected and 2 million people in the black rural areas of South Africa; 10 million people in the RSA/Namibia are at risk of developing bilharzia.[4] As bilharzia is not a notifiable disease in South Africa, the prevalence figures quoted are rough estimates.

Conditions favouring endemicity:

(1) The presence of the intermediate hosts, the *Biomphalaria* and *Bulinus* species of freshwater snails.

(2) The availability of water and favourable environmental temperatures. The presence of schistosomiasis is favoured by the warm humid environment of low-lying, densely populated, well-watered areas where people with unhygienic excretory habits constantly reinfect unprotected water resources. Those water collections especially dangerous because of the high concentrations of cercariae are small dams, reservoirs and stagnant pools in rivers. Fresh water, warm enough to harbour the bilharzia-carrying snails, and fringed with grass on which the snails live, is essential for the propagation of bilharzia. The prevalence of schistosomiasis increases as more land is brought under irrigation by the building of dams.

(3) Worm-rich individuals maintain the infection in the community. It is the small percentage of 'worm-rich' individuals that should be identified (by counting eggs in excreta and rectal biopsies) and treated. Testing the urine for blood and protein holds much promise and saves time when doing epidemiological surveys of schoolchildren. In highly endemic areas the 'worm-rich' group forms only about 10 % of the population.[1]

The peak incidence of schistosomiasis is between the ages of 7 and 15 years when heavy infections predominate; light and moderate infections are found in the older age groups.[5]

Intensity of infection[1]

This indicates the number of egg-laying worms and the density of eggs in the tissues, i.e. those not in the process of being excreted. As the intensity cannot be measured directly, the number of eggs excreted is used as an index of the worm and tissue egg-load of the body. Intensity of infection is expressed as the number of eggs counted per 10 ml urine or per gram stool.

Criteria of heavy intensity of infection

More than 1 200/10 ml urine in *S. haematobium* infections

More than 400/gram stool in *S. mansoni* infections

The tissue egg-load causes the symptoms of bilharzia: haematuria, hepatomegaly as well as the sequelae: hydronephrosis, portal fibrosis. Bilharzial disease is found in 'worm-rich' individuals.

The *Schistosoma*

The *Schistosoma* is an internal metazoal parasite (blood fluke) which causes schistosomiasis (bilharzia) in man. The *Schistosoma* is known as a blood fluke because its habitat in man is in blood vessels — the venous plexuses of the urinary bladder and the female genital organs, as well as the portal and mesenteric veins. Within the blood vessels the thread-like female worm, 20 mm long, lies in a cleft in the body of the male fluke.

There are two main kinds of *Schistosoma* in South Africa:

▪ Schistosoma haematobium causing urinary bilharzia;

▪ Schistosoma mansoni causing mainly intestinal bilharzia.

Note:
(i) Schistosoma mattheei causes bilharzia in cattle, sheep, antelope and occasionally rectal and urinary bilharzia in man.
(ii) Schistosoma japonirum is the main kind of blood fluke in the East.

The definitive host of the human *Schistosoma* is man in whom sexual reproduction by adult male and female flukes (worms) takes place. The intermediate hosts of the worm (*Schistosoma*) are several species of freshwater snails in which asexual development of the fluke larva takes place to a form which is infectious to man.

The snail intermediate hosts of the *Schistosoma*

The *Bulinus* species host the *S. haematobium*. *Bulinus africanus* is little bigger than a large peanut and has a truncate shell with pointed apex.

Biomphalaria species host the *S. mansoni*. The *B. pfeifferi* is a flat orbed snail as big as a 5c piece.

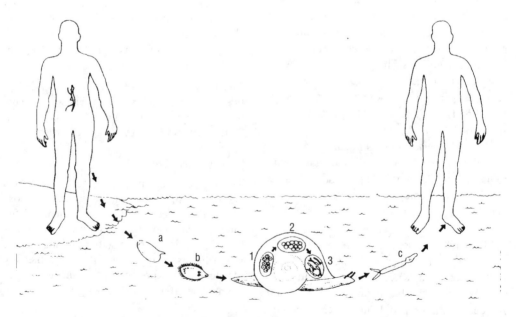

Figure 35.1

Life cycle of the *Schistosoma*

(a) Ovum (few minutes); (b) Miracidium (16 hours); (c) Cercaria (1–3 days)

The endemic area for *B. africanus* is more extensive than for *B. pfeifferi*, but most natural streams and rivers in the endemic region are infested with both species. Man-made collections of waters, e.g. small and large dams, open earth-lined canals and reservoirs can become heavily infested with snail eggs brought by aquatic birds and flying insects. Once introduced, they flourish in the absence of natural snail predators. The snails in the dams become readily infected with miracidia which hatch from the eggs deposited in human excreta. Small dams may give rise to heavy human infections when people swim in them. Irrigation dams in endemic areas increase the risk of spread of schistosomiasis as they are often used for domestic and recreational purposes.

Snails lay eggs on floating material and under surfaces of stones. At times they float upside down and are carried for some distance in flowing water. They prefer open, sunny stretches of water. They will pass alive through pumps and withstand normal concentrations of chlorine in water.

Sexual reproduction of the *Schistosoma* in man

After the cercaria (*Schistosoma* larva) swimming in the water has penetrated the skin of the bather, it reaches the bloodstream via the lymphatics. In the blood the cercariae are known as schistosomulae; they migrate through the heart and lungs[3] and are carried to the liver sinusoids where they begin their growth and maturation for 2–8 weeks after infection. The male and female worms migrate via the portal system to their final location in the mesenteric (*S. mansoni*) or vesical (*S. haematobium*) veins.

In the blood-vessels of man the mobile flukes mate and the female produces approximately 300 sharp-spined microscopic ova (eggs) every few days (more frequently in summer than in winter) for the duration of her natural life span — 5–10 years! The eggs are deposited in the submucous layers of the bladder, lower end of ureter, bowel and female genital tract. A ciliated miracidium develops in each egg within 6 days. Eggs produce enzymes which enable them to pass through the tissues into the lumen of the bowel or bladder, thus causing bleeding.

Asexual reproduction of the larval stage of the *Schistosoma*

Urine and faeces contaminated with schistosome eggs pollute the water supplies of a community when human beings urinate and defaecate either in or on the banks of rivers, canals and dams during the rainy season. If human faeces is deposited on dry land, the eggs may remain alive for 7 days. Viable *S. mansoni* eggs can, therefore, be washed into dams or rivers by rain-water. *S. haematobium* eggs must be deposited directly into water to ensure hatching. Within 15–20 minutes *(S. haematobium)* and 7 days *(S. mansoni)*, the eggs develop into miracidia (first stage larvae) which infect snails in the water, the miracidia being viable for only 16 hours. In the body of the snail, asexual reproduction from primary sporocytes to secondary sporocytes, to cercariae takes place. After 4–5 weeks in summer (6 months in winter), cercariae (free-swimming larvae) emerge from the snail between 10h00 and 14h00 and remain active and viable in the water for 1 to 3 days. When human beings drink or make cutaneous contact with infected water — the slow-moving water on the edge of the river or dam — the cercariae pierce the skin or mucous membrane, causing bumps and petechiae, and gain entry to the bloodstream via the lymphatics. This is called the stage of cercarial invasion.

Clinical stages

There are three distinct clinical stages in schistosomiasis:

(a) An invasive stage with cercarial dermatitis and a generalised itch, 'swimmer's itch', where the cercariae enter the skin to cause petechiae, urticaria and swellings. This stage appears within 5 minutes of making contact with contaminated water and usually lasts a couple of days.

(b) A toxaemic stage in which there is larval (schistosomulae) migration via the lymph nodes and vessels, veins, right heart and lungs to the liver sinusoids where the worms mature, the female lying in the cleft of the male body. From here the mature worms migrate to the veins and venous plexuses of the pelvis, especially the mesenteric and renal, and the female worms start ovipositing. This is almost a continuous process at the rate of 300 sharp-spined eggs every few days for the duration of her life: 5–10 years. Patients may react in different ways to stages (*a*) and (*b*). (See below.)

(*c*) Chronic schistosomiasis stage. The lesions of this syndrome are related to the presence of eggs in the tissues. The adult *Schistosoma* worms, while alive, do not harm the body, apart from the fact that they produce eggs.

Schistosomiasis is essentially an immunological reaction (to the antigenic enzyme secreted by the ova in order to escape from the tissues into the lumen of their target organ). The disease syndromes of chronic schistosomiasis are caused by granulomatous inflammation around viable eggs in the tissue with subsequent fibrosis and constriction, e.g. of the ureters (and eventual hydronephrosis). Calcified and immature ova elicit no host response. There is no local reaction to live worms inside the blood vessels. Dead worms give rise to vascular thrombosis and inflammation.[14]

Acute schistosomiasis (Katayama fever)

In disease-free visitors to the dams of bilharzia-endemic areas and in children not previously affected, bilharzia may, however, cause an acute illness. In these patients the invasive stage is very severe and urticaria may appear periodically for 6–8 weeks.

The toxaemic stage of the disease is very acute and is called **Katayama fever.** It has its onset during the migration of the larvae, approximately 3 weeks after infection. It is characterised by late afternoon and early evening pyrexia and sweating — even rigors and delirium — for about 8 weeks, with normal temperature in the morning. There is loss of appetite and mass, some mild CNS symptoms, alternating diarrhoea and constipation, arthralgia and tender splenic and caecal areas. There is a dry, unproductive cough with wheezing.

Katayama fever is ascribed to a severe allergic reaction to the presence of the developing worms as they migrate through the body. Although the patient may have recrudescences (new outbreaks) of acute schistosomiasis for some years, ovipositing and the appearance of blood in the stools or urine about 2 months after

initial infection indicate the beginning of the chronic, granulomatous stage of schistosomiasis, the pathogenesis of which is the body's immune response to the antigen secreted by the live ova in the tissues. (See Chapter 26: Immunology.)

Clinical features of chronic schistosomiasis

There are five distinct clinical manifestations of bilharzia.[5]

1. **Urogenital schistosomiasis** due to *S. haematobium* infection.

This starts with terminal haematuria (which may be microscopic) due to the extrusion of ova by contraction of the bladder wall. Rural black children often pay no heed to this sign, but start complaining when they experience dysuria and burning on micturition felt in the urethra.

Disease caused by ova in the tissues may be either active or inactive. In urogenital schistosomiasis, the most common form of bilharzia:

(1) The *early active stage* occurs mostly in children and young adults. Polypoid lesions due to inflammation and granuloma are seen on excretory urography in the bladder and distal ureters. Extra-urinary involvement of the rectal mucosa with *S. haematobium* ova, related to the intensity of infection, is found in 76 % of these patients.[5] Viable ova are found in the urine and in rectal biopsy specimens. Ova released into the circulation die and release antigen. This causes eosinophilia and systemic symptoms, including pyrexia.
Sequelae: Obstructive uropathy. This resolves spontaneously, but with treatment improvement is more rapid and marked.

(2) The *late inactive* stage in older persons with collagen deposition and fibrosis. There are no viable ova in urine, calcified ova being found in the urine and rectal tissue. On X-ray, calcifications in the bladder/ureters are seen.
Sequelae: Functional obstructive uropathy in which strictures are more apparent than real.
There are some indications that squamous cancer of the bladder is associated with schistosomiasis.
Renal glomerular function is well preserved

in both active and inactive urogenital schistosomiasis.

Note: Reinfection does occur in endemic areas, causing both active and inactive features of schistosomiasis to be present simultaneously.

2. **Hepatic schistosomiasis** due to *S. mansoni* infection. Its mild manifestation in the RSA is characterised by hepatomegaly with or without splenomegaly. Children with an acute attack sometimes have dysentery and moderately abnormal liver function and anaemia. It is diagnosed by doing a liver biopsy.

3. **Intestinal schistosomiasis** due to *S. mansoni*. It is a self-limiting dysentery (mimicking shigellosis and amoebiasis). Diagnosis is made on stool examination, sigmoidoscopy and rectal biopsy.

4. **Neurological lesions** due to *S. haematobium* and *mansoni*. The patient may develop transverse myelitis through granuloma formation in the spinal cord; this may remit or deteriorate to cause paraplegia.

5. Bilharzia of the **female genital tract**, the cervix being the organ most frequently affected.[14]

Diagnosis of bilharzia

Correct diagnosis is important in order to exclude unnecessary treatment with antischistosomal medicines and also to ensure that infected persons are treated before severe damage to the liver and the urinary tract has taken place.

Apart from a clinical diagnosis of the signs and symptoms based, in the case of visitors, on exposure to infected water and increasing eosinophilia after one month of infection, a decisive diagnosis can be made only by finding eggs in stools and urine or in biopsy or surgical tissue specimens,[6] *S. mansoni* after 5–8 weeks and *S. haematobium* after 10–15 weeks. The laboratory must report on the intensity of infection and on whether the infection is active, i.e. on the presence of viable ova. At least three stool specimens or three midday urine specimens are examined.

Collecting urine samples

The following method of collecting urine samples is recommended. As the greatest number of

eggs appears in the urine in the late morning and early afternoon, i.e. 12h00–15h00, the patient is instructed to empty his bladder at 10h30 and to discard this urine. Urine samples taken after 12h00 should always include the first and the last portion of the urinary flow. The midstream urine may be discarded.

Exercise before taking a urine specimen is unnecessary.

Apart from microscopic tests done to detect ova, urine can also be tested for protein and blood by means of reagent strips.[6] This test, which is useful for the screening of large numbers of people, e.g. schoolchildren, is highly sensitive if the two findings are read in combination according to a simple statistical model.[6]

If these tests are negative and patients who have been exposed to infection have a number of the other signs and symptoms of schistosomiasis then skin tests and, if necessary, schistosomal serological tests are done.

Skin tests (see p. 628) are of little value in the early stages of infection, but are invaluable in carrying out surveys to determine the incidence and geographical distribution of schistosomal disease.[3]

Serological tests first give positive results from 3–5 weeks after infection.[3] The following tests can be done, although they are not specific for type of *Schistosoma* and do not distinguish between present and past, or active and inactive disease.

(1) Bilharzia complement fixation.

(2) Immuno-fluorescent antibody test (IFAT).

Primary prevention

Schistosomiasis in South Africa is steadily increasing, especially in the Transvaal lowveld among the African population. The control of schistosomiasis is, therefore, assuming increased importance. Research has been carried out by the SA Medical Research Council by means of the Research Institute for Diseases in a Tropical Environment (RIDTE) stationed at Nelspruit, Mpumalanga, on large irrigation farms in the most practicable measures of control. Some of the findings are summarised below.

1. Molluscicides

The application of molluscicides (snail poisons) is not practicable. Not only are the molluscicides very expensive but they kill fish as well.

In other parts of the world, however, snail control measures are based on the destruction of snails, both by the application of molluscicides and by the selective application of herbicides (plant-killers) to destroy certain aquatic plants, thereby starving the schistosome snail hosts. Biological agents to reduce snails, e.g. ducks on dams, have little success.

Note: In the RIDTE's bilharzia control project[4] water contact points of the project sample were sprayed with a chemical (molluscicide) to kill the host snails. The researchers claim that this chemical is harmless to man and does little damage to the environment.

2. Environmental control measures

The most heavily infected African villages in the Transvaal lowveld are dependent for their water supplies on the nearest stream, canal or dam. These sources are highly polluted with *S. haematobium* and *S. mansoni*. The most important principle in the fight against schistosomiasis is, therefore, water management to provide the population with unpolluted water adequate for domestic and recreational purposes, including swimming-baths for the children at schools.

(1) All water must be piped from its source and supplied on a communal basis. If possible, the piped water must be purified, or 24 hours must elapse between the time the water is drawn from its source and the time it is used.

(2) Screens must be used on inlet pipes to prevent snails from entering swimming-baths.

(3) If possible, human access to rivers near African villages must be barred and canals running through villages must be covered.

(4) A small water filter, e.g. the Aquapur, can filter and sterilise a litre of water in 12 minutes, for drinking and medical purposes.

(5) Swimming-pools should be provided to communities to obviate the need to swim in a dam or river.

(6) All houses and huts near dams and rivers should be provided with enough latrines to encourage sanitary elimination habits.

See Department of National Health and Population Control pamphlet: *Bilharzia: Beware!* for preventive measures which can be applied at resorts on large dams within the endemic area.

Secondary prevention

(1) *Case-finding*, using an epidemiological survey to discover:
   (a) The incidence of new cases. Intradermal skin testing with antigen is useful in primary screening; if this is negative, serological tests, e.g. IFAT, are done. In the positive reactors, parasitological tests are done. In this way, early detection of schistosomiasis is possible. Urine tests for blood and protein can be used for the same purpose.
   (b) The prevalence of infection as confirmed by the presence of eggs.
   (c) The intensity of infection; for this, quantitative parasitological tests are essential.
   (d) The morbidity produced.
(2) *Clinical management of bilharzia*[5]
   (a) Active disease with viable ova in tissues: Antischistosomal chemotherapy
   (b) Inactive disease: No antischistosomal chemotherapy, as only lesions of active disease respond to drug therapy.

Schutte and Cooppan[6] recommend the following. All patients presenting with symptoms or complications, regardless of the intensity of infection, as well as those without symptoms and complications but with moderate to heavy infection, should receive chemotherapy.

Patients with light infections or those who do not excrete ova but are found to be positive on rectal biopsy only, should not receive chemotherapy.

Patients with hepatic schistosomiasis should receive chemotherapy (praziquantel) in a divided daily dose, irrespective of activity of disease.

Antischistosomal chemotherapy

In 1982 a new wonder drug against all species of bilharzia was developed. It is called praziquantel (Biltricide; Cysticide) and a curative course consists of one oral dose 40 mg/kg body weight. The drug has no dangerous side-effects on the patient, the transient side-effects being: dizziness, nausea and gastro-intestinal upset which can last for 36 hours after taking the extremely bitter tablet.

It must, therefore, be taken during or after a meal.

Praziquantel is contra-indicated for children under the age of 1 year and for pregnant women during the first trimester of their pregnancy.

Praziquantel is thought to be effective against all stages of all types of *Schistosoma* in the human host. After eradication of the worm, existing lesions will regress.[6]

Ova can be excreted for up to 4 months after a curative dose, but most are non-viable. The cure rate, determined after 6 months, is approximately 97 % for both types of *Schistosoma*, but reinfection can take place if the water hazard remains.

Despite excellent drugs, bilharzia can only be conquered permanently if the entire population of the RSA has access to reticulated, chlorinated water supplies.

Treatment with praziquantel can only be considered ineffective if, after 6–8 months, the patient excretes viable ova and there has been no chance of reinfection.

In this case, another good antischistosomal medicine, oxamniquine (Vancil), is given. It is effective only against the *S. mansoni* adult worms.[6] It is given twice daily for two days, the daily dose being 15 mg/kg body weight.

Note:
(1) Patients with haematuria before treatment will continue to pass blood in the urine for 2–3 weeks.
(2) Praziquantel is also a cysticide used in cysticercosis. It must be used with great care and in lower, divided doses in cases of neurocysticercosis, as the antischistosomal dose may cause a fatal cerebral oedema (see p. 632).

Treatment of Katayama fever (acute schistosomiasis)

Antischistosomal drugs have no immediate effects on the course of the acute disease.[13] Evans *et al.* recommend steroids and symptomatic treatment during the acute illness, after which praziquantel is the drug of choice to kill the mature worms and their ova — the true purpose of the drug.

HYDATIDOSIS

Hydatid disease is a zoonosis caused by the tapeworm of dogs, *Echinococcus granulosus*.

Its distribution is world-wide, especially in sheep-raising areas. Hydatidosis is characterised by single or multiple, unilocular cysts in the liver, lungs, brain, retro-ocular space, kidneys, bone and heart. Sixty per cent of all cysts occur in the liver and 20 % in the lungs.[7] In bone multilocular cysts form.[8] The cysts are surrounded by an inflammatory, fibrotic area, and the patient suffers from general allergy with eosinophilia. The cysts take many years to develop to the stage where they cause pressure symptoms and may burst to give rise to daughter cysts.

The tapeworm of dogs

The tapeworm of dogs *(Echinococcus granulosus)* causes *hydatid disease* (hydatidosis) in man. The worm varies in size from 1 mm to 6 mm and lives during its mature phase in the intestines of dogs; the immature encysted larval phase is spent in the connective tissue and serous membranes of some other mammals: man, sheep and cattle. Dogs become infested by eating contaminated offal of sheep and cattle at slaughterhouses. The ovum of the cestode is ingested in invisible particles of dog faeces, usually by handling the coat of the dog. From man's intestine, the liberated embryos are carried by the blood to the liver, lungs, brain and retro-ocular space where they develop into cysts which slowly enlarge.

Note: There is no danger of spread of hydatidosis from man to man.

Primary prevention

The dog is the main source of human infection. Hydatidosis can be avoided by:

(1) preventing children from having close contact (oral) with dogs, or by regularly deworming pet dogs;
(2) by not feeding dogs the raw, infected viscera of cattle, sheep and pigs. Proper meat inspection will reveal infected offal.

Secondary prevention

Hydatidosis must be diagnosed and treated.

Laboratory diagnosis

Laboratory diagnosis is carried out when the disease is suspected because of pressure symptoms accompanied by allergy:

(1) Casoni's intradermal test. A positive result is a raised, red area at the site of the intradermal injection of sterile hydatid fluid.
(2) Serological tests, e.g. complement fixation.
(3) X-rays and ultrasound scanning.
(4) Histological examination of the removed cyst.
(5) Hepatic and pulmonary daughter cysts may be coughed up; they resemble grape skins. Coughing up of cysts constitutes a natural cure.

Treatment of hydatidosis

(1) Surgical removal of located cysts in their entirety. The special danger of a hydatid cyst is rupture or leakage of hydatid fluid with severe toxicity culminating in anaphylaxis and sudden death. Spillage of a small amount of fluid will cause the formation of multiple new cysts. Natural bursting of *in situ* cysts can also give rise to multiple cysts.
(2) Conservative treatment with large oral doses (50 mg/kg/day) of mebendazole[9] for 4 months, partly as an in-patient and partly as an out-patient. The mebendazole is given with a fatty meal to increase absorption.
The patient's condition is monitored regularly with blood counts, estimates of electrolytes, urine, creatinine, liver function tests, blood sugar tests and urinalysis, and the shrinking of the cyst is diagnosed by ultrasonic scanning. This treatment is of value in patients for whom surgery is contra-indicated.

INTESTINAL HELMINTHIASES

Intestinal helminthiases have an endemic distribution in South Africa. Some, for example cestodes (e.g. tapeworms), need an intermediate host to complete their life cycle while the nematodes are easily spread from man to man; nematode infestations can, therefore, assume epidemic proportions where there is poor environmental hygiene.

Helminths are parasitic worms which cause intestinal infestations. In South Africa the main helminthic diseases are caused by the *cestodes* (flat- or tapeworms) and the *nematodes* (roundworms, hookworms, whipworms and pinworms).

The majority of these worms cause infestation by being ingested, the exception being the hookworm which may enter the body, and finally the duodenum, through the skin. Either the eggs or the larvae of worms are taken in through contaminated food and water or through oral contact with contaminated hands.

Preventive measures:

(a) efficient excreta disposal by provision, either by farmers for their labourers or by local authorities for their citizens, of adequate sanitary facilities;
(b) meat inspection to prevent the sale of measly meat; where this service is not available, e.g. on farms, all suspected meat must be thoroughly cooked to ensure destruction of larvae;
(c) attention to personal hygiene, i.e. handwashing before meals and after the use of the toilet to prevent auto-infestation.

A high infestation rate with intestinal parasites (nematodes) is a sign of poor living standards and sanitation.

Treatment

All intestinal infestations can be cured by *anthelmintic drugs* which are taken orally and paralyse or kill the worms and facilitate their expulsion.

Some modern anthelmintic drugs are effective against a number of the common intestinal worms, e.g.:

(1) Those effective against the hookworm, pinworm (threadworm), whipworm and roundworm:
(a) Mebendazole (e.g. Vermox) 2 tablets daily on 3 consecutive days. This standard dosage applies to all age groups from children to adults. If necessary, the course can be repeated after 3 to 4 weeks.
A single 500 mg dose (5 tablets) treatment is effective in children.[10]

(b) Pyrantel pamoate (e.g. Combantrim) dose according to body mass.

(c) Piperazine — for thread- and round-worms only — dose according to age.

(2) For the tapeworms, somewhat stronger therapy is needed to dislodge the adherent scolices, e.g.

(a) Mebendazole, 2 tablets daily for 6 days. It is poorly absorbed.

(b) Dichlorophen, 12 tablets on 2 consecutive days.

(c) Niclosamide, 1–4 tablets in a single dose (depending on age) on an empty stomach.

The pork tapeworm (*Taenia solium*)

The *Taenia solium* causes both **taeniasis** (intestinal worms) and **cysticercosis** (cysticerci in the tissues) in man.

Pigs form the intermediate host of the tapeworm when they graze on pastures contaminated with tapeworm eggs in human faeces. The eggs (ova) develop into embryos which are carried by the bloodstream to the tissues, especially the muscles of the pig. There they become encysted (cysticercus) and can be seen as little measly lumps in the meat. The ova can also be ingested by man to cause systemic human cysticercosis.

When man eats imperfectly cooked measly pork, the cysticerci are liberated in the small intestine, the scolex (head of the worm which has suckers and hooks) evaginates (turns from the inside to the outside of the cyst) and attaches itself to the mucosa. The head is the size of a

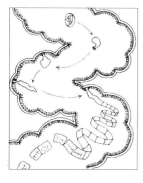

Figure 35.2

The tapeworm attaching itself to the mucous membrane of the jejunum

pinhead and ingests the food intended for the host. It grows a segmented body, 3 metres long and consisting of 800 to 1 000 segments (strobila). The tapeworm takes 3 months to mature and can live up to 25 years, being firmly attached to the small intestine. The terminal segments which contain ova (i.e. are gravid) continually break off and are discharged in the stool, being visible as flat, whitish rectangular pieces. The human host is usually thin with a good appetite and his blood shows an eosinophilia. If sanitary facilities are poor, contaminated faeces may be deposited on pastures and infect pigs.

Cysticercosis

Cysticercosis means the invasion of the body by the larvae of *T. solium*. Cysticercosis is endemic in South Africa and is a widespread disease.

Mode of infestation

Although auto-infestation of the patient with intestinal *T. solium* disease by eggs shed in his faeces, i.e. the anal-hands-oral route, or by eggs regurgitated from the small intestine into his stomach, is possible, the most important mode is the ingestion of eggs in water or food contaminated with faecal matter. In the latter case the patient need not have an intestinal infestation, the source of infestation being someone else. The ingested eggs hatch in the stomach and multiple embryos (ciliated larvae) enter the bloodstream via the small intestine, to disseminate to various parts of the body where they develop into cysticerci (single scolex enclosed in a cyst). Some cysts remain live and active and may become expanded, while others disintegrate to become sterile nodules or calcifications. Multiple cysts can be found especially in skeletal muscle and neural tissue, but also in bone marrow, subcutaneous tissue, eye (vitreous cavity, anterior chamber, sub-conjunctiva), heart muscle, lungs and rarely in the liver and vertebrae.

Diagnostic aids

(1) CT scan of the brain for active and calcified cysts and hydrocephalus (ventricles blocked by cysts).

(2) Anticysticercus antibody (ELISA) test which is strongly positive in cysticercosis.

(3) A positive histological finding on biopsies of subcutaneous nodules.

(4) Radiography of skull and muscles for nodular opacities and calcifications.

(5) Radio-isotope scanning for intense local tissue reaction which accompanies cyst disintegration.

Cysticercosis of the central nervous system is the form that causes the greatest morbidity and mortality. It is usually diffusely spread in neural tissues, but isolated cysts may occur.

The disease presents in a variable manner, sometimes being asymptomatic despite heavy infestation, and sometimes manifesting months or years after initial infestation.

Onset may be sudden or insidious. The clinical features will depend upon the number of parasites, the major site of localisation of the cysts, and on whether the cysts are alive or dead, disintegrating cysts causing tissue reactions. The clinical features of neurocysticercosis may be: epilepsy, either focal or generalised. This is the commonest manifestation of neurocysticercosis. The disease may also be characterised by hemiplegia, headaches, dementia and cranial nerve dysfunctions, such as facial paralysis and diminished vision and hearing.

Treatment of neurocysticercosis[11]

(1) Epileptic seizures are controlled with IV diazepam and phenytoin. Oral phenytoin is continued throughout the illness.

(2) Mebendazole for 3 days followed by

(3) Prednisone daily for 3 weeks

(4) From the third day of steroid treatment praziquantel is given for 15 days.

This treatment regimen should bring about complete resolution of the cystic lesions after about 3 weeks.[11]

The beef tapeworm (*Taenia saginata*)

The *Taenia saginata* causes only **taeniasis** — intestinal worms, in man.

Cattle form the intermediate host of the tapeworm when they graze on pastures contami-

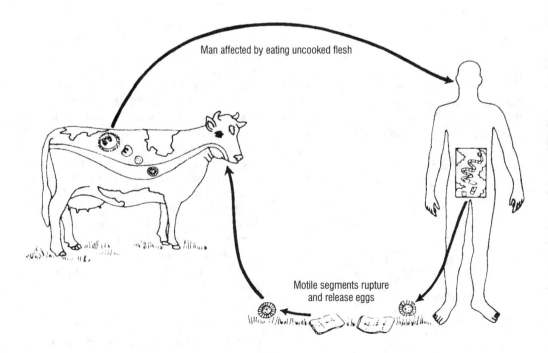

Figure 35.3
Life cycle of *Taenia saginata*

nated with ova released by the gravid segments of the worm. As in the pig, the ova develop into embryos which are carried by the bloodstream to the muscles where they become encysted to form measly beef. Auto-infestation is practically unknown.

When man eats uncooked measly beef, the cysticerci are liberated in the small intestine, the pinhead scolex attaches itself with its suckers to the mucosa of the jejunum and ingests the food intended for the host. It matures within 10 weeks and lives for up to 25 years. The *T. saginata* grows to a length of up to 10 metres, with 1 200–2 000 segments, shedding the gravid terminal segments in the stools. The human host is usually thin with a good appetite and his blood shows an eosinophilia. If sanitary facilities are poor, contaminated faeces may be deposited on pastures and infect cattle.

The roundworm

The roundworm (*Ascaris lumbricoides*) is a uni-host, human intestinal parasite which resembles the earthworm in size (i.e. approximately 200 mm in length) and shape and develops into male and female adult worms in the intestines. Multiple infections by these worms, either by auto-infestation or by ingesting faecally contaminated water and food, is called **ascariasis**. After ingestion, the fertile, embryonated ova enter the small intestine where the embryos (larvae) are liberated. The embryos penetrate the mucosa and enter the lymphatics and

venules from where they are transported by the bloodstream to the heart and lungs. In the lungs they migrate into the alveoli — causing pneumonitis — and ascend the respiratory tree, to be swallowed when they reach the pharynx. After many moultings, they eventually reach the large intestine as mature male and female worms. After conjugation, the female worm produces fertile eggs which are passed in the faeces. These ova mature to the embryonated form in 1 to 2 weeks and remain viable in the soil for months to years.

Adult worms may be vomited and passed in the stool, as adult worms live for only 10 to 12 months in the large intestine. Adult worms can cause obstruction or perforation in the intestines (if infestation is severe) and the bile ducts. The embryos, while in the bloodstream and tissues, can cause allergy, eosinophilia and pneumonitis.

Disseminated ascariasis, in which round-worms spread to the lungs, heart, liver, appendix or pancreas, is a serious condition which may be fatal. Bronchospasm may be caused by larval migration through the lung.

The *Ascaris lumbricoides* has a world-wide distribution, but severe infestations occur in peoples with poor sanitation and poor hygiene habits. The habit of fertilising above-ground vegetables, e.g. lettuce, with night soil, promotes ascaris infestation.

Endemic ascariasis must be controlled by repeated community-oriented chemotherapy.

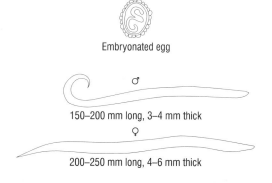

Embryonated egg

♂

150–200 mm long, 3–4 mm thick

♀

200–250 mm long, 4–6 mm thick

Figure 35.4

Ascaris lumbricoides

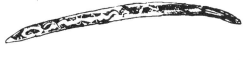

Figure 35.5

The hookworm

The hookworm (*Ancylostoma duodenale*)

Myriads of tiny bloodsucking hookworms attach themselves to the walls of the duodenum and cause chronic anaemia. Eggs are discharged in the faeces and hatch to larvae in warm, dark, damp soil, especially down in the mines where the bucket system of sanitation is used. The larvae can penetrate the skin and also thin shoe soles and infestation commonly takes place when use is made of infested latrines.

Northern KwaZulu is the most heavily infested area in the RSA.[12]

Pinworms or threadworms (*Oxyuris* or *Enterobius vermicularis*)

Infestation occurs by the ingestion of eggs, the worm living in the caecum for 4–6 weeks. At night they crawl out on to the perianal area, lay their eggs and cause irritation. Infestation commonly occurs in children, especially auto-infestation when children scratch the perineum and perianal area, get the eggs on their fingers and bring their hands to their mouths. The dust in the room may become contaminated with eggs and in this way cross-infestation may occur.

Without continuous reinfection, enterobiasis becomes sporadic as the parasite survives only 6 weeks in humans.

Specific hygiene measures:

(1) Infected children must wear protective underwear and night-clothes so that their fingers cannot make contact with the perianal area.

(2) Regular washing of perineum and perianal area.

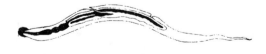

Figure 35.6

The threadworm

Whipworm (*Trichuris trichiura*)

The whipworm causes trichuriasis, an intestinal infestation of man which may be asymptomatic but occasionally causes severe diarrhoea. Different animals have their own species of trichuris, i.e. the disease is not spread from animals to man. Trichuriasis is common in certain coastal areas of the RSA, i.e. Cape Town and Durban. The whipworm has a whiplike appearance. Female are 4–5 cm long and males are shorter. Eggs are 0,5 mm long, i.e. almost invisible.

Man becomes infested orally by soiled hands or by ingestion of egg-contaminated foods or soil. Eggs hatch to larvae in the ileum, mature in a month and then pass to the caecum. Adult worms may live from 2–7 years. Stools are contaminated with eggs and spread the disease.

REFERENCES

(1) Schutte CHJ. Die epidemiologie van bilharzia in die Republiek van Suid-Afrika. *S Afr J Cont Med Educ* 1983; **1**: 45–49.

(2) Walker ARP. *S Afr Med J* 1977; **51**: 541.

(3) Gear JHS, Miller GB, Reid FP. Bilharzia contracted in small dams and while canoeing with special reference to its early stages. *S Afr J Epidemiology and Infection* 1986; **1**: 38–43.

(4) SAMJ News. *S Afr Med J* 1988; **73**: xv.

(5) Cooppan RM. Clinical features of schistosomiasis in the RSA. *S Afr J Cont Med Educ* 1989; **7**: 162–169.

(6) Schutte CHJ, Cooppan, RM. Diagnosis and chemotherapy of schistosomiasis *S Afr J Cont Med Educ* 1989; **7**: 149–156.

(7) Du Toit DF, Loxton AJ, Laker L, Dreyer JF. Hydatid cyst of the pancreatic tail. *S Afr Med J* 1984; **66**: 781–782.

(8) Rollinson PD, Geytenbeek RJ. Hydatid disease of bone. *S Afr Med J* 1987; **71**: 727–728.

(9) Kayser HJS. Treatment of hydatid disease with mebendazole at Frere Hospital. *S Afr Med J* 1980; **58**: 560.

(10) Evans AC, Hollman AW, Du Preez L. Mebendazole 500 mg for single-dose treatment of nematode infestation. *S Afr Med J* 1985; **72**: 665–667.

(11) Sirkin LL. Neurocysticercosis. *S Afr J Cont Med Educ* January 1988; **6**.

(12) Schutte GHJ, *et al*. Intestinal parasitic infections in black scholars in northern KwaZulu. *S Afr Med J* 1981; **60**: 137.

(13) Evans AC, Martin DJ, Ginsberg BD. Katayama fever in scuba divers. *S Afr Med J* 1991; **79**: 271–274.

(14) Friedberg D, Berry AV, Schneider J. Schistosomiasis of the female genital tract. Supplement to *S Afr Med J* 1991, 3 Aug.

TEST OF KNOWLEDGE

The student has benefited from studying this chapter if he/she can answer the following questions:

(1) Define the following:
   - trematode
   - enterobiasis
   - hydatidosis
   - helminthiasis
   - anthelmintics
   - schistosomulae
   - metazoonosis
   - miracidia
   - vermifuge
   - ascariasis
   - nematodes
   - metazoa
   - molluscicide
   - ovipositing

(2) Write notes on the following:
   (a) Anthelmintic medicines.
   (b) The life cycle of the *T. solium* and the difference between *T. solium* and *T. saginata* disease patterns.
   (c) The concept 'worm-rich' persons with trematode and nematode infections and their danger to the community.
   (d) The meaning and characteristics of the stage of cercarial invasion in bilharzia.
   (e) The medicine praziquantel.

(3) Discuss in a comparative way hydatidosis and cysticercosis.

(4) Make an annotated drawing of the life cycle of the bilharzia trematode through man and snail. Indicate at which points the life cycle of the *Schistosoma* may be interrupted by bilharzia eradicating measures.

(5) How would you make an assumptive diagnosis of bilharzia in an ailing person who visited a bilharzia endemic area some weeks previously? How may a decisive diagnosis be made by a doctor?

36

Enteric (Bowel) Infections

OBJECTIVES

The purpose of this chapter is to introduce the student to infections of the bowel, which are important in community health programmes.

Infective enteric conditions are caused by the ingestion of contaminated food and water. Their prevalence is, therefore, an indication of the environmental and personal hygiene standards of a community.

Cholera, the dreaded scourge of Third-World countries, invaded South Africa in 1980 and caused six epidemics. It is once more under control due to the effective surveillance and health educative methods applied by the Department of National Health and Population Development.

Enteric infections are also discussed elsewhere: diarrhoeal diseases of infants in Chapter 24 and food poisoning in Chapter 10.

IN THIS CHAPTER

SALMONELLA INFECTIONS

Salmonella infections can be divided into the enteric fevers and *salmonella* food poisoning (salmonellosis). The salmonelloses are zoonoses, i.e. primarily diseases of wild and domesticated animals and birds and only secondarily the cause of acute diarrhoeal disease in man. Spread of salmonellosis is via the faecal-oral route, with animals acting as carriers. (See p. 166.)

Enteric fever

The enteric fevers are a group of intestinal diseases caused by the *Salmonella typhi* (typhoid fever) and by the *Salmonella paratyphi* A, B and C (paratyphoid fever). Enteric fever favours warm climates with a high rainfall, e.g. the Transvaal lowveld, and affects mostly children and young people (5 to 25 years); it is much more prevalent during the first than during the second half of the year, coinciding with the peaks and troughs of the rainfall. Incubation period: 10–14 days.

Typhoid fever

Typhoid fever is an acute generalised infection with bacteraemia, which is essentially a waterborne infection, although the spread can be more direct in communities where typhoid is highly endemic, i.e. from faeces and urine, via fingers and flies to food and water and from there to the mouth and intestinal canal of the person about to be infected.

The *S. typhi* can survive freezing and drying and can therefore be found in ice and shellfish obtained from polluted water.

Typhoid may present in an epidemic form, especially if the water supplies of a community have become contaminated with infected sewage or if a carrier with poor personal hygiene habits has worked with the milk and food supplies of a large number of people, e.g. the outbreak of 69 cases in Cape Town in 1978, the source of infection being a carrier. Typhoid fever is a disease of underdeveloped countries with poor hygiene standards, especially with regard to the disposal of human and animal excreta, the control of flies and the provision of piped water for domestic use. Water laid on within the home is a most important factor in the control of enteric infections.

Epidemiology

Typhoid fever is the fourth most prevalent infective disease in South Africa at present. It is rife in many rural areas, i.e. Gazankulu, Lebowa, Transkei, Kwazulu/Natal. In 1989, 348 cases were notified in the 7 health regions of the RSA, and 1 900 in the 10 former black homelands (national states).

The majority of notifications are of sporadic cases. Infection is probably acquired through the consumption of contaminated water from natural water supplies. In areas of low endemicity, e.g. Cape Town, notifications come from mini-epidemics.

The provisional findings of the typhoid epidemic in Botleng near Delmas (far East Rand) in November 1993 are that contaminated water from the nearby squatter camp was entering the township borehole, as the borehole was built in

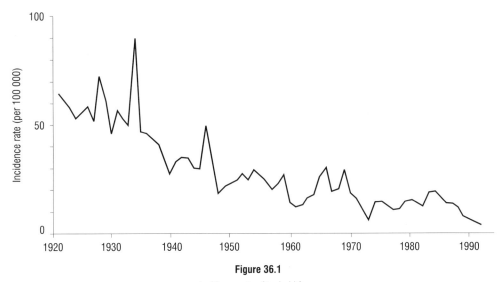

Figure 36.1
Incidence rate of typhoid fever
Source: *Epidemiological Comments* 1994; **21** (3)

dolomite rock which corrodes easily in heavy rain.[10]

Urban patients may acquire the disease while visiting rural areas where the disease is endemic. The number of cases notified annually in South Africa during the past fifty years has remained in the region of 3 000, but as the population has more than doubled, this number represents a greatly reduced incidence.

The *Salmonella* organisms, ingested in infected food and water, are absorbed by the lymphoid tissue (Peyer's patches) of the ileum. From there they are transported by the lymphatics to the liver, spleen and mesenteric lymph glands where the microbes incubate and multiply for 10–14 days.

Signs and symptoms

At the stage of invasion, the microbes enter the bloodstream (bacteraemia) and cause the early signs and symptoms of typhoid fever (pyrexia, headache, malaise). The microbes attack the gallbladder and the Peyer's patches, causing necrosis of the latter, and are excreted in the urine and faeces. The body forms antibodies (agglutinins) against the *salmonella,* which eventually overcome the infection.

Diagnostic tests

First 2 weeks: blood culture will be positive for *Salmonella* (bacteraemia).

Second week (7th to 10th day): on the 10th day a rash (rose spots) appears on the abdomen. The Widal agglutination test will be positive.

Note: This test is based on the formation of antibodies (agglutinins against H and O antigens) which cause agglutination of the microbes. A specimen of blood is taken in a plain tube. The serum is diluted to various strengths (called titres) and each specimen is mixed with a microbial suspension of fixed strength. The higher the titre of the serum, e.g. 1:100, the greater will be its dilution. The highest titre at which agglutination takes place is taken as the Widal result.

Interpretation. A low titre is found in persons recently inoculated against typhoid fever and is of no significance. A fourfold rising titre on specimens taken daily indicates a steadily increasing amount of antibodies in the blood and is diagnostic of enteric fever.

High titres are usually present at the beginning of the second week but may be present during the first week.[1] If patients are admitted late, the Widal is already positive (1:200) and not likely to rise fourfold — the usual diagnostic criterion. Chloramphenicol also depresses the titre.

A titre of 1:160 or more is often interpreted as being indicative of infection. The Widal test is, however, not a reliable diagnostic aid, especially in endemic areas.[2] Bacteriological confirmation must always be obtained before a definitive diagnosis of typhoid can be made.

Third week: During this week the *Salmonella* is found in the urine and stools.

Typhoid fever is characterised by the carrier condition in that nests of *S. typhi* remain alive in the body, especially in the gallbladder, and are intermittently excreted in the faeces. Carriers may, therefore, be difficult to detect as they appear well and their excreta are free of *Salmonella* organisms at times. Carrier states come into being either after a clinical or a subclinical attack of the disease and may offer some resistance to eradication.

Primary prevention

(1) Personal hygiene must be taught to people whose standards of hygiene are such that they become an easy prey to infection or, if they are carriers, they contaminate food and water for drinking with unwashed hands (after defaecation). Hygiene education, especially with regard to hand-washing before the preparation and serving of food, to schoolchildren is especially important. They, in turn, carry the information home.

(2) Carriers must be detected and controlled (see p. 487). Carriers must be registered and kept under close supervision with regard to food handling. They must be advised to accept chemotherapy at an institution and, if that fails, cholecystectomy.

(3) The provision of pure, piped communal water supplies cannot be stressed enough.

This is one of the main methods of controlling typhoid in endemic areas. Until this service is available, drinking water should be chlorinated.

(4) There must be health inspection of places where food is prepared and provided for public consumption.

(5) The standards of household hygiene and environmental hygiene must be such that sewage and refuse are satisfactorily disposed of, and that fly-breeding hazards are eliminated. This is a very important approach in endemic areas.

(6) Prophylactic immunisation is not practised generally, as immunity following vaccination is weak and of short duration and may give a false sense of security. It is useful, however, to protect workers exposed to infection, especially while an epidemic is raging or after a natural national disaster when environmental hygiene practices are disrupted and epidemics of various communicable diseases threaten. Typhoid immunisation is, however, widely used in the Transvaal lowveld,[3] where the disease is endemic.

(7) Breast-feeding must be encouraged.

Secondary prevention

(1) Notification of cases.

(2) The source of the infection and its mode of transmission must be traced and eliminated by health inspectors who do the local investigations. The source may be a carrier who works with public food supplies or a case whose excreta are disposed of in such a manner that the water supply of the community is contaminated. Specimens of water, milk, food and human excreta will be tested free of charge at the SAIMR. Carriers are found via rectal swabs and urine specimens.

(3) Isolation care of the patient.

(4) Treatment of the patient with specific antibiotics such as chloramphenicol, amoxycillin or ampicillin. In endemic areas, certain strains of *Salmonellae* may acquire resistance to chloramphenicol, in which case co-trimoxazole is used. Chloramphenicol is a bacteriostatic drug which does not, in any case, prevent the incidence of relapses and the chronic carrier state. Co-trimoxazole, being bactericidal, is more effective in doing this.

(5) Carriers must be treated, as they are the cause of sporadic and mini-epidemic cases. There are two types of carriers:

(a) Convalescent carriers immediately after the disease. The patient has recovered clinically but continues to excrete the *S. typhi* in stools or urine for several weeks. For this reason no patient should be discharged until his stools and urine have been certified clear of *S. typhi* by a laboratory.

Treatment is by an antibiotic which was not used for the treatment of the disease. The carrier condition implies that the patient has become resistant to the antibiotic used for therapy.

(b) Chronic carriers — persons who excrete, usually intermittently, *S. typhi* in their stools or urine, over a period of many years without showing systemic effects of the disease. Many carriers have had the disease in a subclinical form and are left with a chronic inflammatory nidus (nest) in the gallbladder or billiary tract, or in the urinary tract.

After the diagnosis of the carrier condition, usually by chance during an epidemiological survey, the patient is legally compelled to submit to a curative course of amoxycillin, ampicillin or cotrimoxazole.

CHOLERA

Cholera is an active, epidemic disease, caused by the *Vibrio cholerae*, which is spread by faecal contamination of food and water. It is a disease of tropical and subtropical countries in which people live under crowded and unhygienic conditions. Cholera is endemic in India and the Middle East and epidemics flare up from time to time. Calcutta (India) is a hyperendemic area; epidemics have occurred recently (1977) in a number of countries in the Middle East from where the infection was carried to Tanzania. Cholera does not spread in areas with high standards of sanitation and personal cleanliness, but it thrives in countries in which diseases related to poor hygiene are endemic, especially diarrhoeal diseases.

Cholera has become an endemic disease in certain areas of the Transvaal, Natal and KwaZulu. These rural areas are characterised by lack of the basic amenities taken for granted by developed communities, viz. safe reticulated water supply and proper disposal of wastes.

The history of cholera in South Africa

Until recently cholera was not endemic in South Africa. It was declared a notifiable disease in 1965, however, as it was endemic in Malawi, Angola and Mozambique and was thus a potential threat. In 1973 there was an outbreak on the South African gold-mines as a result of the southward spread of the disease by migrant mine labourers from declared cholera-affected countries, i.e. Angola and Mozambique. A surveillance programme was instituted in November 1973 and through this the outbreak of cholera was actually anticipated by the detection of

Vibrio cholerae in a main sewer of a gold-mine, 10 days before the first case of cholera occurred. Prompt prophylactic (chemotherapy and vaccination) and therapeutic measures were taken to contain the local outbreak which affected 32 recognised carriers and 37 cases. There were no deaths and the disease did not spread beyond the confines of the gold-mines.

To control this threat, cholera regulations were passed in 1974.

Epidemiology of cholera

The introduction of cholera into a country is difficult to prevent — even the USA has had sporadic cases — but cholera will only cause problems and become endemic in areas where diarrhoeal diseases are endemic due to contaminated, unprotected water supplies in dams and rivers and poor sanitation. Industrial urban areas in the RSA with a purified water supply which is conveyed to its users by pipes, are not likely to experience a cholera epidemic, although sporadic imported cases may occur.

South Africa had its first cholera epidemic in 1980/1981, peaking in mid-January 1981. The vibrial strain is the *El-Tor* — a relatively mild vibrio. It is suspected that this outbreak was triggered by carriers from Mozambique where 4 000 cases of cholera were notified in 1979, and that it is an extension of the seventh cholera pandemic which started in 1961. The epicentre of the South African outbreak was the eastern Transvaal, the original source of infection being water from the Crocodile–Malelane canal.

Before 1980 cholera was not endemic in South Africa. It is now an endemic disease. Since 1980 there have been six full cholera epidemics, the sixth one being a minor one. Only 3 cases of cholera were notified in 1989, 14 in 1992 and 94 in 1993.

In 1993 there was an outbreak of cholera in the Hlabisa Health Ward of KwaZulu, in an area that was previously not affected. Although only 46 cases were confirmed, many more people were affected. By prompt intervention the outbreak was soon controlled. This incident points to risk of cholera outbreaks in traditional rural areas where access to safe water and the use of toilets is low.

Estimates of the total case-load per epidemic cholera I, II, III, IV, V and VI, RSA 1980–1986[6]

	I 30/9/80 to 31/7/81	II 1/8/81 to 5/8/82	III 6/8/82 to 31/7/83	IV 6/8/83 to 27/7/84	V 28/7/84 to 27/7/85	VI 28/7/85 to 25/7/86
Number of bacteriologically proven cases	3 786	11 141	7 638	1 977	568	134
Suspect cases treated	30 000 (estimated)	50 000 (estimated)	20 000 (estimated)	5 434 (counted)	1 717 (counted)	1 267 (counted)
Per cent proven cases	12,6	22,3	38,2	36,4	33,1	10,6
Reported deaths[*]	42	218	62	20	4	2
Case-fatality rate %[†]	1,1	2,0	0,8	1,0	0,7	1,5

[*]Not all proven to be due to cholera.
[†]Based on proven cases.

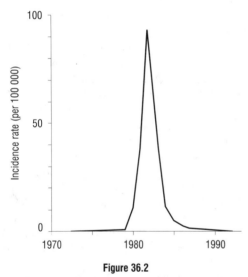

Figure 36.2

Incidence rate of cholera
Source: *Epidemiological Comments* 1994; **21** (3)

The spread and contraction of cholera

Cholera is contracted by drinking, or bathing and washing in, water containing human faecal matter, from food prepared by the unclean hands of carriers and from fruits and vegetables washed in contaminated water. In the gold-mines outbreak,[4] *Vibrio cholerae* was found on the floor of the acclimatisation room which had been contaminated with profuse perspiration from the perianal region of the carriers. Isaäcson

et al. suggest that profuse sweating and physical exertion may play an important role in cholera epidemiology, especially in the tropics and during hot seasons.

Special problems in traditional rural areas that favour spread

In some African countries, the controlling action of community health measures is hampered by local medicine men who sell home-made body ointments as protection against the disease, thereby causing people to ignore precautions and basic hygiene measures.

Traditional habits and poor hygiene favour the spread of the disease, viz. washing contaminated clothes in rivers and children swimming nearby; communal use of a bowl of food or a pot of beer. Rural people often object to the taste of chlorinated water, or believe chlorinated water supplied free by the SADF to be poisoned and rather buy water from vendors carrying water from contaminated rivers. There is often not enough fuel to boil water.

Raw vegetables and fruit (contaminated by water and hand in a cholera-endemic area) and mussels and oysters from endemic areas must be regarded as being potential cholera carriers. Flies play a relatively small role in transmitting the vibrio, except if they abound and have access to faeces in infected areas.

The vibrio does not survive on dry surfaces for more than two days. Dry, solid food will, therefore, not be infected.

An investigation into the survival of *V. cholerae* in water in the environment found that plastic drums and undamaged metal drums least allowed for maintenance of *V. cholerae*. Damaged corroded metal drums release iron and this seems responsible for multiplication of the vibrio. *V. cholerae* passes through the porous material of clay pots, thus the water inside can become contaminated if the pot is handled with infected hands and vice versa.[5]

Infectiveness

In South Africa, a cholera case is defined as a person excreting *V. cholerae*, even though he is asymptomatic and, therefore, a healthy or subclinical carrier of the disease. Being mobile, these carriers are the important spreaders of the disease. For every case sent to hospital there are five or more carriers without symptoms or only mild diarrhoea, who will spread the disease. This is a special problem with the El-Tor vibrio strain. The disease remains endemic and active because sporadic cases occur in the winter to transmit the disease from man to water to man.

Incubation period: Very quick — up to a few days.

Infection confers immunity; in an endemic area, most children acquire an immunity. The main anti-cholera measures advocated by the WHO are: surveillance, environmental sanitation, health education, including the establishment of a well-informed public. These principles were embodied in the anti-cholera campaign of the Department of National Health and Population Development.

Primary prevention of cholera

(1) The supply of pure water and adequate sanitation. People in infected areas without adequate sanitation and water must either chlorinate their drinking water or boil it for 10 minutes (see p. 175).

(2) Tourists in cholera areas are advised to drink only carbonated, bottled water or to carry chlorine or iodine disinfectants to treat water where bottled water is not available; to peel all fruit themselves and not to eat any food which has not been thoroughly cooked and promptly served.

(3) Prophylactic inoculation of the population at risk is 50 % effective, but relative immunity lasts for only two–six months; it is not compulsory for international travel. Travellers to certain parts of Africa, Asia and the Middle East should be vaccinated one month before departure or every six months while resident in the cholera-endemic area. People at risk are travellers to a cholera endemic country, e.g. travellers to Mecca. In endemic areas with regularly recurring seasonal incidence, prophylactic inoculation may be carried out at the beginning of the epidemic period. This is done in Mozambique.

Inoculation does not, however, prevent the carrier state nor the spread of the disease, nor is it of any value in stopping the sudden outbreak of the disease.

Inoculation is not practised in the RSA, as the authorities feel it may create a false sense of security and, in so doing, detract from the importance of the three essential prophylactic measures: adequate waste (including sewage) disposal, safe water supply and personal hygiene, especially with regard to the washing of hands before preparing and eating food and after use of the toilet. Moreover, the person who has been vaccinated could still be a cholera carrier, as the vaccine does not affect the vibrios in the gut.

(4) Prophylactic chemotherapy of direct and family contacts with antimicrobial drugs, e.g. tetracyclines, 1 g/d for 5 days. Chemotherapy is also given to special high-risk groups where an outbreak is imminent, e.g. on the gold-mines in South Africa in 1973, to prevent the spread of infection. Generalised prophylaxis is not likely to be effective in endemic areas where there are many opportunities for reinfection.

Where an acute epidemic is raging, all contacts of patients should be treated with tetracyclines. Where the patient has been treated in his community at a rehydration centre, it is usually easy to get his co-operation to be the vehicle for contact therapy.

The adequate antibiotic treatment of contacts (as well as education of the population in the prevention of cholera) soon brings an epidemic to a halt.

(5) Health education. Massive health education campaigns were conducted by the Department of National Health and Population Development to make the people at risk aware of the dangers of contaminated natural water supplies in rivers and dams and to persuade them to boil or chlorinate drinking water, to apply personal hygiene and to dispose of faeces in proper latrines. In rainy seasons people are advised to collect rainwater to replace the infected source from rivers. The people are persuaded not to drink from streams or rivers, free water being supplied during epidemics from tankers in many areas (see below).

Since the beginning of the cholera epidemics there has been close liaison with the mass media so that the public has been kept informed about the nature of preventive measures, the progression of the epidemic, as well as the containment measures applied. This was part of the health education drive of the department which also included health education bills, pamphlets, posters, books and audio-visual teaching material. Local initiative by private individuals and groups was encouraged and assisted. In the more remote areas of Natal, the anti-cholera publicity campaign was conducted with the aid of a light aircraft and a public address system.

Secondary prevention of cholera

Early recognition of a cholera outbreak is accomplished by: surveillance of all diarrhoeal cases in cholera endemic areas. Known cases are notified to the Department of Health. Community health workers should keep records of all cases of diarrhoea. A record must be kept of any increase in the number or severity of cases, or severe dehydration, or death from diarrhoea in a person over 10 years of age. If cholera is suspected, stool specimens or rectal swabs from suspected cases must be sent to the laboratory for confirmation. In cholera endemic areas all gastro-enteritis cases should be treated as potential cholera cases.

Signs and symptoms

Patients and carriers should be promptly referred for treatment. Cholera is characterised by violent diarrhoea of sudden onset with 'rice-water' stools (without faecal odour, blood or pus), amounting to approximately 10 litres or more per day (as much as 1 litre per hour), muscular cramps, effortless vomiting and rapid dehydration with low urinary output, sunken cheeks and eyes, diminished skin turgor, hypotension and rapid, weak pulse. The temperature is normal and there is no bacteraemia. The patient suffers from acidosis, hypotension, hypokalaemia and haemoconcentration. Without treatment the duration of non-fatal cholera is 3–5 days.

The great outpouring of fluid is due to a vibrial enterotoxin formed in the small intestine; there is no acute inflammatory reaction and the bowel wall is not damaged. The vibrios can be detected in the faeces and a specific serum agglutination test will confirm the diagnosis.

If the dehydration is adequately treated (e.g. intravenous isotonic saline and sodium bicarbonate) and the hypokalaemia controlled, the patient soon recovers. Tetracycline (40 mg/kg/d for 2 days) and oral fluids are administered as soon as the patient stops vomiting. Mortality is high, up to 20–80 % when medical facilities are inadequate, but with rapid treatment the death-rate can be reduced to 1 % (as was the case during the South African epidemics). Before 1930 cholera epidemics regularly claimed more than 300 000 lives per year in India.

Cholera carriers, i.e. asymptomatic or subclinical infected cases, should be isolated and treated with a tetracycline until rectal swabs are negative. The long-acting tetracycline, doxycycline, was used in the gold-mines outbreak. It was given, one daily, for 5 days. Doxycycline concentrates in the bile and faeces and is minimally excreted by the kidneys — an advantage in hot climates where dehydration takes place due to heavy sweating. Other antimicrobial agents used are: chloramphenicol, co-trimoxazole.

Medical measures taken to cope with cholera epidemics in rural areas in Natal (1981–1983)

The onslaught against the cholera epidemics was waged as a co-operative effort between the health departments of the three tiers of government.

As in any major disaster, the help of the SA Defence Force Medical Services was called in. National servicemen, including doctors, rendered emergency services.

Emergency hospitals using army tents were set up in KwaZulu. Half the many thousands of cholera cases were treated in emergency rehydration centres by nursing staff of the health departments of the RSA and KwaZulu. It was seldom necessary to hospitalise patients as early rehydration meant early discharge (same day) from the centres. Health teams went into the community to locate all suspected cholera cases so that they could be taken to the rehydration centres before they became dangerously dehydrated. Treated patients, in turn, brought their ill contacts for treatment, or treated their unaffected contacts with tetracyclines (issued by the rehydration centres).

Primary health care teams at one stage manned 680 cholera points in Natal. Pockets of infection were thus cleared up, enabling the rehydration centres to move to new localities where the disease was rampant.

Every available school in the afflicted areas was turned into a clinic. There were also a number of mobile clinics which could be moved rapidly to areas where they were needed. Pharmacists and army doctors were called in to help the State Health teams man the emergency rehydration centres and dispense chlorine and health-educative aids.

Staff members protected themselves solely by good personal hygiene and by avoiding contaminated water and food.

DYSENTERY IN OLDER CHILDREN AND ADULTS

(For Acute Infantile Diarrhoea, see Chapter 24.)

Dysentery is defined as diarrhoea with blood and mucus in the stools, the large intestine being the site of pathology.[7] Blood and mucus does not always accompany the diarrhoea.

Causes of dysentery

Infective

Bacterial

- *Shigella* — the cause of the so-called bacillary dysentery (shigellosis).

  The cause of severe bacillary dysentery is the *Shigella*, either *Sh. dysenteriae* or *flexneri*; mild bacillary dysentery in temperate climates is caused by *Sh. sonnei*. Shigellosis is characterised by the carrier conditions in *Sh. flexneri* and *sonnei* infections.
- *Salmonella*, usually *S. typhimurium*
- Entero-invasive *Escherichia coli*
- *Campylobacter jejuni*
- *Yersinia enterocolitica*. Only 5 % of cases have dysentery, the main locus of infection being the terminal ileum.

Parasitic

- *Entamoeba histolytica* (amoebiasis)
- Bilharziasis (see p. 624).

Non-infective

- *Inflammatory bowel disease* (Crohn's disease, ulcerative colitis)
- *Neoplasms* of the large bowel
- *Purgative and irradiation colitis*

Common signs and symptoms of bacterial dysentery

Following a variable incubation period there is pyrexia and tachycardia. Within 24 hours the patient has moderate diarrhoea, with tenesmus and colic and sometimes vomiting. Blood and mucus in stools is present in less than half of cases.

In severe cases mucosal sloughs may be passed and the patient become dehydrated and prostrated.

Serious complications are rare: paralytic ileus and toxic dilatation of the colon (megacolon), perforation and haemorrhage.

Most cases of dysentery are mild and self-limiting within a week.

Spread

The prevalence of infective dysentery gives an indication of the standard of hygiene and sanitation of a community. The infection is disseminated by water, fomites, flies, fingers, from the faeces of the carrier or sufferer, to the mouth of the person to be infected. Poor toilet facilities in, for example, schools can be the cause of epidemics. Because the hand/oral route of infection is of paramount importance in bacterial dysentery, the washing of hands before touching food or drink is the most important single measure to prevent infection.

Diagnostic tests common to all bacterial dysenteries:

(1) Microscopic examination of stools including culture.
(2) Proctoscopy and rectal examination.
(3) Where the diagnosis is in doubt, a sigmoidoscopy with biopsy of rectal mucosa is done.

Treatment of bacterial dysenteries

(1) Oral rehydration.
(2) In uncomplicated cases food is not withheld.
(3) Inhibition of intestinal motility with either diphenoxylate (Lomotil) or loperamide (Imodium).
(4) Most cases do not require antimicrobial therapy, but in severe cases the following antimicrobial agents may be prescribed.
    – Shigellosis: ampicillin, tetracycline or co-trimoxazole.
    – *Campylobacter jejuni:* erythromycin.
    – *Yersinia enterocolitica*: tetracycline or co-trimoxazole.
(5) Shigellosis carriers must be identified and treated.

Reiter's syndrome

This post-dysenteric syndrome has been associated with *Shigella, Yersinia* and *Campylobacter* infections.

It comprises:

▨ Ocular inflammation (either conjunctivitis or anterior uveitis) which may precede the dysentery.
▨ Arthritis of large proximal joints, frequently only one. Arthritis suddenly follows the dysentery and resolves slowly and completely over months.
▨ Urethritis.

Reiter's syndrome may possibly be due to an auto-allergic hypersensitivity.

AMOEBIC DYSENTERY (AMOEBIASIS)

Amoebiasis is an infection with the *Entamoeba histolytica*, either in a latent or a clinical form.

The *Entamoeba histolytica* is a protozoan whose sole host is the human being. Human beings become infected by ingestion of the cystic form of the parasite — four nuclei enclosed by a tough cyst wall. In the small intestine, excystation takes place, i.e. four trophozoites are liberated when the cyst wall breaks down. In the large intestine, the trophozoites invade the bowel wall and cause ulceration. Some are absorbed and taken to the liver and lungs. In the lumen of the bowel trophozoites reproduce themselves by binary fission. Some are passed in diarrhoea stools and are soon destroyed, while others encyst in the bowel, i.e. they secrete tough cell walls and two consecutive mitoses produce four nuclei — the future trophozoites. In this cystic form amoebae are passed in semi-formed and formed stools. The cystic form of the amoeba, therefore, is infective when it is excreted in the faeces; it remains viable for a month in a damp medium, e.g. water.

The usual three sites where the amoeba may be found are in the lumen and in the wall of the large bowel, and in the liver.

Pleuropulmonary and pericardial amoebiasis is also known and is secondary to an amoebic liver abscess which extends through the diaphragm to thoracic organs. Only carriers and sufferers who are asymptomatic when the disease is in remission are infectious as they excrete the resistant cystic form of the amoeba in their faeces. Amoebae in the stools of patients with diarrhoea and bowel ulceration, called trophozoites, do not encyst; they die rapidly when liquid stool is passed. The sick patient is, therefore, not an infection hazard. Amoebic cysts survive for 5 minutes on the skin, for 45 minutes under nails and for weeks in water, even if it contains a normal level of chlorine.

The cysts, which give rise to amoebiasis when ingested, are spread by:

(1) carriers with poor personal habits who handle food;
(2) water contaminated by infected sewage;
(3) vegetables contaminated by:
    (*a*) infected night soil applied to crops just before harvesting;

(*b*) raw salads washed with contaminated water;

(4) flies and cockroaches which can contaminate food with their excreta and vomitus;

Note: Man is infected only by human faeces.

(5) direct person-to-person transmission in the family group and in closely associated neighbours.

Prevalence: Amoebiasis occurs in 10 % of the world's population, all over the world, irrespective of climatic conditions. It predominates in the tropics merely because that is where most of the developing nations live, with poor conditions of hygiene and sanitation and polluted water supplies. Epidemics are caused by gross contamination of water supplies with faeces of carriers and non-symptomatic patients who excrete the cysts of the *entamoeba histolytica.*

Primary prevention

(1) As for all enteric infections: improved standards of personal and environmental hygiene with regard to sanitation, water supplies and pest eradication.

(2) Sero-epidemiological surveys should be done in endemic areas to trace pathogenic *E. histolytica* excretors and subject them to treatment.[9]

(3) Known carriers and patients in remission must be prevented from handling food for public consumption and contaminating the water supplies of the community.

Secondary prevention

1. Early detection

Early detection of carriers and sufferers and asymptomatic infected persons. Diagnosis is confirmed by:

(1) A serological test (e.g. Serameba, Ames). A positive test indicates that the amoebae have been or are in the bowel wall.

(2) Motile amoebae containing red cells; they are found in the warm, fresh, liquid stools of patients with dysentery; trophozoites may be found in faeces or in cytology of biopsy specimens.

(3) Cysts found in the formed stools of patients in remission. The stool must be fresh and warm, preferably taken at the laboratory. As the cysts are excreted intermittently, many specimens of stool may need to be examined.

(4) The pus from a liver abscess may or may not contain amoebae (trophozoites). To confirm diagnosis of amoebiasis, stools must be examined at the same time.

(5) Liver scan to detect a liver abscess (by radioisotope, CT or ultrasound).

(6) Sigmoidoscopy to detect amoebic ulcers in the sigmoid colon and rectum. In fulminant dysentery ulcers are confluent and covered by a black slough. The bowel is very friable and perforates easily.

Patients with amoebic dysentery present with the following symptoms. Chronic dysentery with blood and mucus in liquid stools with minimal systemic upset; this may last a few days to several weeks, simultaneous diarrhoea and pyrexia being intermittent. Dysentery may be followed by hepatitis and liver abscess — sometimes characterised by the coughing up of bloodstained purulent ('anchovy sauce') sputum. The disease may be fatal, due to complications.

Causes of death: perforation of the colon, ruptured liver abscess with peritonitis, fulminant amoebic colitis with necrosis of caecum.

2. Prompt referral

Prompt referral and adequate treatment of patients with dysentery in order to ensure complete elimination of amoebae from the intestine, thus preventing the development of the carrier condition or of complications.

Treatment will attack the three sites (lumen, bowel wall and liver) where amoebae are found:

(1) Amoebicides such as metronidazole, tetracycline, chloroquine and tinidazole (Fasigyn).
   – Metronidazole (e.g. Flagyl) is given either orally for 5 days or by IVI where oral therapy is not possible.
   – Metronidazole plus tetracycline are currently used in amoebic dysentery; metronidazole plus chloroquine are used in amoebic liver abscess.

(2) A liver abscess is aspirated; an effusion into the pericardial sac is aspirated before suppuration takes place.

Note the role of emetine in amoebiasis. Emetine is the oldest amoebicide; it is a highly effective tissue amoebicide but is severely toxic to the myocardium. In combination with metronidazole, it is given intramuscularly for no longer than 10 days (as a single course) for severely ill patients, under ECG control and at complete bed-rest. Emetine may also be combined with chloroquine.

Dosage schedule of drugs used for amoebiasis[8]

DRUG	ROUTE	ADULT DOSE	CHILDREN'S DOSE
Metronidazole	Oral	800 mg t.d.s. for 5 days	50 mg/kg/day in 3 divided doses for 5 days.
Tinidazole	Oral	2 g/day for 5 days	60 mg/kg/day for 5 days.
Emetine hydrochloride	Intramuscular	60 mg/day for 10 days (max. daily dose)	1 mg/kg/day for 10 days.
Chloroquine	Oral	300 mg base b.d. for 1 day followed by 150 mg b.d. for 20 days	10 mg/kg/day for 21 days.
Tetracycline	Oral	250 mg q.i.d. for 10 days	Should not be used.

REFERENCES

(1) Sommerville PC, *et al.* The Widal Test in the diagnosis of typhoid fever in the Transvaal. *S Afr Med J* 1981; **59**: 851.

(2) Küstner HGV, Van Wyk JE, Steinberg WJ, Collie A. Widal testing for typhoid. *S Afr Med J* 1987; **72**: 511.

(3) Jacobs MR, *et al. S Afr Med J* 1978; **54**: 434.

(4) Isaäcson M, *et al. S Afr Med J* 1974; **48**: 2557.

(5) New Directions. *The Wits Review.* April 1989.

(6) Department of National Health and Population Development. *Epidemiological Comments* Oct. 1986; **13**: 10.

(7) Solomon EJ. Dysentery. *S Afr J Cont Med Educ* 1983; **1**: 19–22.

(8) Simjee AE. Amoebiasis. *Medicine International* July 1984.

(9) Gathiram V, Jackson TFHG. A longitudinal study of asymptomatic carriers of pathogenic zymodemes of Entamoeba histolytica. *S Afr Med J* 1987; **72**: 669–672.

(10) *Fast Facts.* South African Institute of Race Relations April 1994, No 4.

TEST OF KNOWLEDGE

The student has benefited from reading this chapter if he/she can answer the following questions:

(1) Define the following:
  – Salmonellosis
  – Amoebiasis
  – Reiter's syndrome
  – Shigellosis

(2) Write notes on the following:
  – The carrier condition in typhoid fever.
  – The Widal agglutination test.

(3) Discuss the manner of spread and the primary preventive measures which the following disease conditions have in common: typhoid, cholera, bacterial dysentery, amoebic dysentery.

(4) Discuss the history and epidemiology of cholera in Southern Africa.

37

Vector-borne Diseases

INTRODUCTION

In this chapter tropical diseases, some of them zoonoses and others, e.g. malaria, human diseases, are discussed. All have in common the fact that they can be spread by bloodsucking arthropods such as mosquitoes, lice, fleas and ticks. Some of the diseases, e.g. pneumonic plague and viral haemorrhagic fevers (VHFs), can also be spread directly from man to man or from animal carcasses to man.

The VHFs are highly contagious, do not respond to chemotherapy, and have a high fatality rate, but do not give rise to carrier conditions in man; they lend themselves, moreover, to stringent control by isolation. To date epidemics have been avoided by so-called 'containment' nursing. Passage of the virus through man (who can be secondarily infected) attenuates it, i.e. causes the disease in a mild form.

The student is introduced to the concept of stringent isolation by full containment nursing of viral haemorrhagic diseases which constitute medical disasters; the student is referred to Norma Paverd's comprehensive protocol for nursing patients with Crimean-Congo haemorrhagic fever (one of the VHFs) in a hospital setting. Hospitalisation in academic hospitals with special facilities for containment nursing is mandatory for all patients with VHFs.

Some of the diseases discussed in this chapter, viz. plague, trypanosomiasis, yellow fever, typhus fever, relapsing fever, Lassa fever, Dengue fever and Ebola fever do not occur in South Africa at present; they are included because most of them are none the less notifiable medical conditions; their arthropod vectors are endemic to South Africa; therefore the possibility of their occurrence exists. Constant vigilance is necessary to prevent outbursts of these diseases.

On the other hand, malaria is posing a well-nigh insuperable control problem in the north-eastern Transvaal and northern KwaZulu/Natal, despite a most comprehensive malaria control programme maintained by the Department of Health. The problem is caused by the 'importation' of infected mosquitoes and migrant workers as well as strains of chloroquine-resistant plasmodia from beyond South Africa's northern borders. Malaria differs from the VHFs in that it is not a zoonosis but a human disease. A chronic human carrier population with parasitaemia exists in Africa south of the Sahara. The anopheles vectors of the plasmodium know no international barriers. For the eradication of malaria the co-operation of all countries in the world in which it is endemic is needed. Eradication is one of the aims of the World Health Organisation (WHO).

IN THIS CHAPTER

TABLE 1
Vectors: their agents and resulting diseases

VECTORS[2]	INFECTIOUS AGENTS	DISEASE

Anopheles mosquito
  gambiae
  funestus
  arabiensis
	Plasmodia	Malaria

A. funestus	*Wuchereria bancrofti* (a filiarial worm)	Filiariasis (elephantiasis)
Culex mosquito	Bunyavirus (arbovirus)	Rift Valley fever
Aedes aegypti mosquito *Aedes albopictus*	Flavivirus (arbovirus) Flavivirus (dengue type I)	Yellow fever Dengue fever
Tsetse fly (glossina)	Trypanosomes	Sleeping sickness (Trypanosomiasis)
Rat flea	Yersinia pestis Rickettsia	Bubonic plague Endemic (murine) typhus
Body louse (Pediculus humanus)	Borrelia recurrentis Rickettsia prowazekii	Relapsing fever Epidemic typhus
Hard ticks Hyalomma (bont-legged)	Bunyavirus (arbovirus)	Crimean-Congo fever
Amblyomma	Rickettsia (rickettsii)	Rocky Mountain spotted fever (tick-borne typhus)
Tick larvae	Rickettsia conorii	Tick-bite fever
Soft ticks	Borrelia duttoni	Relapsing fever

VECTOR-BORNE DISEASES

A vector is an arthropod which transfers an infectious agent (arbovirus, protozoon, rickettsia or bacterium) from an infected to a susceptible host.[1]

Source of definition: Centres for Disease Control, Atlanta, Georgia, USA.

An arthropod is a small animal with segmented body and jointed limbs, e.g. insects (mosquitoes, biting flies, fleas, lice) and arachnida (spiders, ticks, mites).[1]

MALARIA

Malaria is an acute tropical, protozoal disease which is a major health hazard in developing countries. Malaria has been a notifiable medical condition in the RSA since 1956, notification being based on microscopic proof.[3]

Eradication measures have been successful in 36 developed countries with a population of 193 million. Developing countries like those of Africa do not have the means to initiate extensive eradication programmes. In Africa malaria continues to be the most widespread infection; it is estimated to affect 88 million Africans south of the Sahara at one time and cause a million

deaths a year, mainly among infants and young children. Malaria is a serious handicap to socio-economic progress in Africa.

When DDT was introduced in 1942, a very successful mass malaria control programme was undertaken by the Union Health Department so that malaria was nearly eradicated from South Africa between 1960 and 1966. Large tracts of rich farm lands in the north-eastern Transvaal were opened up and attracted thousands of workers. Since 1967, however, malaria has once again become endemic in these areas, the malaria problem being exacerbated by the influx of infected refugees and workers from Mozambique, good rainy seasons and the large-scale irrigation of crops.

As it is virtually impossible to eradicate malaria in South Africa, large-scale malaria control measures will remain permanently in operation, becoming more and more extensive in order to cover the areas from which migrants come. Patients are presenting themselves for diagnosis and treatment at medical centres far removed from the malaria endemic districts. Malaria sufferers can be found in any part of South Africa, but a history can usually be elicited of a recent visit to an endemic area. The

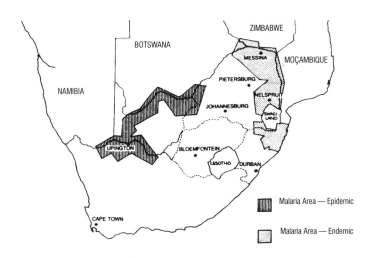

Figure 37.1

Epidemic and endemic malaria-infected areas in the RSA

patient will sometimes admit that his malaria prophylactic measures were not carried out as recommended but at other times these measures have been followed conscientiously, failure being due to the resistance of the plasmodium to chloroquine. Movement of people in and out of malaria areas, especially migrant African workers from neighbouring uncontrolled areas, as well as the unintended transportation of infected mosquitoes in vehicles coming from these areas, make the task of the health educators and the anti-malaria workers an extremely difficult one.

Epidemiology of malaria in the RSA

Endemicity

Malaria is endemic (present throughout the year) in the warm, humid, low-lying areas of the north-eastern corner of the RSA (northern and eastern Transvaal) as well as in the coastal areas of northern KwaZulu/Natal, north of Richard's Bay. Sporadic, small outbreaks may also occur in the Upington-Kakamas area and around the Kuruman and Molopo rivers in the Northern Cape, north of the Orange River.

In endemic areas, clinical malaria is confined to young children, as adults are usually immune with asymptomatic, low-grade parasitaemia (prevalence of 25 %) and enlarged spleen. If attacks of malaria occur in adults, they are mild. People with parasitaemia (either relatively immune carriers or untreated patients with mild or acute attacks of malaria) form the reservoir of infection. Untreated patients remain infective for a month after they are clinically free of malaria. Acquired immunity is mediated by immunoglobulins (antibodies) which are also found in the blood of neonates of an immune mother for the first few months of life.

The malaria endemicity of a region is found by obtaining the prevalence rate as follows:

(1) The percentage of children aged 2 to 9 years with enlargement of the spleen. This is called the spleen rate.

(2) The prevalence of parasitaemia by age (age-specific rates). This is done by counting the parasites on stained thick blood smears from each person in the sample. These rates are high in young children (who have not yet developed immunity) and fall off to a rate of 25 % in adults.

Incidence

The incidence rate of malaria in blacks (1987) in endemic areas is three times that of whites.

Most endemic areas have a clear seasonality with highest prevalence from November to May and lowest in the period June to September.[3] Prophylaxis is advisable from December to

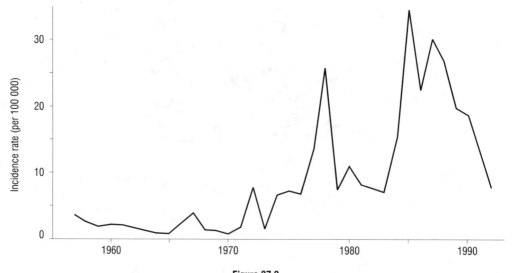

Figure 37.2

Incidence of malaria
Source: *Epidemiological Comments* 1994; **21** (3)

June. The case-fatality rate (CFR) in the RSA is less than 1 % per annum.[3]

Epidemics of malaria occur when the environmental temperature is correct (optimum 27°C), the air is humid and there are pools and streams of water.

Malaria epidemics in endemic areas occur regularly. They started in 1972 with 1790 notified cases, the number increasing annually to reach 7 103 in 1978, 11 358 in 1985, 10 449 in 1987, 6 880 in 1989 and 11 574 in 1993. In the northern Cape, after unusually heavy rains in 1988, 37 cases were notified; during the previous 17 years only 66 cases had been reported in this area.[4]

Many cases of malaria are imported into the region of notification, e.g. Free State, Gauteng, Cape. Migrant labourers from Mozambique form approximately one third of the cases notified in the north-eastern parts of the RSA.

Other causes of the steady upsurge of malaria is the increased drug resistance of the Plasmodium spp. to chloroquine and the increasing inability to control vectors (mosquitoes). *An. arabiensis* remains susceptible to DDT, but because it also bites outdoors, contact with the insecticide is reduced.

The plasmodium

Malaria is caused by a protozoon, the plasmodium, of which there are four kinds: the pernicious, *P. falciparum* and the benign *P. vivax, P. malariae* and *P. ovale*. The vector of the plasmodium is the *anopheles* mosquito.

Over 98 % of South African malaria infections are due to the *P. falciparum*[3] which is the aetiological agent in cerebral malaria and black water fever. The benign forms of malaria, rarely seen in South Africa, may be either tertian (sudden rise of temperature with rigor every 48 hours) or quartan (the same signs every 72 hours). These acute manifestations of malaria coincide with the entry of millions of parasites into the blood from the lysed (burst) erythrocytes. The periodicity of falciparum temperature peaks vary. In mixed plasmodia infections the patient may have a rigor every day while infection lasts.

Falciparum malaria may flare up after apparent recovery if therapy is ineffectual (see

chloroquine-resistant infections). This flare-up is called recrudescence. The benign forms of malaria may relapse, i.e. occur again after clinical cure at a time when the patient's immunity is lowered, if a radical cure has not been effected (see next page).

Life cycle of the plasmodium

In its life cycle, the parasite passes through different stages: the *asexual stage* takes place in human blood and the *sexual stage* in the body of the anopheles mosquito. The immature sporocytes of the plasmodium are injected into man when the mosquito bites him to suck his blood. During the incubation period of malaria, the sporocytes multiply in the liver and change into primary schizonts (schizogony) which mature and rupture, each one releasing hundreds of merozoites. These enter the erythrocytes and multiply there, 20 % of erythrocytes being affected thus in severe infections. Multiplication, which lasts 2 to 3 days, once more includes schizogony, the mature schizonts rupturing to release merozoites which in turn invade other erythrocytes. The breaking up of the mature schizonts releases substances which cause the characteristic attacks of pyrexia. The characteristic structure of the merozoite in the erythrocyte is the annular (ring-shaped) schizont, the presence of which is diagnostic of malaria when a blood smear is examined under the microscope. Some merozoites (of the *P. vivax, P. malariae* and the *P. ovale*) return to the liver to form the source of infection during a relapse at a later stage. This does not occur in *P. falciparum* infections.

The insect vector of the plasmodium is the *anopheles* mosquito which serves as the definitive host for completing the sexual reproductive cycle of the plasmodium. Untreated patients with parasitaemia infect the bloodsucking female mosquito. In the stomach of the mosquito the male and female gametes mate to form oocytes which give rise to sporocytes. These in turn migrate to the salivary glands of the mosquito to be injected into man, the intermediate host, when the mosquito sucks blood.

Chloroquine resistance in *P. falciparum*

Chloroquine is the most commonly used anti-malarial drug. Until 1984, South African-acquired malaria was 100 % sensitive to chloroquine treatment and prophylaxis, although drug-resistant plasmodium mutants had appeared north of its borders for some years. These resistant strains are now (1990) present in 14 % of malaria patients in northern KwaZulu/Natal. The resistant strain was brought in by migrants from Mozambique. In north-eastern Transvaal the problem is much smaller — less than 1 % of falciparum infections. The benign forms of plasmodia have not yet developed resistance to chloroquine.

The chance of South African mosquitoes being infected with drug-resistant strains by migrants is very great. Chloroquine-resistant falciparum malaria is a serious community health problem. Chloroquine-resistant infections respond to a single dose (3 tablets) of Fansidar (pyrimethamine-sulphadoxine) which is, however, used only for therapy, i.e. not for prophylaxis, because of the danger of severe or fatal skin reactions.

Note: Chloroquine resistance is suspected if a visitor to an endemic area develops malaria despite satisfactory chloroquine prophylaxis.

The mosquito vectors

Malaria infection is carried from man to man by the anopheles mosquitoes. The formerly common mosquito vectors, *A. gambiae* and to a lesser extent *A. funestus*, are endemic in tropical and subtropical climates with a liberal summer rainfall, viz. the north-eastern Transvaal lowveld, coastal areas of northern KwaZulu/Natal and in Africa, south of the Sahara. Changes have recently taken place within the vector community. The *A. gambiae* has been replaced by the *A. arabiensis* as the main vector of malaria. The *A. gambiae* has almost been eradicated by the spraying of huts in endemic areas with DDT.

In contrast to the *A. gambiae*, the *A. arabiensis* bites as readily outside as inside huts and houses.[7] Although its period of contact with DDT is reduced, it remains fully susceptible to DDT.

The female *Anopheles* mosquitoes feed on the blood of humans and, to a lesser extent,

animals, some preferring to rest on the inside of human dwellings and others habitually resting outdoors. The breeding habits of the mosquitoes differ, *A. gambiae* laying their eggs in warm pools left by summer rainstorms and *A. funestus* preferring the reed-shaded water along banks of rivers. Less is known about the habits of the *A. arabiensis*.

The *Anopheles* female mosquito lays single eggs which hatch in 2 to 3 days in warm weather into larvae, also called wrigglers because they actively jerk their bodies through the water. They feed on small plants and animals that live in the water and breathe through a tube-like siphon situated at the rear of their bodies, the opening projecting slightly above the surface of the water. When breathing, their bodies lie parallel to the surface (thus distinguishing them from the larvae of the *Culex* mosquito). They grow quickly and moult four times in 4–10 days after which they change into pupae. A pupa looks like a comma and is mobile, breathing through a trumpet-shaped tube which protrudes above the surface of the water. It does not eat and changes into an adult mosquito in 2 to 4 days, when the pupal shell splits to allow the mosquito to creep out. An adult mosquito flies for short distances only, usually within a radius of 1,6 km from the place where it was hatched. The *Anopheles* mosquito rests in the tail-in-the-air position, in contrast to the *Culex* mosquito which rests with its body parallel to the surface. The female of the *Anopheles* must suck blood before she can lay eggs that will hatch. The female *A. gambiae* rests inside dwellings for 2–3 days after sucking blood while digesting the blood and developing a new batch of eggs. This gives ample time for DDT to act. Females may live 30 days or longer but the males which feed on vegetable matter live for only 10 to 20 days.

Vector control

Anti-malaria measures are the following.

1. Eradication of larvae

The eradication of mosquito larvae and pupae in high-density living areas where water suitable for breeding is limited.

(1) Insecticides which are relatively non-toxic, e.g. organophosphorus compounds, are applied weekly to kill larvae present at the time of application.

   Note: DDT and BHC are not used for this purpose, because of the danger of environmental pollution. Their use for this purpose is prohibited.

(2) Originally oil, combined with spreading agents, was sprayed weekly on breeding water surfaces (dams, tanks, banks of rivers) to suffocate the larvae and pupae. Oil is no longer used for mass vector control.

   Note: Weekly larvicidal control measures are not always feasible in rural areas.

(3) Breeding places can be destroyed by filling in the hollows in rocks near river banks and draining swamps to reduce the size of breeding sites.

2. Killing of mosquitoes

Mosquitoes are killed by spraying the inside of walls and roofs of dwellings with residual insecticides. Residual contact insecticides are the chlorinated hydrocarbon chemicals (DDT, BHC) that remain effective for 3 to 6 months when they dry on surfaces and are ingested by the mosquitoes which die at a later stage. Spraying is very effective in endemic rural areas where one million structures are sprayed annually, sometimes twice and even three times in certain areas if and when the need arises.

Adult mosquito control is practised throughout the year. It is the most important preventive measure in view of the growing resistance of the plasmodium to chemotherapy.

The type of insecticide used, its strength and the type of wall surface determine the duration of its effectiveness, e.g.:

Organochlorides. DDT at 2g/m^2 metre lasts 6–12 months. BHC at 0,3 g/m^2 lasts 3 months.

Organophospates. Malathion at 2 g/m^2 lasts 3 months. Fenitrothion at 0,7 g/m^2 metre lasts 2–3 months.[9]

Spraying teams of the Department of Health visit every house and hut in malaria endemic areas regularly to maintain effective vector control. Before a dwelling is sprayed on the inside, all household belongings must be removed. This applies especially to food and cooking utensils.

Ingestion of chlorinated hydrocarbon (organochloride) insecticides has potentially dangerous long-term effects on human beings as they are indestructible. For this reason they are not procurable for ordinary household purposes. The insecticides are used only inside the huts and under the eaves.

DDT is used on wattle-and-daub huts and houses and organophosphates on 'western-type' houses.

Householders can use safer 'knock-down' pyrethrum insecticides to free a room of mosquitoes during periods of risk.

Resistance of the *A. gambiae* to organochloride insecticides has been encountered in most malaria regions of the world. In the RSA, control based on DDT house-spraying continues to be satisfactory.[10]

The spraying of dwellings does not completely destroy the mosquito population because the mosquitoes which feed on man and animals outdoors are not eradicable as they cannot be reached by the insecticides.

Note: The *An. arabiensis* feeds on human beings inside and outside the dwellings.

The human factor is very important in malaria control measures; unenlightened persons who are relatively immune to malaria and do not fear the disease because they get it in a mild form, do not take necessary precautions to keep mosquitoes from biting them, thus reinfecting the mosquito population and maintaining the life cycle of the plasmodium.

Spraying teams have found that in huts infested with bedbugs, this pest becomes a greater nuisance after spraying with DDT which merely irritates the bug. Some people react by replastering their DDT sprayed walls to eliminate the effects of DDT (see p. 161), or they sleep out of doors. Thus spraying may have a negative effect in combating malaria if the bedbug problem is not eradicated by Karbaryl spraying.

If the transmission of malaria can be interrupted for several years, the parasite reservoirs will become depleted, i.e. relatively immune persons with parasitaemia will get cured of their parasitaemia by their own immune responses and reinfection will not occur.

3. Exclusion of contact

Contact of mosquitoes with the human skin is excluded by:

(1) mosquito-screening of dwellings;
(2) sleeping under mosquito nets;
(3) wearing clothes which cover the body as much as possible when going out at night, e.g. long-sleeved tops and trousers;
(4) not being outside in the dark without taking suitable precautions to ward off mosquitoes — the evening braai can be dangerous;
(5) using mosquito repellents on the naked skin if direct contact with mosquitoes is inevitable;
(6) mosquito insecticidal coils and vapour mats containing pyrethrum can be used indoors to release the insecticide continuously;
(7) perfumes and the wearing of light-coloured clothing should be avoided when going outside after dusk.

Malaria Control Programme (MCP)

This programme is run by the Department of Health.

The National Institute of Tropical Diseases (NITD), based in Tzaneen, Transvaal, acts as the central co-ordinating authority of the Department. Malaria research is conducted by the MRCs Research Institute for Diseases in a Tropical Environment (RIDTE) in Durban.

The Malaria Control Programme comprises five different strategies:[14]

(1) residual insecticide spraying;
(2) active surveillance;
(3) larviciding (larvae killing);
(4) epidemiological investigations;
(5) chemoprophylaxis.

The aim of the MCP[3] is to:

(1) prevent deaths from malaria and to reduce morbidity;
(2) anticipate and avert local outbreaks (epidemics) of malaria;
(3) reduce the amount of malaria in endemic areas.

The MCP's ultimate aim is to eradicate malaria. Theoretically eradication can be attained by finding all infected persons, treating them to render them non-infected at a particular point in time. Should this aim be achieved, anopheline mosquitoes would no longer be dangerous to man.

Note: The mosquito is not 'sick' with malaria. It merely carries the plasmodium from sick man (as the source of infection) to infection-susceptible man (man as victim), because the female mosquito needs blood for the maturation of her eggs. This she obtains by biting man and animals and, in so doing, introducing contaminated salivary gland secretions into the victim as she sucks his blood. Animals are not susceptible to the plasmodium, i.e. they are not a source of infection.

The organisation of the Malaria Control Programme

There are a number of subregions in endemic areas in which this programme operates.

Each subregion employs teams of field workers. Each team is supported and supervised by a field official (field officer) who also organises epidemiological investigations. The field officials are supervised by health inspectors who administer the MCP as part of their other duties. The MCP is financed by the Department of Health. The field teams are generally stationed on farms in high-risk areas and also in game parks. The teams are, therefore, domiciled in the community they serve and are able to visit high-risk areas 2–3 times per week. Transport is facilitated by the use of bicycles, the field officials using trucks to carry bulk materials and people. The field teams carry out the following duties: active surveillance, insecticidal spraying, larviciding, and epidemiological investigations.

Surveillance of malaria

This is a very important strategy of the MCP, the data thus obtained being used to introduce more effective ways of combating malaria. The term *active surveillance* refers to the screening of the population at risk for infection. Screening is done by house-to-house visits by field workers for case-finding, i.e. those with fever or a history of fever and newly arrived migrant workers have thick blood smears taken. If no 'cases' are found, some routine smears are taken from healthy persons to detect asymptomatic malaria carriers who can initiate an outbreak of malaria. Smears are examined by trained microscopists at the nearest laboratory, half a million blood smears being examined annually. Positive cases are entered into the malaria register. The case is reported to the field officer and notified to the regional health office by telephone or telex and from there by mail to the Epidemiology Unit in Pretoria.

The field officer will initiate an epidemiological investigation to determine the source of infection in each case. The cases suspected by the field workers of having a malaria infection are given presumptive treatment at the time of the first blood smear. This consists of four Darachlor (pyrimethamine plus chloroquine) tablets. After confirmation of positivity, a full course of 10 Darachlor tablets is given over a period of 4 days. A follow-up smear is done after 1–2 months to check the success of treatment. In this way chloroquine-resistant cases are detected and treated.[14]

The officer in charge of the field teams of a region (health inspector) moves from area to area inspecting laboratory reports on smears sent in by clinics and hospitals. This is called *passive surveillance*.

Epidemiological investigation[14]

This is initiated in response to a positive blood smear found on active or passive surveillance. By means of a Case Investigation Report, each case is questioned in detail to determine his/her movements prior to diagnosis, in order to pinpoint the probable place of infection, and whether it is local or imported.

Note: The regional health office in the endemic area where a patient contracted malaria must be notified if a patient is diagnosed outside an endemic area.

During an epidemiological investigation blood smears are taken of all inhabitants of adjacent dwellings. A knockdown vector count is also done on the house of the suspected source of infection as follows: the inside of the dwelling is sprayed with pyrethrum and all dropped insects are caught on a sheet spread on the floor. In this way a count of all resident insects is obtained. These insects are identified by the NITD. If anopheline mosquitoes are found in residual-insecticide-sprayed houses, the cause is sought. It will be due either to destruction of the layer of insecticide (see handling by inhabitants of bedbug nuisance) or to vector resistance to the insecticide used.

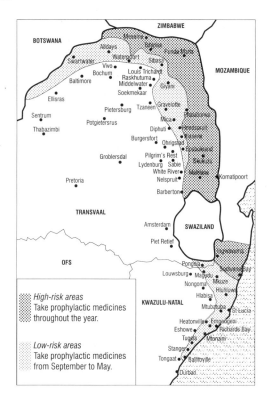

Figure 37.3

Areas where prophylactic medicines must be taken
Source: *Epidemiological Comments* 1994; **20** (4)

Prophylactic chemotherapy

No prophylaxis is ever completely safe. People who travel in endemic areas and are not taking prophylactic drugs for some reason or another, should carry stand-by treatment — a prescribed therapeutic dose of quinine (600 mg) or Fansidar (see p. 660) (3 tablets) so that they may treat themselves if they develop symptoms (fever, headache, backache or abdominal pain) of malaria where medical help is not immediately available. Medical help must be sought without delay.

Note: Porphyrics and those sensitive to sulpha drugs may not take Fansidar.

Visitors should take adequate precautions, especially at night, to prevent mosquito bites. The malaria transmission season is from September to May and even throughout the year. Visits should be arranged, where possible, for the dry seasons. The risk of contracting malaria

Suggested chemoprophylaxis for travellers within the RSA and to neighbouring African countries, 1993

Area	Malaria prevalence	Recommended drugs
Kruger Park Northern and Eastern Transvaal Lowveld Northern Natal Northern KwaZulu (except Ingwavuma and Ubombo districts)	*Low* During dry seasons (mainly June to October) and in years when rainfall is very low *High* During hot, wet seasons (mainly November to May)	High-risk persons: chloroquine Others: nothing chloroquine
Ingwavuma and Ubombo district	Throughout the year	chloroquine & proguanil (if available) doxycycline (if appropriate) mefloquine (on prescription only) nothing*
Swaziland	Throughout the year in lowveld areas	chloroquine & proguanil (if available) mefloquine (if appropriate and available) nothing*
Zimbabwe	Mainly November to June in areas below 1 200 m and throughout the year in Zambezi Valley	chloroquine & proguanil (if available) doxycycline (if appropriate) mefloquine (if appropriate and available) nothing*
Angola Comoros Kenya Madagascar Malawi Mozambique Zaire	Throughout the year	chloroquine & proguanil (if available) doxycycline (if appropriate) mefloquine (if appropriate and available) nothing*
Botswana	Mainly November to June in the northern parts of the country (e.g. Okavango)	chloroquine & proguanil (if available) doxycycline (if appropriate) mefloquine (if appropriate and available) nothing*
Namibia	Mainly November to June in northern rural areas (e.g. Ovambo, Kavango & Etosha)	chloroquine & proguanil (if available) doxycycline (if appropriate) mefloquine (if appropriate and available) nothing*
Zambia	Mainly November to June but throughout the year in the Zambezi Valley	chloroquine & proguanil (if available) doxycycline (if appropriate) mefloquine (if appropriate and available) nothing*
Seychelles	No malaria	
Mauritius	Only benign form of malaria in rural areas in the north	Prophylaxis is usually not necessary. Chloroquine may be recommended if travelling to rural areas.

* In situations where the risk of contracting malaria is low, (e.g. in cities, air-conditioned hotels or when rainfall has been low, etc.) the traveller may be advised to take no drug prophylaxis but stand-by treatment must be carried out unless medical care is readily available.

Note:
• The drugs are not necessarily in order of priority. Drug selection depends on each individual person's situation.
• If travelling to areas where no medical help is available, especially if no chemoprophylaxis is taken, travel with stand-by malaria treatment. If symptoms of malaria develop before leaving the malarious area, take stand-by treatment and seek medical help as soon as possible.

Source: Department of National Health and Population Development, *Malaria Prophylaxis — the South African Viewpoint*, January 1993.

is greater in the bush than in the towns, especially during the rainy season.

People who live in malaria endemic areas usually practise chemoprophylaxis only during periods of increased risk of contracting malaria.

Examples of high risks:

(1) occupation which involves being outside at night;
(2) good rainfall between February and April;
(3) poor physical health.

A mass chemoprophylaxis campaign for a particular community resident in an endemic region is carried out only if the community is at particularly high risk. It should be done in a limited period of time and 70 % of the population must be reached during the campaign.[3]

The global spread of drug-resistant *P. falciparum* has complicated malaria prophylaxis and treatment.

The table on p. 658 shows the malaria prophylaxis recommended for South African travellers.

The recommended dose of chloroquine is taken once a week, starting one week before entering the area, and continuing while in the area and for four weeks after leaving the area. Proguanil is taken daily instead of weekly, starting one day before entering the area and continuing as for chloroquine. Mefloquine is taken like chloroquine.

Pregnant women should be advised not to visit a malaria endemic area, especially not during the rainy season.

Breast-fed infants must be given their own oral prophylaxis.

Persons at high risk for severe malaria are pregnant women, babies and young children, the immunocompromised, the splenectomised and the elderly. High-risk persons should be advised not to visit malarious areas. Epileptic patients should be warned that drug prophylaxis may interfere with seizure control.

Measures to prevent mosquito bites remain the mainstay of prophylaxis, as no drug is 100 % effective.

Summary: MCP intervention measures

1. Man as the source of infection (secondary prevention)

(1) Case-finding by active surveillance.
(2) Confirmation of diagnosis by blood smear microscopy; 400 000 slides are examined annually by MCP microscopists to diagnose patients and asymptomatic carriers.
(3) Rendering the patient non-infectious by prompt and effective chemotherapy.
(4) Extending case-finding around the index patient.
(5) Epidemiological investigation of the source of infection.
(6) Screening all immigrants and treating those infected.
(7) Monitoring:
   – by active and passive surveillance;
   – locally acquired and imported infections;
   – of resistance to chloroquine and other antimalarials.
(8) Reducing the residual infectious load in winter months.
(9) Localised mass blood smear surveys.

2. The mosquito vector (primary prevention)

(1) Residual contact insecticide spraying of inside of dwellings.
(2) Targeted killing of mosquito larvae, especially near dwellings.
(3) Entomological (insect) surveillance by monitoring other possible vectors.
(4) Monitoring of vector resistance to DDT and effectiveness of larvicides.
(5) Potential breeding sites should be eliminated in and around human habitations, e.g. empty tins, pools of water, old gutters and tyres.

Man as victim (largely primary prevention)

(1) Health education — Education is aimed at making people aware that malaria is a preventable disease and they can take measures to protect themselves. Their co-operation with the malaria field teams is encouraged, especially with the case-finding teams.
(2) Protection against bites:
out of doors: long sleeves and trousers at night, rub-on repellants;
indoors: insect repellant sprays, gauzed windows and doors, mosquito nets for sleeping.

(3) Prophylactic treatment for all visitors from non-endemic areas.

(4) Prompt treatment when indicated.

(5) Monitoring of resistance to chloroquine and other antimalarials.

(6) Pregnant women: the disease is far more dangerous in pregnancy because of the depressed immune state. Prophylactic chloroquine when visiting an endemic area is, therefore, mandatory.

(7) Mass chemoprophylaxis only in emergencies, e.g. threat of a massive outbreak.[3]

Incubation period of malaria: 8–11 days.
It can be as long as: 4–6 weeks.

Diagnosis

The diagnosis of malaria should be considered in every person who has been in a malaria area for 10–30 days (incubation period) and is suffering from flu-like symptoms.

The signs and symptoms of malaria may resemble a number of pyrexial diseases. Pyrexia, rigor and headache are the usual presenting symptoms, but myalgia, arthralgia, jaundice, gastro-intestinal symptoms with dehydration and prostration, acute renal failure, delirium and coma, may confuse the picture and cause misdiagnoses to be made, especially if the patient is first seen by a doctor at some distance from a malarious area. The periodic fever, typical of tertian and quartan malaria, may be preceded by continuous fever for several days.

The temperature peaks of 40–41°C are followed within several hours by severe sweating and a fall in temperature. *P. falciparum* causes a pernicious (destructive) type of malaria infection, while the other kinds of plasmodium which rarely occur in South Africa are more benign.

Where there is any likelihood that a person has been exposed to infected mosquitoes, blood smears (one thin and one thick) — taken preferably when a patient is having a rigor — should be examined for the annular (ring-shaped) forms of the plasmodium. As these forms disappear periodically, a negative result does not mean that the patient is free from malaria; smears should be repeated several times a day, if the first results are negative.

A quantitative estimate of parasite density, by counting the parasites on stained thick blood smears, is made to help the doctor prescribe drug therapy wisely, e.g. quinine in cases of hyperparasitaemia. Parasitaemia is also monitored during therapy to assess the patient's response. If parasitaemia is not drastically reduced within 24–48 hours, the plasmodia are resistant to the antimalarial drug and therapy must be changed.

Therapeutic chemotherapy

If malaria is diagnosed early and effective treatment is started immediately, it is unlikely to progress to a life-threatening disease.

The aims of treatment are:

(1) to destroy all parasites in the blood and liver;

(2) to relieve the blockage of capillaries (e.g. of the glomerulus) in the malignant forms of the disease;

(3) to treat the anaemia.

Falciparum malaria, the cause of 98 % of malaria infections in the RSA, causes greater morbidity and mortality than the benign malarias which are, however, inclined to relapse if radical treatment is omitted. This may occur in mixed infections in which benign plasmodia are not diagnosed, e.g. *P. ovale* infections in Natal.

Serious complications (see p. 661) and chloroquine resistance cause major therapeutic problems.

Treatment of chloroquine-resistant malaria (see p. 654). In this case the schizonticides (drugs destroying the asexual schizonts) of choice are quinine (with or without antibiotics) and Fansidar.

In severe malaria where vomiting, coma or shock may preclude oral therapy, intravenous quinine is given, i.e. quinine dihydrochloride 600 mg in 500 ml saline or glucose by constant infusion over 4 hours, i.e. slowly. This is repeated every 8 hours until the patient can swallow. Then oral quinine sulphate 600 mg is given 8 hourly for 10–14 days.

The dose of intravenous quinine for children is 8–10 mg/kg, diluted in 10 ml fluid per kilogram. This is also run in over 4 hours and given 8-hourly.

Side-effects of quinine: cinchonism with deafness, tinnitus, giddiness, headache, blurred vision. These symptoms do not necessitate the stopping of therapy. Quinine may, however, cause many other adverse side-effects if used in toxic doses; moreover, rapid intravenous administration may lower the blood sugar drastically and cause death.

Note: Tetracycline and other antibiotics with weak antimalarial effects can be combined with the quinine.

Fansidar (pyrimethamine and sulphadoxine) three tablets together and once only, taken with lots of fluid, can be used as the sole drug in chloroquine-resistant malaria or be combined with quinine. It has many side-effects and is potentially lethal due to fatal cutaneous reactions.

Standard therapy of non-chloroquine-resistant malaria

This includes all types of malaria, i.e. pernicious and benign.

Adults:

Oral chloroquine base 600 mg (4 tablets) immediately, followed by 300 mg base (2 tablets) 6 hours later. This dose (2 tablets) is repeated daily to a total of 1 500 mg (10 tablets) after the initial large dose.[13]
OR
Oral chloroquine: 4 tablets on Day 1 and 2; 2 tablets on Day 3 in suitably divided doses.

Parenteral chloroquine: IMI 200–300 mg every 6 hours or IVI (over a period of not less than an hour) to a maximum of 800 mg in the first 24 hours, with conversion to oral therapy as soon as possible.[15] This is seldom necessary as quinine is the IV drug of choice.

Children:

Oral chloroquine: 25 mg base on days 1 and 2 and half this dose on day 3.[15]
Oral Darachlor: (pyrimethamine plus chloroquine).
Adults: 10 Darachlor tablets over a period of 4 days.[14]
There are many potential adverse effects of chloroquine, but serious problems are unlikely to occur.

Nausea, vomiting and diarrhoea are avoided by taking the drug with food and avoiding alcohol.

A regular parasitaemia check is kept. If the latter fails to abate, the patient is treated with either quinine and tetracycline or Fansidar.

Note: After successful treatment with chloroquine, *P. falciparum* takes 2 days to be cleared from the circulation.

The following medicines should be avoided in the treatment of severe falciparum malaria: steroids, dextran, heparin, urea, mannitol, prostacyclin, adrenaline.[13]

Radical cure of benign malaria

Falciparum infections are radically cured after effective treatment with chloroquine, quinine or Fansidar, but the benign infections caused by *P. vivax*, *P. malariae* and *P. ovale* develop resistant forms of merozoites during the course of the disease, which remain dormant in the liver while the antibodies and anti-malarial drugs are active against the parasites in the blood. The above drugs effect a clinical cure only and the dormant merozoites are responsible for recurrent malarial attacks (i.e. relapses) when the patient's resistance is lowered for some reason or another. Patients with benign infections must, therefore, receive primaquine in combination with the chloroquine, to eradicate all forms of the plasmodium and thus effect a radical cure. This medicine is a **malaria eradicating medicine**. The adult dosage is 15 mg primaquine (an 8-aminoquinoline) daily for 14 days.

Complications of falciparum malaria with hyperparasitaemia (5–10 %)[13]

As these serious complications may be fatal, the basic management is with intravenous quinine. The patient is often chloroquine-resistant and has not responded to chloroquine therapy.

(1) Cerebral malaria. The patient with malaria becomes lethargic and confused and lapses into coma. Depending upon which part of the brain has been affected, the patient may develop aphasia, paralysis or convulsions. Anticonvulsants and intensive nursing care are required. It carries a mortality of 20–50 %.

(2) Haemoglobinuria (black water fever). This is caused by massive intravascular haemolysis, blockage of the glomeruli, renal failure, jaundice and anaemia. Rehydration and blood transfusions may be neces-

sary; in cases of renal failure, dialysis is required.

(3) Acute pulmonary oedema occurs especially in pregnant women and those with cerebral malaria. The fluid balance must be maintained. Raising the head of the bed, diuresis, 100 % oxygen with positive pressure ventilation may be life-saving.

(4) Acute tubular necrosis with anuria. Fluid restriction and dialysis may be required.

(5) Hyperpyrexia must be treated by cooling the body and with non-aspirin antipyretics such as paracetamol.

(6) Severe haemolytic anaemia (haematocrit below 20 %) requires a packed cell transfusion or fresh whole blood with furosemide to prevent pulmonary oedema.

(7) Disseminated intravascular coagulopathy is treated with a platelet concentrate or transfusion of fresh frozen plasma.

(8) Gram-negative septicaemic shock ('algid malaria'). The patient becomes shocked and hypotensive. The shock may be due to massive blood loss (from a ruptured spleen) or hypoglycaemia but if these causes are excluded, the Gram-negative septicaemia probably arises from the gastro-intestinal

tract. Resuscitation and appropriate antibiotics may be life-saving.

PLAGUE

Plague is a zoonosis of wild rodents caused by the *Yersinia pestis*. It is transmitted from the infected rodents to man by the rat or wild rodent flea. Man is an incidental host in whom plague may spread rapidly if the route of transmission changes to an airborne one (pneumonic plague). The incubation period is 5–6 days.

Plague is well controlled in South Africa. The most recent plague epidemics in southern Africa occurred as follows:

- Ovamboland in 1963;
- Uitenhage district in 1967 (minor epidemic);
- Lesotho in 1968;
- Coega, Port Elizabeth, 1982.

In March 1982 there was an outbreak of bubonic plague at a missionary settlement of 80 people of Coega near Port Elizabeth. An *ad hoc* anti-plague committee of local, railways and state health authorities under chairmanship of the RD was formed to contain the epidemic. Health inspectors discovered a number of diseased rats in the settlement. Eighteen cases were notified

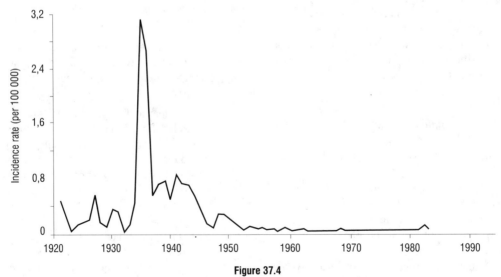

Figure 37.4

Incidence rate of plague
Source: *Epidemiological Comments* 1994; **21** (3)

and one man died of the disease. The entire settlement was placed under quarantine; houses were treated for fleas. The confinement of the plague epidemic to Coega by these prompt measures was a success.

Plague is, however, endemic (i.e. it is enzootic) in localised areas in southern Africa and in different parts of the world where there are pockets of wild rodents. These natural foci can give rise to sporadic cases in man and, if the population of domestic rats and mice in a city is not controlled, there is always the danger of an epizootic (epidemic amongst animals) which could pose a health threat to the human city-dwellers.

Three forms of plague occur:

(1) **pneumonic plague** spread by droplets from infected man to man;

(2) **bubonic plague**, characterised by bubos — swollen, infected regional lymph glands which drain the area where the *Y. pestis* has been introduced by the bite of the blood-sucking flea;

(3) **septicaemic plague** which rarely occurs and is a complication of bubonic plague.

The *Y. pestis* was responsible for the great epidemics which decimated the populations of Europe in the Middle Ages, e.g. the Black Death which raged in Europe from the fourteenth to the seventeenth century, and wiped out one-quarter of the European population in 1348. The epidemic of plague which raged in England in 1665 killed the inhabitants of entire villages and one-tenth of London's population of 460 000. The Fire of London, 1666, put an end to this epidemic, probably by killing off the black rats that were responsible for the epidemic.

Bubonic plague need not be a fatal disease today as it is easily curable with modern chemotherapy, especially the tetracyclines.

Unless an epidemic is raging, however, the diagnosis may be missed. An epidemic of fleas and dead rodents lying about, or a sudden decrease in rodent activity, should alert community health personnel to the possibility of an outbreak of plague, especially if the area in which it occurs is endemic for plague.

Primary prevention

Long-term control

(1) The endemic foci of plague must be kept under surveillance by community health authorities. A periodic rodent survey can be done to note the rate of natural rodent deaths and to detect the presence of *Y. pestis* in samples of the rodent population. Human serological surveys are done by collecting blood from a random sample of persons living in the endemic area, for plague antibody assays. The incidence of plague antibodies in a population gives an idea of the subclinical plague infections that occur in apparently healthy people. The higher the percentage of people with plague antibodies in an endemic area, the higher the population immunity and the less likely is the probability of an outbreak of plague.

(2) Vermin extermination forms part of a surveillance programme. In cities with 'rodent officers', rodents are controlled with rodenticides (Warfarin) and fleas with insecticides. In endemic areas, fleas are exterminated in gerbil burrows near human habitation, with zinc phosphide and DDT.

Note: A gerbil is a small wild rodent — a persistent source of plague infection.

(3) In cities and in endemic areas, dwellings must be rat-proofed and rubbish likely to harbour rodents must be removed.

Short-term control during an epidemic

(1) Anti-flea measures by the population, e.g. by the dusting of places where fleas congregate, e.g. carpets, with organophosphates, e.g. malathion.

Fleas usually remain on their natural hosts, i.e. different kinds of fleas infest dogs, cats, man and rodents, only the rat flea — and other closely related fleas found on wild rodents in Africa — transmitting plague. Fleas breed by laying small, white, oval eggs in the fur of the host animal. Eggs are shed and roll into tiny crevices where they hatch into tiny larvae which feed on scraps of organic matter. If the weather is damp and there is much food, the larvae pupate in 2 to 3 weeks, adult fleas emerging 2 weeks later, if the weather is hot. The rodent flea feeds on the blood of its host; if the host is infected with plague, the germs lie in its crop. When the rodent dies, the flea seeks a new host, which may be a human being if no rodents are available. It pierces the skin of its new host and vomits the bolus of germs which enter the bloodstream of the host, thus transmitting infection. Only then can the flea feed on the blood of its new host.

(2) Prophylactic treatment of people at risk in affected areas by:

  (a) daily sulphonamides until 1 week after the last contact with an infected person;

  (b) immunisation, the first dose of the vaccine being repeated after 10 days. The effects of immunisation last for 6 months.

Secondary prevention

Plague is still a notifiable disease.
Case-finding and diagnosis. Prompt hospitalisation and treatment of patients with antibiotics, e.g. tetracycline. Pneumonic plague is a man-to-man infectious disease which requires strict isolation care to prevent an outbreak of epidemic proportions.

TRYPANOSOMIASIS (SLEEPING SICKNESS)

Trypanosomiasis is an acute, formidable epidemic tropical disease, caused by the trypanosome which is not endemic in South Africa. The disease is endemic in tsetse fly areas, e.g. Angola, Zimbabwe and other tropical African countries. The last notified case of trypanosomiasis in the RSA was in 1982. It is no longer notifiable.

Trypanosomes are blood flagellates with a single flagellum (whip-like appendage) with which they propel themselves. Reproduction of the trypanosome in both the tsetse fly and man is by binary fission.

Tsetse fly

The biological vector of the trypanosome is the tsetse fly (glossina) which feeds only on blood which it sucks in large amounts from animal hosts, sucking up parasites and passing them to other animals. The tsetse fly is a brown fly which folds its wings scissorwise over its abdo-

men. It lives within the shelter of the forest and bush where it is shady, warm and dark. The female does not lay eggs but hatches one egg at a time in her uterus, the maggot growing within its mother's body for two weeks. The female deposits the large white maggot in a shady spot where it forms an oval pupa. The adult tsetse fly emerges from this pupa within a month. A female gives birth to eight maggots in her lifetime.

The *Trypanosoma brucei* causes nagana in animals but does not infect human beings.

The *Trypanosoma brucei rhodesiense* attacks both game and human beings; game, therefore, serves as a reservoir for the trypanosome.

The *Trypanosoma brucei gambiense* is a riverine species which attacks only human beings and, therefore, has no animal reservoir; man is the reservoir host, and man-to-man transmission occurs.

Sleeping sickness may be congenital and could possibly be spread by coitus, but its usual method of spread is by the bloodsucking tsetse fly.

The bite of the tsetse fly usually causes a chancre with a necrotic centre to form locally where the injected trypanosomes proliferate. The trypanosomes are disseminated by the bloodstream and attack the tissue spaces in all the organs, especially the lymph nodes, causing lymphadenopathy. During the early stages of trypanosomiasis the clinical picture resembles that of tick-bite fever with severe headaches, malaise, pyrexia, rash (morbilliform and/or petechial) and hepatosplenomegaly.

There is leucopenia with relative lymphocytosis. Eventually, in untreated cases, these symptoms may clear up and the patient relapse later or he may become drowsy — a sign that the trypanosomes have penetrated the blood-brain barrier to cause cerebral trypanosomiasis (sleeping sickness) which progresses to stupor, coma and death, if the patient is not treated.

Primary prevention

(1) Destruction of the insect vector, the tsetse fly. This can be done by means of aerial insecticidal spraying of bush harbouring game and domestic animals which are the hosts of the tsetse flies.

(2) Control of game in trypanosomal endemic areas. Animals can be confined either to farms or game parks where there would be more chance of eradicating the tsetse fly.

(3) Protection of people in endemic areas against the bite of the tsetse fly by: sleeping indoors in fly-proof dwellings; not camping in the open without a mosquito net surround.

(4) Prophylactic injections of either pentamide isethionate or suramin (trypanocides) every 3 to 6 months for people at risk in endemic areas.

Secondary prevention

(1) Case-finding and diagnosis of patients with chronic trypanosomiasis in endemic areas. A tentative diagnosis is confirmed by finding the trypanosomes in the blood or aspirated tissue fluid, e.g. of lymph nodes.

(2) Treatment of patients, not only to cure them but also to prevent the infection of the tsetse fly population. Treatment is done with either pentamide or suramin in the early stages of the disease before there has been involvement of the central nervous system. As these medicines do not cross the blood-brain barrier, cerebral trypanosomiasis is treated with trypanocides that do, e.g. the arsenical compounds, tryparsamide and melarsoprol. These are dangerous medicines and the comatose patient must be hospitalised.

YELLOW FEVER

Yellow fever is an acute, haemorrhagic fever caused by a virus (arbovirus), which can be controlled by primary preventive measures (immunisation and vector control) as the biological vector of the virus, the *Aedes aegypti* mosquito, is known. The yellow fever virus was the first virus ever to be incriminated as a cause of human disease.

Yellow fever is a formidable epidemic disease subject to International Health regulations. Cases must be notified to the WHO by the Health Administration of a country.

Vaccination against yellow fever is required by certain countries for international travel, the vaccination being carried out by centres designated by the WHO in order to obtain an interna-

tionally recognised certificate. For example, in South Africa vaccination can be done by the medical officer of health of a city health department.

Yellow fever is endemic in the tropics of Central Africa and Central and South America and used to occur in devastating epidemics. In Africa it has never been found south of the Zambezi valley. It is also present as an enzootic in the forest monkeys of Brazil and cases of human jungle yellow fever in the tropical parts of the Americas still occur.

The infected mosquito vector of yellow fever remains infected throughout its life and is easily transported by plane, ship and car from country to country; yellow fever can, therefore, be spread along routes of communication. Planes that fly over tropical Africa are required to land initially at a sanitary international airport in South Africa, e.g. Johannesburg International Airport, where they are boarded by the hygiene team and sprayed for mosquitoes.

Urban yellow fever in the cities of tropical Africa and America, where man-to-man transmission of the virus used to take place through the agency of the domesticated *Aedes aegypti* mosquito, had been so well controlled that a case of yellow fever was a rarity. There are signs, however, that yellow fever is again becoming a threat. West Africa (Ghana and Nigeria) recently (since 1969) had epidemics of yellow fever and the Caribbean was affected in 1979. Yellow fever is, therefore, still endemic in tropical countries and the risk of an epidemic is ever present. Because of the ubiquitous presence of the *Aedes aegypti* mosquito, a traveller with yellow fever viraemia can start an epidemic in a new area; hence the need for continuous vigilance by countries far removed from the theatre of past epidemics of this formidable epidemic disease.

Primary prevention

(1) Vaccination against yellow fever for international travel across Africa. Travellers who cannot show acceptable evidence of vaccination on arrival at a sanitary international airport, are required to submit to a period of quarantine in a state isolation hospital. The yellow fever vaccine is one of the most

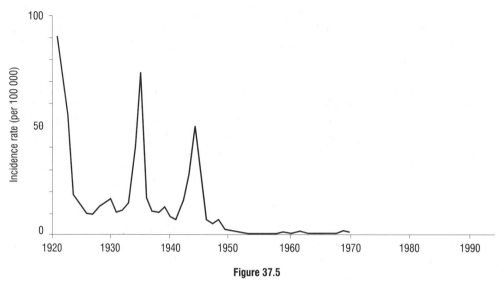

Figure 37.5
Incidence rate of the louse-borne typhus
Source: *Epidemiological Comments* 1994; **21** (3)

effective vaccines ever developed. It is made from a live, attenuated (weakened) strain of yellow fever virus, 17D. A booster dose of the vaccine is required every ten years.

(2) Aeroplanes flying across Africa, to and from Europe, are inspected and sprayed on arrival at a sanitary airport in case they harbour infected *Aedes aegypti* mosquitoes.

THE RICKETTSIOSES

The rickettsioses are a group of rickettsial diseases which are transmitted to man by lice, fleas and ticks. The rickettsiae gain entry through skin lesions, i.e. bites or scratches. In South Africa the following types of rickettsial diseases are of importance.

Epidemic, louse-borne typhus fever

This is caused by the *Rickettsia prowazekii*. It is a notifiable epidemic disease with high mortality before the antibiotic era. The vector is the common human (body) louse which is carried from man to man in overcrowded conditions. Louse infestation of human beings is associated with poverty and unhygienic living conditions, when people are crowded together under conditions of filth, in city slums, in armies and in gaols.

Lice

The sucking louse is species-specific, man and animals hosting different species. Lice live parasitically on the human body by sucking blood, but can remain alive away from the body, e.g. in clothes. Lice do not jump like fleas and are usually transmitted from person to person through close contact. The female lays from 100 to 200 eggs called nits, the nits being attached to hairs with a glue-like substance. The head louse and the body louse interbreed, but human and animal lice never change hosts. Eggs hatch within 4 to 7 days, the small louse (nymph) resembling its parent. It moults 3 times in 10 days, during which time it is growing to maturity. The life span of a louse is 10 days.

Outbreaks of typhus fever have occurred in all parts of South Africa at various times, but since World War II when DDT was discovered, outbreaks of the disease are easily controlled by effective insecticidal control of the louse vectors of typhus. Primary prevention in overcrowded communities threatened by typhus can also be obtained by immunisation against typhus, and secondary prevention of an outbreak assuming epidemic proportions can be achieved by the treatment of sufferers with tetracyclines or chloramphenicol. Thus typhus fever is no longer a community health problem in South Africa, provided the odd cases that still occur are promptly notified so that immediate steps can be taken to stop the spread of the disease. Once a patient has been disinfested he is no longer infectious. No cases of typhus (epidemic or endemic) have been reported in the RSA since 1981.

Endemic, murine, rodent flea-borne typhus

This is a mild form of the louse-borne typhus fever and is also notifiable. Attention to poor living conditions, destruction of mice and rats and application of insecticides to kill off the fleas in the homes of affected people, should bring an outbreak under rapid control. The treatment of murine typhus is as for louse-borne typhus fever.

Tick typhus

This is the collective term for all forms of tick-borne rickettsial disease. The type of tick typhus commonly found in South Africa is called tick-bite fever. It is clinically a typhus-like disease.

Tick-bite fever

It is caused by the *Rickettsia conorii var, pyperi* which is introduced into man by the bite of the larva of the common veld tick, *Amblyomma hebraeum*. At the point of entry a lesion with black centre (eschar) is formed. Tick-bite fever is characterised by pyrexia and severe headache which usually starts 10 days after a day spent in the open. It responds to tetracyclines. As tick-bite fever is neither a contagious nor an epidemic disease, no community prophylactic health measures are warranted. One attack confers immunity if the disease has run its full course, i.e. without tetracycline therapy. Fatalities are not known to occur, but the patient may develop thrombosis and disseminated intravascular coagulopathy (DIC) with a tendency to bleed from mucous membranes.

Gear[16] (quoted by Findlay) discovered that there are animal reservoirs of infection, viz. rodents and domesticated dogs with latent or overt infections. He also discovered that the bite of a tick is not essential for the transmission of the disease, infection being possible through a squirt of blood from an engorged tick into the conjunctival sac of a human being while detick-ing a dog. The rickettsia can also be transmitted

from generation to generation of ticks which, therefore, also form a reservoir of infection.

Ticks

Ticks are important parasites of wild and domestic animals but none is a human parasite; some species, like the *Amblyomma hebraem*, do attack man when the opportunity presents itself. Some ticks attach to their animal hosts and feed continuously for several days; when engorged with blood they drop off. The female lays her eggs in a mass and dies. Six-legged larvae (nymphs) hatch from the eggs, crawl up on blades of grass and wait for a suitable host, usually a small animal, to pass by; they attach to it, have a blood meal and detach again to fall to the ground. They then moult to become eight-legged nymphs which repeat the cycle of the six-legged nymph. These nymphs repeat the breeding cycle and when they drop off after a blood meal, they moult into adult males and females. Adults can live up to three years without food and water and repeat the breeding cycle when they come across a suitable host. The hard ticks described carry Rocky Mountain spotted fever, Q fever and Crimean Congo fever. Soft ticks, which differ slightly in their breeding habits, are the vectors of spirochaetal Borrelia relapsing fever.

Relapsing fever

Relapsing fever is not a notifiable disease. It is caused by spirochaetes of the genus *Borrelia*. Its biological vectors are human lice (carrier of *B. recurrentis*) and soft-bodied ticks (carrier of *B. duttoni*).

Louse-borne relapsing fever

This occurs in epidemics and requires a human reservoir. It is transmitted to man through contact of crushed lice with abraded skin or mucous membrane. It is endemic in north-east Africa, Asia and South America and is not found in the RSA.

Tick-borne relapsing fever

This has an almost world-wide distribution. It is hosted by rodents and transmitted by the bite of a tick. The spirochaete can also be transmitted from generation to generation of ticks, thus obviating the need for a human or rodent reservoir. The disease used to be endemic in KwaZulu and Transvaal, but seldom occurs at present due to the insecticidal spraying of insides of huts and houses to eliminate ticks (and malaria mosquitoes).

Signs and symptoms

Non-specific fever of sudden onset, rigors and many accompanying symptoms. This attack lasts 3–5 days and is repeated after an afebrile period of 4–10 days. In the louse-borne disease there are 3–4 relapses, while in the tick-borne disease there may be up to 13 relapses. During pyrexial episodes the spirochaete is seen in stained peripheral blood smears.

Therapy

Therapy with antibiotics is aimed at a gradual clearance of the spirochaetes from the blood.

VIRAL HAEMORRHAGIC FEVERS OF AFRICA

These dangerous diseases are notifiable as a group, the recent notification figures being: 10 in 1988 and 12 in 1989 (cases of Crimean-Congo Haemorrhagic Disease — CCHD). Viral haemorrhagic fevers (VHF) of importance in South Africa are Rift Valley fever, Marburg virus fever and Crimean-Congo haemorrhagic fever. Three others included in the VHF notification list, Lassa fever, Ebola fever and Dengue fever have occurred in South Africa but are not at present endemic.

Many infectious diseases are accompanied by a bleeding tendency which may culminate in severe haemorrhages from mucous membranes, injection marks and into the skin. Thus, for instance, there is a haemorrhagic form of tick-bite fever. Bleeding is caused by thrombocytopenia with or without DIC (disseminated intravascular coagulopathy), or endothelial cell dysfunction affecting platelets, or decreased production of clotting factors due to liver failure. The infective agent may be either bacteria, rickettsiae, viruses or protozoa, e.g. typhus, bacterial septicaemia. These diseases are not, however, included in the category 'Viral Haemorrhagic Fevers' (VHF).

The VHFs are an entity with many common features: they can be vector-borne but not necessarily so; they are caused by viruses; they can be deadly as a primary disease, but are less malignant when infection is secondarily spread from man to man. The host of the virus is mainly man and animals, but the virus causing Rift Valley fever has even been found in an ostrich. The tick can also be a host of a tick-borne virus as it can transmit the virus to its offspring biologically.

These highly contagious, dangerous new diseases are mainly zoonoses endemic to Africa, although the natural reservoir of some has not yet been identified with certainty. They are characterised by a flu-like onset (i.e. pain in head and muscles, pyrexia, etc.) followed in some cases by an erythematous maculopapular rash. The extreme virulence of the infection causes bleeding from mucous membranes and injection pricks. Necrotic hepatitis and kidney damage add to the likelihood of a fatal outcome.

The contagious viral haemorrhagic fevers are a serious hazard to medical and nursing personnel in attendance as well as to veterinary surgeons who do post-mortems on infected animals. In one Sudan hospital, 76 staff members became ill and 41 of them died from Ebola virus disease.[17]

No prophylactic vaccines have been developed for most of these diseases and there is no chemotherapeutic cure. The patient either dies or recovers within two weeks. The only specific treatment is the administration of convalescent (hyper-immune) serum. Treatment is essentially supportive.

At the International Conference on Disaster Medicine (1979) in Johannesburg, Professor Prozesky, Director of the National Institute for Virology, pointed out that viral haemorrhagic fevers (VHF) are important medical disasters because of high mortality rates, high infectivity, the absence of effective treatment and vaccines, and the panic they induce.

Viral haemorrhagic fevers (VHF) are suspected if:

(1) the source of primary infection can be traced to recent travels in eastern, central or western Africa;

(2) there has been contact with the raw flesh and blood of animals, during an epizootic of domestic animals;

(3) the patient was stung by mosquitoes (*Culex* or *Aedes*) or bitten by ticks or handled carcasses within the incubation period;

(4) the patient has had contact with a sufferer from VHF within the incubation period. Secondary infection, i.e. infection acquired by man from man, is not as serious as primary infection, as the virus becomes attenuated by passing through a human being. Transmission of the virus from man to man probably occurs through small breaks in the skin, the conjunctiva or respiratory tract, or through sexual contact.

If the diagnosis of a VHF has been confirmed by laboratory tests at the National Institute for Virology, Johannesburg, the identification of the source and the tracing of other cases become an urgent necessity to prevent an outbreak (epidemic). Healthy contacts are not isolated after decontamination. Special high security containment facilities for the nursing of VHF patients (see p. 671) are available at some of the academic hospitals, e.g. Johannesburg and Tygerberg, as the virus can be transmitted from man to man.

Patients with arboviral infections must be nursed in a vector (mosquito) free environment during the acute phase of the illness.

Lassa fever

Lassa fever is caused by an arenavirus. Its vector is unknown; spread may be by direct contact with the secretions or body of the animal host. Infection may be airborne. Lassa fever is associated with rodents. Gear[18] states that the mouse *Mastomys natalensis* has recently been proved to be the reservoir of Lassa virus in West Africa.

Prevention: Lassa fever is extremely contagious and containment nursing is practised. Other preventive measures are control of rodents and prevention of food contamination by rodent excreta.

Dengue fever

Dengue fever has been practically unknown in the RSA since an epidemic occurred in Durban in 1926–1927. As it has appeared in southern Africa since then, it could possibly spread to the RSA. In 1983 three pilgrims returning from India and Saudi Arabia developed dengue fever. As imported cases could infect our *Aedes*

aegypti mosquitoes, the principal vectors of the virus, the early diagnosis and isolation of infected persons is mandatory.[19]

Ebola fever

Ebola fever is, like Marburg disease, also very contagious and dangerous. In 1976 a member of the US Peace Corps contracted Ebola virus disease in Zaïre and was flown for stringent isolation care to Johannesburg. By very meticulous barrier nursing an outbreak of this highly contagious disease was averted; the patient recovered. The natural reservoir of the virus is unknown. At present (1995) an epidemic is raging in Zaire.

Marburg virus disease

Marburg fever hails from East Africa and the original (1967) outbreak occurred in Germany when 25 laboratory workers developed the disease; 7 died. The infection was traced to tissues of vervet monkeys imported from Uganda.[20] Travel in the African bush may be responsible for the first case of an outbreak; subsequently the disease is very contagious, i.e. it spreads directly from man to man (secondary infection). Such was the history of the first Marburg fever outbreak in Johannesburg. The first patient with the disease died and two contacts contracted the disease from him but survived. They were stringently isolated and barrier nursed and so further spread of the disease was prevented.

Marburg virus disease starts as an attack of influenza. Between the 5th and 7th day a rash develops and then bleeding starts. Massive haemorrhages into the intestine and lungs may cause death. The mortality rate is high.

Pathology: Necrosis of liver, spleen and lymphoid tissue, DIC and acute tubular necrosis with kidney failure.

Diagnosis is confirmed by the presence of the virus and antibodies. Swabs can be taken from the excreta and throat; blood smears are tested; tissue samples post mortem are used for virological studies.

Incubation period: 7–8 days. There is a high risk of secondary infection in attendants and household contacts.

There is not yet clarity about the reservoir (animal) hosts of the disease (primary source of infection) and its mode of transmission. The above case originated in South Africa, therefore the source of a potential epidemic is present in the RSA.[21]

Rift Valley fever (RVF)

Rift Valley fever is a very important arthropod-borne arbovirus (bunyavirus) disease affecting man and his domestic animals in Africa, including South Africa. It is transmitted to animals by the bite of an infected mosquito, principally the *Culex theileri,* and causes epizootics. Man is secondarily infected by handling the carcasses of animals that have died from the disease or by inhaling infected aerosols (droplets). Infection of man by mosquitoes is possible.

Epidemiology

There were major epizootics amongst cattle and sheep in South Africa in 1951, 1953 and 1975,[19] after heavy rains in the sheep and cattle farming areas of the Cape and OFS. The heavy rains encouraged the breeding of mosquito vectors (*Aedes* and *Culex*). These epizootics were accompanied by human epidemics of RVF. In 1975 seven fatal cases occurred in humans as a result of gastro-intestinal haemorrhages; farmers suffered large stock losses. Two cases were notified in 1989.

In man the incubation period is 2–6 days.[22] The patient develops a severe flu-like illness which usually clears up after a week. The disease may, however, be complicated by a haemorrhagic state with DIC and thrombocytopenia developing on the 4th day. This may cause death. Other complications are: retinitis (with defective vision) which occasionally causes a detached retina, and meningo-encephalitis with intense headaches, cortical dysfunction and cerebral haemorrhage with hemiparesis. The outcome may be fatal but partial or full recovery is probable.[22]

RVF is preventable by the vaccination of selected persons at greatest risk during an epizootic, i.e. farmers, farm labourers and veterinary surgeons who are likely to handle infected carcasses. The best protection, however, lies in the vaccination of stock to prevent an epizootic.

Careful isolation procedures must be applied when handling infected human beings or infected carcasses, including the wearing of protective clothing and goggles.

Crimean-Congo haemorrhagic fever (CCHF)

CCHF is a zoonosis caused by an arbovirus, the bunyavirus, which affects man, cattle, sheep, goats, migratory birds and the ticks that feed on these animals and birds. CCHF is the most prevalent of the VHFs in the RSA, notified cases being listed under the heading, Haemorrhagic Fevers.

Infectiveness

Direct infection of man by the blood of infected animals leads to severe and often fatal infections. The infection is also spread indirectly from animals to man by the arthropod vector, the bontlegged hard tick, Hyalomma. Once man has contracted the disease, he is highly infectious to caretakers and contacts as well as to laboratory personnel who are unaware of the highly infectious nature of his blood specimens. Spread of the virus from the primary case to others in his environment is called secondary infection and further spread from the secondary case, tertiary infection. The virus becomes attenuated by passage through the human body, therefore tertiary infection is usually mild. The virus is found in the blood of the affected person by the 4th day of the illness and antibodies, a sign of the body's resistance, a few days later. The blood of convalescent patients is the source of hyperimmune plasma which is used for therapy and prophylaxis but is in extremely short supply. Primary infection occurs mostly in those exposed to infected animals (farmers and farm workers) and secondary infection in their caretakers and other contacts. Secondary infection is the clearest indication of the highly contagious nature of CCHF.

Note: CCHF does not cause clinical symptoms in animals, but antibody titres to CCHV in cattle are widespread in the RSA.[24]

Epidemiology

CCHF has caused epidemics in Africa, Asia and Europe. An epizootic occurred in the RSA in 1974/1975 affecting farm animals. In 1981 a

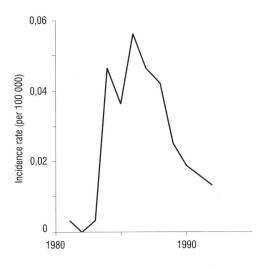

Figure 37.6

Incidence rate of the CCHF
Source: *Epidemiological Comments* 1994; **21** (3)

school boy picked up the disease in the Bloem-hof district from a bontlegged tick and sub-sequently died. This was the first human case in South Africa. From 1981 to 1984 only 8 sporadic primary cases were notified countrywide. In 1984 there was a nosocomial outbreak of CCHF at the Tygerberg Hospital, the index patient being a railway worker from Darling (Cape). By the end of 1988 over 80 sporadic cases had been notified, the incidence rate at present (1989) being 10 to 20 cases annually.[23] Primary CCHF is almost exclusively rural in its distribution, endemic areas stretching in a broad band from the northern Cape in the West to northern Transvaal and Natal in the East.[23] Four cases have occurred in the southern Cape. The association with a farm and contact with animals in the endemic areas appears to be the main risk factors in primary infections. To date no Asians in the RSA have been affected, the highest incidence rate occurring amongst whites, followed by coloured persons.

Incubation period: 5 days with a range of 2–10 days.

Diagnosis is made on the history and clinical picture and the presence of the virus and its antibodies in the blood, as proven in the laboratories of the National Institute for Virology, Johannesburg. Blood samples are highly in-fectious and should be handled only by the Special Pathogen Unit of the Institute. The disease starts as a flu-like illness, muscular pains being severe. Bleeding starts occurring 3–5 days after onset of the illness. It is characterised by petechial or purpuric haemorrhages in the skin and bleeding from mucous membranes (epistaxis, haemoptysis, haematemesis, melaena, haematuria). The conjunctivae are red and the face flushed; the tongue is dry and often covered with blood. Blood loss may be massive causing peripheral vascular collapse (shock) and, in fatal cases, cardiac arrest.

Secondary preventive measures

(1) Early recognition of a case on clinical and epidemiological evidence, i.e. without taking the risk of submitting a blood specimen to an ordinary unsuspecting laboratory which is at high risk of disseminating the infection. In the special containment unit of an academic hospital to which the suspect case is admitted, blood specimens will be submitted with special precautions to the National Institute for Virology in Johannesburg.

(2) Notification of the nearest regional director of the Department of Health to obtain directions for admission to a special high security containment unit maintained at some of our academic hospitals. Admission is authorised on suspicion and is not deferred until the case has been proven.

(3) Where available, hyperimmune plasma of a convalescent CCHF patient is given to mitigate the symptoms of severe infection or to prevent the development of a fulminating illness. Other treatment is symptomatic and supportive.

(4) Complete and early isolation of a suspected case of primary CCHF to prevent the development of secondary cases and large numbers of contacts. Healthy contacts are not placed in quarantine, but they are traced and monitored for early symptoms.

Isolation with full containment procedures

This kind of management is mandatory for patients with RVF, yellow fever, CCHF, Lassa fever and Marburg and Ebola viral infections.

For these very contagious, haemorrhagic fevers primary preventive measures are dependent on containing the infection by strict isolation of patients. Vaccination against Rift Valley fever is confined to high-risk workers. Responsibility for preventing the spread rests with the Department of Health at its special containment units. Isolation is started even before the disease has been diagnosed in case the patient is suffering from viral haemorrhagic fever (VHF). The main principles of *secondary prevention* by stringent isolation and barrier nursing ('containment nursing') are as follows:

(1) Contacts must be traced. High-risk contacts are placed under surveillance for early signs of the disease, temperature and blood counts being monitored.

    Low-risk contacts are examined daily by a doctor who wears protective clothing; contacts must monitor their own temperatures.

(2) The patient is flown to the central isolation hospital in a Trexler-Vickers transport isolator (if he is first seen at a distance from this hospital) and transferred by special connector to a Trexler-Vickers bed isolator in which he will be nursed. The negative pressure bed isolator is placed in a special isolation ward, in the isolation complex, quite separate from the rest of the hospital and with facilities for staff and for autoclaving disposable and non-disposable nursing equipment, as well as excreta and other waste.

    Patient negative pressure isolators are complicated, modern pieces of equipment which allow the patient to be effectively sealed off from his environment. Thus the patient can be transported and nursed without endangering the lives of doctors and nurses. Special high security (containment) laboratory facilities are also available for safeguarding the health of the technicians dealing with biological specimens from the patient. Blood and urine are sent to the laboratory for electron microscopy, white cell and platelet counts, serological tests, coagulation studies, etc.

(3) All excreta, waste and utility articles leaving the bed isolator, effectively wrapped in several layers of plastic, are immediately autoclaved in an adjoining room. After that, disposables, including crockery and cutlery, are incinerated in the hospital incinerator, and the sterilised excreta and waste water discarded in the sewer.

(4) The patient must wear either disposable clothing or clothing that can be autoclaved.

(5) Staff who have been in direct contact with the patient must be quarantined in the isolation complex with him, but staff who have taken proper precautions against direct contact with the patient and his discharges and fomites from the beginning, can return home after a spell of duty, after taking suitable decontaminating measures. While attending to the patient, staff must wear special exchanged, protective clothing, gloves, plastic overshoes and a full face mask. A Trexler-Vickers positive-pressure half-suit is also available for staff in the absence of the isolator unit.

(6) Terminal disinfection includes fumigation and thorough washing of the room and isolator, sterilisation of non-disposable equipment and incineration of disposables.

For a protocol for control and containment of Crimean-Congo Haemorrhagic Fever, study the article by Norma Paverd in *Nursing RSA Verpleging*: part 1 in Volume 3 No. 5, May 1988, part 2 in Volume 3 No. 6, June 1988, part 3 in Volume 3 No. 7, July 1988.

REFERENCES

(1) Department of National Health and Population Development. *Epidemiological Comments* January 1985; **12** (1).

(2) Department of National Health and Population Development. Synopsis of vector-borne diseases. *Epidemiological Comments* June 1983; **10** (6).

(3) Department of National Health and Population Development. Malaria: Problems new and old. *Epidemiological Comments* January 1988; **15** (1).

(4) Department of National Health and Population Development. Malaria in the Northern Cape Health Region. *Epidemiological Comments* May 1988; **15** (5).

(5) Spracklen FHN. Management of acute malaria. *S Afr J Cont Med Educ* 1989; **7**: 117–121.

(6) Hansford CF & Pammenter MD. Diagnose en profilakse van malaria. *S Afr J Cont Med Educ* 1989; **7**: 138–145.

(7) Gear JHS. Malaria in South Africa: Its history and present problems. *The Southern African Journal of Epidemiology and Infection* 1989; **4**: 63–66.

(8) Hansford CF. Prophylaxis and treatment of falciparum malaria. *S Afr J Cont Med Educ* 1989; **7**: 1440–1443.

(9) Gear JHS, Hansford CF, Pitchford FJ. *Malaria in Southern Africa*. Pretoria: Department of Health and Welfare, 1981.

(10) Technical Report Series 655: *Resistance of vectors of disease to pesticides*. Geneva: World Health Organisation, 1980, p. 16.

(11) Department of Pharmacology, UCT Medical School. *S Afr Med J* 1989; **75**: 255–256.

(12) Sharp BL, Freese JA, Schutte CHJ. Suggested malaria prophylaxis for South African travellers. *S Afr Med J* 1989; **76**: 285.

(13) Spracklen, FHN. Management of acute malaria. *S Afr J Cont Med Educ* 1989; **7**: 117–121.

(14) Department of National Health and Population Development. The epidemiology and control of malaria, Nelspruit subregion, 1980–1985. *Epidemiological Comments*. May 1986; **13** (5).

(15) Drugs in practice — Chloroquine. *S Afr J Cont Med Educ* 1988; **6**: 94.

(16) Findlay, FH. South African tick-bite fever (1931–1981). *S Afr Med J* 1982; **61**: 801.

(17) Editorial. *S Afr Med J* 1977; **52**: 626.

(18) Gear JHS. *S Afr Med J* 1978; **53**: 236.

(19) Blackburn NK, Rawat R. Dengue fever imported from India. *S Afr Med J* 1987; **71**: 386–387.

(20) Gear JHS. Haemorrhagic fever. *S Afr J Cont Med Educ* 1984; **2**: 41–49.

(21) Rippey JJ, Schepers NJ, Gear JHS. The pathology of Marburg virus disease. *S Afr Med J* 1984; **66**: 50–54.

(22) Department of National Health and Population Development. *Epidemiological Comments* April 1988; **15** (4).

(23) Department of National Health and Population Development. CHF-update. *Epidemiological Comments* May 1988; **15** (5).

(24) Pefanis SM. Infectious diseases in the RSA transmissable from animals to man. *S Afr J Cont Med Educ* 1986; **4**: 91–95.

TEST OF KNOWLEDGE

The student has benefited from studying this chapter if he/she can answer the following questions:

(1) Define the following:
 – Vector
 – Zoonosis
 – Clotting factors
 – Arthropod
 – Arbovirus
 – Gerbil
 – Fansidar
 – Trypanosomiasis
 – Epizootic
 – Black water fever
 – Plasmodium
 – The Black Death of the Middle Ages
 – Thrombocytopenia
 – Larviciding and larvicides
 – Enzootic
 – DIC
 – Malaria Eradicating Medicine
 – Viraemia and parasitaemia
 – Chemoprophylaxis
 – Organophosphates

(2) Write notes on:
 (a) Chloroquine-resistant plasmodium (malaria)
 (b) Active surveillance in the malaria control programme (MCP)
 (c) Epidemiological investigation of a malaria case
 (d) The diagnosis of malaria
 (e) The role of quinine in the treatment of malaria
 (f) *Anopheles arabiensis*
 (g) The use of organochlorides in the MCP.

(3) (a) Discuss the role of biting flies, fleas, lice and ticks in the spread of infections, with special emphasis on the rickettsioses.
 (b) Write a note on yellow fever and its vector.

(*c*) What primary preventive measures can be taken against the introduction of yellow fever into a country?

(4) Distinguish between infections accompanied by a bleeding tendency and the group of diseases known as 'Viral Haemorrhagic Fevers' (VHF). What are the features common to the VHFs which would raise the suspicion that someone is suffering from a VHF?

(5) How may Rift Valley fever (RVF) be spread? What primary preventive measures may be taken in RVF?

(6) (*a*) What is meant by primary, secondary and tertiary infection in Crimean-Congo Haemorrhagic Fever (CCHF)?

(*b*) Discuss the infectiveness and epidemiology of CCHF.

(*c*) What secondary preventive measures can be taken in CCHF?

38

Some Zoonoses

INTRODUCTION

The zoonoses are infections which man and the vertebrate animals have in common. Many infections and parasites are transmissible between man and animals, but the most important reservoirs of zoonoses are domesticated animals as man is in constant contact with them and their products and is thus liable to acquire their infections. In rabies the black-backed jackal and the yellow mongoose are the commonest reservoirs of the virus in South Africa, yet the usual transmitter of the disease to man is the dog that lives in close proximity to man and may become infected by wild animals.

The zoonoses discussed in this chapter are not vector-borne; they are spread by direct contact between the infected animal and man. Thus, the flesh of the infected animal may be eaten, his secretions and excretions ingested, the dander from his skin inhaled or man's wounded skin may become contaminated by his infected secretions or excretions.

Anthrax and brucellosis are zoonoses of sheep, goats and cattle; they are very important as they cause serious losses to animal husbandry and pose a hazard to the health of people who drink contaminated milk and of workers who handle the animals alive and after slaughter.

IN THIS CHAPTER

BRUCELLOSIS (MALTA FEVER, UNDULANT FEVER)

Brucellosis — a notifiable disease — is a protracted incapacitating disease which occurs throughout the world, but especially in warm climate countries. It is a most damaging zoonosis as far as human health and wealth are concerned. In animals it attacks especially the genital organs and the udders and interferes with reproductive functions. The microbe is excreted for a variable period in the milk of the affected animal. In human beings it is an occupational disease.

Brucellosis is caused by the *Brucella*, an intracellular bacillus:

- *Br. melitensis*, the more virulent species, causes infection of sheep and goats;
- *Br. abortus* of cattle causes septic abortion. This disease is enzootic in the RSA.

The disease is transmitted to man by direct contact of the infected material with man's mucous membranes and abraded skin. Infected material includes discharges from animal genitalia (during abortion, or calving, kidding and lambing), milk and carcasses. Veterinary surgeons, farmers and abattoir and dairy workers

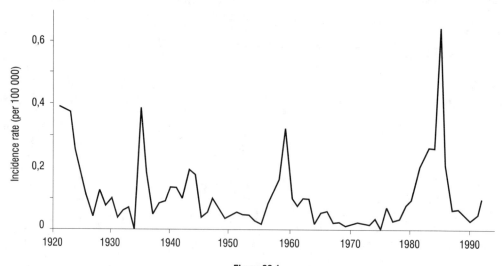

Figure 38.1

Incidence rate of brucellosis
Source: *Epidemiological Comments* 1994; **21** (3)

are specially at risk, but people who drink un-pasteurised and unsterilised infected milk will also become infected. Transmission between human beings does not occur.

Br. melitensis has been found amongst sheep and goats in north-west Cape and north-west Transvaal. Isolated human cases occur amongst karakul farmers.

Br. abortus is very common in cattle throughout most of the RSA.[1] The incidence (notification figures) of brucellosis varies between 20 and 40 per annum. *Br. abortus* infections are by far the commonest cause of brucellosis in the RSA.

Incubation period: 1–4 weeks.

In man the disease is difficult to diagnose, often presenting as a pyrexia of unknown origin. Periods of pyrexia may last for weeks, alternating with periods of apyrexia — a pattern which may continue for months and even years if the disease is not diagnosed and treated. The patient also gets severe attacks of polyarthritis.

Blood cultures taken early in the course of the disease may demonstrate the presence of the *Brucella* in the blood; specific agglutination tests with rising titre provide serological evidence for the presence of the disease.

Primary prevention

(1) Pasteurisation of all milk for human consumption, especially milk sold by a dairy which obtains its milk supplies from several dairy farms.

(2) Regular inspection of the dairy farms which supply milk for public consumption, to exclude the possibility of brucellosis infection in the milk animals. Inspection also applies to goats used for milking.

(3) Abattoir workers need suitable protective gloves, masks and glasses.

(4) Immunisation of dairy and beef herds with a live attenuated vaccine against the *Brucella*.

(5) At-risk workers can be immunised against brucellosis.

Note: Dairy herds supplying raw milk for human consumption or fresh milk for pasteurisation are required to be Brucella- and tubercle-free (Act 54, 1972).

Secondary prevention

(1) Prompt notification of the disease in human beings as soon as it is diagnosed.

The disease starts with fever, malaise, myalgia and diarrhoea. It is characterised by extreme fatigue, recurrent episodes of pyrexia relieved by drenching sweats. Hepatosplenomegaly may develop. The duration of brucellosis is from two weeks to several months.

Notification should be followed by prompt investigation by a community health team, to trace the source of infection and institute appropriate measures to end the threat to human health. The animal reservoir must be treated and the infection eliminated. This is done by co-operation between the local authority and the Veterinary Services of the Department of Agriculture.

(2) The human sufferer is treated chemotherapeutically with tetracyclines for 5 weeks and streptomycin for 10 days (different schedules are tried).

ANTHRAX

Anthrax is a zoonosis of domestic animals (sheep, cattle, pigs and horses), of herbivorous wild animals and also of ducks and ostriches. There are anthrax endemic areas — mostly in rural environs — in most parts of the world, but especially where the veterinary services are poor. Sporadic cases occur in South Africa. Anthrax is caused by the *Bacillus anthracis*, an aerobic, spore-forming organism which forms resistant spores when exposed to the air. Spores may survive for several years in pastures or animal products, e.g. bone meal, wool, bristle. The *B. anthracis* secretes an antigenic toxin against which the host produces antibody. It is usually spread from animal to man in the spore form, the spore germinating at its point of entry into the body. Entry is gained through a break in the skin (forming a 'malignant' pustule — a bluish black necrotic mass), by the ingestion of under-cooked infected meat and by the inhalation of infected hide dander. The pneumonic form is called woolsorter's disease. Eating the flesh of animals that have died from anthrax causes severe haemorrhagic gastro-enteritis.

Untreated infection may result in septicae-mia and death. Infection can also spread from man to man through contact with the malignant pustule.

Incubation period: 1–5 days. It is a rare disease and no cases have been notified in the RSA recently.

Diagnosis: *B. anthracis* is found in smears from skin lesions. It is found in the blood and spleen aspirate of animals soon after death. In-fection of hides can be detected by a serological test.

Note: It is legally prohibited to cut open the carcass of an animal with suspect anthrax. The risk of animal anthrax remains in the RSA. When anthrax occurs in animals, the entire herd should be quarantined for two weeks after the last case. All the animals in the herd should be vaccinated.

Primary prevention: control in endemic areas

(1) Free or low-cost vaccination of livestock with a live vaccine must be done at regular intervals, which may be twice a year in heavily infected areas.

(2) Human beings who handle potentially con-taminated meat, wool or hides can be pro-tected by a vaccine made of the toxin anti-gen. Frequent boosters are necessary.

(3) Workers with wool, hides and carcasses must wear protective clothing, including masks and gloves.

(4) The control of anthrax in animals depends upon the local facilities for diagnosis of anthrax and safe disposal of infected ani-mals. The carcasses of animals that die of suspected anthrax must either be incinerated or deep-buried if there are no facilities for burning the animal. The depth of burial is important as the spores remain alive for many years and if later exposed by digging in the superficial layers of the soil will be a source of infection for generations. Before disposal of the carcass, a diagnosis should first be obtained. Only blood, hide and spleen aspirate may be obtained for this purpose. No post-mortem may be per-formed because of the danger of releasing *B. anthracis* into the surrounding aerobic atmosphere which is growth-promoting for this aerobic bacillus.

Secondary prevention

(1) Notification of cases and prompt investiga-tion by a community health team to trace the source and institute prophylactic measures: the treatment of the human sufferer from malignant pustule or destruction of the in-fected animal.

No cases were notified in the RSA since 1988.

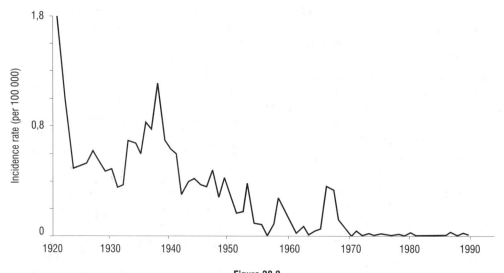

Figure 38.2

Incidence rate of anthrax
Source: *Epidemiological Comments* 1994; **21**(3)

(2) Anthrax in human beings is treated with penicillin and tetracyclines.

RABIES (HYDROPHOBIA)

Rabies is an acute viral encephalomyelitis which is usually fatal and is transmitted to man by the bite of a 'mad' (rabid) animal. The virus is transmitted in the saliva and penetrates broken skin and intact mucous membrane.

Rabies is a zoonosis of canines (dog family), felines (cat family), mongoose (red meerkat) and bats. The black-backed jackal is the biggest reservoir of rabies in the Transvaal and countries to its north-west, and the yellow mongoose in the OFS, northern Cape and parts of Natal. The dog is, however, the main transmitter to man because of their close association.

Rabies in man

Incubation period: From 15 days to 6 months or longer. This will depend upon the site of the bite, the extent of the wound and its degree of contamination. If adequate post-exposure vaccine treatment has been given, the patient may be considered safe 90 days after the bite. Ingestion of meat of infected cattle does not pose any risk.

If the incubation period is less than 21 days, failure of vaccine treatment can be expected.

There are two clinical types of rabies:

(1) Furious rabies: Premonitory signs are of cerebral irritation, muscle pains, pyrexia and vomiting. Later the voice becomes husky, swallowing is difficult with drooling of profuse saliva. The patient then becomes excited and has recurrent spasms of deglutitory muscles, triggered by suggestion of water or swallow-

Human rabies cases confirmed in South Africa since 1984 (as on 25 August 1992)[12]
The geographical distribution of the total number of cases by year

Region	1984	1985	1986	1987	1988	1989	1990	1991	1992	Total
KwaZulu/Natal	10	7	6	15	23	9	11	20	14	115
Cape Province	0	0	0	1	0	0	0	0	1	2
Transvaal	0	0	2	0	0	0	0	0	0	2
Orange Free State	4	0	0	0	2	0	0	0	0	6
KaNgwane	0	1	0	0	2	0	0	0	0	3
Transkei	0	0	0	1	2	0	0	0	0	3
Non-SA	0	0	1	2	1	1	0	1	0	6

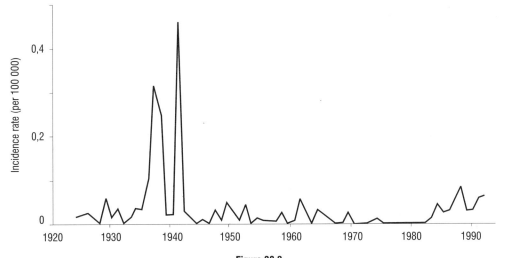

Figure 38.3

Incidence rate of rabies
Source: *Epidemiological Comments* 1994; **21** (3)

ing (hence: hydrophobia — fear of water). The patient may die in a convulsion with opisthotonus. If not, he develops flaccid paralysis and dies in a coma.

(2) Paralytic rabies: The premonitory signs and symptoms are followed by an ascending myelitis in the affected limb, followed by flaccid paralysis and death.

Treatment: The patient is placed under heavy sedation and analgesia to relieve the pain and terror. Recovery is possible with intensive symptomatic and cardiopulmonary resuscitative treatment. Survival will then depend on the severity of the acute encephalomyelitis.

Rabies in animals

Although dogs and meerkats are commonly associated with rabies, abnormal behaviour and an unprovoked attack by any animal, even cows, should be reported, especially if this occurs in a rabies enzootic area.

In animals the clinical picture is also due to a progressive encephalomyelitis. Incubation period in an animal after a bite by an infected animal is 2 to 8 weeks. The furious form — the typical 'mad dog' form — presents as follows:

- excessive itching and scratching;
- dilation of pupils giving the eyes a bright, glinting appearance;
- excessive salivation;
- initial greed, then a depraved taste for stones and wood;
- no feeling of pain;
- a bark which turns to a throaty howl; and
- irritability when disturbed.

Hydrophobia does not occur, but dysphagia may prevent drinking. The dog then becomes excitable and goes berserk. It runs around aimlessly, strays away from home and bites at any object; it attacks moving objects with extreme viciousness. Finally ascending paralysis, coma and death supervene.

If possible, the biting animal must not be killed; it must be captured though and kept under observation for 5–10 days, under the care of a state veterinarian or stock inspector. If it remains healthy for this period, the anti-rabies treatment of the victim is stopped. If the animal dies or has to be killed because it cannot be restrained, the brain is removed and preserved and sent to Onderste-

poort for examination. The fluorescent antibody test and histopathological sections are done. If the tests are negative, the cause of death of the animal is not rabies.

Primary prevention

(1) Control of stray dogs, by destruction if necessary, through the efforts of the SPCA and the government.

(2) Immunisation of all dogs in an area in which a known or suspected case of rabies has been reported. A vaccine given at 6 months will protect the dog for 3 years. Domesticated dogs must be registered and licensed. In order to organise this successfully, the full co-operation of dog owners is essential.

(3) Pre-exposure prophylactic vaccination: persons at risk of possible rabies exposure at diagnostic and research laboratories, veterinarians, stock inspectors, farmers, butchers. The Department of Health is not financially responsible for the free-of-charge supply of vaccine for pre-exposure prophylaxis.

Employers (including other government institutions) are responsible at own cost for the protection of at-risk personnel against rabies.

Dosage: 1,0 ml HDCV (Human Diploid Cell Vaccine) intramuscular injection in the deltoid muscle (upper arm) on day 0 and day 28 (4-week interval), followed by a booster dose one year later. Further booster doses are only necessary every third year.[11]

(4) A dog suspected of having rabies must be isolated for at least 5 days. If it remains healthy after this period, it is released as it does not suffer from rabies. Wild life rabies can be controlled only by eradication of the suspected animals, e.g. jackals and mongooses. Vampire bats cannot be controlled to the same extent. Cats seldom get rabies.

(5) Surveillance programmes of enzootic areas should be continuous. Random samples of wild carrier animals are subjected to laboratory investigation at regular intervals, and all dogs should be immunised against rabies.

(6) Dogs and other carrier animals imported into a country must remain in quarantine at their place of entry into the country until

their freedom from rabies has been ascertained.

(7) The public, and especially children, must be made aware that, apart from dogs, monkeys, squirrels, fruit bats and the other small animals can be carriers of rabies, and that it is dangerous to touch a strange and seemingly paralysed small animal.

Rabies has never been known to spread from man to man or to occur in epidemics. Special **therapeutic measures** are taken in the case of each person bitten or scratched by a rabid animal or one merely suspected of being rabid.

Post-exposure treatment

1. Local treatment of the wound

Prompt treatment is essential. Wounds are allowed to bleed. The soft tissues around the wound are infiltrated with local analgesia. This helps to prevent the transmission of the virus in nerve tissue. The wound is washed and flushed with an antiseptic solution.

The patient is given antibiotics and anti-tetanus vaccine to prevent tetanus and bacterial infection.

Anti-rabies hyper-immune serum (Rabies Immune Human Globulin, 20 IV/kg body mass) is given to severely exposed persons as soon as possible, but preferably within 72 hours. Half the dose is infiltrated into the tissues surrounding the wound and the rest is given by deep intramuscular injection.

A little serum is also allowed to run into the wound after cleansing.[11]

2. Parenteral anti-rabies treatment with HDCV vaccine

The victim of a rabid animal is given prompt, specific anti-rabies treatment until the danger of contracting the disease is past or until it can be proved that the biting animal does not have rabies.

The vaccine is supplied free of charge by the Department in cases where genuine exposure to rabies has occurred. Mere contact with rabid animals (such as handling) offers no risk. The rabies virus does not pass through intact skin but is introduced primarily as the result of a rabid animal bite. Persons who have a pre-existing wound, not more than 24 hours old, contaminated with saliva from a rabid animal or who receive such saliva in the eyes, mouth or other mucous membranes must, however, receive the vaccine.

Dosage

(a) In the absence of pre-exposure immunisation: 1,0 ml HDCV intramuscular injection in the deltoid muscle (upper arm) on day 0, 3, 7, 14 and 30. A repeat dose on day 90 is only necessary if rabies-antiserum (Immune Human Globulin) was administered.

(b) After adequate pre-exposure immunisations: 1,0 ml HDCV intramuscular injection in the deltoid muscle (upper arm) on day 0 and 21 (3 week interval).[11]

TOXOPLASMOSIS

Toxoplasmosis is caused by the *Toxoplasma gondii*, a small obligate intracellular protozoon. It multiplies by fission (endodyogeny) of trophozoites (the amoeboid vegetative form of the protozoon) in endothelial cells, muscles, central nervous system and retina. The host cells burst to release merozoites into the blood. Infection occurs in wild and domesticated animals (especially cats) and in man. The *Toxoplasma* may occur in either the vegetative or cystic form. The disease is spread to man by cysts (collections of merozoites enclosed within tough, resilient thin walls) in raw meat (including biltong) and cat faeces, or transplacentally from a pregnant woman with clinical toxoplasmosis to her foetus.

Toxoplasma infection is widespread throughout the world, including the RSA. Serological studies done in the RSA[2, 3] showed that a very high percentage of the population (ranging from 9 % in San Bushmen to 58 % among some Indian groups) gave a positive *Toxoplasma* indirect fluorescent antibody test result.

The definitive host of the *Toxoplasma* in nature is the cat, oocysts being excreted in cat faeces. Tissue cysts form in infected persons and persist for life.

In human beings the disease is rare in comparison with the prevalence of *Toxoplasma* antibodies. The three major clinical syndromes are the following.

1. A benign acquired toxoplasmosis with lymphadenopathy

In the majority of cases, it resolves spontaneously within a month. Most cases are mild and self-limiting and do not require chemotherapy. Sometimes there is persisting extensive lymph node enlargement and incapacity, enough to be confused with lymphoma or infectious mononucleosis. This 'glandular fever syndrome' requires prolonged chemotherapy, as it may be resistant to treatment.[4]

Most cases of toxoplasmosis in man are subclinical, infection conferring immunity which can be confirmed by serological testing. These cases are not treated.

2. Acute acquired toxoplasmosis

This potentially lethal form of the disease occurs in immunocompromised patients and is characterised by fever, rash, pneumonia, myocarditis and meningo-encephalitis.

Treatment:

(1) In acquired symptomatic clinical infections, e.g. toxoplasmic uveitis which may progress to blindness or severe lymphadenopathy, chemotherapy must be given.
(2) Laboratory workers who have been accidentally exposed to infection, require prophylactic chemotherapy.
(3) Patients with life-threatening toxoplasmosis or advancing blindness can be successfully treated with clindamycin, with due regard for the dangers of drug induced pseudomembranous colitis.

3. Congenital toxoplasmosis

Congenital toxoplasmosis is acquired by the foetus of an asymptomatic or mildly affected mother with parasitaemia. This is the most serious form of toxoplasmosis. It results either in intra-uterine death or in congenital disease in which the CNS and retina are partially destroyed. The foetus will not be affected if the mother had the disease before the conception and subsequent pregnancies will not be affected if the mother no longer has the disease.

Congenital toxoplasma infection of the foetus occurs at any time during pregnancy, depending upon when the mother becomes infected. The severity of foetal infection is greatest during the first trimester.

Prevention of toxoplasmosis in the pregnant woman (especially if she is seronegative)

(1) Great care must be exercised when handling raw meat, e.g. hands must be washed afterwards and before preparing raw salads;
(2) biltong should not be eaten;
(3) close contact with cats and their litter trays should be avoided, or hands should be washed after such contact;
(4) raw vegetables likely to be contaminated with cat faeces should be washed before consumption;
(5) adequate cooking of meat.

Note: Poor hygienic living standards contribute to the prevalence of toxoplasmosis.

Diagnosis of toxoplasmosis[5]

(1) Direct microscopy of *Toxoplasma* in tissues or body fluids.
(2) Serological tests:
    (a) Methylene blue dye test to indicate *Toxoplasma* antibodies.
    (b) Complement-fixation test to supplement the dye test (CFT).
    (c) Direct haemagglutination test (DA).
    (d) Indirect fluorescent antibody test (IFAT).
(3) The intradermal skin test probably remains positive throughout life. It is used:
    (a) to determine the infectivity rate of a population;
    (b) as a screening test in uveitis and early pregnancy;
    (c) to determine the role of *Toxoplasma* in the aetiology of lymphadenitis.

The management of women who have contracted toxoplasmosis in the early stages of pregnancy:

(1) Termination of pregnancy in cases where early foetal infection has been demonstrated.
(2) Continuing pregnancy with the risk of severe foetal damage. The following treatment of the infected woman during pregnancy reduces the likelihood of congenital transmission: daily spiramycin from the mo-

ment of diagnosis (true or assumptive) until the end of pregnancy.[9] If foetal toxoplasmosis is confirmed and pregnancy is continued, pyrimethamine, sulphonamides and folinic acid supplements are given to the mother to the end of pregnancy, thereafter to the neonate. These drugs cannot reverse damage already done, but are given to limit further tissue damage.[9]

Toxoplasmosis is dangerous for immunocompromised patients, particularly for those with AIDS, cerebral toxoplasmosis being a common opportunistic infection, usually of endogenous origin.

HISTOPLASMOSIS

Histoplasmosis is a zoonosis of bats, the fungal spores being excreted in their guano. Histoplasmosis is caused by the fungus *Histoplasma capsulatum*, the spores of which are found in bat-containing caves, and in soil inhabited by chickens and birds. It is commonly called 'cave disease' by speleologists (cave explorers).

Histoplasmosis is endemic in the Americas, central Africa and parts of Asia. In southern Africa it occurs in Zimbabwe and Transvaal.

Infection occurs from inhaled spores. The infection is usually mild, resembling a cold or flu; it therefore often goes unrecognised.

Incubation period: Two weeks. The spores may be dormant in an urban environment and give rise to an epidemic.

Histoplasmosis occurs in acute and chronic forms and may be confined to the lungs or disseminate throughout the body if the patient is immunocompromised. Acute, benign, pulmonary histoplasmosis is the common form; it occurs when a previously non-exposed cave explorer inhales a moderate dose of spores, and it lasts from 4–6 weeks, the patient recovering without treatment. Disseminated histoplasmosis is treated with IVI amphotericin B.

Clinical signs and symptoms: Unproductive cough, dyspnoea, anorexia, fever, lassitude, chest pains and headache.

Diagnosis is confirmed by chest radiographs. Histoplasma antibody tests gradually become positive.

Prevention advice to visitors to possibly infected guano caves:[6]

(1) do not raise dust;
(2) wear a respirator or other mask to prevent the inhalation of dust;
(3) wash all clothing and equipment thoroughly after leaving the cave.

Exposure to the *Histoplasma* stimulates antibody formation and cell-mediated immunity.

LEPTOSPIROSIS

Leptospirosis is a zoonosis caused by leptospira (spirochaetes), of which there are many serogroups and serotypes, with varying effects on man. Leptospirosis is not a common disease and diagnosis may often be missed. In 1981 one case was notified and since then, none.

Leptospirosis is transmitted to man through accidental contact of mucous membranes or abraded skin with animal excreta, usually rat urine but also the urine of other animals, especially dogs. Infection is either direct or indirect by bathing in contaminated water, as the leptospira can survive in water for a month.

- *Incubation period:* 7 to 12 days.
- *Distribution:* World-wide. There are no seasonal variations.

Main varieties:

(1) Weil's syndrome caused by the *Lept. icterohaemorrhagiae* and other serotypes. It is spread mostly by rats.
(2) Canicola fever caused by the *Lept. canicola*, is spread mostly by dogs.

These two leptospira and the many other serotypes may cause either a mild or a serious disease which can be fatal if not diagnosed and treated early; the disease can, however, be self-limiting. Every organ in the body can be affected by the leptospira.

Primary prevention

(1) Protection of workers at risk by the wearing of protective clothing and the adequate treatment and isolation of wounds and abrasions. High-risk occupations are: sewage workers, refuse collectors, dock and farm workers, abattoir workers, fish handlers.

Most cases (60 %) reported in the USA to the Atlanta Center for Disease Control were, however, children, students and house-wives.[7]

(2) Eradication of rodents.

(3) Sick dogs should be adequately diagnosed and treated.

(4) Immunisation of livestock and domestic animals.

Secondary prevention

Early diagnosis and treatment with antibiotics (penicillin and tetracyclines), i.e. within 48 hours of onset of symptoms before renal failure supervenes. Diagnosis is difficult as the disease is uncommon and, therefore, not suspected, often being confused with viral hepatitis.

Diagnosis is made by:

(1) Serological tests. Large agglutination titres give an indication of the infecting serotype. A large increase in agglutination titres in blood taken at two-weekly intervals is con-firmatory evidence of leptospirosis.

(2) Isolating leptospira from any clinical speci-men such as urine, blood or CSF. This is seldom possible.

(3) Signs and symptoms which are those of a pyrexial illness with myalgia, conjunctivitis and jaundice. One or more of the organs may be affected to give a variable picture with signs of myocarditis and/or nephritis, and/or hepatitis, and/or aseptic meningitis, and/or gastro-intestinal disturbances. There is a haemorrhagic tendency.

Q-FEVER[1]

Q-fever is caused by a rickettsia, *Coxiella burnettii*. It is an important but innocuous zoonosis of cattle, amongst others. The rick-ettsia is secreted in the milk and in this way spreads to humans who drink unpasteurised milk. It can also be spread by dust and tick faeces. Q-fever infection in man is characterised by recurrent fever, severe headaches and retro-orbital pain: some patients develop pneumoni-tis. Symptoms are mild and may go unnoticed.

Note: 'Q' is an abbreviation of 'query' — referring to the erstwhile doubt about the aetiology of this disease (Sted-man's Medical Dictionary).

PSITTACOSIS[10]

Psittacosis is caused by the Chlamydia psittaci, an obligate intracellular parasite. It is a zoonosis of the parrot family and other birds and in the RSA infection is carried mainly by budgerigars and cockatiels. Outbreaks amongst birds have been associated with imported parrots and Aus-tralian finches.

Psittacosis is widespread in the RSA and diagnosis can be made on its presenting symp-toms of fever, a dry cough and a history of close association with birds.

Psittacosis was made a notifiable disease in 1979 and in the following 3 years only 4 cases were notified. Notification was rescinded in 1989, the year in which 3 cases were notified.

Diagnosis

Infection in man may be asymptomatic or re-semble an attack of flu with severe headache, muscle pain, fever and an irritating cough (pneumonitis). If no treatment is given, the dis-ease continues for 3–4 weeks and the patient may develop the following complications: pneumonia, hepatitis and gastro-enteritis.

Diagnosis is confirmed by a complement fixation test which shows a marked rise in anti-body titre and by culture of the chlamydia in sputum and blood.

Treatment

Specific treatment with tetracyclines is curative. In undiagnosed and untreated cases the outcome may be fatal.

Prevention

(1) The disease in birds
People dealing with pet birds should be fa-miliar with signs of infection in birds. Im-ported birds may sicken with psittacosis while kept in a crowded environment during transport, despite being kept in quarantine for the regulation period in their country of origin. Infection of a flock of birds, or those in quarantine, can be eradicated by feeding birds on seeds soaked in a solution of tetra-cycline.

(2) Early signs in human patients must be diag-nosed so that timeous therapy with tetracy-

cline will prevent the severe forms of the disease.

REFERENCES

(1) Pefanis SM. Infectious diseases in the RSA transmissible from animals to man. *S Afr J Cont Med Educ* 1986; **4**: 91–95.

(2) Jacobs MR, Mason PR. Prevalence of toxoplasma antibodies in southern Africa. *S Afr Med J* 1978; **53**: 619.

(3) Mason PR, Jacobs MR, Fripp PJ. Serological survey of toxoplasmosis in the Transvaal. *S Afr Med J* 1974; **48**: 1707.

(4) Jacobs P. Toxoplasmosis as an unusual cause of massive lymph node enlargement. *S Afr Med J* 1981; **60**: 784.

(5) World Health Organisation. *Toxoplasmosis*. Tech. Report Series No. 431, 1969.

(6) Craven SA, Benatar SR. Histoplasmosis in the Cape Province. *S Afr Med J* 1979; **55**: 89.

(7) Maze SS, Kirsch RE. *S Afr Med J* 1981; **59**: 33.

(8) Department of National Health and Population Development. Rabies on the rise. *Epidemiological Comments* June 1985; **12**: (6).

(9) Editorial. Toxoplasmosis — an often unrecognised danger. *S Afr J Cont Med Educ* 1988; **6**: 78–80.

(10) Gear JHS, Miller GB, Woolf M, Patz IM. Psittacosis in the RSA. *S Afr Med J* 1986; **69**: 689–693.

(11) Departmental policy — Administration of rabies vaccine. *Epidemiological Comments* 1991; **18** (10).

(12) Rabies Update. *Epidemiological Comments* 1992; **19** (8).

TEST OF KNOWLEDGE

The student has benefited from studying this chapter if he/she can answer the following questions:

(1) Define the following:
   - Malta fever
   - *Bacillus anthracis*
   - *Toxoplasma gondii*
   - Psittacosis
   - Woolsorter's disease
   - Hydrophobia
   - *Histoplasma capsulatum*
   - Leptospirosis

(2) Give a short account of the zoonoses transmitted to man through animal excreta.

(3) Give a short account of the zoonoses transmitted to man through infected milk.
   How is this community health problem controlled?

(4) Enumerate the primary preventive measures in human rabies.

(5) Discuss toxoplasmosis in pregnancy — its possible effect on the foetus, its prevention and the management of a pregnant woman who contracted the toxoplasmosis during the first trimester of pregnancy.

Part 6

IMPAIRMENT AND DISABLEMENT
AS COMMUNITY HEALTH PROBLEMS

39

Hearing Impairment

INTRODUCTION

Deafness causes vocational and social disability through its effect on communication. The early detection of a severe hearing handicap is an important task of the community nurse involved in maternal and child health care.

The normal child learns to discriminate sounds during his first year of life and listens for language during this time; he has a special aptitude to learn to distinguish sounds. At the age of 3 years this special human ability to distinguish new sounds diminishes until, after the age of 7 years, it becomes impossible for a child who hears sounds for the first time to discriminate between them, i.e. to learn speech by hearing others speak. As many children who are born deaf have some residual hearing capacity which can be augmented with the aid of automatic volume-control hearing aids, early detection and alleviation of a handicapping hearing deficit is imperative to ensure the development of a vocabulary. The learning of a language is especially important for the development of inner speech on which thinking and ideation depend. The person who has no knowledge of language and speech cannot develop his full intellectual potential and is severely handicapped socially and vocationally.

As there is no 'deaf' pension, it is expected of deaf adults to seek employment in the open labour market. For purposes of employment, deafness can be defined as 'the lack of sufficient hearing to understand conversational speech with or without hearing aid, since birth or from the formative years of childhood'.[2] Deafness causes different degrees of vocational adjustment disability depending on the personality and intelligence of the deaf person. Thus there are: exceptional deaf people who secure professional and managerial positions in the field of computer programming, engineering, architecture and accountancy; retarded deaf people who cannot achieve vocationally; psychologically disturbed deaf people who are failures in school, work and society, not because of lack of intelligence, but because of disturbed family relationships and early emotional trauma. In the silent world of the deaf, use must be made of the other senses to compensate for sensory deprivation. The hearing-impaired are denied the enjoyment of some of man's greatest pleasures, the world of music and the human voice. As sensory stimulation is essential for intellectual and psycho-social development, hearing and visually impaired persons are sensorily deprived of the full richness of the human experience and are, indeed, disabled people.

IN THIS CHAPTER

HEARING IMPAIRMENT AND DEAFNESS

Impairment of hearing may range from slight deafness (enough to make it difficult for the deaf person to follow a conversation), to total inability to hear. Deafness may be uneven in that certain tones, usually the high ones, cannot be heard, while the perception of lower tones is unimpaired. If one ear is totally deaf, only 10 % to 15 % of hearing is lost.

Deaf-mutism means an inability to hear and speak. It is caused by sustained profound deafness which is present at birth or is acquired before speech is learned. Deaf-mutes can be taught to lip-read and to speak, but as they cannot be taught to modulate the voice, speech will sound metallic and monotonous and will be indistinct, due to articulation defects.

Deafness may be due either to a fault in the conduction of sound waves to the inner ear or it may be due to a fault in the perception of sound due to the destruction or non-development of the sensori-neural (inner ear, auditory nerve) apparatus. The fault in the hearing apparatus may be anywhere along the auditory tract, from the external ear to the auditory centre in the temporal lobe of the brain.

Conductive deafness can be distinguished from perceptive (sensori-neural) deafness by the response to a tuning fork held against the skull. The waves emitted by the fork can be perceived as sound in cases of conductive deafness. Conductive deafness can usually be re-lieved by surgery and, if the operation is unsuccessful or refused, a hearing aid (which amplifies sound waves and facilitates their conduction via the mastoid bone to the inner ear) serves to restore useful hearing.

According to a survey done by the Department of Genetics, University of Cape Town, more than 10 000 children in the RSA have a significant degree of hearing loss. Some attend ordinary schools, some get no schooling, while only 3 000 attend special schools for the deaf.

The prevalence of deafness in South Africa is difficult to assess. At a rough estimate, in line with the statistical norm for other disabilities, from 1 % to 5 % of the general population may have a hearing impairment.

Deafness is generally regarded as a very serious handicap, especially in the young child, as it affects intellectual, emotional and social development. The deaf person's communication skills are affected to a greater or lesser extent, poor communication being the greatest handicap.

In South Africa there is no Deaf Person's Act and no Deaf Pension, qualification for a disability grant for a deaf person depending upon additional handicaps which make it impossible for the deaf adult to earn a living.

An early childhood hearing deficit, especially one that has not been detected and treated to prevent the complications of muteness and social alienation, is much more serious than deafness acquired later in life. A hearing deficit in childhood prevents scholastic achievement, language comprehension and expressive skills.

The very important handicaps in congenital deafness and in being hard of hearing (partial deafness) are defective communication and social alienation which may lead to distortions of the personality. The development of personality and the ability to interact socially and thus to feel part of a group depend upon communication skills. A deaf person is often suspicious of others, fearing that he is being discussed in a derogatory way, and is inclined to withdraw from people.

Amongst themselves, the deaf communicate by means of sign language. At present there is no uniformity in the signs used throughout the RSA.

The causes of deafness and related communication problems

1. In children

Deafness may be either specifically genetic or it may be familial; it may also be acquired. The incidence of inherited and acquired deafness is approximately the same.

Note: Deafness which is present at birth (congenital) may be either an inherited or an acquired condition.

There are a large number of inherited disorders — specific genetic syndromes — with deafness as one of the features, e.g. Waardenburg syndrome. Familial deafness, on the other hand, occurs in families without any other associated abnormalities, being transmitted from generation to generation in any of the monogenic modes of inheritance (see p. 117). Deafness may be acquired in one of the following three ways:

(1) Prenatally through the teratogenic effect of drugs or viruses in the maternal circulation which penetrate the placental barrier.

    (*a*) Maternal rubella is the most important cause of prenatally acquired deafness, especially when it occurs during the second and third months of pregnancy. The deafness may be unilateral and varies in severity; it results from arrested development of the inner ear. The infection persists in the inner ear during infancy (see p. 572).

    (*b*) Congenital abnormalities of the outer and middle ear may be present due to absence or deformities of bony structures.

(2) Perinatally by birth trauma and anoxia and by neonatal jaundice with hyperbilirubinaemia. The mild deafness in the latter results from damage to the cochlear nuclei by deposition of bilirubin pigment (kernicterus). Neonatal jaundice may be due to prematurity and to erythroblastosis foetalis (rhesus incompatibility).

(3) Postnatally by:

    (*a*) Meningo-encephalitis may precipitate deafness by causing inflammation of the labyrinth or auditory nerve.

    (*b*) Ototoxic drugs, such as streptomycin, may damage the auditory nerve permanently.

    (*c*) Complications of otitis media, such as unhealed perforation of the drum and destruction of the ossicular chain, may result in deafness, usually unilateral. All septic conditions of the ear likely to give rise to conductive deafness involve the middle ear at some stage.

    (*d*) Serous otitis media, which may cause partial deafness in babies and toddlers during the crucial time for speech development, may escape detection as the child does not appear to be ill. It is a non-infective condition.

2. In adults

The causes of deafness in adults are as follows:

(1) Over-exposure to noise, e.g. occupational noise in industry (see p. 66) and acute acoustic trauma due to intense sound.

(2) Senescence is accompanied by presbycusis (deafness of old age) which is due to degeneration of the auditory nerve.
The normal hearing loss which occurs with advancing age usually develops after the age of 65 years and may be partially physiological, but exposure to noise caused by social living probably contributes to its development. Social noise, especially that generated in a city, is difficult to eliminate, but the occupational noise to which workers are exposed in modern industries can be curbed.

(3) Acute labyrinthitis and Ménière's disease.

(4) Otosclerosis — a familial disease which starts manifesting in adulthood. There is progressive hardening of the bony wall of the labyrinth causing the membranous openings between the middle and inner ear to be closed off by the thickened bone and the footplate of the stapes to become fixed in the oval window.

(5) Ototoxic drugs and sepsis as in childhood.

Prevention of deafness and communication disorders

Primary prevention in children

Deafness in children may be prevented by:

(1) Genetic counselling to prevent the specific genetic syndromes with which deafness is associated.

(2) Prevention of maternal rubella (see p. 572) and therapeutic abortion in cases of proven rubella during the first trimester of pregnancy.

(3) Prevention of erythroblastosis foetalis by injecting anti-D immunoglobulin into an Rh negative mother within 72 hours after the birth of an infant, to prevent erythroblastosis and the danger of neonatal jaundice in subsequent pregnancies.

(4) Exchange transfusions in infants with severe neonatal jaundice (hyperbilirubinaemia) and phototherapy for neonatal jaundice of haemolytic origin, phototherapy being started when blood bilirubin levels reach 8 mg % in preterm infants and 12 mg % in full-term infants. These measures prevent kernicterus, which may cause high-tone hearing loss, apart from other damage to the brain.

(5) The use of antibiotics in meningitis will reduce the incidence of deafness due to infection of the labyrinth and auditory nerve.

(6) The delivery of at-risk pregnant women in hospitals with good obstetric facilities to prevent birth trauma and neonatal anoxia.

(7) The hearing of any child on long-term ototoxic drugs must be tested at frequent intervals so that timeous precautions can be taken to prevent deafness.

(8) Early medical treatment for otitis media. The insertion of grommet tubes in children with serous otitis media is an important prophylactic measure.

Primary prevention in adults

Preventive measures are as follows:

(1) Precautions should be taken in adults on ototoxic drugs, as for children.

(2) Hearing conservation programmes in industry are important. See p. 67 for the legal enforcement of such programmes.
Education of the worker in the proper use of protective equipment and in the dangers of exposing himself to excessive noise is important in order to get his co-operation in carrying out the requirements of the law.

(3) Young people should be warned about the dangers of excessive exposure to the loud music which is characteristic of discothèques.

Secondary prevention

Secondary prevention aims at the early detection of deafness and at the prevention of the communication problems of the congenitally deaf or hard-of-hearing child. In some cases, deafness can be cured by expert medical attention.

1. Case-finding

Case-finding by screening for hearing problems in infancy and early childhood should be done on a national basis for all racial groups. Hearing screening services should, therefore, be the responsibility of health authorities, with teachers and nurses playing a major role in the screening process. Screening can be done as follows:

(1) on all neonates in maternity hospitals; an apparatus which determines hearing ability in neonates younger than 7 days was recently (1986) invented in the RSA (*Nursing News*, July 1986);

(2) on all infants attending the general mothercraft services at well-baby clinics;

(3) in crèches, on babies and toddlers not covered by the screening services of the well-baby clinics;

(4) on children from the age of 3 years at pre-primary schools;

(5) after viral infections, e.g. measles.

Training of pre-primary teachers and community health nurses, school nurses and midwives to do audiological screening tests in order to use them in mass screening programmes is essential. Some community health nurses are trained in the use of audiometers in their CHN course.

In babies and toddlers hearing ability can be assessed by observation of the reflex and other physiological responses of the child to a variety of sounds: known and strange; loud and soft; the normal and the whispered voice. Even the smallest hearing, awake infant will show some response to a tinkling bell or a hand clap, sometimes by blinking the eyes or frowning, sometimes by stopping an activity, e.g. stopping crying when he hears his mother's voice; or sometimes by momentarily holding his breath when someone makes a noise outside his range of vision; or sometimes even crying when he hears a loud noise which frightens him. Poor responses to noise stimuli at this early age need not necessarily indicate a hearing deficit, as other factors may be responsible for the child's apathy.

Audiological screening tests used on infants and toddlers are not accurate, but they do give an indication of which children have normal hearing and, therefore, require no further screening tests. Those children who could possibly have a hearing problem could then be put on a 'High-Risk Register' for retesting at intervals, especially at the ages of 6 to 7 months and 3 years. Only those children whose screening tests persist in giving results which suggest a hearing deficit are sent for further testing to a specialised audiological unit at a hospital or a university which trains speech and audiology therapists. Where these units are not available and parents can afford to pay, ear, nose and throat specialists can do a thorough audiological examination and audiometric tests. The doctor or the audiological units prescribe a suitable programme of training in language and speech, making use of the child's own residual hearing, augmented by hearing aids.

By doing the simple screening tests described above, most hearing problems in babies and toddlers can be picked up and managed before the age of 2 years, i.e. before permanent damage to the acquisition of language and speech occurs. Hard-of-hearing and deaf babies can be fitted with hearing aids from the age of 6 months. Thus they are enabled to use any residual hearing for sound discrimination and the learning of speech. These children can be sent for special training to special centres for the deaf and hard of hearing, from the age of 3 years. The child and his parents need to be involved in a training programme in which they get the utmost encouragement from a trained speech therapist and/or teacher of the deaf. Parents of deaf children need guidance from speech therapists and social workers in the handling of their handicapped children.

2. Restoration by surgery

Some remediable hearing problems, e.g. serous otitis media, can be picked up by referral to medical specialists at this early age and these children can have their hearing completely restored by surgery. In adults conductive hearing problems can often by restored by operation.

Example: the deafness of otosclerosis is treated by stapedectomy, the fixed stapes being replaced by an artificial one which transmits the sound vibrations from the incus to the refashioned oval window. In middle ear disease or anomalies of the ossicular chain, the operation of tympanoplasty can be done. In serous otitis media, hearing is restored by inserting a grommet tube in the drum to drain the middle ear.

Hearing is restored by replacing the missing parts of the ossicular chain with tantalum wire, polythene, teflon or nylon materials and by constructing a new eardrum from the inside of the ear canal itself.

3. Hearing aid

Some persons with conductive as well as those with sensori-neural hearing handicaps manage very well with the use of a hearing aid which amplifies sound; the former often prefer this method of coping with their handicap to surgery.

4. Schooling for the deaf

In South Africa there are 26 schools for the deaf. These schools accommodate more than 3 000 children. Some schools are run privately and are subsidised by the state.

Amongst the less enlightened people, workers with the deaf still come across completely uneducated deaf children of all races whose parents refuse to admit their deaf children to a school for the deaf.

There are some special schools which cater for the hard-of-hearing children, e.g. Sonitus School in Pretoria, the Mary Kihn School in Cape Town and the Open Air School in Durban for both the physically handicapped and hard-of-hearing child, from the pre-school class to matriculation.

The education of the hearing impaired child is the most specialised type of education in the world. The combined method of communication (i.e. sign language and verbal) is used as medium of communication. The oral system is employed in order to give the deaf child a large vocabulary and teach him good articulation so that he will be understood in the world of the hearing. He is also taught to speech-read (lip-read).

5. Early detection and pre-school habilitation of the hearing impaired child[1]

The most important advances in the management of the congenitally deaf or hard-of-hearing child has been the screening of infants for hearing loss, the full assessment of those found to have a deficit at special paedo-audiological centres and the early pre-school habilitation of the hearing-impaired infant and toddler.

The objectives of this approach are to help the child acquire sufficient language and speech to develop intellectually and emotionally; the child is thereby enabled to fit into the conventional educational system. Consequently he will be able to adjust to his society and compete in the professions and in the open labour market.

Communication for young deaf children is made possible by the use of powerful electronic hearing devices which augment the sound transmitted to the inner ear to stimulate any residual hearing potential. These devices bring out hearing that in extreme cases cannot be measured by audiometric techniques. Practically all deaf-born infants have some degree of hearing. It is possible to test the hearing of a baby at the age of 7 months (and even earlier). This is the age at which community health nurses test the hearing of infants at well-baby (family health) clinics. This is also the age at which treatment for any significant hearing loss should be started, because at this age the child becomes aware of the mother as a separate person and is set to listen and to respond to her. After the age of 3 it becomes increasingly difficult for the child to develop the listening attitude and to acquire speech. The deaf infant whose hearing is partially restored by a powerful modern hearing aid will learn speech in the same way as a hearing child, provided his mother or caretaker speaks to him continuously while he is awake. The requirements for the adequate acquisition of speech are: the hearing of normal sounds, including the mother's continuous 'patter', at the

early age (i.e. up to the age of 3 years and even longer) of readiness to listen and speak. Any hearing child who is deprived of this early experience will exhibit poor verbal ability for the rest of his life; this applies equally to the hearing-impaired child.

The mother of a hearing-impaired infant who has been fitted with a powerful hearing aid should be involved in a pre-school habilitation programme. In this way, a deaf child can learn to speak just as clearly and intelligibly as a hearing child and can often be educated in the conventional school system.

Some pre-school, primary and high schools have a special unit for hearing-impaired children. Children from the unit are integrated into normal classes when they are ready to do so, where this is at all possible. Only if the child cannot cope within the unit is he sent to a special school for the deaf. Social integration in the conventional school system is difficult and needs special attention. These facilities are offered only at some private schools and a few provincial schools in the Cape and Natal.

Du Toit[1] states that in Denmark, where pre-school habilitation programmes have been in use for 20 years, 50 % of children with hearing aids attend ordinary primary schools, 20 % the same schools but in small classes that cater for their special needs, and only 30 % attend state schools for the deaf. In the RSA the law still requires the white deaf child to go to a special school under control of the Department of National Education.

Pre-school habilitation is comparatively new in the RSA, being offered at the Universities of the Witwatersrand and Pretoria and at the Provincial Paedo-audiological Centre, Tygerberg Hospital. The latter centre extends its programme to children as far away as Port Elizabeth and East London.

COMMUNICATION BETWEEN HEARING AND HEARING-IMPAIRED PERSONS

Lip-reading (speech-reading) is a skill acquired by some hearing-impaired persons.

Lip-reading is only possible under certain conditions:

(1) The person speaking must speak clearly (without exaggerated lip movements) and fairly slowly.

(2) The speaker's lips must be visible to the listener, well lit and not obscured by smoke or shadows.

(3) Hands must not be used for gesticulating near the speaker's face.

(4) Distracting visual stimuli, e.g. brightly coloured clothes, make lip-reading more difficult.

If these conditions are met, face to face communication for trained hearing-impaired persons is possible.

Deaf persons communicate with one another by sign language (signing), but few persons with normal hearing can communicate with them in this way. The method of signing is not uniform. Schools teach the deaf to speak, but where speech is difficult they usually make use of writing.

Assistive devices are important as a support system of hearing-impaired persons. The most important device is the hearing aid, but newer devices include household environmental aids (such as visual alarm signals for doorbell, baby cry), as well as telephone and television devices.[3]

Hearing aids have their limitations: amplified sound is not as 'true' as that perceived by the normal ear; hearing aids are expensive to maintain and they are inclined to amplify environmental sound; this sometimes 'drowns' speech.

Successful use of a hearing aid is dependent upon acceptance of its limitations and a willingness to learn how to gain the most benefit from it.

Sign language is occasionally used to broadcast church services by SATV, either the minister himself or an interpreter translating the spoken word into hand signs. Films with subtitles are a boon to the hearing-impaired, but at present only foreign-language films are clarified thus, and for all viewers.

VOCATIONAL PROSPECTS OF DEAF WORKERS

It is estimated that 20 % of employable deaf persons are unemployed.[2] Hearing-impaired persons are expected to find employment in the open labour market and receive no state subsidies or disability pensions, unless their deafness is part of multidisabilities, e.g. Waardenburg syndrome.

Vocational counsellors assist young deaf persons to reach vocational habilitation by pre-vocational training. Deaf children are cut off from mainstream society and learn little about the work-a-day world around them. The young deaf person who leaves the protected atmosphere of the School for the Deaf is forced to join the outside world in quest of a means of livelihood. He needs to be told by the counsellor about his own strength and weaknesses, what vocations are open to him and what is expected of an employee.

Many deaf school-leavers are socially immature and ignorant and need to be taught the basics of good relationships with colleagues.

Training of the deaf worker

Because of communication problems, deaf trainees cannot attend courses geared to the hearing population. Many deaf workers, therefore, have to learn on the job. For those wishing to follow an academic career, there are no special facilities for the deaf at any South African university. They either go to Gallaudet College for the Deaf in Washington, DC or attend UNISA or a local university without the services of an interpreter.

The technical college at Worcester offers a variety of practical courses with the help of a teacher from the local School for the Deaf. Bursaries for higher education are available through the Department of Manpower (Labour).

In the Transvaal, technical colleges do not cater for the deaf apprentice. Since 1986 the Department of Manpower has subsidised short training courses in welding, basic hand skills and for motor repair-shop assistants at the Chamdor Group Training Centre in Krugersdorp. Several young deaf men have received a training with the assistance of the Witwatersrand Association for the Deaf.

Another successful training course, supported as above, is a 2-week computer course with Nixdorf Computers. In this course use is made of a full-time interpreter who translates the content of the course into sign language.

Job placement and creation of job opportunities

The vocational counsellor or social worker needs to help with job placement to the extent of accompanying the deaf person for the initial job interview. The deaf employee often needs ongoing support during the period of adjustment to his first job. Parents are also called in to assist in the creation of job opportunities. They are assisted by Schools for the Deaf, Associations for the Deaf and the Department of Manpower (Labour).

THE SOUTH AFRICAN NATIONAL COUNCIL FOR THE DEAF

This is a registered, voluntary welfare organisation, based in Johannesburg, on which the deaf themselves are liberally represented. Representatives of the various special schools for the deaf serve on committees of the council, of which the most important are:

(1) Welfare committee which controls social welfare services (see below).
(2) Committee for pre-school clinical facilities for preparing deaf children for school. Clinics have been established for the pre-school deaf child at Port Elizabeth, Lenasia (Johannesburg), East London and Durban; these are affiliated to the council. In addition, clinics to overcome the problems of the pre-school deaf child are functioning well at the Witwatersrand University and Tygerberg Hospital.
(3) Technical committee comprised mostly of doctors, concerned with noise pollution (research and influencing legislation) and the quality and distribution of hearing aids.
(4) Committee for the spiritual help of the deaf.
(5) Non-white affairs committee to negotiate with the authorities with regard to schools and job opportunities.
(6) Education committee composed mostly of teachers who investigate deaf education trends and make recommendations.

(7) Committee composed solely of deaf members with special status and access to the executive committee.

Some of the objectives of the council are:

(1) To assist in and encourage the formation of local associations and societies for the deaf, and to guide and co-ordinate the activities of such societies. At present (1987) nine societies are affiliated to the council; they are located at various centres in the RSA and cater for all race groups. These societies provide, *inter alia*, for recreational facilities; the deaf need their own clubs where they can mix with other deaf persons as they are somewhat lost in a hearing crowd. The associations have full autonomy and do not operate as a division of the national body.
(2) To act for the protection of the interests of the deaf and to promote their well-being.
(3) To obtain statistics regarding the deaf, particularly of children of schoolgoing and pre-school age.
(4) To be the official channel which may be required for communication between members of the council and the state, provincial and other authorities; to co-operate with the state and other authorities in all measures for the welfare of the deaf.

The council is a welfare organisation (NGO) which appeals to the public for funds and which receives government subsidies for the salaries of social workers. Social welfare services are, therefore, an important part of the services rendered by the National Council for the Deaf.

At present (1987) there are twenty-four social workers and three social worker supervisors, specially trained to deal with deaf people, in the service of the council. The council employs its social workers throughout the RSA.

The functions of the social workers are the following:

(1) Counselling of parents of very young deaf children.
(2) Counselling of hearing children of deaf parents.
(3) Counselling of families of deaf children still at school.
(4) Social workers help with the establishment of clubs which are run by the deaf themselves.

(5) Social workers give after-care services — just as at any family care agency — and deal with marital and unemployment problems. They make use of the services of sheltered employment workshops for their multiple handicapped deaf patients and apply for disability pensions for their unemployable charges. Generally, however, employment is found for the deaf in the open labour market.

(6) The social worker is also employed as a community worker to educate the public to see the deaf as fully productive people.

REFERENCES

(1) Du Toit CJ. The implications of early detection and preschool habilitation of the hearing-impaired child. *S Afr Med J* 1981; **60**: 851–855.

(2) Ross E. Strategies for improving the vocational prospects of deaf workers. *Rehabilitation in SA* 1986; **30** (3).

(3) Ross E. Assistive devices: A supportive system for hearing-impaired persons. *Rehabilitation in SA* 1988; **32** (4).

TEST OF KNOWLEDGE

The student has benefited from studying this chapter if he/she can answer the following questions:

(1) Define:
- deaf-mutism
- otosclerosis
- tympanoplasty
- presbycusis
- sero-mucinous (serous) otitis media
- stapedectomy

(2) Distinguish between:
- conductive deafness/perceptive deafness
- specific genetic deafness/familial deafness

(3) (a) What are the greatest handicaps of the deaf person (besides deafness)?
    (b) Discuss the ways in which the hearing-impaired person communicates with other human beings.

(4) (a) What are the after-effects of occupational noise in industry? How is this controlled? (Refer to Chapter 5.)
    (b) Discuss the ways in which deafness may be acquired in childhood and the role of the nurse in primary prevention of deafness.

(5) (a) What is the role of the nurse in the early detection of the hearing-impaired child?
    (b) Why is early case-finding such an important secondary preventive measure in deafness?

40

Visual Impairment

INTRODUCTION

Severe loss of visual acuity is a disability which handicaps the blind person in all spheres of life. Children who have been blinded before they learned to read and know their world are at a tremendous disadvantage when it comes to social adjustment. A congenitally blind child walks much later than a child with normal vision. The unrehabilitated blind person is virtually helpless and dependent upon others; he lives a very restricted life and is unable to realise his human potential.

A large number of bodies, some voluntary, some state-subsidised, have been formed in South Africa to care for the blind and partially sighted and to habilitate and rehabilitate those who have never been able to see and those who have lost their sight.

The Blind Person's Act controls the care and training of the blind child and sees to the general welfare of visually handicapped persons.

The Social Assistance Act allocates disability pensions to registered blind persons who are needy.

The South African National Council for the Blind (SANCB) co-ordinates and organises voluntary blind welfare work (in partnership with the state) and is especially geared to promote the education of the blind and to ensure that eye-care medical services are carried to the remotest parts of the RSA, e.g. by the eye-care (PHC) train.

There are special schools for the education of the visually handicapped. At some, basic education is extended to include vocational training to enable the blind young person to earn his living in the open labour market.

The important South African Blind Workers Association has as its prime objective the placement of blind workers in open labour. There are a number of Societies to Help the Civilian Blind in all the large centres.

The Enid Whitaker Rehabilitation Centre for the Blind in Johannesburg caters especially for the newly blinded person.

This facility has been extended to the Optima Training Centre in Pretoria.

A Directory of Services for visually handicapped South Africans in English and Afrikaans is obtainable from SANCB headquarters in Pretoria.

According to the Chairman of the SANCB (29th Biennial Report, 1987–1989), facilities for education and training of visually handicapped people have increased tenfold over the past 60 years and employment opportunities have diversified to such an extent that 82 occupations are currently (1989) practised by blind people in South Africa. Yet only 25 % of the 103 000 blind people in the RSA have received any special education to help them adjust to the world of the sighted. The educationally neglected blind live in the rural areas where services have generally been poor. In order to reach all corners of the RSA, several affiliated societies of the SANCB have established basic rehabilitation programmes — called community-based rehabilitation — whereby the necessary assistance and training are decentralised and use is made of 'skills developers' and indigenous resources. In 1989 the Committee for Rehabilitation and Training of the SANCB had two community development workers appointed in black communities to use the Indigenous Resources Approach which encourages self-help projects to grow from within the community. These are small beginnings of the national target to reach all blind people by the year 2000. This work is extended by the Eye Care Services of the Bureau for the Prevention of Blindness of the SANCB.

IN THIS CHAPTER

EPIDEMIOLOGY

There are approximately 40 million blind people in the world, i.e. nearly 1 % of the world's population is blind.[1] Trachoma claims 50 million victims, the greatest prevalence of this chlamydial infection being in the Middle East. Twenty per cent of affected people are likely to become totally or partially blind. In India there are 15 million blind persons, most of them blind from avoidable causes, nearly 5 million from trachoma.

Eighty per cent of the world's blindness occurs in the developing countries of Asia, Africa and Latin America.[1]

In 1987 there were 3,57 legally blind people per 1 000 of the population, but as registration is a voluntary act, this number may not reflect the true number of blind persons in the RSA. In 1989 there were at least 103 000 visually handicapped people in the RSA.

Note: Avoidable blindness[1] includes both preventable blindness (e.g. blindness from trachoma) and remediable blindness (e.g. blindness from cataracts). Rowland[1] states that at least 80 % of the world's blindness is avoidable.

Bilateral cataracts, trachoma and xerophthalmia are the major causes of avoidable blindness in the world and as such should receive priority in world health programmes.

The World Health Organisation established an International Agency for the Prevention of Blindness (IAPB) in 1975 to co-ordinate the work of international ophthalmic organisations, governments and blind welfare bodies.

CAUSES OF VISUAL IMPAIRMENT

In children blindness is commonly due to congenital and hereditary factors, adults being more likely to acquire blindness than children.

Congenital blindness

Blindness which is present at birth or in the neonatal period (though not necessarily recognised at this stage) may be due either to hereditary factors or to intra-uterine factors which affect the developing eye. These factors include rubella and the ingestion of teratogenic drugs during the first three months of pregnancy.

(1) *Non-development or rudimentary development of the eyes.*

(2) *Bilateral cataracts, either hereditary or due to intra-uterine rubella virus infection.*

(3) *Buphthalmos (ox-eye).* This is congenital glaucoma with gross enlargement of the globe of the eye due to increased intra-ocular pressure.

(4) *Chorioid albinism* — a pigment deficiency in the chorioid layer of the eye due to an inborn error of melanin synthesis. Persons with this condition are not blind but have poor vision, usually accompanied by nystagmus and photophobia. Pigment is also lacking in the skin and the hair.

Progressive hereditary blindness

This kind of blindness develops insidiously and may be complete at any age.

(1) *Optic atrophy.* This is not always a hereditary condition, as the conducting function of the optic nerve may be affected by any intracranial disease which causes pressure on the nerve.

(2) *Retinal dystrophy and degeneration caused by progressive myopia.* Elongation of the globe of the eye increases as the child grows older, causing the stretched retina to degenerate due to defective nutrition.

(3) *Macular degeneration* with loss of central vision.

(4) *Retinitis pigmentosa* (tapetoretinal degeneration) (see p. 132). Chronic inflammation of the retina with pigmentary infiltration causes progressive retinal atrophy.

(5) *Corneal dystrophy* — defective nutrition of the corneae causing corneal opacities to form in the absence of inflammatory lesions.

(6) *Retinoblastoma* — a malignant tumour of the eye arising from immature retinal cells. Retinoblastoma may be uni- or bilateral and manifests itself by the age of 3 years.

Acquired blindness

(1) *Trauma* which destroys either part of, or the entire eye, and enucleation of a destroyed or cancerous eye.

(2) *Pathological conditions of the retina*:
  (a) retrolental fibroplasia;
  (b) vascular lesions of the retina and papilloedema in hypertension;
  (c) retinitis;
  (d) retinal detachment;
  (e) diabetic retinopathy (of vascular origin);
  (f) senile macular degeneration.

(3) *Optic atrophy* and pathology of the occipital cortex of the brain.

Note: Blindness in one eye is due to pathology of the eye or its optic nerve. If damage occurs to one optic tract distal to the optic chiasma, or to the optic cortex of one cerebral hemisphere, there will be blindness of half of each retina (hemianopsia).

(4) *Pathological conditions of the cornea*:
  (a) keratoconus and keratoglobus;
  (b) corneal scarring;
  (c) keratomalacia due to vit. A deficiency;
  (d) climatic droplet keratopathy due to long-standing UVL damage in outdoor workers.

(5) *Glaucoma.*

(6) *Bilateral cataracts.*

(7) Malnutrition causing *xerophthalmia* (conjunctivitis arida). The extreme dryness causing destruction of the conjunctiva and cornea is due to lack of tears caused by vitamin A deficiency (see p. 213).

(8) *Infection*:
  (a) Intraocular infections may occur during the course of intraocular operations. This may cause chorioiretinitis and panophthalmitis with total loss of vision in the eye affected.
  (b) Ophthalmia neonatorum, especially that caused by the *N. gonorrhoeae* (see p. 704) which is accompanied by keratitis.
  (c) Trachoma chlamydial ophthalmia can also be contracted at birth.

Note: Trachoma is a chronic conjunctivitis caused by the *Chlamydia trachomatis*. Frequently a secondary bacterial infection, superimposed on the chronic chlamydial infection, causes acute ophthalmia. Infection does not confer immunity and reinfections take place (see p. 457).

(9) *Infestation caused by the filaria worm —* onchocerciasis. Onchocerciasis is a generalised parasitic, non-fatal but crippling disease, estimated to affect approximately 20 million people, mainly in tropical Africa (i.e. not in South Africa). It is caused by a filaria worm carried from person to person by small bloodsucking blackflies. The infestation affects the skin, causing nodules and unbearable itching, as well as the eyes (cornea, retina and optic nerves) and may eventually lead to blindness. Onchocerciasis is often called 'river blindness' as it is endemic near river water in which the blackflies breed.

Mahoney[2] states that although microfilariae infiltrate the eye, blindness is uncommon. He would prefer the disease to be called 'river eye disease' and not 'river blindness'.

Systemic drugs can be used to cure the disease, but reinfection occurs. Established blindness is untreatable but loss of vision can be arrested. Effective control of the disease is by insecticidal attack on the larval stage of the flics.

DEFINITION OF BLINDNESS

The South African National Council for the Blind (SANCB) includes the following definition of blindness in its constitution: 'totally, partially or intermittently deprived of sight'.

The Blind Persons Act 26 of 1968, as amended by the Blind Persons Amendment Act 16 of 1971, includes the following description of blindness: '. . . if his acuity of vision is so restricted that he is unable to perform work for which eyesight is essential' (i.e. if he is visually handicapped).

THE BLIND PERSONS ACT 26 OF 1968

The aims of the Blind Persons Act are **rehabilitation**, the care and training of the blind child and the general welfare of blind persons. In furthering these aims, the Act relies heavily on the functions of the South African National Council for the Blind to help with:

(1) medical care;

(2) accommodation of the adult blind, if necessary in hostels;

(3) employment opportunities;

(4) extension of training facilities for the blind beyond the school.

State grants-in-aid are authorised by the Act to registered associations or approved institutions for the provision and maintenance of, for example, hostels, workshops and other places where registered blind persons can be rehabilitated, trained or employed. The state also subsidises the augmentation of the wages of registered blind workers.

The Blind Persons Act was partly replaced by the Social Assistance Act 59 of 1992 which controls the allocation of disability pensions to registered blind persons. The objectives of the Blind Persons Act remain the same, however.

Pensions for the needy blind and visually handicapped are issued to whites, blacks, Indians and coloureds under the provisions of the Social Assistance Act 59 of 1992. The means test is leniently applied, only half the blind person's earnings being taken into account.

Conditions for pensions for the blind as laid down by the Social Assistance Act 59 of 1992 are:

(1) the applicant must be registered as a blind person in terms of the Blind Persons Act 26 of 1968;

(2) no one is entitled to a pension for the blind if he, *inter alia*,

   (*a*) is required by law to attend a school;

   (*b*) is a person in respect of whom a grant is already paid in terms of the Child Care Act;

   (*c*) refuses to submit to medical examination or treatment;

   (*d*) refuses to register for employment if so directed;

   (*e*) refuses to accept employment which is within his capacity.

REGISTRATION OF THE BLIND ('LEGALLY BLIND' STATUS)

Registration as a blind person is voluntary and qualifies a blind person for a pension. It carries no stigma; moreover, it facilitates the rendering of services, either by the state or by welfare organisations.

Note: Even where persons cannot be legally registered, societies affiliated to SANCB will render services to such persons.

An applicant for registration shall be deemed to be blind if:

(1) Visual acuity is so restricted that he is unable to perform work for which sight is essential.

(2) Visual acuity is below 3/60 Snellen.

(3) Visual acuity is above 3/60 Snellen, but below 6/60, and field vision is reduced to 50 % of the normal field; provided visual defect is not long-standing, e.g. albinism or myopia.

(4) Visual acuity is 6/60 Snellen or better and the visual field is contracted to 25 % of the normal field and the lower part of the field to 50 % of normal; provided that he does not suffer from homonymous or bilateral hemianopia while retaining 6/18 Snellen or better.

A medical certificate for registration must be filled in by a doctor who shall:

(1) determine acuity of vision by means of the Snellen's test;

(2) in light of not less than ten foot-candles;

(3) determine the best direct vision of each eye separately, as well as both eyes together.

Forms requesting registration must be filled in by the applicant and, together with the above certificate obtained from a general practitioner, must be submitted to the local magistrate or district surgeon.

THE SOUTH AFRICAN NATIONAL COUNCIL FOR THE BLIND (SANCB)

The South African National Council for the Blind is the body which co-ordinates and organises voluntary blind welfare work and works in partnership with the state. The council co-ordinates the work of 43 affiliated organisations and liaises with 50 associated organisations and 9 state departments, as well as the Departments of Social Welfare of the Provincial Administrations. No handicapped person in the RSA is better catered for than the blind person, yet 75 % of the visually disabled people in the RSA are not reached by any existing service.[3]

Head Office is in Pretoria, regional offices in Cape Town and Durban.

The SANCB administers a subsidy from the state of 20 % of running costs and serves as a channel for communication with the various state departments for the subsidisation of the Optima Training Centre, 19 workshops and 6 hostels. Eighty per cent of the SANCB running costs is obtained by fund raising.

Some of the associates and facilities affiliated to the council are: a large number of Civilian Blind Societies and clubs in many of the larger towns and cities in the RSA, the South African Blind Workers' Organisation in Johannesburg and Port Elizabeth, Tape Aids for the Blind in 8 cities, workshops and homes for the blind in Worcester, the South African Library for the Blind in Grahamstown, the SA Guide Dogs Association for the Blind in Johannesburg and Durban and 8 schools for the blind.

The production of braille is undertaken by Braille Services — a department of the SA Blind Workers' Organisation in partnership with the SANCB. Nearly half a million pages of braille are produced annually in Afrikaans, English, Sotho, Zulu and Xhosa, important braille publications being textbooks and periodicals.

The *SA Library for the Blind* helps blind students to obtain textbooks in braille and on tape.

Training in the use of guide dogs and of the long cane is offered by the *SA Guide Dogs Association for the Blind*. The aim of providing a blind person with a guide dog is to give him some mobility and independence. Blind people are making increasing use of this service which entails not only the training of the guide dogs and their blind owners but also after-care work. This association is not state-aided and relies on the support of the public.

The SANCB provides direct services in our major cities. These direct services are:

(1) The Bureau for the Prevention of Blindness (see later).

(2) Rehabilitation centres in Johannesburg and Pretoria (see later).

(3) Placement in employment. The council's employment offices assist with the assessment and selection of candidates for specific jobs and persuade employers to make opportunities available, etc. The visually handicapped are employed in open labour and in sheltered workshops.

(4) Sales depot for visual aids. These aids include white canes, braille frames, labels and watches, as well as electronic equipment (Optacon), CCTV reading systems, light probes for telephonists and pocket calculators. The Blindiana library also issues audio-visual materials and deals with queries and requests.

(5) Statistics.

(6) Blindiana Library — a research facility — was started in 1977 at headquarters in Pretoria. This library is a source of information about all aspects of blindness for the members of professions, for those providing direct services to the visually handicapped, for the general public and for the visually handicapped themselves.

(7) A resource centre where prospective buyers can try out equipment before making a purchase.

(8) Education of the public in the prevention of blindness, especially by running the annual Eye-Care Awareness Week.

THE PREVENTION OF BLINDNESS IN SOUTH AFRICA

Primary prevention

(1) *Genetic counselling* of parents and children with familial poor sightedness, especially where children are in schools for the blind or partially sighted children. Here young people who carry defective genes for sight live in close social contact and are likely to choose marriage partners who also carry defective genes, thus increasing the likelihood of producing blind offspring. Although two blind people cannot be prevented from marrying each other, full knowledge of the dangers for their offspring may cause them to decide not to have a natural family.

(2) *Avoidance of oxygen therapy in premature neonates* to prevent retrolental fibroplasia. If the premature neonate desperately needs oxygen, the ambient oxygen concentration must never be higher than 50 %.

(3) *No drugs of known or doubtful teratogenicity* should ever be given to pregnant women during the first three months of pregnancy and rubella should be avoided during this period by prophylactic inoculation. At the present time some of our public health authorities have started on widespread rubella inoculation campaigns which include school girls.

(4) *Ophthalmia neonatorum.* Routine eye prophylaxis is practised. Antiseptics are instilled into the swabbed eyes of infants immediately after birth, e.g. silver antiseptic drops or erythromycin ophthalmic ointment.

Note: Erythromycin ophthalmic ointment is preferred as it is effective in preventing both gonococcal and chlamydial ophthalmia.

(5) The prevention of *xerophthalmia* and *keratomalacia* is theoretically simple:

(a) the diet of at-risk children must be corrected by effective education of mothers to include yellow and green vegetables in the family diet;

(b) the large-scale use of vitamin A fortified foods such as sugar and maize products;

(c) the mass distribution of vitamin A capsules can be done by schoolteachers to children at-risk in areas with suboptimal nutrition. Even the intermittent administration of vitamin A will prevent xerophthalmia as the vitamin is stored in the liver.

(6) *The prevention of trachoma is by health education, the supply of piped water to households, and by raising the standards of personal and environmental hygiene,* especially the combating of the fly menace.

The success of any community health project depends upon whether the community accepts the scientific (essentially the Western) definition of the aetiology of trachoma and therapy based thereon. All blacks in the Northern Province know trachoma, but they explain its aetiology according to their magico-religious beliefs. Unless they can be reached intellectually by scientific health education principles, they are not likely to co-operate in therapy. The traditional blacks believe every child must go through a stage of discharging eyes in order to be able to see in later life. For this reason they do not take their infected children to the clinics for eye treatment. They also believe that the sequelae of trachoma are caused by evil spirits going from hut to hut to inflict entropion, trichiasis and blindness. Trachoma is, therefore, considered inevitable in the young and caused by 'fate' in the elderly. Few people come of their own volition to hospital for treatment, only about 3 % of those with entropion seeking operative relief.

Sutter and Ballard[4] found that only people from the community can change people's attitude to the disease. Westerners who attempt to educate the people find to their dismay that the people simply laugh at scientific explanations. Sutter and Ballard devised a successful way of applying primary and secondary preventive treatment in a circumscribed area in the northern Transvaal by letting the community look after itself, under the supervision of the central hospital and clinic staff and social workers. Through their efforts 'Care Groups' (community health workers) came into existence.

Secondary prevention

The secondary preventive measures to restore sight include the following:

(1) Prompt treatment of *acute glaucoma* and effective maintenance treatment and supervision of *chronic glaucoma* by an ophthalmologist.
(2) Effective *topical chemotherapy in trachoma* and corrective surgery to the scarred eyelids in cases of chronic trachoma to cure trichiasis and prevent the progress to complete blindness due to scarring of the cornea.
(3) *Lens extraction* for the cure of cataract with adequate correction of vision.
(4) *Corneal transplantation* for the cure of blindness due to pathological conditions of the cornea.
(5) *Photocoagulation* to prevent the progression of diabetic retinopathy.
(6) *Removal of diseased vitreous* (vitrectomy) when diabetic retinopathy causes blindness due to fibromuscular membranes and chronic haemorrhage.
(7) *Argon laser photocoagulation* to prevent progression of macular disease which causes blurred central vision and impairment of colour vision.

The work of the Bureau for the Prevention of Blindness of the SA National Council for the Blind (SANCB)

The headquarters of the Bureau are at the National Eye Centre in Pretoria. The Bureau functions with the aid of the Department of Health and other authorities.

The Bureau works mainly by conducting field tours of areas where there are no facilities for regular eye care. The Bureau for the Prevention of Blindness, through its five (now four) mobile units, carries eye-care services to the remotest parts of the RSA and into neighbouring states. Thousands of patients are examined, minor operations are performed in the field, spectacles and treatment are prescribed and provided free of charge; more serious cases are referred to larger centres and even transported there.

The teams which visit remote areas in mobile units consist of an ophthalmologist, field officer (in charge), registered and enrolled nurses and, at times, an optometrist.

Note: Spoornet's Eye-care train in the Transvaal visits inaccessible rural areas and has been transformed into a fully-fledged PHC mobile clinic.

The mobile units work as follows:

(1) The Colin Anderson Eye Unit visits only the black rural areas, where there is the greatest need for preventive eye care, viz. Bophuthatswana, Transkei, Lebowa, QwaQwa, KwaZulu and Namibia. The responsible authorities provide a subsidy for the service. This unit undertakes 10 tours of 12–20 days each per year.

 The unit does research work on glaucoma amongst the Pondo people of Transkei, where glaucoma is a significant cause of blindness. Extension of this unit will make it possible to do extensive epidemiological and incidence studies as well as screening campaigns, e.g. for trachoma.

(2) The St. John Eye Unit has the same staff complement and work output as the above unit, but confines its activities to rural areas nearer the towns, particularly the coloured and Indian communities in which eye-care facilities are inadequate.

 The unit works in close collaboration with provincial hospital services. Each area requiring this service is usually visited once in three years, a deficiency which can only be made good by increased resources.

(3) The SAB Sight Savers Project/Regular Treatment Clinics. The object of this unit is to hold three- to four-day treatment clinics once every two months at specified remote hospitals. This service has been started at Jubilee Hospital (Hammanskraal), Groothoek Hospital (Lebowa), Elizabeth Ross Hospital (QwaQwa), Ngwelezana (KwaZulu), Donald Fraser Hospital (Venda) and Rietvlei Hospital (Transkei). The unit is staffed by a guest ophthalmologist and optometrists, as well as ophthalmic nurses and a field officer drawn from the above two units.

Cataract is the greatest national (South African) eye problem; 16 000 more people in rural areas could have their sight restored annually if eye-care services were adequate. To make this a reality, the Bureau is taking a more advisory and training role in the prevention of blindness.

Apart from the training of ophthalmic sisters in the local eye (Sight-Savers) centres, they are training Ophthalmic Medical Assistants (OMAs) to provide primary health care at clinic level. Besides giving simple PHC, they are taught to treat minor eye ailments and to screen patients for specialist care. The first trained OMAs are expected to be ready by the end of 1994. The training of OMAs is complementary to the establishment of permanent eye care (Sight Savers) centres.

The centres are being established in the regional or district hospitals of communities of high need and population densities in rural areas. Public health authorities and NGOs are expected to supply the ophthalmic drugs and surgical requirements in their own areas, thus making them partners of the Bureau in eye-care programmes.

A Sight Savers unit will visit these centres and train the local nursing staff in theatre and eye clinic procedures. Subsequently, a Bureau-approved volunteer ophthalmologist and assistant (e.g. an optometrist) will visit such a centre whenever the local staff feel they have sufficient referrals to warrant such a visit. This makes it unnecessary for an entire mobile unit to visit the centre.

At the end of 1991, four Sight Savers centres had already been established in some of the former black national states. For the future it is hoped to get sponsorship for ophthalmologists to perform eye-care duties at the centres for extended periods, e.g. two weeks at a time.

Local medical officers will be sent to larger centres for ophthalmic training as cataract surgeons to deal with this great eye problem. Trained OMAs will be placed at clinics serving the Sight Savers centres to enhance the eye-care programme.

Statistics show that, despite the reduction in the mobile units of the Bureau (from 5 to 4), eye-care work (screening, supply of spectacles, eye operations) has maintained its level of service from 1989–1993, in the face of great economic pressures.[5]

An important step towards the fulfilment of the ideal of eye care for all by the year 2000 is the training of ophthalmic sisters on the model of the training course offered at Elim Hospital in Gazankulu.

The work of 'Care Groups' in the prevention of trachoma in the Northern Province

'Care Groups' (community health workers) are assembled, trained and required to work as follows.

Professional staff (doctors, community health nurses, social workers) elicit the help of chiefs and headmen to bring together groups of people held in esteem in the community. These groups meet with members of the professional health care team and are informed about the nature of the endemic eye disease and the role the community can play in combating it. Volunteers are asked to help fight the disease and to form themselves into 'care groups'. A care group consists of twenty volunteer women who receive no pay for their work. Some are motivated because of their concern for others, while some join the group because the chief may exempt the 'carers' from compulsory village work.

'Carers' must be an example to the rest of the community with regard to making use of community preventive health services, e.g. their children must have been immunised and attend the 'under-fives' clinic regularly, and the family must own a pit privy. Teachers often join the care groups but illiterate mothers also do so, getting their children to do the writing work for them.

The care group meets with a professional health instructor every 14 to 21 days and is taught the facts about trachoma: methods of transmission, especially the role of the communal face-cloth and flies; methods of diagnosing trachoma (e.g. how to evert the upper lid to spot the granular appearance of the conjunctiva) and method of inserting the antibiotic ointment. They are also taught how to recognise other common endemic disorders, especially malnutrition, and to refer such cases to the clinics or hospital. By these means, esteemed but medically non-professional members of the community are doing primary health care amongst their people. They also help the clinic sisters trace TB defaulters and keep an eye on discharged kwashiorkor patients.

Special emphasis is placed on teaching care groups personal and environmental hygiene as they will be expected to teach these primary preventive measures to their clients: the combating of flies by the building of pit privies, the washing of cooking utensils immediately after use and the disposal of refuse by burning or, where possible, by making compost. They are taught how to wash hands without contaminating the washing water (e.g. by pouring water over soaped hands) and how to bath babies (to make them less attractive to flies). They are also taught how to make vegetable gardens for a continuous supply of fresh vegetables which are so important for the prevention of xerophthalmia. They help with the teaching of child nutrition, especially the promotion of breast-feeding at the 'well-baby' clinics.

The 'care group' workers, when trained, are expected to go into the huts of the people for case-finding and to teach the principles of good hygiene and nutrition. The mothers of infected families are issued with tubes of antibiotic ointment (either tetracycline or chloramphenicol) by the 'care group' workers and are taught how to use it. Care group workers are expected to supervise the method and frequency with which the ointment is used and to keep and submit records of their cases and visits and tubes of ointment issued. The WHO recommends the following regimen of ointment application to the population at risk: five times a day for one week each month, continued for a year, after which the patient is placed under surveillance. The work of the 'care groups' is constantly supervised by professional health workers from the clinics or central hospital.

This scheme has been very successful and a large number of volunteer groups is operating in the field, taking treatment into the homes of families infected by trachoma.

EDUCATION AND REHABILITATION

Education of the blind

In order to increase the quality of life for the visually handicapped person, adequate training in the substitutive use of the other special senses, especially touch, is essential. For the blind or nearly blind child this entails training at a special school for the visually handicapped.

The first **Schools for the Blind** were the Worcester Pioneer School for whites and the Athlone School, Bellville, for coloured and black children. Since then, thirteen more schools for the blind and partially sighted children have been established. Some of these schools provide secondary education and six schools are teaching pupils at matriculation level. Over the past sixty years, seventy visually handicapped matriculants have been trained in London as physiotherapists. Pretoria University recently admitted its first partially sighted physiotherapy student. The SANCB started a Student Advisory Service in 1988.

The rehabilitation of children with severe visual problems must be started early in life — as soon as the problem is recognised. The nurse can be of great help to the affected family by bringing to their attention the facilities for helping the blind which are available in the community. She can stress the importance of early referral to and contact of parents and blind child with a suitable school, so that the handicapped child and his family will be prepared for the separation when the child reaches schoolgoing age, which may be necessitated by his attendance at the special school.

Children with severe visual problems are sometimes sent to ordinary schools as they seem to be fairly independent and mobile, and visual acuity is deemed to be adequate on superficial testing of vision. The strain which myopia (especially if the condition is progressive), eye fatigue, restriction of field of vision and accompanying muscle abnormalities such as nystagmus and strabismus impose in the classroom situation, makes it virtually impossible for such a child to learn. It is, therefore, important to recognise the visually handicapped child's problems and to recommend referral to an ophthalmologist for full investigation and expert advice about the necessity of special education.

In order to help a blind person obtain a professional qualification, the SA Blind Workers' Organisation makes available bursaries and interest-free loans to blind university students. They aid in the provision of brailled lectures and textbooks. Tape Aids for the Blind and the SA

Library for the Blind supply books on tape, free, on request.

Tape Aids for the Blind provides free loan recorder/play-back machines for deserving students. Postal services for braille and tape materials are free, provided they are clearly marked 'Literature for the Blind' and sent by or addressed to an officially recognised institution for the blind. This concession does not apply to library books returned to Blindiana Library.

The Enid Whitaker Rehabilitation Centre of the SANCB for all race groups

This is a department of the SANCB and is mainly a social rehabilitation centre for the newly blinded adult. It is able to offer three-month courses for nine persons at a time. A new rehabilitation centre, attached to the Optima Training Centre in Pretoria, offers social rehabilitation courses to 25 blinded persons. Accommodation is provided during the course.

1. Techniques of daily living

A completely furnished flat is provided for training housewives in housekeeping, including cooking and recognising the contents of the grocery cupboard. The blind person is taught to care for himself without help and to identify clothing.

Women are taught the art of make-up. Clients are taught to recognise different denominations of money.

2. Independent mobility

The newly blinded adult is also taught mobility, i.e. how to move around independently with the aid of the long cane, the principal means of mobility for the blind.

3. Communication skills

The newly blinded must also learn how to read and write by means of:
(1) braille;
(2) the Optacon, an electronic reading device;

Recently the Optacon, an electronic device the size of a small tape recorder, was invented, to enable the blind to read an ordinary printed book, albeit rather slowly, where brailled books on specialised subjects are not available. The Optacon scans a printed page and converts ordinary print into minute raised rods in the shape of individual letters which can be 'read' through the fingertips of the trained blind person.

(3) low-vision aids, e.g. magnifying apparatus and CCTV;
(4) dictaphone typing.

The social work services, transport and workshop facilities of the Civilian Blind Societies are available to those undergoing rehabilitation training. While the breadwinner is being trained for new employment, a social worker will take care of him and his family.

The **Optima Training Centre** opened in Pretoria in 1985. It is run by the SANCB, being its most important and largest training centre. It is an extension of the Enid Whitaker Rehabilitation Centre.

The Optima centre is comprised of two sections:

(1) The social rehabilitation training centre mainly for newly blinded persons. Here they learn skills of independence: techniques of daily living, orientation and mobility, communication (reading braille and typing).
(2) Optima College for vocational training. Here blind and partially sighted students learn secretarial, telephonic, Optacon reading, computer and word processor skills.

The college also trains 'skills-developers', who, though not highly trained teachers of the blind, will fill the need for home visiting and low-cost community-based rehabilitation training of the vast majority of blind people who are not able to attend expensive centrally based rehabilitation courses.

Optima College assesses persons with low vision from the College and the local community, with the help of volunteer ophthalmologists and optometrists. Optima's O&M (Orientation and Mobility) instructors train the partially blind person how to make the best use of residual vision, and stimulate the use of functional vision.

In 1993 a Small Business Development Unit was opened on Optima premises. A major priority in the SANCB's future work is independence training and assisting people in engaging in economic activities, especially in the townships and rural areas. This empowerment will make the life of visually disabled people more meaningful and productive.

Societies to help the Civilian Blind run **sheltered workshops** where blind people make cane furniture, tennis nets leather goods etc., and string tennis rackets. These societies for the blind help all racial groups. Successful contract work has made some of these workshops viable factories able to pay good wages.

The Department of Manpower (Labour) subsidises workshops of the SANCB.

Employment of the blind and partially sighted

People who need employment can contact the placement/employment section of the SANCB which works within the SA Blind Workers' Organisation and the Department of Manpower (Labour). Placement of the visually handicapped person is an onerous task. The Department of Manpower (Labour) subsidises the salaries of three placement officers attached to the SA National Council for the Blind. The workplace most suitable for an applicant is determined by his abilities and may be either a workshop or the open labour market.

Much remains to be done to enable blind persons to hold down jobs in a competitive labour market and to live as normal a life as possible, despite their handicap. The South African Blind Workers' Organisation has as its prime objective the placement of blind workers in open labour, especially in the careers of telephony, piano tuning and repair, typing and arts and crafts, and lately as computer programmers and word processor operators.

In 1990, 82 occupations were practised by blind people in South Africa. The SANCB promotes the employment of blind people by the education of the public and especially of employers about the abilities of blind people.

Education of the public in the prevention of blindness

The Eye-Care Information Centre of the Bureau for the Prevention of Blindness arranges an Eye-Care Awareness week during October each year. Each Awareness Week deals with a specific eye theme.

Some publications of the SANCB

The SANCB issues an official publication, *Imfama*, every second month. *Imfama* and the ra-dio programme 'In Touch' bring new developments to the attention of the public and visually handicapped persons. *Imfama* is also available in braille and on tape. *Blindaba* is an English braille magazine for black youth.

Directory of Services for Visually Handicapped South Africans (English and Afrikaans).

Early Years: A Guide for Parents of a Partially Sighted Child.

REFERENCES

(1) Rowland W. *Curationis* 1978; **1**: 5.
(2) Mahoney JL. Management of onchocerciasis. *S Afr Med J* 1982; **61**: 50.
(3) McKendrik B. New approach to development. *Imfama* 1989; **29**: 8–11.
(4) Sutter EE, Ballard RC. *S Afr Med J* 1978; **53**: 622.
(5) Rowland W. Executive Director's Report. *31st Biennial Report*. 1991–1993. South African National Council for the Blind.

The author acknowledges with gratitude the help of the South African National Council for the Blind (SANCB) through information obtained from *Imfama* — the official journal of the SANCB — and biennial reports of the council (1989–1991 and 1991–1993).

TEST OF KNOWLEDGE

The student has benefited from studying this chapter if he/she can answer the following questions:

(1) Define the following terms:
- avoidable blindness
- buphthalmos
- nystagmus
- retrolental fibroplasia
- myopia
- retinitis pigmentosa
- glaucoma
- chorioid albinism
- keratomalacia
- cataract
- keratoconus, keratoglobus
- onchocerciasis
- hemianopsia
- retinoblastoma
(2) Write an account of trachoma under the following headings:

(a) Definition and pathology

(b) Epidemiology

(c) Natural progression of the disease

(d) Prevention

(e) The work of 'Care Groups'.

(3) Write notes on:

(a) The definition, prevention and treatment of xerophthalmia

(b) Ophthalmia neonatorum

(c) Diabetic retinopathy.

(4) (a) Why is registration of a blind person recommended?

(b) What procedure is followed to obtain registration?

(c) What are the conditions for registration?

(d) What are the aims of the Blind Persons Act and how are these aims executed?

(5) Name the objectives of: the SANCB, the SA Blind Workers' Organisation, the Enid Whitaker and Optima Rehabilitation centres.

41

Psychiatrically and Mentally Handicapped Persons
The Brain-Damaged Person

INTRODUCTION

'Psychiatric' implies personality and behavioural disturbances, and 'mental' (as used here) intellectual or cognitive disturbances. If mentally handicapped, the person is backward or retarded due to a deficit in his ability to learn and retain what he has learned, to make sound judgements, to conceptualise and to take care of, and responsibility for, himself and others.

Psychiatric and mental can be used alternatively for describing the behaviourally disturbed person, but the term *mental* has pejorative (deprecatory) connotations and is thus not generally used for labelling the functional psychoses, e.g. schizophrenia.

There are many different kinds of psychiatric disturbances, but chronic schizophrenia has been chosen for inclusion in Part VI because it is a chronic disabling condition causing social dependency. The modern trend in psychiatric hospitals is early discharge of schizophrenic patients on antipsychotic medication to keep the acute symptoms at bay. This has placed the responsibility of caring for the chronic patient on the community. The nature of schizophrenia is such that the patient finds it difficult to socialise and hold down a job. He is dependent on others yet does not acknowledge this dependency because he withdraws into his own world. He is thus a cause for great concern for his caretakers (community psychiatric services) who feel responsible for the regularity with which he takes his medication, his living conditions, his attempts at socialising and his employment. If these skills break down, his sickness relapses and he has to be temporarily readmitted to hospital. This constitutes the 'revolving door syndrome' which, if repeated on many occasions, suggests that rehabilitation is not complete. Intractable dependency is sometimes conceded by admitting the patient to 'halfway houses', e.g. Gordonia in Johannesburg, or to LifeCare Group contract hospitals. Both schizophrenia and mental retardation are the concerns of the SA National Council for Mental Health and its many member associations which run state-subsidised institutions for these dependent members of society.

Day Care and Stimulation centres run by Mental Health associations are a great boon to working parents of mentally retarded children from the lower socio-economic strata of society.

The neurologically (brain) damaged person discussed in this chapter includes epileptic and head-injured patients with neurotrauma.

The chapter thus deals with damage to the brain from many causes. This damage cannot be cured, although certain lesions causing continuing irritation and nervous discharge (epilepsy) can be surgically removed. Generally, though, a damaged brain causes intellectual, emotional, social and vocational disability — the ingredients of chronic dependency and family disruption and despair.

Clinical neuropsychological testing helps to highlight problem areas in neurotrauma, thus enabling highly skilled neuropsychologists to work with problems related to memory, problem solving and attentional activities, among others. These modern services are not generally available; moreover, the intellectually severely impaired person responds poorly to therapeutic efforts.

Many brain-damaged persons have serious work limitations. This results in feelings of powerlessness and helplessness in managing their own lives, let alone taking responsibility for the lives of others.

The student is made aware of the measures taken to prevent brain damage, whatever the cause, especially in children whose learning ability may thus be grossly handicapped. Epilepsy is a very important community health problem which requires optimal nursing intervention on a primary health care level. In a study done at a day hospital in one of Cape Town's low socio-economic areas, a group attending a clinic for adult epileptic patients was assessed for quality of care. The findings were: drug compliance poor (55 %); seizure control poor; 50 % of seizures were precipitated by tension, anger and similar stressful emotions. Thirty-eight per cent of the patients had post-traumatic epilepsy. The majority of the clients were not rehabilitated, 62 % receiving a disability pension and only 11 % being self-supporting. These results were obtained despite a comprehensive approach to the management of the epileptic patient, including liaison with SANEL. Psychosocial stress and a high incidence of post-traumatic epilepsy predispose to poor drug compliance and seizure-promoting emotional factors, hence poor seizure control.

VOCATIONAL REHABILITATION OF THE CHRONIC SCHIZOPHRENIC PATIENT

Schizophrenia is a psychiatric condition which is not curable; it runs a chronic course with relapses (usually due to non-compliance with medication) which require hospitalisation for restabilisation on psychotropic medicines. The schizophrenic out-patient receives lifelong medication, often in so-called halfway houses with protective workshops. Some are permanently cared for in LifeCare Group rehabilitation hospitals under contract to the government. Many, however, live semi-independently in a supervised flat with other schizophrenic patients or with relatives. The semi-independent schizophrenic person needs supervision in the community by the community psychiatric nurse.

Pre-vocational rehabilitation

Because the nature of the disability often precludes the ability to hold down a job and find vocational fulfilment, much pre-vocational preparation may be necessary before successful placement can be made, either in the open labour market or in training and work centres (sheltered employment factories) of the Department of Manpower (Labour).

The schizophrenic 'personality' is generally characterised by:

(1) Lack of energy and drive and lack of vocational goals; low productivity level.
(2) Lack of initiative and creativity.
(3) Passivity and dependency.
(4) Poor ability for self-maintenance.
(5) Lack of self-confidence and sense of adequacy.
(6) Poor concentration.
(7) Moodiness and poor ability to form interpersonal relationships; the schizophrenic person lives in his own world and is inclined to withdraw from people. He is extremely sensitive (e.g. to good-natured ragging), and cannot take criticism from those in authority over him.
(8) Poor sense of responsibility; he does not take responsibility for his behaviour.
(9) Inability to be punctual because he lacks a time sense.

The purpose of rehabilitation of the schizophrenic person is integration into social and vocational life and prevention of the deadening effects of understimulation in an environment that makes no demands. In such an environment time and place mean nothing. When life loses its meaning, human beings withdraw into themselves and stop communicating. The 'burnt out' schizophrenic needs to have a meaningful occupation and to form relationships. The negative personality factors and poor work record make work placement a difficult task for the social worker. It is important to keep the chronic schizophrenic person out of hospital where he is likely to develop the Hospital Dependency Syndrome with complete social breakdown and personality deterioration which is not a direct result of the treatable acute schizophrenic condition. The vocational counsellor (Department of Labour) can run pre-vocational rehabilitation groups of schizophrenic persons to make the latter aware of the requirements of the role of an employee, thus helping them to join the world of work.

Group counselling for rehabilitation[1] is considered the most suitable therapeutic measure. In the shared experience of the group, the client is helped to maintain healthy interpersonal relationships — a prerequisite for successful vocational adjustment. Group therapy helps clients to comply with medication and thus prevents rehospitalisation.

In the group sessions acceptable and non-acceptable working habits are communicated by the counsellor and solutions are found to problems in the work situation. Group members gradually develop a more positive self-image with enhanced feelings of self-worth. The therapist sets out to encourage communication amongst group members and focuses attention on the interpersonal relationships resulting from communication. Once motivated, the group member is taught the basics of the requirements of the work role, viz. personal care, punctuality, self-discipline, relations with superiors and colleagues, co-operative efforts in the work situation and many more. Extreme dependency is changed as the client is gradually confronted with more difficult situations for which he must take responsibility. It is hoped that the insights thus gained will carry over into the work situation.

Pre-vocational rehabilitation of the schizophrenic person needs the services of a highly skilled counsellor. The rehabilitation process is concerned essentially with the building up of a personality structure which is outer directed so that the schizophrenic person no longer withdraws into his own world.

MENTAL RETARDATION

The term *mental retardation* is used for a person with defective or subnormal intelligence. A mentally retarded person is one who, because of arrested or incomplete development of the mind, has a marked lack of intelligence (i.e. low IQ) and inadequate ability to adapt to his environment and is, therefore, mentally handicapped. The onset of mental retardation is before the age of 18 years.

The IQ is, however, only a rough guide to the degree of intellectual deficiency; inability to profit from education provided for the subnormal in special classes by the subnormal child with an IQ above 55, or inability of the adult of like intelligence to live independently, is used as an additional criterion for applying the label of mental handicap. Using these criteria, the Van Wyk[2] Committee found that 4 out of every 1 000 white South Africans are mentally handicapped.

The following children may appear to be mentally retarded when, in fact, their retarded-like behaviour is due to remediable conditions: severe emotional disturbance (pathological withdrawal, depression, physical abuse), lack of stimulation, severe perceptual problems, severe learning disabilities.

In assessing the intelligence of retarded children, use is made of standard intelligence scales customarily used on normal children, e.g. Griffiths Mental Development Scale for the first eight years of life and the Fick Scale (Old SA Individual Scale).

The American Association on Mental Deficiency places the upper age limit of mental development at 18 years, i.e. the chronological age (CA) used in the calculations must never exceed 18 years.

Intelligence quotient (IQ) is the ratio of a person's intelligence (as measured by tests of mental competency to supply a mental age, MA) to the average or normal intelligence for his age (which is called the chronological age (CA)), viz.

$$\frac{MA}{CA} \times 100 = IQ$$

Example:

$$\frac{MA\ 6\ years}{CA\ 5\ years} \times 100 = IQ\ of\ 120$$

In normal children under normal conditions, the IQ remains constant throughout the developmental period as the mental age rises concomitantly with the chronological age. Lipman (1974)[3] points out the danger of using the IQ as an indicator of a retarded child's potential; the rate of mental development of the retarded child is much slower than that of the normal child, therefore, mental age will lag behind CA. The retarded child's IQ at 5 years does not predict what his IQ will be at the age of 12 years; the IQ tends to become lower as the retarded child grows older.

Lipman advocates the use of special tests for placement in an environment (special schools or institutions) where retardates can develop whatever abilities they have to acquire skills which will help them function as adequately as possible in family and community situations. It must be remembered that retardates are not a homogeneous group and exhibit variability in motor and verbal skills, e.g. the brain-damaged child is likely to have better verbal skills than motor skills, whereas the culturally deprived child will be the opposite.

Causes of mental retardation

(1) *Primary causes*
   (a) Specific genetic and chromosomal syndromes with associated retardation. Examples: phenylketonuria (PKU), Tay-Sachs disease and Down's syndrome.
   (b) Multifactorial causation, both polygenetic poor intellectual endowment and unfavourable nurture in a culturally (and emotionally) and economically deprived home. These familial retardates form the largest aetiological group and their intellectual impairment is not pronounced, usually above IQ 55.

(2) *Secondary causes:* i.e. damage to the fertilised ovum, foetus, newborn or young child. Damage may be caused by infection (virus), chemicals, physical trauma, anoxia, hormonal and nutritional deficiencies at any of the following developmental stages:
   (a) Intra-uterine (antenatal) stage: congenital rubella and syphilis, cytomegalovirus and herpes infection of the foetus, developmental aberrations, e.g. microcephaly probably caused by teratogenic agents, cretinism, smoking and malnutrition leading to small-for-date infants, prematurity, cerebral palsy, alcoholism (foetal alcohol syndrome).
   (b) Perinatal stage: anoxia and cerebral haemorrhage, especially in premature infants, hypothermia, hypoglycaemia, kernicterus.
   (c) Postnatal stage: meningitis, encephalitis, head injury; child abuse is an important cause of mental retardation.

Primary prevention of mental retardation — genetic counselling

Measures can be taken to reduce the incidence of mental retardation by preventing a birth which is thought likely to produce a defective child. These measures are possible only if health education has been effective in bringing to the notice of the public the causes of mental retardation and the types of parents who are at risk.

Parents-at-risk who are sufficiently concerned will take the following steps to prevent the birth of a defective child:

(1) If a specific gene or chromosomal aberration is suspected in a family, the expecting parents should undergo the relevant tests at a cytogenetic and tissue culture laboratory (SAIMR). *Examples:* karyotyping for possible carrier status (translocation trisomy 21 — Down's); biochemical tests on cultured leucocytes for detection of carrier status in diseases like Tay-Sachs. (See Chapter 8.)

(2) Amniocentesis of a woman who is pregnant if she has had a child with either Tay-Sachs disease or Down's syndrome or neural tube disorder (e.g. anencephaly). (See Chapter 8.)

(3) Termination of pregnancy if the foetus is suspected of being damaged, e.g. positive amniocentesis, rubella early in pregnancy, ingestion of teratogenic drugs, dangerous exposure to radiation early in pregnancy. (See Chapter 8.)

(4) Sterilisation operation or attendance at a family planning clinic to prevent further pregnancies if the risk of producing abnormal children is high. (See Chapter 20.)

(5) Multiparous women of low intelligence who cannot control their reproductive potential and cannot cope with a large family, should be persuaded to undergo a sterilisation operation. (See Chapter 20.)

Genetic counselling can be done by the family doctor, a paediatrician or a clinician with special knowledge of inherited disorders.

Nurses who are aware of the genetic causes of mental retardation (see p. 131) can play a very important role in primary prevention by referring patients to genetic counsellors and by making sure that patients understand the advice given by the counsellors.

Note: Good antenatal and perinatal care remains the most important primary preventive measures. Heavy smoking and drinking during pregnancy adversely affect brain development in the foetus.

Secondary prevention of mental retardation

Parents with mentally retarded children sooner or later bring their affected child to a doctor for diagnosis, especially if the child has neurological disabilities. Ideally they should be referred to a Mental Assessment Clinic of a Children's Hospital. The clinic is usually run by a paediatrician or a neurologist, assisted by a multi-disciplinary team consisting of a social worker, clinical psychologist, community health or domiciliary nurse; the family doctor and minister of religion can be co-opted to the team at a later date.

A full investigation is instituted to establish the cause and extent of the intellectual deficit. Investigations include:

(1) detailed relevant history of the family and the child, including details of pregnancy, birth and postnatal disorders and accidents;

(2) physical and neurological examination of the child;

(3) psychometric assessment to establish the mental age and IQ of the child;

(4) assessment of sight, hearing and speech (if the child is old enough);

(5) chromosomal studies and other chemical blood tests if an inherited disorder is suspected.

At the interpretation ('follow-up') interview, the empathic leader of the team attempts to help the parents understand their child's problem and accept him despite his handicap. Parents may react to the confirmation of their suspicions by rejection of the child and by self-blame and guilt that the child has been sent by God as a punishment (for some real or imagined sin).

It is important that the parents be told the extent of their child's intellectual deficit to prevent unnecessary 'shopping around' for further opinions and setting unrealistic standards of achievement for the child.

Help for the parents of the mentally handicapped child

Help for the parents of a mentally and/or physically handicapped child is preventive care, in that it promotes the mental health of the defective child and other children in the family. The parents are helped to work through their problems: their guilt and fear of blameworthiness, their anger at the child and death wishes towards him, their anger at fate and their need to blame someone for the burden placed upon them. If the parents can work through these negative emotions, they will be able to accept and love their child — a prerequisite for an effective helping relationship and involvement in the child's progress.

The parents are encouraged to keep their child at home; even with his intellectual deficit, a retarded child is entitled to mothering and to the best possible education and training which are available in the larger centres. The helping team (if one is available) takes over from the paediatrician in helping the family cope with their problem. A retarded child who is institutionalised at an early age will not develop his full potential because he will lack the stimulation normally provided by parents and siblings. The world-wide trend is to institutionalise (in state or private homes) only the severely mentally and physically handicapped children whose presence in the home constitutes a threat to the physical and mental health of the family.

Note: The interaction of mother and baby enables the baby to attain a level of attentiveness in which he can respond to stimulation. Thus the retarded infant can be helped to develop to his fullest potential.

In the beginning, a member of the team, e.g. the community health nurse, should visit the home regularly to support the family in their crisis. If the parents feel supported, they will be less likely to get rid of the child by sending it to a home. If the mother can be helped to try to look after her handicapped child, she will be less likely to feel guilty if later it becomes necessary to place the child in a home, either permanently, or for a holiday period or during school terms, with the concurrence, or on the advice of the team. The aim of the team should be to get families to maintain their child at home either permanently or as long as possible, and to assist them with institutionalisation, if this becomes necessary. The latter becomes necessary if the harm done to family life by the presence of the child is greater than the good done to the handicapped child by home care.

The team brings to the notice of parents the existence of the Division for the Mentally Retarded of the South African National Council for Mental Health. This division co-ordinates all voluntary societies which aim at the welfare of the mentally retarded and their families. It encourages the parents to join small voluntary groups of parents for mutual support, or the mothers of mentally retarded pre-school children to form play groups for their children and mothers' groups in which they receive counselling in the handling and training of their retarded children. Supportive community agencies are most important for the family and their handicapped member during the early formative years of the defective child's life.

Foster homes can be used to supply holiday relief for the mother who bears the brunt of the burden of caring for the child.

Residential Care Centres, e.g. the Woodside Sanctuary in Johannesburg, and Care and Rehabilitation centres take children temporarily while their parents go on holiday.

DSM-III Classification of mental retardation

Categories of retardation

IQ	Category
71–80	Borderline
50–70	Mild retardation (80 % of retardates)
35–49	Moderate retardation (12 % of retardates)
20–34	Severe retardation (7 % of retardates)
Below 20	Profound retardation (1 % of retardates)

Educability of retardates

IQ	Educability
55 and up	educable to read and write in special class
30–55	ineducable but trainable
below 30	untrainable

Mentally handicapped persons in South Africa are cared for by the public and the private sector. Mental handicap may be associated with physical handicap; therefore, habilitation of the child may require a range of caring services. As far as possible the handicapped person should remain in the community, either at home or in licensed or registered residential homes and hostels. The state subsidises its mentally handicapped citizens in some way or another.

TRAINING AND CARE OF THE INEDUCABLE MENTALLY HANDICAPPED PERSON

The profoundly retarded person (IQ under 20)

The most profoundly handicapped (adults and children) and those with a lesser degree of mental retardation but with physical handicaps and psychotic disturbances, are hospitalised in 'Care and Rehabilitation' centres, large institutions of which there are seven; they are run by health departments. Here nursing, medical and paramedical services are available. Due to shortages of facilities, the state has entered into contract with the LifeCare Group to provide accommodation and care for thousands of mentally handicapped (as well as psychiatrically ill and frail aged) persons. The state pays this company a daily tariff comparable with state costs of caring for these patients. Private organisations (residential care centres) also care for the profoundly retarded person, e.g. Woodside sanctuaries.

The severely retarded person (IQ 20–34)

The severely handicapped person who does not live at home is accommodated in care centres (homes and hostels) in the community, which are subsidised (to the rate of a single care grant per child) by departments of health which licence and inspect them. Many of these care centres are run by welfare organisations under the aegis of the South African National Council of Mental Health, or churches or private organisations (e.g. Avril Elizabeth Homes).

It is realised more and more that good, intensive habilitation programmes will produce optimal self-sufficiency and quality of life in those with a mental handicap. The important goal of a habilitation programme is to socialise the child so that he can live amongst and get along with other people. This facilitates his integration into society. Those who are capable of so doing are encouraged to live in the community with their families or in group homes.

The moderately retarded person (IQ 35–49)

They fall within the ineducable but trainable group and can be taught many skills.

Special training centres for children often have hostels attached to them, thus providing accommodation during school terms. Special training centres cater for the 3–16 year age group and may be run either by the government (departments of education) or by the private sector (e.g. The Hamlet and the Camphill schools).

Private training centres are heavily subsidised. The top age of 16 may be extended. Some training centres run by Departments of Education and Culture are situated in the grounds of Care and Rehabilitation centres. There should be liaison between the special training centres and protective workshops so that the child in training may be prepared for effective functioning in the protective workshop to which many are referred when they reach the age of 16. Some private organisations make provision for the transition from training to vocational facilities within their organisation. Although essentially geared to train the trainable retarded child, the training centres will also teach those capable of learning to read and do simple arithmetic.

Information on educational facilities may be obtained from the SA National Council for Mental Health.

Although definite IQ cut-off points are laid down for the various grades of educability, e.g. above 55 — can be taught to read and write; below 30 — untrainable to care for himself, in practice this is not the case. Thus a child who is ineducable 'on paper' may very well learn to read and do simple arithmetic, while a so-called untrainable child may learn to care for his body if he has a patient and loving teacher, especially if this teacher is his own mother who is able to accept him in spite of his handicap. Intelligence is not a static quality, hence the importance of giving every child the opportunity to develop to his full potential.

Training centres therefore take in both trainable and untrainable children and assess their progress frequently in order to step up stimulation and demands for achievement. Likewise, they have facilities for teaching the 3 Rs and no child is denied the opportunity to develop his skills to the full.

In the special training centres for retarded children, the educational programme should encourage the development of gross-motor, fine-motor (hand), perceptual, linguistic, musical and scholastic abilities — learning experiences which are meaningful to retarded and physically handicapped children. This educational programme is carried out by a multi-disciplinary team consisting of pre-primary and primary schoolteachers and speech, occupational and physiotherapists. These teachers and therapists must be infinitely patient people who are committed to their work, as success with retarded children does not come easily.

The atmosphere must be one of permissiveness and children persuaded to conform to required standards by the use of incentives, e.g. praise and adult approval, for tasks accomplished. The child is allowed to work at his own pace, as any pressure applied may cause overwhelming anxiety and a stubborn refusal to do anything, due to feelings of inadequacy which these children undoubtedly incorporate into their self-image.

When young retarded children have been exposed to a suitable educational programme with maximal stimulation for some time, the rate of their intellectual growth (note, their intelligence quotient is not used for this purpose) can be assessed from yearly psychometric tests. Thus their educational potential can be correctly diagnosed. This enables their teachers to place them correctly in classes (for adult career training), according to ability and aptitude.

If the child is ineducable but trainable, training can be done either by the mother at home (if there is no training centre in the vicinity) or in a group setting in day-care or residential training centres. If the mother does the training, she must be of good intelligence and receive guidance, if any success is to be achieved.

Skills in personal care and daily living

Although moderately and severely retarded children are unable to acquire cognitive skills, they can be taught and will retain skills in personal care and daily living. The child must be helped to become as self-sufficient and independent as possible. The following skills will help the child to become integrated into the family:

(1) toilet training, dressing skills, personal hygiene and tidiness with regard to his clothes;
(2) table manners, good posture and the use of cutlery and crockery; this will ensure that the child is not a source of embarrassment to his family;
(3) the ability to make simple choices, e.g. between wearing a blue frock or a pink frock;
(4) the control of emotions, e.g. temper tantrums: firm but loving holding during such an attack gradually gives the child the idea of control;
(5) the acceptance of limits: the child must be taught that certain antisocial acts are not permissible;
(6) the doing of simple chores about the house.

After the above skills have been mastered, the child is helped to acquire more difficult skills:

(1) The value of money (e.g. by going on shopping expeditions with an adult), the roles of commonly encountered public servants (e.g. policemen) and the rudiments of the rules of the road.
(2) Speech training according to the child's potential. The child's imagination is stimulated by stories and pictures and general knowledge is supplied by TV and by taking the child to places of interest, e.g. a fire station.
(3) Social manners. Some retarded children can be very difficult behaviourally. Aggressiveness and destructiveness are generally not tolerated and need to be controlled by parents who understand the reason for this behaviour, viz. aggression may be due to pressure being put on the child to achieve; lack of insight and the need to experiment may be the cause of a child destroying his toys. Instead of punishing this so-called 'naughty' behaviour, a loving, understanding parent will encourage conformity by playing with her child or letting her retarded child play with normal siblings, thereby affording him the opportunity to copy their behaviour. Retarded children are encouraged to conform, even though they cannot grasp the reason for the acceptable behaviour.

Retarded children must be taught from an early age what kinds of behaviour are acceptable in private (e.g. masturbation if they resort to this — a very common occurrence) and what is inappropriate behaviour in public (e.g. nose-picking or masturbation in public). Thus they are taught discriminatory behaviour.

Some retarded children, especially those with Down's syndrome, are very affectionate and will hug and kiss strangers. This must be strongly discouraged so that affectionate interchanges within the circle of family and friends acquire some significance. Adolescents should not be taught about the dangers of rape — which they are unlikely to grasp. The safety of girls from this ever-present danger can only be ensured by lifelong inculcation of discriminatory behaviour towards strangers and non-strangers. Thus the retarded girl, who is often the target of conscienceless males, learns to resist any accosting stranger. (See law with regard to abortion after rape, incest or unlawful carnal intercourse where the woman has a permanent mental handicap — p. 348.)

(4) Sex instruction is given from an early age, beginning with grooming skills and teaching body parts and their names and functions, only to the level at which the child is able to understand.

(5) Manipulative skills are taught and include simple handicrafts and domestic chores. The child may progress from here to some form of pre-industrial training to equip him for sheltered employment at protective workshops or state-run sheltered employment factories (see p. 775). Employment facilities for the moderately and severely retarded adults are insufficient but do exist, for example, the Cluny Farm School in the Transvaal which offers residential care and employment for whites over the age of 16 years, and 'The Village' at Kalbaskraal, Cape, run by the Camphill organisation.

Note: Day Care and Stimulation Centres are run by regional mental health societies for intellectually handicapped children who are ineducable but trainable and for whom there are no residential or adequate home services for socio-economic or political (e.g. inadequate services for blacks) reasons.

PROTECTIVE WORKSHOPS AND WORK CENTRES FOR ADULTS

Many adults are taken up in protective workshops and after-care hostels after they have completed their training in a children's training centre.

Protective workshops are not legally defined and are established by welfare organisations to provide adequate accommodation and work facilities for adults. Every inmate is trained to his maximum capacity so that he may find vocational fulfilment. Unfortunately the demand for protective workshops and live-in facilities is greater than the supply.

It is not enough, however, just to supply work and accommodation. The retarded person also needs the opportunity to relax and mix socially. Healthy social adjustments in the protective workshops include co-operation with colleagues and staff and the acceptance of authority and discipline. Sporting and recreational facilities are essential to enrich the monotonous life-style of the retarded person.

Where mildly retarded persons educated at special schools for the mentally handicapped or in special classes of normal schools are able to function in subsidised sheltered employment (training and work centres), they become the responsibility of the Department of Manpower (Labour). From here some of them progress to the open labour market. The disability pension falls away if the mentally handicapped person is gainfully employed. For training and work centres (Sheltered Employment Factories) see p. 773.

PREVENTION OF PROCREATION BY THE MENTALLY RETARDED PERSON

Females must be guarded against inadvisable pregnancies. A family planning clinic will advise in this regard. The responsibility for contraception must, however, be borne by a responsible person.

Sterilisation is permissible if the retarded adolescent or adult is not accountable for the fruits of coitus.

Steps to be taken for the legal sterilisation of a retarded adolescent or adult by a referral centre

The male is first sent to a urologist and a female to a gynaecologist for a physical check-up.

A social worker then interviews the family requesting help and takes a family history. If necessary the candidate for sterilisation is referred for psychometric assessment; this is unnecessary if there is profound retardation.

After this, one psychiatrist and one doctor assess all the gathered information and, according to their judgement, submit a request for sterilisation to the Minister of Health, who gives the necessary permission.

Note: See the law with regard to the sterilisation of the mentally handicapped (p. 346).

The age at which sterilisation is done will depend upon the temperament of the adolescent or adult and the kind of control he/she has. If a female cannot cope with menstruation, then a hysterectomy may be recommended.

A mentally retarded male is usually impotent, i.e. he cannot reach orgasm, and may masturbate excessively. Despite fears to the contrary, boys are usually not sexually precocious.

Where there is danger or the problem of rape, the advice of a urologist should be sought. Vasectomy, the usual procedure applied for male sterilisation, does not stop rape.

STATE AID TO THE MENTALLY HANDICAPPED

The following grants and pensions are payable in respect of mentally retarded persons.

Single care grants

An allowance may be paid by the Department of Health to the person entrusted with the care of a person who is certified as a state patient under the Mental Health Act, and who is under the age of 16 years. Application should be made to the magistrate's office.

The parent/guardian must submit himself/herself to a means test and on receiving the grant is named the responsible person caring for that child. This grant is not payable for persons in state or state-aided Care and Rehabilitation Centres.

Disability pensions

A disability pension is payable to a physically or mentally handicapped person over 16 years of age who is not capable of supporting himself. It is paid to the person himself, whether he is in the care of parents, a private institution or protective employment, but not to persons in state or state-aided Care and Rehabilitation Centres, or to persons who are still attending school.

Application should be made to the magistrate's office.

Approval of a disability pension is subject to a means test. An attendant's allowance can be granted to the mentally handicapped person who requires the continual care of another person.

THE SOUTH AFRICAN NATIONAL COUNCIL FOR MENTAL HEALTH

The South African National Council for Mental Health was established in 1920, following the efforts in Cape Town and Johannesburg to copy the American Mental Health Movement which was fathered by Clifford W. Beers. The South African National Council is a foundation member of the World Federation for Mental Health.

The South African National Council for Mental Health (called the 'Council' for short) is the only nationally organised mental health welfare organisation in South Africa and has its headquarters in Johannesburg, from where it co-ordinates the work of its 16 constituent mental health societies with their 24 mental health clinics, situated throughout the RSA.

The Council is the official public body to make representations to the government and provincial and local authorities on mental health matters.

It is governed by an executive committee and consists of members of the public, representatives from each constituent mental health society and from affiliated organisations, i.e. organisations concerned with mental health work, e.g. child guidance clinics, as well as advisory representatives of government departments. In the interval between meetings of the Council or its executive committee, the affairs of the Council and of its Division for the Mentally Retarded are governed by a Standing Committee; executive power is vested in a director who is assisted by full-time staff to carry out the functions of the Council. Since 1974 the Council has received a government grant to cover a small percentage of the administrative expenses of mental health societies.

The achievements of the Council

It has played a significant role in public education on matters of mental health and in mental health reforms.

It co-ordinates mental health projects initiated by the community. It helped to initiate child guidance clinics and in 1934 was directly responsible for the establishment of the Rand Epileptic Association, now the Epileptic Employment Association.

Indirectly, through its pleas for an enquiry into mental health services, it was responsible for the new Mental Health Act 18 of 1973 with its emphasis on Community Psychiatric Services, in line with the Third Mental Health Movement.

In 1960 a **National Division for Mentally Handicapped Children** was formed and in

1977 the Council appointed a full time co-ordinator of this division to expand its activities. It is now known as the **Division for the Mentally Retarded** as it deals with the problems of all retarded persons, irrespective of age or race. To it are affiliated more than 50 welfare organisations specialising in the care of the mentally retarded, with more than 60 homes and training centres.

Note: Mental health is here used synonymously with psychiatric health.

Functions of the SA National Council for Mental Health

(1) Formulation of a national policy regarding psychiatric health.
(2) Mental health promotion and the prevention of psychiatric illness.
(3) Promotion of improved treatment services for the psychiatrically ill.
(4) After-care and rehabilitation of the psychiatrically ill.
(5) Promotion of co-operation among scientific and professional groups contributing towards the advancement of mental health.
(6) Promotion of research in the field of mental health.
(7) Promotion of high standards of training for mental health professionals.
(8) Collaboration with all government and private agencies in connection with mental health matters.

Direct services operated by constituent mental health societies and other affiliated organisations may take the following form:

- Psychiatric out-patient clinics operated jointly with the Departments of Health.
- After-care hostels and halfway houses for discharged patients and for those who cannot function independently in the community.
- Child guidance clinics.
- Counselling services for people with problems of an emotional nature.
- Hostels, training centres and workshops for the mentally retarded.
- Public education.

Examples of projects of mental health societies (psychiatric and mentally handicapped):

(1) Day Care and Training as well as Stimulation Centres for intellectually handicapped children who are ineducable but trainable. The societies are striving towards the establishment of more protective workshops for their handicapped pupils once they reach the age limit of 16 years (or even older).
(2) Toy libraries for handicapped children in conjunction with a counselling service for the mothers.
(3) In Johannesburg in 1980 the Witwatersrand Mental Health Society (WMHS) established a halfway house — the Gordonia Residence and Protective Workshop — for discharged psychiatric hospital patients. Here the residents can live within the community and develop their remaining skills, thus increasing their self-esteem and their chance of one day entering the open labour market. These halfway houses are also being established in other centres.
(4) The Threshold Foundation (founded in July 1978) is a day centre also run by WMHS to enable schizophrenic adults to socialise and gain occupational skills for future gainful employment.
(5) POWA (People Opposing Woman Abuse), established in March 1980, is affiliated as a branch of the Witwatersrand Mental Health Society. This organisation is run entirely by women volunteers. They assist women and girls who have been raped or otherwise physically abused by men.

Finance

The South African National Council for Mental Health is a registered welfare organisation and as such receives part of its funds from the state. It does, however, rely on the public to provide a considerable portion of its money, which it raises by means of film premières, letter appeals and so forth.

Information has been supplied by the South African National Council for Mental Health.

THE BRAIN-DAMAGED PERSON

Two subjects will be discussed under this heading: epilepsy (often caused by brain damage) and the post-traumatic syndrome.

Epilepsy

Epilepsy is a fleeting, periodic, excessive neuronal discharge of energy by groups of brain cells, the brief interruption of function being known as a 'fit', 'ictus' or a 'seizure'. The brain disturbance develops suddenly and ceases spontaneously. Epilepsy is not a disease — it is a disease symptom which has a cause. Its main feature is its recurrent paroxysmal character, the attacks of seizures being interspersed with periods of normality.

Any organic lesion of the brain and some metabolic states may cause an epileptic seizure, but sometimes no aetiological factor can be found; such a disorder is then designated 'idiopathic' or 'cryptogenic' (of hidden origin). In practice it is impossible to exclude the possibility of an organic lesion as the cause of epilepsy and all recurring epileptic seizures, whether 'symptomatic' of an organic lesion or 'idiopathic', are treated with anticonvulsive drugs (anti-epileptics).

Epileptiform seizures (convulsions) may occur in childhood and adulthood without causing epilepsy, being distinguished from the latter by the absence of recurrent attacks. A child who has a convulsion in certain situations only does not suffer from epilepsy.

The terms 'epilepsy' and 'epileptic' are used only for those cerebral attacks which result from excessive discharge of hyperexcitable neurons. Other causes of seizures, such as metabolic disorders or alcoholic withdrawal symptoms, must be excluded (by CT scan, X-ray, EEG) before the diagnosis of epilepsy can be made and continuous therapy instituted.

Leary[6] states that 6 % to 8 % of the population experience one or more convulsions during childhood. Neuronal dysrrhythmia is relatively easily induced in the immature brain.

Approximately 1 % of South Africans (more than 300,000) suffer from one kind of epilepsy or another.

Status epilepticus

Status epilepticus refers to the persistence of a seizure (partial or generalised), either because of its lengthy duration or because repeated attacks occur at such short intervals that inter-ictal recovery is impossible. Generalised status epilepticus may be due to metabolic disorders, tumours, drug overdosage or uncontrolled hypertension with encephalopathy. In treated epileptics it may be caused by poor therapeutic compliance, change in anticonvulsive therapy, intercurrent infections, metabolic abnormalities and alcohol abuse. Status epilepticus may terminate fatally.[7]

Causes of epilepsy

(1) *Genetic factors.* There is considerable evidence for the genetic aetiology of some cases of primarily generalised epilepsy (idiopathic). It is possible that only the tendency to epilepsy is inherited with unknown precipitating factors causing the overt seizures. Epileptic disease is thus not inherited as such — only the predisposition or abnormal susceptibility to develop seizures. A first convulsion in a school-age child suggests idiopathic epilepsy.

(2) *Brain lesions*, usually as a result of perinatal insult or postnatal brain injury. Seizures occur in 25 % to 50 % of cerebral palsy children with hemiplegia and quadriplegia. Cerebral hypoxia can cause convulsions at birth and give rise to epilepsy years later.

(3) *Intra-uterine infections*, e.g. by toxoplasma, cytomegalovirus.

(4) *Tuberous sclerosis with epilepsy — epiloia*, characterised by small multiple sebaceous adenoma on the face in infancy or childhood. It is a genetic condition (autosomal dominant inheritance) accompanied by mental retardation.

(5) *Functional instability of the temporal lobe* (detected by EEG) is associated with epilepsy and deviant behaviour patterns (through a defective personality structure), perceptual, speech and psychomotor disorders. Prolonged febrile convulsions may be a cause of temporal lobe epilepsy (TLE) which may exhibit first in the school age.[8]

(6) *Evoked or reflex epilepsy.*[9] Many epileptic seizures do not occur spontaneously (i.e. they are not of central origin), but are evoked by afferent impulses which may be defined by careful history taking.

Examples:

(a) A flickering light ('photo-epilepsy') e.g. by watching television or driving along an avenue of trees.

(b) Music with or without affective impact. Musicogenic epilepsy is a type of TLE. The seizure may be triggered by a specific passage of music.

(c) Repetitive stroking of the skin.

(d) Stress with hyperventilation.

(e) Overtiredness.

(f) Reading.

(g) Certain movements.

(7) *Brain tumours and operations*, especially supratentorial operations which involve cortical interference and brain injury (excluding postnatal).

(8) Neurocysticercosis (see p. 632). Naidoo *et al.* found neuro-cysticercosis to be present in 30 % of a random sample of black epileptics of all ages.[10]

(9) Cerebro-vascular damage in the aged.

Primary prevention of epilepsy

(1) *Genetic factors.* Parents who suffer from epilepsy must be counselled about the likelihood of children inheriting the susceptibility to epilepsy. The risk to offspring is as follows:

Both parents with primary generalised or idiopathic epilepsy: 25 % (1:4).

Parent with tuberous sclerosis: 50 % (1:2) chance of the child having tuberous sclerosis.

(2) *Perinatal factors.* Good obstetric practice is important in the prevention of epilepsy.

(3) *Immunisation.* Vaccines can cause a susceptible child to run a high temperature. No child should be given a pertussis vaccine after the age of 2 years as there is increased danger of encephalopathy with seizures and brain damage.

(4) *Febrile convulsions.* A high temperature may cause a convulsion in susceptible children between the ages of 6 months and 4–6 years. Although one brief convulsion may not do any harm, prolonged (status epilepticus) and repeated febrile convulsions may cause cerebral anoxia with subsequent chronic temporal lobe epilepsy.

The prevention of *recurrent attacks* of febrile convulsions (where this is likely) is by continuous medication with phenobarb or sodium valproate until the dangerous stage (6 years) has passed.

Status epilepticus in the child with a high temperature is controlled by means of the following first-aid treatment:

(a) tepid sponge and fan to correct hyperpyrexia;

(b) IMI paraldehyde or IVI diazepam by continuous infusion;

(c) correction of electrolyte imbalance and hypoglycaemia;

(d) antibiotics for the infection causing the hyperpyrexia.

(5) *The prevention of head injuries from motor cycle and car accidents.* Grant[11] states that from 5–15 % of patients with closed head injuries and from 15–45 % of those with more severe injuries will subsequently develop epilepsy. The wearing of crash helmets by cyclists and safety seat belts by motorists are attempts to prevent head injuries.

Secondary prevention of epilepsy

This is done by early diagnosis of epilepsy and by the efficient management of the epileptic patient. Some patients with focal epilepsy can be cured by surgical removal of the epileptogenic focus.

Anti-epileptic medication is dispensed and controlled at epileptic out-patient (seizure disorder follow-up) clinics run by most provincial hospitals, in order to maintain the patient in the community.

Although most children with epilepsy go to normal schools, special schooling is available for those children who need extra help.

The diagnosis of epilepsy

A complete and detailed history must be taken. Both the patient and eyewitnesses of seizures should be questioned. It is possible to over-diagnose epilepsy and to restrict a person to the life of an epileptic when, in fact, he does not suffer from epilepsy. It is also possible that the diagnosis of minor epilepsies can be missed. *Petit mal* absences may well be the cause of poor school achievement in the child accused of being lazy, inattentive and prone to day-dreaming. The absences may go unnoticed by the teacher and by the family.

RECOGNITION OF EPILEPSY IN CHILDHOOD

(1) Electro-encephalography. This test is not essential for the management of a child. Abnormal electrical activity of the brain, when measured by EEG, indicates instability of brain function. Fifteen to twenty per cent of children show an abnormal EEG without suffering from seizures. Interseizure records show focal paroxysmal bursts, spikes or sharp waves. Fifteen per cent of epileptics have a normal EEG record. The EEG may be helpful in *petit mal*, psychomotor epilepsy, if due to cortical damage, and in salaam spasms, but it is not diagnostic of these conditions. For this purpose, clinical data are more important. When epileptic firing is deep-seated, e.g. mesial temporal area, scalp EEG recording will not reflect the abnormal brain waves.

(2) In the neonate, the seizure may be a tonic spasm of one hand or a twitching of part of the face. The tonic component is prominent and leads to cyanosis.

(3) Careful physical examination for a likely cause of convulsions.

(4) Psychomotor or TLE may be difficult to diagnose. The child may be frightened due to alarming auras. The limbs may stiffen and there may be posturing and post-ictal confusion. There may be transitory impairment of consciousness and behaviour which is inappropriate to current activity.

(5) *Petit mal* must be distinguished from fainting and hysterical attacks.

(6) Skull radiograph for confirmation of lesions, or calcifications (toxoplasmosis), or calcified cysts of tapeworm (cerebral cysticercosis).

(7) Sometimes a CT scan, ventriculography or isotope studies are resorted to if there are localising physical signs, raised intracranial pressure or marked EEG evidence of a focal (e.g. Jacksonian) lesion. CT scanning may reveal a slow-growing tumour or a lesion due to cerebro-vascular damage.

(8) Biochemical tests are done if a metabolic cause is suspected.

RECOGNITION OF EPILEPSY IN ADULTHOOD

This is essentially a clinical matter, plus a history of recurrent, sudden, brief episodes which reflect transient disturbances of brain function and/or disturbances of consciousness. The patient can describe what happens at the onset and end of an attack and the missing data can be supplied by witnesses. On admission to hospital a fit can be induced by artificial means.

Clinical features are:

(1) Sudden fits, day or night, without apparent cause. They often occur in clusters with intermissions, sometimes before or after waking. In women there may be a link with menstruation.

(2) Tonic-clonic convulsions with foaming at the mouth, biting of the tongue (tooth marks on the side of the tongue) and a hangover.

(3) Temporary, retrograde amnesia lasting several hours. Memory is recovered later. This occurs in certain types of TLE.

(4) Confused automatic behaviour, during or after attacks — fumbling with clothes, looking or wandering around aimlessly. There is amnesia for such events.

(5) A characteristic aftermath (post-ictal state) after a severe generalised attack — automatic behaviour, headaches, nausea or vomiting, mental dullness, aching limbs, soreness of tongue, drowsiness, sleep.

The immediate treatment of a seizure

GRAND MAL (TONIC-CLONIC)

The first-aid treatment of a patient having a grand mal seizure. Once a seizure has begun, it must run its course. First aid is, therefore, not directed towards aborting a seizure, but towards ensuring the safety of the unconscious patient. He must not be forcibly restrained. Safety is ensured by removing objects in the patient's vicinity, which may possibly injure him. Any tight clothes around the patient's neck and chest are loosened and he is turned on his side. The mouth must not be forced open (in an attempt to prevent the patient from biting his tongue), as this may cause more injury. The patient must not be 'revived' by giving him anything to drink. The patient is allowed to rest after a seizure and inquisitive crowds, who may embarrass the patient, are kept away.

A patient who has just had a seizure should not be allowed to drive a car until he has recovered completely, usually after a sleep. If the patient insists on going home, he should be accompanied. A doctor or ambulance is called only if the seizure lasts longer than 10 minutes. Status epilepticus is a dangerous condition which needs expert medical attention.

STATUS EPILEPTICUS

Although drug therapy must be commenced as soon as possible, the unconscious patient must be examined for head injury and a tentative diagnosis established by reading his Medic Alert bracelet and obtaining a short history from a companion. The patient is admitted to hospital and the above first-aid principles observed. In the ambulance O_2 is given and an IV saline drip commenced.

IV diazepam or clonazepam, bolus dose of 10 mg (repeated after careful titration against the patient's response) is given by the doctor to control the acute seizure. If the status persists, thiopentone is given. Intubation and ventilation may be necessary.[7] A maintenance anti-epileptic drug for long-term seizure control, e.g. phenytoin, is started immediately.

The management of epilepsy

1. In the child

(1) *Drug treatment.* An early age of onset and prompt seizure control are factors associated with the lowest recurrence rate. EEG is of limited value in predicting recurrence. Anticonvulsive (anti-epileptic) drug therapy is based on mass and surface area.

Large combinations of drugs (i.e. more than 2) should not be used; 2–3 doses/day are required. Monotherapy is a modern trend. Drug dosage can be accurately worked out according to laboratory methods for serum level determination. Therapeutic ranges have been computed on the basis of mass. The arbitrary dosage with resultant polypharmacy if the dosage is not correct, is

no longer tolerated. The serum drug content is established if good control is not achieved after several weeks — the dosage is then adjusted. This method in combination with mother compliance ensures good control in 80 % of children.

(2) In those who cannot be controlled with drugs, a ketogenic diet is given: Fat: CHO 4:1. This ensures metabolic ketosis. Strong maternal motivation is needed for this diet to be a success.

(3) When recurrent seizures are due to a localised lesion, surgery may be curative, if the focus lies in non-essential areas, e.g. anterior temporal lobe.

The prognosis in well-controlled childhood epilepsy is good. As a child grows older, he becomes more resistant to seizures. If the control is good, many children will be free of attacks in adulthood. It is difficult to decide when to discontinue medication — usually after four years without fits, provided the risk of relapse is low, i.e. in children with a normal EEG and in those with primary generalised epilepsy.

EDUCATION OF THE EPILEPTIC CHILD

Unrecognised *petit mal* seizures are a cause of a learning disorder in children. The attacks last from 5–15 seconds during which time the child is unconscious (with eyes wide open) and unaware of the ongoing lesson. The absences may be unnoticed. The cause of the so-called daydreaming, mental dullness and conduct disorder is eventually uncovered by a typical EEG finding. Neither the child nor his parents may be aware of brief *petit mal* attacks. The scholastic achievement of the child with *petit mal* can be improved on anti-epileptic medication.

Where possible, epileptic children should attend normal schools.

Some children with epilepsy are mentally retarded, however, the brain damage which caused the epilepsy being severe enough to cause a mental deficit. These are the children who need special education, preferably in schools for epileptics, or, if they suffer from cerebral palsy, in special schools for cerebral palsied children.

Special schools for epileptics are the Jan Kriel School and Bel-el Centre at Kuils River in the Cape, the Transvalia School for Epileptics in Pretoria and the WK du Plessis School for Epileptics in Springs.

Children are admitted to the special primary school on reaching schoolgoing age and in the secondary school are prepared for a commercial career or are taught handicrafts. The neurological status of all the children in these schools is regularly monitored and all receive anti-epileptic medication as prescribed by the physician who attends at the school. A psychologist assesses maladjusted children. These schools have residential hostels in which the children are closely supervised. Hostel accommodation is necessary because the special facilities for epileptic children are available in only four centres in the RSA. Social workers maintain the link between the hostel child and his family. The social worker also finds suitable work for school-leavers.

Attention must be paid to all the social, educational and other problems, to allow as full and normal a life as possible and to promote the fullest development of the child's potential. In the schools for epileptics, paramedical staff attend to physical and speech problems of children. Restrictions of activities and unhealthy attitudes of caretakers may be far more crippling than the condition itself. Help involves help to the family.

2. In the adult

(1) Removal of any cause wherever possible, e.g. brain scars and tumours, especially in certain cases of temporal lobe epilepsy.
(2) Avoidance of evocative stimuli.
(3) The control of seizures by medical means can be effective in 70 % of cases. Only about 10 different anti-epileptic medicines are in regular use, although approximately 20 are known. The patient must be observed for side-effects. It is important to balance seizure control with side-effect control. Complete suppression of seizures at the cost of drug intoxication is not successful therapy.
(4) Therapeutic drug monitoring. Non-compliance of patients with the prescribed drug regimen in epilepsy is an important cause of poor seizure control. Non-compliance and underdosage can be detected by measuring the plasma concentrations of anti epileptic

drugs of out-patients. By comparing the obtained results with expected therapeutic levels, adjustments can be made to drug therapy (in cases of underdosage) and compliance with prescribed dosages can be obtained by appropriate health education and, in some cases, by simplifying the drug regimen, for example, from multi-drug to single-drug therapy. This type of therapeutic change-over will depend upon the presence of side-effects from the consequent higher doses of a single drug. Blood level measurement of anti-epileptic drugs can thus contribute to the successful management of an epileptic patient.[12]

MANAGEMENT OF ADULT EPILEPSY AT A PRIMARY HEALTH CARE CLINIC

(1) Patients and their families are educated about epilepsy and its treatment. Apart from impressing upon patients the need for compliance with anti-epileptic drug therapy, the health educator must also warn about the epileptogenic effects of alcohol and the danger of using another epileptic patient's medicine.
(2) Relatives are encouraged to accompany patients, supervise medication and keep a record of seizures.
(3) Social problems must be given attention and occupational therapy arranged for those unable to work.
(4) Employment opportunities are created by liaising with a SANEL or Department of Manpower (Labour) work centre.
(5) Medic-Alert discs must be arranged for patients.

Tertiary prevention — rehabilitation of the epileptic person

The handicaps of epilepsy

These handicaps are psychological, social and economic.

PSYCHOLOGICAL AND SOCIAL HANDICAPS

The diagnosis of epilepsy is always a shock and elicits much anxiety. Parents are afraid that they may in some way be responsible for their child's condition and, if epilepsy runs in families, parents may feel guilty because they took the risk of producing epileptic children.

Epilepsy may cause severe emotional problems because of the uncontrolled nature of seizures and the avoidance at school of children who display *grand mal* seizures. Social attitudes to epilepsy are often of a rejecting nature. People with epilepsy have great difficulty in finding gratifying employment and are socially handicapped in many other ways, e.g. children are not allowed to swim if their seizures are not well controlled.

All these factors play a role in causing personality problems. Except for temporal lobe epilepsy and the dementia caused by uncontrolled fits and status epilepticus episodes, epilepsy *per se* does not have any effect on the growth of the personality or the intelligence. If epilepsy in the child is due to brain damage, the latter will have an adverse effect on the intelligence, not the epilepsy itself if seizures are well controlled.

Although it is constantly iterated by the health professionals that there is no such a thing as an epileptic personality, some persons with epilepsy undoubtedly have personality and behavioural disturbances characterised by loss of drive, delayed reaction time, religious fanaticism, irritability. Some patients with post-traumatic epilepsy may have violent temper outbursts and become physically violent.

People with epilepsy are usually not allowed to drive a car; in England someone who has been free of seizures while awake during the previous 3 years is allowed to hold a driving licence. Further, if they have only had attacks while asleep over a period of more than 3 years, they are also allowed to drive. The greater the success with the control of seizures, the greater the chance a person with epilepsy has for social rehabilitation and adaptation. The public must be made to realise that epilepsy is a treatable condition; in this way attitudes and prejudices based on long-held myths will be changed in favour of helping the person with epilepsy to live a normal social and vocational life. SANEL has set itself the task of educating the public towards healthier and more enlightened attitudes towards people with epilepsy.

EMPLOYMENT HANDICAPS

Many epileptics have difficulty in finding suitable employment; they find employment in the open market only if their seizures do not create hazards for themselves and others.

Employment of the epileptic person is, therefore, conditional.

Public prejudice which persists despite public education, contributes to employment problems as do some patients' own 'felt' stigma about their handicap which makes them hide the fact that they suffer from epilepsy. This secrecy causes a high level of anxiety and tension. They feel socially undesirable and often act accordingly, thus eliciting negative responses from others.

The needy, unemployable epileptic persons who cannot adjust to society and who receive state disability pensions comprise approximately 25 % of all persons with epilepsy.

Employment in the open market is often a problem for the epileptic person, but nevertheless a goal to be striven for in rehabilitation.

Employment opportunities for epileptic persons who are not employable in the open market, or who are in the process of being rehabilitated for work in the outside world, have been created by the Department of Manpower (Labour) assisted by two voluntary societies, SANEL and REEA, whose sole interest it is to promote the welfare of people with epilepsy.

THE SOUTH AFRICAN NATIONAL EPILEPSY LEAGUE (SANEL)

Only persons with epilepsy are admitted to SANEL. They must be 18 years of age or older and not fit for work in the open labour market. SANEL was founded in 1967 under the aegis of the South African National Council for Mental Health. The National Council of SANEL with head office in Edenvale, Transvaal, supplies specific information about the diagnosis, management and any other matters regarding epilepsy, such as those concerned with employment and rehabilitation. R & C Pharmaceuticals recently introduced a specialist epilepsy-oriented library information centre at SANEL's head office. This library contains information for the lay public as well as for the medical and related professions.

SANEL arranges lectures and seminars for the concerned public to eliminate the prejudice against epilepsy caused by ignorance. SANEL teaches that many epileptic persons can lead a normal, useful life if their seizures are well controlled. SANEL also advises epileptic persons about improving their lives.

SANEL is financed by the Department of Health and by the Western Cape Community Chest. SANEL also appeals to the public for funds. The National Council of SANEL has regional branches in Cape Town, Durban and Pietermaritzburg. SANEL is an important link between state services and concerned members of the public who wish to provide services for disabled epileptic persons.

SANEL has established a number of centres with workshops for epileptic persons throughout the country. Each centre's Management Committee falls under the umbrella of the National Council of SANEL. The first one was established in 1973 in Springs to assist epileptic persons from all racial groups with accommodation and employment. A number of old buildings were acquired in Springs and transformed into hostels and workshops. This complex has a halfway house and an aged home.

Residents at centres must be self-supporting; they are placed in a work situation in which they are required to work according to their capabilities in various trades. Some of the men work in the gardens. Ladies are suitably employed, some even being trained as nursing assistants. All employees are paid a salary. Medical, social, psychological and recreational needs are catered for. In these SANEL work centres the needy epileptic person can live a fulfilled life.

The SANEL work centres are also rehabilitation centres for placing suitable candidates in the open labour market. Social workers, subsidised by the state, provide a service to work centres by assessing and referring clients, counselling their families, promoting their rehabilitation and providing a follow-up service to encourage and guide those who have been placed in open market employment.

THE RAND EPILEPTIC EMPLOYMENT ASSOCIATION (REEA)

REEA was established in Johannesburg in 1934 on the initiative of three doctors who believed that men severely afflicted by epilepsy were employable.

Today the Association is run by a council comprising voluntary members of the public. It provides meaningful employment mainly for white male epileptic persons in a large modern nursery in Craighall Park which is under the supervision of trained professional staff. The three centres of the Association are a Men's Hostel, a Women's Centre (where women live and perform contract work for outside organisations) and a married settlement comprising cottages for white male married epileptic persons and their families.

Each centre has the services of social workers and nurses. Patients are seen regularly at clinics by the district surgeon and where necessary are counselled by a psychiatrist. REEA is semi-independent financially; it gets assistance from the Department of Health and from the public through regular donations, street collections and other fund-raising activities.

THE DEPARTMENT OF MANPOWER (LABOUR)

People of all races with epilepsy may apply to the Department of Manpower (Labour) for work. As in the case of all disabled persons, the abilities of the epileptic person will be evaluated by trained staff.

The following factors will be considered in placement: ability, training, interests, as well as the possibility of injury to self and others and damage to machinery and apparatus caused by uncontrolled attacks.

If disability is such that competition on the open market is precluded, the epileptic person can be placed in one of the department's 'Service Products' factories (Training and Work Centres) (see p. 773), which cater for many different kinds of disabled persons.

There are some epileptic persons who cannot be rehabilitated to any state of independence and who are cared for by the state.

Psychotic epileptic persons are certified inmates of psychiatric hospitals and severely mentally retarded epileptic persons are certified inmates of state Care and Rehabilitation Centres. Epilepsy is certifiable under the Mental Health Act when the epileptic person is a danger to himself or others or is incapable of managing himself or his affairs.

This section was compiled from information obtained from:

■ Minde, M. History of mental health services in South Africa. *S Afr Med J* 1975, **49**. 1568.

- Die Sanel Sentrums. *Rehabilitation in SA* March 1982.
- Epilepsy. *Rehabilitation in SA* September 1981.
- *Rehabilitation in SA* June 1988; **32**(2).

The neuropsychological sequelae in head-injured patients — the post-traumatic syndrome

The majority of head-injured patients suffer no permanent after-effects. Some, however, may be left with physical disabilities, e.g. blindness, hemiplegia. Others may appear physically normal but develop a factitious (non-genuine) disorder especially if the pre-trauma personality was inadequate or if environmental factors at work or at home were (and still are) unfavourable. These unfavourable factors include uncongenial work and marital discord. These patients need counselling.

For a small percentage of non-paralysed patients, return to a pre-trauma state of mental health is not possible despite adequate social and psychological rehabilitative care. These patients are victims of the post-traumatic syndrome.

Behaviour after consciousness has been regained

The brain-damaged patient may regress to a more primitive stage of functioning, emotionally, socially (morally) and physically. The superego may, therefore, not be able to control sexual and aggressive impulses. Psychological functions that developed last, i.e. control of primitive id impulses by the ego and superego are always the first to be lost when the cortex is damaged. The nurse will notice that conscious head-injured patients are often coarse and violent — given to the use of abusive language. This trend is also noticed when people become intoxicated. The thin veneer of civilised behaviour disappears when the higher cortical centres can no longer exert their controlling function.

When the onset of an organic brain lesion is acute, the patient may find it very difficult to adjust to the psychological deficit. This may lead to the development of a very poor therapeutic relationship between the patient and the therapeutic team. The nurse who understands the reason for her brain-damaged patient's 'impossible' behaviour, will attempt to establish a therapeutic alliance with him in which the patient does not attempt to resist his caretakers as if they were his tormentors and persecutors.

These patients are often unable to attend to the therapist's directions, to remember instructions or to co-operate in medical procedures. If the nurse is aware of these psychological deficits, she will be less likely to resent her difficult charges who need great understanding and patience. It is always remarkable how the reprehensible behaviour of an organically damaged patient improves once the underlying organic defect has improved, in cases where the damage is reversible. Nowhere is this of greater applicability than in the nursing of head-injured patients.

The dramatic success of active resuscitation programmes in the acute phase of a head injury may keep alive patients who are disabled to such an extent that they need constant life-long care or support.

The post-traumatic syndrome[13]

This syndrome describes the lasting effects (sequelae) of brain damage. Some patients develop temporal lobe epilepsy. In others the ictus may not be apparent. The following incapacitating disabilities may be present.

Disturbances of speech: dysphasia

This is a speech impairment resulting from injury to the dominant hemisphere. Dysphasia may be either expressive or receptive.

EXPRESSIVE

This causes problems with communication; it can be alleviated to varying degrees by speech therapy.

RECEPTIVE

This means the inability to comprehend speech (spoken and written) properly. The patient appears to be confused and cannot read. As a result of the verbal input deprivation and interpersonal isolation, the patient deteriorates intellectually and becomes psychiatrically disturbed to such a degree that rehabilitation is impossible.

Disturbances of sensation

In rare instances, sensory areas may be affected to cause loss of temperature, pain and position sense; cortical injury may cause loss of fine discriminatory sensation in the hand. Loss of sensation in a limb, which may lead to denial of its presence, may prevent a patient from using a paralysed limb again.

Disturbances of the body-image and spatial orientation

These are very disabling traumatic disasters and may prevent a patient with an injury to the non-dominant hemisphere from caring for his body.

Disturbances of the personality

The personality may be adversely affected by residual temporal lobe epilepsy and by damage to intellectual and emotional functions. The latter disturbances correlate with the duration of post-traumatic amnesia, i.e. the period for which the head-injured patient has no memory. The longer the post-traumatic amnesia, the worse the prognosis will be.

Cortical damage may exhibit as a frank mental deficit, or its ravages may be more subtle: the patient may appear normal but he cannot cope with his previous job. He may have lost drive, initiative, persistence, ambition and speed; he may suffer from poor memory and need constant reminding. His concentration span and ability to grasp new problem-solutions may be reduced and his distractibility increased.

Some patients are given to violent temper outbursts and may even become physically violent — a manifestation of post-traumatic epilepsy. On the other hand, the patient may withdraw into himself and lose interest in the world around him.

Inability to hold down his previous job, lowered earning capacity and accompanying loss of a sense of responsibility usually lead to domestic and social problems.

If the patient has insight into his mental and personality deterioration, he may become anxious and depressed. Depression causes loss of motivation to work hard at rehabilitation.

Patients with traumatic brain injuries may lose their self-esteem, become confused and mistrust self and others. These feelings undermine intimate relationships and working life.

Rehabilitation

With the recent emergence of a new branch of clinical psychology, viz. clinical neuropsychology, brain injury rehabilitation therapy groups have been established in Durban and Johannesburg.

The Head Trauma Rehabilitation Programme[14]

The aim of the programme: to return the brain-injured person to the mainstream of life. By the time the so-called 'trainees' enter the programme, they have attained maximum benefit from a conventional physical, occupational and speech therapy programme, yet they are not functionally autonomous in daily living, nor can they hold down a job.

Family counselling is important to maintain an adequate support system for the patient. An in-depth neuropsychological assessment is made to pinpoint the neurological processes that have been damaged irrevocably and those that have been spared. In training sessions the patient is helped to gain insight into his impairments, to improve his residual abilities and to use them for overcoming his problems. Independence in coping with the day to day activities necessary for survival is fostered. Finally, employment possibilities are investigated by means of work trials. He is assessed for the kind of work he can do and at what levels, i.e. whether he can seek employment in the open labour market (competitive work) or whether he is capable of doing 'sheltered' work only.

The Head Trauma Rehabilitation Programme is based on an identification of intact behavioural functions and strengthening these functions to help the patient adjust socially and emotionally and to prepare for employment by, if necessary, educational and vocational training. This is a long and arduous programme and its success is not guaranteed. It does, however, offer some hope for the victim of a head injury in that it gives him insight into the nature of his problems, enhances his self-esteem, removes confusion and helps him compensate for lost abilities.

In 1983 a Head Injuries Association named **Headway** was established (with headquarters in Johannesburg and branches in all the major centres in the RSA) to assist the head-injured person to function at maximum capacity. Headway acts as a support group for the patient and his family. It plans to establish rehabilitation units and day care centres for head-injured patients where they will be stimulated as soon after the injury as possible in order to readjust to their altered perception of reality.

Head injuries in young children[14]

The child's brain is incompletely developed at birth and grows and develops rapidly in the first seven years. This process comprises dendrite growth, the establishment of countless connections (synapses) between neurons and the myelination of nerve fibres. Injury to the brain which is severe enough to cause loss of consciousness during this crucial developmental period will have very serious effects on the later functioning of the child in his environment.

Although brain-damaged children may recover speech and locomotor functions, emotional control and intelligence are invariably adversely affected. Moreover, the child may suffer from post-traumatic epilepsy. Some head-injured children later have learning and personality problems with uncontrollable temper outbursts and need special schooling.

Preventable causes of childhood head injury

(1) Motor vehicle accidents in which the child is usually a pedestrian. His short stature causes his head to take the impact of the vehicle.

(2) Falls at home, e.g. when a baby or toddler rolls from a bed or table or is dropped.

(3) Child abuse which may be compounded by the recurrence of assaults to the head.

The management and rehabilitation (or habilitation) of those children who survive severe brain damage are costly and require specialised hospital care and the concerted efforts of a team of therapists.

REFERENCES

(1) Crafford E. Aspekte van die beroepsrehabilitasie van skisofrene. *Rehabilitation in SA* 1986; **30**: 56–59.

(2) *Report of the Committee of Enquiry into the Care of Mentally Deficient Persons.* Government Printer 1967.

(3) Lipman L. *S Afr Med J* 1974; **48**: 2241.

(4) Levin A. The state's responsibility to the mentally handicapped person. *Rehabilitation in SA* 1987; **31**: 9–11.

(5) Botha G. The role of an early intervention service centre for the Down's syndrome child. *Rehabilitation in SA* 1987; **31**: 33–35.

(6) Leary PM. *S Afr Med J* 1987; **53**: 197.

(7) Fritz VU. Convulsions. *S Afr J Cont Med Educ* 1988; **6**: 40–46.

(8) Dunstead C, Lindsay L, Norman RM. In *Clinics in Developmental Medicine* 15, Heinemann Spastics Society, London, 1966.

(9) Ames FR. The evoked epilepsies. *S Afr Med J* 1982; **61**: 661.

(10) Naidoo DV, Pammenter MD, Moosa A, *et al.* Seventy black epileptics. *S Afr Med J* 1987; **72**: 837–838.

(11) Grant RHE. Responsibilities in the management of epilepsy, p. 179. In: *Epilepsy Today — Management and Guidelines for the Practitioner.* David Lewis Centre for Epilepsy, Alderley Edge, Cheshire.

(12) Miller R, *et al.* The role of therapeutic drug monitoring in the case of epileptic patients. *S Afr Med J* 1982; **62**: 512.

(13) Tollman S. The role of human clinical neuropsychology in rehabilitation after head injury. *Rehabilitation in SA* September 1989.

(14) Peacock WJ. Head injuries in children. *S Afr Med J* 1984; **66**: 789–790.

TEST OF KNOWLEDGE

The student has benefited from studying this chapter if he/she can answer the following questions:

(1) Distinguish between the following pairs of concepts:
  – psychiatric/mental
  – educable/trainable
  – care centres/training centres (for the mentally handicapped)
  – single care grant/disability pension

(2) Discuss the personality structure of the chronic schizophrenic patient who is likely to be seeking employment. What pre-voca-

tional therapy is sometimes available to ensure vocational rehabilitation (or habilitation)?

(3) Define the following terms:
- IQ
- POWA
- familial retardate
- halfway house
- Division for the Mentally Retarded
- moderately retarded person

(4) Discuss the secondary causes of mental retardation and the role of the nurse in prevention.

(5) Compare the functions and control of protective workshops with that of training and work centres (as discussed in Chapter 44).

(6) (a) Discuss the sterilisation of a mentally retarded adult with special reference to Chapter 20.

(b) How may an adult woman who is severely retarded be protected against an unwanted pregnancy, apart from sterilisation?

(7) Define the following terms:
- ictus
- febrile convulsion

- status epilepticus
- sequela
- epilepsy
- neurotrauma
- photo-epilepsy
- REEA

(8) Describe the immediate treatment of:
(a) a *grand mal* (tonic-clonic) seizure;
(b) status epilepticus;
(c) febrile convulsion.

(9) Discuss the causes of epilepsy and their primary prevention.

(10) Epilepsy is an important community health problem, especially in the lower socio-economic population group. What measures can be taken at a PHC epileptic clinic to ensure good seizure control?

(11) (a) What is meant by the post-traumatic syndrome after head injury?
(b) Why can the post-traumatic syndrome be considered a community health problem?
(c) What are the preventable causes and sequelae of head injuries in young children?

42

Disablement through Alcohol and Chemical Substance (Drug) Abuse

INTRODUCTION

The United Nations Organisation has declared the years 1991 to 2000 as the decade of combating drug abuse and international illicit drug trafficking. In South Africa, the Abuse of Dependence-producing Substances and Rehabilitation Centres Act (4/1971) has been replaced by two acts; Drugs and Drug-trafficking Act (140/1992) and Prevention and Treatment of Drug Dependency Act (20/1992).

Tobacco, alcohol and dependence-producing medicines and other chemical substances are discussed in this chapter.

Smoking and drinking are two popular social customs, some people enjoying their relaxing effects without any visible harm to health. Whereas smoking always harms the body, unlike moderate consumption of alcohol, it does not have the same adverse social consequence as chronic alcohol abuse.

Alcohol abuse is difficult to control as alcohol is freely available and there is no social stigma attached to its moderate consumption. Most white South Africans use some alcoholic beverage at some time or another. This habit is becoming more prevalent amongst the other racial groups who are, at present, more abstemious in their social drinking patterns (HSRC survey[4]).

When it comes to the abuse of alcohol, however, blacks, coloureds and whites are equally affected by the ravishes of its effects on the person drinking excessively and on others, especially the family. Alcohol abuse causes more human misery than any other indulgence man is capable of in his quest for happiness and peace. Substance (drug) abuse has the same destructive potential, but as drugs are not freely available and their use for non-medicinal purposes is legally controlled, their impact on society is less obtrusive.

The drug problem in South Africa, especially the use of cannabis (dagga) which grows with weed-like ease in South Africa, is none the less a serious health problem, especially among the youth who are not aware of the dangers when they yield to peer group pressure to experiment with mind-altering substances.

Drug dependants who inject themselves are also exposed to the new scourge of humanity: HIV infection causing AIDS is spread by shared needles and syringes.

Addictive substances become a vicious master to their addicted slaves whose escape is, however, possible by lengthy therapy in a treatment centre. Prevention of drug abuse by involving the youth in educational programmes is the only way of dealing with this problem effectively.

IN THIS CHAPTER

SUBSTANCES OF ABUSE

The term 'substance' is used to describe a wide range of chemical substances which are taken into the body for the effect they have in altering the level of consciousness, the mood or the perceptions.

Abused substances invariably produce psychological and/or physical dependency and may thus be called dependence-producing substances. All substances of abuse act readily on the central nervous system (CNS) to alleviate unpleasant feelings, thereby causing a false sense of security and happiness (euphoria). Some stimulate the brain and cause wakefulness, self-confidence and euphoria and these also suppress the appetite. They are colloquially referred to as 'uppers'. Others cause sedation, reduce anxiety (i.e. tranquillise) and cause withdrawal from the surroundings. They are called 'downers'.

Uppers and downers may be used in a complementary fashion. A third kind of substance may be either sedative or stimulant, but its main effect is to distort perceptions, thereby causing hallucinations. The hallucinating individual loses contact with reality, as well as his ability to visualise his own body.

According to Act 20 of 1992, 'drugs' means any medicine or substance prescribed by the Minister after consultation with the Medicines Control Council, established by section 2 of the Medicines and Related Substances Control Act 101 of 1965, and includes alcoholic liquor.

Substances abused are **classified** either according to their:

- procurability,
- their action (see p. 746), or
- legal controllability (see p. 752).

(A) Procurability

(1) Illegal (prohibited or illicit) drugs in the RSA:
- dagga
- methaqualone (Mandrax)
- LSD (mind-expanding drugs)
- cocaine
- opium
- heroin
- amphetamines
- phencyclidine (PCP)
- psilocybin
- mescoline (Peyote cactus)

(2) Prescription medicines:
- opioids (derivatives of opium)
- barbiturates

- benzodiazepines (Mogadon, Halcion)
- other CNS depressants (e.g. mepro-bamate)
- anti-cholinergics, e.g. biperiden (Akine-ton)
- appetite suppressants
- methylphenidate (Ritalin)
- anabolic steroids

(3) Over-the-counter (OTC) medicines:
  - cough mixture containing sedative
  - appetite suppressants (S2)
  - analgesics

(4) Household solvents:
  - volatiles (glue)
  - petrol
  - volatile organic nitrites
  - plant materials, e.g. datura stramonium seeds (malpitte, stinkblaar); morning glory seeds.

(5) Tobacco (see Chapter 15), (not included in Act 20/1992); alcohol.

According to a Drug Advisory Board report to MASA recently (1994), alcohol is the most abused drug in South Africa, alcohol abuse being twice as common as dagga addiction. The report further states that South Africa is the world's largest consumer of Mandrax. South Africa is being used as a transit country for cocaine and heroin. Since 1990 the abuse of cocaine has increased by 400 per cent (by 1994).

USE OF ALCOHOL

Alcohol is a central nervous system depressant which may have a stimulating, convivial effect initially, hence its almost universal use since time immemorial for festive occasions and religious rituals. Larger doses of alcohol will eventually cause muscular incoordination, dizziness, drowsiness and sleep; the drunken person may vomit and thus get rid of some of the poison. On the other hand, retention of a poisonous overdose may lead to depression of the vital centres, coma and death. This is known as alcoholic poisoning.

The use of alcohol as medicine and for traditional cultural practices is accepted throughout the world; there is no law against the buying of alcohol nor stigma attached to its use in moderation. The drinking of wine with a meal is considered the height of good taste in affluent societies and the communal use of a calabash of sorghum beer is an essential element in some tribal ceremonies. Communion wine is used by most Christian religions. Thus, approximately 90 % of people will use alcohol for religious and social occasions during the drinking age of a population, estimated to be between 15 and 70 years.

The drinking pattern of adult South Africans was as follows in the 1982 HSRC Survey.[4] The percentage denotes the number of people using alcohol.

	Male	Female
White population	91 %	76 %
Coloured population	60 %	28 %
Black population	54 %	22 %
Indian population	45 %	4 %

The white, First-World, population group shows a near saturation point in terms of alcohol usage.

ABUSE OF ALCOHOL

The use of alcohol lends itself to abuse; people may drink poisonous amounts. The abuse of alcohol may cause a tremendous amount of human misery and ill-health; it has created the greatest social problem in South Africa. The seriousness of this problem exceeds that of drug abuse. It has been estimated that over half a million people in the RSA abuse alcohol.

Alcohol abuse is manifested either in the acute form as alcoholic poisoning which may be fatal, or in the chronic form.

Chronic alcohol abuse, problem drinking, (chronic alcoholism) manifests itself as recurring compulsive bouts of excessive drinking, e.g. over weekends (dipsomania) or as continuous, compulsive drinking relieved intermittently by periods of sobriety when the alcoholic is too sick to continue drinking.

Problem drinking

Some 27 % to 30 % of the drinking population periodically abuse alcohol in an irresponsible way. They are the 'problem drinkers' who experience alcohol-related problems in the form of damage to physical and psychological/emotional health, accidents, loss of employment through drinking, criminal acts and family disruption. These periodic abusers are heavily influenced by environmental conditions; their numbers increase during times of stress, especially unemployment and separation from normal family life.

Alcoholism

Chronic alcoholism (alcohol addiction, alcohol dependence), on the other hand, is a physical disease in that the addict experiences an uncontrollable urge to drink alcohol, the urge being rooted partly in his body chemistry, assumed to be caused by a biogenetic factor.

The alcoholic is physically and psychologically dependent on the alcohol. Approximately 6 % to 8 % of the drinking population are likely to become physically dependent on its use; these are the chronic alcohol addicts who are powerless over their addiction to alcohol. Total abstention is their only weapon against alcoholism.

The number of alcoholics in South Africa (1990) is estimated to be 353 000.

EFFECTS UPON THE HUMAN ORGANISM OF HABITUAL ALCOHOL ABUSE

Alcoholism eventually causes malnutrition with protein and vitamin deficiencies. This leads, for example, to cirrhosis of the liver, gastritis and gastric ulceration, peripheral neuritis and cardiomyopathy.

The brain may be affected, resulting in intellectual deterioration (dementia), Korsakoff's psychosis, acute alcoholic psychosis and delirium tremens.

Alcoholic psychosis (alcoholic hallucinosis)

This hallucinatory paranoid state, which results from chronic alcohol abuse, is characterised by subacute delirium. The patient suffers from delusions and auditory illusions and hallucinations which are not accompanied by a thought disorder or a discrepancy in affect; thus this condition can be distinguished from schizophrenia. It may be accompanied by signs of Korsakoff's psychosis (see below). The patient must be hospitalised in a psychiatric ward or hospital and alcohol must be withdrawn completely. Delusions and hallucinations usually disappear rapidly and, in the absence of organic involvement (Korsakoff's), intellectual functions are re-

stored. Recurrent attacks occur if the patient does not abstain from alcohol.

Note: In black psychiatric hospitals, alcoholic psychosis comprises 60 % of acute psychiatric admissions; hospitalisation for this condition is of short duration.

Delirium tremens — 'the horrors'

The condition of DTs is a psychosis of chronic alcoholism characterised by an acute, short episode of delirium which requires intensive medical care. It is caused by an acute nutritional deficiency of the vit. B group when the alcoholic has starved himself of food (but not alcohol). The delirium with visual hallucinations may come on after emotional or physical stress or after the sudden withdrawal of alcohol. Apart from the hallucinations (usually of quickly moving, small animals) the patient's hands, head and tongue exhibit a coarse tremor. The animals may be seen as threatening and cause the patient to become terror-stricken. The restless, delirious patient who may injure himself and may even die from heart failure, usually sinks into an exhausted sleep after 3 to 7 days of feverish activity (if not treated), after which he is fully recovered from the attack. In some alcoholics, attacks may become habitual.

Korsakoff's syndrome or psychosis

This is an organic psychosis characterised by polyneuritis and permanent selective memory loss, caused by the severe malnutrition with vitamin deficiency which accompanies chronic alcoholism.

The nutritional state of the patient is poor and there are signs of peripheral neuritis with muscular weakness and impaired sensation.

Korsakoff's psychosis is characterised by confusion and severe impairment of memory, especially for recent events, for which the patient compensates by confabulation to fill in the gaps. Korsakoff's psychosis may accompany or follow delirium tremens or alcoholic hallucinosis, the disturbance of memory becoming evident as the hallucinations subside.

The prognosis is poor, the patient becoming an economic liability to the family or the state.

Note:
(1) Whereas the symptoms of delirium, e.g. hallucinations and clouding of consciousness, are temporary, the memory disorder in Korsakoff's psychosis is perma-

nent as it is caused by destruction of brain cells which cannot be replaced.
(2) Dementia and peripheral neuritis indicate organic damage to neurones; the damage is irreversible. Damage to other organs (liver, stomach) is reversible if not too far advanced as epithelial and connective tissue can regenerate.

Epidemiology of alcohol abuse

Alcoholism is a growing problem in rural and urban blacks. In traditional black societies, alcoholism was rare, as the use of beer with low alcoholic content (2–3 %) was institutionalised and beer was used mainly on festive occasions and in a group setting. This does not mean that people never got drunk, the fortification of beer being practised by some, but the amount of alcohol consumed was never enough to cause a dangerous alcohol addiction. The modern trend in both urban and rural areas is for black people to drink strong liquor (e.g. brandy with alcoholic content of 43 %) in addition to their traditional beer.

'Hard tack' is freely available as more and more bottle stores open in the black urban townships and in the rural areas. Brandy and methylated spirits (with ethyl alcohol content of 94 %) have a quick effect; they are therefore preferred by people who use alcohol mainly for its mood-altering effects — in fact, by those who are set to abuse alcohol. The alcohol-abuse problem is becoming especially severe in urban hostel inmates who drink when they come back from work, instead of eating. The subsequent malnutrition is commonly manifested as alcoholic psychosis, pellagra and beriberi cardiomyopathy.

The coloured community also has a severe alcohol problem, the favourite beverage of the Cape coloured being wine, with which they were often supplied by the farmers. The incidence of alcoholism amongst the coloured people is of the highest in the world. The incidence of alcoholism amongst the whites is also very high. A recent trend has been the rising incidence of alcoholism amongst women.

The following data are given by Dr S de Miranda:[4]

(1) Over 50 % of all traumatic injuries are alcohol-related.
(2) Over 50 % of all fatal traumatic injuries are alcohol-related.

(3) 10 % of chronic psychiatric hospital bed occupancy is alcohol-related.
(4) Over 60 % of acute psychiatric hospital admissions of black patients are alcohol-related.
(5) In many black hospitals 30 % of medical beds are occupied by patients with alcohol-related diseases.
(6) A large number of motor vehicle and pedestrian traffic accidents are alcohol-related.

Alcohol abuse and its related problems adversely affect industry and commerce in the RSA to the extent of some R1 200 million per annum.

Causes of chronic alcoholism (or alcohol-related problems)

(1) Individual psychopathology, including loneliness (alienation from people), boredom, depression and feelings of gross inadequacy which are relieved by alcohol. Individual sensitivity to alcohol predisposes to addiction.
(2) The easy availability of drink with high alcoholic content and the pressure of friends who seek drinking companions. The temptation of the shebeens in the black townships, that cater for all black social classes and provide an opportunity for men to drink together, away from their spouses and the conflicts and demands of family life, is an insidious and bad influence on family life.
(3) Social causes which affect large numbers of people, e.g. poverty, miserable living conditions, frustration in the work sphere, lack of recreational facilities and break-up of stable family life, e.g. migrant labourers who live away from their families in hostels, for long periods of time.
(4) Exposure of the youth to alcohol is an important aetiological factor, i.e. the influences of the already existing prevalence of alcoholism in a community on the youth. In children exposed to the abuse of alcohol in the home, especially in communities where it carries no social disapproval, the example of parents and their friends exerts a powerful effect on the life-style of the growing child. Alcohol abuse may become a way of life perpetuated from one generation to another.

This has been the trend amongst the rural Cape coloured, especially those exposed to the 'tot' system.

(5) Excessive stress, especially in the work situation.

Alcohol dependence in alcohol-sensitive persons causes disintegration of the personality; this results in chronic feelings of guilt and depression, suspiciousness (paranoia), social withdrawal and alienation, as well as lack of social responsibility, especially towards spouse and children. Many alcoholic men do not feel it incumbent upon them to support their wives and children, spending most of their earnings to feed their addiction.

Suspicious signs of alcohol abuse, often seen in patients coming to clinics for other complaints, are:

(1) enlarged, tender liver;
(2) dusky blue colour and puffiness of the face;
(3) the shakes, i.e. tremor and anxiety; these symptoms plus sweating are due to alcohol withdrawal and may warn of impending delirium tremens;
(4) bloodshot eyes;
(5) peripheral neuritis of legs and feet: the patient seems to be 'walking on eggs';
(6) signs of malnutrition: the chronic alcoholic may suffer from pellagra and beriberi.

Social consequences of habitual alcohol abuse

(1) Family tensions and child neglect and abuse; relationship difficulties and negative self-image.
(2) Family disorganisation and disintegration, often resulting in the institutionalisation of the children at state expense.
(3) Loss of job and employment leading to poverty, malnutrition and dependency on a state subsidy for the upkeep of the family.
(4) Desertion, separation and divorce.
(5) Economic loss to the community through absenteeism, inefficiency and disablement of skilled workers, and industrial accidents.
(6) Vagrancy (hoboism) and begging.
(7) Crime and prostitution.
(8) Mental ill-health of children exposed to violent family relationships; children may become aggressive and antisocial and/or exhibit signs of emotional deprivation, especially if disintegration of the family leads to their institutionalisation.
(9) Social blighting of the neighbourhood in areas where alcoholism is rife and homes neglected.

Primary prevention of alcohol abuse

(1) Improvement in the socio-economic circumstances of economically depressed, frustrated ethnic groups, e.g. the coloured people in the RSA, is the most effective way of combating alcoholism on a large scale. If people can be uplifted socially and economically and given a pride in their homes and their jobs, the mass misery which finds alleviation in the mind-dulling effects of alcohol can be eased. Poverty and misery result from alcoholism but they also give rise to alcoholism; this vicious cycle can be broken only by large-scale community projects launched by the government. People who have something to live for are not likely to persist in behaviour which threatens their survival. The social upliftment of the children in a blighted community by social agencies, either state or voluntary, plays an important role in preventing widespread alcoholism.

(2) Health education to encourage people to drink in moderation and to take the necessary precautions when they attend a party where alcohol is served, to ensure that they do not drive home in an intoxicated state. The SA Medical Association, SANCA (see p. 756) and the SA Nursing Council have made concerted attempts to stop the advertising of alcoholic products on the broadcasting and television media, by making representations to the governors of the SABC, so far without success.

Information services of SANCA help in the prevention of addiction. A comprehensive information service has been built up to provide the correct facts regarding alcohol and dependence-producing drugs, the cause and nature of alcoholism and drug-dependence and treatment facilities available. This information is distributed by way of appropriate literature, press and radio and personal consultation with industrial leaders, employers, doctors and ministers of religion. Information offices for blacks and whites have been opened in all cities and major towns in the RSA and some of the rural areas, free services being offered to any group or person.

(3) Social care of people alienated by urbanisation, industrialisation and immigration in order to help them adapt to their new social circumstances and overcome their loneliness and boredom, without recourse to alcohol.

(4) It is incumbent upon the nursing, medical and other health professions to warn people about the danger of becoming dependent upon alcohol where they come across early signs of alcohol abuse in the execution of their duties. (See the beginning of the left side of the 'Chart of Alcohol Addiction and Recovery', p. 743.)

Note: Prohibition of the sale and production of alcohol is impracticable and likely to cause problems rather than alleviate them. Prohibition was attempted in the USA from 1920, but instead of curing the alcoholism problem, it gave rise to bootlegging (liquor smuggling) and the establishment of the great crime syndicates which still flourish in America today.

Secondary prevention of alcohol abuse

Deterrent measures

(1) Legislation to serve as a deterrent to drunken driving. It is compulsory for every driver suspected of being under the influence of alcohol (because of smell of breath, behaviour or because of involvement in an accident) to submit to a blood test for alcoholic content. The danger level is deemed to be 0,08 mg/dl. This test must be carried out by the district surgeon, nurse or other doctor and sent to the SAIMR as soon as possible after suspicion has been aroused, before the alcohol can be excreted from the body. Sentences are imposed and drivers' licences suspended or cancelled by the presiding magistrate in accordance with the severity of the crime, i.e. endangering or taking the lives of people on the road.

(2) Nurses who come on duty in an intoxicated state are subject to disciplinary action by the SA Nursing Council; not only might they endanger the lives of their patients by faulty drug administration but they also damage the good name of the nursing profession. The danger of losing a means of livelihood and the social disgrace should be sufficient to deter nurses from such reprehensible behaviour.

Therapeutic measures

1. Detoxification therapy — short-term medical intervention, 5–7 days

The alcoholic can be brought into remission by admission to hospital or clinic with in-patient facilities. The patient is nursed at bed-rest for a week and stops the intake of alcohol. To prevent delirium tremens (withdrawal psychosis) from occurring, he is sedated during this time and given massive parenteral doses of vitamins to build up the organs (liver, CNS, heart) damaged by vitamin depletion of the body.

The benzodiazepines (e.g. diazepam) are of value as tranquillisers, hypnotics and anticonvulsives.

During this drying out period, a high glucose diet is also given to help restore the health of the liver and the nervous system. Thiamine is always given in conjunction with glucose. After this period of intensive care, the ambulant patient continues on a high energy, high protein, high vitamin diet and is put on either tranquillisers or antidepressant drugs.

Chronic alcoholic subjects with withdrawal symptoms can be treated with 100 % oxygen or with oxygen and nitrous oxide mixtures, in addition to routine detoxification therapy. Only light sedation is necessary. The gases are administered with a dental analgesia machine as follows:

- Pure O_2 at 8 litres/min is given for 20 minutes, followed by
- N_2O plus O_2 given for 20 minutes, followed by
- Pure O_2 given for 20 minutes.
- N_2O is given to reverse affective depression, and is titrated according to need.

Within the first 24 hours, this procedure can be repeated if the physical symptoms recur.

2. In-patient (residential care) of 3–6 weeks duration

The detoxified patient is given psychotherapy, either individual or group, and is involved in physiotherapy and/or occupational therapy. He is given a tremendous amount of protection, support and understanding to help him strengthen his resolve to quit drinking. Out-patient after-care is essential for the rehabilitation process.

3. Out-patient therapy

The short in-patient clinic treatment is not likely to 'cure' years of physical, psychological and social deterioration caused by alcohol dependency. The abstaining alcoholic is at this stage only in remission and backsliding frequently occurs. Should this happen, the patient is encouraged to try again and is reassured that backsliding does not mean permanent failure.

Abstaining alcoholics are advised to take disulfiram (Antabuse) 1 tablet (200 mg) daily to strengthen their resolve. Disulfiram therapy is not likely to be successful unless the patient wants to stop drinking and willingly undertakes the treatment. Patients on disulfiram are under medical care and, if necessary, their doctor will prescribe tranquillisers and antidepressants temporarily for anxiety and depression.

Disulfiram is rapidly absorbed but slowly eliminated so that 1/5th of a dose may still be present in the body after a week. It potentiates both barbiturates and paraldehyde and these drugs should not be given concomitantly. Should a patient on disulfiram therapy imbibe alcohol, the effects of the interaction start manifesting themselves after 10 to 15 minutes. The patient experiences facial and conjunctival flushing, throbbing headache, tachycardia, throat irritation and vertigo. If he drinks more than 50 ml the patient may vomit and perspire and collapse due to a marked fall in blood pressure. The effects gradually wear off and after a sleep the patient feels well again.

Note:

(1) In order to give the patient an experience of the effects of disulfiram, he is sometimes given disulfiram daily for a week while in hospital. On the fifth day he is given a test dose of alcohol (10 to 15 ml) and his physical reactions are monitored. The alcohol may be increased until the reaction is severe enough to create a lasting aversion in the patient's mind. The patient is advised to take a daily dose of disulfiram in the morning and to register as an out-patient at an alcoholic clinic which he attends monthly (or more often) for encouragement and control, and for supply of disulfiram tablets.

(2) The effectiveness of disulfiram therapy is only as good as the patient's resolve to take his medication every morning. He must never be given the drug secretly, e.g. by a well-meaning spouse. The contra-indications to disulfiram therapy are: cardiac failure, CHD, pregnancy, psychosis.

(3) Patients who are likely to default are required by SANCA clinics to call for their daily dose of disulfiram every morning. In this way ineffective therapy regimens are controlled.

The alcoholic in remission is further helped by fellowship with ex-alcoholics through organisations such as Alcoholics Anonymous (see p. 756) and Christian Alcoholic Services.

Long-term follow-up (after-care) is essential during the period of readjustment to family and community life and to the work situation to help the patient grow and develop.

After-care on an out-patient level is carried out by most in-patient clinics. The patient is encouraged to maintain contact with the clinic and its therapists.

The period of after-care varies from clinic to clinic and should not be shorter than six months. The patient must, at some stage, be weaned from the clinic in order to function as an independent human being with self-esteem.

After-care contact with the clinic is maintained and therapy given by one of three methods:

(1) telephonic contact;

(2) contact by correspondence for those living at a distance from the clinic; and

(3) personal contact, i.e. either individual or marital therapy for those living near the clinic.

The problem areas likely to retard full rehabilitation, which can be handled by contact are: depression caused by inability to find a fulfilling job; marital misunderstandings and non-acceptance; problems with socialising and consequent isolation; problems with guilt feelings and self-acceptance.

SANCA (see p. 756) provides facilities for the comprehensive treatment of alcoholics and

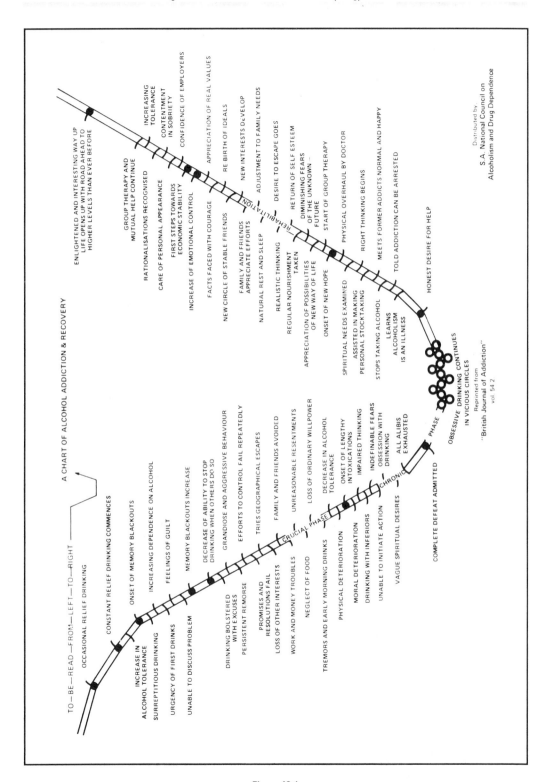

Figure 42.1

A chart of alcohol addiction and recovery

drug dependants. SANCA's in-patient and out-patient clinics provide the following:

(1) Medical detoxification treatment mainly for treating withdrawal symptoms, administering vitamins for the build-up of the system and medication for the relief of anxiety and tension.
(2) Psychological, social and spiritual assistance. Psychiatrists, clinical psychologists, social workers, ministers of religion and recovered alcoholics render valuable services. Where possible the family of the patient also participates in the treatment.
(3) After-care services.

If patients can afford to, they pay for these services at a subsidised fee.

The goals of treatment are:

(1) Interruption of the repetitive pattern of drinking.
(2) Substitution of constructive attitudes and activities for disruptive and destructive patterns of living.
(3) Development of self-knowledge and inner resources to cope with problems without recourse to alcohol.
(4) Improvement of interpersonal relationships.
(5) Solid establishment of sobriety, not as an end in itself, but as a means to a greater end. Abstention from alcohol must be for a lifetime; one drink after 40 years' abstention can restart the compulsive drinking.

There are a large number of SANCA out-patient clinics for whites, blacks, Indians and coloureds on the Reef, Pretoria, Vaal Triangle, Pietermaritzburg, eastern and northern Transvaal, Klerksdorp, KwaZulu, Durban, Bloemfontein. In Port Elizabeth and East London there are halfway houses (hostels) where single alcoholics can live while they are rehabilitating. In-patient clinics are in Durban, Boksburg, Klerksdorp, Roodepoort, Pretoria, Bloemfontein.

McCabe[2] considers alcoholism amongst township blacks not only a national problem but a national emergency. She found that the black alcoholic retains insight into his illness and often asks for help. SANCA services (educative, preventive and therapeutic) are established in many black townships. A Black National Development Advisor at headquarters (Johannesburg) is responsible for the co-ordination and development of these services throughout the black townships of the RSA.

Other welfare organisations which run in- and out-patient clinics for alcoholics and drug dependants are affiliated to SANCA, for example:

Elim Clinic (Railways) for Problem Drinkers in Kempton Park.

Rand Aid clinics in Wedge Gardens (Sandton).

Crossroads Salvation Army Rehabilitation Centre in Muldersvlei, Cape.

Clinics of the Dutch Reformed Church in Parow East, Pretoria and Welkom.

The LifeCare Clinics (Pty) Ltd run the only private recovery treatment centre for alcohol and drug dependants in the RSA, Riverfield Lodge Alcohol and Drug Treatment Centre, north-west of Johannesburg. Treatment is costly, involving a team of therapists (medical practitioners, psychologists, social workers, occupational therapists).

The treatment programme consists of medical detoxification followed by a one-month in-patient programme, a family participation programme and a 23-month follow-up programme. The family, employer and other significant people are encouraged to take part in the treatment and follow-up programmes.

The problem of alcohol abuse has been steadily increasing in the RSA over the past few years. It is a national problem which is receiving the attention of the government. A National Plan for the Prevention of and Combating Alcohol Abuse in South Africa has been formulated. The objectives of this plan are:

(1) to prevent alcohol abuse and alcoholism;
(2) to set up an effective treatment service for alcohol abusers and alcoholics;
(3) to co-ordinate measures for the prevention and combating of alcohol abuse and alcoholism.

If treatment by the above measures is not successful and the alcoholic is a danger to himself and others, he can be committed by the courts to a treatment centre (see p. 753). Care in a treatment centre can also be given on a voluntary basis.

THE ABUSE OF DRUGS
(dependence- producing chemical substances)

Note: The term 'drug' is used in this section to refer to 'dependence-producing substances' as defined by Act 20/1992 and detailed in Schedule 2 of Act 140/1992.

Large-scale drug misuse has recently emerged as a social problem affecting mainly the adolescent group. In adolescence the symptom of drug abuse may be a sign of either a transient personality maladjustment or a severe personality disturbance which has its roots in personality development during the early years of life. The severe personality disturbance may be in the form of a neurosis, or a personality disorder, or a borderline or true psychosis (placed in order of severity from mild to severe). The stresses and strains of adolescence may merely accentuate a problem which has existed since childhood.

Definitions of terms used

To be 'hip' is jargon used by members of the drug subculture. It means to be an initiate, an experimenter with drugs. Many teenagers are 'hip', i.e. they go through a phase when it is considered to be smart to use drugs. Fortunately the more stable personalities are able to exchange the 'hippie' culture for a more socially acceptable way of life.

The 'junkie' is the person who is drug dependent and who lives in degradation and squalor, either by his wits, or by prostitution, or as a peddler of drugs. His right to live in this way is not recognised by society and therefore he is persecuted by the law and by the indignant citizenry.

The World Health Organisation (WHO) Expert Committee on Addiction-producing Drugs (1964) adopted the following definitions:

Drugs: Any substance that, when taken into the living organism, may modify one or more of its functions.

Drug abuse: Persistent or sporadic excessive drug use inconsistent with or unrelated to accepted medical practice.

Drug dependence: A state, psychic and sometimes also physical, resulting from the interaction between the living organism and a drug, characterised by behavioural and other responses that always include a compulsion to take the drug on a continuous or periodic basis

in order to experience its psychic effects, and sometimes to avoid discomfort of its absence.

Tolerance may or may not be present. A person may be dependent on more than one drug.

Psychological dependence: A psychic drive which requires periodic or chronic administration of the substance for pleasure or to avoid discomfort.

Physical dependence denotes a craving for a drug which is caused by the physical symptoms of withdrawal illness when the drug has been withdrawn. Only certain drugs, e.g. narcotic analgesics and the barbiturates, cause physical dependence.

Tolerance refers to the resistance which the body builds up to the action of certain drugs, usually nerve poisons such as the opiates. With prolonged use of these drugs, dosage must be increased in order for the drug to exert the same effects.

In psychological dependency, tolerance for the drug has been established in the central nervous system while in physical dependency, tolerance has been established in the peripheral nervous system. Some experts believe that any drug taken excessively over a long period will cause physical withdrawal symptoms when its use is suddenly discontinued.

Addiction refers to a state of dependence on a drug. This term was formerly used for dependence on drugs producing physical dependence, but this distinction is no longer valid. The WHO Expert Committee on Addiction-producing Drugs (1964) recommended that the old terms 'Habituation' and 'Addiction' be replaced by 'Drug Dependence', the practitioner specifying on which drug the subject is dependent.

The dependence-producing drugs which form the subject-matter of this chapter, alter mood, perception or consciousness and it is this alteration of the psyche which is responsible for chronic use (misuse). Drug dependence implies the compulsive use of a drug to alleviate a craving. The person who is dependent on the above-mentioned medicines is usually called a drug addict.

(B) Classification of the main drugs of dependence, classified **according to their action** (see p. 736 for classification according to procurability):

1. Central nervous stimulants

(1) *Cocaine* — 'snow' which produces only psychological dependence.
(2) The *sympathomimetic amines*:
   (a) Ephedrine, given by injection.
   (b) The *amphetamines* ('speed') taken either in the form of pills or by injection (IMI or IVI), the latter being called a 'shoot'. One of the newest crazes is 'ice' — translucent crystals of methamphetamine which are 'smoked'.
(3) Methyl phenidate (Ritalin). This is used therapeutically in children with MBD.
(4) Diethylpropion (Tenuate Dospan).

2. The narcotic analgesics

These are arbitrarily known as the 'hard' drugs because they are drugs which cause physical and psychological dependency, usually taken by injection. The potential dependent takes them for their euphoric effects.

(1) *Opium derivatives:*
   (a) Morphine and Cyclimorph (morphine with an anti-emetic);
   (b) Omnopon (which contains morphine) (total opium alkaloids);
   (c) Chlorodyne (chloroform with morphine): this is taken by mouth;
   (d) Diamorphine (heroin);
   (e) Codeine.
(2) *Synthetic drugs:*
   (a) Pethidine; Pethilorfan;
   (b) Methadone (Physeptone);
   (c) Dipipanone (Wellconal).

3. Hypnotics and sedatives

(1) The barbiturates, e.g. Seconal ('pinks'); special combination: Vesparax.
(2) Non-barbiturates:
   (a) Methaqualone, an ingredient of Mandrax;
   (b) Potassium Bromide;
   (c) Hyoscine (Scopolamine);
   (d) Dextrometorphan Hydrobromide in the cough suppressant Romilar;

   (e) Dihydrocodeine bitartrate, (e.g. Paracodin, DF 118);
   (f) Chlordiazepoxide (e.g. Librium ('libbies')); diazepam (Valium);
   (g) Tranxene, Equanil.

4. *Cannabis sativa l.*

Dagga, marijuana, hashish, pot, grass, reefers.

5. The hallucinogens

Mescaline, LSD and LSD-25, psilocybin, bufotenine, harmaline. These drugs do not give rise to dependence, but they are misused because their use in South Africa, for whatever purpose, is prohibited by law.

6. Glue and various solvents (e.g. benzene)

These substances are inhaled (sniffed) and produce an anaesthetising action on the CNS. The brief dulling of the senses causes a feeling of intoxication. Sniffing is a common form of addiction among deprived children who cannot obtain other drugs; it may cause physical damage to the body.

Although there are pan-dependants — people who use any drug they can lay their hands on — drugs are generally not used indiscriminately, the drug of choice depending on the emotional need requiring satisfaction. The mentally healthy adolescent with an adequate personality is not likely to become drug dependent; dependence develops in those emotionally immature persons who are deficient in character strength and who are so emotionally disturbed that they are unable to adjust to society. During adolescence, the resurgence of childhood conflicts, guilts, anxieties and depressions makes the young adult especially vulnerable to the effects of mood-altering drugs. Thus it is that we find this age group prone to the drug-craze which is sweeping the Western world at present. Chemotherapeutic substances are very much a part of the phenomenal advance in modern medicine, which even seeks to cure unhappiness with mood-altering drugs.

The emotionally balanced adolescent often experiments with drugs, especially speed pills and dagga, but sooner or later relinquishes the habit, or uses drugs only on special occasions, in favour of development and active mastery of the social environment. An adequate person who is able to form satisfying human relationships is not likely to become enslaved to drugs; in contradistinction to the chronic user of drugs, healthy adolescents are able to reduce psychic distress by their own efforts; they like to achieve independence.

Dependence on narcotic analgesics is not as common among the adolescents as dependence on Mandrax. Narcotics are more difficult to come by and are generally taken by injection.

In the drug subculture, their use is generally considered the ultimate way of life to which the initiate is gradually introduced. Once an addict has become 'hooked' by the 'hard' drugs, his chances of a cure from dependence are very remote.

Dipipanone (Wellconal), supplied in tablet form for oral use, is an efficient analgesic. It has given rise to a severe drug problem. It is crushed, dissolved in water and injected intravenously. Apart from this dangerous administration technique, lethal overdosage is a common occurrence.

Dependence becomes a way of life which sets the addict apart from the rest of society. This way of life is in part a revolt against organised society in which the disturbed adolescent does not feel accepted. Drugs are, therefore, not taken in secret, except in so far as it is necessary to escape prosecution. Society is very much aware of the drug problem and addicts are poorly motivated to seek a cure.

Narcotic drugs are taken not only for the sensuous pleasure the user experiences after injection, in the form of a psychic disturbance described variously as a 'rave', a 'kick' or as being 'high' (euphoric), but also because of the capacity of the drug for blotting out anxiety, relieving emotional stress and making the user feel adequate, full of self-confidence and happy. Normal, relaxed, self-assured people are not likely to experience the euphoric effects of the drug and are therefore not likely to want to repeat the experience, unless they require the drug for analgesic purposes — its true purpose. The danger of dependence lies not so much in the drug itself as in the psychic disturbance of the potential dependent which is corrected by the drug. Unfortunately for the dependent, chronic abuse of narcotic analgesics aggravates the original personality disturbance.

Both the central and the peripheral nervous systems develop tolerance to narcotics, tolerance being responsible for the psychic (central) dependence and the physical (peripheral) dependence. Once dependence on the narcotic has become established, the victim has developed a new drive system which needs to be satisfied. The narcotic hunger is infinitely more demanding than the bodily drives of hunger and thirst. The dependant's whole life centres around satisfaction of his craving for drugs: where to get a 'fix'; how to evade the law; where to get the money to buy the drug on the black market. The craving for drugs is so demanding that the dependant will stop at nothing to get his supplies; thus he will resort to stealing, lying, graft and even murder. He loses interest in life, becomes constipated, anorectic and impotent and is constantly drowsy. Drug tolerance causes the need for an ever-increasing dose which merely serves to increase the dependant's physical misery.

Narcotic dependants sometimes take stimulants to counteract the numbing effects of the depressant. Thus a concomitant dependence on cocaine or amphetamines may arise. The stimulants are physically more damaging than the depressants. Dependants become neglectful of their physical needs and their health deteriorates through malnutrition, exposure and unhygienic living. The use of infected syringes and needles leads to the formation of abscesses, serum hepatitis, AIDS and septicaemia, which may have fatal consequences. Drug dependants die either from suicide, or from general ill-health or end their days in a mental asylum because of dementia.

The physical affliction which is feared more than anything else by the dependant is **physical withdrawal sickness**. If the drug is withdrawn abruptly, either in prison or in an effort to effect a cure by exposing the dependant to a condition known as 'cold turkey', or if an intravenous injection of the narcotic antidote Lorfan or Lethidrone is given, the following clinical picture will arise. At first the patient feels very sick and weak; there is excessive sweating and discharge from the eyes, nose and salivary glands. Yawning then sets in and may become violent. The skin becomes cold and the arrector pili muscles contract, causing goose flesh, hence the name 'cold turkey'. The whole body shakes with cold and muscle twitchings. Violent peristalsis causes severe diarrhoea with colic and vomiting; the patient becomes dehydrated because of fluid loss and inability to take in fluids. Painful muscular cramps prevent sleep and rest. Suffering is acute for a week; the symptoms then abate, leaving the patient weak and dehydrated and in a highly nervous condition. An injection of the withdrawn drug at any time during the withdrawal sickness will restore the patient almost immediately to comfort and comparative health. The cure of the physical craving does not cure the drug addiction, as the psychic dependence on the drug remains.

More humane ways of effecting gradual withdrawal of the drug of addiction obviate the agony and physical dangers of 'cold turkey'. In one method the daily dose is cut down gradually and restlessness and anxiety are counteracted with tranquillisers and sedatives. The patient is given massive doses of vitamins and a nourishing diet. Sometimes the drug of dependence, e.g. morphine or heroin, is replaced by a less incapacitating addictive drug, such as methadone. This drug satisfies the craving and enables the addict to hold down a job.

Amphetamines — the so-called 'speed' or 'pep' pills — are generally taken by exhausted housewives and adolescents, people who may feel bored and under-stimulated. They act almost exclusively on the central nervous system and have little peripheral effect.

Amphetamines are central nervous stimulants which produce alertness, euphoria and self-confidence. They are also anorectic and were frequently prescribed for this purpose. The subject under the influence of 'speed' becomes active, restless and subjectively competent, but judgement and accuracy are diminished; people driving under the influence of the amphetamines, taken in an effort to ward off the fatigue of long journeys, may become accident-prone. Sometimes dissociation takes place: when the mind becomes extremely active and productive of thoughts, yet the latter cannot be expressed in appropriate motor activity. A split takes place between thinking and doing, for example students writing examinations under the influence of amphetamines may imagine themselves writing a brilliant paper, yet produce only doodling. Afterwards there is no recollection of the split

because complete dissociation took place between the mind and the body.

The toxic effects of amphetamine overdosage are central, i.e. fatigue, mental depression, hypertension, respiratory failure, disorientation, hallucinations, convulsions and death.

Dependence follows on chronic use of the drug and may lead to a psychosis which resembles schizophrenia with ideas of reference (the feeling that completely unrelated people are making derogatory remarks about one), delusions of persecution and auditory and visual hallucinations. Withdrawal symptoms are not a feature of amphetamine dependence as they have so little peripheral effect, but may be experienced as depression and exhaustion. The 'speed' pills commonly used for addictive purposes are purple hearts (Drinamyl) and black bombs (Anorexine), but 'mainline' drug takers who inject the drug intravenously use methylamphetamine for this purpose. Methylamphetamine is supplied in ampoules of 20 mg/ml; addicts may use up to 1 g per daily shot. When dependence has progressed to this extent, life expectancy is less than two years.

Cannabis sativa indica is found in the flowering tops, seeds and leaves of the female Indian hemp plant. It grows in South Africa in the wild state or is cultivated illegally with the greatest of ease. For use, the leaves and flowers are dried and crushed and smoked in short cigarettes or pipes (bottle necks).

The use of dagga is forbidden in most countries, the penalties for being in possession of the drug being especially heavy in the USA and South Africa, where a person convicted of being in possession of more than 115 grams of dagga (see p. 757) is deemed by law to be dealing in drugs.

Dagga acts almost exclusively on the central nervous system and, unlike alcohol, has no deleterious effects on the peripheral nervous system, hence the chronic user does not develop physical tolerance nor does he suffer physical withdrawal symptoms. This does not mean, however, that dagga is a safe drug to use, as psychic dependence does develop; the continued use of dagga is habit-forming. Acute dagga intoxication causes mental disorientation — a temporary hallucinatory psychosis which leaves no permanent after-effects, but may cause dangerous, irrational behaviour for a period of days.

The immediate physical effects of dagga smoking are very characteristic and obvious: reddening of the conjunctivae, dryness of the mouth, tachycardia, lowering of body temperature and a voracious appetite. Dagga sharpens the wits and causes moderate euphoria. Although dagga increases the imagination, it reduces concentration, alters perception, impairs co-ordination and therefore causes a driving hazard. Dagga releases the inhibitions which normally hold drives and impulses in check — it reveals the true personality. Because personalities differ markedly, it is obvious that dagga will not have the same effect on everyone. Thus it acts as an aphrodisiac (sex stimulant) in some people, it releases aggression in others, it makes some assertive while others become cool, calm and relaxed. Some people become paranoid while others are sadly sentimental under its influence. Some show an enthusiasm for work in an effort to please the 'boss', while others become indolent. Chronic users may lose all motivation to work, and become loafers. Dagga and alcohol potentiate each other and their simultaneous use may cause loss of control which makes the user a danger in his community. Irrational crimes of violence may be committed under the influence of dagga.

In small doses, dagga and alcohol have similar 'stimulating' effects, relieving anxiety and producing euphoria, but in larger doses the similarity disappears: the pleasurable effects of alcohol soon reach a climax after ingestion and then rapidly decline, while the effects of dagga remain 'high' for 8 to 10 hours. High-dosage alcohol causes greater intellectual disorganisation than dagga, which may, however, cause hallucinations and depersonalisation.

All the indigenous races of South Africa have eaten and smoked dagga since before the white man settled here, and do not believe that the moderate use of the drug is harmful. It is a fallacy, however, that continuous use of the drug is harmless. A person who smokes dagga, like a person who drinks alcohol, is not necessarily dependent on the drug. Dependence can, however, develop in the same way that alcohol dependence develops.

Dagga smoking tended to take the place of alcohol drinking at adolescent parties, the young people preferring the softer effects of dagga to the harsher, more explosive effects of alcohol. The dagga smoker can never indulge his habit in secret: the acrid fumes of the weed are poorly concealed by the burning of incense and the smoker's body exudes the odour of the burning weed. There is a stigma attached to the smoking of dagga in addition to the danger of prosecution.

Responsible medical opinion is that there should be a total restriction on the use of dagga; it is dangerous to the user and to the community; its use may lead to addiction to mainline drugs, amphetamines and hallucinogens.

It has no medicinal value.

The original **hallucinogen**, mescaline (LSD) — an alkaloid of the Mexican peyote cactus — has been used by the American and Mexican Indians for many centuries for the purpose of producing a mystical trance state which is an important religious experience.

LSD-25 is a synthetic substance with powerful hallucinogenic action, even in minute doses of 50 µg (micrograms). Up to 200 µg are used for a full 'trip'. LSD is the most commonly used hallucinogen or mind-expanding drug — it is the most powerful mind-altering drug known to man. Because it is a synthetic substance, it can be manufactured by any organic chemist if he has the correct apparatus and ingredients. The precursors of LSD are related to ergometrine, obtained from fungus-infected rye. Such minute quantities are used that the smuggling of the drug into the country, in the form of powders, tiny pills or impregnated blotting paper, is a relatively simple matter. Although the illicit use of LSD is prevalent in South Africa, especially in the artistic and intellectual circles in which dagga has found favour, its use for therapeutic and experimental purposes is illegal and importation is prohibited. LSD has been used overseas for psychotherapy, but as its use requires the presence of an expert therapist for many hours at a stretch, it is not a very popular technique for treating psychiatric disturbances.

LSD is taken by mouth, takes effect within an hour and is effective for 4 to 8 hours. There may be a recurrence of hallucinations for some time afterwards. Although LSD has such a profound effect on the brain, it causes only slight objective signs in the subject: goose flesh, exaggerated tendon reflexes and enlarged pupils. Its major effects are on the sensory and interpretative functions of the brain: perception (especially vision), imagery, beliefs and memory. All sense impressions become exaggerated as the brain becomes incapable of filtering irrelevant sensory input. There is intensification of colour and depth and the most insignificant sounds become clearly audible. Sense impressions, however, become unrelated and unintegrated. These sense impressions appear novel because it appears that the learning of perceptions which has taken a lifetime has become obliterated. Learned patterns of behaviour also break up, the subject feeling that he has lost control over his actions. If loss of control under normal circumstances would be frightening for the subject, he will become extremely paranoid and experience a terrifying 'trip'. If the state of unintegration fulfils a psychological need, or if loss of control is normally not anxiety-provoking, a 'trip' will be a glorious experience.

An LSD 'trip' is essentially a psychotic experience, delusions and hallucinations being a prominent feature. These hallucinations may either be taken to be real images, in which case the experience becomes real for the subject, or their hallucinatory nature may be appreciated. 'Trips' are usually taken in the company of other people, preferably one trusted companion. As all inhibitions are lost under the impact of LSD, people become intensely aware of one another to the point of psychic fusion when all the barriers which normally separate people are broken down. This can be a most satisfying experience for the borderline psychotic who normally feels isolated from people. Time sense becomes distorted and a minute may seem like an hour. Memories which have been repressed into the unconscious can be released and relived, the subject remaining aware of them after the effects of the drug have worn off.

The dangers of LSD are, firstly, the emotional effect of a bad (i.e. paranoid) 'trip', which may precipitate a neurotic or psychotic breakdown if the subject is left to experience his terror by himself, and if the predisposition to breakdown exists; secondly, uncontrolled behaviour

(leading to suicide or murder) where hallucinations and delusions are taken to be real, the subject therefore being unaware of the real dangers in the environment.

Although the LSD state mimics the schizophrenic state, these states are not equivalent. Whereas the hallucinations of schizophrenia are largely auditory, i.e. the hearing of voices, LSD hallucinations are visual as a rule. The schizophrenic patient is withdrawn, while the LSD subject on a good 'trip' is gregarious and euphoric. The LSD experience can be gratifying and mind-expanding (enlightening) to a normal person who understands what is happening, and who is neither unduly disturbed by the uncovering of childhood memories nor by his lack of control over his own feelings and perceptions. The schizophrenic, on the other hand, may show an exacerbation of symptoms, while the borderline schizophrenic may regress to the florid schizophrenic state.

Drug abuse is an alarming social problem in medically advanced countries. Ours is a drug-oriented society; most discomforts can be alleviated by swallowing a pill or having an injection. Our children grow up accepting the practices of their elders; therefore drugs do not hold any terrors for them.

Throughout the Western world, mood-altering drugs are prescribed to combat the effects of anxiety. People who are emotionally (or spiritually) starved or isolated and who experience an emptiness, or a fear of rejection within themselves, are placed under a great temptation to fill the void or to ease the anxiety by recourse to mood-altering drugs.

Although drug abuse is a major community health hazard, the drug problem has not assumed the enormous proportions that the alcohol problem has, because drugs are not as freely available as alcohol and, although used for medicinal purposes, have not become integrated into traditional cultural practices. Drugs are procured either legitimately on a doctor's prescription (the doctor being ethically and legally bound not to prescribe for non-therapeutic addictive purposes) or illegally on the black market from pushers and criminal drug rings — both buyer and seller committing a criminal offence during the transaction.

Whereas the abuse of alcohol cannot be concealed for long — the demeanour and facies of the patient, his slurred speech and the smell of his breath revealing his 'secret' — concealment is common amongst drug abusers and medical help is seldom sought. When confronted with a suspicion, the addict will vehemently deny his addiction. The personality deterioration is much greater in the drug addict when he eventually submits to treatment than in the alcoholic; therefore, institutionalised treatment of the drug dependant is much more protracted.

Dagga is nearer to alcohol in the ease with which the addict can be identified (smell and physical signs of red conjunctiva, tachycardia, thirst and ravenous appetite), but it is not a drug of physical addiction and dependence is fairly easily broken.

It is a much milder drug than the other drugs of dependence. It is, moreover, easy to procure as it grows luxuriantly in South Africa.

The **dependence on hard-line drugs** such as opiates (e.g. heroin and morphine) and pethidine, to which members of the helping professions can become addicted because of the accessibility of the drugs to them, can sometimes be picked up when there are signs of drug toxicity or when supplies are unprocurable and the addict suffers withdrawal symptoms.

In 1982 a man was jailed after he was caught trying to sell opium in Hillbrow (Johannesburg). This was the first time someone had tried to introduce opium on a large scale on the Reef drug market.

Despite their total prohibition for medicinal purposes, the amphetamines, which are obtainable only on the black market, are still used by drug dependants.

The psychedelic (mind-expanding) drugs, dagga and LSD in the form of microdots, are commonly used, despite the heavy penalties for possessing them. They are used mainly by the younger generation as part of the expression of their revolt against established society (which represents authority). Mind-expanding drug dependence is fairly common amongst adolescent scholars and students and may cause school and university drop-outs. At present nothing is known with certainty about the permanent effects of dagga. Its immediate effects on mood,

perception and psychomotor co-ordination affect driving skills to a serious extent. Benzene and glue (used by sniffing) belong to this group of drugs and are used more commonly by deprived children.

The rebellious young people, especially those who use LSD, attempt to obtain spiritual freedom by a mystical experience ('high') which lifts them far above the common earth-bound mortals.

Trends in drug abuse have changed drastically.

In the 1960s substances such as cough mixtures and cannabis, together with alcohol, were abused.

In 1973/74, Mandrax, a drug causing physical and psychical dependence, was introduced and joined cannabis as a much sought-after drug. From the 1970s children as young as 12 years started experimenting with dangerous drugs.

In 1976, opium, morphine and Wellconal were introduced and addicts started 'spiking'.

The intravenous use of drugs has become common practice among drug abusers in South Africa. It is called 'spiking'. According to Dr De Miranda (quoted in the *Rand Daily Mail,* June 1984) the addicts — those who cannot survive without their 'fix' — reach such a level of desperation that they will happily maim themselves just to get a needle into a vein that has not already collapsed.

Prolonged dependence on the dependence-producing drugs causes personality deterioration from which it is very difficult to recover, even though there is no organic brain deterioration (dementia). In-patient therapy in a treatment centre may last for months and even years.

Primary prevention of drug dependence

(1) It is important to educate children and adolescents in the dangers of drug abuse.

(2) All dangerous and potentially dangerous dependence-producing drugs should be strictly controlled so that they do not fall into the hands of unauthorised persons.

The registered nurse has a grave responsibility for the safe-keeping of drugs and for guarding against their misuse. The administration of medicinal substances is controlled by the *Medicines and Related Substances Control Act 101 of 1965*. Controlled medicines are listed in nine schedules.

The Act lays down that some drugs, i.e. those listed in schedule 8, e.g. cannabis sativa-indica, amphetamines, coca leaf, Mandrax, LSD and heroin, are totally prohibited as medicines and that the other dangerous and potentially dangerous drugs of dependence may be obtained by the public only on a doctor's prescription.

The conditions for issuing of drugs are also prescribed in the Act and failure on the part of the medical profession to comply with the proscriptions of the Act is punishable by heavy fines.

Secondary prevention of drug dependence

In 1971 an Act known as *The Abuse of Dependence-producing Substances and Rehabilitation Centres Act* was passed (Act 41 of 1971). This Act was replaced in 1992 by two new Acts: Act 20/1992 and Act 140/1992 (see p. 753). One of the main objectives of these Acts is the deterrent use of criminal prosecution for being in unlawful possession of dependence-producing drugs, as listed in the schedules of the Act. Drug-trafficking is prohibited in South Africa on the penalty of imprisonment and confiscation of property. Socially disturbing drug and alcohol abuse are treated by legal committal to treatment centres.

The government is attempting to cope with the problem by severely repressive anti-drug legislation.

(C) Classification according to legal controllability

Dependence-producing substances are listed in Parts I, II and III of the Schedule of the non-repealed part of Act 41 of 1971.

Part I: Prohibited dependence-producing drugs

- Amphetamine
- Bufotenine
- *Cannabis sativa indica* (dagga), the whole plant or any portion or product thereof
- Coca leaf
- Dexamphetamine
- Diethyltryptamine
- Dimethyltryptamine
- Harmaline
- Harmine
- Heroin (diacetylmorphine)
- Lysergide (LSD, LSD 25)
- Mescaline
- Methamphetamine
- Dimethoxyamphetamine
- Phenmetrazine
- Prepared opium
- Psilocin
- Psilocybin
- Tetrahydrocannabinol
- Methaqualone, including Mandrax, Isonox, Quaalude or any other preparation containing methaqualone
- Methylene-dioxyamphetamine (MDA)

Part II: Dangerous dependence-producing drugs

- Benzphetamine
- Chlorodyne (Tincture of Chloroform and Morphine)
- Cocaine
- Codeine (methylmorphine)
- Dextromoramide
- Diphenoxylate
- Dipinanone (e.g. Wellconal)
- Ecgonine
- Ethylmorphine
- Fentanyl
- Levorphanol
- Methadone
- Methorphan
- Methylphenidate (e.g. Ritalin)
- Metopon
- Moramide
- Morphine, except preparations containing not more than 0,2 % morphine
- Opium
- Pethidine
- Phenadoxone
- Phendimetrazine (e.g. Obex)
- Pholcodine
- Proheptazine
- Properidine
- Sufentanil

Part III: Potentially dangerous dependence-producing drugs

- Amobarbital, cyclobarbital, pentobarbital, secobarbital
- Diethylpropion (e.g. Tenuate)
- Glutethimide (e.g. Doriden)
- Pentazocine (e.g. Sosegon)
- Phencyclidine
- Tilidene (e.g. Valoron)

SUMMARIES OF THE NEW DRUG ACTS

Prevention and Treatment of Drug Dependency Act 20 of 1992

Note: The 'drugs' covered by this Act include alcohol and the drugs listed in the Schedule of Act 41 of 1971 — Abuse of Dependence-producing Substances and Rehabilitation Centers Act. A shortened version of this schedule is given on p. 752.

This Act provides for:

(1) The establishment of a Drug Advisory Board consisting of nine members, including a chairman and executive committee who have special knowledge of the problems relating to the abuse of drugs and who will advise the Minister (one or several decided on by the State President) on any matter affecting the abuse of drugs.

(2) The establishment of treatment centres. The Minister may establish, maintain and manage **treatment centres** for the reception, treatment and training of referred patients/persons.

(3) Procedure for bringing a suspected person before a magistrate. These patients/persons are either voluntary (see p. 754) or found eligible for admission by any persons, including any social worker, because they are dependent on drugs and/or on alcohol and in consequence thereof squander their means or injure their health, or endanger the peace, or in any other manner do harm to their own welfare or the welfare of their families or fail to provide for their own support or for that of any dependant whom they are legally liable to maintain. A police officer shall be authorised to serve a summons on non-voluntary persons to appear before a magistrate, or the magistrate may issue a warrant of arrest of persons eligible for admission to a (registered) treatment centre, after he has obtained from a social worker a report as to the social circumstances of the person concerned. All the provisions of the Criminal Procedure Act shall apply in respect of warrants of arrest and summonses issued under this section, as well as the court proceedings governing criminal trials in magistrates' courts.

(4) Committal of persons to a (registered) treatment centre. The magistrate may direct that the person on trial be examined by a medical officer, psychiatrist or clinical psychologist, forcefully if necessary. If it appears to the magistrate that the person on trial is likely to benefit by the treatment and training provided in a (registered) treatment centre, or that it would be in his own interest or that of his family and the community, he may order that the person be thus detained (committed).

The magistrate may also order that such person be detained in custody, or released on bail or warning until such time as effect can be given to the order.

Programmes for prevention and treatment of drug dependency

The Minister may cause to be established programmes which are aimed at:

(*a*) the prevention of drug dependency;

(*b*) information to the community on the abuse of drugs;

(*c*) the education of the youth in regard to the abuse of drugs;

(*d*) the observation, treatment and supervision of persons who have been placed under supervision of a court;

(*e*) the rendering of assistance to the families of persons detained in a (registered) treatment centre.

Volunteer workers, stringently selected and registered by the Director-General, may be appointed to carry out the above programme. Remuneration of volunteers is conditional.

The patients of a treatment centre are there to undergo treatment, including training, and to perform such duties as the authorities may determine. Treatment may be physical, psychological, spiritual or social. Treatment centres may be:

(a) newly established;

(b) rehabilitation centres established previously by the state under Act 41 of 1971;

(c) institutions registered as treatment centres. Registration must be applied for and must comply with certain conditions before a registration certificate will be issued. Such registration can be amended or cancelled, but may not be transferred.

The Minister (state, including provincial administrations) may establish, maintain and manage **hostels** or use those already in existence for the purpose of providing homes for:

(a) patients who have been released on licence or granted leave of absence, from treatment centres;

(b) discharged patients;

(c) voluntary patients and those eligible for admission to a treatment centre;

(d) persons who are undergoing treatment for dependency in any approved institution.

Institutions outside those owned by the state, may apply for registration as a hostel.

Registered treatment centres and hostels may be inspected by a social worker or medical officer if so directed by the Director-General or magistrate. The Director-General shall appoint for every treatment centre a social worker, medical practitioner, psychiatrist, clinical psychologist or nurse as superintendent. Except for voluntary patients, patients/inmates may be transferred to and from prisons and treatment centres, to and from children's homes, schools of industries or reform schools and treatment centres, to serve the best interest of the person with a drug (including alcohol) dependency problem, before he is returned to the community. Retransfer may occur if such a person has proved to be unsuited to or is not likely to benefit from the kind of treatment and training provided in the treatment centre.

A patient from a mental institution may be transferred to a treatment centre if he is likely to benefit by a particular kind of treatment and training. He is then discharged from the provisions of the Mental Health Act (1973). Likewise, a patient committed to a treatment centre

by a magistrate may be transferred to a mental institution if it is thought that he will benefit from such a transfer. Patients from treatment centres may be granted leave of absence (conditionally) or may be released on licence (conditionally). Both leave and licence may be revoked if the patient cannot adjust himself properly to the normal life of the community. If there is any resistance to readmission, the patient may be arrested without warrant by any police officer, social worker or member of the staff of any treatment centre.

Voluntary patients

Any person may be admitted to a treatment centre on application to its superintendent and the submission of a report by a social worker and, if necessary, a medical and/or psychiatric report. The voluntary patient may be subsidised by the state if necessary. The person with a drug problem will be detained as a patient for not longer than six months, but absconding penalties will not apply to him.

The Minister may pay allowances to patients of treatment centres, under prescribed conditions.

Discipline in treatment centres will be maintained by prescribed disciplinary steps. A record of punitive proceedings, with written statements by the superintendent and the patient, are submitted to a magistrate who will decide on a just outcome.

On discharge from treatment centres, the 'dry' alcoholics who have problems with finding work in the open labour market can be accommodated in The Department of Manpower's Training and Work Centres (Sheltered Employment Factories) (see Chapter 44).

Drugs and Drug Trafficking Act 140 of 1992

This Act deals with the 'dealers' and 'traffickers' in drugs and the illicit manufacturers of drugs. It is a criminal Act. In this Act, a 'drug' refers to:

(1) any dependence-producing substance;

(2) any dangerous dependence-producing substance, or

(3) any undesirable dependence-producing substance.

It does not include alcohol (as in Act 20, 1992). Schedule 1 of this Act lists substances useful for the manufacture of drugs, e.g. ephedrine, ergotamine, lysergic acid, acetone, ethyl ether, piperidine. These are called scheduled substances. Schedule 2, Parts I, II and III, lists any substance or any plant from which a substance can be manufactured. Some 200 drugs have been listed in Schedule 2 (not included here). The Minister may consult with the Minister of National Health about the inclusion or deletion of drugs.

Act 140/1992 provides for the prohibition of the use or possession of, or the dealing in, drugs and of certain acts relating to the manufacture or supply of certain substances; the acquisition or conversion of the proceeds of certain crimes; for the obligation to report certain information to the police; for the exercise of the powers of entry, search, seizure and detention in specified circumstances; for the recovery of the proceeds of drug trafficking.

'Sell' in relation to a drug includes to offer, advertise, possess or expose the drug for sale, to dispose of it for consideration or otherwise or to exchange it.

'Minister' in this Act means Minister of Justice.

Illegal acts (relating to scheduled substances)

Manufacture. No person shall manufacture any scheduled substance or supply it to any other person knowing or suspecting that any such scheduled substance is to be used in or for the unlawful manufacture of the drug.

Use and possession. No person shall use or have in his possession:

(a) any dependence-producing substance; or
(b) any dangerous dependence-producing substance or any undesirable dependence-producing substance unless he is a patient or other person who has acquired it legally for medicinal use, or other recognised use.

Reporting of information and investigations

Any person may disclose to any attorney-general such information necessary for the prevention of combating of a drug offence.

Obligation to report certain information to the police

If a person in charge of a place of entertainment has reason to suspect a person to be a user or dealer in a 'drug', he must report his suspicions to any police official on duty and furnish him with particulars. The same applies to a manager of a financial institution or stockbroker who suspects business is the proceeds of a defined crime.

A police official must investigate the suspected 'drug' crime. The magistrate may issue a warrant of arrest and detention of the suspected 'drug' offender.

Any person held on this charge shall as soon as possible be examined by a district surgeon and at least once every 5 days be visited by a district surgeon who reports to the magistrate.

Presumptions relating to (a) possession and to (b) dealing in drugs

(a) the drug is found in the immediate vicinity of the accused

(b) 115 grams of dagga or any undesirable dependence-producing substance was found in possession of the accused.

(c) any dangerous dependence-producing substance was found in the possession of the accused in or on any school grounds or within 100 metres of the school grounds; or on a vehicle used by the accused, it shall be presumed that the possessor is a drug dealer.

(d) the growing of dagga plants will also incriminate the grower.

Any person convicted of an offence under this Act will forfeit to the state all the drugs in his possession, and any container or vehicle used for its storage or transport. This also applies to immovable property.

Proceeds of drug trafficking

'Drug trafficking' includes any act in or outside the RSA which constitutes a drug offence or an economic offence. A person has benefited from drug trafficking if he has received any payment in connection with drug dealing by him or any other person.

If a court finds that a dealer has benefited from drug trafficking, it may impose a confiscation order to cover the dealer's gains in addition to any punishment which the court may impose. It is presumed that any property held by him at any time since his conviction was as a payment or reward in connection with drug trafficking.

A restraint order may be made by a superior court, which prohibits any person from dealing in any manner with any property to which the order relates. The property may be seized by a police officer and become the responsibility of the superior court. Legally the case may be taken much further and entail international law and foreign confiscation orders.

The following laws have been repealed: Act 41 of 1971 and its five amendment Acts. They have been replaced by Act 140 of 1992 and Act 20 of 1992.

REHABILITATION OF PERSONS DEPENDENT ON ALCOHOLIC LIQUOR OR DEPENDENCE-PRODUCING DRUGS

Rehabilitation of the alcoholic should be commenced while the patient is still undergoing detoxification therapy. Many recovering alcoholics attend as out-patients at either hospital or SANCA and its affiliated clinics which employ social workers to help the alcoholic with social problems, such as employment, housing or accommodation and reconstructive services to the family.

Great use is made of the services of the organisations, **Alcoholics Anonymous (AA)** and **Narcotics Anonymous**. Members of these organisations are invited by SANCA and affiliated clinics to come and talk to their detoxified in-patients for the purpose of giving them guidance regarding abstinence, as well as acceptance and emotional support.

Al-Anon helps the families of alcoholics help their sick member. (See p. 757.) During the rehabilitation process, and even after full rehabilitation, the chronic alcoholic may never touch a drop of alcohol again as this may re-establish his craving. Rehabilitation, therefore, implies lifelong abstention from alcohol.

THE SOUTH AFRICAN NATIONAL COUNCIL ON ALCOHOLISM AND DRUG DEPENDENCE (SANCA) (WO 1955)

SANCA is a welfare organisation concerned with the prevention of ill-health and social pathology caused by alcohol and dangerous dependence-producing substances ('drugs') and

with the rehabilitation of addicted persons. Drug dependence came within the ambit of SANCA only in 1969. SANCA serves the whole South African population.

SANCA is subsidised by various state departments responsible for the welfare of the white, black, coloured and Indian populations and is further supported by donations from the public, commerce and industry. It acts within the framework of Act 20 of 1992 — Prevention and Treatment of Drug Dependency Act, 1992.

The main objectives of SANCA

SANCA's main objectives are:

(1) To gain recognition, by all sections of the community, of the fact that alcoholism as well as drug dependence is to be regarded as a disease, with physical, psychological, social and spiritual components in its origin and development, which can and should be treated.

(2) To extend its facilities for the treatment of alcoholics and drug dependants.

(3) To help those who require counselling.

(4) To disseminate information regarding alcoholism and drug dependence to all groups and sections.

(5) To obtain increased support from the public, commerce and industry, state and provincial authorities, for this important work.

(6) To co-ordinate activities in the field of alcoholism and drug dependence.

The majority of organisations concerned with substance abuse liaise and co-operate with SANCA. Particulars of additional sources of help may, therefore, be obtained from SANCA.

ALCOHOLICS ANONYMOUS (AA)

AA is a brotherhood (and sisterhood) of ex-alcoholics who help one another and welcome anyone from any ethnic group to join them. The only requirement for AA membership is a desire to stop drinking. New members are referred to a SANCA or hospital clinic if they require medical treatment, e.g. sedation or detoxification.

AA accepts no charity or donations from outside, every group being entirely self-supporting. Field and other workers give their services on a voluntary basis and will visit people in their homes or in a SANCA clinic, if they have had the call to do so, or if the need arises. Group meetings take place on a weekly basis at a fixed venue. Members remain anonymous to one another, being known only by first names; no registers are kept of patients, except those who are giving their services and need to be contacted to go on a mission. Members always maintain personal anonymity at the level of the press, radio and films.

Although workers are non-professional (as far as the work of AA is concerned), service centres may employ special workers.

AA does not involve itself in any outside activities and members express no opinions about outside issues, as they do not want to become involved beyond AA activities. They do no welfare work in the community: the common welfare of AA members comes first.

The spiritual philosophy of AA

The primary aim of AA is a spiritual one, but no specific religious tenet is embraced. Both Moslem and Christian can find spiritual harmony in its teachings of a Supreme Being — a power greater than themselves that can restore them to sanity. They seek through prayer and meditation to improve their conscious contact with God — as they understand Him, praying only for knowledge of His will for them and the power to carry it out. When they achieve a spiritual awakening, they try to carry this message to other alcoholics who are still suffering, and practise these principles in all their affairs. Anonymity is the spiritual foundation of all their traditions, which places principles above personalities.

Al-Anon

Al-Anon is an associated (but separate from AA) fellowship and caters for the families and close friends of alcoholics. The main purpose of this group is to help the family understand alcoholism as a disease and themselves in relation to the alcoholic in their midst. Members get a form of group therapy which helps them adjust to the presence of an active drinker in the home and to help the alcoholic when he is attempting the rehabilitation struggle.

Al-Anon is a world-wide organisation with branches in most of the bigger centres in South Africa.

REFERENCES

(1) Lichtigfeld FJ, Gillman MA. The treatment of alcoholic withdrawal states with oxygen and nitrous oxide. *S Afr Med J* 1982; **61**: 349.

(2) McCabe EMI. Alcoholism — its emergence in the black townships of South Africa. *S Afr Med J* 1982; **61**: 881.

(3) Editorial. *S Afr Med J* 1981; **59**: 583.

(4) De Miranda S. Alcohol — the incidence, treatment and rehabilitation. *Rehabilitation in SA* 1988; **87**: 32-84.

(5) Zaayman HM. Nasorg met die probleemdrinker na behandeling by Elimkliniek. *Rehabilitation in SA* 1988; **32**: 92–94.

TEST OF KNOWLEDGE

The student has benefited from studying this chapter if he/she can answer the following questions:

(1) Give an account of the effects of habitual (chronic) alcohol abuse on:
   (*a*) the body;
   (*b*) the brain;
   (*c*) society.
(2) Discuss the care of the alcoholic in remission until full rehabilitation appears to have been reached.
(3) Discuss the legislation to curb the illegal use of dependence-producing substances.
(4) Write on:
   (*a*) Withdrawal sickness in: (i) the alcoholic, (ii) the morphine addict.
   (*b*) Give the causes and treatment of withdrawal sickness in each case.
(5) Define the following terms:
   – dependence-producing drugs
   – 'spiking'
   – amphetamines
   – an LSD 'trip'
   – drug addict
   – chronic alcoholism
   – problem drinking
   – psychological dependence on drugs
   – tolerance to drugs
   – hallucinogen

(6) Write an essay on the problem of *Cannabis sativa indica* abuse in South Africa and the attempts which are being made to curb the problem.

(7) Define 'treatment centres' as used in Act 20/1992 and describe the committal procedure to such an institution.

(8) Discuss the work done by Alcoholics Anonymous and Al-Anon in helping the chronic alcoholic and his family.

(9) Give reasons for the inclusion of this chapter in Part VI of this manual, 'Impairment and disablement as community health problems'.

43

Physical Disablement and Cerebral Palsy

INTRODUCTION

Physical handicaps included here are afflictions of the skeleto-muscular system which prevent the full mobility and functioning of the affected person, causing him to be 'lame' and disabled. The brain may be affected, especially in congenital conditions, and this may affect speech and intellectual functions. The physical handicap may be either congenital, e.g. cerebral palsy, a defect which is present at birth, or secondary to disease or injury, e.g. paralysis due to poliomyelitis, deformities due to TB of the spine, traumatic paraplegia and quadriplegia, and amputations. A 'cripple' is a person with a physical defect or injury, who is partially or completely disabled.

The aim of medical rehabilitation is to restore the crippled person to the fullest possible physical, mental, vocational and economic independence and usefulness. Because of the involvement of the skeleto-muscular system in cripples, medical rehabilitation is achieved through the co-operation of a professional team of medical and paramedical personnel and nurses. Surgical correction of the defect is made by the orthopaedic surgeon

and orthopaedic technicians and prosthetists who make and fit splints and prostheses (artificial parts of the body). Function is further restored by the specialised therapy given by physio-, speech and occupational therapists.

The physiotherapist uses exercises to promote co-ordination and strengthening of muscles and teaches correct movements, postural sense and walking patterns. The occupational therapist corrects visuo-motor co-ordination difficulties and teaches activities to improve muscle co-ordination and hand and finger dexterity. She also trains the physically handicapped person in the skills of daily living.

The speech therapist gives brain-damaged children, and others with defective speech, specialised training in the co-ordination and use of the muscles involved in respiration, feeding and speech.

The orthopaedic community nurse plays an important role in caring for the physically handicapped person in his home, after discharge from the hospital for corrective surgery. Cripples receive a tremendous amount of help from the community in South Africa.

IN THIS CHAPTER

PERSONAL (SELF-CARE) REHABILITATION OF THE PHYSICALLY HANDICAPPED

(With special reference to paraplegia and quadriplegia)

There are approximately half a million physically handicapped people in South Africa; of these 200 000 are in wheelchairs. The majority of wheelchair users are either paraplegic or quadriplegic and many owe their disability to violence. Paraplegics and quadriplegics (tetraplegics) can be taught self-care activities to preserve physical health and independence.

The first step in the rehabilitation of the paralysed person is to establish the site of the spinal cord lesion; this gives an idea of which sensory and motor functions have been lost and which functions can be strengthened in order to give the person a measure of autonomy.

Examples: middle cervical lesions lead to tetraplegia; the person will need help with moving and care of the body, including toilet, dressing, feeding, bowel and bladder functions. He will always be dependent on the help of other people.

If the lesion is at C6, however, the paralysed person will be able to use his shoulders, elbows and wrists; thus he will be able to grasp and hold objects and be more independent as regards feeding and dressing himself as well as operating a wheelchair. If the lesion is at C7, the person is able to do much more with his hands, the height of achievement being the driving of a hand-controlled, automatic car.

If the lesion is in the thoracic and lumbar regions, the person is paraplegic; he has not lost his ability to use his upper extremities. These can be strengthened to enable him to become mobile and to care for himself.

The higher the lesion in the thoracic spinal cord, the poorer will be the person's ability to breathe strongly because of paralysis of intercostal muscles. In lesions above T1, breathing is diaphragmatic. With low thoracic and lumbar lesions, the person can become a functional crutch walker; the higher the lesion the weaker the muscular control will be. In cord lesions through L5 to SI, the person will be able to walk with short leg braces.

Persons with complete section of the cord below T12 are impotent, i.e. males cannot manage coitus. If the lesion is at T12, the male may be potent but cannot achieve orgasm or ejaculation.

Self-care activities

The community nurse who works amongst paraplegics and tetraplegics must be able to counsel the disabled person and/or his family on his ongoing physical care. Incontinence of urine and faeces and pressure sores on the buttocks of wheelchair users are constant problems.

Faecal incontinence

Faecal incontinence will be a problem which can be overcome, however, if a bowel training programme is followed, e.g. bowel action is brought about every morning at a fixed time by inserting a laxative suppository followed by digital stimulation. Colostomy is not advised.

Incontinence of urine (spontaneous voiding)

The main cause of incontinence is the neurogenic bladder when lesions of the spinal cord abolish voluntary control over micturition. Any cord lesion above the voiding reflex arc (S1–S4) will cause a spastic neurogenic bladder.

The neurogenic bladder is caused by both traumatic (severed spinal cord) and non-traumatic (spina bifida with myelomeningocele, multiple sclerosis) lesions of the spinal cord which result in paraplegia or tetraplegia.

The management of the neurogenic bladder is aimed at preserving renal function because the patient's life span is dependent on renal competence.

Early management during the acute stage is usually by regular or continuous bladder drainage by means of a catheter inserted with strict aseptic precautions.

Long-term management can be tried in consultation with the disabled person by the establishment of an *automatic bladder*. This means bladder training in order to be free of the catheter and for micturition to be under voluntary control of the paraplegic. It is accomplished by regulating fluid intake and assessing at what capacity the bladder is likely to void spontaneously. Spontaneous voiding is then anticipated and precipitated by using certain triggering stimuli, e.g. straining, slapping the thigh, traction on a pubic hair, suprapubic compression at regular intervals. Once voiding starts, no further stimulation is required. Heavy pressure over the bladder must be avoided. Just enough pressure must be exerted to start the bladder contracting. The efficiency of the bladder reflex activity is judged by the amount of residual urine. Voiding is considered satisfactory if the residuum is less than 10 % of bladder capacity. Bladder control is never complete as any rise in abdominal pressure caused by movements may cause expulsion of urine. Leakage of urine and soiling of clothes is controlled by using one of the following methods:

(1) the wearing of an absorbent pad;

(2) condom and tube attached to the penis and draining into a leg bag.

If the automatic bladder cannot be established, *intermittent (3–4 hourly) self-catheterisation* may be carried out.

Catheterisation is done with special rubber or stainless steel catheters, washed with soap and water after use, thoroughly rinsed and

shaken dry and stored in a clean self-sealing bag which can be carried in a handbag.

The woman washes her hands and vulva and if she is capable of sitting on a toilet, the procedure is done in this position, initially with the aid of a mirror. The catheter is lubricated with KY jelly and pushed up the urethra into the bladder for 8 cm. The urine will flow into the pan. The bladder is emptied completely, by suprapubic pressure if necessary. If this position cannot be managed, the woman sits on a bed or chair and receives the urine in a receiver. Children can be helped by adults at first but must be taught to become independent as soon as possible.

Males usually use a Nelaton size 12 or 14 FG catheter. Utmost cleanliness must be observed, hands and glans penis being sprayed with Savlodil or other antiseptic after washing. The catheter tip is lubricated with KY jelly and inserted to its full length into the bladder. When the flow of urine slows, the catheter is slowly withdrawn while applying pressure suprapubically.

Although a sterile procedure is not followed, strict cleanliness is necessary and the apparatus may be handled by one person only. It has been found that bacteria introduced into the bladder via a catheter will not cause infection if the blood supply of the bladder is good, if there is no infection (from the bladder or from bedsores) and if the quality of the blood is good. Clean intermittent self-catheterisation will not cause infection. This does not apply if the bladder becomes overfilled, thus causing pressure on blood vessels and consequent diminution of blood supply.

The doctor may prescribe medicines to keep the urine acid.

Some paraplegics and tetraplegics never gain bladder control. In this case the bladder is managed as follows:

(1) *Condom drainage in a male.*

(2) *Permanent indwelling catheter.* A Foley catheter is inserted and a closed system drainage bag is attached to the catheter, using a strict aseptic technique. The catheter is fixed to the person's thigh. The fixing of the catheter via a looped portion of the connecting tubing is most important to prevent pull

on the catheter and balloon of the Foley catheter *in situ*. Pull causes irritation of the mucosa and may even dislodge the balloon.

It is advisable for the penis to be strapped to the abdomen to prevent the formation of a penile ulcer (between the base of the penis and the scrotum) as a result of kinking of the catheter in the urethra should the penis hang down. The person must drink liberal quantities of fluid and the urine must be kept acid. If alkaline (and infected), the doctor will prescribe mandelic acid with ammonium chloride and acid sodium phosphate. The genitalia and the catheter where it leaves the body must be kept scrupulously clean.

In exceptional cases where none of the above methods of managing incontinence in the paraplegic and tetraplegic persons can be managed, a surgical operation is done to divert the urine to a *colonic or ileal conduit*.

Pressure sores and their prevention

The problem of pressure sores arises in paraplegic and tetraplegic persons confined to a wheelchair who cannot feel the pain caused by ischaemia. This can be a great problem as the constant sitting thins the fat and muscle pad over the ischial tuberosities, thus increasing their pressure potential. The best way of preventing any pressure sore is to relieve pressure on pressure parts.

Pressure-relieving manoeuvres

(1) The use of soft cushions filled with air, water or sponge. Cubex (S&N) cushions are filled with shifting globular polystyrene beads 2–5 mm in diameter which mould to the user's body and distribute pressure over a large area. A seat made of sponge rubber with holes over the ischial tuberosities and perineum is also effective.
(2) The paraplegic wheelchair user is taught to lift his buttocks off the chair five times every half hour by pressing with hands on the armrests of the chair.

The health of the skin over pressure parts is preserved by keeping the skin dry and clean, in the case of incontinence or heavy sweating, and by regular deep massaging with alcohol or pow-

der which has a drying effect. Massage helps to promote the circulation if done often enough (4-hourly) by means of deep kneading movements.

The paraplegic should have a course of muscle strengthening exercises to enable him to use the functioning muscles of the upper limb and shoulders to compensate for the loss of function of paralysed muscles.

Paraplegics are taught maintenance of their wheelchairs, how to move from the bed to the wheelchair and to the toilet. Dressing, undressing and personal hygiene, including bathing, are well within the activities the paraplegic can master if his arm and shoulder muscles are strong.

Paraplegics are taught to walk with calipers and crutches or walking frames. Although most paraplegics will use the wheelchair for daily activities, the exercise of walking is important to prevent contractures of lower limbs, pressure sores on buttocks and osteoporosis. Swimming is encouraged once the paraplegic has control of his bladder.

Sexual counselling, usually done by a doctor or a psychologist, especially in males, is important as residual sexual functions will depend upon the site of the spinal cord lesion.

Mechanical aids to mobility

Mobility of the physically handicapped person is essential in rehabilitation. The most popular aid for those with limited mobility is the wheelchair.

Wheelchairs may be self-propelled or motorised and many different models are available. Self-propelled wheelchairs are used for competitive sporting activities.

Motorbikes can be modified to the driver's requirements and to carry a wheelchair. The acme of luxury is a modified car for manual driving with a hoist for a wheelchair which is accommodated on the roof. The whole procedure of getting the wheelchair *in situ* and the car in motion can be done single-handedly by the paraplegic. This is an expensive luxury. Vans supplied with ramps and large doors are used by agencies to transport multiple wheelchairs and their occupants.

Aids to independent living

Independent living (IL) has been facilitated recently by the establishment of IL resource centres in Cape Town and Johannesburg where persons with restricted mobility and dexterity, their families and professionals can view modified equipment and aids to modern living. Specially adjusted stoves, baths, toilets and kitchen gadgets (especially for arthritic hands) are demonstrated and clients referred to suppliers. The IL Centre in Johannesburg provides a counselling and advisory service for the physically disabled. They also liaise with architects concerning the construction of new buildings in order to make them more accessible to wheelchair users. Modified kitchens and bathrooms are expensive, but where they can be afforded they enable a disabled person to cope alone in a dwelling.

CEREBRAL PALSY

Molteno *et al.*[1] refer to cerebral palsy as 'a group of conditions which are characterised by a disorder of movement and posture due to a defect or lesion of the immature brain' (p. 823). In cerebral palsy the aetiology of the movement disorder is in the brain. Clinical types of cerebral palsy:

Note: Palsy (paralysis) is used here to indicate partial paralysis or paresis.

(1) Spastic (68 %): hemiplegia, quadriplegia, diplegia (double hemiplegia) with greater involvement of legs, mono/triplegia.
(2) Dyskinetic (18 %):
   (*a*) pure athetoid and choreo-athetoid;
   (*b*) dystonic (with sustained spasm of muscles resulting in abnormal posture) athetoid;
   (*c*) tremor.
(3) Ataxic.
(4) Hypotonic with diminution or loss of muscular tone. This may lead to stretching of muscles beyond their normal limits.
(5) Mixed group, usually spastic plus athetoid types.

In spastic palsy, affected muscles are hypertonic (stiff and hard) and their movements are limited. Spasticity is due to upper neuronal lesions. Muscle reflexes are increased.

In dyskinetic palsy, movements of the face, head and limbs are coarse and jerky when the child tries to execute a single purposive movement. Dyskinesis may vary from athetoid movements to tremor. Choreo-athetoid movements combine the spasmodic jerking and abrupt involuntary movements of chorea with the constant, slow writhing involuntary movements of athetosis. It is due to lesions of the basal ganglia and is commonly caused by kernicterus.

In ataxic palsy there is loss of co-ordination in executing purposive movements. Jerky and waving movements indicate lesions of the cerebellum.

The following is an extract of the findings of Molteno *et al.*[1] on 389 coloured cerebral palsied children in Cape Town, born between 1964–1975.

Main causes of cerebral palsy and characteristic type

▨ Prematurity usually causes spasticity, especially diplegia; perinatal asphyxia may cause either spasticity or dyskinesis.
▨ Kernicterus causes dyskinesis.
▨ Foetal deprivation (bleeding during pregnancy, infarction of the placenta, toxaemia, small-for-date infants, maternal diabetes) causes spasticity.

Associated handicaps

Associated handicaps occurred in 91 % of the cerebral palsied children studied by Molteno *et al*. Of these handicaps, 67 % were mental retardation (IQ below 70) and 30 % were epilepsy. The other associated handicaps were: perceptual and conceptual problems; microcephalus and hydrocephalus; bilateral hearing loss; blindness or partial sightedness; strabismus; behavioural disorders (hyperkinesis, distractibility).

The physical handicaps were graded as follows:

(1) mild 9 % (no or minimal disability);
(2) moderate 54 % (ability to carry out age-specific activities is interfered with);
(3) severe 37 % (inability to carry out normal activities).

Cerebral palsy is a multi-handicap condition necessitating assessment and treatment in comprehensive clinics and special schools.

Aetiology and primary prevention of cerebral palsy

The causes of cerebral palsy may be either congenital or acquired, the latter either perinatally or postnatally. In a study to find out if cerebral palsy is a preventable disease, McManus et al. (Canada) analysed 96 cases and came to the conclusion that 38 % of the cases could have been prevented by better perinatal care.[2]

The infants especially at risk during the perinatal period are Rh negative infants who develop kernicterus, low birth mass (below 2 500 g), including preterm babies and those with the respiratory distress syndrome. Birth trauma is another important cause of cerebral palsy. McManus et al.[2] found that the 5-minute Apgar score correlates well with the incidence of neurological sequelae; for this reason, rapid and adequate ventilation of asphyxiated infants is essential. All infants with asphyxia should be referred to an intensive care unit for resuscitation almost immediately after birth as there is no way of determining at birth which infants will recover fully and which will develop cerebral palsy. In the prevention of cerebral palsy, the prevention of neonatal asphyxia with cerebral hypoxia is the ideal to be aimed at (see p. 378 for the aims of antenatal care).

McManus et al.[2] found that 7 % of cases of cerebral palsy were postnatal in origin, due especially to encephalitis and trauma. A study done by Arens et al.[3] found that poor socio-economic conditions play a role in the aetiology of acquired cerebral palsy.

Secondary prevention of cerebral palsy

A large number of motor and sensory functions are affected in the cerebral palsied child. It is important in secondary prevention that the condition be identified in infancy, so that early physiotherapeutic intervention can be undertaken to strengthen and educate the balance reflexes, to normalise muscle tone and to enable the child to experience kinaesthetic feedback from the movement of muscles.

Early detection is facilitated by:
- History of gestational and perinatal risk factors.
- Abnormal movements and postures.

Diagnosis can be made soon after birth if at-risk infants are referred to Assessment and Treatment Clinics, of which there are a number on the Witwatersrand and in Cape Town and at schools for the cerebral palsied.

Habilitation of the cerebral palsied child

Physiotherapy uses specialised neuro-developmental techniques (e.g. those of Doman-Delacato). These techniques have a neurophysiological basis, i.e. they aim to give the child more normal sensori-motor experiences than his damaged brain would naturally afford him. Treatment must start from the age of 5 months or even earlier, before the infant has experienced abnormal patterns and developed contractures. The results will depend on the extent of the brain damage (including mental retardation) and the time when therapy is commenced, as well as the co-operation and motivation of parent and child.

The SA Neurodevelopmental Therapy Association was established in 1976. Members are speech, occupational and physiotherapists. Courses in the Doman-Delacato technique are run annually under the aegis of this Association for speech, occupational and physiotherapists who work with cerebral palsied children.

The aim of treatment is to improve the functioning of the cerebral palsied child. Even mildly affected cerebral palsied children can benefit from therapy to help improve the motor skills (handwriting, sports). Disabilities in these areas become more obvious as the non-treated child gets older.

Severely handicapped children with spastic quadriplegia can be improved by physiotherapeutic techniques which improve posture to help the child sit propped up. Improved posture helps with basic nursing care and with the prevention of scoliosis, dislocated hips, contractures and painful joints. All cerebral palsied children should be supervised by a neurodevelopmental assessment and therapy clinic.

It is also important to teach the infant correct feeding methods with a special NUK teat; the spastic infant is held forward with limbs and neck flexed and is made to suck his feed, instead of having it poured into the mouth while flopping backwards in the typical extended cerebral palsy posture. The establishment of correct feeding routines is important not only to ensure good nutrition but also to lay the foundations for speech. Early training of muscles and feeding methods always involve the mother who is encouraged and supported to accept the child. Although the mother is involved in the child's therapy, she must never replace the therapists; her main task remains that of the mother of normal children — the establishment of a focused (bonded) mother–child relationship.

At a later date, therapy needed may not only be conservative but also surgical, e.g. lengthening of tendons to relieve a crippling deformity. Special education, in which the remedial teacher plays an important role, is necessary in special schools for cerebral palsied children and physio-, speech and occupational therapy are continued, the child being the focus of a multidisciplinary team.

In the habilitation of the cerebral palsied person, the goals of therapy and education are to promote competence in functional activities which are needed to carry out self-care — dressing, feeding and walking. Schooling is geared to provide the child with education which is realistic and will prepare him for vocational self-sufficiency and to play his part in society to the best of his ability.

At present (1990) there are forty-three special schools for cerebral palsied children of all races, throughout the country.

These schools are really treatment and education centres. Medical and paramedical services are recognised as part of the school curriculum. All the special facilities for educating and training the CP child and for meeting his special needs are available, e.g. medical supervision and corrective surgery (done at provincial hospitals by panel doctors who visit the school), physiotherapy, speech therapy, occupational therapy and academic education by teachers with special skills. These schools have a strong medical bent. The cerebral palsied (CP) child is accepted for enrolment for special therapy from the age of 3 months, and his parents are trained to do ancillary treatment at home to promote his development.

In cerebral palsy schools, children are often assessed and treated by psychologists and families are given guidance in the handling of their children. Most CP schools have hostels to cater for children from outlying areas.

Although some cerebral palsied children improve sufficiently to go to ordinary schools and later compete in the open labour market, many require sheltered employment in adulthood. Special facilities are available, e.g. Forest Farm in Johannesburg. Psychological adjustment may be poor and depends very much upon the degree of competence attained and the extent to which the child feels accepted by his family and the wider community.

Note: The incidence of cerebral palsy is decreasing due to improvements in obstetric care.

STATE PRESIDENT'S MESSAGE TO THE NCPD OF SOUTH AFRICA

The State President declared 1986 as the 'Year of Disabled People' in the RSA.

Below is an extract from the State President's message to the National Council for the Physically Disabled (NCPD) of South Africa, of which he is the Patron-in-Chief.

(From the *Jubilee Report* of the NCPD of SA, 1989)

'Research undertaken during that time brought to the fore the alarming fact that 16,3 out of every 1 000 people of the population are physically disabled. Based on the 1985 Census it represents 450 000 people. Out of this massive total only some 10 000 people, excluding those cared for in hospitals, are supported from state funds in their difficult day to day existence. . . . It is a fact that South Africa has only 2 spinal units — at the H F Verwoerd Hospital in Pretoria and at the Conradie Hospital in Cape Town — each of which has to deal with between 400 and 500 patients per annum.'

The State President goes on to say that the following principles for the care of disabled have been accepted (by the government):

(1) the creation of a physical and social environment within which each could develop to his full potential;

(2) less institutionalisation and more positive community involvement so that the disabled can live his or her life to the full.

WELFARE ORGANISATIONS FOR THE PHYSICALLY DISABLED

Welfare organisations play an important role in making state help available to the disabled and in extending this kind of help in areas not covered by state help. The associations for the physically disabled help the disabled not only to obtain maximal material help from the state — the Council (for care of disabled) always negotiating with the authorities for better disability pensions — but also through rehabilitation, to earn as much as possible on the labour market, either open or sheltered.

A welfare organisation means a non-government organisation registered under section 13 of the National Welfare Act 100 of 1978.

THE NATIONAL COUNCIL FOR THE PHYSICALLY DISABLED IN SOUTH AFRICA (NCPD)

(Henceforth referred to as the 'Council'.)

The Council is the central co-ordinating body of a large number of autonomous regional bodies (Associations for the Physically Disabled or Cripple Care Societies) which work in defined areas in the RSA providing direct services to disabled individuals of all races and all ages. Some bodies are affiliated to the regional associations, e.g. Avalon Association, St Giles Association, Happiness for the Handicapped Organisation, Cheshire Homes. These affiliated bodies are autonomous, but their social workers are subsidised by the Department of Health and they exchange information with the NCPD.

A National Cerebral Palsy Division comes within the framework of the Council. The Council liaises with state, provincial and local authorities.

The Patron-in-Chief of the Council is the State President and amongst its officers are many prominent doctors who may be special members of the Council. The ordinary members of the Council are representatives of the regional associations for the physically disabled. Special members have special qualifications and representative members are appointed by various state departments, the Compensation Commissioner, the provincial administrations and municipal associations and all nationally organised bodies interested in the care of the disabled.

The work of the Council is carried out by a director and an executive committee. The Council is affiliated to Rehabilitation International New York.

Apart from co-ordinating and funding the work of the regional societies, the Council is concerned with research into physical disablement and the preventive aspects of physical disablement and disability. Example: the Council's Scoliosis Committee persuaded several centres to extend school screening programmes for early detection of scoliosis.

The Council brings 'facts' about physically disabled persons to the notice of authorities, in this way influencing legislation pertaining to improved conditions for the disabled.

Example: To give the physically disabled greater freedom of movement in the community, especially those in wheelchairs, the Council persuaded the authorities to make *national building regulations* which will specify the provision to be made for the physically handicapped in all buildings used by the public to eliminate architectural barriers, thus making it possible for the handicapped to enter buildings and use public toilets. Some public buildings are already bearing the sign (figure 43.1) which indicates 'accessibility of building'. It is important that the public be educated to the extent that they are aware of the need to have a 'barrier-free' city, especially for its paraplegic citizens.

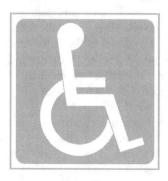

Figure 43.1
International symbol of accessibility of building

The international symbol of access for the handicapped can be displayed if the building has:

(1) an entrance with a ramp;
(2) doorways and entrances at least 80 cm wide;
(3) toilet facilities accessible to wheelchair users with room to turn around inside;
(4) lifts wide enough to admit a wheelchair.

Education of workers is an important task of the Council, as trained personnel are essential for the specialised work done with the disabled. Examples:

(1) Recently a symposium for physically disabled care social workers was held in the RSA as part of in-service training.
(2) The Council has bursary and scholarship schemes for workers, i.e. social workers, physio-, and occupational and speech therapists and orthopaedic technicians, as well as for black orthopaedic nurses who have no orthopaedic training school in their area.

Although the salaries of social workers and orthopaedic nurses in 'approved' posts are paid by state health and provincial hospitals, the Council pays the salaries of a large number of workers in unsubsidised posts. For example, the Council supplies social workers for cerebral palsy schools which have no approved posts for social workers. Social workers work with the families of the CP child.

The funding of voluntary physically disabled care work is done by fund-raising campaigns launched by regional associations for the physically disabled. Most of the funds come from the Easter Stamp Fund campaigns conducted by the regional societies every year.

The *regional associations for the physically disabled* give direct services to the physically disabled.

(1) Detection and discovery of physically disabled, especially in rural areas where medical services may be poor. Early referral to medical rehabilitation centres is an important secondary preventive measure.
(2) Meeting the needs of physically disabled with regard to:
    (a) Treatment and nursing care. Care given varies from region to region, e.g. amongst the rural Zulu, patients are put into POP after surgery at the urban centres, and sent home. They then go to the clinics for check-ups. Associations for physically disabled employ social workers and orthopaedic domiciliary nurses to visit physically disabled out-patients in their homes. These workers ensure that the patient gets to the clinic and they also make arrangements for transport and for accommodation if necessary. Social workers investigate and handle family problems and apply for disability pensions. Social workers also help the physically disabled cope with the great frustration which his/her dependence creates.
    (b) Training and education.
    (c) Accommodation and transport. Transport is provided to get children to school. Transport is also needed to get adults to and from work. Physically disabled care transport is often sponsored by motor companies. Accommodation may be a problem if a disabled person is placed in employment away from his family. Hostel accommodation for adult disabled persons is a physically disabled care priority. There are several homes for crippled children.
    (d) Employment for the severely handicapped in protective workshops (training centres). These workshops, of which there were 18 in the RSA in 1988, are subsidised by the Department of Health and are run by Physically Disabled Cripple Care.
    (e) Material aid in the form of loans and grants must often be given to the disabled who do not qualify for aid from the state to help them function in the community; some may need cars specially adapted to their disability, while others may need a wheelchair to move about independently or semi-independently outside the home. Physically disabled care social workers help clients of all races who qualify for state aid with their applications for permanent wheelchairs.

Social workers employed by Associations for the Physically Disabled do community work, particularly public education, by giving talks to professional groups and women's organisations.

Beyond subsistence

One of the aims of physically disabled care (cripple care) is to create a better and wider awareness of the physical, emotional and social needs of disabled persons. Within the physically disabled care voluntary organisation, there has been a growing awareness of these needs and an acceptance of the principle of employing disabled workers as members of staff of physically disabled care agencies at all levels, e.g. even as speech therapists, and to bring disabled people on to committees.

There has been a world-wide tendency to integrate the disabled into the life of the community and to help them lead useful, satisfying lives.

Sport and recreation are necessary activities for the full rehabilitation of the physically disabled person. The South African Sports Association for the Physically Disabled has been established to meet the need for organised sport for the physically disabled. The association is an independent sports body run by voluntary members; it has a national council and executive, regional councils and local sports clubs. It is a member of, *inter alia*, the SA Sports Federation for Youth and Sport, the SA National and International Olympic Games Association and the International Stoke Mandeville Games Federation (for polio victims and traumatic tetraplegics and paraplegics) and other sporting bodies to cater for the different groups of physical disabilities.

Members compete in a large number of games according to their medically determined class and group, both nationally and internationally.

REFERENCES

(1) Molteno CD, Arens LJ, Marshall SR, Robertson WI. Cerebral palsy in Cape Town. *S Afr Med J* 1980; **57**: 823.

(2) McManus P, *et al. Obstet & Gynec* 1977; **50**: 71.

(3) Arens L J , *et al. S Afr Med J* 1978; **53**: 319.

The author acknowledges with gratitude the help of the National Council of the Physically Disabled of South Africa and its National Cerebral Palsy Division through information obtained from their journals, *Towards Independence* and *SA Cerebral Palsy Journal.*

TEST OF KNOWLEDGE

The student has benefited from studying this chapter if he/she can answer the following questions:

(1) (*a*) Discuss the causes of cerebral palsy and the role of the nurse in preventing this condition.

    (*b*) How can the young cerebral palsied child be habilitated?

(2) (*a*) Name the functions of the NCPD of SA.

    (*b*) What services are rendered to the physically disabled by the regional associations of the NCPD of SA?

(3) (*a*) What are the architectural conditions for displaying the international symbol of access on a building?

    (*b*) Why is the symbol important for the physically handicapped person?

(4) State how you would teach a traumatic paraplegic patient to:

    (*a*) gain control of micturition;

    (*b*) prevent pressure sores over the buttocks.

(5) Define the following terms:

    – welfare organisation (NGO)

    – cerebral palsy

    – diplegia

    – tetraplegia

    – choreo-athetoid movements

    – kernicterus

    – Doman-Delacato technique

    – protective workshop

44

State Aid to Disabled Persons
Rehabilitation of Handicapped Persons

INTRODUCTION

In South Africa, 1986 was declared the year of disabled people by the government. By this declaration South Africa participated in the Decade of Disabled People (1983–1992) proclaimed world-wide by the United Nations Organisation.

Excerpt from the UN *Declaration of the Rights of Disabled Persons*:

'Disabled persons have:

(1) the same civil and political rights and the same right to respect for human dignity as other human beings;
(2) the right to medical and other services which will enable them to develop their capabilities and hasten their social integration;
(3) the right to obtain and retain employment and to become as self-reliant as possible;
(4) the right to live with their families, or to living conditions as close as possible to normal.

(5) Disabled people shall be protected against treatment of a discriminatory, abusive or degrading nature.'

To these rights the underdeveloped people, amongst whom the majority of disabled people are found, would add: 'The right to develop' (see p. 775).

The philosophy underlying the care of the disabled is that every impaired person has the right to independence and that it is in the economic interest of a country to ensure that its handicapped citizens attain as high a level of self-sufficiency as possible. 'The meaningfulness of a person's life is largely determined by the measures by which that person deploys his/her talents in society, particularly in a work situation. In the case of a handicapped person research indicates that meaningful employment is a cardinal factor determining both quality of life and rehabilitation.'[1]

IN THIS CHAPTER

INVESTIGATION OF DISABILITY IN THE RSA[1]

The Department of National Health and Population Development and the Human Sciences Research Council (HSRC) investigated all aspects of the care of disabled people in a joint research project which lasted two years. Their report was published in 1987 for consideration by the Cabinet.

Important findings of the investigation:

(1) Approximately 3,5 million, 12,7 % of the population of South Africa, are handicapped (physically, mentally and/or sensorily). In 1994 it was estimated that South Africa has 5 million disabled persons.

(2) The state spent R942,7 million on the care of disabled people in the financial year 1985/1986. The total expenditure, public and private sector, is estimated at R3 000 million.

(3) There is a serious lack of co-ordination amongst the services for the care of disabled people.

(4) The database for care is inadequate in many respects.

(5) The services are limited mainly to metropolitan areas and are largely inaccessible to disabled people in rural areas.

(6) The development of an 'own industry' as part of the 'disabled care armamentarium' is badly needed.

Recommendations of the researchers:

(1) A comprehensive national policy on care of the disabled.

(2) A structure, viz. an intersectoral council for care of the disabled, for the co-ordination of all care activities in South Africa.

(3) The establishment of one-stop assessment units for every development region where disabled people in need of care can be reported.

(4) A multiprofessional and multidisciplinary approach to the prevention of disability and the treatment, the development and the care of disabled people.

(5) Important recommendations were also made with regard to housing, transport, accessibility and legislation to alleviate the problems and needs of disabled persons.

World statistics on disablement[8]

There are 500 million disabled people in the world; of these, only about 2 % have had any formal education. Therefore, the majority of disabled people are uneducated and underdeveloped.

DEFINITIONS

▪ *Impairment* is any loss or abnormality of psychological, physiological or anatomical structure or function.

▪ *Disability* is any restriction or lack of ability (due to an impairment) to perform an activity in the manner considered normal for a human being.

▪ *Disabled person* is any person who has attained the age of 16 years and is, owing to his physical or mental disability, unfit to obtain from any service, employment or profession, the means needed to enable him to provide for his maintenance. A disabled person is one who has not been rehabilitated or is unrehabilitable and is, therefore, entitled to a disability pension.

■ *Handicap* is the social and environmental consequence of impairments and disabilities. It is an individualised disadvantage that limits or prevents the fulfilment of a role that should be achievable.

STATE AID TO DISABLED PERSONS

Departments of Health Services (provincial) run protective workshops (training centres), e.g. Forest Farm, for adults who are not employable in the open labour market or in Training and Work Centres (sheltered employment factories) of the Department of Manpower (Labour). These training centres are sponsored by various welfare organisations (NGOs).

The state helps with the maintenance of 'disabled persons' by giving social aid, i.e. social pensions and grants.

Social assistance by the state had been covered by a large number of Acts which individually provided for the needy: e.g. Aged Persons, War Veterans' Pensions, Blind Persons, Disability Grants, Abuse of Dependent-producing Substances and Rehabilitation Centres, Mental Health, Social Pensions, National Welfare, Child Care, Pension Laws Amendment, Community Welfare and Social Aid Acts. The social assistance sections of these Acts have been repealed and concentrated in one Act — the Social Assistance Act (59/1992) — one which covers all government social assistance — to individuals as well as to NGOs. All population groups will get the same social allowances; the maximum amount for old age, disability and parent grants will be R 390 per month (1994).

The Social Assistance Act 59 of 1992

(See p. 429.)

This act provides for social assistance by the state to aged and disadvantaged persons and to National Councils and Welfare organisations (NGOs) which render organised activities and social welfare programmes regarding:

(*a*) (i) family care;
(ii) care of the aged;
(iii) social security;
(iv) care of the disabled;
(v) alcohol and drug dependency;
(vi) care of the offender.

(*b*) Any organisation which has the care of mentality or psychiatrically disabled persons as one of its objects.

The following conditions obtain for the granting of a disability pension:

(1) The physical or mental disability is permanent.

(2) No one is entitled to a disability pension if he is, *inter alia*,
(*a*) legally required to attend a school;
(*b*) a person to whom an allowance is paid in terms of the Child Care Act;
(*c*) refuses to subject himself to medical examination or treatment;
(*d*) refuses to be registered with the Bureau of Labour should he be requested to do so;
(*e*) refuses to accept employment which is within his capacity.

Implicit in the granting of a disability pension is that provision be made for the **rehabilitation** of the assisted person, so that he may qualify for entry into the labour market, either open or sheltered. State welfare relief therefore incorporates both material relief and rehabilitation of the disabled person.

Note: As the disability pension is a social pension it is subject to residential qualifications and the means test as for all social pensions.

An attendant's allowance can be granted to the physically disabled person who requires the continual care of another person.

No social pension or allowance is payable to a person who is maintained by the state in an institution, prison or treatment centre (see p. 755).

Medical care is provided gratis by state health (by district surgeons and nurses) for persons eligible for a disability pension — as for all social pensioners.

Maintenance grants can be obtained for disabled persons with children and a *single care grant* for disabled children under the age of 16 years, in terms of the Child Care Act.

The Department of Manpower (Labour) is involved in:

(1) The prevention of disabilities by the Occupational Health and Safety Act (85/1993).
(2) Support of the occupationally disabled person: Compensation for Occupational Injuries and Diseases Act (130/1993) and the Unemployment Insurance Act.
(3) The training of disabled people through the Manpower Training Act of 1981, National Readjustment Committee and Vocational Board.
(4) The guidance and placement in employment of handicapped work seekers: Guidance and Placement Act 62 of 1981.

Guidance and placement centres

The Department of Manpower (Labour) plays a very important role in the rehabilitation of the unemployed in the RSA, including the employment of disabled people, through its Special Job Creation and Training Programme. The Guidance and Placement Act 62 of 1981 requires the Department to establish guidance and placement centres where:

(1) persons may receive vocational guidance;
(2) a register of work seekers is kept;
(3) work seekers are placed in jobs. Work seekers must be above the age of 15 years.

Disabled people, including ex-prisoners and rehabilitated alcoholics, also qualify. At present there are 36 centres with job placement services and at 22 of these the services of vocational counsellors are available for the assessment of the potential of the work seekers and for counselling. (For location, addresses and telephone numbers of these centres, see the back page of every copy of *Rehabilitation in SA*.)

Assessment is done by:

(1) the interview;
(2) aptitude and personality testing and an interest questionnaire;
(3) a medical report, social worker's report and school record may also be required.

The special job creation and training programme[1]

Launched in 1985 for unemployed persons, it offers training with extra skills to facilitate entry into the labour market. The programme employs 372 training contractors to train its registered workers in approved courses. The service is available to all work seekers who may legally seek employment in the RSA, including the handicapped who do not require special attention or the use of special apparatus. Finding jobs for handicapped people often proves very difficult, as there is no labour market for the handicapped — it must be created. The responsibility rests with the handicapped person himself to prove that he can be used. The employer expects the handicapped work seeker to offer work skills, a positive outlook on life and that his salary expectations should be realistic.

The Department of Manpower (Labour) also runs programmes for training severely handicapped persons who may require transport, medical and paramedical services, mobility, communication and special equipment. These handicapped persons are usually the victims of accidents. Training takes from 3–48 weeks and is contracted out to private training centres. At present (1985) 6 centres are involved in the scheme, 4 in Port Elizabeth, 1 in Randburg and 1 in Durban. The following courses are offered: secretarial skills and business administration, technical skills such as computer programming, sewing, knitting, carpentry, toy making.

Inducements to employ handicapped persons

The Department of Manpower (Labour) attempts by various means to persuade employers to employ handicapped workers.

(1) *By appealing to their humanity and compassion*. The handicapped deserve employment because 'they are reliable and responsible people; their rate of absenteeism is low; with the correct aids many handicapped can attain full production and when selectively placed, the handicapped worker can hold his own in the labour market' (p. 72).[3] Over a thousand handicapped workers are selectively placed in jobs annually in the open labour market.
(2) *By the Wage Subsidy Scheme for Handicapped Work Seekers*.[3] Unrehabilitated alcoholics, drug dependants and 'work-shy' people do not qualify for subsidised labour.

Subsidies are paid for 3 years only: the government contributes 80 % of the real wage of the handicapped employee for the first 12 months of uninterrupted service with the same employer, decreasing to 60 % and 40 % in the second and third years. There are conditions to this 3-year period of subsidisation.

(3) *By competition for the Amtronix Recognition Award.*[4] NOSA (National Occupational Safety Association), in conjunction with the firm Amtronix, sponsor regional competitions for the handsome Amtronix floating trophy, for firms employing handicapped persons as part of their labour force. The firms must also run NOSA-safety programmes so adapted to accommodate handicapped employees.

Bursaries

(1) The Development Fund for Disabled People. The objective of this fund is to provide bursaries to deserving handicapped people for training purposes and to fund assistive devices essential for training and employment. Applications are invited from members of the seven member organisations of the SA Federal Council for Rehabilitation of Disabled People.

A Board of Trustees of the Development Fund meets once a year to consider applications and distribute the funds.

(2) Study bursaries for higher education of the Department of Manpower (Labour).[1, 2] Large sums of money are voted for this purpose every year. The bursaries are administered by the Readjustment Committee and Vocational Board. The purpose of the bursary is to enhance the placement possibilities of handicapped persons. Tertiary study at a university, technikon or technical college must, therefore, be vocationally directed.

Conditions for the granting of a bursary:

(a) Applicants must be disabled and not have the necessary funds for further study.

(b) Applicants must have the potential for higher education and have a good academic school record.

(c) They must be older than 16 years, be South African citizens and live in South Africa.

(d) Applicants are subjected to psychometric testing and interviewing.

Placement in Training and Work Centres

(Formerly called 'sheltered employment factories'.)

Handicapped workers who cannot be placed in the open labour market are considered for placement in a training and work centre, of which there are thirteen in the RSA. The state finances the centre by subsidising working losses.

Handicapped work seekers are interviewed by a placement committee and those considered able to meet the demands of the work are accepted. At present there are waiting lists at most of the centres.[5]

Note: Seriously disabled persons are placed in protective workshops which are run by Cripple Care associations subsidised by the Department of Health Services. Seriously disabled persons are referred for a disability pension by the placement committee (see p. 771.)

Training and work centres (Service Products) are run by the Department of Manpower (Labour) through Management Committees and managers. Country-wide these centres employ over 2 000 handicapped persons.

Type of worker: Apart from the physically disabled, training and work centres accept schizophrenics, dry alcoholics and youngsters over the age of 16 from special schools (retarded). Once in employment they lose their disability pension, if they had one. They are taken on trial for 3 months and earn R117–R152 per week (1988).[5] Light meals are subsidised and they live independently in hostels or at home. They work 40 hours per week, 5 days per week. They are entitled to sick leave and holidays.

Type of work: They do contract work for state departments, making garments, hospital linen, greatcoats for the Army, knitted, leather and canvas goods; bind books and make tubular steel furniture. Their woodwork includes desks and bookshelves. Artisans are employed to teach and supervise the work. Work is assessed every year and those with great output are rewarded.

Medical, first aid and psychiatric services are available in the factory and a community nurse supervises the taking of medication.

Reasons for discharge:

(1) Progress to a job in the open labour market. This is encouraged and assistance is given. They can be re-employed in the work centre within 3 months if the venture into the open market is unsuccessful.

(2) Old age which entitles them to an old age pension.

(3) Unsuitability for the work required. If they are unable to be productive, the disability pension can be reinstituted. However, if they have given of their best, they will retain employment at the centre.

(4) Intractable alcoholic. A disability pension will not be given; sheltered employment is the state's last attempt to rehabilitate the alcoholic outside rehabilitation centres.

REHABILITATION OF HANDICAPPED PERSONS

Rehabilitation is an important aspect of tertiary intervention. Rehabilitation can be defined as the restoration of the ability to function in a normal or near-normal way, following disease or injury, i.e. the management of disability. The more comprehensive WHO definition reads as follows:[6]

'The combined and co-ordinated use of medical, social, educational and vocational measures for training or retraining the individual to the highest possible level of functional ability.'

Rehabilitation aims at training a disabled person to make the best use of his remaining capacities to earn a living, to care for his own body, to participate in social relationships and to enjoy pleasurable activities.

Habilitation requires similar training in functioning, but in this case there has been no loss of function, only an absence of function due to early injury or congenital anomalies, e.g. cerebral palsy, deafness. For the purpose of this chapter, no distinction will be made between rehabilitation and habilitation, which is called 'preventive rehabilitation' by some authorities. The aims of preventive rehabilitation are early detection of incapacity and preventing its development.

The first South African Rehabilitation Council

This council was established in 1955, with the following functions:

(1) to formulate a uniform national rehabilitation policy;

(2) to advise the Minister of Labour on the usefulness of certain rehabilitation services;

(3) to initiate the creation of certain rehabilitation services which involve a number of national bodies and government departments, e.g. Access College in Gauteng — a commercial tertiary education college which runs business and computer classes;

(4) to distribute information on rehabilitation (this gave rise to the publication of the journal, *Rehabilitation in SA*);

(5) to review all aspects of vocational guidance and retraining pertaining to placement in the open labour market and sheltered employment and to encourage follow-up services;

(6) to endeavour to establish legislation to promote the interests of all disabled people and to accomplish better co-ordination of existing legislation.[2]

The aim of the journal *Rehabilitation in SA* has been:

(1) to disseminate information concerning rehabilitation;

(2) to illustrate the integration of the disabled as a source of manpower;

(3) to remove prejudice against the disabled;

(4) to promote the employment of the disabled.[2]

Aid to the handicapped by welfare organisations (NGOs)

Welfare organisations have attempted to co-ordinate their activities by forming the South African Federal Council for Rehabilitation of Disabled People. The Federal Council is comprised of the following member organisations:

■ SA National Council for Mental Health, PO Box 2587, Johannesburg, 2000;

■ SA National Council for the Blind, PO Box 11149, Brooklyn, Pretoria, 0011;

- SA National Council for the Deaf, Private Bag X04, Westhoven, Johannesburg, 2142;
- National Council of Physically Disabled in SA, PO Box 10173, Johannesburg, 2000;
- SA National Tuberculosis Association, PO Box 10501, Johannesburg, 2000;
- SA National Epilepsy League, PO Box 200, Springs, 1560;
- Disabled People South Africa (DPSA), PO Box 39492, Booysens, 2016.

MAIN REHABILITATION MOVEMENTS

The student will notice two different value bases, used by society and accepted by handicapped persons, underlying the rehabilitation of the physically and visually disabled. These value bases give rise to two ways in which rehabilitation services are rendered to persons with these disabilities.

The Western Rehabilitation Movement is based on a 'medical' model. It came into prominence during World War II with the awareness of the medical profession that treated, but still maimed, war casualties had to recover confidence when resuming vocational and social life. Rehabilitation requires the help of a team of paramedical professionals, headed by a medical doctor. In this frame of reference the disabled person is seen as a patient who plays the 'sick role'. The patient is dependent on his caretakers and looks to them for help in adjusting to society. The care-taking team decides on his treatment, his work potential and the state helps to look after him, e.g. guides and places him in employment and, if necessary, subsidises his work and creates work opportunities. Inherent in the 'sick role' are the following exemptions and obligations: normal activities and responsibilities are not expected from the patient, nor is he expected to take responsibility for his 'sickness'. He is not expected to cope with life through his own efforts, but is expected to seek help and to co-operate with the care-taking team in improving his situation. The 'patient' in this frame of reference can put the blame for his problem on his disability. This model is inclined to foster dependency. The state and society generally accept the Western rehabilitation movement and have created an extensive infrastructure to implement its principles. This model

needs extensive funding which can be afforded only by developed countries.

The self-help independent living movement (ILM) started in South Africa in 1979[7] and is developing rapidly. It is proving to be a strong force in the rehabilitation of persons with physical disabilities and is based on the need felt by underdeveloped people for the **'right to develop'**. 'The purpose of self-help organisations is the empowerment of their members through a process of development.' (Rowland)[8] Empowerment means that the socially and vocationally powerless, handicapped person is enabled to take control of his own life with the help of professional development workers.

The self-help independent living movement (ILM)

This modern approach to physical disability is away from the focus on the physical limitations of the disabled; it espouses the idea that both society and the disabled must make adjustments for the benefit of both.

The underlying value base of the Independent Living Movement (ILM) has the following components:

(1) The location of problems experienced by the physically disabled person lies largely within his physical and social environment. Social prejudices against disabled persons cause inadequate supporting services as well as economic and architectural barriers, e.g. inaccessibility of buildings to wheelchairs. The disabled person is thus handicapped because he is discriminated against as an 'impaired' citizen. Consequently he is not given the social and physical amenities given to 'normal' citizens.

(2) The physically disabled person does not want to be relieved of familial, occupational or civic responsibilities in exchange for a child-like dependence. He wants the right to participate in the life of the community as consumer, policy-maker and planner in order to change society's attitudes and the physical environment.

(3) The management of medically stabilised, physically disabling conditions should be 'demedicalised'. The professional rehabilitation team and the disabled person should become partners; management of disabili-

ties should primarily be a personal matter, e.g. self-management of incontinence and prevention of pressure sores. The disabled person should be able to 'ask' for help where necessary and accept this help. In order to do this comfortably, good interpersonal relationships with non-disabled society is essential.[7]

Disabled people South Africa (DPSA)

A national coalition of self-help groups, 'Disabled People South Africa' (DPSA), has been formed and is a member of the SA Federal Council for the Rehabilitation of Disabled People.

This organisation, composed of disabled South Africans, irrespective of colour, age or culture, has as its objective, 'to work for equal opportunity and participation in the society in which all belong'.[7]

Self-help factories[9]

The ILM has given rise to the establishment of self-help factories which were started by blacks in Soweto. These factories are not subsidised by the government and give employment to disabled people outside the open labour market. It is helped by the private sector as it falls into the category of developing black business. The Self-Help Association of Paraplegics (Soweto) (**SHAP**) was launched in 1981 by 100 paraplegics who wanted a better future for themselves. They focus their efforts on self-employment in order to earn a decent living. They gradually built a factory (community sponsored) in Soweto by doing work on a subcontract basis for industry. Fund raising by the private sector is necessary for the purchase of capital items such as equipment, vehicles and building extensions. SHAP in 1989 housed 130 employees. The self-help factory aims to be economically viable and to pay viable wages. Although it is unlikely that a self-help factory could compete with other factories, its performance should not fall below 75 %. The idea of self-help factories has spread amongst blacks. The DPSA hopes to expand to other townships and to black rural areas. SHAP differs from the Department of

Manpower's sheltered employment factories (training and work centres) (see p. 773) in that:

(1) they are run by the disabled people themselves with all staff responsible to an executive committee of disabled people;

(2) the disabled workers are capable of economic production.

REFERENCES

(1) Fourie JD. Address by the Director-General of Manpower. *Rehabilitation in SA* 1989; **33**: 83–85.

(2) Editorial. *Rehabilitation in SA* 1987; **31**: 1.

(3) Dillman H. Die indiensplasing van gestremdes deur die Departement van Mannekrag. *Rehabilitation in SA* 1989; **33**: 72–76.

(4) Editorial. The Amtronix Award. *Rehabilitation in SA* 1989; **33**: 53.

(5) Editorial. Training and Work Centres for the Disabled. *Rehabilitation in SA* 1988; **32**: 7.

(6) World Health Organisation. *Technical Report Series No. 419*. WHO, Geneva, 1969.

(7) Hoffman W. Practice paradigms in service delivery to persons with disabilities. *Rehabilitation in SA 1986;* **30**: 26–29.

(8) Rowland W. CBR and/or empowerment. *Imfama* 1989; **29**: 7–9.

(9) Du Toit M. An indigenous response to the unique circumstances of black disabled people in South Africa. *Rehabilitation in SA* 1989; **33**; 86–90.

TEST OF KNOWLEDGE

The student has benefited from studying this chapter if he/she can answer the following questions.

(1) (*a*) What are the characteristics of the 'sick role' often ascribed to the physically disabled patient?

(*b*) What is meant by the Independence Living Movement (ILM) in rehabilitation?

(*c*) How does the basic philosophy underlying the ILM differ from that of the Western Rehabilitation Movement?

(*d*) What is the relationship between SHAP and the DPSA?

(2) Discuss the 'rights' of disabled people, especially in the context of the 'Independent

Living Movement' recently started by underdeveloped people.

(3) (a) Define 'disabled person'.

(b) Under what conditions is a Disability Pension likely to be granted?

(4) (a) What is a 'training and work centre' of the Department of Manpower (Labour)?

(b) What type of employee is likely to be accepted in such a centre?

(c) What are the reasons for discharge from such a centre?

(5) Discuss the Department of Labour's special Job Creation and Training Programme. How can a handicapped person benefit from this programme?

Part 7

A MISCELLANY OF SUBJECTS

45

Accident Prevention

INTRODUCTION

As famine and infectious diseases have responded to the advances of medicine and technology in First-World communities, the importance of trauma as a cause of death and disability has gained ascendancy.

The main causes of trauma are accidents, natural and man-made, and person-on-person violence.

Accidents are unintentional acts causing injury and damage.

Natural disastrous accidents, such as floods, fires and earthquakes, will not be discussed in this chapter.

Man-made accidents, the subject of this chapter, occur mainly through hazards in the home to which unprotected children are exposed, through dangerous modern machines in industry and through motor vehicle collisions. Although the accident may be unintentional, it is usually preventable and therefore accidents are an appropriate topic in community health.

The incidence of accidents in our modern, technologically advanced society is very high. According to the WHO, up to the age of 45 years accidents claim more victims than heart diseases, cancer or cerebro-vascular diseases — accidental death takes place more commonly than death due to sickness in people below the age of 46 years. Home accidents occur four and a half times more often than industrial and road accidents. The greatest toll in deaths and serious disablement occurs among young people in their twenties — reckless fiery youth who often throw safety precautions to the wind. Research has shown that the large majority of accidents are caused by human failure.

IN THIS CHAPTER

HOME ACCIDENTS

It is estimated that 10 000 children in the Cape Peninsula are injured each month, some lightly and others fatally.[1] Accidents can be considered a serious community health problem.

Accidents are also the main cause of death in childhood,[1] accounting for 47 % of deaths in the age group 5–14 years in blacks and coloureds and 1–14 years in whites. The age of greatest risk in all population groups is 1–5 years, the age at which children start exploring their environment but are not yet able to act responsibly and knowledgeably.

The possibilities for **home accidents** are legion. Hazards are inherent in electricity, gas, paraffin, fire, roofs and windows, doors and floors, toys and firearms and the swimming-pool. Every mother should know the first-aid treatment of home accidents. The community health nurse can do no better than to make sure every mother who attends her clinic knows the contents of a first aid book on Home Accidents.

Child Safety Centre

A Child Safety Centre was established at the Red Cross Hospital in Cape Town in 1978. This centre operates within the ambit of the Department of Paediatric Surgery. Its aims are to investigate the cause and to promote the prevention of accidents in children and to make adults aware of their responsibility for the safety of children. The Safety Centre has established an ongoing epidemiological survey of accidents to children with the aim of influencing lawmakers and producers of potentially hazardous equipment and substances to cause the environment to be less dangerous for children. The protection of young children against harming themselves is an important task of parents. More than 500 children drown each year in South Africa. It is important for children to be supervised by adults while swimming.

Poison Information Centre

There is a computerised Poison Information Centre at the Johannesburg Hospital which has gathered data in collaboration with the Poison Centre of the Red Cross Children's Hospital of Cape Town. This centre can be contacted for advice in all cases of poisoning, no matter what its nature or the age of its victim. (See Emergency Services, main Telephone Directories.)

Accidental burns

In a study on burns in children, done by De Wet et al.[2] in Cape Town, it was found that over-crowded living conditions, e.g. in squatter camps, and inadequate bathing and cooking facilities among the lower socio-economic groups are the main contributory factors to the precipitating causes of burns. Children were just not sufficiently protected against fires, hot water and cooking food. The exigencies of living made it impossible for parents to exert the necessary control and supervision to safeguard their children. Moreover, the struggle to survive and the heavy demands made on parents of large impoverished families are not conducive to a positive involvement of parents with their children. The usual recommendations made for safety in the home apply to middle-class homes and would be irrelevant in a shack, i.e. safety screens for stoves, the use of hot-water geysers, the use of closed stoves and separate rooms for different activities.

In these cases, therefore, accident preventive measures are aimed at the contributory causes rather than at the precipitating causes of burns, viz. better housing and smaller families through effective family planning, to prevent overcrowding and to help the mother be more effective in protecting her young children.

The South African Burn Society has made a great contribution towards the education of the public in the first-aid treatment of burns through the publication of its booklet, *First Aid in Thermal Injury* (1981) by Geoffrey Campbell, a plastic surgeon of the University of Natal.

First-aid treatment in burns is a very important secondary preventive measure; its principles are as follows:

(1) A burning person must be flung on the ground so that he will not inhale fumes. Any flames present (e.g. if clothes are on fire) are smothered with a blanket or by rolling the burn victim in nearby sand (if outside) until the flames are extinguished.

(2) Cooling by water. Iced water and ice-packs are ideal but cannot be used if the burns are large, in infants and small children, or in ill patients, as the sudden cooling of the body by ice is too shocking. As a general rule the whole person or a burnt limb is placed as soon as humanly possible in a bath of cool water. This cools down the burned tissues and prevents further thermal damage to healthy contiguous tissues. Cold also relieves pain. Cooling by water should not be practised for longer than 20 minutes.

(3) Analgesics for pain. Pain contributes to shock which inevitably follows burns. Medical aid must be sought as soon as possible; the doctor will prescribe a safe analgesic.

(4) Removal of burnt clothing. Burnt clothing must be removed while in the water and the patient or burnt limb gently dried and wrapped in a clean sheet on removal from the water. Articles of adherent clothing must under no circumstances be ripped off as this may damage tissues with a potential for healing. They are gently cut away.

(5) Chemical burns of skin and mucosa are rapidly irrigated with water. Acids and alkalis are neutralised with sodium bicarbonate (2 tablespoons to a litre of water) and vinegar, 50 % respectively, in order to halt the burning process. If the chemical has been ingested, the patient is made to drink as much water as possible. Campbell[3] states that vomiting in the first hour is of no consequence and may be beneficial. Later, in hospital (within 4 hours) and under general anaesthesia, endoscopy (oesophagoscopy and gastroscopy) will be carried out to assess the damage to the mucosa and to irrigate the oesophagus and stomach with saline or mild buffer solutions.

(6) The severely burnt person must be conveyed to a hospital as soon as first-aid treatment has been given and in less than 24 hours after the accident to avoid the occurrence of complications of oedema of limbs and mucous membranes during transportation over a long distance. If early transportation cannot be managed, burnt limbs should be elevated and the patient intubated by a doctor before embarking on the journey. A trained first-aider should accompany the patient to the hospital.[3]

MOTOR VEHICLE ACCIDENTS

Motor vehicles include the following: motor cars, motor cycles, taxis, buses, minibuses, motorised freight carriers.

If everyone were to drive responsibly, there would be very few motor vehicle accidents. Road traffic collisions are essentially preventable causes of trauma, i.e. the purely accidental nature of these catastrophes are questioned by many.

Brown[4] quotes the following figures for the RSA in 1971: killed — 8 400; seriously injured — 18 400; less seriously injured — 45 000. For every person killed, at least one is so badly injured that he will require continued nursing and other medical treatment for the rest of his life.

The 1980s started the era of the 'black taxis' in South Africa. Although a boon to urban communities, accidents have exacted a heavy toll in morbidity and mortality.

Epidemiology of MVAs

The following extracts were made from *Epidemiological Comments* **16** (3).[5]

In 1986, 9 343 persons were killed in road accidents, the number of vehicles involved being 622 522. Compared with the annual total in

Table 1
Trends of casualty, accident and death-rates
from 1976–1986 (11 years)

	A Casualties per 1 000 vehicles involved	B Casualties per 1 000 accidents	C Accidents per 1 000 vehicles registered	D Deaths per 1 000 casualties
1976	165	345	82	102
1977	167	354	69	85
1980	162	333	79	85
1981	157	324	87	88
1985	165	334	69	80
1986	180	361	68	83

Note: *Casualty (deaths or injuries) is not the same as accident (damage to a vehicle). The damage need not include passengers or pedestrians.*

the RSA of all deaths, MVAs accounted for 3,6 %.

In table 1 (above) both A and B rates have increased from 1976 to 1986. Between 1981 and 1986, B rose by about 3 % p.a.; D has dropped by about 2 % p.a. since 1976, but has remained fairly constant at 80–85 since 1977. B increased by about 2 % p.a. from 1981 to 1986. The authors[5] conclude that, though the accident rate (C) has decreased, probably due to various intervention strategies applied to prevent MVAs, the casualty/1 000 vehicles and casualty rate since 1977 is relatively constant. More casualties and a constant number of deaths are, therefore, arising from fewer accidents (see p. 787).

The following statistics for 1985 were supplied by the Central Statistical Service.[5]

- Vehicles (all types) involved in accidents: 619 559
- Accidents: 307 665
  Injured: 102 686
  Killed: 8 972

Percentage of MVA deaths by population group (1986):

- Asians 3 %
- Whites 18 %
- Coloureds 11 %
- Blacks 68 %

Deaths due to MVA per status of road-user (1986):

- Drivers of vehicles 20 %

- Cyclists 7 %
- Passengers 27 %
- Pedestrians 46 %

Percentage of pedestrian deaths by population groups (1986):

- Asians 2 %
- Whites 3 %
- Coloureds 15 %
- Blacks 80 %

It is estimated that the expenditure incurred as a result of MVAs in South Africa in 1986 was over 4 billion rands, almost the same as the total health budget of the public sector for the entire country.

Causes of injuries and fatalities

Causes of injuries and fatalities due to MVAs as stated by the National Road Safety Council are:[6]

(1) Reckless and negligent driving, the person behind the wheel overestimating his skill and judgement.
(2) Misuse of alcohol and stupefying drugs.
(3) Injudicious speed; bad road manners.
(4) Disregard for traffic signals and road signs. (The Accident Investigating Unit of the CSIR has found that 9 out of 10 accidents in urban areas are linked to violations of traffic regulations.)
(5) Following the vehicle in front too closely; this may give rise to chain reaction crashes.
(6) Driving cars that are not roadworthy.

Other factors which contribute to MVAs are:

- uncontrolled epileptics who may suddenly have seizures while driving;
- inattention of the driver due to sleepiness, overtiredness or preoccupation;
- incompetence of driver resulting from inadequate training or inadequate testing;
- reduced visibility due to darkness or inclement weather;
- jaywalking and children playing in the streets; and
- crossing the road at night, especially if the pedestrian is under the influence of alcohol or drugs.

Persons who are psychiatrically disturbed and have poor judgement, the aged with severe sensory losses and locomotor disability, as well as those with poor vision should not drive cars. It can be very difficult for the authorities to detect such persons until they become involved in accidents. It is incumbent upon family members, in consultation with the family doctor, to persuade disabled persons to give up driving for their own good and the good of society.

The bad-risk driver

When it became necessary in 1973 for the government to introduce fuel-saving measures, speed limits of 60 km/h were imposed in urban areas. This measure and traffic police surveillance caused a general improvement in traffic accidents. Whereas road accident head injuries had always carried a poor prognosis, both the severity and frequency of head injuries diminished during the first six months after imposition of speed restrictions. At the time this seemed to solve the problem of road safety. During 1975, however, the number of fatal car accidents again rose.

Excessive speed (speeding) is, however, generally considered to contribute greatly to the severity and frequency of road accidents, hence restrictive legislation.

The causes of fatal MVAs point to the importance of the personality of the driver as the main aetiological factor. The typical accident-prone individual who has a history of accidents may be impulsive and lacking in control. Accident proneness increases once the blood-alcohol concentration of the driver goes above the 0,05 % level. Cheetham[6] discusses the correlation between road safety and mental health and comes to the conclusion that emphasis must be placed on 'the personality type involved in repeated, serious traffic accidents or offences, with aggressive and antisocial attitudes, or influenced by alcohol and drug dependency, and a possible connection with organised crime'. He calls for regular examination of those involved in repeated accidents or offences and recommends 'medical treatment and suspension or cancellation of licences in specific instances'. In the RSA it is suspected that 10 % of drivers are responsible for 90 % of traffic accidents. Not until an accident register is kept will these drivers be traced and rendered harmless.

The *personality variables of the bad-risk driver* include: lack of responsibility, antisocial attitudes and poor control of aggression. These symptoms are pathognomic of the immature personality. In the age group 15 to 24 years, three-quarters of deaths are by violence, almost half this number being the result of road accidents in most Western countries.

Alcohol consumption is intimately related to road deaths. High blood-alcohol drivers who are problem drinkers are viewed by some authorities as either immoral or mentally sick, as deduced from the fact that they are not even deterred by severe legal sanctions such as fines, imprisonment or both. The law prohibits drivers from being on the roads while under the influence of either alcohol or drugs. In road accidents, a large number of drivers have a blood-alcohol concentration (BAC) of 0,05 % or higher, 0,05 % being the lowest concentration at which the brain is affected and driving problems arise, although the lowest level at which legal prosecutions may be instituted is 0,08 % (80 mg/dl).

The average person of average mass reaches the 0,08 % BAC after: 4 metric tots of spirit (25 ml each), *or* 5 cans of beer (standard size).

It is generally accepted that drivers in 50 % of serious road accidents have been affected by alcohol (Cheetham). The National Institute for Transport and Road Research (NITRR) found that alcohol was a contributory factor in 42 % of the driver and 53 % of the pedestrian accidents studied over a number of years in Pretoria, Durban and Cape Town.[7] Mr Justice Tebbutt states that alcohol is involved in 60 % of South African road deaths.[8]

Patients who attend casualty departments after an accident due to drunken driving often get off scot-free as casualty officers are not obliged to take medico-legal specimens of blood, and are hesitant to do so, as it may be viewed as a breach in the doctor-patient relationship.

Uken[12] describes the **current law-enforcement practices** as follows:

'A driver who has been drinking and who drives in a tell-tale manner, may be stopped by a traffic officer. Before a blood sample can be taken, the suspect will have to be taken to a police station where the traffic officer will have to convince the police constable that a test is really necessary. After a charge has been laid, the suspect has to be accompanied by the traffic officer and a policeman. They have to go to a district surgeon, or more recently since the amendment of the Criminal Procedure Act has been promulgated, to any recognised hospital where any medical officer or any registered nurse on his instruction, may take a blood sample — test cases in Pretoria have shown that this sequence of events cannot be concluded in less than three hours per case. The suspect, therefore, stands a good chance of sobering up before the blood test can be conducted.' (p. 16)

Some of the **recommended procedures** are:

(1) Evidential breath testers, e.g. the Breathalyser, which has been tested for accuracy according to SABS specifications, should be used. These screening devices are based on the chemical oxidation of exhaled alcohol in breath.

(2) It should be an offence to be driving with a BAC of 0,08 % as measured in breath.

(3) With the correct use of regularly calibrated evidential breath testers, the trained traffic officer can do the screening test more promptly than the doctor in the procedure detailed above.

(4) Provided social acceptance can be obtained, the pedestrian should also be subject to this sort of control on the public roads, the permissible BAC in this case being 0,15 %.

Cheetham[6] is of the opinion that harsher penalties are not likely to reduce the carnage on South African roads. 'More attention should be paid to education, public awareness, positive identification and the prevention of road accidents.'

Primary prevention of road accidents

(1) Deterrent legislation against driving while under the influence of alcohol and drugs. Convictions for drunken driving should also entail psychiatric assessment or treatment or both, especially if the misdemeanour is repetitive.

(2) Patients with severe psychiatric illness are unfit to drive a car and this should be brought to the attention of the authorities or of the family of the sick man.

(3) More school and family education of children in road manners is required to prevent pedestrian accidents involving children.

(4) More pedestrian education is necessary, especially education of blacks. They should be made aware that if they walk across a dark road at night they are poorly visible. The introduction of fluorescent clothing for night wear will be an advantageous innovation; motorists must have good, wide-spreading headlights in dark areas and speed must be reduced at night.

(5) There are many patients with physical disabilities who should not be allowed to drive a car, viz. patients with severe hypertension, alcoholics, uncontrolled epileptics, brittle diabetics who are prone to hypoglycaemic attacks, deaf people who are unaware of auditory danger signals from the environment and the rigid aged who lack judgement and insight.

(6) Full use should be made of the mass media to sell the idea of road courtesy; interschool teenage competitions can be, and have been, organised on SATV to make the future drivers of the country conscious of the principles of road safety.

(7) Better and safer cars should be built and roads made as safe as possible. Much is done in South Africa on an official level to combat road accidents. The Accident Investigating Unit of the NITRR (National Institute

for Transport and Road Research) investigates:

- the safety of cars;
- the safety of roads;
- violations of traffic regulations;
- qualifications for a licence.

(8) Employers should teach employees who have recently arrived in a city from the black rural areas about traffic rules and the traffic dangers for pedestrians.

(9) Intervention strategies aimed at reducing injuries and deaths should include compulsory breaks and maximum driving hours for long-distance haulage drivers, stringent training courses for all bus drivers, regular and compulsory inspection of buses for roadworthiness.

(10) Improvement in the driving standards of licensed drivers.

The observation that more casualties and a constant number of deaths are arising from fewer accidents suggests that more persons are at risk when an accident occurs, probably because of the increased use of buses and minibuses. The drivers of these vehicles take the responsibility for many more lives than an ordinary car driver. Their proper training and control are of the utmost importance.

The human factor is a major reason for South Africa's high death toll on the road. A poor standard of driving may be due to personality factors, alcohol consumption, or it may be due to inefficient driving. To be a good driver, good training is needed at a certified driving school which teaches correct procedures under all driving conditions, e.g. driving at night; driving in heavy rain. Some countries legislate for the compulsory attendance at driver training courses before a candidate may present himself for the driver's licence test. This is not applicable in South Africa, although the trend appears to be in this direction.

An **Institute of Driver Instructors (SAIDI)** was founded in 1977, under the aegis of the National Road Safety Council. Its aim is to improve the standard of driver training. The institute, when fully functioning, will unite on a professional level driving schools and driver instructors, and elevate the standard of training where necessary. This should promote road safety.

The National Road Safety Council (NRSC) — an advisory and public educating body — was abolished in 1992. The Director-General of Transport took over the functions of the NRSC.

The following are some of the aspects of road safety in urban areas, treated as priorities by the Director-General, on which he makes recommendations to the Minister of Transport:

(1) legislation and more effective law enforcement against drunk drivers and pedestrians;

(2) elimination of hazardous places and the promotion of better pedestrian facilities. Example: the use of 4-way stop streets at dangerous intersections.

Note: Members of the public are encouraged to bring hazardous places and other dangers to the attention of the Director-General of Transport.

Secondary prevention of the hazards of motor vehicle accidents

Secondary prevention aims at reducing or preventing the harmful effects of road accidents. Secondary preventive measures include first-aid treatment of casualties and the wearing of safety seat-belts, i.e. restraining devices for occupants of motor vehicles.

First-aid treatment at the site of the accident

Victims of accidents who die in the early stages invariably do so as a result of head injury. Other fatal injuries are rupture of the aorta and acute fracture-dislocation of cervical spine. For the salvaging of severely injured persons a good ambulance service with trained paramedics is essential. Over holiday periods the main roads are patrolled on ground and from the air; it is often possible to summons help during the crucial first hour.

In the care of the head-injured patient the provision of a good airway is essential in order to maintain adequate ventilation for oxygenation of the brain. External bleeding must be stemmed and hypovolaemia corrected (in the case of severe bleeding or the hypotension found in high cervical spinal injury). Unless ventilation and blood pressure can be artificially restored, the head- and neck-injured patient has little hope of surviving as a functioning human being.

Safety seat-belts to prevent head and neck injuries

There are several types of safety seat-belts:

(1) The harness type supports the whole upper part of the body; they are used in sport and racing cars.

(2) The lap belt fits only across the lap. It does not protect the wearer against injuries but is useful for restraining a padded carrier cot with a baby in it on the back seat.

(3) The combined shoulder and lap belt (three-point seat-belt). This is standard equipment in all cars.

The legal requirements with regard to **safety-belts** are:

(1) As from 1 December 1977, all occupants of the front seats of cars which were registered for the first time after 1 January 1965 will have to wear their seat-belts, which must comply with the specifications of the South African Bureau of Standards and bear the mark of the SABS.

(2) The legislation does not apply to light trucks or heavy vehicles, but only to motor cars which were registered after 1 January 1965.

(3) Anyone seated on the front seat of any vehicle described in (1), which is fitted with seat-belts and moving on a public road, must be properly belted up with the fitted seat-belt.

(4) The legislation does not apply to a vehicle driver who is reversing or parking his vehicle.

(5) Any person above the age of 13 who fails to comply with the regulations will be guilty of an offence.

(6) A vehicle driver who fails to ensure that a child under the age of 14 complies with the regulations will be guilty of an offence.

(7) Exemption from the provisions can only be granted on medical grounds, and then only by the authorities.

French research has shown that out of over 12 000 persons involved in road accidents, 54 % were wearing seat-belts. Among these persons the death-rate was 1,92 %, whereas amongst those not wearing a belt the rate was 4,24 %. Amongst seat-belt wearers, nobody died who was going at a speed of under 90 km/h.

It is sometimes necessary, however, for a patient to get an exemption certificate from a doctor if it is felt that the seat-belt may do more harm than good. Exemptions may be given either on physical or on psychiatric grounds (claustrophobia). Although the doctor must decide on the merits of each case, some concede the following contra-indications:

(1) the person who wears a pacemaker;

(2) the person with a renal transplant;

(3) previous injuries to the thoracic cage.

Pregnancy is not a contra-indication because of the supposed danger of uterine rupture; if the belt is properly adjusted so as not to compress the abdomen, there is little risk to the foetus.

Drivers of cars would, however, not be considered for an exemption certificate by a doctor who is generally guided by the truism that any person who is fit enough to be in charge of a vehicle, is fit enough to wear a seat-belt.

Seat-belts must be properly anchored so that they will not come away from the bodywork of the vehicle when a sudden force is exerted on the belt. Corrosion of the bodywork (e.g. at the coast) can weaken the anchorage points.

Since January 1987, the fitting of rear safety-belts (seat-belts) for passenger vehicles (excluding M2 vehicles, e.g. combis) has been compulsory in South Africa.[11]

It is important that seat-belts be worn correctly to prevent damage.

If the belt is too loose, it is not only ineffective but the driver can smash his/her sternum or ribs against the steering wheel. Correct wearing of the belt is ensured when the shoulder part of the belt fits tautly over the upper part of the body, without causing discomfort. The lap part of the belt must fit firmly over the lower part of the abdomen with the buckle on the hip. The belt should pull the wearer slightly into the seat.

Child car-restraints

Children are prohibited from sitting in the front passenger seat of a car. If for any reason the child must travel in the front of the car, he must be restrained in some safe way (safety seat-belt or safety-seat). Current research[11] indicates that if there is no appropriate child restraint on the back seat the child is safer restrained on the front seat by an adult belt than left loose at the back.

The unrestrained child is five times more likely to be injured than a restrained child.

It is dangerous to take a neonate home cradled in his mother's arms as the infant can be crushed by his mother in the event of a collision.[10]

Compulsory specifications for child car-restraint were introduced in July 1986. The South African Bureau of Standards lays down the following guidelines for the use of child safety restraints:[10]

(1) Infants from birth to 6 months: an approved carry-cot restraint properly installed on the back seat, and covered by a safety net. All cars manufactured since 1987 have rear seat-belts.

(2) Infants from 6 months to 4 years: an approved safety-seat, rearward- or forward-faced, bolted to the car.

(3) Children from 4–10 years: an approved child harness used with an approved booster seat.

(4) Older children: adult seat-belts used with a booster seat if necessary.

Note: (i) Hook-on, screw-on and dog-leash type restraints should not be used for children, as they can be lethal in the event of an accident.
(ii) Stocks of SABS-approved child restraints are held at all the branches of the Automobile Association.

INDUSTRIAL ACCIDENTS

Industrial hazards will depend on the nature of the industry, e.g. mining, production of heavy machinery, the use of saws, and other dangerous implements, excessive noise and air pollution. Occupational hazards are kept to a minimum by constant inspection and legislation (see p. 48).

The National Occupational Safety Association (NOSA) states[12] that each year in the RSA injuries at work claim approximately 2 000 lives, while 32 000 people are permanently disabled; 330 000 accidents causing injury are reported annually, the majority causing no permanent damage.

NOSA was established in 1951 by major employer associations in conjunction with the Compensation Commissioner. It is financed largely by the Compensation Fund (see p. 53) to which employers contribute according to the number and severity of staff accidents. Occupa-tional safety is the concern of major employers of labour who realise the immense benefits that result from accident prevention and loss-control measures.

NOSA advises management on techniques of accident prevention. It runs six different safety training courses and conducts safety promotion campaigns (field-work) by means of educational literature and a five-star grading system (MBO system). NOSA operates mainly in industry and state mines; privately owned mines constituting the Chamber of Mines have their own safety organisations.

NOSA operates in 6 000 industries. It has regional offices in the larger centres. Field staff conducting safety promotion campaigns obtain their information on accidents from the Compensation Commissioner to whom all accidents are reported. NOSA field staff work out a safety programme for each industry requiring help because of high accident rates according to the following data: the number and frequency of serious accidents and the size of the work-force.

NOSA safety training courses concentrate mainly on the training of management because safety-conscious management will introduce safety measures not only to protect the workers but also to control losses.

Managers can also follow the national diploma correspondence course in safety management offered by technikons.

NOSA has introduced the MBO (Management By Objectives) system which leads to five-star grading (with regard to accident prevention) for compliance with a list of 76 accident prevention measures which are common to all types of industry. The programme involves all members of staff, from the floor walker to the manager. MBO means the process whereby all grades of staff jointly identify the common goals of the organisation.[12]

REFERENCES

(1) Heavens J. Letter to the Editor (22 August 1981) *S Afr Med J* **61**: 305.

(2) De Wet B, Davies MRO, Cywes S. *S Afr Med J* 1977; **52**: 969.

(3) Campbell G. *First Aid in Thermal Injury*. SA Burn Society 1981.

(4) Brown DD. *Car* June 1971.

(5) Department of National Health and Population Development. Motor vehicle accidents
in SA 1975–1986. *Epidemiological Comments* 1989; **16**(3).

(6) Cheetham RWS. *S Afr Med J* 1974; **48**: 167.

(7) Odendaal JT. *NITRR Report RU/8/76*. Pretoria, 1976.

(8) Tebbutt PH. *Rand Daily Mail*, 8.10.1982.

(9) Uken EA. *Robot* 1978; No. 99.

(10) Pieterse SH. (NITRR, CSIR) Child restraints in motor vehicles. *S Afr Med J* 1987;
72: 646.

(11) Razis N. Child car-restraints — the facts. *S
Afr Med J* 1988; **74**: XIX.

(12) Van Pletsen. *Informa* 1983; **30**(5).

TEST OF KNOWLEDGE

The student has benefited from studying this
chapter if he/she can answer the following questions:

(1) What advice would you give to a group of:
   (*a*) middle-class mothers;
   (*b*) mothers from a squatter camp;
in the prevention of accidents, including burns,
which may occur in the home and its immediate
surroundings?

(2) What first-aid treatment would you give to
a 6-year-old child who fell over a brazier of
glowing coals during an epileptic seizure?

(3) (*a*) What are the reasons for South Africa's
falling accident rate and constant death-
rate from MVAs during the past decade
despite an increasing casualty rate?
What intervention techniques are being
used to remedy the reasons given?

   (*b*) Discuss the bad-risk driver and the possible measures that can be taken to curb
his harmful driving practices.

(4) (*a*) What safety advice would you give to a
mother with regard to the transport by
car of her newborn baby and 4-year-old
son?

   (*b*) Discuss the circumstances under which
the administrator may grant exemption
from wearing a safety seat-belt.

(5) Describe the importance of NOSA in industry.

46

The Epidemiology and Prevention of Cancer

INTRODUCTION

Cancer is a frightening, emotionally stressful illness which requires traumatic treatment and always holds the threat of recurrence or untimely death.

This chapter deals with the epidemiology of cancer and its primary prevention, by education and PAP testing, secondary prevention by early detection and support after ablative cancer surgery.

M E Vlok, *Manual of Nursing* II carries a chapter on cancer which deals with the diagnosing and staging of neoplasms, treatment modalities and some aspects of the care of the terminal cancer patient.

The division of the cancer nursing material is somewhat arbitrary, in line with the themes of the two books, community nursing and hospital nursing.

It is important for nurses to receive a wide education in cancer so that they may fulfil their role as health educators. Because 80 % of cancers have environmental causes (genetic predisposition accounting for the other 20 %), the prevalence of cancer is closely associated with cultural practices and lifestyle, especially with regard to diet and the habits of smoking and the drinking of alcoholic beverages. Nurses as health educators are in a position to influence people who, through ignorance, adopt destructive lifestyles. Perhaps the nurse's major preventive role is to increase public awareness of the early self-detection of cancer which makes it possible for the patient to seek early treatment and cure.

Some non-governmental organisations (NGOs) are important in the fight against cancer.

1. The National Cancer Association of South Africa (NCA of SA)

The NCA of SA plays a very active role in combating cancer by its involvement in:

(1) Anti-cancer research, sponsoring research projects by universities and the SAIMR.

(2) Public education by distributing literature to bring the facts of cancer to public notice, e.g. the leaflet, *Conquest*, as well as professional information to the medical profession, e.g. *Cancer Bulletin*.

(3) Patient services, by running interim houses which provide free accommodation for ambulant cancer patients undergoing treatment, and Hospicare Home Services which support and teach caretakers of terminal cancer sufferers being nursed at home.

2. The International Union Against Cancer (UICC)

This is a world-wide association of 254 organisations in 84 countries.[1] These organisations include voluntary and professional societies and ministries of health. The UICC holds international cancer congresses.

Among the programmes operated by the UICC is professional education. In 1978 the Cancer Nursing Education Project was established by a South African nursing leader as a component of the Professional Education Programme.[1] Its goal is to provide information and support which will prepare nurses, especially those in developing countries, for a more active and effective role in cancer care. The Cancer Nursing Education Project thus created a speciality of cancer nursing and has published a manual, *Basic Concepts in Cancer Nursing,* which has been translated into Afrikaans.

The South African Cancer Registry

The South African Cancer Registry was established in 1986. It is a central place where all cases of cancer are reported by laboratories on a voluntary, co-operating basis. The Registry holds and distributes epidemiological data which are essential for the goal-directed fight against cancer. Before the central Registry came into being, data were gathered piecemeal by small research studies and local Registries for specific cancers, e.g. cancer of the cervix in the Transvaal. From 1979 to 1989 primary malignancies of the bronchus, lung and pleura required compulsory notification to the Department of National Health and Population Development, but this practice was discontinued in 1989.

Cancer is a malignant neoplasm, its malignancy referring to its ability to kill the host. In cancer there is an uncontrolled multiplication of cells (neoplasm) which invade surrounding tissues by direct infiltration and destroy them and which have a tendency to spread by blood and lymph to distant sites where they form secondary growths (metastases).

IN THIS CHAPTER

THE NATIONAL CANCER ASSOCIATION OF SOUTH AFRICA (NCA OF SA)

The National Cancer Association of South Africa is a voluntary organisation which plays an important role in the prevention of cancer by its extensive educational, welfare and research programmes. The Association is centred in Johannesburg but has branches throughout the country:

- Gauteng Branch: PO Box 32979 Braamfontein. This branch has 8 area offices.
- Western Cape Branch: PO Box 186 Rondebosch. This branch has 8 area offices.
- Kwazulu/Natal Branch: PO Box 2662 Durban. This branch has 3 area offices.
- Northern Province Branch: PO Box 275 Pretoria.
- Free State Branch: PO Box 1686 Bloemfontein.
- Namibia Branch: PO Box 3271 Windhoek.

Each branch has one or more information officers. Some of these are nursing sisters who are essential for the education programme for women, for the taking of smears and for screening projects.

NCA services

(1) The epidemiology and basic **cancer research projects** of the National Cancer Association of South Africa include the following:
   - Maintaining the Association's Cancer Research Unit, at the South African Institute for Medical Research.
   - Research into chemical agents and their use in cancer (medical oncology).
   - A comparative study of the haematologic malignancies in African and Indian children in Natal.
   - The irradiation of tumours with deep hypothermia.
   - Diet and other risk factors in breast cancer in South African inter-ethnic women.

(2) **Cytology laboratories** of the Association are in Durban and serve the whole country. The Association offers a free service for those people who cannot afford private services. In addition, the Association pays the salaries of some cytotechnicians in various laboratories. Cytotechnicians are trained in the Durban Laboratory.

(3) Branches of the Association launch **cancer screening** and **education projects**, e.g. the

Mobile Uterine Cancer Detection Unit of the Western Cape.

(4) The Association makes available to the **public free educational pamphlets** as well as films to educational bodies for showing to the public or to students. This material can be used by the health educator as aids in her educational programme.

(5) The Association sponsors various voluntary societies for the Rehabilitation of Cancer Patients:
  – 'Reach for Recovery' for post-mastectomy patients
  – 'Ostomy Association' for bowel and urinary cancer patients
  – 'Lost Chord Club' for laryngectomees
  – 'Candlelight Club' deals with cancer in children
  – The 'Let's Face it' groups are for those who have had disfiguring operations for cancer of the face and mouth

(6) An **Advisory Nursing Service** of the Cancer Association (Hospicare Home Service) assists cancer patients who are dying at home and are cared for by their relatives. At present this service is available only in the larger centres, but its extension into the rural areas is envisaged.

This free service is run by nursing sisters employed by the NCA. The sisters do not do the actual nursing of domiciliary patients; they are concerned with counselling and teaching the family how to cope. They help the family to control pain by means of analgesics.

Some special hospitals, e.g. Karl Bremer Hospital in Cape Town, have a hospice section where quality care is given to terminal cancer patients. Hospicare patients receive holistic care by a team of caregivers headed by an NCA-appointed physician and including nurses, occupational therapists, volunteers and ministers of religion.

AETIOLOGY OF CANCER

The cancerous growth is initiated by a cancer-generating (cancerigenic, carcinogenic or oncogenic) substance which reacts with a sensitive or susceptible host cell. Different carcinogenic agents may interact with one another to increase the likelihood of a malignant change occurring

in the body cells, e.g. the cigarette smoker who is exposed to asbestos dust is more likely to get lung cancer than the person who is exposed to only one of these carcinogens.

Sir Richard Doll, Regius Professor of Medicine at Oxford University, averred in 1986 that the steady discovery of new causes of cancer now brings the total to more than forty. Cancer risks change with the passage of time and with migration from one part of the world to another.

Carcinogens and co-carcinogens (co-factors)

Viruses play a role in the aetiology of some cancers, e.g. Burkitt's lymphoma; the virus is not infectious. In 1977 Dr Gwen McNab of the SAIMR and Dr Jennifer Alexander of the Virology Department demonstrated the presence of viral antibodies in the culture medium of a human liver malignant cell line. This was a momentous achievement in cancer research. It demonstrated that a virus was present in the cancer cells themselves. Since then the hepatitis B virus has been proved to be the cause of 80 % of liver cancers throughout the world.[2] Vaccination, especially of black children, against hepatitis B-virus infection with the new genetically-engineered vaccine should prevent the infection in childhood and the subsequent development of liver cancer in adulthood. Scientists are still working on a way to prevent liver cancer in carriers of the hepatitis B virus. The human papillomavirus (HPV) and herpes simplex virus (HSV) are widely accepted as important aetiological factors in cancer of the cervix[3] (see p. 596).

The actinic (electromagnetic) — ultraviolet — rays of the sun may cause genetic mutation in skin cells exposed excessively or over long periods to sunlight. This may sometimes lead to skin cancer, especially in old age.

Ionising radiations from radioactive materials may be carcinogenic to certain organs in the body of man, especially the lymphatic and haematopoietic tissues. This is especially hazardous if the whole body is irradiated, e.g. the foetus *in utero*. It is thought that one diagnostic antenatal X-ray to the uterus could have carcinogenic effects on the child many years later.

When the whole body is exposed to radiation for diagnostic or therapeutic purposes, the low dosage used does not cause visible destruction of the skin, but the combined effects can be serious on radiosensitive organs inside the body.

Attendants in radiology departments and radiotherapy wards who absorb small daily doses of ionising radiations over long periods are also at risk. Under normal conditions of vigilance there should, however, be no exposure to ionising rays. It is important for the attendants to observe the official protective measures against such radiation.

Hormonal imbalances and certain physical states of the vulnerable organ: lack of skin pigment, keratoses, leukoplakia and cryptorchidism, predispose to cancer. Cancer may also arise in burn wounds and bilharzia-scarred bladders.

Diet plays an important role in the aetiology of cancer, 50 % of cancers in males and 75 % of cancers in females being linked to diet, either too much of certain nutriments or too little of others. Diet is an important risk factor in breast and colon cancers.[4]

Genetic and immunological factors also predispose to certain cancers, e.g. cancer of the breast. The effect of the carcinogen in the body will depend upon host resistance. If resistance is good, the initial cancer cells may either be destroyed outright or the population of cancer cells kept low so that the disease remains latent (cryptic) or becomes recognisable but remains localised and essentially curable. Loss of host resistance for whatever reason, or the introduction into the body of a powerful carcinogen, causes a rapid proliferation of cancerous cells and the dissemination of malignant cells (metastases) via the lymphatics and blood-vessels to other parts of the body, to cause advanced, incurable cancer. The degree of host resistance probably accounts for the fact that despite communal exposure to carcinogens some people get cancer and others do not. Heredity plays a role in host resistance.

The nature of the cancer cell

Although much is known about the aetiology of cancer, the way in which the cancerous change takes place in the body cells is not understood despite a number of credible theories. These are tied up with the micro-structure and function of the cell — with the life process itself.

It has been possible to compare the intimate physiological and biological details of those changes occurring within the malignant cell to changes which appear to take place in the normal cell by growing cells in the laboratory in culture.[5] Cancer cells behave abnormally and the malignant process involves several biochemical systems of the affected cells, e.g. respiration, glycolysis, etc.

The histological picture of malignant tissues is specific for cancer type and location and is used as the main criterion.

In normal cells which are proliferating, half the daughter cells mature to become the functioning cells of the organ. These mature cells lose their ability to divide, leaving cell division to the other half. The number of cells which can divide, therefore, remains constant and supplies just enough new cells to replace those destroyed by wear and tear. In a cancerous cell, the control of maturation is disturbed, both daughter cells proliferating to cause a tremendous increase in the total population of cells. These abnormally proliferating cells are immature and cannot carry out normal cell functions. No one has as yet discovered how a carcinogen and a susceptible host cell interact to trigger the abnormal proliferation and functioning. The abnormal cancer cells act as antigens, thus eliciting an auto-immune reaction and the production of antigen-specific antibodies. This reaction has not yet been demonstrated in every type of cancer.

Terms which describe abnormal tissues

Dysplasia: abnormal tissue development, e.g. dysplasia of cervical epithelium may regress or progress over a long period to carcinoma.

Anaplasia: a reversion of a cell to an immature type with marked ability to proliferate. This is characteristic of most cancer cells.

Metaplasia: the abnormal transformation of one tissue into another, e.g. the transformation of glandular epithelium into stratified squamous epithelium. A metaplastic cell constitutes a premalignant cell. A PAP smear may reveal metaplastic cells, thus warning that a carcinoma *in situ* is likely to develop in the cervix. This is reported as a dysplasia.

THE EPIDEMIOLOGY OF CANCER

**The annual global incidence
of the 8 most common types of cancer**

Site	New cases per year world-wide
1 Stomach	680,000
2 Lung	590,000
3 Breast	540,000
4 Colon-Rectum	510,000
5 Cervix	460,000
6 Mouth-Pharynx	340,000
7 Oesophagus	300,000
8 Liver	260,000

Source: WHO

The WHO has estimated that 60 to 90 % of all human cancers are associated with environmental carcinogens; 90 % of all lung cancer patients are smokers. Because all the known human carcinogens are environmental in nature, use can be made of epidemiological studies to establish an association between cancers of unknown aetiology and specific carcinogens for the purpose of cancer prevention. Epidemiological observations either confirm the validity of laboratory findings — experiments are of necessity done on animals — or point to possible carcinogens which can be subjected to experimental tests on animals.

The epidemiology of cancer is a very exciting subject for study in South Africa because the cancer pattern in whites and in urban and rural blacks differs, the urban black pattern approximating the white pattern to an increasing degree. The group differences are due to environmental factors such as diet and customs, as well as to genetic differences. Epidemiological cancer research purports to gather information about the aetiology of cancer by studying man: the nature of the geographical area in which the population group to be studied lives, the way of life of the people concerned and the age, sex and parity (in women) of cancer sufferers.

Skin

Skin cancers are very common amongst whites, especially males, because of long exposure to the sun through outdoor activities, but occur much less frequently in blacks because the melanin pigment filters out the actinic rays of the sun. Johannesburg and the Transvaal highveld have one of the highest rates of skin cancer in the world in whites.[6] Solar radiation does affect blacks, however, albinos being even more liable to skin cancer than whites. In blacks, the majority of skin cancers are grafted on to pre-existing lesions such as scars and ulcers. Malignant melanoma incidence rates are the same in blacks and whites, but there are topographical differences in that in blacks 90 % of melanomas occur in the feet whereas in whites the distribution is more general.

For the prevention of solar keratoses and skin cancer in whites, refer to Chapter 14.

Lung

According to Yach,[7] 'Cancer of the lung accounts for between 8 % and 17 % of deaths in the RSA.' In 1984, 3 015 lung cancer deaths were registered. Lung cancer is the most common cancer among white, coloured and Asian males and the second most common cancer among black males and white females. Between 1969 and 1984 lung cancer rates have increased in virtually all population groups, the rate of increase being highest among coloured females (344 %), followed by coloured males (144 %), white females (129 %) and white males (53 %).

That cigarette smoking is the major cause of cancer of the lung has been established with certainty. Approximately 10 % of lung cancers occur in non-smokers, however.

Smoking causes an elevenfold increase in risk of contracting lung cancer.

In the USA smoking has been incriminated as a factor in 30 % of cancers, viz. lung, lip, pharynx, larynx, oesophagus, bladder, pancreas.

(Refer to Chapter 15 for the role of smoking in lung cancer.)

Paranasal sinuses

Whereas cancer of the paranasal sinuses (antral cancer) is fairly common amongst rural blacks, probably because of the type of snuff they use, its incidence is low amongst whites and urban blacks.

Gastro-intestinal system

Whereas in whites cancer of the gastro-intestinal system occurs mostly in the stomach and colon, in blacks primary liver cancer and oeso-phageal cancer predominate

Colon and rectum

Cancer of the colon and rectum is ten times more common among the whites than among the blacks, probably because of the difference in intestinal bacterial flora which is diet-de-pendent. Because of their refined diet, whites are inclined to be constipated and suffer from colonic stasis and diverticulosis.

The death-rate among Johannesburg Jews from colon cancer is twice that for other Johan-nesburg whites and four times that of Jews in Tel Aviv, according to the South African Institute for Medical Research.

Stomach

The incidence and mortality rates from stomach cancer have approximately halved in the RSA in the past twenty years, except in coloured males.[8,9] World-wide it remains the single com-monest cancer, salted and smoked foods, low in vit. C, contributing to its pathogenesis.

Liver (hepatocellular cancer)

Primary liver cancer is rarer in whites, affecting mainly the elderly, but is the most common cancer in the young black South African male, in whom it runs a much more acute course than in whites. In 80 % of cases, primary liver cancer is associated with cirrhosis of the liver[10] which is caused by either chronic alcoholism or chronic hepatitis B-virus disease.

Oesophagus

Although oesophageal cancer was found among the whites before World War II, it appeared among South African blacks only since that time. Its highest incidence used to be amongst the Xhosa of Transkei, where it assumed epi-demic proportions in the early fifties. It ap-peared in other parts of South Africa in descend-ing chronological order going from south to north. Oesophageal cancer became a clinical problem in the northern Transvaal only about 1967.[6]

In a study done at Baragwanath Hospital in 1982, it was found that the incidence of oeso-phageal cancer in the men and women of Soweto is higher than in Transkei,[11] although it is the most frequently reported cancer in Tran-skei.[12] A report published in *Epidemiological Comments*[13] states that in black males cancer of the oesophagus is now the leading cause of cancer deaths. Except for Asians, the rates in urban areas are higher than those in rural areas.

While cancer of the liver is found in children as well as in adults, cancer of the oesophagus affects only adults, predominantly males, but of a younger age group in blacks than in whites.

Of prime importance in epidemiological studies of cancer of the gastro-intestinal system are the oral habits (eating, diet, drinking, chew-ing) and agricultural and food-storage practices of the high cancer incidence population groups. For example, epidemiological research reveals that oesophageal cancer is also rife in other parts of the world where the soil is poor and plants suffer from deficiency diseases (as they do in the Transkei) and heavy fungal (mycotoxin) infection.

The connection between poor agricultural practices and oesophageal cancer seems obvi-ous, but cannot be made with scientific certainty in man because other factors such as the inges-tion of noxious plants used medicinally in these areas also seem to play an aetiological role. Moreover, oesophageal cancer is associated with niacin deficiency associated with an unfor-tified maize diet, and with a deficiency in trace elements and minerals.

Cancer of the oesophagus is also associated with smoking and alcohol intake. There appears to be a synergism between alcohol and tobacco.

Breast

In white women in most Western countries can-cer of the breast is the commonest malignancy, the incidence of breast cancer being twice as high as that of uterine (corpus and cervix) can-cer.

The annual death-rate from cancer of the breast ranges from 26 to 22 per 100 000 of the population in Western countries, the Nether-lands having the highest rate; the South African rate is 23 per 100 000 in white women, while in Japan it is only 4 per 100 000 and in Vietnam 1 per 100 000.[14] Emigration of the latter to Western countries and adoption of their dietary habits cause an increase in the incidence of breast cancer in these low-incidence peoples. In South Africa the incidence of breast cancer among the affluent whites is very much higher than amongst blacks who generally consume a low fat diet.

A high fat intake appears to play an important role in the high prevalence of cancer of the breast, colon and prostate in affluent Western societies, just as it does in the high prevalence of coronary heart disease. In people who live on a very low fat diet, e.g. the Japanese, the prevalence of gastric carcinoma is very high, but the prevalence of breast and colon carcinoma is low.

Parity and lactation do not appear to be correlated with cancer of the breast, the statistics suggesting that environmental factors, including socio-economic circumstances, play an important role in the incidence of breast cancer. Of particular importance is the intake of diets high in fat content in the post-menopausal woman who is rather obese and who has always enjoyed a typical Western diet.[14, 15]

The presence of endogenous oestrogens has been found to be important in the genesis of post-menopausal breast cancer. After the menopause, both the high fat diet and adipose tissue give rise to the production of oestrogens; moreover, delayed menopause and the prolonged presence of endogenous oestrogens in the body are associated with increased risk of breast cancer.[14] Different factors appear to be operative in pre- and post-menopausal breast cancer. Other risk factors are a genetic predisposition (the highest risk factor), chronic psychogenic stress[15] and ionising radiation.

Immunological mechanisms are also important (as in all cancers) in permitting the action of most of the aetiological factors.[15]

There is no proof that the exogenous oestrogens (e.g. the 'pill' and Premarin) cause breast cancer, but in pre-menopausal women the growth of an existing breast cancer can be stimulated by low-dosage, long-term oestrogens.[14] No woman who develops benign breast pathology on exogenous oestrogens should continue with this medication, as there is a risk of a benign disease becoming malignant.

Cervix uteri

Carcinoma of the cervix is the commonest malignancy in all black women, irrespective of tribal affiliation or rural-urban habitat. Among the blacks, for every breast cancer today there are nearly four cervical cancers.[16]

The lower incidence of cervical carcinoma in whites probably has to do with their lower parity and genital infection. Early marriage and childbirth and promiscuous sexual intercourse are important causal factors. Male cleanliness with coitus is believed to be important in the prevention of cervical cancer.

Bladder

The epidemiology of bladder cancer in South Africa suggests that bilharziasis is a predisposing factor in its aetiology, but not necessarily the cause. The incidence of bladder cancer is highest in areas where bilharziasis is endemic, with a preponderance of males being affected.

Occupational

The modern industrial environment has given rise to occupational cancers through the repeated exposure of workers to dyes, nickel, chrome, chemical substances, lead in petrol fumes and asbestos fibre dust (amongst miners and insulation workers).

Age

Age also plays an important role in carcinogenesis, age distribution patterns varying from one type of cancer to another. Some cancers are specific to childhood, e.g. Wilms tumour, while others are more likely to appear in the aged, e.g. skin cancers. Although cancer affects all age groups, being the second greatest killer in white children, there is generally an increased incidence with age as the result of the cumulative effects of repeated exposure to carcinogenic agents which sheer length of life causes in the aged.

When exposure to a specific carcinogen stops, the risk of cancer ceases to rise but remains operative for many years. It probably takes 10 to 15 years for the person who has stopped smoking cigarettes to return to pre-smoking levels of risk of contracting lung cancer, though the risk diminishes rapidly after five years.

Urban/rural cancer in blacks

Generally it has been found that there are urban/rural differences in the distribution of cancers among blacks, pointing to the probable influence of westernisation. In a study by Robertson et al.[16] on the cancer patterns of black males in the Transvaal lowveld (1962–67), it was found that cancer of the liver was the most prevalent kind of cancer, followed by cancer of the bladder, the oesophagus, the skin and bone and connective tissue. There were tribal differences in the distribution of cancers, showing the influence of tribal customs. Amongst Johannesburg black males cancer of the liver also predominated, followed by cancer of the oesophagus, prostate, mouth and pharynx, with a low incidence of bladder cancer. In the females of both regions, half of the cancers were of the cervix and breast (with a mean ratio of 4:1). Both the cervical and breast prevalence rate is much higher in Johannesburg, however. The incidence of liver and oesophageal cancer is much lower for the women of both regions than for the men.[17]

Note: These surveys were done before 1967 and there is a time interval of 10 years between the two surveys. It is a well-known fact that black cancer patterns have been changing over the past 20 years. Liver cancer is decreasing in frequency in Johannesburg.

THE SOUTH AFRICAN CANCER REGISTRY

The registration of cancer is of great national importance. The Cancer Register was established on 1 January 1986, and is housed at the SAIMR in Johannesburg. It is controlled by an executive committee and funded by the Department of Health.

Cancer registers yield a supply of accurate incidence data fed to them from diagnostic centres country-wide. Accurate data require the full co-operation of contributors. The registering centre stores and collates the data.

The South African Cancer Registry is at present pathology-based and will register all malignant tumours diagnosed in all South African histo-pathology and haematology laboratories.[18] When an expanded infrastructure has been developed, clinically and radiologically diagnosed malignant tumours will be included in the Register. In the mean time under-reporting of malignant tumours necessarily occurs, particularly in the case of cancer of the lung. The returns from the contributing laboratories are submitted monthly. If full co-operation is obtained, incidence rates will be accurate and meaningful. The first report of the SA Cancer Registry — 1986, was released in 1988.[19] This was one of the most significant events in the epidemiology of, and research on, cancer in the RSA. The Registry report contains the details of the number and types of cancer recorded for the year 1986, and includes information on age, sex and ethnic group.

To quote the executive committee, 'Up to now, the general picture of cancer occurrence in the different ethnic populations had to rely on studies of death rates, hospital admissions and a few limited incidence studies.'[19]

In the first year (1986), 32 000 cancer diagnoses were recorded.

TABLE 1
The incidence of cancer and recovery rate in all the populations groups in South Africa[24]

Number of cancer notifications per 100 000 per year	Cancer Register 1986	Recovery rate	Special conditions in whites
450	White	95 %	with skin cancer
300	White	50 %	without skin cancer
250	Black	25–30 %	
250	Coloured	30–35 %	
300	Indian	40 %	

Although the data generally confirmed earlier assessment of cancer occurrence, the new data underline the following: 'the excessively high rates for oesophageal cancer in black males and cervical cancer in black females. In blacks, stomach, colorectal, skin, pancreas and breast cancer rates are low.

The total rates for cancer in blacks are nearly half the rates for whites. With the exception of skin cancers, the overall rates for most cancers in South Africa are lower than those in most populations in other countries.

The cancer rates of the South African Indians are much lower than those of whites. The coloured population has a much lower total cancer rate than do the whites due to the very high skin cancer rate in whites. Compared with whites, coloureds have high rates for oesophageal, stomach and cervical cancers, but lower rates for prostate and bladder cancer as well as for the leukaemias.'[19]

THE PREVENTION OF CANCER

Although the early detection of cancer plays an important role in the control of the disease, it is not as effective as primary preventive measures; approximately half of all solid tumours develop metastases while the growth is as yet hidden.

Primary prevention

Primary prevention of cancer is, therefore, of prime importance in the fight against the disease. Prevention is based on the knowledge of aetiological factors, knowledge gained by epidemiological studies. The recognition and avoidance of carcinogens are of prime importance in the fight against cancer. We know today that cigarette smoke causes lung cancer, that prolonged exposure to sun and wind gives rise to solar keratoses and pterygium of the conjunctiva — both pre-cancerous conditions — and that contact with certain chemicals and asbestos fibre causes occupational cancers. Avoidance of these known environmental carcinogens will diminish the incidence of cancer.

Pre-cancerous conditions of the cervix, pigmented moles which start enlarging and leukoplakia (irregular white patches on mucous membranes) can be treated to prevent the development of cancer.

At present a possible breakthrough has been made in the prevention of primary liver cancer through the prevention of hepatitis B by means of a vaccine. A connection has been established between cancer of the liver and B hepatitis virus (HBV) by the research of McNab and Alexander and by more recent international studies involving Johannesburg scientists. See p. 566 for a discussion of B. hepatitis.

Secondary prevention

This includes early detection of cancer which is aimed at the treatment of cancer while it is in the first stage or in the pre-invasive stage with dysplasia of cells in high-risk areas of the body such as the cervix uteri.

Diagnosing malignant neoplasms

Signs and symptoms of malignant growths are often so insidious that the pathological process is far advanced before medical advice is sought. At other times pathological signs may be obvious, yet arouse no suspicion of malignancy because they cause no discomfort. By the time cachexia and pain are experienced the disease may be advanced beyond human aid.

Procrastination may be caused by the fear and horror which the thought of cancer evokes in the lay mind. A diagnosis of cancer is emotionally unacceptable because tradition teaches that it is incurable and causes unbearable pain. (This is a misconception, however.) These are some of the reasons why patients so often seek advice when it is too late to help them.

Early diagnosis and early cure are very important principles in the handling of malignancy. For this reason, every nurse and every lay person should be familiar with the following signs and symptoms of cancer.

The seven danger signals of cancer
(1) A sore which does not heal.
(2) A lump or thickening of the breast or elsewhere.
(3) Extraordinary bleeding or discharge.
(4) Change in a wart or a mole.
(5) Persistent anorexia, indigestion or dysphagia.

(6) Persistent hoarseness or cough.

(7) Any deviation from normal bowel habits, e.g. increasing constipation alternating with bouts of diarrhoea and abdominal colic are early signs of carcinoma of the colon.

A persistent pain in a bone may be an early symptom of osteogenic sarcoma.

The warning signs in children are:[24]

(1) Bruising or bleeding easily; purpuric spots

(2) Unexplained fever that does not subside

(3) Pallor — prolonged or of sudden onset

(4) Regular pain that does not subside

(5) A mass or swelling anywhere

(6) Change in balance, gait or personality

(7) Development of a squint or other eye signs

(8) Facial distortion

The diagnosis of cancer is confirmed by:

(1) The physical examination in which the doctor inspects and palpates the skin, abdomen, breast, rectum, mouth, pharynx and does a routine gynaecological examination.

(2) Radiography, including mammography and computerised tomography (CT scan). Mammographic screening techniques for the early detection of breast cancer are available to women at risk.

(3) Radio-isotope scanning.

(4) Ultrasonography.

(5) Colour thermography.

(6) Endoscopy which usually includes biopsy.

(7) Cytology (exfoliative). The cells are obtained in a number of ways, e.g. scrapings and brushings of cervix when taking the PAP smear; fine needle aspiration. Cytological screening programmes are well known in the fight against cervical cancer.

(8) Histological examination of a biopsy specimen obtained by punch, excision or big needle aspiration.

(9) Blood and bone marrow specimens for leukaemia.

(10) Surgery, e.g. diagnostic curettage and laparoscopy.

Late signs and symptoms of cancer

(1) Cachexia, a condition of physical exhaustion, due to the absorption of toxic substances from the necrotic cancerous tumour, and from lack of nutrition. It is recognised by loss of weight, emaciation and sunken eyes; dry, loose and yellowish skin (sallow complexion).

(2) Excruciating pain, sepsis and tissue necrosis which give the patient a characteristic unpleasant smell.

The community nurse must be able to define the population at risk of developing certain types of cancer and apply health-educating measures to encourage people to:

(1) avoid exposing themselves unnecessarily to known carcinogens, e.g. cigarette smoking;

(2) become aware of the seven warning signs of cancer and seek timeous medical aid (the community nurse must explain to her patients the danger of delaying the seeking of medical help by, for example, first consulting quacks and folk healers);

(3) undergo screening tests, where these are available, in order to detect cancer in the curable stage.

This is especially important in cancer of the cervix uteri, breast and rectum.

Screening at-risk populations for cervical cancer

The *Canadian Medical Association Journal* in 1976 published a report by a task force who investigated a Canadian cervical cancer screening service and recommended that this report be widely distributed to bring its contents to the notice of the public.

These excerpts have been quoted from an editorial of the *S Afr Med J* 1977; **51**:

'... squamous carcinoma of the cervix lends itself to control by means of a cytological screening programme because invasive carcinoma is preceded by a spectrum of disease extending over many years which may be recognised at the stages of dysplasia and carcinoma *in situ*.'

In Canada screening programmes have been effective in reducing mortality from cervical cancer. In South Africa, cervical cancer is the most common cancer in black women and the second commonest cancer in white women. Fragoyannis *et al.*[20] detected a high incidence of positive smears (31 per 1 000) in cervical cytology studies on 6 756 initial cervical smears of Tswana women in the cytology laboratory at Ga-Rankuwa Hospital. Half had moderate to mild dysplasia (age range 16–63 years), while the rest ranged from severe dysplasia to invasive carcinoma (age range 18–72 years).

The Canadian report further recommended that 'the initial smears should be obtained from all women over 18 years who had had sexual intercourse, and that if the initial smear is satisfactory a second one should be taken within 1 year. Provided these two smears and all subsequent ones are satisfactory, further smears may be taken at approximately 3-year intervals until the age of 35 and thereafter at 5-year intervals, until the age of 60. Women at continuing high risk should be screened annually.'

Cervical cancer is the commonest type of cancer amongst women of the lower socio-economic classes, especially if they start having coitus at an early age. The smegma of men has been mooted as the carcinogenic source; a herpes-type virus and the papillomavirus are also thought to be the cause. Other contributory factors are chronic infection of the vagina and sexual promiscuity, especially if standards of hygiene are poor in the male sexual partners. There has been much controversy over a possible relationship between cancer and the use of oestrogens, especially their long-term use for menopausal symptoms. The American College of Obstetrics and Gynaecology declared in its October 1976 Bulletin: 'At the present time, no firm conclusions are warranted regarding the carcinogenicity of oestrogens . . .'[21]

To sum up, in some developing populations the rates of cervical cancer are up to 8 times those in most Western populations.

The risk factors include:

(1) Early age at first sexual intercourse.

(2) Low socio-economic status which may be the cause of poor hygiene standards.

(3) Promiscuity, i.e. multiple sexual partners.

(4) Being widowed or divorced (implying many new casual sexual partners).

(5) Having a husband who has, or has had, multiple sexual partners.

These risk factors point to the strong probability that cancer of the cervix is a sexually transmitted disease (see p. 597). Generally two infecting viruses are suspected: the herpes simplex virus (HSV) and the human papillomavirus (HPV).

The human papillomavirus (HPV)

The HPV is a venereally transmitted microbe causing squamous cell lesions (flat, inverted and papillomatous condylomas) in the uterine cervix of mainly young, sexually promiscuous females, but also in black women whose normal family life has been disrupted by the migrant labour system and who live in poverty.

The human papilloma-(wart) virus is one of the causes of cancer of the cervix.[20] This virus has been found in most cases of serious cervical pathology as revealed by PAP tests. The HPV is probably only a potential oncogenic agent in the genital tract. Markowitz *et al.* reported a 100 % association between HPV infections and CIN III (ca *in situ*).[3] HPV infection is linked with cervical intra-epithelial neoplasia (CIN), invasive cervical cancer and similar changes in the vulval and vaginal epithelium. Genital warts also occur in males. No fewer than 40 types and subtypes of HPV are known, each with a site of predilection. Examples: the deep plantar wart, the common wart and genital condylomas (exophytic condyloma acuminatum on the vulva and perineum) and a variety of flat warts affecting the uterine cervix. Some of the latter are at high risk of malignant transformation.[20]

It is probable that the human papillomavirus causes cancer only in the presence of a co-factor, the three most frequently implicated being herpes simplex virus (HSV), smoking and a 'male factor'. A large number of women have asymptomatic HPV infection; there is a long latent period before the development of an invasive cancer. HPV and HSV are, theoretically, important co-factors which operate only in certain women.[22]

If HPV infection is found on PAP testing, the following guidelines are recommended:[22]

(1) The patient is made aware of the potential danger and is advised to practice responsible and safe sex, i.e. with one partner and, where indicated, with a condom.

(2) If HPV infection is present and persists for longer than 6 months, a colposcopic examination for lesions is indicated.

(3) All abnormal lesions should be excised. This also applies to mild lesions such as CIN I and II.

(4) Routine follow-up visits to the gynaecologist.

(5) The male sexual partner should be investigated for flat scrotal and penile warts and/or cytological smears taken from the urethra as the man could serve as a reservoir for reinfection of the female.

South Africa and Namibia have the highest prevalence rates for HPV and CIN (pre-malignant lesions) yet recorded in the world, viz. 66 % and 55 % respectively.[3] This is tantamount to a 'wart virus epidemic' and argues for the free availability of cytological screening (PAP smears) of all women at risk.

The screening for cervical cancer

The PAP cell test is a screening test for cervical cancer.

PAP smears are taken not only in private practice but also at most municipal family planning clinics by sisters of the NCA who visit groups of women who request the service and as an adjunct to services for women at antenatal clinics and gynaecological OPDs. The state family planning department does not budget for large-scale PAP laboratory expenses. PAP smears are generally subsidised by the National Cancer Association of SA; they run a large laboratory in Durban, which can examine up to 80 000 PAP smears a year. State family planning clinics do supply this screening service if they are situated near government laboratories.

All family planning nurses are taught to take PAP smears during their training course. Therefore, if a sister holds a family planning certificate, she is qualified to take a PAP smear.

The PAP cell test in exfoliative cytology

Exfoliative cytology is the study of epithelial cells, shed from the body, for abnormalities which may warn of early malignant changes, one to two years before there are any clinical signs of malignancy.

The term PAP refers to Papanicolaou, the man who originally described a smear of the posterior fornix where endometrial cells (for the diagnosis of uterine cancer) are likely to pool. The term, PAP, has stuck and is generally used for cervical smears obtained to diagnose precancerous lesions of the cervix.

Cervical smears may be taken from the ectocervix (vaginal portion of the cervix covered by squamous epithelium) — the usual smear for diagnosing cervical cancer — and also from the endocervical canal (covered by columnar epithelium) to gather TZ material (see p. 804) from the crypts of the endocervix. Overlap of these smears ensures inclusion of the squamocolumnar epithelial junction. A third smear is sometimes required of the posterior fornix of the vagina for endometrial cells, if uterine cancer is suspected.

Note:

(1) For routine screening of an asymptomatic woman, only one ectocervical smear is necessary. The endocervical and posterior fornix smears are taken only on special indication.

(2) The required number of smears should be taken in conjunction with every vaginal examination.

The first test is done two years after sexual intercourse has started; it is repeated after a year and, if both tests are negative, the woman should have a PAP smear taken routinely every three years, irrespective of her marital status or parity, until she reaches the age of 60 years.

Equipment

Examining couch, torch or other source of light, spray fixative such as hairspray, clean glass slides with frosted ends for marking details with a soft lead pencil.

Sterile Cusco vaginal speculum, Ayre cervical spatula (wooden) or an ordinary wooden tongue spatula split lengthwise in half, swab-holding forceps and swabs, cotton-wool swab, or Cytobrush, gloves and warm saline (for warming the speculum and for its lubrication).

Technical procedure

The woman is placed either in Sims' or lithotomy position and the Cusco speculum passed. With swab and swab-holding forceps, any mucus plug from the external os of the cervix is removed. As three smears will be made, either three glass slides are used or one slide is divided into three parts.

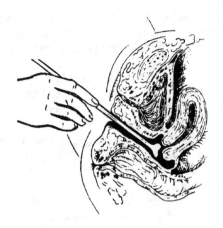

Figure 46.1

Technique for vaginal and cervical cell collection
(speculum not illustrated)

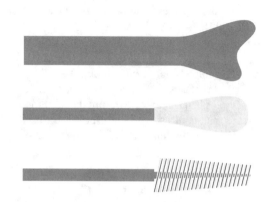

Figure 46.2

Instruments for taking a PAP smear:
(1) Ayre cervical spatula; (2) Cotton-wool swab;
(3) Cytobrush

The ectocervical scraping is taken of the cervix in the following way: the narrow tip of the spatula is placed in the cervical canal, the spatula is then gently rotated a full 360° to obtain a scraping from the cervix at the level of the external os.

Then the endocervical specimen is taken by rotating the saline-soaked swab or the Cytobrush in the cervical canal. Even smears are now made of this material on their respective slides or on portions of one slide by gently stroking the slide with the scrapings in both directions. A third smear is made by lightly scraping the vaginal wall of the posterior fornix with a split wooden spatula.

As soon as the smears have been made they are fixed by spraying with fixative and allowing the smear to dry for 15 minutes while the slide remains on a flat surface. It is important that smearing and fixing should be done almost in one motion as a minimum of air drying of the specimen is required. Some authorities hold the ectocervical specimen until they have taken the endocervical specimen and then make both smears in quick succession.

Note:

(1) For reliable cervical cytology a representative smear is of the greatest importance. The routine combination of ectocervical and endocervical smears is the best guarantee that the smear contains cells from the transformation zone (TZ) (see p. 803). This is used only where specially indicated.

(2) The spray must be held at least 20 cm from the slide to prevent the cells from being washed off, or freezing and bursting, thereby causing a negative result.

(3) Some cytological laboratories prefer an alcohol fixative for PAP smears. The rule about fixing the smear immediately applies here as well. A solution of ether 50 % and alcohol (95 %) 50 % in a small wide-mouthed jar with a fluid depth of at least 6 cm can be used, keeping the lid on. Two slides at a time can be placed back to back in the jar for 15 minutes after which they are removed and allowed to dry. For the protection of the smear, they should be coated with spray fixative before being packed carefully and sent to the laboratory.

The following data accompany the smears:

Biographical details of the patient, date of onset of last menstrual period, date of last pregnancy, history of hormone therapy or contraceptives, history of radiation therapy, gynaecological complaints and significant medical conditions.

The following results of PAP smears are likely to be received from the laboratory:

Micro-organisms: Trichomonas, Candida, Schistosoma, viruses, e.g. human papillomavirus and the herpes simplex virus.

Cells derived from cervical lesions

(1) Metaplasia — young cells changing from columnar to squamous epithelium and thus more vulnerable to carcinogens.

(2) Dysplasia. Dysplastic cells (CIN — cervical intra-epithelial neoplasia) are the forerunners of carcinoma of the cervix.
(3) Epidermoid carcinoma *in situ* (CIN 111).
(4) Invasive epidermoid carcinoma.
(5) Adenocarcinoma of the endocervix.

Note: The exact site at which dysplastic cells (CIN) develop has been defined and is called the transformation zone (TZ); it is situated on the ectocervix, but may also extend into the crypts of the endocervix. The entire TZ has neoplastic potential. CIN can be diagnosed by PAP smear (cytological examination) and the diagnosis confirmed by the histological examination of a small punch biopsy. Colposcopy defines the site of CIN.

Treatment of dysplasia (CIN)

(1) CIN grade I (mild dysplasia). No treatment is given but cytological colposcopic examinations are done at 3–6 monthly intervals to watch for progression or regression — both being possible.
(2) CIN grade II and grade III (carcinoma *in situ*).
  (*a*) Complete hysterectomy is advised in women who have completed their families.
  (*b*) Younger patients who wish to have children can expect a 90 % cure by colposcopic out-patient treatments which destroy the TZ:
    (i) Cervical conisaton (cone biopsy) to excise the TZ.
    (ii) CO_2 laser vaporisation.
    (iii) Electrocoagulation diathermy.
    (iv) Cryosurgical destruction with a cryoprobe cooled to –89 °C.
    In the last three instances colposcopic conservation methods are applied unless there is invasive carcinoma.

If the patient is pregnant, monthly PAP smears are taken instead until delivery which is either *per vaginam* or by Caesarean section. Six weeks later a biopsy is done and the PAP smear is repeated at yearly intervals.

Survival after treatment for cancer of the cervix

Screening for cancer of the cervix by using the PAP test to detect the pre-malignant stage of the disease has markedly reduced the cervical cancer incidence and mortality rates in Western populations.[21] Patients whose disease is diagnosed and treated in Stages I and II survive far longer than those detected in a later stage. Black Sowetan women of all stage detection succumb much earlier than matched patients in Western populations. Studies done in the USA suggest that poverty plays a role here.

Cancer of the cervix is likely to remain a very serious public health problem as the risk factors, except smoking, do not lend themselves to real change. Sexual behaviour is a personal matter which is tied up with inculcated cultural values and with a person's emotional, social and economic needs.

In South Africa nation-wide screening programmes are impracticable.[23] Selected groups, e.g. those attending family planning clinics, could benefit from regular PAP testing as this group is at high risk of developing cancer of the cervix. Medical opinion is in favour of screening all women of childbearing age who attend clinics.

The screening for breast cancer

In Western countries cancer of the breast is the most common cancer in women. It can affect the pre-menopausal as well as the post-menopausal woman. Every lump in the breast does not signify cancer — the final diagnosis must be made on histological grounds — but in the post-menopausal women it usually does. It is disastrous to adopt the 'wait-and-see' attitude towards any lump in the breast.

Carcinoma *in situ* of the breast is highly curable; it may be multiple and it may become invasive. Mammography, xerography and thermography are new diagnostic techniques for detecting small tumours at a pre-invasive stage. The useful screening technique is, however, not within the reach of every woman, as is the PAP smear which detects carcinoma *in situ* of the cervix. Mammography may be used to diagnose carcinoma of the breast if there are suspicious symptoms without palpable lumps such as: thickening of the skin and nipple retraction, swollen axillary glands. It can be used to reassure cancerophobic women or those from a carcinogenic family.

Early detection of carcinoma of the breast

Mass screening techniques for carcinoma of the breast are not practical in South Africa as only 1:200 women screened at random is likely to have breast cancer. Screening for breast cancer by mammography (and aspiration cytology in positive cases) has been adopted (1987) in the UK. Screening is targeted at women aged 50–64 years, and takes place at 3-year intervals. Suspicious lesions require specialist radiological localisation and excision. This very expensive scheme may reduce deaths from breast cancer by a third or more.

It is doubtful if this type of First-World preventive medicine is of application in South Africa where health budget priorities are the establishment of effective primary health care services.

The following selected 'women-at-risk' should, however, be subjected to lifelong follow-up regimens:

(1) after mastectomy;
(2) those with a family history of breast cancer;
(3) those who have had benign breast pathology, especially fibroadenosis, nipple discharge and gross papillomatosis;
(4) those with cancer of the endometrium.

Follow-up regimen for women at risk:

(1) Regular clinical examination every three to six months.
(2) An exfoliative cytology examination should be done on nipple discharge.
(3) A biopsy should be done on any suspicious lump discovered on palpation.
      Pre-menopausal women may have lumps for many reasons other than adenocarcinoma. The woman, therefore, needs to have her mind set at rest by a negative biopsy finding.
(4) Fine needle aspiration cytology and mammography if a lump is discovered.
(5) Monthly examination of the breast for lumps. Breast examination is done by inspection and palpation.

Inspection by an examiner

(1) Both breasts should be equal in size. While the patient is sitting with arms stretched above the head, the examiner looks for:

–   Skin retraction (i.e. dimpling)
–   Orange peel (*peau d'orange*) appearance of skin

These are late manifestations of cancer when the lymphatics are blocked and the cancer has become invasive.

(2) Nipples: pointing in the same direction and protruding equally (normal); scaling and desquamation; discharge — serous, bloody.

Palpation of the breast by an examiner

The woman lies on her back, arms extended above her head and a pillow under her shoulders.

Palpation is done with the entire flat of the hand pressing down firmly on the breast tissue in a slow rotatory movement. The characteristic of a cancerous lump is that it is firm to hard, but not necessarily so. Lumps may be multiple. Often the lump is not tender but a painful lump does not exclude cancer. The lump may be fixed to breast tissue or to the skin, in which case there will be skin dimpling.

Palpation of the axilla for affected lymph glands.

With the forearm of the patient resting on the examiner's arm the axilla is palpated gently along the margin of the pectoralis major muscle. The skin and underlying tissues are gently depressed against the thoracic cage. Any lumps are gently rolled under the finger and compared with the absence or presence of a similar lump in the other axilla.

Note: Innocent lymph nodes may be palpable; unilateral lumps are suspicious.

Self-examination of the breast (see p. 807)

Monthly examination of the breast for lumps can also be done by the woman who has been suitably instructed at family planning clinics, at pre- and postnatal clinics and by private doctors. Women in white South African society, who are much more likely than black women to get breast cancer, have become very breast cancer conscious; moreover, the greater majority of early diagnosis (i.e. 90 %) are made by women themselves through auto-palpation. It is, therefore, worthwhile to direct a health educational programme to auto-palpation of the breast in both black and white women.

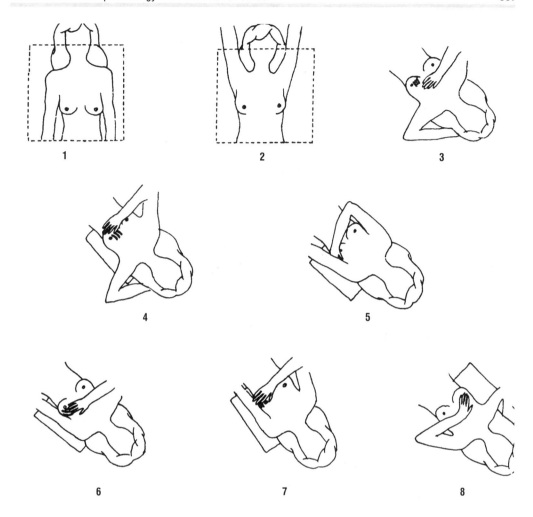

Figure 46.3

BREAST SELF-EXAMINATION

1. Sit or stand in front of your mirror, with your arms relaxed at your sides, and examine your breasts carefully for any changes in size and shape. Look for any puckering or dimpling of the skin, and for any discharge or change in the nipples.

2. Raise both your arms over your head, and look for exactly the same things. See if there's been any change since you last examined your breasts.

3. Lie down on your bed, put a pillow or a bath towel under your left shoulder, and your left hand under your head. (From this step to step 8, you should feel for a lump or thickening.) With the fingers of your right hand held together flat, press gently but firmly with small circular motions to feel the inner, upper quarter of your left breast, starting at your breastbone and going outward toward the nipple line. Also feel the area around the nipples.

4. With the same gentle pressure, feel the lower inner part of your breast. Incidentally, in this area you will feel a ridge of firm tissue or flesh. Don't be alarmed. This is perfectly normal.

5. Now bring your left arm down to your side and, still using the flat part of your fingers, feel under your armpit.

6. Use the same gentle pressure to feel the upper, outer quarter of your breast from the nipple line to where your arm is resting.

7. And finally, feel the lower outer section of your breast, going from the outer part to the nipple.

8. Repeat the entire procedure, as described, on the other breast.

With acknowledgment to the American Cancer Society, Inc.
Used here with kind permission of the National Cancer Association of South Africa.

Testicular self-examination

Men should feel very gently around each testis for inequality in size and texture.

SUPPORT FOR CANCER PATIENTS TREATED BY ABLATIVE SURGERY

The National Cancer Association has sponsored a number of associations of cancer ex-patients who are in need of emotional support and practical help in rehabilitation.

Although the founding of these associations was initiated by members of the medical profession, they are run almost entirely by patient members and their families. The main associations are the following.

The South African Ostomy Association

This association was formed in 1969 and has its headquarters in Johannesburg. Correspondence can be addressed to:

> The Honorary Secretary
> SA Ostomy Association
> PO Box 2000
> Johannesburg 2000

Some of the objects of the Association are:

(1) to operate as a non-profit health service agency and to provide a central organisation to compile, publish and distribute information for the better rehabilitation of persons who have lost the normal function of their bowel or bladder, necessitating colostomy, ileostomy, ileal bladder or ureterostomy surgery;

(2) to encourage and maintain an exchange of ideas and methods for the promotion of the rehabilitation of these persons;

(3) to promote and assist with research concerning the management of ostomy and the prosthetic equipment and appliances connected with it, by assisting and co-operating with qualified persons in the pursuance of such research and study;

(4) to disseminate information for public education as to the nature of ostomy, thereby eliminating job and insurance discrimination;

(5) to establish a liaison service with institutions and hospitals in the Republic of South Africa, where ostomy operations may be performed, or ostomy patients nursed.

Membership: all ostomy patients shall be entitled to automatic membership of the Association; members' spouses may be admitted as members of the Association.

The Lost Chord Club of South Africa

This club is run under the auspices of the National Cancer Association of South Africa for persons who have undergone laryngectomy for cancer (or other incurable disease) of the larynx. Such persons are called laryngectomees or neck-breathers and their neck stoma, a tracheastome. The only functions affected are breathing, coughing and speech. Laryngectomees cannot do physical labour which requires powerful movements of the arms and shoulders as they cannot fix the thorax after a deep inspiratory movement by closure of the vocal chords. Bearing down movements are, however, possible by momentary digital closure of the tracheastome. Taste and smell are likely to be lost for some time, but should return once oesophageal speech is learned.

The Medic Alert Foundation will assist all laryngectomees by issuing them with disc bracelets to warn first-aid personnel of the artificial airway when respiratory resuscitation may be necessary.

Laryngectomee volunteers, members of one of the regional Lost Chord Clubs, will visit patients before the operation in order to encourage them and assure them of friendship and help after the operation. Nurses who wish to contact such volunteers, can obtain information from:

> The National Cancer Association of South Africa
> PO Box 2000
> Johannesburg 2000

Members of the Lost Chord Club are encouraged to help others; each one has been helped by an older member and it is expected of each one to help a new member. Every novice laryngectomee is afraid of losing his job and his friends and the only real reassurance to the contrary can come from those who have successfully overcome their difficulties.

Speech therapy is usually started before the operation in order to facilitate mastery of oesophageal speech after the operation. In oesophageal speech, air trapped in the oesophagus is expelled to produce a low-pitched sound which can be articulated into words by the tongue, lips, teeth and palate. The learning of oesophageal speech may be a very arduous task requiring much encouragement, best obtained by attending club meetings of laryngectomees who are in different stages of mastering audible speech.

From an introduction to the booklet, *Your New Voice*, by William F Waldrop and Marie A Gould, the following extracts have been taken:

'Here you are with no voice. You will not develop your new voice by feeling sorry for yourself. The going is rough but each day of practice will have its accomplishments . . . At first you will probably be quite concerned, especially about coughing but you will soon realise that you have a normal throat . . . Your sense of smell will begin to return as your speaking improves . . . Your job is to be cheerful, begin mingling with your friends . . .'

Although speech is never perfect — the oesophagus cannot hold as much air as the lungs can — some laryngectomees have resumed careers in which it is essential to use speech.

For those who are unable to master oesophageal speech, there are electronic substitutes which produce a low quality sound adequate for communication purposes. The electrolarynx is placed against the throat and emits a buzzing sound which can be articulated into words by the tongue, lips, teeth and palate.

The 'Reach for Recovery' Volunteers

(Rehabilitation after mastectomy)

Although radical mastectomy for carcinoma of the breast is hardly ever practised today, even a simple mastectomy followed by radiotherapy may be a very traumatic experience for a woman. It is for this reason that a number of 'Reach for Recovery' Volunteer Groups have been formed in some of the larger centres of the Republic, under the auspices of the National Cancer Association of South Africa.

In the pamplet *Reach for Recovery*, issued by this organisation, their objects and operational methods are clarified:

'The 'Reach for Recovery' Volunteers came into being as a direct result of a visit to South Africa by Mrs. Terese Lasser from New York. Mrs. Lasser, a mastectomy patient herself, has devoted the years since her operation to helping other women who have had to undergo a similar experience. Her organisation in America is known as 'Reach for Recovery'. Her lectures in the Republic resulted in the formation of eager and hardworking Groups for the rehabilitation of mastectomees.

Objects
Briefly, the objects of the Group are: 'To encourage and promote the post-operative rehabilitation of mastectomy patients in consultation with, and under the general direction of, their medical attendants.' The 'Reach for Recovery' Volunteers feel very strongly from their visiting experience, that the problem is only partly a physical one. Important after effects following mastectomy may be mental and emotional upheavals. Instead of the shrinking and secrecy with which a patient tends to surround herself, it is considered she should be shown how to face up fearlessly and openly to her problems.

The importance of obtaining the doctor's permission before attempting this, or any other programme for recovery, is always stressed.

The doctor's advice must be followed first and foremost and the efforts of the volunteers are directed to supplement the doctor's instructions, and are not intended as a 'cure', but to relieve endless hours of doubts and fears.

Volunteer organisation
The organisation is a non-profit group and mainly comprises volunteers who have themselves undergone the operation, and can thus offer help and guidance from their own personal experience. They are trained to visit patients in hospitals and at home. Their aim is to co-operate with the respective surgeons and not do or say anything which may be contrary to the surgeon's wishes.

Operational methods
The rules to be followed by the volunteer, guided by the committee of the 'Reach for Recovery' Volunteer Group are as under:
(1) The first visit is made to the patient in the Nursing Home or Hospital.
(2) The volunteer takes along a pack, which contains a temporary prosthesis for immediate use, and a suitable length of rope required for the exercises which the volunteer will demonstrate.
(3) Careful explanations for each exercise are given and a booklet, with the fullest information, is handed to the patient.
(4) Explanations of various prostheses and suggestions for personal needs are given, together with a list of sources of supply of such prostheses.
(5) A frank and free discussion of individual personal needs and problems take place, and a carefully phrased 'Letter to Husbands' is made available.
(6) Further visits are arranged in the interests of the patient, often at her home if more convenient.
(7) The necessity for periodic check-up visits to the doctor is stressed.

Personal relationship
The volunteer, who has by this time established a personal sympathetic relationship with the patient, gives the latter her telephone number and address and makes herself readily available whenever her services are needed.
The volunteers went through the same period of doubts and worries which the patient is now facing and hope to ease this period by passing along the carefully developed and proven

results of their own experience, in 'non-professional' and distinctly 'womanly' terms.

At first there may be disbelief that the volunteer has undergone a similar operation. However, the morale-building is extremely effective when the patient discovers that this is true indeed and the volunteer shows her the extent to which she can move the arm on the affected side and the efficiency of the prosthesis she is wearing.

A series of questions usually follows and these are frankly answered — the whole interview is designed to implant the unspoken thought — 'Well if she looks as she does and moves her arm so well, surely I shall be able to do the same in time.'

Doctor–volunteer relationship
Great care must be taken never to make the initial visit to the patient without the doctor's permission. The Volunteer Group has yet to find the most satisfactory way of acquainting busy doctors and surgeons with the service offered and the advantages which can accrue to them and their patients. There are many doctors and patients who have not had time nor the opportunity to acquaint themselves fully with the Group's aims and methods and, in some instances, there may be the erroneous feeling that volunteers are trespassing in the surgical and medical fields.

Help for nursing staff
Staffs in nursing homes and hospitals have become familiar with the service. They get to know the volunteers and appreciate the post-operative help offered. Matrons and nursing sisters have been extremely co-operative in bringing the work to the notice of patients and surgeons. The best recommendation is by word of mouth but, excellent as it is, it is a slow process.

The Volunteer Group is fortunate in that it has at its disposal volunteers of all age groups and that the most compatible volunteer is always sent to each individual patient. This is an important factor in establishing common ground and instilling in the patient the wish to see the volunteer again.'

Further information may be obtained from:
The National Cancer Association of SA
PO Box 2000
Johannesburg
2000

Coping with the stress of a cancer diagnosis

The disclosure or non-disclosure by the doctor of the diagnosis of cancer has been a controversial subject for many years. Some people would rather not hear what, for them, is a death sentence. Members of the public are, however, becoming more and more enlightened about medical matters, especially about cancer and the possibility of successful therapy. This is conducive to the formation of an alliance between the doctor and his patient in which the diagnosis is disclosed and the treatment and prognostic possibilities outlined. In this way it is hoped to gain the confidence of the patient and his family and their co-operation in the sometimes lengthy and traumatic therapy.

Once the doctor has enlightened the patient and his family, the nurse must follow his decision with regard to treatment strategy.

Different people have different coping skills to reduce anxiety and stress, which they use when faced with a life-threatening disease. The nurse who relates to her patient empathically will soon pick up his/her coping strategies and thus be able to help the patient by her understanding and compassionate handling.

The following coping skills meet the needs of different people.

(1) The ego defensive mechanisms used by those who have not yet formed a relationship of trust with professional caregivers:
(a) denying that there is any cause for distress by ignoring symptoms, e.g. failing to keep a medical appointment for a check-up;
(b) projecting anger by blaming others, e.g. caregivers for lacking concerned caring;
(c) giving meaning to their suffering (rationalising) and hereby finding relief from the terror their illness inspires;
(d) displacing their anxiety about their own condition onto concern for others, thus forgetting their own worries.

(2) Seeking information about cancer, its causes and treatment, thereby allaying fear of the unknown and maintaining a sense of control over own destiny. Anxiety and insecurity can be reduced in the patient who uses this adjustive strategy if he is well-informed and understands the nature of his therapy. He will adopt the hopeful attitudes of his professional caregivers and thus the quality of his life is enhanced.

(3) Anticipating the course of the illness and mentally rehearsing it. This is a self-reassuring way of coping with anxiety through knowing the course of the illness.

(4) Some people with cancer turn to family and friends for emotional nurturing and are able to find comfort in dependency. This may cause uncomplaining, overcompliant, passive behaviour because of fear of displeasing those upon whom they feel dependent. Passivity and dependency may, however, be a source of distress to the normally assertive type of person who is forced into a position

of dependency because of the severity of his symptoms.

REFERENCES

(1) Greene P. The Cancer Nursing Education Project of the International Union Against Cancer. *Nursing RSA* 1990; **5**: 34–35.

(2) SAMJ News. *S Afr Med J* 1989; **75**: xvi.

(3) Markowitz S, Leiman G, Margolius KA. Human papillomavirus and cervical intra-epithelial neoplasia in an African population. *S Afr J Epidemiology and Infection* 1986; **1**: 65–69.

(4) Levin L. The dietary influences in breast and colon cancer. *SA Cancer News* 1982; **3**: 3.

(5) Harington JS. Cancer research workers and projects supported by the NCA of SA in 1984. *SA Cancer Bulletin* 1984; **28**: 268–272.

(6) Keen P. The epidemiology of cancer in Africans in Southern Africa. *SA J Surgery* 1975; **13**: (3).

(7) Yach D. Lung cancer study group meeting. *S Afr Med J* 1988; **73**: 261.

(8) Walker ARP. Cancer prevention, detection and survival — how hopeful is the outlook? *S Afr Med J* 1987; **71**: 376–380.

(9) Walker ARP, Madden MV, Dent DM. Gastric cancer. *S Afr Med J* 1987; **72**: 30–33.

(10) Kew MC. Primary liver cancer. *S Afr J Cont Med Educ* 1984; **2**: 21–32.

(11) Kneebone RL, Mannell A. Cancer of the oesophagus in Soweto. *S Afr Med J* 1985; **67**: 839–842.

(12) Jaskiewica K, Marasas WFO, Van der Walt PE. Oesophageal and other main cancer patterns in four districts of Transkei, 1981–1984. *S Afr Med J* 1987; **72**: 27–30.

(13) Department NHPD. Cancer of the oesophagus in the RSA. *Epidemiological Comments* 1986; **13** (7).

(14) Thomas DB, Lilienfeld AM. (1976) Geographic, Reproductive and Sociobiological Factors. In: A Stoll (Ed) *Risk Factors in Breast Cancer*. London: Heinemann Medical Books.

(15) Papaioannnou AN. (1974) *The Etiology of Human Breast Cancer*. New York: Springer–Verlag.

(16) Robertson MA, *et al*. Observations on cancer patterns among Africans in South Africa. *Brit J Ca* 1971; **25**: 377.

(17) Higginson J, Oettle AG. Cancer incidence in the Bantu and 'Cape Coloured' races of South Africa: Report of a cancer survey in the Transvaal. *Jnl Nat Ca Inst* 1953–5; **24**: (3).

(18) Simson IW. The National Cancer Registry. *S Afr Med J* 1986; **69**: 2–3.

(19) Executive Committee, South African Cancer Registry 1986. *S Afr Med J* 1988; **74**: 259.

(20) Fragoyannis S, *et al*. *S Afr Med J* 1977; **52**: 493.

(21) Editorial. *S Afr Med J* 1977; **43**: 1105.

(22) Bloch R, Dehaeck CMC. Human papillomavirus and the squamous epithelium of the female genital tract. *S Afr Med J* 1987; **72**: 557–558.

(23) Walker ARP. Cancer of the cervix. *S Afr Med J* 1985; **68**: 316–320.

(24) Lee NC. *A new look at cancer*. MASA 1990.

TEST OF KNOWLEDGE

The student has benefited from studying this chapter if he/she can answer the following questions:

(1) Define the following terms:
  – carcinogen
  – oncogenic
  – dysplasia
  – carcinoma *in situ*
  – exfoliative cytology
  – transformation zone of cervix
  – ablative surgery
  – solar keratosis
  – human papillomavirus
  – metaplasia
  – Ayre spatula
  – aspiration cytology
  – *peau d'orange*
  – cachexia
  – leukoplakia

(2) Write notes on:
  (*a*) Auto-palpation of the breast
  (*b*) The NCA of SA
  (*c*) The South African Cancer Registry
  (*d*) The UICC

(e) The Cancer Nursing Education Project
(f) Hospicare Home Service of the NCA of SA
(g) The aetiology of primary liver cancer
(h) The three main characteristics of a malignant growth
(i) The aetiology and epidemiology of oesophageal cancer
(j) The aetiology and epidemiology of breast cancer

(3) Write an account of cancer of the cervix under the following headings:
(a) Causes and risk factors
(b) Epidemiology
(c) The reading of a PAP smear for possibility of abnormalities and the treatment of any positive findings.

(4) What are the causes and epidemiology of skin cancer in the RSA; how can skin cancer be prevented?

(5) (a) What are the causes and epidemiology of lung cancer?
(b) Name other cancers in which smoking plays an aetiological role.

(6) Discuss the role of diet in the aetiology of cancer.

47

Geriatric Problems

INTRODUCTION

Geriatric problems arise mainly from the social structure of the community which determines its laws, customs, values, beliefs and attitudes. The independence of the nuclear family has made the role of grandparents redundant except as peripheral supportive figures. Grandparents generally need the support of their children and to maintain the emotional ties of the extended family. When adult children migrate to far-off places, parents are usually left behind, bereft of their support system at a time when their powers are waning and inflation cuts deeply into their savings.

Few aged are economically productive and a large number receive social pensions. This is paid for by the younger productive sector of the population. At present the proportion of aged is increasing rapidly: the financial burden of large numbers of dependent old people will place an increasingly large financial burden on the working sector.

The ageing of the populations of westernised countries is due to:

(1) the decline in the fertility rate so that the ratio of old to young people increases;
(2) improvement in living standards and medical technology causing more people to survive to old age.

There is a tendency in advanced societies to segregate and socially isolate the elderly from the young. Many elderly people resent losing their independence and often prefer to live by themselves. Thus, unless there are very strong emotional bonds in the family, old people may find themselves isolated — uninvolved in their community, socially unrecognised and forgotten, emotionally and economically insecure and with a deflated sense of worth which leads to depression and feelings of despair and hopelessness. What is more, old people often do not recognise the seriousness of a physical complaint and may deteriorate physically, unattended and uncared for. Much can, however, be done to meet the needs of old people for independence, for something to do and something to live for by providing suitable assistance.

Not all old people experience geriatric problems. In some communities in the RSA a good network of health care for the needy aged exists, although no national plan is operative as yet. Middle-class aged, mostly whites, who can afford the costs, are increasingly buying houses in retirement villages where their needs for security, compatible human companionship and frail care (when necessary) are taken care of.

The CHN will come across many unsolved geriatric problems in her ageing clients, however. These problems may be economic and psychosocial in nature. A decline in physical health is the most important problem of old age. Clients with problems require expert geriatric care. Geriatrics is a subdivision of medicine; preventive geriatrics has to do with primary prevention of diseases, the promotion of health by health education and social therapy (clubs, service centres), secondary prevention (curative treatment), and rehabilitation after illness, especially after prolonged hospitalisation.

The main aim of this chapter is the improvement of the quality of life in old age of those persons experiencing geriatric problems.

IN THIS CHAPTER

THE DEMOGRAPHY OF THE AGED IN SOUTH AFRICA

The WHO gives the following definition of old
age:

- Middle age ends at: 59 years
- Elderly: 60 to 74 years
- Aged: 75 years and above

The last two are also known as 'senior citizens'.

The number of senior citizens in the RSA
(more than 1 million in 1989) is expected to
grow to 5 million by the year 2030; the majority
will be women.[1] In the year 2000 the total
population above 65 years will be 2,5 million.[2]
Of this age group 15 % show signs of waning
independence and increasing infirmity. Apart
from the cost of illness in the elderly, the economic burden of pensions is likely to be stag-
gering. In 1980 the following percentages of
each population group were over 65 years of
age:

- Whites: 8, 1 %
- Blacks: 3 %
- Asians: 2,1 %
- Coloureds: 3,4 %

(See Population Pyramids, p. 81.)

**Projected growth in geriatric persons (over 60 years) for three
population groups[3]**

Year	Whites	Coloureds	Blacks
1980	515 840	129 600	814 480
2000	698 500	198 000	1 870 000
% increase	35 %	53 %	129 %

There are, at present, proportionately more aged
whites over the age of 65 years than aged blacks,
coloureds or Asians. People below the age of 15
and above the age of 65 are economically dependent, i.e. they generally do not do productive
work which brings in an income. The whites
have a lower dependency rate than any of the
other population groups because of their much
lower birth-rate. Because the whites are economically advanced, a fairly large proportion of
white elderly are economically self-sufficient.
In 1970 only 42 % of all aged whites received
old-age pensions, whereas 99 % of the coloured
and 88 % of the Asian aged received old-age
pensions. In blacks, coloureds and whites there
are many more aged females than males, while
amongst Asians aged males predominate; the
latter trend is changing, however.

PHYSICAL AND PSYCHOSOCIAL PROBLEMS OF WHITE AGED

In white society, achievement is important for
the allocation of role and status and ageing
involves increasing exclusion from family life,
as children leave the home to start their own
nuclear families.

The needs of the aged are frustrated by the changing social values relating to the closeness of family ties. The nuclear family has become independent of the extended family and often does not feel obliged to take the responsibility for the older generation, responsibility being relegated to the state and community services.

Quite often children migrate to distant countries in search of a better life and either abandon their old parents or require them to uproot themselves. In a new environment the worth of the old persons may not be recognised; they need familiar people to affirm their worth. Old people often find it difficult to accept their waning strength in a society which emphasises the importance of efficiency and money-earning capacity. Old people fear the computer age and the fact that their skills are redundant.

Death of spouse and retirement from productive work cause social and psychological isolation. Because of the long life expectancy in whites (65 years for males and 73 years for females), the extent of physical and psychiatric infirmity amongst the aged is increased.

Thus the special needs of the white aged are to re-establish meaningful social relationships (outside the family) and to be cared for physically.

SOME SPECIAL PROBLEMS OF THE BLACK AGED

Amongst the traditional blacks with their extended family structure and ancestor worship, aged females no less than aged males play a very important role in the family and are likely to be cared for and feel wanted and needed; they are involved in the life of the family and the society. Traditionally, power was in the hands of the elderly who commanded respect and obedience from the young. The aged in traditional black society would, therefore, be relatively secure were it not for the gross poverty which affects the rural blacks more than the urban blacks.

Urbanisation and industrialisation have caused dramatic changes in the role, status and security of the black aged. The extended family structure is breaking down, family bonds are becoming weak as the social structure is changing. Because of the high rate of illegitimacy amongst urban blacks, families with a woman at the head are becoming common.

Age and sex are no longer bases for status, although the black male still retains his privileged position as head of the household in complete families. In line with Western values, status is now dependent on achievement. For this reason the aged are becoming increasingly insecure, both socially and economically.

Degradation, alcoholism and malnutrition, especially beriberi and pellagra, and ill-health are fairly common amongst the aged blacks in communities, both urban and rural, in which the traditional attitudes to the aged are no longer held. Few female pensioners are able to live independently and alone in the two-roomed houses in the townships which have been set aside for pensioners who have no relatives with whom to live. Old black people have seldom saved for their old age, nor have they prepared themselves for retirement; the aged woman is usually not skilled in housekeeping because traditionally the daughter-in-law did this, and is inclined to neglect herself and her environs, especially if the loneliness and isolation cause depression.

The attitude of blacks to the maintenance of health in old age is negative — death is often welcomed. Chronic illness may be ascribed to earlier bewitchment, hence the fatalistic attitude of many blacks to their physical sufferings. Medical care is sought merely for the relief of symptoms, not for cure of the condition. Some physically able female aged make a career of child-minding and even rearing. Children whose mothers work in the cities are sometimes sent to the country — 'the farm' — to be reared by their grandmother who is paid insufficiently to feed, clothe and educate the child properly. Both in the cities and in the country, child-rearing by poor and ill-informed grandmothers can play havoc with the health of children who do not get proper food and medical care.

Old people who live with their children in the townships do not necessarily fare any better. Unless the affectional bonds in the family are very close, their presence in impoverished families living in overcrowded conditions can cause much interpersonal friction.

Most poor families expect their aged to buy food for the family from their pension money, but to the aged it may be more important to pay their monthly instalments to the undertaker.[4]

Being assigned to a pauper's grave is indeed a fate many old people are not prepared to risk.

The hospital may be used as a place where the old people go for terminal care, as satisfactory total body care cannot be given in the townships where children often assume responsibility for the care of their aged relative. The domiciliary nursing services available in some white communities are not as yet operative in black townships. Therefore, overcrowded black hospitals may find themselves burdened by sick and frail old people who could be looked after in the community if adequate facilities — old-age homes with nursing services, home helps, district nurses — were available.

By October 1976 the South African National Council for the Care of the Aged had established twelve old-age homes for blacks. Lekgetha and Robertson[5] state that these homes, some of which are situated in isolated areas, have not been popular as the old people feel lonely, being cut off from their relatives and friends. They resent the restriction on their movements and the change in their life-style. Various misunderstandings with the management cause friction and unhappiness.

It would seem that the black aged, no less than the white aged, like being involved in their communities and like being free and able to make their own decisions. Community help to enable the aged to live independently in their own homes appears to be the best way of ensuring a happy and fulfilled life for the aged population.

CONTROL OF CO-ORDINATED HEALTH SERVICES FOR THE AGED

The Health Act 63 of 1977 established the legal means by which services for the aged can be controlled and co-ordinated. The Act made provision for the establishment of a National Health Policy Council under the Minister of National Health and Population Development and a Health Matters Advisory Committee.

The Health Matters Advisory Committee has appointed a subcommittee of Health Services for the Aged; this subcommittee delegates responsibility for care of the aged to a national network of regional co-ordinating committees, consisting of members of the various health authorities. The latter co-ordinate the work of the people who actually work with the aged, either voluntary organisations (NGOs) or official authorities.

Social welfare services, both private (voluntary) and state, and including those concerned with the welfare of the aged, are governed by the National Welfare Act 100 of 1978.

The National Welfare Act provides for the establishment of a SA Welfare Council and regional welfare boards and committees under the control of the Department of Welfare.

The main objectives of the Department of Welfare for the elderly are:

(1) Old-age homes planned for the future are to accept only those who need frail care.
(2) The elderly must be kept out of old-age homes and in the community, as far as possible.
(3) Support services for the elderly in the community must be continuously extended.

The support services are provided mainly by voluntary organisations (NGOs) for the aged. Most of these services are co-ordinated by the South African National Council for the Care of the Aged (SANCCA). There is close liaison between the government and SANCCA with regard to the welfare of the aged and the provisions of the National Welfare Act.

PRIMARY PREVENTION OF GERIATRIC PROBLEMS

Ageing and retirement from work are inevitable in those who live long enough to reach old age. Ageing need not be a traumatic experience, however, if the wear and tear of the body occur gradually without causing unusual physical suffering and if the roles lost as a result of ageing are replaced by other equally satisfying roles, e.g. that of grandparent or that of absorbed hobbyist, leisure-time user, sportsman or friend. Primary prevention is aimed at preventing geriatric problems caused by inability to adapt to: the ageing process, enforced retirement, loss of a spouse and reduced income.

Counselling on health promotion and the early detection of disease

Examples:

(1) The health benefits of regular exercise: swimming, brisk walking, gym, sports.
(2) Regular checking for preventable disease:
    (*a*) in women, breast palpation; PAP smears are seldom done after the age of 60 years;
    (*b*) in both sexes: blood pressure and blood cholesterol checks, rectal examination, especially when there is periodic diarrhoea and/or blood in the stools;
    (*c*) the benefits of a well-balanced diet and avoidance of obesity;
    (*d*) the use of oestrogens in menopausal women to prevent osteoporosis and pathological fractures.

Retirement

Many people are unprepared for retirement and have few resources. Most people find a purpose in life through their jobs and the rearing of their children. They may believe that retirement is a time for sitting back and resting. For these constricted personalities, the future, when they give up work, can mean loneliness and misery — an existence without meaning and purpose. These retired people may deteriorate mentally and become depressed and a burden to the community. In 1977 the Minister of Social Welfare and Pensions appointed a Committee of Inquiry into Preparation for Retirement.

Formal education does not prepare a person for retirement and many people feel useless and redundant when demands are no longer made on them by their children and their jobs.

Those with many resources who, through lifelong, continuous education have equipped themselves with the best tools available — not only for earning a living but also for enjoying life to the full — have no retirement problems and can look forward to a happy and fulfilled old age with life remaining meaningful to the end.

The retirement association

At a conference in Johannesburg in 1966, representatives of industry, commerce, education and medical and social services, investigated ways of helping South Africans prepare for retirement. This led to the formation of the Witwatersrand Retirement Council — a non-profit project. The success of the council — now called the Retirement Association — has led to the establishment of a number of affiliated Retirement Councils in various centres of the RSA.

The Retirement Association comprises some 70 member companies from the mines, industry and the business sector. Their employees benefit from the 'Design for Living' courses run by the Association and financed by the employer companies. The educational courses cover Mental and Physical Health, Nutrition, Development of Mental Potential, Extension of Interests Into the Arts and Sciences, Finance in all its Aspects, The Need for Continued Education, A Place to Live, An Occupation, Travel. The courses cater primarily for Employer Member nominees, but individuals wishing to attend in a private capacity may do so on the payment of a fee. Employers send their employee nominees to these courses at intervals, from 15 years onwards before retirement is due.

The following are some of the special services run by the Association:

(1) an Employment Bureau — free to the general public over the age of 60;
(2) an Advisory Bureau — a voluntary service staffed by voluntary workers;
(3) painting courses.

The function and purpose of the Retirement Association are primarily to promote physical and mental health by health education and the prevention of ill-health.

Geriatric screening clinics

Geriatric screening clinics are located either in Community Health Centres or in service centres and should be run by the health departments of local authorities.

Screening clinics are an out-patient preventive service by which the aged likely to be at risk, i.e. the group of 65 to 70 and older, can be physically and mentally assessed and treated at the first signs of pathology before illness and disability set in. The prevention of suicidal depression is especially important, as depression wreaks havoc in the lives of a great many of our senior citizens.

Primary prevention by health supervision of the old person in his own home is an important function of the community health nurse who works in close liaison with the general practitioner and the geriatric screening clinic of the local authority.

Geriatric clinics attached to Preventive (Family) Health Centres of local authorities have recently been established in some urban areas; the clinics cater not only for the health needs of the aged but also act as referral agents to state health services and welfare agencies.

A podiatry service (subsidised) can be arranged by the CHN for interested clients who make timely appointments and pay a reduced fee.

Health education of the elderly is an important task of the CHN, not only with regard to the necessity for taking medication regularly and to go for medical check-ups, when there is progression of the disease process, but also with special emphasis on nutrition, accident prevention, personal hygiene, cultural stimulation and maintenance of social relationships.

She does regular periodic follow-up visits to her geriatric out-patients and becomes their confidante and the person they will turn to in times of crisis and need. These home visits, if carried out regularly, obviate the necessity for repeated visits to the geriatric clinic with consequent overloading of medical services.

Research into geriatric problems in the community

To find out the extent of the geriatric problem and what the needs of the aged in the community are, especially in overcrowded, blighted areas, requires research by the health department of the local authority. Community health nurses (CHN) usually do the field work, going from door to door in the densely populated areas to find out the whereabouts of elderly people, especially those above the age of 65 years. Some old people live in back rooms or in cheap flats, uncared for, unwanted and unknown.

In the course of the research study, the CHN interviews the old people she comes across in her door-to-door search and tries to obtain the following information which is relevant for the formulation of a geriatric policy by the local authority:

(1) the adequacy, accessibility and cleanliness of the accommodation;

(2) the social circumstances under which the aged person lives, e.g. his contact with people and his mobility to and from his abode;

(3) the source of income and the economic status of the old person, e.g. independent means, social pension;

(4) the community facilities, e.g. services, clubs and concessions, used by the aged;

(5) the state of independence, e.g. capacity for self-care, ability to do domestic chores and shopping;

(6) the needs and wants of the old person;

(7) the health status of the elderly person. This is assessed by the CHN and by a medical officer.

In the place of abode, the CHN records the medical history and habits (e.g. smoking, appetite, sleep, bowels, drinking) of the aged person and does a cursory (screening) examination of his nutritional and mental state, his special senses, his skin, mouth, tongue and teeth, his breathing, cough, pulse and blood pressure, haemoglobin, oedema of legs, varicose veins and the breasts of a woman.

At the geriatric clinic, a full medical examination is carried out by a medical officer on all the old people found to be in need of medical care by the screening examination of the CHN.

When all this information has been collated, a register can be compiled of all the old people in need of community care and a geriatric policy formulated according to the needs of this population.

During the 1980s the SENSORG (SENCARE) project was carried out by the Department of Community Health, University of Stellenbosch, at the request of welfare organisations experiencing problems with the placement of frail elderly in suitable old-age homes.[1]

The main findings were:

(1) There is a tremendous lack of knowledge of available services for the aged.

(2) The membership of, and attendance at, service centres (see p. 826) are poor.

(3) Goal-directed, co-ordinated planning of old-age care, as one of the goals of service centres, is lacking.

Conclusions:

(1) Good care is given in homes for the aged, but social workers are not used adequately.

(2) For the aged who become frail in the community, there is difficulty with placement in an old-age home due to the fact that too many healthy, mobile elderly occupy these homes.[1]

Care of the healthy, mobile aged in and by the community

The community services, to help old people remain an integral part of a healthy community, are:

(1) Giving senior citizens, especially those in the cities, full information about the health and supporting social services available to them, e.g. in Johannesburg and Cape Town booklets on the concessions and amenities available to senior citizens are freely procurable. The booklets contain a wealth of information about: bus, cinema and buying concessions, podiatry services, clubs, employment, home helps, holidays and entertainment, medical services and geriatric clinics, subsidised meals, housing, social pensions and homes for aged, preparation for retirement, etc.

(2) Specially planned housing programmes, e.g. cottages, flatlets and rooms, to ensure a normal social environment for people of limited means who want to live independently. Provision should be made in these homes for bath handles, hand-rails in corridors, and ramps beside steps to accommodate wheelchairs. Steps must be shallow and wide. There are subsidised government, municipal and voluntary organisation housing schemes which cater specifically for the aged.

Regional associations for the care of the aged, e.g. JAFTA in Johannesburg, will supply information about the availability of subsidised housing.

(3) Service centres (see p. 826).

SECONDARY PREVENTION OF GERIATRIC PROBLEMS (DIAGNOSIS AND CARE)

Secondary prevention concerns those geriatric patients who are experiencing physical and/or psychiatric problems, or problems with their capacity for 'activities of daily living' (ADL) and ability for self-care. The problems may require decisions to be made with regard to the placement in homes for the aged or with regard to hospitalisation. On the other hand, the problem may be handled by admitting the patient to a day care centre (see p. 826) to prevent the admission to hospital of the aged with chronic diseases. Another way of handling this problem is to make use of domiciliary nursing services and home visiting by community health nurses (CHN). State district nurses on the staff of the district surgeon are allowed to do domiciliary nursing on social pensioners who are not out-patients of a provincial hospital. In the latter case the patient can be attended to by provincial district nurses attached to the provincial hospital.

Community health services must pay special attention to those aged who have been discharged from hospital. The infirm elderly who live alone must be visited by family and friends, social workers and CHNs. Domiciliary services must be arranged for them to prevent relapses.

Where infirm aged live with their families, continued stay should be encouraged by offering families some relief from caring duties, e.g. by institutionalising the infirm aged person for a period while the family goes on holiday.

If available, a day care centre (see p. 826) plays an important role in keeping the sick and incapacitated aged at home with their families. Beyers[6] describes clinic and community care at the Geriatric Clinic at Tygerberg Hospital and Goodwood Aftercare Hospital, of patients who come for help. The target of the geriatric team is to keep 90 % of patients over the age of 75 years free from physical and mental disabilities.

The comprehensive health team consists of:

(1) Professional personnel (doctors, nurses, paramedical staff, social workers). They are trained in geriatric diagnosis — for the early prevention and treatment of disease and disability — and in health promotion and rehabilitation.

The community sister is taught to do a full clinical evaluation of the geriatric patient. She visits patients in the whole catchment area of the clinic and trains the family to care for the patient. She can call on the services of team members, e.g. physiotherapists and social workers.

(2) The community rehabilitation team (the family as well as neighbours, friends and members of the congregation) is motivated to render social services and to create a friendly, caring environment. Spiritual problems are dealt with by the patient's own minister of religion. Economic problems are referred to the community helping agencies.

The geriatric clinic and the geriatric CHN

The (geriatric) community health nurse (CHN) plays an important role in secondary prevention, both in the community and in the geriatric clinic of the hospital or the local authority.

In the community she is the first health worker to contact the old person in need of care. This contact is made possible either through her own door-to-door search or through referral by concerned persons in the community. The CHN takes a medical and social history and assesses her client's psychiatric and physical state; she decides whether he needs further medical examination either at home by the patient's own general practitioner or at the geriatric clinic. She assesses her client's social, spiritual, domestic, recreational and economic needs and liaises between the old person and geriatric welfare agencies.

The weekly geriatric clinic is a very important component of the preventive geriatric services of the local or provincial authority. The medical officer of health attached to the clinic makes a comprehensive assessment and a definite diagnosis of the physical, economic, social and psychiatric abnormalities of the patients brought in for special attention from the community by the CHN. The doctor may refer the patient for treatment to a hospital or welfare agency and decides whether the old person is capable of looking after himself or requires institutionalisation.

Medical examination for physical diagnosis

At the weekly geriatric clinic, the CHN assists the medical officer with the physical examination of the patients she has brought into the clinic for more extensive medical examination.

The common physical problems are: hypertension, chronic coronary artery disease and CCF, arthritis and rheumatism, bronchitis and emphysema, neoplasms and poor sight and hearing.

Geriatric patients are often referred to the doctor when the disease is already far advanced. The sick old person may suffer from multiple pathologies and many diseases at the same time, which are difficult to diagnose because of their atypical presentation. Some old people take a long time to recover from their illness; on the other hand, it is quite remarkable how a desperately sick, dehydrated old person recovers when fluid and electrolyte balance has been restored.

Note: Social pensioners in need of medical care are referred to the district surgeon if they need domiciliary care.

The CHN measures the height, mass, blood pressure and haemoglobin. She arranges for voluntary workers from the community to support patients, to create a social atmosphere for them at the clinic and, if necessary, to escort them to the general or day hospital for more specialised diagnostic procedures, prostheses and treatments. It is the task of the CHN to educate the voluntary workers in elementary health principles regarding old people so that they, in turn, can help them lead healthy lives within the limitations imposed by their age and socio-economic circumstances.

Curative health care for the aged (geriatric medicine) has lacked the status and excitement that other branches of medicine hold for doctors and nurses. Yet it is a speciality which requires different skills and knowledge because disease in the elderly may present in different ways to disease in the young. Old people are not as aware of their bodies as younger people, some symptoms being masked and others not considered important enough to warrant seeking medical aid. Old people do not feel pain in the same way as younger ones, e.g. coronary infarction and fractured femur may occur without causing much suffering. Difficulty in walking because of painful feet and joints, painful muscles due to 'rheumatism', bone diseases causing postural difficulties, tiredness because of anaemia and chronic heart failure and non-vascular, degenerative senile dementia with memory loss may be accepted by the old person and his family as the inevitable accompaniments of old age.

Deafness and defective vision are disabilities which preclude enjoyment of life but which, in some cases, can be improved by suitable aids. Physical handicaps such as dizziness and poor postural control, which cause falling with the danger of sustaining fractures, and poor memory, increase with age, eventually causing an old person to become dependent on others for his day-to-day care. Ability of old people to care for themselves and live independently will depend on their mental ability, their continence of urine and faeces, mobility, ability to communicate verbally, hearing and visual acuity, and their ability to feed themselves and keep their bodies clean. Completely dependent old people must be cared for by others, either by relatives or in homes for the aged.

Assessing functional capacity for ADL

The community health nurse can assess the geriatric patient's functional capacity for 'activities of daily living' (ADL).

The results of this questionnaire (filled in by the family) are very important in deciding whether the patient needs nursing care in a frail care centre or can remain in the community with the help of domiciliary services, the family and district nurse.

The aged who are considered for placement in subsidised old-age homes are classified as follows:

- Group I: Healthy and mobile
- Group II: Semi-frail and senile
- Group III: Very frail and bedridden

Assessing the patient's social ability

A social worker is attached to the geriatric clinic to investigate and assist with all social problems encountered amongst old people, and to arrange for a social pension and other economic aid if necessary. The social worker can advise the family on:

(1) whether to have the patient declared incompetent and apply to the courts to have a *curator bonis* appointed to look after his affairs; and

(2) whether to prevent the patient from driving a car.

The social worker plays a very important role in institutional placement of patients who are no longer capable of caring for themselves with help in the community. The social worker and the nurse must work as a team to facilitate placement in institutional care. The community

A method of assessing functional ability[7]

Activity of daily living	Requires no assistance	Requires some assistance	Totally incapable without assistance
Bathing			
Dressing			
Toileting			
Mobility			
Feeding			
Continence	Fully continent	Occasional accidents	Incontinent, catheter required or supervision helps control
Bladder			
Bowels			
Mark appropriate spaces X.			

nurse who knows the patient persuades him to accept this care and thus presents a motivated, co-operative patient to the social worker who may be a total stranger to him. The old person, who may be very suspicious and somewhat resistant, must be prepared for the visit from the social worker who is investigating the case.

Assessing the patient's mental ability

The finding and treating of old people who are suffering from psychiatric illness at an early stage, especially depression and dementia, are important secondary preventive measures practised by the CHN. The community health nurse can assess the patient's mental status by using Goldfarb's Mental Status Questionnaire for estimating a cognitive defect characteristic of dementia.[8]

(1) Where are we now?
(2) Where is this place located?
(3) What is the day of the month?
(4) What month is it?
(5) What year is it?
(6) How old are you?
(7) When is your birthday?
(8) In what year were you born?
(9) Who is the State President of South Africa?
(10) Who was the State President before him?

Score

8–10   Absent/mild chronic brain syndrome
5–7   Mild/moderate chronic brain syndrome
2–4   Moderate/severe chronic brain syndrome
0–1   Severe chronic brain syndrome

This questionnaire tests memory and orientation. Patients with low scores are less able to cope with the demands of life and are, therefore, anxious. These persons may be referred to a psychiatrist or psychogeriatric clinic for final diagnosis and advice as to management.

Psychogeriatrics

The psychiatric problems of the aged may be either *acute short-term confusional states and depression* or they may be *chronic long-term organic states with dementia of insidious onset.* Gillis[9] states that dementia is present in 3 % of persons over the age of 60 years, in 13 % of persons over the age of 75 years and in over 20 % of those over the age of 80 years.

Senile degenerative dementia is a progressively deteriorating organic disorder of the brain due to cerebral atrophy. The damage to brain cells is permanent and there is a steady reduction of intellectual processes. Memory becomes progressively impaired, with recent-memory gaps which may be filled in with fabrications (lies).

The old person eventually becomes confused and disorientated for time and place, a condition known as 'senility'. The senile person is suspicious, hoards rubbish, is slovenly, dirty and incontinent, apathetic or restless, in which case he may wander away from home. As he loses contact with reality, he develops a senile psychosis.

For a description of Alzheimer's disease consult *Manual of Nursing Volume 2* (Vlok).

The long-term care of demented persons will depend upon the severity of their condition and the presence of other pathological states, e.g.:

(1) *Physically ill patients with some dementia but with no behavioural problems.* These patients need special medical and nursing care and can usually be managed by a physician-geriatrician if available — in a general hospital or nursing-home.

(2) *Persons with a mild degree of dementia.* They could be managed in the community with the aid of community social and health services. The majority of these persons need not go to hospital, but they need someone to help care for them. The following possibilities for care are generally available:

(*a*) residential care in an old-age home with nursing facilities and with group activities to stimulate the withdrawn and to combat depression;

(*b*) living in supervised accommodation for the aged, e.g. the Flower Foundation, residential clubs — villages and housing projects for the over 60s;

(*c*) help to families caring for their aged members by: regular visiting by nurses and partial or periodic hospitalisation, 'granny watchers', home helps, and day care centres organised by the regional bodies affiliated to SANCCA.

(3) *Persons with a severe degree of dementia* (senile psychosis) need continuous nursing care, either in a frail care home or in a psychogeriatric ward of a psychiatric hospital. These senile, incontinent patients need bed care and sedation if they exhibit behavioural symptoms.

Depression in old age is a common illness, reactive depression being due to social isolation, physical ill-health and retirement. It is characterised by feelings of uselessness, of being unwanted and in the way and fear of loneliness. It leads to social withdrawal, lack of motivation for self-care and self-neglect, malnutrition and suicide.

In psychogeriatrics, the main function of the psychiatrist is to make an **accurate assessment** of the behavioural disturbances in the elderly, in order to ensure that the aged patient receives the best possible care without resorting unnecessarily to admission to a psychogeriatric unit of a psychiatric hospital. The latter placement may prejudice the old person's chances of later gaining admission to an old-age home. There are, however, always some psychogeriatric patients whose behavioural disturbances are such that they will be acceptable only to a psychiatric hospital, e.g. paranoid old people may become very aggressive and their severe behavioural disturbance cannot be controlled within the community. In 1969, 3,7 % of all white admissions to psychiatric hospitals in the RSA were psychogeriatric patients. Psychiatric assessment can be made either at the home of the geriatric patient or in psychogeriatric assessment units.

Domiciliary assessment

When a geriatric patient is referred for admission by the family, a domiciliary assessment service is available at some of the major centres. The assessment team should consist of a psychiatrist, social worker and a psychiatric community nurse (PCN). Often, by giving effective help and support to the family, admission to hospital can be avoided. The PCN does follow-up care and helps the family in crisis situations. The PCN brings to the attention of the family all the community social and medical services they can call upon for help. In this way, unsuitable

placement in a psychiatric hospital can be avoided for many dependent old people who can, if necessary, be diverted to more suitable placement, i.e. homes for the aged with full nursing facilities.

Assessment in short-stay psychogeriatric assessment units

The first psychogeriatric assessment unit in the RSA was established at Valkenberg Hospital, Cape Town, in 1976. Assessment units with approximately ten beds for patients over the age of 60 years are attached to either psychiatric or general hospitals. Ambulatory patients with behaviour disturbances are admitted (on a voluntary basis) to the wards of the assessment unit for no longer than four weeks. If the patient is obviously grossly disordered, he will be admitted to the long-term wards of the hospital.

Assessment units offer a full range of psychiatric, medical, nursing and diagnostic facilities needed to make a correct diagnosis and to decide on the correct placement, medication, and continuation care of psychogeriatric patients who may also have medical, social and occupational problems. Investigation consists of:

(1) physical examination;
(2) biochemical and psychological tests;
(3) investigation of family and social circumstances.

A multidisciplinary team decides on the management of each patient. Assessment units function in close co-operation with long-term hospitals and out-patient departments, community services for the aged and old-age homes; therefore they are enabled to effectively handle the multidimensional problems of old people with acute and chronic psychiatric conditions. Depression, especially if accompanied and exacerbated by physical illness, often improves rapidly with medical, pharmacological, occupational and social treatment during the short-term admission for assessment; thus the patient could be discharged after four weeks either to a residential home or to his family.

The assessment unit serves as a liaising body between the depressed, dementing, confused and dependent, frail aged and the various hospital and community caring services with and for whom the multidimensional team establishes contact and counselling services. Community psychiatric nurses from the assessment unit visit discharged patients at home or remain in contact with them if they are cared for in old-age homes or hospitals. They also deal with the families who need help in caring for their aged, e.g. by arranging for day care or temporary readmission of the old person in order to relieve the burden of the family.

TERTIARY PREVENTION — REHABILITATION OF THE AGED

Many disabilities and diseases in old people are remediable; the potential of the old person can be restored after an illness. Rehabilitation of the disabled old person by a health care team is often attempted at service centres and at special after-care hospitals and geriatric out-patient departments with facilities for occupational and physiotherapy to help with the restoration of function. At these centres a social worker is in attendance to help with the resettlement of the old person in the community. The aim of rehabilitation is thus to restore the old person who has been sick or disabled to his home in as healthy and active a state as possible. Reactivation refers not only to physical mobilisation but also to the remotivation of the depressed patient who has become lethargic and passive, withdrawn into his own miserable inner world.

INSTITUTIONAL (RESIDENTIAL) CARE OF THE AGED

In the developed world with its high proportion of aged persons, of people over the age of 65 years, 50 to 60 % have normal health, 20 to 30 % are physically infirm and 10 to 25 % are extremely frail.

The general opinion of people who work with the aged is that old people should be admitted to a home only when they have become so frail that they can no longer maintain their independence, even with the aid of domiciliary community services. Old-age homes do, however, cater for the physically able as well as for the frail who need assistance with dressing and bathing. The majority of homes have nursing facilities which cater specially for the frail and infirm who need a fair amount of nursing and

for the extremely infirm chronic sick who need a great amount of nursing care.

The South African National Council for the Care of the Aged (SANCCA) is of the opinion that mentally frail old people should be cared for in homes for the aged, as they become senile.

Beyers[6] found 40 % of all psychogeriatric conditions to be due to indigence and lack of proper care. Stimulation and activity counteract the symptoms of senility.

The Department of Health Services has compiled a manual on the care of the aged and, jointly with the Department of National Education, runs a correspondence course for the training of the staff of old-age homes. The department supervises the standard of nursing in homes and provides free medical services by district surgeons.

Recently the SA Nursing Council approved a syllabus for the training of nursing auxiliaries in geriatric care. In South Africa there are over half a million (1980) whites over the age of 65. Most of these old people live independently or with their children. Retirement villages are a boon to many senior citizens.

Approximately 8 % of white aged are accommodated in homes for the aged.

The large majority of these homes belong to welfare organisations and are subsidised by the Department of Health. The residents, the majority of whom draw the old-age pension, pay for board and lodging according to their means.

Homes may be either economic or subeconomic, the latter for those with an income of less than R450 per month.

A survey[2] of admissions to old-age homes in Cape Town showed that 50 % of referrals were due to psychiatric factors, *inter alia*, confusional states, senility and depression: social and physical factors (frailty, incontinence, etc.) account for the rest. The residents of these old-age homes were older, poorer and more isolated than the aged in the community.

In state-subsidised homes, approximately half the residents are classified as frail and dependent on nursing care. Old-age homes are, therefore, fast becoming nursing homes for the infirm, frail aged, i.e. Group II and Group III (see p. 821) and are, therefore, an essential part of health services.

All homes for the aged fall under the jurisdiction of the Aged Persons Act.

THE PROTECTION OF THE AGED BY THE STATE

The Aged Persons Act 81 of 1967 has in part been replaced by the Social Assistance Act 59 of 1992, which controls old-age pensions and supplementary allowances for attendants, paid by the state. The Minister may also make financial awards to welfare organisations for care of the aged. The objectives of the Aged Persons Act remain unchanged, however, viz. the protection and welfare of certain aged and debilitated persons.

'1. Definitions under this Act include the following:

    (i) 'aged person' means a white person, a coloured person, an Asian, Chinese or black person who, in the case of a male, is sixty-five years of age or older, and in the case of a female, is sixty years or older;

    (ii) **'debilitated person'** means a white person, a coloured person, an Asian, a Chinese or a black person who is sixty years or older and, by reason of old age or a physical or mental defect or illness, unable to care properly for his person or his interests, but does not require constant care by a medical practitioner or a qualified nurse;

    (vii) **'home for the aged'** means any institution or other place of residence maintained mainly for the accommodation and physical care of aged or debilitated persons;

    (xv) **'registered home for the aged'** means a home for the aged registered in terms of section 3;

    (xvii) **'social welfare officer'** means an officer who is employed in the professional division of the public service and who in the performance of his official duties is mainly engaged in welfare work;

2. The Minister may, in consultation with the Minister of Finance and out of moneys appropriated by Parliament for this purpose, and subject to the provisions of this Act —

    (a) establish and maintain homes for the aged ...'

Note: If such a person lives in a subsidised home for the aged, provincial hospital or hospital for the chronic sick, an attendant's allowance is not paid.

'**3.** (1) No person shall manage a home for the aged (except such a home maintained by the state), unless such home has been registered under this section.

    (2) If any person desires to manage a home for the aged he may in the prescribed manner apply to the Minister for registration thereof.

4. (1) A social welfare officer may at any time visit and inspect a registered home for the aged, and interview any aged or debilitated person accommodated therein, and, either with or without the assistance of a medical practitioner, there enquire into the welfare of any such person.

5. (1) If a social welfare officer submits or makes a written statement under oath to a Public Prosecutor, and in such statement it is alleged that any person within the area of jurisdiction of the magistrate's court to which the Public Prosecutor is attached —

    (a) accommodates or cares for an aged or debilitated person in a place other than a registered home for the aged in circumstances or in a manner likely to be injurious to his physical or mental well-being; or

    (b) presumably takes advantage of an aged or debilitated person by receiving excessive remuneration, by way of money or goods, for the accommodation or care of such a person in a place other than a registered home for the aged: the first mentioned person may be summonsed to appear before a magistrate.

6. (1) Subject to the provisions of this Act every aged person shall be entitled to receive an old-age pension or a war veterans' pension under certain conditions ... A means test is applicable to old-age pensions and war veterans pensions.'

Note:

(1) The means test is not applicable to persons above the age of 100 years.

(2) The residential requirements for pensioners are as follows:

    (a) they must be resident in the RSA at the time of application;

(*b*) they must be South African citizens; or

(*c*) must have lived in the RSA for five years before application and, according to the Aliens Act of 1937, qualify for local residence.

Old-age pensions are notoriously inadequate, being set at a marginal subsistence level. In 1993 old-age pensions for South Africans of all races were equalised at R370 per month. This was raised to R390 in October 1994 and R410 in 1995. The state seems to be expecting people to take responsibility for their own economic requirements in old age. The state is encouraging such responsibility by making tax concessions on contributions to pension funds.

THE SOUTH AFRICAN NATIONAL COUNCIL FOR THE CARE OF THE AGED (SANCCA)

In 1956 the South African National Council for the Care of the Aged was formed to assume the major responsibility for the care of the aged in South Africa. The council looks after blacks, whites and coloureds.

The SA National Council for the Care of the Aged is a voluntary welfare organisation which plans and co-ordinates services to the aged. It works through various affiliated regional bodies, e.g. the Johannesburg Association for the Aged (JAFTA), Howick and District Care of the Aged, Cape Peninsula Welfare Organisation for the Aged.

There is a need for close co-operation between welfare organisations rendering domiciliary and non-domiciliary services to the aged and medical services (local authority, provincial and state) to promote effective care of the discharged geriatric patient.

The main problems of the aged which are the concern of the council are: economic stress caused by reduced income and rising cost of living, increased ill-health, especially in those over the age of 65 years, restriction of mobility caused by fractures, rheumatoid and osteo-arthritis, and loss of interest and companions, the causes of isolation, loneliness and depression.

Private (voluntary) social welfare services

These services may be either domiciliary (i.e. in the home of the aged person) or in the community, outside the home.

Domiciliary services

Home helps obtainable from a regional affiliated body of SANCCA, Red Cross, St John, etc. These home aids assist the semi-dependent aged in the community with bathing and personal care, cleaning, cooking, washing and shopping. Their wages are paid either by service centres or by the aged, if they can afford to.

Laundry services for pensioners living alone by regional bodies or welfare societies. The linen is supplied free and a nominal fee is charged for the weekly laundering.

Meals on Wheels (usually by church organisations). Low-cost hot meals are delivered to the homes of house-bound elderly people, and those unable to cook for themselves.

Public library 'shut-in' free service for home-bound people. Friendly visiting schemes are comprised of volunteers who befriend one or more elderly people, visit them regularly and even do their shopping and take them for drives.

These services make it possible for the aged to manage at home.

Non-domiciliary community services

Employment agencies which either advise the elderly (e.g. retirement councils) or find employment for them, e.g. women as home aids or companions.

Holidays for aged through the Holidays for Aged Association or clubs, e.g. Rotary.

Clubs for the aged run either by regional Councils for the Care of the Aged, Red Cross, municipal recreation centres, church and bowling and other recreational clubs. At the clubs, the elderly are entertained and meet other people on a friendly social basis.

Day-care centres. These centres care for the sick or incapacitated aged (living in the community) during the day while their caretakers, e.g. their families, are working. Only a few have thus far been established, attached either to a service centre or an old-age home. There is a great need for the extension of this service which provides social, occupational, rehabilitative, medical and nursing care.

Service centres are 'clubs' for the healthy, mobile aged who live in the community. The service centres supply a variety of services and are run mainly by affiliates of SANCCA, but also by many welfare organisations which care for the elderly. Service centres can get a government subsidy if they render a certain minimum number of services. The subsidy is applied for every year and will also depend on the number of registered members and the actual daily attendances.

One service centre may have up to 500 members who pay a monthly subscription fee of approximately 50 cents. Service centres augment their subsidies by appealing for donations from the public. In charge of a service centre is a social worker who deals with the needs of members. Some of the geriatric problems the social worker deals with are: advice on pensions, admission to old-age homes, personal and family problems, how to obtain medical and other assistance.

At the service centre members can enjoy companionship and social activities. They may once more feel that they belong to a group and develop a group identity. They are provided with a health advisory service, recreation and a sheltered workshop.

They can also buy low-cost groceries, second-hand clothing and a daily hot meal at low cost. Service centres may have health clinics with physiotherapy and occupational therapy facilities. They may also have podiatry and hairdressing services.

A modern trend is the provision of geriatric screening clinics (run by the local authorities) in service centres to promote primary prevention and maintain the elderly in the best possible health. Some service centres may be attached to homes for the aged.

Service centres are open daily during the week and provide occupation for the retired and lonely; they also assist in rehabilitating the disabled. They give old people the opportunity to meet others and make friends in a social club atmosphere. Through the social service centres, many of the elderly can be kept in the community, free from the loneliness and insecurity which can lead to ill-health and admission to hospital.

REFERENCES

(1) Wicht LL, Prinsloo FR, Skibbe CJ, *et al.* Ondersoek na die gesondheidsdienste en behoeftes van bejaardes (SENSORG). Supplement to *S Afr Med J* March 1989; **7** (9).

(2) Meiring P de V. A system for rendering comprehensive health services to the elderly. *S Afr J Cont Med Educ* 1989; **7:** 1137–1148.

(3) Watermeyer GS, Bourne DE. Demographic imperatives in geriatrics in South Africa. *S Afr J Cont Med Educ* 1984; **2:** 21–25.

(4) Pollack H. *Race Relations News* **39** (June 1977).

(5) Lekgetha AN, Robertson B. *SA Nursing Journal* March 1978.

(6) Beyers BC. Health care of the elderly at Tygerberg Geriatric Clinic and Goodwood Aftercare Hospital. *S Afr Med J* 1980; **57:** 492.

(7) Meiring P de V. A method of geriatric assessment. *S Afr J Cont Med Educ* 1984; **2:** 27–32.

(8) Gillis LS, Elk R. Physical and mental incapacity in elderly white persons in Cape-Town. *S Afr Med J* 1982; **59:** 147–149.

(9) Gillis LS. *S Afr Med J* 1971; **49:** 149.

(10) Verrier-Jones P, *et al. S Afr Med J* 1978; **54:** 113.

(11) Wicht CL. *S Afr Med J* 1977; **51:** 440.

(12) Trichard O, Zabow A, Gillis LS. Elderly persons in old-age homes. *S Afr Med J* 1982; **61:** 624.

TEST OF KNOWLEDGE

The student has beneflted from studying this chapter if he/she can answer the following questions:

(1) Compare the economic and psychosocial problems of white and black (traditional and urban) aged persons in South Africa.

(2) Write an essay on the primary prevention of geriatric problems amongst middle-class South Africans.

(3) What community and state measures can, in your opinion, be taken to relieve the plight of the indigent and isolated white and black social pensioner?

(4) *(a)* What is meant by 'activities of daily living'?

(b) On what grounds would you recommend the admission of an old person to a frail care home?

(c) Why should healthy aged persons not be admitted to an old-age home? What other arrangements for accommodation can they make?

(5) Write notes on the following:
   – Old-age pensions
   – Service centres for the aged
   – Domiciliary services as social welfare services for the aged
   – SANCCA
   – Day care centres for the aged

(6) (a) What is meant by dementia?

(b) How could a nurse assess dementia in an aged person?

(c) Describe the main psychogeriatric conditions.

(d) What role does the social worker play in psychogeriatrics?

Index